Family Medical Guide.

Better Homes and Gardens®

Family Medical Guide

Edited by Donald G. Cooley

Art Direction by Paul Zuckerman

BETTER HOMES AND GARDENS BOOKS

NEW YORK • DES MOINES

FOREWORD

The Family Medical Guide has been in preparation over a period of several years by a corps of medical men which includes several of America's most distinguished specialists and authorities.

We've designed the book to supplement the counsel of one's own personal physician, who alone is competent to diagnose and treat conditions in individual patients. Advances in medicine make it more than ever necessary that intelligent persons have some understanding of body structures and processes of health and disease which doctors can rarely take the time to explain fully to us.

The Better Homes and Gardens Family Medical Guide is a reference to which you may turn for authoritative information about health problems that arise from time to time in your family and personal life, as well as about practical matters of appropriate home care, prevention of disease, maintenance of health, and recognition of illness leading to prompt treatment by a physician who has the great resources of modern medicine at his and your disposal. The illustrations illuminate the wondrous mechanisms of the body and they identify structures concerned with particular conditions. We explain unfamiliar technical terms; none have we avoided, as many "doctor's words" are now part of the common language.

Eminent physicians have demonstrated their belief that such a book is desirable by taking time from their practices and from their academic duties to contribute chapters on their special fields of medicine. We invited each contributor to discuss his topic as if he were speaking across his desk to an intelligent and concerned patient and with all the time in the world to give counsel and to dispel misconceptions. Some of the topics are discussed by different specialists. Cross references throughout the book direct you to more extended discussions. If this book helps to make you a more understanding patient, then it's surely the indispensable complement to an understanding doctor.

Acknowledgments

Howard C. Baron, M.D. Instructor in Surgery, New York University; Director of Surgery, Jewish Memorial Hospital (New York).

Samuel M. Bluefarb, M.D. Professor of Dermatology, Northwestern University Medical School; Attending Dermatologist, Cook County Hospital; Senior Attending Dermatologist, Chicago-Wesley Memorial Hospital.

Albert N. Brest, M.D. Associate Professor of Medicine; Head, Section of Vascular Diseases and Renology, Hahnemann Medical College and Hospital.

William J. Darby, M.D. Professor and Chairman of the Department of Biochemistry and Director of the Division of Nutrition, Vanderbilt University School of Medicine; Member, Food and Nutrition Board of the National Academy of Sciences.

Vincent J. Derbes, M.D. Professor of Dermatology and Director of Division of Dermatology and Allergy, Tulane University School of Medicine; Member, Subspecialty Board of Allergy of American Board of Internal Medicine, 1954-59.

Charles A. Doan, M.D. Dean Emeritus and Professor Emeritus; Director, Division of Hematology, Department of Medicine, Ohio State University; President, American Society of Hematology, 1962-1963; Master, American College of Physicians, 1961.

* Lewis J. Doshay, M.D. Associate Attending Neurologist, Presbyterian Hospital, New York (ret.). Formerly Director, Parkinson Laboratory, Columbia Presbyterian Medical Center; Chairman, Medical Advisory Board, National Parkinson Foundation.

Robert H. Fagan, M.D. Clinical Staff, UCLA Hospital, Los Angeles; Senior Staff, Hospital of the Good Samaritan, Saint John's Hospital, Hollywood Presbyterian Hospital.

Robert H. Felix, M.D. Dean, St. Louis University School of Medicine; past Director, National Institute of Mental Health; Recipient, Rockefeller Public Service Award for distinguished service in the field of science.

Adrian E. Flatt, M.D., F.R.C.S. (England). Associate Professor of Orthopedics, State University of Iowa; Consultant to Veterans Hospital, Iowa City.

R. H. Flocks, M.D. Professor and Head of the Department of Urology, State University of Iowa College of Medicine; Urologist-in-Chief, University Hospitals (Iowa).

James Graham, M.D. Chairman, Department of Surgery, Springfield Clinic (Illinois); Fellow, American College of Surgeons.

Robert B. Greenblatt, M.D. Professor and Chairman, Department of Endocrinology, Medical College of Georgia; Chief of Endocrine Clinic, University Hospital (Augusta).

Morton M. Hunt. Distinguished writer in fields of mental health; Recipient, Family Service Association Award, 1963; Author, "Mental Hospital" and "The Talking Cure."

Robert G. Kesel, D.D.S. Professor and Head of the Department of Applied Materia Medica and Therapeutics, University of Illinois College of Dentistry.

Ronald W. Lamont-Havers, M.D., F.R.C.P. (Canada). Associate Director for Extramural Research and Training, National Institutes of Health; past National Medical Director, the Arthritis and Rheumatism Foundation.

Robert Landesman, M.D. Associate Clinical Professor of Obstetrics and Gynecology, Cornell University Medical School (New York).

Ted F. Leigh, M.D. Professor of Radiology, Emory University School of Medicine; Director, Radiological Society of North America; Fellow and Chancellor, American College of Radiology.

Milton I. Levine, M.D. Associate Professor of Clinical Pediatrics, Cornell University Medical College; Attending Pediatrician, New York Hospital; Consulting Pediatrician, New York City Department of Health.

* Perrin H. Long, M.D. Professor of Medicine and Chairman, Department of Medicine, State University of New York College of Medicine; Chief, Department of Medicine and Attending Physician, Second Medical Division, Kings County Hospital Center (New York).

Daniel G. Morton, M.D. Professor and Chairman, Department of Obstetrics and Gynecology, University of California at Los Angeles; Assistant Dean and Chief of Staff, UCLA School of Medicine.

John H. Moyer, M.D. Professor of Medicine and Chairman, Department of Internal Medicine, Hahnemann Medical College and Hospital (Philadelphia).

J. Arthur Myers, M.D. Professor Emeritus of Medicine, Preventive Medicine and Public Health, University of Minnesota School of Public Health; Past President,

National Tuberculosis Association and American College of Chest Physicians.

Thomas M. Peery, M.D. Professor of Pathology and Chairman of the Department, George Washington University School of Medicine (Washington, D.C.); Chairman, Planning Committee for Clinical Exhibit Laboratory at annual meetings of American Medical Association.

J. Alfred Rider, M.D. Assistant Clinical Professor of Medicine, Gastrointestinal Clinic, University of California Medical Center (San Francisco).

Albert P. Seltzer, M.D. Associate Professor of Otolaryngology, University of Pennsylvania Graduate School of Medicine; Chief of Department of Otolaryngology, Philadelphia General Hospital and Albert Einstein Medical Center, southern division.

* Howard B. Sprague, M.D. Former Lecturer on Medicine, Harvard Medical School; Member of Board of Consultation, Massachusetts General Hospital; Past President, American Heart Association; Past President, Massachusetts Heart Association.

Madison H. Thomas, M.D. Associate Clinical Professor of Neurology, University of Utah Medical School; American Epilepsy Society (Salt Lake City).

Derrick Vail, M.D. Professor and Head of Department of Ophthalmology, Northwestern University Medical School; Attending Ophthalmologist and Director of Department of Ophthalmology, Cook County Hospital.

Charles Weller, M.D. Director, Diabetes and Metabolic Research Unit, Grasslands Hospital, Valhalla, N. Y.; President, New York State Society of Internal Medicine.

Artwork by Designs for Medicine, Inc. Paul Zuckerman, Medical Artist, President, Buffalo, Chicago and New York.

* Deceased

Table of Contents

Chapter		Page
1	Home Care of the Patient	11
2	Infectious Diseases	33
3	The Heart and Circulatory System	77
4	Blood-Forming Organs and Their Disorders	139
5	The Skin and Its Disorders	177
6	The Lungs and Chest in Health and Disease	207
7	The Nervous System	241
8	Kidneys and Genito-Urinary Tract	281
9	The Endocrine Glands	313
10	Pregnancy and Childbirth	357
11	Infant and Child Care	389
12	Special Concerns of Women	427
13	The Digestive System	451
14	Nutrition	493
15	The Teeth and Their Care	521
16	The Eyes	551
17	Ears, Nose and Throat	583
18	Bones and Muscles and Their Disorders	615

Chapter		Page
19	Arthritis and Rheumatism	653
20	Allergies and Hypersensitivity	671
21	Emotional and Mental Illnesses	707
22	Your Operation	721
23	X-Rays and You	781
24	Laboratory Tests	793
25	Medical Genetics	803
26	Cancer	811
27	Drug Use and Abuse	815
28	First Aid for Your Family	821

So that you can get *First Aid* information quickly, this
section is tabbed with a red cross.

Illustrated Encyclopedia
of Medical Terms

	Page
Words Your Doctor Uses	873
Encyclopedia of Medical Terms	880

INDEX

HOME CARE OF THE PATIENT

by DONALD G. COOLEY

GOOD NURSING HABITS

Giving Medicines • Communicable Diseases • Sickroom Routines • Sanitation • Moving the Patient in Bed • Comfort with Pillows

SICKROOM EQUIPMENT

The Patient's Bed • Footrests and Backrests • The Nurse's Gown • Ventilation • Furnishings

COMMON NURSING PROCEDURES

Handling Dishes and Linens • Taking the Temperature and Pulse • Making an Occupied Bed • The Patient's Bath • Bed Baths • Backrub • Bedpan • Bedsores • Hot Compresses • Steam Inhalation • Croup Tents • Paraffin Packs • Cold Applications • Enemas

SPECIAL DIETS

Convalescent Diet • Bulk-forming Diet • Bland Diet • Low-sodium Diet

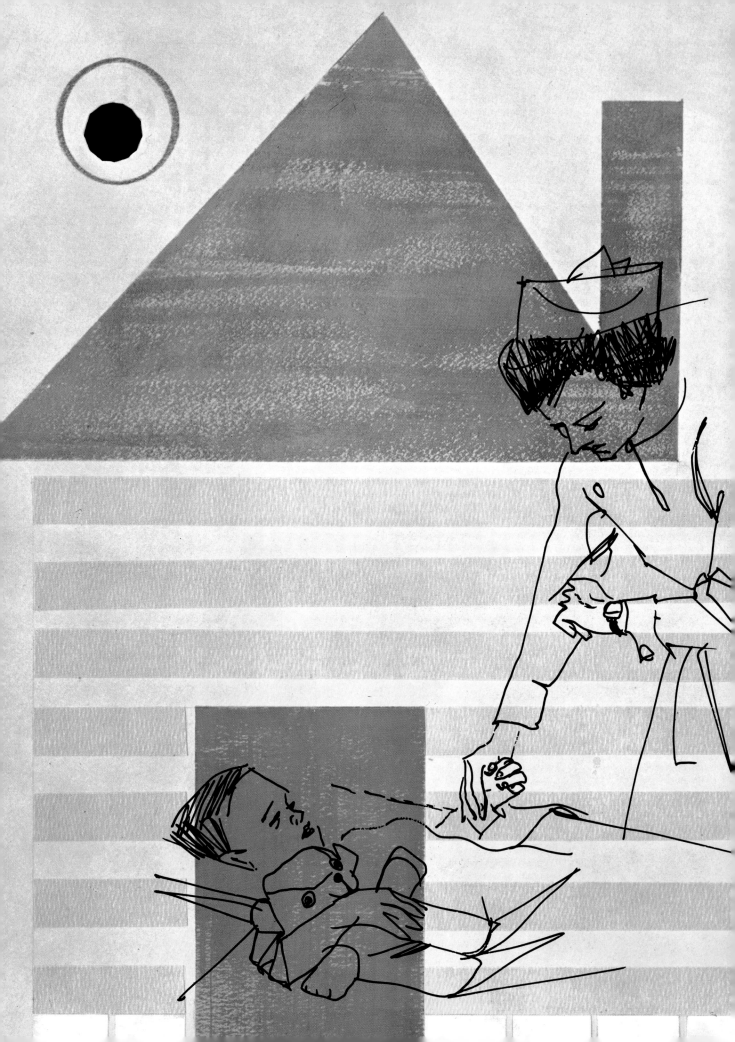

HOME CARE OF THE PATIENT

by DONALD G. COOLEY

To every family there comes a time when someone who is ill or injured or convalescent must be, or could be, taken care of at home. An illness may be so trivial and fleeting that no special nursing skill is needed, other than placating an irritable and grumpy patient who isn't sick enough to be tractable. Other illnesses may be chronic, prolonged, require rearrangement of a room of the house, perhaps some special equipment, and unremitting care of a bedfast patient. For many illnesses, of course, hospital care is mandatory, at least in the acute stages.

Things to Consider

A decision to undertake home care of a patient for any extended time is not to be made lightly. Yet home care is often feasible and in the best interests of the patient, if there is someone who cares and can give care. There is increasing emphasis on "co-ordinated home care" or "extended medical care in the home," for patients who do not need fulltime medical attention in hospitals. This tendency is accelerated by earlier discharge from the hospital of both surgical and medical patients, and by shortages of hospital beds in some communities.

There are other cogent reasons for home nursing care. It is almost always less expensive than hospital care at $75 a day or even more. Perhaps more important, the ill and convalescent usually are happier and get well faster in familiar surroundings. This is especially true of children.

If prolonged care of a chronically ill or disabled or handicapped person who needs fairly constant attention is involved, remember that a decision to take care of the patient at home is not easily reversible. Be realistic; anticipate what lies ahead. It may be advisable to employ a housekeeper or practical nurse to help ease the burdens that could eventually "wear down" a lone home nurse, no matter how devoted.

It is presupposed that patients cared for at home are under the supervision of a physician. The other essential ingredient is a capable home nurse. Talk matters over with your doctor before assuming the responsibility of nursing care for any considerable length of time. Get a clear idea of what you will have to do for a particular patient, write down the doctor's orders, and keep written records as he directs.

This chapter describes some common nursing procedures, sickroom equipment, and "know-how" which make care easier to give or more comforting to the patient. Not every measure will apply to every patient, of course. An ordinary patient with an ordinary minor upset can be kept in his ordinary bedroom in an ordinary way. But keep watch for *fever, vomiting, prostration, pain,* which may indicate that the illness is not ordinary at all and that the doctor should be called.

There are better ways of becoming an accomplished home nurse than by reading a book. It is a splendid idea for someone in the family to take a home nursing course such as is given by the Red Cross in most communities. Usually mother is elected, but mother can get sick too, and a father or son or daughter who can give some minimum niceties of attention is nice to have around the house.

Assistance may be available. Visiting nurses associations in many communities provide trained nurses who come to the home to give aid and attention where need exists. Some voluntary health groups have mobile therapy units. Loan or rental of equipment may sometimes be arranged through local sources. Your doctor and local health department can inform you about services that may appreciably ease the burdens of home care.

Good Nursing Habits

Regardless of the nature of the patient's illness, certain nursing practices should become so automatic that you apply them routinely as a matter of habit. Other measures which apply to specific situations will be discussed later.

Handwashing. Wash your hands — preferably under running water—before and after attending the patient. Work up a good lather with soap and water. Rub hands together vigorously and work between the fingers and around the nails. Nurses keep their fingernails trimmed closely (imagine being backrubbed with clawlike nails). Wash above your wrists. Rinse well. If running water is not available, pour clean water from a pitcher over your hands. Repeat the lathering and rinsing. Rinse the bar of soap after each use.

Dry your hands well with a clean towel or paper towel. A combination of moisture and cold predisposes to chapping. You can use a hand cream or lotion to help keep the skin supple.

Gown. Some sort of gown for the home nurse looks professional and protects the clothing. If your patient has a minor "in one day, out the next" upset, an apron or launderable cotton dress may be most practical. If he has a communicable disease (see below) the doctor may recommend a gown to be worn and kept in the sickroom.

Waste disposal. Dispose of the patient's bowel and bladder discharges immediately. Provide a container for soiled tissues and bandages. Line it with a paper bag which can be closed without touching the contents. Place it where the patient can reach it. Pick up soiled materials through a fold of newspaper or use tongs. Provide paper tissues for nasal and throat discharges.

Dishes. It is a good idea for the patient to have dishes and eating utensils separate from the family's — perhaps a set of a different color. However, hot water and soap, hot water rinsing and drying, remove or destroy most germs. Your usual dishwashing methods will be adequate unless the patient's illness requires special precautions. Mechanical dishwashers which use water at temperatures higher than human hands can stand are excellent. Dirty dishes of course should be washed promptly. Scrape the patient's food scraps onto a newspaper, wrap, and put in the garbage can.

Linens. Collect soiled sickroom linens in a bag or newspaper and wash the batch in your usual way. After washing, the linens may be dried and ironed along with the rest of the family laundry, unless other orders have been given.

Giving Medicines

Check the label and directions each time you give a medicine (you could be mistaken about lookalike bottles). Measure the amount exactly. Ask the doctor whether tablets can be crushed and given in orange juice or something palatable to a child. Or whether capsules can be opened and the contents mixed with jelly to "get it down" a small child. Set an alarm clock to be sure that medicines are given at specified times. Ask the doctor whether a patient should be awakened at night to take his medicine. Sometimes this is necessary, sometimes not. Medicines, and the doctor's reasons for prescribing them, differ a great deal, and it is important for the nurse to get clear directions, to write them down, and to keep a record of doses she gives.

If the Patient Has a Communicable Disease

A "catching" or communicable disease requires extra nursing precautions. If at all possible, the sickroom should be isolated and removed from the flow of family traffic. While it is true that members of the family may have been exposed to the patient's germs during the incubation stage of his disease, it is best to have a separate sickroom and to keep family members, pets, and visitors out of it. Transmission of infection works both ways. A visitor may "pick up" the patient's germs, but the patient may also acquire some of the visitor's germs, which, on top of those he already has, may complicate his illness.

A *coverall gown* for the nurse is practically mandatory. This can be any suitable light garment which covers the clothing and arms — a housecoat, full apron, long smock. Preferably, it should fasten at the back. Hang it on a clothes tree inside the sickroom. Put it on when you go in and take it off when you go out.

Think of the inside of the gown, next to your clothing, as the clean side, the outside as the contaminated side. Wash your hands before you put it on. Grasp the inside of the gown and work your arms into the sleeves without touching the outside. Fasten. Wash your hands before removing the gown, slip your arms out of the sleeve, and put it on its hanger with the inside in. Just remember: inside clean, outside contaminated.

Dishes should be kept separate from the family's. Soak them in boiling water for about ten minutes, immediately after use, then wash with soap or detergent. Paper dishes are convenient; they can be wrapped in a newspaper, food scraps and all, for immediate disposal.

Linens may need boiling for ten minutes before laundering. Some diseases may require special handling of bowel discharges. Your doctor will give any special directions that may be necessary. He will also tell you what local health regulations may require, and whether or not it is necessary to keep family members out of school or work.

Cleanup of the Sickroom

The final cleanup of the sickroom after the patient has recovered is, in essence, little more than good housekeeping. Fumigation is almost never practiced any more, except in special circumstances, such as ridding premises of ticks and mites. Sunlight and dryness destroy most germs in a short time.

Launder everything washable in your usual way. Non-washable things such as mattresses, thick rugs, pillows, and overstuffed toys should be given an all-day outdoor airing in bright sunshine. Non-boilable rubber equipment should be washed in soap and water, dried, and aired in the sun. Wash down the floors, woodwork, doorknobs, bathroom, and unupholstered furniture with soap and water. Air the room for several hours on a dry, sunshiny day.

Don't Give House Room to Staph Germs

Staphylococcus germs are common inhabitants of the skin and nasal passages. Some strains of these germs cause little trouble, and if they do, are controllable by common antibiotic drugs. The worst strains are called "resistant staph" because common drugs have little if any effect on them. Sometimes they are called "hospital staph" because the resistant varieties tend to proliferate under hospital conditions. Strenuous aseptic techniques and housekeeping measures have done a great deal to reduce epidemics of hospital staph.

But resistant strains are sometimes unknowingly carried into the home. What happens then may not be recognized as due to staph germs. A baby may have impetigo, an older brother, nasty crops of styes. Father may have boils, mother, a severe fingernail infection, sister, a bad sore throat. There may be minor troubles that clear up without medical attention. The illnesses may come weeks or months apart, and probably will not be attributed to a common cause: a bad strain of staph germs at loose in the house. Even doctors may not recognize an epidemic situation, if impetigo is treated by a pediatrician, boils by the family doctor, styes by an ophthalmologist. Suspicion may be aroused by a plague of infections, with different manifestations, which seem to run through the family.

Hygienic measures, some of them quite simple, others calling for a little more effort or alertness than usual, can do a great deal to interrupt chains of staph transmission. Here are some recommended precautions if your doctor confirms that bad-acting staph germs are being passed around in your house:

Take showers instead of tub baths.

Give everybody his individual towel and washcloth. No common towel.

Don't share brushes, combs, toilet articles.

Keep washbowls, toilet seats, bathrooms and fixtures scrupulously clean.

Use disposable tissues instead of handkerchiefs. Put paper towel dispensers in the kitchen and elsewhere. Drop these soiled disposable articles into a paper bag, close the top and burn or discard promptly.

Wash the hands before eating and after handling dressings, bandages, or contaminated clothing of an infected person. Germicidal soaps and liquid germicidal detergents that have longer-lasting germ-suppressing action on the skin than ordinary soap are widely available.

After laundering towels and linens, iron with a dry iron.

Comfort with Pillows

There is immense comfort to the bed-fast patient in the artful positioning of pillows. They "doeth good like a medicine." The human body has joints, bony prominences, and curves that are pleasing to the eye but ill-designed for lying in flat planes on a flat surface. In principle, "pillowmanship" is the art of giving cushiony support to body parts that are in a state of tension or pressure and of keeping the parts in comfortable alignment. A patient in bed needs frequent changes of position not only for comfort but to help sustain good muscle tone and spread the labor fairly among different structures.

In addition to pillows of conventional size, there should be one or two smaller ones. Pillows for support need not necessarily be regular pillows. You can put a small cushion into a pillowcase, or roll a blanket to make a long bolster, or fold cloth pads to any desired shape and thickness.

There are no hard-and-fast rules about positioning pillows. You'll know you've done right if, after tucking a pillow in place, the patient says "that feels good."

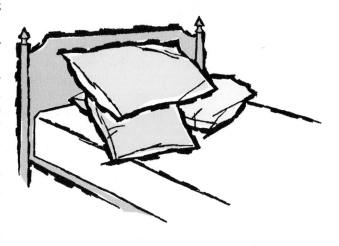

Three pillows arranged as shown give stable support for a patient lying on his back in a partial sitting-up position. Adjust to give support to upper shoulders and small of the back.

Common sense will guide you if the patient has a sore spot, a bandaged leg or some local area of injury or discomfort. We will discuss some common situations and some well-tested ways of dealing with them.

Lying on back. If only one head pillow is used when the patient lies on his back, it should be pulled down enough to support the upper shoulders and base of the neck where many tensions begin. Don't

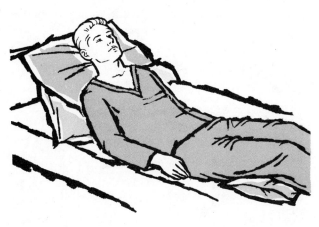

For comfort of legs stretched out straight when the patient lies on his back, bend the knees slightly and tuck a small pillow or blanket roll under them. This also helps to keep him from slipping toward the foot of the bed.

put the pillow so high that the patient's chin is pushed down toward his chest.

With three pillows, you can make a comfortable nestlike arrangement that is quite stable. Place two pillows like an inverted V pointing to the top of the bed, with one pillow overlapping the other. The inside corners where the V spreads should be fairly close together. Put a third pillow crosswise over the bottom

two. Or the order can be reversed, with the horizontal pillow on the bottom.

The legs of a patient lying on his back will be most uncomfortable if stretched out straight for any length of time (try it yourself — a good way to become an understanding nurse). Bend his knees a little and tuck a small pillow or folded roll under them. If his legs tend to roll outward, a pillow or blanket roll on the outer side of each leg will give support. Another way is to put a pad or blanket under the patient's legs and roll each projecting end inward to make a cushion. (See footrests).

Lying on side. The side-lying patient curves like a comma. A pillow at the abdomen gives something to "curl on." Another pillow at the small of the back gives something to lean on. Tuck the pillow edges under the body just enough to give resilient anchorage. Use a head pillow giving shoulder support.

In lying sidewise the lower leg naturally is slightly bent and extended to a comfortable position. The upper leg should be bent more upward and forward, like a buttress to keep the trunk from rolling. Put a pillow under the upper leg to support and elevate it a little from knee to foot. If the patient wants

In side-lying position, give comfort and support with a pillow at the small of the back and another in front of the abdomen — tucked in close enough so the patient has something to lean on. A pillow under the flexed knee of the upper leg (or between the knees) is also comforting. If ankles rub together another pillow can be placed between them.

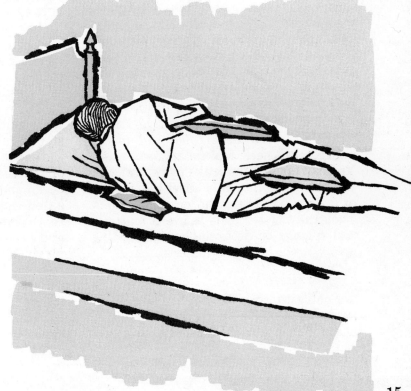

to lie with one leg on top of or close to the other, put a pillow between the legs to prevent knee and ankle from rubbing.

Lying face down. Some people like to sleep on their "stomachs." There is nothing the matter with this position (babies often prefer it) and no reason why a patient can't take it for a change unless his illness forbids it. It is a good position for a backrub. Besides a head pillow, the patient's arms and chest may need support — a second pillow may be needed for an outflung arm to curl around, another to tuck along the ribs.

Sitting up in bed. Some sort of backrest slanted against the head of the bed is necessary when the patient sits up. Put pillows on the backrest to support head and shoulders, perhaps at the sides to rest elbows and forearms, and at the small of the back.

Backrests can be bought or improvised. Inexpensive wedge-shaped backrests are stuffed with firm material; some kinds have armrests. These are good for reading in bed any time. You can improvise a backrest from a card table (legs folded), or a piece of plywood, tied at a slant to the headboard of the bed. A carton made of stiff corrugated cardboard can be made into a wedge-shaped backstop. Cut the carton ends diagonally. You will then see how, with a little cutting and bending, the parts can be taped together to make a box with triangular sides, straight back, and slanted front. Cover with cloth. You can remove the legs from a suitable chair and use it as a backrest.

One trouble with sitting up in bed is that one tends to slide down and footward. A pillow or blanket roll placed under the knees makes a good brake. You can anchor the brake more firmly by wrapping a pillow in a sheet like a piece of taffy and twisting the loose sheet ends. Tuck the twisted ends between mattress and springs or tie to the bedrail.

Foot Supports

Footrests serve two purposes. They keep upper bedding from pressing heavily on upturned toes, and they give

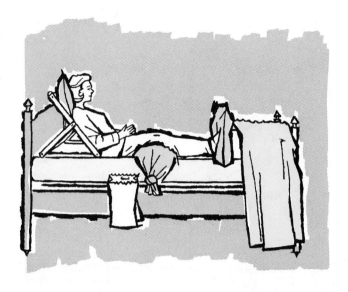

The Complete Patient: backrest, pillow support for shoulders, knee support, footrest, "bumper" at foot of mattress to prevent slipping, waste bag pinned to mattress within easy reach.

the patient something to brace his feet against. It is very uncomfortable for a patient who lies on his back to have his feet pulled down by a tight topsheet that leaves no room to wiggle. In time this may cause a floppy condition known as foot-drop.

It's quite simple to give footroom to a bedridden patient. All that is necessary is to elevate top bedding an inch or two higher than the patient's upturned feet. You can do this in a variety of ways.

You can place a fat roll of blanket, or stuff a couple of pillows, under the tucked-under topsheet at the foot of the bed. A piece of plywood, a fold of thick foam rubber, or cushions from upholstered furniture can be placed between the end of the mattress and the footboard of the bed. A bumper of proper size can be made by cutting and taping a corrugated paper carton. If the bed has no footboard, a piece of wood can be nailed and braced at right angles to a piece of plywood which fits between mattress and springs. The plywood can be tied to bedrails if mattress pressure does not hold it firmly enough. Drape the top bedclothing over the footrest to give the patient space for toe movements.

When the patient sits up there may be a gap between his feet and the footrest. Close it with pillows, cushions, a weighted box, so that the soles of his feet are comfortably braced. When making the bed, pinch the top bedclothing together in a pleat or two so it can "give" and afford kickroom.

Moving the Patient in Bed

Always let the patient move or help to move himself if possible. If he is helpless he will need aid. Tell him what you are going to do before you do it. Remove or pull down top bedding for freedom of movement. *Roll* and *slide* the patient gently; do not lift unnecessarily. Think of the hips and shoulders as "pivots" of the body. The patient should be fairly close to the edge of the bed so the nurse doesn't have to bend awkwardly.

Turning from back to side. Put the patient's ankles together and straighten his legs. Keep your knees against the edge of the bed. Reach across and put your right hand around and partly under his far shoulder near the arm joint. Put your left hand similarly around and under his hip. Roll him toward you with an upward-pulling motion until he is on

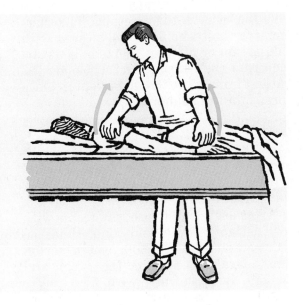

To turn patient from his back to his side, straighten his legs, grasp shoulder and hip firmly, and roll him toward you as shown.

his side. Arrange his arms comfortably.

You can also put your hands under his near shoulder and hip and roll him away from you. But it is usually easier to pull than to push.

If there is a drawsheet under the patient, you can loosen it, grasp its far edge and pull up and toward you to roll the patient on his side. A drawsheet may also be used to pull the patient toward the foot or head of the bed, or to roll him from a face-down position onto his side or back.

Turning from side onto back. Reverse the above procedure. Standing at the patient's back, put your hands on his near hip and shoulder and roll him downward and toward you.

Helping the patient to sit up. Curl one arm under and entirely around the patient's shoulder so that your flat hand will have a good grasp around the arm-shoulder joint. Let your other forearm lie along the patient's chest so he can situate his arm under your armpit and grasp the top of your shoulder. At "ready" signal, lift up and forward. The patient can use his free arm as a brace to prop himself. Keep your arm high enough around his shoulders and neck so his head doesn't flop backward.

If the patient is to get out of bed, into a chair brought to the bedside, help him to sit up and support him while you swing his legs around to hang over the bed. Keep supporting him until any momentary dizziness passes. A patient's chair should be sturdy and have arms that he can grasp to help himself out of bed. If the patient cannot help himself you may need assistance to get him safely into the chair. An ironing board as a bridge between bed and chair helps the patient to slide over.

How to Take the Temperature

Body temperature varies slightly through the day and in different parts of the body. Skin is cooler than internal organs. Average normal temperature taken by mouth is 98.6° F. A range of 98° to 99° is not particularly significant.

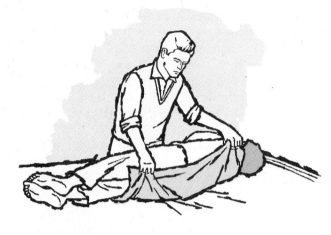

When a drawsheet is used, the patient is easily turned from his back to his side by rolling him toward you in the sheet, as shown. If there is no drawsheet, lean over the patient, grasp under shoulder and hip, and roll him toward you.

But fever—excessively high temperature —is significant, and a subnormal temperature may also have meaning. Whether a fever fluctuates, increases, disappears and returns, subsides or does not subside after taking medicines, or has other characteristics, may be important for a doctor to know. Frequently the doctor asks a home nurse to take the patient's temperature at certain times or intervals. If so, follow his directions faithfully and be sure to keep an accurate written record of the time and reading.

The clinical thermometer is the familiar instrument for taking temperatures. There are two general types, *oral* and *rectal*. The latter has a somewhat fatter bulb (the part that holds the mercury). The thin glass tube of the thermometer, about three and a half inches long, has a triangular shape, with short and long lines that look like markings on a ruler on one side of the triangle, and figures beginning with "94" and ending with "110" on the opposite end.

You "read" the thermometer by holding the end opposite the mercury bulb in your fingers, in good light, and looking through the peak of the triangular glass toward the flat base. There is a little bubble where the clear glass joins the bulb. Rotate the thermometer slowly; the bubble appears to widen. Above it you should see a flat silver ribbon. If you

don't, rotate the thermometer a very little one way or the other until the ribbon appears. It disappears completely if the viewing angle is slightly changed.

The end of the silver ribbon marks the temperature reading. The long lines of the ruler-like markings correspond to degrees of temperature on the other side of the triangle. The short lines are fifths of a degree (or two-tenths). An arrow points to the 98.6° mark, and above this the markings are usually in red, indicating fever.

Temperatures are most commonly and conveniently taken by mouth. Be sure the mercury is shaken down to around the 95° mark. To shake it down, hold the thermometer firmly between thumb and fingers by the end opposite the bulb and give two or three sharp downward flicks of the wrist, like cracking the whip. Read the thermometer to be sure that the mercury is actually shaken down.

Place the thermometer bulb well under the patient's tongue, and keep it there at least three minutes. He must keep his lips closed and not talk or bite on the stem. Do not take the temperature immediately after taking a hot bath, smoking, or eating hot or cold foods.

Rectal temperature is about one degree higher than mouth temperature. For various reasons, such as dry or inflamed mouth, or nasal congestion with mouth-breathing, it may be necessary to take the temperature rectally. The thermometer bulb should be lubricated with cold cream or oil and inserted about one inch into the rectum, preferably by the patient himself. It should be kept in place three minutes or more.

Sometimes the temperature is taken by placing the thermometer in the armpit, with the arm well pressed against the body for five minutes or more. Normal armpit temperature is one degree lower than mouth temperature.

After use, clean the thermometer with cool or tepid water and soap. Hold the thermometer by the top, wet a cotton wipe, wrap it around the stem and wriggle it downward with firm finger pressure. Rinse with clean water. Repeat the same operation, dry the thermometer, put it in its container. It is not necessary to use powerful antiseptics. Do not hold the thermometer under very hot running tap water, or in a basin of hot water. The mercury might expand enough to break the instrument.

If you cannot read the thermometer, put it away until someone else can. The silver ribbon will stay where it is until it is shaken down.

What happens if a clinical thermometer breaks in the mouth and some of the mercury is swallowed? Nothing much. Salts of mercury are poisonous but metallic mercury is inert.

kinds of necessary or desirable equipment will be described later. The main thing is that accumulated equipment should be kept tidily (and some pieces, inconspicuously) in a closet of the sickroom, or the bathroom, or neatly arranged on a table or shelves, so that steps are saved when the nurse needs them.

A few things are essential. Give the patient some means of summoning you— a bell, a buzzer, even a tin pan to be struck like a gong. There should be a bedside table within the patient's reach, to hold a glass of water, paper tissues, perhaps a book or magazine or clock. The

Oral and rectal clinical thermometers are shown below. The oral type has a relatively long bulb that holds the mercury; the rectal type has a fatter bulb. Rectal temperature is about one degree higher than oral temperature.

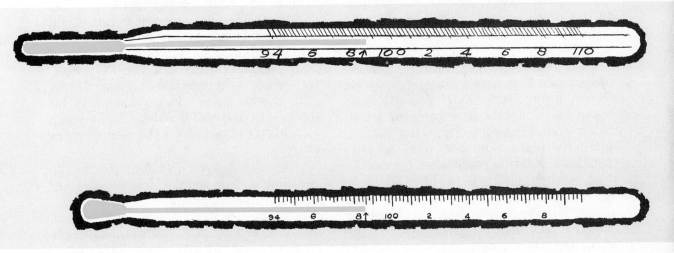

The Sickroom

The ideal sickroom is cheery, light, quiet, uncluttered, well ventilated, and has an adjoining bathroom. A room on the ground floor, where the kitchen is, saves the home nurse much tiring stairclimbing. Also, a ground floor room is usually closer to household activities and easier to get to when an unattended patient calls for attention. You may have to compromise. An upstairs room may be quieter and easier to isolate. If there's a choice, select a room that is close to a bathroom. Place the bed to avoid dazzling light or shiny reflections.

Equipment. Needs of patients vary. Some need bedpans, some don't. Various

doctor may allow a table radio, a joy to shut-ins who are not too ill. An ordinary night table may be too small to accommodate desired items. A table like a teacart on casters, with a shelf, is quite practical and can be rolled aside for bedmaking.

There should be a waste can lined with newspapers or a paper bag to drop used tissues and dressings into. A paper bag, rolled at the top to make a rim that keeps it open, can be pinned to the side of the mattress within easy reach of the patient.

Furnishings. Don't strip the sickroom to prison-like bareness. Leave some of the amenities that soften harshness and cheer the patient. His emotional attitudes are important to his getting well.

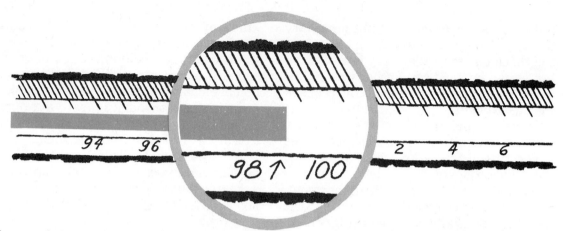

94 96 98↑ 100 2 4 6

Closeup of clinical thermometer registering normal temperature of 98.6 degrees, marked by arrow. To read the thermometer, hold the end opposite the mercury bulb, look through the peak of the triangular-shaped glass stem toward the base, rotate slowly until the ribbon of mercury comes into view.

A rug or carpet that covers most of the floor may be left where it is. But remove small scatter rugs that are invitations to tripping.

Leave everything that is easily laundered — curtains that soften glare, dresser covers, doilies. Mainly, get rid of excesses that give a cluttered look or impair nursing efficiency. You will need a table — a sturdy card table or something comparable — for wash basins, pitchers, trays, and the like, so that articles are within reach when needed.

A comfortable chair for the patient, if he can sit up, is essential. Add a plain chair for the nurse, another chair or bench if visitors are permitted and the room is large enough. Removal of a big upholstered chair may leave room for a couple of plain ones, and give the room a more airy look. A footstool which helps the patient to get out of bed also serves as rest for his legs when he is sitting in a chair.

Check the position of room lamps so they do not glare at the patient. A sick person should not look at a lamp with part of a bare bulb visible — nor a well person, either. A switch for turning on a lamp at night should be reachable by the patient in bed.

Dust the room with a damp cloth or oil mop. Keep a carpet-sweeper for the rug in a nearby closet. Dry-dusting and sweeping stir up dust. The woodwork and exposed floors can be washed down occasionally with water and soap or detergent.

Room ventilation. In cool weather, the room temperature should be kept evenly around 72 to 75 degrees in the daytime and three or four degrees lower at night. Fresh air is not necessarily cold air. A cold sleeping room is not ideal for everybody, and certainly not for ill people. Babies put snugly to bed in a warm room with a wide open window may kick off the covers and suffer severe chills when cold blasts of air drop the temperature sharply.

Keep the sickroom free of drafts. To ventilate a room when it's cold and windy outside, open opposite windows a little way at the top to create a gentle cross-flow of fresh air. You can put a deflector on the sill of a partly open window, or muffle incoming drafts by standing a folding screen in front of it. If drafts are inevitable, the patient can be protected by placing a couple of chairs on the drafty side of his bed and draping a blanket over them.

Room air is practically always too dry when heating systems are on. This dries nasal membranes and may irritate respiratory passages and cause breathing discomfort. You can increase the sickroom humidity gratifyingly, and comfortingly, by using a humidifier, vaporizer, shallow pans of water on a radiator, or letting vapor from the hot shower tap in an adjacent bathroom permeate the room.

People get sick in hot, muggy weather as well as in winter. Excessive heat is a great physical burden on the heart, actually a form of strenuous exercise even though one is lying still in bed. If the house has an air-conditioned room, obviously this is the room of choice for the patient who is ill during a heat wave. Fans do not cool the air, but move it. Air moving over the skin assists the evaporation of perspiration, and feels cool. However, a properly placed fan can draw cool night air into the house, or a single room.

For instance, you can place a good-sized fan directly in front of an open window of the sickroom, to push air *out* of the room. Close the sickroom door and open another window through which cool night air can come in to replace muggy room air that is being blown out.

Cooling part of the body cools the whole of it. A good "body cooler" is a basin of cool water in which the patient submerges his hand and wrist or entire forearm. This is practical for a patient in bed. A cool sponge bath is also comforting.

The Patient's Bed

For a brief illness, the bed the patient is accustomed to is quite satisfactory. For more extended home care, choice of a bed that saves the nurse's energies is more important. A single or twin bed is easier to make, and walk around, than a double bed, and the patient is more accessible. If the patient is completely bedridden and requires care for a long time, it may be wiser to rent a hospital type bed from a hospital supply company. Equipment is sometimes loaned by community agencies. Ask your doctor.

The mattress should be firm and resilient. Foam rubber mattresses are good. The patient should not sink into a too-soft or saggy mattress. If bedsprings sag, a piece of plywood between mattress and springs will give stiffness.

Ordinary beds are lower than hospital beds. This makes little difference if the patient is in and out of bed frequently, sits in a chair, goes to the bathroom. But a little extra bed height saves much wear and tear on the home nurse, is kinder to her back, and reduces stressful bending and reaching, if the patient needs considerable bed care for considerable time. Some height can be added by putting a second mattress on top of the first. Or the legs of the bed can be raised by putting them into tin cans filled about two-thirds full with sand or gravel, with the cut-out end of the can, or something flat and firm, placed on top of the sand. Cement blocks, wood blocks, or firmly tied stacks of newspapers can also serve as "elevators."

Place the bed so that neither the sides nor foot are against a wall.

Bedmaking

Obviously, the patient should be kept warm and comfortable and free from drafts while his bed is being made. If he has a communicable disease, observe the special precautions mentioned elsewhere.

The usual sequence of bedding, from the mattress up, is as follows:

Mattress pad
Bottom sheet
Waterproof pad *if necessary*
Drawsheet
Topsheet
Blanket and spread

Sheets should be wide and long enough for generous amounts to be tucked under the mattress to hold the sheet smoothly and firmly. Contour sheets with boxlike corners that fit around the mattress leave few wrinkles, if of the proper size.

If the patient needs bedpan care, is incontinent, perspires profusely, or if the aridity of the mattress is otherwise imperiled, a pad of moisture-resistant material is clearly indicated. But it is best omitted if it serves no real purpose. Rubber sheets and similar materials tend to make the patient feel uncomfortably warm (and humiliated). Washable waterproof materials with a cloth covering can be purchased. Oilcloth or old shower curtains are serviceable substitutes. You can put layers of newspapers inside plastic garment bags. These have the advantage of discardability.

Quilted mattress pads with washable stuffing are standard. If disposability is desired, you can make a good pad from layers of newspapers with old sheeting or cotton cloth laid above and below.

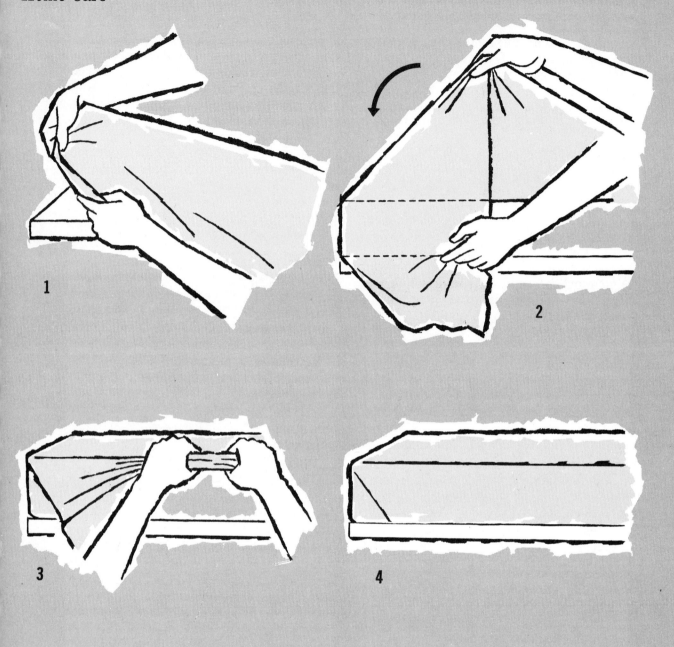

How to make square corners: 1. Spread sheet smoothly over mattress with about 18 inch overhang at head and foot; tuck the ends under. 2. Lift edge of sheet to taut triangular shape as shown, tuck bottom part under mattress. 3. Drape overhang of sheet over edge of mattress. Pull sheet tight, smooth, wrinkle-free. 4. Tuck overhang under mattress as shown.

A drawsheet may or may not be needed. It is simply a short sheet immediately under the patient, extending from the head to the knee region. Smooth the drawsheet and tuck the ends under the mattress sides to hold it securely. A drawsheet may be helpful in turning or moving the patient, and it gives a little extra mattress protection.

Making an Empty Bed

Assemble what you will need — clean linen, a chair or table to hold blankets or spreads that will be re-used, a receptacle for soiled linen. The latter can be a tub or basket lined with newspapers, a laundry bag, or, perhaps simplest of all, newspapers spread on the floor. The corners of the newspapers can be pulled together without touching the soiled linen inside.

Strip the bed. Turn the mattress from head to foot if it seems "lumpy." Put on the mattress pad and smooth it. If you use a contour sheet, apply it, making sure that the sheet and the pad beneath it are tight and smooth. The keynote of good bedmaking is smoothness without wrinkles. Patients are not quite so sensitive as the princess who couldn't sleep because there was a butterfly's wing beneath her eiderdown mattress, but some come close to it.

If you use a flat sheet, spread it over the mattress pad with enough overhang —about 18 inches—at the head and foot. Tuck this under. Now is the time to "corner." If you haven't learned to make "square corners," you should. It separates the nurses from the girls, and is equally good for domestic bedmaking.

The drawing explains the process better than words, which make it sound more complicated than it is. Look at the drawing and directions and practice on any bed. The knack comes easily enough by doing. You can save some steps by making one side of the bed at a time. Corner the bottom sheet on one side and smooth it toward the opposite side. Place the waterproof pad, if you use one, and over this the drawsheet, which can be an ordinary sheet folded in the middle so it's standard width but about half as long. Smooth the drawsheet so the top edge will be under the patient's pillow, and tuck the sides tightly under the mattress.

Unfold the topsheet lengthwise and line its center with the center of the bed. Let the foot end hang over. Smooth the sheet on your side. Place the blanket in the same way. Go to the other side of the bed. Grasp the bottom sheet firmly and pull it tightly and smoothly over the edge of the mattress. Pull diagonally as well as toward you for uniform tautness. Make corners. Smooth out the waterproof pad. Pull the drawsheet tightly and anchor it. Smooth out the topsheet and blanket and tuck under at the foot. Allow for toe room (see *footrests*).

The usual way of putting on a pillow-case, by holding the pillow in one's teeth and pulling the cover over it, is not out-standingly hygienic if there has been nasal or oral contamination. You can fluff out the clean pillowcase, stand the pillow on a chair, and work the mouth of the pillowcase over it a little way. Pinch the edge of the pillow through the pillowcase and pull the covering down without touching the pillow.

Making an Occupied Bed

Have the patient hold the top of the blanket while you pull the top sheet out from under. The rest is not very much different from making an empty bed, except that you roll the patient to one side of the bed to make the unoccupied half, and then roll him back again to make the other. Meanwhile keep him warm in the blanket.

Loosen the bottom sheet and draw-sheet and roll or fold lengthwise against the patient's back. Place a clean bottom sheet on your side of the bed with the unused half folded lengthwise at the center of the bed. Smooth the sheet, pull it tight, make corners and tuck under. Place and anchor the drawsheet with the unused part folded similarly. Roll the patient over the folded or rolled material to the clean side of the bed. Go to the other side, remove soiled linen, draw the bottom sheet tight and make corners. Smooth the drawsheet and tuck under. Roll the patient on his back and straighten the blanket that covers him. Place a clean topsheet over the blanket. While the patient holds the topsheet, pull the blanket from under it and spread it on top of the sheet. Smooth blanket and topsheet and tuck them under the foot of the mattress.

The Patient's Bath

A quick bath stimulates circulation, is refreshing, and of course cleansing. A daily bath for the patient is customary. But use judgment. More frequent baths may be necessary if there is much soiling. On the other hand, too frequent, too prolonged baths can be fatiguing and may

How to make an occupied bed: 1. Pull topsheet from under while patient holds top of blanket. 2. Roll blanket-covered patient to one side of bed. Loosen bottom sheet and drawsheet and tuck these along patient's back. Make unoccupied side of bed. 3. Roll patient over soiled linen to other side of the bed. Strip off soiled bottom sheet and drawsheet. Pull exposed edge of clean bottom sheet and drawsheet toward you and make rest of bed. 4. Place topsheet and blanket and straighten pillows.

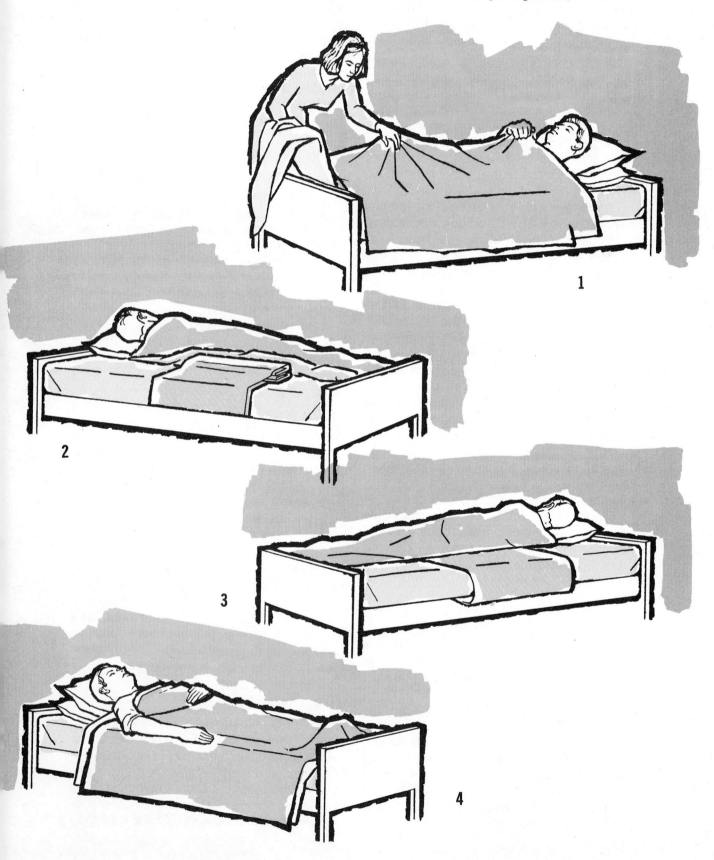

even cause slight macerations of the skin. The skin of elderly patients is often dry, and too much soap and water too frequently applied may cause itching and other discomforts. If the patient has a skin rash, eruptions, sores, ask the doctor about bath precautions.

You may want to change the bed linen when you give the bath. The sickroom should be warm and free of drafts. Keep the patient covered except for parts of the body that are being washed.

Tub Baths

Patients who are not too ill may take a tub bath if the doctor permits. The mild activity can be helpful. Fill the tub to the

simple general principles in mind:

Protect bedding with towels or blankets. Wash each part quickly, rinse off the soap, *dry thoroughly*, cover and proceed to the next area. Dry skin creases and folds particularly well. Let the patient help to wash himself, if only the face and hands, if he is able to.

Assemble what you need: wash basin, bath towels, bath blankets, washcloths, soap, toilet kit. If the sickroom is not near a bathroom, provide an extra washbasin for clean rinse water, a pitcher of warm water, and a pail for waste water.

It is good to have two lightweight cotton bath blankets. Put one of them on top of the bed blanket, have the patient hold it, and strip bed blanket and top

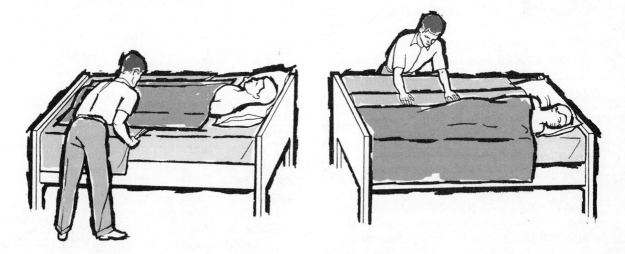

How to use lightweight bath blankets when bathing a patient in bed: 1. Put one bath blanket on top of bed blanket. While patient holds bath blanket, strip off bed blanket and topsheet. 2. Roll patient, covered by bath blanket, to one side of bed. Spread bath blanket on unoccupied side with loose edge rolled at patient's back. Move patient back onto bottom blanket. Straighten top and bottom bath blankets.

desired level with water a little warmer than body temperature (100° to 105°). Have all the essentials — soap, towels, fresh nightclothes — handy. Do not leave the patient alone in the bathroom with the door locked. Keep within earshot outside and speak to him occasionally. Never leave a small child alone in a bathtub.

Bed Baths

The art of bathing a patient in bed is not very complicated if you keep some

sheet from under. Move the covered patient to one side of the bed. Spread the second bath blanket over the bottom sheet with the loose edge folded along the patient's back. Move the patient back onto the bottom blanket and smooth it out on the other side of the bed. Remove nightclothes.

You can also put a bath towel strategically under an arm or leg as you wash it.

Fold the washcloth over your hand like a mitten so dangling ends don't drip. Wash around the patient's eyes with clear water. Wash face and ears with soapy water, rinse, dry. With patient on back, pull bath blanket part way down, wash chest and abdomen. Work quickly. Re-cover washed parts with blanket or bath towel, as you progress.

Wash arms and hands. Put the wash basin on the bed so the patient can submerge his hands. Wash the legs and feet. Place the basin so the patient can soak his foot. Turn the patient on his side and wash the back of his neck, back, and buttocks.

Leave the genital area to the last. Here the patient should wash and dry himself if he can, but assistance may be needed.

Provide a tray with toothbrush, dentifrice, water to rinse the mouth, and an empty basin, if the patient can sit up to brush his teeth. Drape a bath towel around his neck for protection. If the patient is helpless, use moistened cotton-tipped applicators to swab the inside of the mouth, teeth, gums and tongue — gently.

An occasional shampoo may be needed. The easiest technique, especially with women's long hair, is to rest the patient's head comfortably on an edge of the bed, with bath towels underneath. Put a tub or large basin on the floor, with one end of a shampoo tray, washboard, or baking pan resting in it, the other end slanted upward to rest under the patient's head. Wet the patient's hair with water from a pitcher, work up a lather with the shampoo, rinse and dry. Let the hair stream down the tray so that waste water collects in the basin on the floor.

Backrub

A good backrub can be very comforting in relieving numbness and stimulating circulation. A good time to give one is during or after the bath, before fresh nightclothes are put on. The patient may lie on his side or face down if that is more comfortable.

Wet your hands with warm rubbing alcohol or lubricate them with cocoa butter, and place them flatly on the patient's back. Move your hands to the neck, around and down to the lower spine and buttocks, up and down again for several minutes. Use firm, long, gentle strokes with a kneading motion, a little stronger on the up than the down stroke. Do not remove your hands between strokes. The area at the sides and back of the neck where big muscles connect with the upper shoulder region is a site where muscular tensions often begin. A little extra massage in this area will usually be appreciated by the patient.

Bedsores

Bedsores result from continued pressure, including weight of the body itself, on bony prominences where overlying skin is poorly padded. Vulnerable areas are the hips, elbows, tailbone, knees, shoulder blades, heels, ankles.

Earliest signs of bedsores are tender, warm, slightly reddened skin. Watch for such signs when caring for a patient, and call them to the doctor's attention. In later stages the skin is purplish, broken, raw, circulation is impaired, and treatment is difficult.

The best treatment of bedsores is prevention. Here the home nurse is very important. When bathing the patient, inspect the skin for any unusual redness, breaks, discoloration.

Cleanliness is vital. Moisture from discharges predispose to skin breakdown.

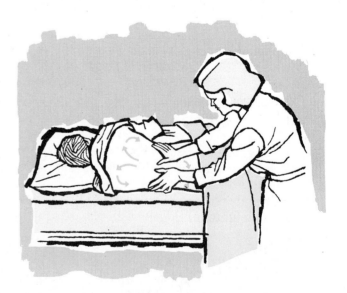

Move hands in directions shown by arrows in giving a backrub. Lubricate hands, do not remove them between strokes, use firm strokes with gentle kneading motion.

Keep the patient's skin dry. Be prompt in attending incontinent patients.

Change the position of the patient frequently. Ease pressures on reddened, tender skin areas (see *Comfort with pillows*). A pad of foam rubber under the pressure area is comforting. Pads of cotton or resilient layers of soft cloth may be bound or taped over a reddened area. Don't use inflated air cushions or "doughnut rolls" unless the doctor approves.

Don't rub reddened, tender skin areas vigorously. Wash the area with warm soapy water, rinse and pat dry, sponge with rubbing alcohol — unless the skin is broken — and cover with large cotton pads unless the doctor advises other measures.

Keep sheets dry, free of wrinkles and crumbs. Be careful to avoid skin friction when lifting the patient onto a bedpan or moving him in bed.

Pulse and Respiration

The doctor may ask you to count the patient's pulse and respiratory rate. If so, keep a written record of the reading, the date and hour. You will need a watch or clock with a second hand.

The pulse is usually counted at the wrist. A little below the base of the thumb, just inside the point where a projection of the wristbone can be felt on the thumb side, an artery runs under the skin of the inner surface of the wrist. Place your fingertips (not your thumb) on this part of the patient's wrist. Press just hard enough for pulsations to be felt. Count for 30 seconds and multiply by two to get the pulse rate. Take the pulse when the patient is quiet. For extra accuracy, count the pulse for two 30-second intervals, a little time apart, and add the two figures to get the rate per minute. The average adult has a pulse rate of 70 to 72 per minute, but this can vary a little in either direction and still be normal. Activity and excitement as well as illness can cause changes in the pulse rate.

The pulse can also be taken in other areas where an artery crosses bone near the skin surface — for instance, at the

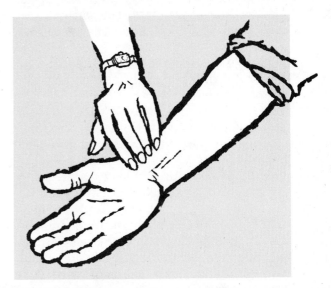

temples, or between the ankle bone and heel on the inner side of the foot.

Respiration, or breathing rate, is best counted when the patient is not aware of what you are doing. Breathing is affected by apprehension, exertion, and other factors. The resting respiratory rate of adults ranges between 14 and 18 per minute, is faster in children, and faster still in infants.

The Bedpan

Whenever it is at all possible, patients are encouraged or aided to get up and go to the bathroom. Useful activity is helpful and the seated posture more natural. However, the bedfast patient requires the ministrations of that utilitarian instrument, the bedpan, and a bell or buzzer to let his wants be known.

It is best to buy a commercial model, but a serviceable bedpan can be improvised from a baking pan with a cloth-covered board for a hip rest. A cover for the bedpan can be made by folding newspapers around it like a sleeve and fastening them with safety pins, or a thick towel may be used. It is expedient to place a large sheet of plastic or other waterproof material under the patient.

When the bedpan is needed, remove the cover and put a towel around the opening, or warm it. A bedpan kept at room temperature may feel warm enough to the hands, but not when sat upon. Unless totally helpless, the patient can assist matters by flexing the knees and digging heels and elbows into the mattress. Put your hand under the small of his back, and at signal help to raise the hips while with the other hand you slide the pan under and adjust it with the open end toward the feet. Cover the patient, leave toilet paper at hand, and give him privacy.

Provide a basin of warm water, soap, washcloth and towel. Patients want to cleanse themselves if they can. Give help if necessary. Empty the bedpan into the toilet unless the doctor instructs otherwise or there is something unusual about the contents. Rinse the pan with cold water, then brush with hot soapy water.

Rinse again, dry, cover the pan and put it away.

If the rim of the pan is chipped, padding is advisable to avoid skin scratches. Be careful to raise the patient high enough so that the skin is not injured by friction when the pan is given and removed.

If the patient can sit up, but no bathroom is nearby, an improvised commode is very helpful. Cut a hole in the seat of an old armchair — edges smoothly sanded, please—and place a pail beneath. Protect the floor with newspapers.

Male patients may need a urinal. This is a deepish bottle with a curved neck and fairly wide mouth. A reasonable facsimile can be selected from the glassware of the average home.

COMMON NURSING PROCEDURES AND EQUIPMENT

Some items of sickroom equipment mainly make it easier to give care to the patient, or make him more comfortable and contented, or both. Here are some useful items to help the patient:

Bed table. This is a flat surface on which the patient's meals are served and which he can use for writing, using coloring books, and other allowable activities when he sits or is propped up in bed. Simple U-shaped tables with long feet that slide under the bed, and a top that projects above the bedclothes, can be bought and are useful pieces of furniture for many purposes. The tops can be tilted and adjusted for height. You may have an ironing board that can be used in a similar way. Or a folding ironing board or padded board may be supported by the backs of chairs pushed against the sides of the bed. With a little cutting, taping, and ingenuity, a stout paperboard carton can be made into a serviceable bed table. Cut holes in opposite sides of the carton, for the patient's legs to fit under.

A bed cradle is a means of keeping the weight of bedclothing off the patient's body. Here, too, a paperboard carton cut with holes that arch over the patient's outstretched body is serviceable. A bed cradle can be made by cutting a barrel hoop in half and tacking lath or wood strips to the half-hoops to make an arched, tunnel-like support. Pad carefully. Often, firm cushions or pillows placed strategically alongside the patient will support sheets and blankets enough to keep him comfortable.

A bed rope gives the patient something to pull on, to help himself sit up or turn in bed, if he is permitted to. Tie a rope, strap, or nylon clothesline securely to the foot of the bed, with the loose end in reach of the patient. Be sure the rope is strong.

Treatments

The important thing in giving simple treatments to patients is to *be sure that you know what you are doing.* A hot water bag to warm a bed is safe enough, but a hot water bag on the abdomen of a patient whose pains are caused by appendicitis can be dangerous. If you have any uncertainty about doing the right thing, ask the doctor for advice.

Heat applications can be of considerable help in many conditions. Heat is soothing, tension-easing, helps to relax muscles and ease many pains. Heat increases the flow of blood, dilates vessels, brings more blood to local areas and thus improves drainage. Heat applications may be *dry* (hot water bag, electric heating pad, infra-red lamp) or *moist* (hot compresses). Dry heat is more superficial, moist heat penetrates more deeply.

Too much heat can, of course, burn. Don't apply anything to the patient's body that is too hot to hold in your own hands, or which feels too warm to the skin of your inner forearm. Check electrical heating devices for broken wires and be sure to follow the manufacturer's directions. Check a hot water bag for leaks. Fill it about half full with hot but not boiling water. Screw in the stopper a little way and squeeze out air so the bag is floppy, not inflated like a tire. Tighten the stopper and hold the bag upside down to be sure there is no leakage. Wrap in a warm towel and apply. Refill with warm water when the bag cools and reapply as often as necessary.

Remember that a comatose or disoriented patient or a baby can't tell you that a hot water bag is so hot that it's inflicting a bad burn. Be very careful in applying a hot water bag to an infant or a patient who is sedated, semi-conscious, or who can't move.

A hot compress furnishes moist heat. Use folded gauze, flannel, or soft woolen fabrics. Hold with tongs and dip into boiling water. Shake off excess water. Or you can lay a towel over the bottom and sides of a basin, place the compress in it, and pour hot water over it. Lift the towel by its ends and twist to squeeze out excess moisture. Test the compress on your own skin. Apply loosely to affected part. A strip of plastic sheeting or heavy waxed paper can be laid over the compress. Cover with a towel or soft cloth, or you can use a hot water bag to maintain heat and hold the compress in place. Replace the compress with a warm one when the first begins to cool. Continue as long, and repeat as often, as the doctor orders.

Steam inhalation is very soothing to congested breathing passages. Inhaled steam helps to soften thick secretions, to ease coughing, hoarseness, and sore throat, and to make breathing easier. Technically, what the patient inhales is not live steam, but water vapor. But this vapor may be hot enough to burn, or a wobbly container of scalding water may be tipped over, so take safety precautions.

An electric vaporizer is a worthwhile investment. Follow the manufacturer's directions. Quite satisfactory steam inhalation can be obtained from simple household equipment. Pour steaming water into a broad-mouthed pitcher or container set in a pan or basin on a table low enough for the seated patient to lean over it. Drape a blanket over the patient's head and shoulders and above the pitcher in such a way that steamy vapor is concentrated for inhalation. Or a paper bag can be slipped upside down over the pitcher, with a hole cut under a top edge to deliver vapor to the patient. A rolled newspaper can be used in a similar way, something like a stovepipe.

A croup tent is simply a means of concentrating warm water vapor for inhalation by an infant. Put a steaming teakettle or other vapor source at the side of the baby's crib. Be sure it is secure and of course out of the baby's reach. Roll newspapers into a funnel which directs vapor into the crib. Any tent-like arrangement which is secure and which confines vapors within the crib space will serve. You might cover the top of the crib with a card table or umbrella and cover the top and sides with a blanket, except the side through which warm water vapor enters the crib.

Paraffin packs may be ordered by the doctor in some special situations, such as comforting a painful arthritic hand. Such packs are, essentially, a means of maintaining heat long enough for quite deep penetration. The treated area should be hair-free, since imbedded hairs make their presence known to the patient when solidified paraffin is removed.

Melt paraffin and some mineral oil in a double boiler. A proportion of 4 pounds of paraffin (the same kind used in sealing jar tops) to 1 cup of mineral oil is about right. Test the melted mixture on your own skin. When the temperature is about right (not over 125°), have the patient dip the part in and out of the paraffin bath. Or you can paint it on with a brush. Let the paraffin harden between dippings. Build it up layer by layer to a thickness of about a quarter of an inch. Cover with aluminum foil or wax paper with a towel over all. Leave on about half an hour. The paraffin will crack off in chunks when the part being treated is moved. It can be washed and re-used.

Cold Applications

Cold compresses may be ordered for comfort, to reduce swellings or bruises, and for other purposes. Cold reduces local circulation, the opposite of heat applications. Check to be sure that cold is what the doctor ordered.

Soak folded gauze, flannel or soft cloth in a basin of ice water. Wring thoroughly so water doesn't drip and apply to the affected part. Replace with a freshly wrung compress when the first becomes warm. Stop if there are signs of chilling.

An ice collar is often advised for patients convalescing from tonsillectomies, and for other purposes. This is an ice-filled, waterproof device which fits around the throat. Check the closure to be sure that no cold water drips out. An *ice bag* can be improvised from any waterproof material, such as plastic sheets, that can be wrapped around ice and sealed tightly, or crushed ice can be poured into a hot water bag to make a cold one of it.

Sponge baths to reduce fevers are often ordered. Rubbing alcohol mixed with water is an efficient cooler because of the evaporative qualities of alcohol. However, alcohol may be inadvisable if the skin is broken, dry, or "weepy" from eruptions, and fumes may be inhaled if rubbing alcohol is used lavishly and frequently in poorly ventilated quarters. Cool but not freezing water (except in emergency treatment of heatstroke) is always safe. Dip cloths in cool water, squeeze out excess moisture, bathe the entire body. Apply moist cool cloths in

"heat pockets" of the armpit and groin. Watch for signs of chilling and stop at once if the patient begins to shiver.

Enemas

Enemas are most commonly given to flush wastes from the lower bowel, but there are other medical purposes, and sometimes medications are included. Soapsuds enemas are irritating to membranes. Unless the doctor specifies some other solution, use plain water.

Prudent considerations — waterproof sheeting, nearness of bedpan, commode, diapers or bathroom — can be left to common sense. Have everything in readiness: enema bag or container, nozzle, rubber tubing with stopcock (if necessary, tubing can be pinched with the fingers to control the flow), and something from which to hang the enema bag about 18 inches above the bed. Unless otherwise ordered, about one pint of solution is standard for adults — and please see that it is considerately warmed.

Fill the enema bag, hang it, and allow the solution to fill the tube. Preferably, the patient should lie on his side with knees partly drawn up. Lubricate the nozzle and insert it gently about two inches into the rectum. The patient will prefer to hold it in place, but give assistance if necessary. Let the solution flow out slowly; stop if the patient complains of pressure. The patient should retain the solution a few minutes, if he can. If there is any doubt the bedpan should be placed before giving the enema.

Disposable enemas containing bowel-cleansing solutions can be bought at the drugstore. These contain a half-pint or so of solution which can be expelled by squeezing a plastic bag. The entire unit can be discarded after use.

Children and infants. Give smaller amounts of enema fluid to children — a half-pint for children, two or three ounces for a baby. Use a smaller rectal tube. To give an enema to a baby, lay him on his back and remove diapers. Protect your lap, table or bathinette with waterproof material. The baby probably will not retain the solution so it is best to have him on a bedpan. A bulb syringe with a soft rubber tip is suitable for infants, or a "baby size" soft rubber catheter or baby enema equipment can be bought at a drugstore. Fill the enema bag or draw the solution into the syringe. Be sure to expel air from the tube or syringe, for air bubbles may cause cramps.

Lift the baby's legs by the ankles. Insert the lubricated nozzle about one inch into the rectum, gently. Let the solution flow out slowly. Press the baby's buttocks with a folded diaper to help hold the solution. Have basin or diaper ready to receive the expelled enema and bowel movement.

SPECIAL DIETS

Sometimes when a child has a minor illness or a patient is convalescing at home the doctor says "give him a light diet" or "a bland diet" and the home nurse may not be exactly sure what foods are suitable. Doctors also prescribe special-purpose diets as part of the treatment of certain conditions. *No one should ever go on a very restricted diet without the orders and advice of a physician.* However, some understanding of various properties of common foods is very helpful in carrying out a doctor's suggestions for the home-feeding of a patient who is not seriously or chronically ill.

Light or convalescent diet

A light, soft, or convalescent diet should furnish appetizing, easily digested, plainly cooked foods limited in coarse roughage. To tempt appetite, serve meals attractively. Don't overload trays.

Beverage: Customary beverage. Nutritious liquid snacks.

Breads, cereal products: Fine white or rye bread or rolls, crackers. Cooked cereals (strain if necessary). Cereal mush with sugar, milk. Rice, macaroni, noodles, spaghetti.

Meats, eggs, cheese: Bacon, tender beef, poultry, liver, lamb chops, fresh fish. Canned salmon or tuna. Soft-cooked eggs. Cream or cottage cheese, cheddar cheese used in cooking.

Fats: Butter, margarine, cream.

Vegetables: Strain if necessary to remove coarse fibers (or use strained vegetables or fruit for infant feeding). Vegetables can be rubbed through sieve and served as purees, used in cream soups. Or fold sieved vegetables into egg white and bake as souffles.

Fruits: Juices, purees, strained fruits, ripe bananas, cooked or canned apples, apricots, pears, peaches (no skins or seeds should be left).

Soups: Broths, clear soups. If you serve cream soups, puree the vegetables.

Desserts and sweets: Sugar, jelly. Plain cake and cookies. Gelatin desserts, custards. Ice cream, sherbet, fruit ices. Rice, tapioca, cornstarch pudding. Fruit whips.

AVOID: Fried foods, batters, rich pastries, fat-rich foods and dressings, doughnuts, nuts, pickles, bran, coarse and raw vegetables.

Bulk-forming (high-residue) diets

A certain amount of bulky material is necessary for normal bowel regularity. Foods that help to correct chronic constipation furnish increased bulk, water, lubricants, sugars and organic acids that have laxative effects. Some foods wrongly believed to be constipating are merely foods that are well assimilated and consequently leave very little residue.

High-residue foods: Whole grain cereals. Fruits as purchased. Leafy green vegetables. Vegetable pulps that are high in fiber content.

Low-residue foods: Finely milled cereals; polished, refined. Fruit juices. Pureed vegetables. Milk. Cheese. Meat, fish, poultry. Eggs.

Bland diets

List below gives some common foods that are soft, smooth, free of rough fibers and seeds, unlikely to cause irritation or to cause any increased secretion of acid juices in the stomach.

Fruits: Remove skin, strain to remove coarse fibers and seeds if present. Raw ripe banana or pear; cooked or canned apples, apricots, cherries, peaches, pears.

Fruit juices: Strain and dilute drinks by mixing with equal parts of water.

Cereals: Finely milled refined wheat, corn, rice, dry breakfast cereals, cooked cereals, macaroni, spaghetti, noodles.

Breads: Enriched white, toast, rolls, crackers.

Milk and milk products: Whole or skim milk, butter, cream, ice cream.

Meat and fish: Scraped or tender beef, lean meat, chicken, turkey, lamb, liver. Fresh fish, canned tuna or salmon.

Eggs: Soft-cooked, poached, souffle, or baked omelet.

Vegetables: Potatoes (baked, boiled, mashed, creamed), cooked or pureed asparagus, beets, carrots, peas, pumpkin, spinach, squash, green beans.

Soups: Creamed soups of allowed vegetables.

Desserts: Gelatin, custards, ice cream, ices, tapioca, rice pudding, prune whip, angel food or sponge cake, plain sugar cookies.

Beverages: Weak tea, milk.

AVOID: Coarse cereals, bran, breads made of scratchy grains, carbonated drinks, coffee, pork, veal, broth, bouillon, meat extracts, chili, highly spiced foods, fried foods, gravy, raw fruits and vegetables, nuts and pickles.

Salt-poor (low-sodium) diets

A rigid low-sodium diet requires medical supervision. Table salt, baking soda, many medicines contain sodium. The following foods are relatively low in sodium:

Fresh vegetables: Asparagus, lima and string beans, broccoli, carrots, cabbage, Brussels sprouts, cauliflower, cucumbers, eggplant, onions, parsnips, potatoes (sweet or white), lettuce, green peppers, tomatoes, turnips, pumpkin, squash.

Eggs: Yolk only.

Fats: Unsalted (sweet) butter or margarine, vegetable oils, shortenings.

Fruits and fruit juices: Apricots, pineapple, grapes, plums, oranges, grapefruit, apples, peaches, pears, figs (fresh or canned), all berries (fresh or canned), all fruit juices.

Meat: Contains sodium but one serving a day for protein is usually allowed. Fresh or frozen beef, lamb, veal, pork, chicken, turkey, fresh fish.

Milk: Contains sodium. Not over one glass daily.

Sweets and desserts: Canned and fresh fruits; rice pudding, gelatin desserts, jellies, applesauce, apple butter, marmalade, maple syrup, sugar (check possible sodium preservatives in jellies).

Cereals: Wheat cereal, farina, oatmeal, buckwheat, rice, puffed rice, puffed wheat, macaroni.

Spices and herbs to make low-salt foods more appetizing: cloves, dry mustard, pepper, onion, vinegar, horseradish, bay leaf, parsley, thyme, garlic, chives, basil, rosemary, marjoram, sage.

INFECTIOUS DISEASES

by PERRIN H. LONG, M.D.

BACTERIAL DISEASES

Pneumonia • Sore Throat • Trench Mouth • Boils • "Strep" Infections • Quinsy • Blood Poisoning • Bacterial Endocarditis • Meningitis • Botulism • Tetanus • Typhoid Fever • Food Poisoning • Dysentery • Gonorrhea • Tularemia • Anthrax

IMMUNIZATIONS

SPIROCHETAL INFECTIONS

Syphilis • Yaws • Rat-bite Fever • Relapsing Fever

VIRAL DISEASES

The Common Cold • Influenza • Yellow Fever • Cold Sores • Shingles • Parrot Fever • Lymphogranuloma Venereum • Colorado Tick Fever • Rabies • Coxsackie and ECHO Virus Infections • Poliomyelitis • Encephalitis Viral Hepatitis • Mononucleosis • Cat-scratch Disease

RICKETTSIAL DISEASES

Rocky Mountain Spotted Fever • Typhus • Q Fever • Rickettsialpox

PARASITIC INFECTIONS

Tapeworm • Trichinosis • Schistosomiasis • Hookworm • Roundworm Infections • Pinworms • Whipworms • Threadworms

PROTOZOAN INFECTIONS

Amebic Dysentery • Malaria • Toxoplasmosis

FUNGUS INFECTIONS

Thrust and Yeast-Fungus Infections • Histoplasmosis • Lumpy Jaw • Coccidioidomycosis

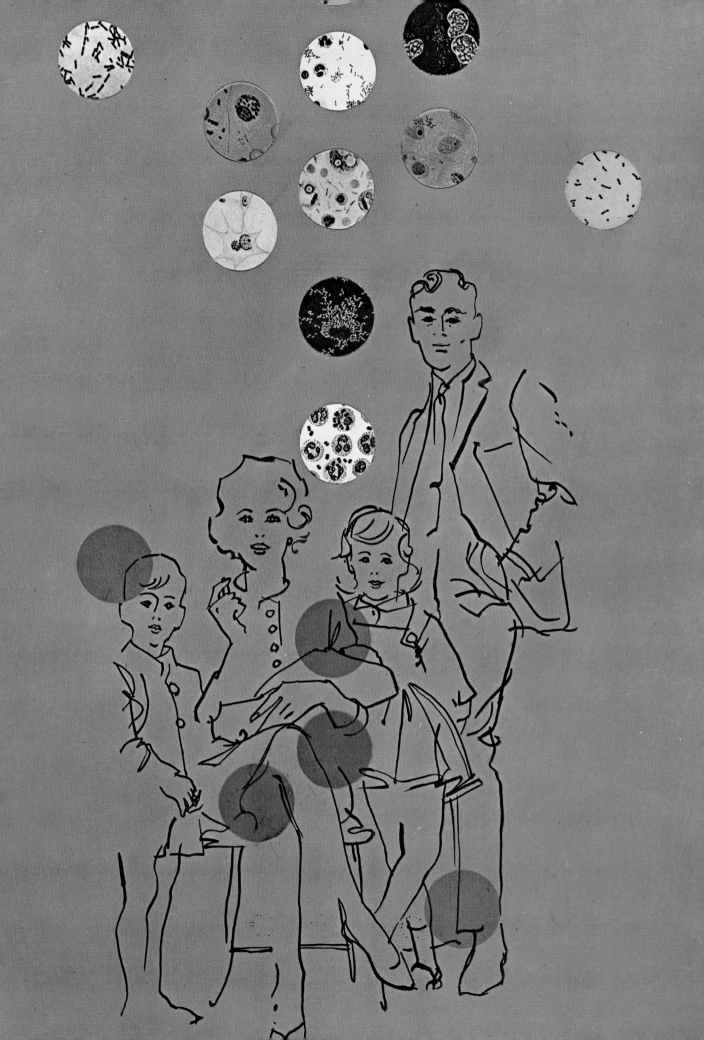

CHAPTER 2

INFECTIOUS DISEASES

by PERRIN H. LONG, M.D.

Everybody knows what causes infections. It is "germs" or microbes. "Germ" is a useful word but it covers an extraordinary variety of organisms which are quite different from each other, as we shall see. There are "good" microbes as well as "bad" ones. In fact, the good ones predominate. Many of the microbes in or on our bodies are harmless and coexist with us quite peacefully, and some, such as those which normally inhabit the intestinal tract, are useful.

"Bad" germs are *pathogenic* (disease-causing) organisms. When they are bad they are very, very bad. It is these that we shall be concerned with in this chapter.

Disease-causing organisms get into the body in various ways. They may be inhaled, or swallowed in food and drink, or be passed from hand to mouth, or from person to person, or be acquired by contact with contaminated materials or infected people, or be injected during the bite of a mosquito or bug, or penetrate the skin through a scratch or wound.

It is impossible to avoid all microbes in this germy world. Good housekeeping, sanitation, personal hygiene, handwashing, soap and water, do a great deal to minimize the number of germs we come in contact with. Public health measures, safe water, milk pasteurization and pure food laws have diminished the toll of infections. Many infections are preventable by inoculations that give immunities. Sulfa drugs, antibiotics, and other chemotherapeutic agents are powerful medical weapons which did not exist a generation ago. Prevention and control of infectious diseases is a great triumph of modern medicine. But infections still occur and are not to be neglected just because there may be some wonder drug that cures them overnight. There may not be.

Fever is the most common symptom of an infection. The way a fever behaves — whether it comes and goes, peaks at certain times, is sudden, insidious, low-grade and so on — sometimes gives the doctor a clue as to the nature of an infection. Sometimes fever is not conspicuous. A chill may precede its onset. An infectious process may cause inflammation, pain, and production of pus. Pus is largely the remains of the dead bodies of protective white blood cells which have engulfed germs. Headache, sore throat, nausea, "all gone" feelings, may accompany infections.

Often a doctor can diagnose an infection quite satisfactorily without going to elaborate lengths. Puzzling infections may require laboratory tests and the taking of cultures to identify specific germs so specific drugs may be prescribed.

Many infectious diseases are popularly named for the organ they primarily affect. Pneumonia, for instance, is a lung infection. But there are several types of pneumonia caused by different organisms. The crux of the matter is, what organisms cause the infection? Bacteria, viruses, protozoa and fungi cause different infections. For purposes of discussion we shall therefore classify infectious

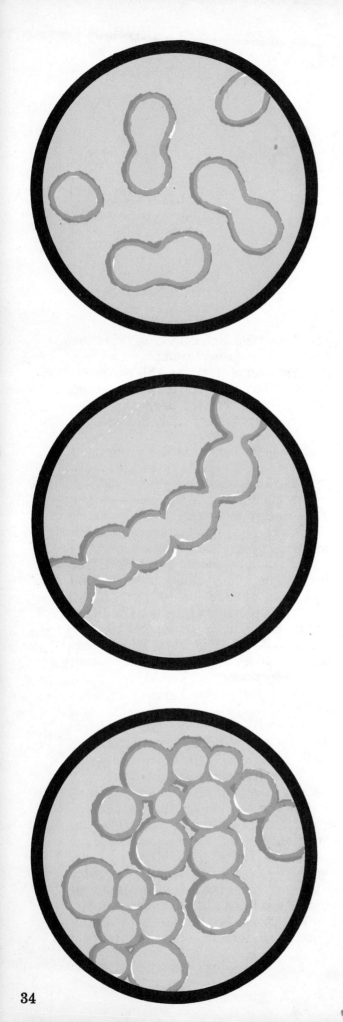

diseases, in a general way, according to the pathogenic organisms concerned.

(For chart of infectious childhood diseases, see Chapter 11.)

BACTERIAL DISEASES

Bacteria are one-celled micro-organisms of the vegetable family. They are the smallest living things with self-contained metabolic processes. The smallest bacteria are barely visible under an ordinary light microscope. It would take about 30 trillion bacteria of average size to weigh an ounce. Bacteria have outer cell membranes enwrapping chemical processes of life as complicated as any that transpire within a single animal cell or any cell of our own.

There are many families of bacteria and strains or "tribes" within families. Some require oxygen in order to multiply and are called *aerobic* bacteria. Others called *anaerobic* will not grow if oxygen is present. Some have whiplike flagellae which permit a certain amount of locomotion. Some bacteria grow at low temperatures, others only at or near body temperature; a few grow in hot springs.

Bacteria have different shapes which are useful in classification. The *cocci* (singular, *coccus*) are spherical. *Streptococci* grow in chains. In popular language, they are "strep germs," as in "strep throat." Some strains are hemolytic (destructive to red blood cells). *Staphylococci* tend to be clumped like a bunch of grapes. Cocci also grow singly and some, like the pneumococci, are paired.

Bacilli are rod-shaped; the name means "little stick." There are spiral corkscrew-shaped bacteria *(spirilla)* and comma-shaped *vibrios*. The diversity of shapes and strains reflects a diversity in capacity for harmlessness or wickedness.

Pneumonia

Pneumonia is an inflammation of the lungs which may be caused by a variety of organisms. Some forms, such as "measles pneumonia," tend to follow or to be complications of diseases which may involve the respiratory tract. The "natural course" of pneumonia in the past was rather sudden or more gradual resolution of the disease, or, sometimes, death. Today, most patients with pneumonia recover quite promptly with timely diagnosis and use of appropriate

Before the development of specific treatment, the disease ran a generally benign course in children but in adults the death rate ran from 10 to 50 per cent, depending on the type of pneumococcus responsible for the infection. There are at least 75 different varieties of the pneumococcus, and before specific treatment came along, infections produced by Type II or Type III germs were most deadly. Even today, Type III pneumococcus pneumonia may be severe and dangerous.

Common complications in the past were pus in the space between the lung and chest wall, pus in the sac enclosing the heart, infection of the heart valves

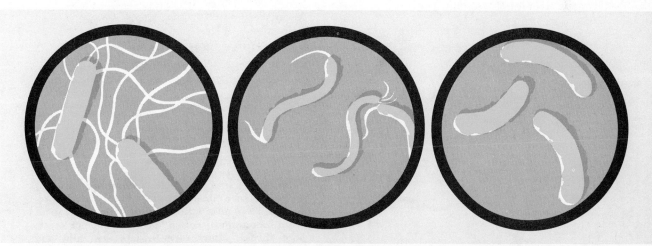

Bacilli are shaped like slender, short, or bent rods. LEFT: Tetanus (lockjaw) bacillus, *clostridium tetani*. "Clostridium" means a microbe that forms spores and lives in the absence of air. CENTER: Typical *spirillum*, or screw-shaped bacillus, with flagellar tufts at each pole which enable movement. RIGHT: Short, bent rods of the comma-shaped bacillus that causes cholera, *vibrio cholerae*.

chemotherapeutic agents. However, some cases of pneumonia are still serious and life-threatening, particularly in debilitated or elderly persons, and early symptoms should never be neglected.

Pneumococcal pneumonia is a quite common acute infection produced by spherical bacteria called pneumococci. These germs are commonly paired, and under a microscope rather resemble two coffee beans put together. The disease typically has a sudden onset, with pain in the chest, fever, chills, bloody sputum or sputum the color of prune juice.

or membranes covering the brain and spinal cord. These are rare today. In 1937-38 about 21 of every hundred patients who entered the Johns Hopkins Hospital with pneumococcal pneumonia died, despite treatment with specific anti-sera. Today the death rate is about five per cent. These deaths occur mostly in older age groups. Penicillin is the drug of choice in treating this disease.

Streptococcal pneumonia. Formerly, from three to five per cent of bacterial pneumonias were produced by Beta hemolytic streptococci. It generally appeared as a complication of influenza or other respiratory tract disease, but not as a sequel of "strep throat" or scarlet fever. Today it is rare. Treatment of the disease with penicillin or one of the tetracyclines is very effective.

Staphylococcal pneumonia. This pneumonia, produced by staphylococcus aureus ("golden staph") is ordinarily quite uncommon, but tends to appear during epidemics of influenza, measles, or whooping cough. It is a serious disease and one which in many instances requires treatment with special types of penicillin because many staphylococci have developed resistance to the killing effects of the original penicillins. Another factor which often makes treatment difficult is the frequency with

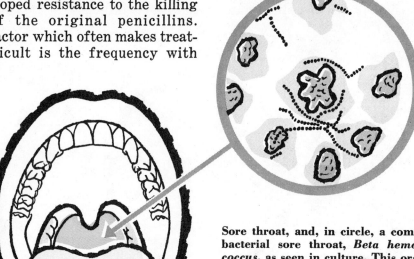

which multiple lung abscesses develop in this type of pneumonia.

Klebsiella pneumonia is an uncommon disease which still has a high death rate, due to the fact that early diagnosis may not be made, and because the disease so frequently occurs in older and debilitated patients. Because the infecting organism (Friedlander's bacillus) produces a great deal of mucoid material, the sputum in this type of pneumonia is very viscid and stringy. Treatment should be begun as

soon as possible with specific antibiotics.

Viral pneumonia (primary atypical pneumonia) is an older term for pneumonia now known to be caused by *mycoplasma* organisms. It sets in gradually, with fever, cough (often very annoying), headache, chilly sensations, a sense of being really ill. The true nature of the disease may not be recognized for several days, or at all, without x-ray films of the chest. While some studies indicate that tetracycline may be effective in treat-

Sore throat, and, in circle, a common cause of bacterial sore throat, *Beta hemolytic streptococcus*, as seen in culture. This organism causes what is commonly called "strep throat" or septic sore throat. Many sore throats are mild and soon over, but others accompany a variety of diseases. If fever is present a doctor should be called. A throat culture may be taken to identify the causative organism.

ment, no one is entirely sure of the value of this antibiotic in this disease. Symptomatic treatment to relieve the cough is important. Prospects of recovery from the disease are excellent.

Sore Throat

Many things, including some that are not germs, can cause a sore throat. Viruses are often responsible. Frequently the throat is sore at the beginning of a common cold or of influenza, and several of the Coxsackie viruses may produce herpangina which results in a pretty sore throat. Probably there are other viral agents which produce a sore throat such as that seen in infectious mononucleosis.

The most common bacterial sore throat, familiarly called "strep throat," is produced by the *Beta hemolytic streptococcus*. Fever is an almost invariable accompaniment. Persons whose tonsils are cleanly removed appear to have fewer sore throats of this nature. Complications of "strep throat" are abscesses of the tonsils, and — if they can be called complications — rheumatic fever and acute hemorrhagic glomerular nephritis. The treatment of choice for a sore throat is penicillin administered as early as possible. The author has never found evidence that other types of streptococci, pneumococci, meningococci or staphylococci produce sore throat.

"Trench mouth." With the exception of diphtheria, the only other bacterial sore throat is *Vincent's angina*, sometimes called "trench mouth" or *ulceromembranous stomatitis*. Although the disease usually affects the gums and mouth tissues, it may at times invade only the tonsillar area and produce a sore throat. It is produced by a mixture of two micro-organisms called *Bacillus fusiformis* and *Borrelia vincentii*. Poor oral hygiene, heavy smoking and other factors may predispose to this disease. This form of sore throat accompanied by fever, painful membranous ulceration in the infected area, and enlargement of lymph nodes in the neck responds rapidly to treatment with penicillin.

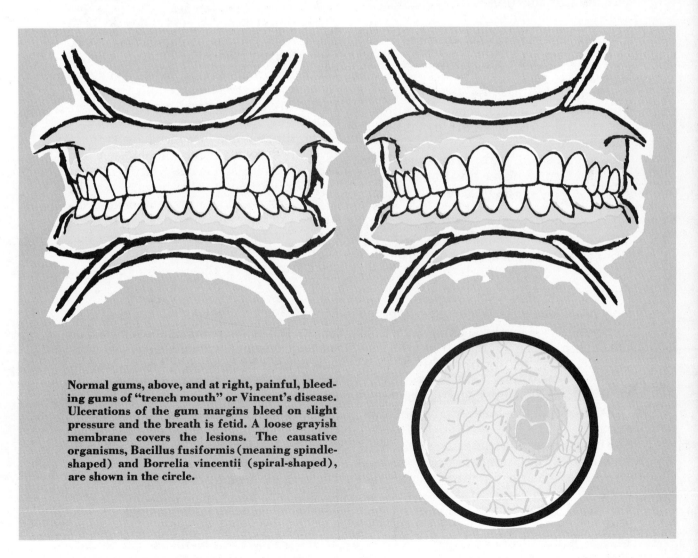

Normal gums, above, and at right, painful, bleeding gums of "trench mouth" or Vincent's disease. Ulcerations of the gum margins bleed on slight pressure and the breath is fetid. A loose grayish membrane covers the lesions. The causative organisms, Bacillus fusiformis (meaning spindle-shaped) and Borrelia vincentii (spiral-shaped), are shown in the circle.

Erysipelas

This disease produced by *Beta hemolytic streptococci* has almost disappeared since the introduction of sulfa drugs in this country. It is characterized by rapid onset, high fever, often a chill, and a curious, hard, deep-red, tender skin lesion which often begins on the nose and spreads over the cheeks on both sides. Rarely, other skin areas may be affected. The organisms gain entrance through breaks in the skin which may be quite invisible. Erysipelas may also start from a surgical incision or burned area. It is essentially a disease of middle-aged persons. Formerly, erysipelas was highly lethal in patients over 60 and in children under two years of age. Now it is easily cured with penicillin.

Quinsy (peri-tonsillar abscess)

As its medical name indicates, this disease is an abscess in and around the tonsil, produced by *Beta hemolytic streptococci*, although some people think the inciting organisms are members of the Bacteroides group. Quinsy is generally a one-sided, sore, tender swelling accompanied by fever and malaise. The swelling may get so large the patient can't swallow. If caught early, treatment with penicillin will cure it, but if pus is present the area should be incised and drained in addition to penicillin therapy.

Boils

A *furuncle* or ordinary boil is a local, inflammatory, pus-producing infection of the skin and surrounding tissues. Usually the infection originates in a hair follicle. A *carbuncle* is a "super boil," really, a closely knit collection of boils which extend into deeper surrounding tissues.

Furuncles and carbuncles are generally caused by *Staphylococcus aureus* and usually occur in areas which the hand can reach and scratch — that is, the face, back of the neck, buttocks, chest, the armpits, in other words where there is hair and/or sweat glands. People who tend to have boils commonly carry staphylococci in their noses, and as they rub and pick at their noses frequently, they contaminate their fingers and nails and by scratching start infection in other parts of their bodies.

As far as boils are concerned, treatment with hot packs to make them "point" as rapidly as possible so they can be incised and drained is the usual treatment. With carbuncles the same general therapy is used, but in certain patients it is good to use a type of penicillin effective against the staphylococcus, as well as the drainage procedure described.

Osteomyelitis

Both *Beta hemolytic streptococci* and staphylococci may produce *osteomyelitis,* which is an infection set up by invasion of the blood by bacteria which settle in the terminal loops of capillaries of the long shaft of the bone. The infection of the bone produces pus. When produced by hemolytic streptococci, and diagnosed early, treatment with penicillin alone will bring about a cure in a relatively short time. When produced by staphylococcus aureus, the pus should be evacuated by surgical means, and treatment with an antibiotic effective against the organisms should be instituted immediately. Fortunately, this disease has become uncommon since the introduction of antibiotic therapy. For fuller description, see Chapter 18.

Blood Poisoning

The terms *bacteremia* and *septicemia* usually signify that bacteria have entered the blood stream from an original focus of infection, and are multiplying and causing symptoms. Almost all kinds of harmful bacteria may enter the blood at one time or another. In general, the finding of bacteria in the blood indicates seriousness of a disease. Certain bacteria, of which the staphylococcus is an excellent example, tend, in the course of a bacteremia, to seed themselves in the body and set up secondary foci for spread of infection. Treatment should be carried out intensively with an appropriate antibiotic or sulfonamide, and as abscesses or pockets of pus develop they should be incised and drained if feasible.

Bacterial Endocarditis

This may occur in acute or subacute forms. In the acute form, bacteria such as hemolytic streptococci, pneumococci, or other germs may, in the course of a bacteremia, settle on a heart valve, where they multiply rapidly and quickly destroy the heart valve. The outlook for a patient with acute bacterial endocarditis is always grave. Treatment is, of course, carried out very intensively with the appropriate antibiotic.

Subacute bacterial endocarditis may be produced by any of a number of bacteria, but is most commonly caused by *Streptococcus viridans* (the modifier means "green") or by other streptococci which are *not* hemolytic. The disease almost always occurs in persons who have had damage to the heart valves from a previous attack of rheumatic fever, or who have arteriosclerosis of the heart valves, or who had heart-valvular

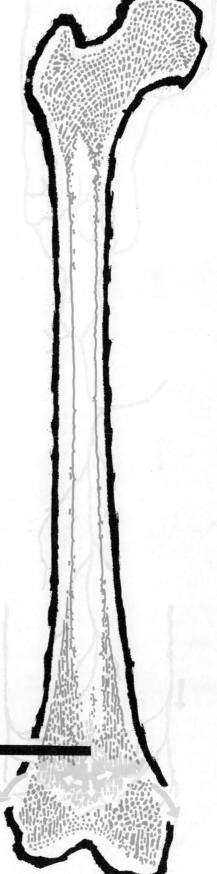

The drawing shows how microbes in the bloodstream produce osteomyelitis. The arrows indicate how bacteria enter bone (in this case a thighbone) from blood vessels supplying bone tissue and spread infection through bone and periosteum, the fibrous membrane of bone surfaces. If not treated promptly, an abscess forms and pressure from pus can destroy large areas of bone. Various organisms cause the infection; hemolytic streptococci are shown in the circle.

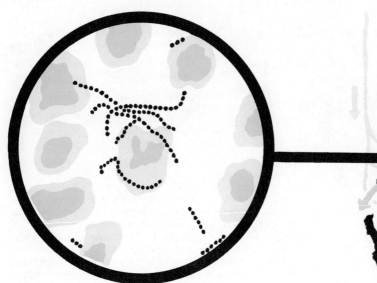

surgery. Where formerly this subacute type of the disease was almost always fatal, now about 90 per cent of its victims have a good chance of recovery when intensive treatment with penicillin and streptomycin is given. Recovery does not confer immunity, however, and an individual may have several attacks of the disease of the heart valves.

Venereal Diseases of Bacterial Origin

Gonorrhea, by far the most common venereal disease, is an infection produced by the gonococcus. Gonorrhea is worldwide in distribution, and while there is considerable variation in individual susceptibility to this infection, immunity is not produced by an attack, and a person may have gonorrhea over and over again.

The great majority of infected persons acquire gonorrhea by having sexual intercourse with an infected partner. Nonvenereal transmission is very, very rare. The principal exception is female infants and children who may acquire the infec-

tion from contaminated hands of other persons. Newborn infants may be infected in passing through the birth canal of an infected mother, and it is routine practice to put drops into the eyes of newborn babies to kill gonorrhea germs that may possibly be present. Tissues of the eyes are very susceptible to blinding damage by gonorrhea organisms.

Initial symptoms occur shortly after intercourse (two days to a week) and in the male consist of a burning sensation on urination which is soon followed by a pussy urethral discharge. In the female, painful urination followed by a vaginal discharge are usually noted, although occasional female carriers of the gonococcus may have no overt symptoms and this tends to spread the infection. Penicillin is the drug of choice for male and female patients who have this disease, and is highly effective. Complications such as meningitis, arthritis, endocarditis and sterility have become rare since penicillin has been used to treat this disease.

The problem with gonorrhea is to treat both sexual partners simultaneously,

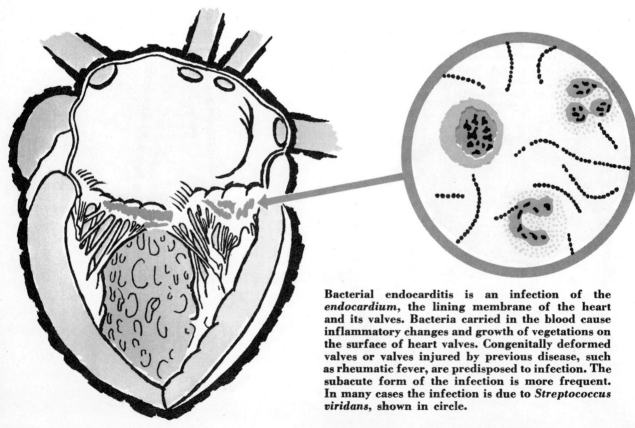

Bacterial endocarditis is an infection of the *endocardium*, the lining membrane of the heart and its valves. Bacteria carried in the blood cause inflammatory changes and growth of vegetations on the surface of heart valves. Congenitally deformed valves or valves injured by previous disease, such as rheumatic fever, are predisposed to infection. The subacute form of the infection is more frequent. In many cases the infection is due to *Streptococcus viridans,* shown in circle.

Initial symptoms of gonorrhea, caused by *gonococci* shown in circle at the left below, are painful urination and pussy discharge (sometimes female carriers may have no overt symptoms). At right, *Hemophilus ducreyi* baccili which produce soft chancre, a venereal disease. The initial lesion is a small red lump, generally on the genitals, which breaks down and forms a painful ulcer.

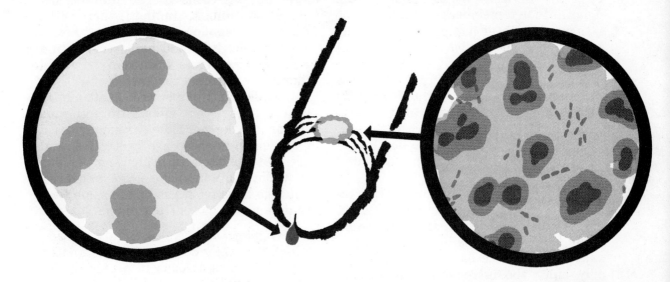

otherwise the cure will not last very long because re-infection will take place promptly.

Chancroid (soft chancre) is a venereal disease produced by the bacillus *Hemophilus ducreyi*. It occurs most frequently in areas in which feminine hygiene is habitually at a low ebb, and in areas where standards of feminine hygiene fall during periods of war. The disease is characterized by the appearance of a little red lump, generally on the genitals, two to 14 days after sexual intercourse. This becomes pussy in the course of a few days, then breaks down, and a tender, usually painful, indolent (slow to heal) ulcer is formed. From a medical point of view, sulfonamides are best for the treatment of chancroid, for although certain antibiotics are very effective, they are equally effective against syphilis and may prevent early recognition of the latter disease. Little or no immunity develops from an attack of chancroid.

Granuloma inguinale is another venereal disease, produced by a coccobacillus, which has a low degree of communicability. It is relatively painless, insidious in onset, and very slowly progressive. The first indication is a pimple or nodule, usually on the genitalia, which slowly progresses to destructive ulceration and granulomatous lesions (tiny red granules

visible in the base of an ulcer). Treatment with streptomycin, chloramphenicol, or one of the tetracyclines is effective. Washing the genitals thoroughly immediately after intercourse, especially with a good liquid soap, greatly reduces the possibility of developing infection.

Meningococcal Infection (Meningitis)

The most common disease produced by the meningococcus is *meningococcal meningitis*, also known as *cerebrospinal fever*, *spotted fever*, or *cerebrospinal meningitis*. The disease occurs sporadically, or it may occur in limited epidemics as in military installations, or in widespread epidemics througout the country. The disease attacks the covering membranes of the brain or spinal cord. One thing that is quite true is that incidence of the disease is always higher in countries engaged in a prolonged war.

Transmission is from person to person by direct contact or droplet infection. Closeness of contact is significant. During one epidemic period the author saw a mother and her three children who had meningitis. All slept in the same bed.

The disease may have a sudden or gradual onset, with fever, headache, stiff neck, a red spotty rash which at times may coalesce into an extensive bluish rash. In patients who have this type of rash the disease may be rapidly fatal. Your author remembers one patient who was drinking beer happily with her husband in a beer garden at 11 p. m. one evening and who died of an overwhelming meningococcal infection at 8 a. m. the next morning. Formerly the death rate in this disease was from 20 per cent to as high as 80 per cent in certain epidemics. In World War I the death rate was 39 per cent, in World War II, around four per cent.

Another type of meningococcal infection, chronic recurrent meningococcemia, used to be seen occasionally. It would recur time after time at varying intervals. Its incidence has decreased markedly since the introduction of specific therapy (sulfanilamide) in the treatment of meningococcal meningitis by your author in 1936-37. Sulfadiazine or penicillin are now the drugs of choice. Equally good results are obtained when either is used, singly or in combination.

In controlled mass populations such as military or other groups, an outbreak of meningitis can be stopped almost in its tracks by administration of two grams of sulfadiazine a day for two days to every member of the group.

Clostridial Infections

These are produced by spore-forming anaerobic (multiplying in absence of oxygen) organisms which create powerful toxins that injure the body.

Botulism results from eating canned foods which have been inadequately sterilized, or which the organism has entered and produced its toxin after sterilization. Botulinus toxin is an incredibly powerful poison. A mere teaspoonful of it, distributed equally in many millions of people, could kill them all. Improperly home-canned foods, particularly non-acid foods such as beans, corns, asparagus, etc., are the prime sources of botulism. Spoiled canned foods and leaky cans should be discarded without tasting the contents. The toxin does not produce a bad taste, or any taste, and there may be no obvious signs of spoil-

age. Boiling foods for 30 minutes destroys botulinus toxin, but if there is the slightest suspicion of spoilage of home-canned food it should be destroyed and not even be given to a pet that you would like to keep around for a while.

Specific antitoxins are available to counter the lethal effects of botulinus toxins on the nervous system. If used early enough, these are protective, and are most valuable in protecting persons in whom symptoms have not yet appeared but who have partaken of the same food that caused a case of botulism.

Gas gangrene is a clostridial infection which generally occurs in contaminated wounds or has a focus in a uterus contaminated with feces at childbirth. There are gas bubbles in tissues, high fever, malodorous discharge from the wound. Generally, treatment is primarily a matter of judicious surgical measures plus gas gangrene antitoxins and administration of penicillin.

Tetanus (Lockjaw)

Tetanus is a serious disease which need never occur and should never be permitted to. The causative organism, *Clostridium tetani*, forms longlived spores which are found in soil, street dirt, and the intestinal tracts of man and animals. These reproductive cells "come to life" only if there is little or no oxygen in their environment. Spores may enter the body through a penetrating wound, burned skin, or an injury so trivial it isn't noticed. In conditions to their liking, such as devitalized wound tissues, the organisms produce tetanus toxin, a powerful nerve poison.

Tetanus has an incubation period of a few days to weeks or months. *The shorter the interval from injury to symptoms, the worse the outlook for recovery.* Onset of tetanus is marked by restlessness, irritability, stiffness of certain muscle groups, and often difficulty in swallowing. Spasm of the jaw muscles may be the first diagnostic sign.

Treatment of tetanus is still unsatisfactory and the immediate outlook grave if but a short time has elapsed between injury and symptoms. Prevention is the best hope, and very effective. That is why tetanus prevention is uppermost in a doctor's mind when he treats a person injured in an accident, a child who has scraped his knee in the street, a home gardener who has pricked his hand while digging, and in many other circumstances.

An immediate injection of tetanus antitoxin may be necessary if the patient has no active immunization. Tetanus antitoxin gives prompt, passive immunity that lasts long enough to prevent infection from developing, if given in time. Unfortunately, some people react badly to horse serum from which the antitoxin is made. Recently antitoxin prepared from human donors has become available in a limited way.

Injection of antitoxin is quite unnecessary if the patient has built up *active* immunity to tetanus. This is easily achieved by *tetanus toxoid* immunization. (See Chapter 11.) Tetanus toxoid is harmless and does not cause any of the bad reactions of antitoxin. The toxoid stimulates the body to manufacture its own neutralizing chemicals against tetanus. But it takes a little time for this protection to become complete.

Tetanus would never occur if everyone were immunized with tetanus toxoid and received a booster dose after each injury in which the skin and muscles were seriously hurt. *Remember that no one should have tetanus. If you haven't been immunized with protection against tetanus, start today. Tetanus produces a painful and horrible death.*

Salmonella Infections

The *Salmonella* (no relation to salmon; they were named after a Dr. Salmon who studied them) are a group of bacilli that produce intestinal diseases.

Typhoid fever is an acute feverish illness, generally gradual but at times sudden in onset. There is sustained high fever, headache, apathy, cough, a pulse slow in relation to the height of the

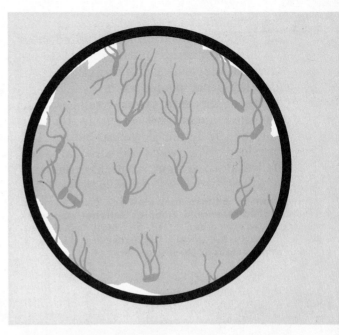

Bacilli *(Salmonella typhi)* that cause typhoid fever. The whiplike flagellae, made visible by special stains, enable the organisms to move about. The germs may remain in the body and be shed unknowingly many years after a patient has recovered from typhoid fever.

fever. Sometimes there is an eruption of little rose-red spots, especially over the abdomen. Major complications are intestinal hemorrhages and/or perforation of the intestine, producing peritonitis.

The typhoid bacillus is a parasite of man and as it is found in the feces can, unless sanitary precautions are taken, contaminate water and food. The major route of transmission is from feces and urine of infected patients and unknowing "carriers." Typhoid fever used to occur in widespread epidemics when organisms contaminated drinking water systems, but outbreaks in this country are now generally localized and result from a typhoid carrier who unknowingly contaminates food consumed by others.

Some persons who recover from typhoid fever continue to shed the germs in their stools for the rest of their lives, and are known as typhoid carriers. They may not know that they are carriers. When recognized, carriers have to observe special sanitary precautions and are barred from food-handling trades. The term "typhoid Mary" for a troublemaker comes from a New York City woman named Mary who was a cook and who, a generation ago, ignited local typhoid epidemics until she was restrained, much to her indignation, from handling other people's food.

The death rate from typhoid fever remained unchanged, eight to ten per cent, for a hundred years before Dr. Theodore Woodward demonstrated in 1948 that treatment with chloramphen-

Pseudomonas in culture and closeup. Bacteria have enclosing membranes and complex internal structures that secrete enzymes and effect chemical transformations essential to the germ's life processes. Antibiotic drugs disrupt certain of these processes.

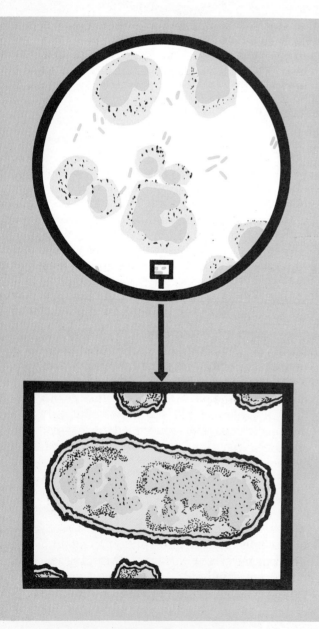

icol and cortisone is very effective. Now the death rate is about one per cent in this country. There is a good vaccine against typhoid fever and everyone leaving the country should be vaccinated. Immunity produced by the vaccine can be broken if the individual receives a very heavy dose of typhoid bacilli in food or water.

"Food poisoning" or acute gastroenteritis can be caused by strains of Salmonellae all over the world. The term "ptomaine poisoning" is very old hat, since ptomaines are too putrid for anyone knowingly to ingest.

Generally the story of bacterial food poisoning is something like this: There is a $100-a-plate dinner for a prominent politician. Something tasty, let us say Hollandaise sauce, is served. Four or five hours after the dinner, guests begin to come down like flies with fever, nausea, vomiting, and severe diarrhea which lasts for four to 16 hours, and then passes off leaving its victims washed-out and weak. It is found that with one or two exceptions, only those who ate the Hollandaise became ill. Some Hollandaise sauce may be left, and from it health authorities grow the Salmonellae and pinpoint the cause.

Treatment consists primarily of trying to replace fluids lost from both ends of the gastrointestinal tract. Attacks are dangerous only to infants, the debilitated, and the very old, who may have to be treated for shock.

A third type of Salmonella infection is produced by so-called hog cholera bacillus (which does not produce hog cholera). The disease somewhat resembles typhoid, fever is fairly high, bacteremia common, and about one out of three patients develops focal lesions from the bacteremia: bronchopneumonia, pus in the joints, pus pockets elsewhere, or meningitis. The infection almost always occurs in persons debilitated by other disease, surgical operations, or malnutrition. Treatment with chloramphenicol may or may not be helpful. If not, treatment is directed toward the symptoms of the infection.

Pseudomonas and Others

A type of bacillus called *Pseudomonas* primarily infects areas which have "corruption" — pus and dead tissue. These infections produce greenish or bluish pus and can best be treated by getting rid of dead tissue and pus by dissolving them with enzymes available for this purpose. Occasionally, the infection is systemic or produces an ulcer in the cornea of the eye, for which special antibiotics should be instituted.

Proteus bacilli are common in infected wounds, and here again the problem is to get rid of the corruption because then these bacteria will disappear. The organism is common in urinary tract infections, especially when stones or obstructions are present. Chemotherapy has not been too successful. One has to get rid of the stone or the obstruction to the urinary flow, usually by surgery.

Coliform bacilli (common inhabitants of the intestinal tract) can cause infections such as peritonitis, bacteremia, urinary tract infections and even peritonitis. Pus if present should be evacuated if possible and treatment with an effective antibiotic instituted.

Bacillary Dysentery

This is the most common form of dysentery. It is caused by different strains of the dysentery bacillus and results from poor sanitation — that is, it is transmitted by the fecal-oral route. Flies expedite its spread in many parts of the world.

Attacks come on abruptly, with fever, nausea, vomiting, abdominal pain and cramps, and diarrhea sometimes so intense that patients go into shock. Blood and mucus are present in the watery stools in severe cases. Untreated, it is a self-limited disease as a rule, clearing up in a week or ten days, but it may become chronic and debilitating and progress to a chronic colitis. Treatment aimed at maintaining salt and water balance is very important. Specific treatment may be carried out with an appropriate antibiotic or sulfadiazine. Complications are very infrequent when specific treatment with medication is begun early.

Cholera

This disease used to travel slowly along trade routes of the world in great epidemic waves, killing millions of people. Now it is confined to parts of India and Pakistan. The last case of cholera in the United States occurred in an immigrant on Ellis Island in 1909.

Cholera is caused by the *vibrio comma*, which in endemic areas is transmitted in food and water. It can also be transmitted by the fecal-oral route. It is characterized by sudden onset, enormous watery stools, sudden and overwhelming dehydration, large vomits, and great prostration. In native areas up to 60 per per cent of those infected die, but with modern treatment the death rate may be lowered to five per cent. Treatment is devoted primarily to salt and water replacement to prevent grave shock. Specific therapy has not proved successful. A fairly good cholera vaccine is available. All people going to Southeast Asia should be vaccinated.

Brucellosis
(Undulant Fever, Malta Fever)

Brucellosis is an infectious disease produced by one of the three species of *Brucella* organisms (named for Sir David Bruce who in 1886 identified certain micro-organisms in the spleens of patients who died of Malta fever). Brucellosis has an acute phase which may start suddenly (when the author had this disease, he was a well man driving past Edgewood Arsenal, Md., and a sick man when arriving at the turnoff to Aberdeen Proving Grounds, Md., on Route 40). There is fever which may be "undulating" (up in the evening, down in the morning), chills, sweating, weakness, pains and aches, and a very depressed feeling. Brucellosis which progresses to a chronic stage is characterized by all sorts of odd complaints which sometimes may cause the victim to be labeled "psychoneurotic," quite wrongly.

The natural reservoir of the disease is in cattle, hogs, and goats, and direct or indirect contact with infected animals or their products is the source of human infection. Butchers, packing house workers, farmers and veterinarians are at special occupational risk of acquiring this disease.

Brucellosis is one of the diseases in which the bacillus invades human cells, lives in them, and probably multiplies in them. Authorities disagree on best treatment. The author on the basis of his experience (personal and otherwise) feels that in the acute form of the disease, large doses of a tetracycline antibiotic should be given daily for one week,

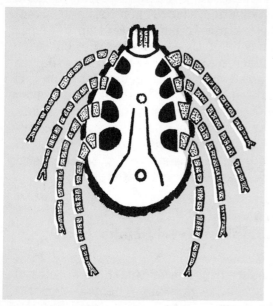

Ticks and mites (like *Acarina* above) can transmit bacterial, protozoal, rickettsial, and spirochetal diseases through their bites. Adult ticks and mites have four pairs of legs, and thus are not insects, which by definition have three pairs of legs.

and then the dose halved and administered daily for another week. (He must say that this is rather spartan treatment, but it seems to work.)

Plague

The fearful plague that killed millions of persons and played a dark part in history is a diminished but not vanished threat to mankind. Plague is a rare disease in the United States, occurring primarily in the West where ground squirrels and other small rodents constitute a reservoir of infection. Don't fuss with dead ground squirrels, gophers, or prairie dogs. They may be infected.

The reason we do not have more plague in this country is that there is no insect that commonly bites both man and infected small rodents. In epidemic areas the black rat carries the infection and the rodent flea passes it along. There is some evidence that the human flea may transmit this disease.

There are two varieties of plague — *bubonic* (the glandular type) which has the lower death rate, and *pneumonic* (the lung type) which has the higher death rate. A fairly good vaccine exists but if vaccinated, frequent booster doses should be given if one is in an area where there is an epidemic. Treatment is best carried out with chloramphenicol or one of the tetracyclines.

Tularemia (Deer-Fly Fever, Tick Fever, Rabbit Fever)

Much of the early work on this disease was done in Tulare County, California, hence the name tularemia. The causative organism, *Pasteurella tularensis,* is thought to be able to penetrate unbroken skin. Tularemia probably occurs all over the world and is destructive to its host animals (keep your hands off dead rabbits).

Man gets into the picture by hunting and killing infected animals which he then cleans and may not cook properly, or by being bitten by a bloodsucking fly or tick, or by drinking contaminated water. In this country many persons develop the disease during or just after the rabbit-hunting season. Others get it in the summer from tick bites. *Preventive measures are to clean and cut up killed wild rabbits with hands encased in intact rubber gloves, and then cook the rabbit thoroughly.*

There are several types of tularemia. A typhoidal type proceeds to generalized disease without local manifestations. Skin lesions such as red spots, little boils, and red lumps may appear anywhere on the body in tularemia. The disease may be superficial with a small lump at the site of a cut. There may be enlargement of lymph nodes regional to the cut and possible suppuration of nodes. Tularemia commonly begins suddenly with headache, chills, fever, and prostration. Ophthalmic tularemia may occur in conjunctival sacs of the eyes. There is a pleuropulmonary type characterized by pneumonia. Oral tularemia occurs in and around the mouth, generally from eating improperly cooked wild rabbit.

Streptomycin is very effective in the treatment of this disease as are chloramphenicol and the tetracycline antibiotics. One final word. *Use great care in handling, cleaning, and cooking wild rabbits.*

Anthrax (Wool-Sorter's Disease)

Anthrax has been known since antiquity and is primarily a disease of herbivorous animals, transmitted from them to man. It is quite uncommon and occurs primarily where raw wool or hides are being processed, or in certain

agricultural areas where the disease exists in cattle and horses. The organism is spore-bearing and spores may survive for many years in the soil. Man to man transmission may occur.

Anthrax may occur in four forms. "Malignant pustule" is characterized by development of a "carbuncle" at the site of infection. Headache, nausea, vomiting, joint pains and fever may be present. Outlook in this type of anthrax is favorable if lesions are not on the head or neck. Malignant anthrax edema is characterized by swelling of subcutaneous tissue, usually without carbuncle formation. Untreated, the outlook is poor in this form of the disease. In pulmonary anthrax, caused by inhalation of anthrax spores, a severe lung inflammation develops which can be fatal in 18 to 48 hours. This is "wool-sorter's disease." Gastrointestinal anthrax follows ingestion of improperly cooked food containing anthrax bacilli and spores. It rarely occurs in this country. It is rapidly fatal in many instances.

The treatment of choice in all forms of anthrax is penicillin in fairly large amounts. The outlook is good in patients treated soon after infection.

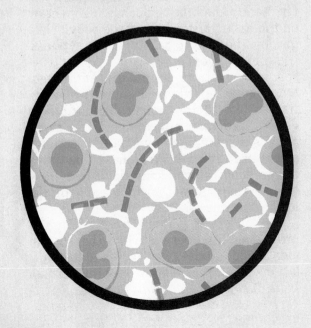

Anthrax bacilli, shown below, are spore-forming germs. Spores are very resistant to heat, drying, and antiseptics, and can live in "suspended animation" in contaminated soil or materials for many years, and "come alive" again when they enter living tissues.

SPIROCHETAL INFECTIONS

A *spirochete* is a spiral micro-organism similar to bacteria. Certain **venereal diseases** are caused by spirochetes, but so are others that are non-venereal. There are several technical subdivisions of the spirochete family, of which the most notorious are the *treponemes* which include the organism that causes syphilis (treponema pallidum).

Many species of spirochetes are completely harmless while others produce some of the most widespread diseases. A characteristic of infections produced by the treponemal group is immunological changes in the infected person. This is the basis for the Wassermann and other "blood tests" for syphilis. Such tests of both partners are required by many states preparatory to issuing a marriage license. However, malaria and

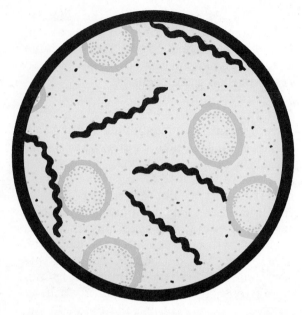

Spirochetes are spiral-shaped microorganisms. Many spirochetes are harmless, but certain venereal infections, rat-bite fever, and other diseases are due to pathogenic members of this germ family.

some other conditions can cause a "false positive" reaction to a Wassermann test, which indicates that a person has syphilis when he does not. The falsity of such a reaction can be proved by a "treponemal immobilization" test, so in doubtful instances there need to be no worry about the validity of a blood test.

Syphilis

This disease, thought by some to have been introduced into Europe by the pilot of the Pinta, quickly became one of the most famous, or one should say infamous, of all diseases in history. If one excepts congenital syphilis, one can say that the disease has a venereal spread by direct contact, usually sexual intercourse. The causative organism, *Treponema pallidum*, is a colorless corkscrew-shaped microbe that moves incessantly under the microscope.

Within a few years after its introduction into Europe, syphilis stepped up its ravages and highly fatal epidemics, abetted by sexual promiscuity, swept the nations. Each country disclaimed proprietorship. To the French, syphilis was the "Italian pox," and to the Italians,

vice versa. Such unpopularity was deserved.

As the years passed, syphilis gradually lost its initial extreme virulence, and by the twentieth century it had become an infectious disease, generalized at first, then becoming localized, which in the long run, if not treated with medication, permanently injured or killed about one out of five of its victims.

Congenital syphilis is present in some newborn babies, but the disease is not inherited from parental germ cells, as traits such as hair and eye color are. Congenital syphilis is transmitted to the fetus by an infectious mother, who may not know that she has the disease. Proper pre-natal treatment can prevent congenital syphilis when it is known that the mother is infected with the disease. That is a reason for the routine blood tests of all pregnant women who receive proper prenatal care.

Symptoms and stages. Syphilis germs are widely disseminated in the body within 24 hours after entrance, and among other things, they promptly initiate something like an allergic mechanism (see Chapter 20). The natural course of *untreated* syphilis is as follows:

The first sign the patient is aware of is a hard chancre or sore at the site of germ entry, usually the genitals, frequently the lips, or perhaps anywhere on the external surface of the body. This marks the *primary* stage of syphilis invasion, promptly followed by the *secondary* stage when disseminated treponemas produce lesions in body tissues of their choice. Typically, a generalized rash appears and is almost always accompanied by small, infectious ulcers in the mouth. At or near this time, the infected person may develop syphilitic meningitis or other forms of syphilis of the nervous system.

The infected person is most highly infectious to others during the stages mentioned above, when exudates of lesions are aswarm with syphilis germs. *With proper treatment, an infectious person can almost always be rendered non-infectious to others within 24 hours.*

Even without treatment, the rash and mouth lesions disappear and the patient goes into the *latent* period which may last for many years. In the past, about 80 percent of such infected persons felt perfectly well and were not bothered by syphilis for the rest of their lives. But the other 20 per cent, after longer or shorter periods of time, would become insane (from *paresis,* or "softening of the brain"), or develop staggering gait and locomotive disability, or severe and fatal heart disease, blindness, or ugly ulcerative lesions in any part of the body.

With timely modern treatment syphilis no longer runs its natural course.

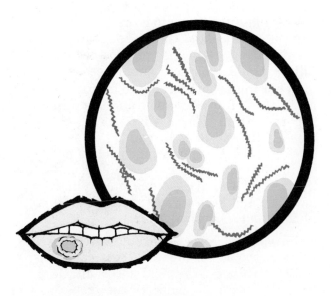

The causative organism of syphilis, *Treponema pallidum,* is colorless and special techniques are necessary to make it visible under the microscope. The first sign of primary syphilis that the patient is aware of is usually a hard sore at the site of germ entry.

Treatment. The earliest effective treatment for syphilis was mercury, which was used as late as 1940. In 1910, Paul Ehrlich of Germany introduced the first of the arsphenamines, famous at the time as "606." The methodical Ehrlich tested and discarded 605 compounds as failures before achieving the one which proved to be successful.

Early treatment with arsphenamine, an arsenic-containing compound, gave the patient a good chance of cure, and also reduced the manifestations of late syphilis if treatment were fully carried out. Treatment of female syphilitics reduced the incidence of congenital syphilis. But arsphenamine treatment required a series of uncomfortable injections over a long period, and when disturbing symptoms were reduced there was a very human tendency for patients to stop treatment before they were fully cured. The great hope of Ehrlich that a single dose of a drug would kill all syphilis germs in the body was not realized until 1943 when the late John Mahoney demonstrated that penicillin cured syphilis.

Currently, it is fair to say that one can cure 99+ per cent of patients suffering from syphilis, in the stage before the rash appears, with proper penicillin therapy. If the rash has made its appearance, 98 to 99 per cent can be cured. If the patient is in the latent stage and receives proper penicillin therapy, the chances that a late syphilitic, heart, artery, nerve, or brain disorder will develop are almost if not quite nil. In realization of Ehrlich's hope, this can be accomplished with a single injection of a long-acting penicillin.

VD—"A RAGING EPIDEMIC"

In the early 1970's, venereal disease, once fairly well under control, burst its bounds and became what many public health authorities call "a raging epidemic." At least 500,000 Americans, according to the U. S. Public Health Service, do not know that they have syphilis and are in urgent need of medical attention. Some of them will progress to insanity, paralysis, blindness, heart and other serious impairments. Upwards of 2,000,000 cases of gonorrhea are treated yearly.

Many factors underlie the epidemic: population mobility, greater sexual freedom, contraception, undue belief in quick cures, unawareness of grave health complications, lack of foolproof chemical or mechanical means of prevention, increasing reservoirs of infectious persons. Teenagers and young adults account for about one-half of reported venereal disease. Many young people are grossly misinformed or uninformed. The public does not realize the full scope or threat of the epidemic situation.

One phenomenon of the present outbreak is that females infected with gonorrhea may have no symptoms whatever, apparently because they build up antibodies in the genital tract. They are symptom-free carriers who can transmit gonorrhea to sexual partners. Ultimately, females who do not know they have gonorrhea may suffer pelvic infection, sterility, septic shock. A quick method of screening for gonorrhea would be a boon. Standard culture tests require some time and usually the expertise of an outside laboratory. An improved test (Clinicult) enables a physician to get a test result in his own office in 24 to 48 hours.

Immunization against venereal disease is not an imminent prospect. Rational approaches to an immunizing or preventive agent against gonorrhea have not been formulated. A satisfactory vaccine against syphilis is still in the experimental stage, and, at the present rate of progress, is not expected to be available for some years.

Other Spirochetal Infections

Yaws is a common tropical disease characterized by early skin lesions followed by lumpy skin eruptions and, in some patients, by late destructive lesions of the skin and bones. Yaws is rarely transmitted by sexual intercourse, but generally by person-to-person contacts or by certain non-biting insects. This tropical disease usually responds promptly to treatment with penicillin.

Bejel is a non-venereal form of syphilis, transmitted by contaminated drinking utensils, which affects natives of the Middle East. In some villages as high as 90 per cent of the inhabitants show evidence of having had bejel. Penicillin is highly effective in treatment.

Pinta is a chronic, endemic, infectious disease in Central and parts of South America, characterized by discolored lumpy skin lesions which eventually become depigmented blotches. Six to 12 months later, pinkish flat spots or small pimple-like eruptions form. These may coalesce and look like lesions of psoriasis. Penicillin therapy is specific and responses are usually dramatic.

Relapsing fever is an acute infectious disease characterized by episodes of fever which subside spontaneously, then recur, over a period of weeks. Fever is accompanied by a bad headache, chills, pains in muscles and joints, often nausea and vomiting, sometimes a bad cough and bronchitis, occasionally by nosebleeds and intolerance to light. Sweating may be profuse and the pulse rapid. As the disease goes on the relapses become milder and milder and finally cease.

Relapsing fever is produced by a spirochete of the *Borrelia* genus and has been reported from nearly all parts of the world. Lice and ticks spread the disease. Treatment with chloramphenicol or one of the tetracyclines gives good results. To prevent the disease one must eliminate lice and keep away from soft ticks of the genus Ornithodornus.

Tropical ulcer is a chronic ulcer involving the lower leg or foot, caused by a spirochete. Tropical ulcer affects great numbers of people in the tropics, destroys tissue rapidly, and is brought promptly under control by injection of long-lasting penicillin.

Rat-bite fever. One variety caused by a bacterial organism is also known as Haverill fever. Streptomycin is effective.

The other variety of rat-bite fever is caused by a spirochete introduced by the bite of a rat suffering from a pussy conjunctivitis caused by this organism. There is a hard ulcer at the site of the bite, a relapsing type of fever, a dusky red skin rash, and enlarged lymph nodes in the region of the bite. In rat-infested areas, babies bitten in their cribs by rats often develop this disease. Treatment for rat-bite fever is best carried out vigorously with penicillin, streptomycin, or one of the tetracycline antibiotics.

Weil's disease, first described in Germany, is characterized by fever, headache, severe muscular pains in the low back and calves, nausea, vomiting and diarrhea. Light hurts the eyes. Hepatitis with jaundice occurs in about 70 per cent of patients and many have a nephritis as well. Relapse may occur three or four weeks after the disease starts. A variety of animals, including mice and rats, become chronically infected with this disease and the organism is found in large numbers in the urine of infected animals. Humans are infected by contact with materials on which infected animals have urinated. There is no uniformly successful specific therapy so the disease must be treated symptomatically.

FEVER AND CHILLS

An attack of shivering or chills followed by fever may usher in a disease process. Forms of pneumonia, malaria, and other conditions are commonly characterized by chills.

Strenuous activity increases body temperature very slightly, perhaps two-fifths of a degree.

Chills—a mechanism for raising body temperature—are usually followed by fever. A doctor considers the patient's age—infant, toddler, pre-schooler, adult—in determining the significance of fever, which can be an indicator of the course of a disease. Treatment is directed to the cause.

Hyperthermic fever is one marked by exceedingly high temperatures of 105 degrees or more.

An *intermittent* fever is one that falls to normal or below during the day, but then rises again.

A *sustained* fever is one in which the average daily temperature remains above normal.

A *relapsing* fever is one that may disappear for a day or several days and then return, in alternating episodes.

Fever may have other causes than infections. Heatstroke, for example, results in high body temperatures.

HEALTH HINTS FOR TRAVELERS

Have a medical checkup before departure and after return. Carry your lens prescription if you wear glasses. If you have diabetes, are allergic to penicillin, or have a condition that may require emergency care, have some identification—a tag or bracelet or card—on your person at all times.

Assemble a small medicine kit with your doctor's help. Useful items might be "starters and stoppers" (a laxative and an anti-diarrheic such as paregoric) ; a pain medicine; tetracycline capsules; an antihistamine; adhesive bandages; thermometer. Medicines should be labeled as to what they are for.

Travelers with chronic illnesses such as diabetes or heart disease should restrict themselves to areas where competent medical advice and drugs are available. They should carry as clear a statement of their health condition as possible with specific information about drugs and doses and should be alert to symptoms warning of flareups.

If you want to find an American or western-trained physician abroad, inquire at an American or British embassy. A directory of English-speaking physicians trained in the U. S. is available free from the International Association for Medical Assistance to Travelers, 745 Fifth Ave., New York, N. Y. 10022.

Special Tips for the Tropics

Precautions against "tourist's diarrhea" are advisable when traveling in "hot countries" or regions outside of Europe and western nations, where sanitary or public health measures are poor if not primitive: All hot vegetables are safe if freshly heated, not warmed over. Any well cooked meat is safe if freshly cooked. Most breads are safe—toast if doubtful. Fruits that you can peel are safe if skins are washed and do not have breaks (do not cut with a dirty knife). Alcoholic beverages and local beers are safe, but local soft drinks may not be (the sugar medium is a good culture for growth of bacteria).

Air Travel

A patient who is under a doctor's care for some condition or illness may wonder if it is safe to travel near or far by air. The question should be asked of one's doctor. But a general rule of thumb is that if a patient is able to walk into a plane under his own power, there is no reason why he shouldn't fly. Special needs of particular patients can be arranged for with the airline.

Airsickness troubles some people. It is easier to prevent than to treat. Take an anti-motion sickness tablet before boarding; no alcohol before or during flight; sit between wings of the aircraft; do not read; do not watch horizon.

IMMUNIZATIONS FOR TRAVEL ABROAD

Some requirements for immunization for foreign travel have been liberalized; optional vaccinations or preventive measures left to the traveler's discretion are important. The patient's health history, his doctor's advice, places to be visited, length of stay, should be considered. Required vaccinations must be recorded on an International Certificate of Vaccination card which will be given with your passport application. Your own physician can give all the vaccinations except the one for yellow fever.

Smallpox. No immunization card required for re-entry to U. S. and travel to Europe and most other countries except a half dozen or so where smallpox still occurs. Dropping the requirement for smallpox vaccination, now that the disease is rare, is quite recent. One's local health office can give current information.

Cholera. Recommended for travelers to India, Burma, Pakistan. Required by many countries if arriving travelers have crossed or been within an endemic area within 5 days.

Yellow fever. Essential for travelers to parts of Africa, South and Central America. Required by many countries of travelers arriving from yellow fever areas.

Typhoid fever. Recommended for every visitor to tropical areas (over 1 year of age) and to areas of questionable sanitation.

Typhus. Recommended for visitors to highlands and interior parts of western coast of Asia, northern India, Burma, Indonesia, Taiwan, Peru, Vietnam.

Plague. Unnecessary, unless advised by local health officers, if travel is to an area, such at Vietnam, where plague is endemic.

Malaria. Preventive measures nowhere required, but all visitors to malarial areas should consult their physicians about precautions and possible need to take antimalarial drugs.

Poliomyelitis, tetanus, diphtheria, measles. Most persons have acquired immunity to these diseases, often through immunization measures given in childhood. It may be desirable to have "booster" shots to sustain immunity at a high level while traveling abroad, or, in the case of children, to complete a routine vaccination program before starting on a trip. Check with your doctor.

Infectious hepatitis. There is no vaccine for this disease, which is common in tropical and other areas of poor sanitation. But many doctors feel that for travel in high-risk areas, an injection of gamma globulin may give some worthwhile protection for three to five months.

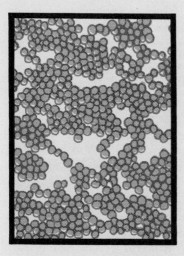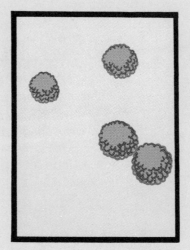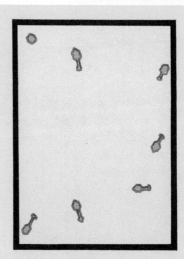

Small viruses are much too tiny to be seen in ordinary microscopes, but the electron microscope has made their varied shapes and forms visible. At left, above, poliomyelitis viruses look like tiny spheres when magnified about 200,000 times. Center, influenza viruses resemble fluffy balls of cotton. Right, T-4 *bacteriophage* (viruses that attack bacteria) have hexagonal "heads" and tadpole-like "tails."

VIRAL DISEASES

How often we say, when we have a sniffle or an intestinal upset, "I must have picked up a virus" — and how often we may be right! The Latin word "virus" means "a slimy liquid or poison." It came to be applied to diseases when it was found that infectious material, passed through porcelain filters so fine that all bacteria were removed, still had the capacity to infect susceptible animals. All known kinds of germs were removed from the filtrate, yet some mysterious poison or virus remained to cause dangerous infection.

Viruses are not at all so mysterious as they once were. True, small viruses are much too tiny to be seen in an ordinary microscope, but when the electron microscope came along with its enormous magnifying power they became visible for the first time — as particles, not mysterious amorphous poisons — to the eyes of man. Polio viruses, for instance, are spheres about a millionth of an inch in diameter, and influenza viruses, about four times larger, look like balls of fluffy cotton. Other viruses, not all of which cause human diseases, are hexagonal, rod-shaped, many-sided. Certain viruses (bacteriophage) which attack bacteria are shaped like tadpoles.

The first pure virus was crystallized more than 30 years ago by Dr. Wendell M. Stanley. It was the virus which causes mosaic disease of tobacco plants. Dr. Stanley's dry, lifeless crystals appeared to be as inanimate as molecules of table salt. Yet when rubbed on tobacco plants they produced characteristic disease. This gave rise to controversies as to whether viruses are alive or dead or are strange particles on the borderlands of

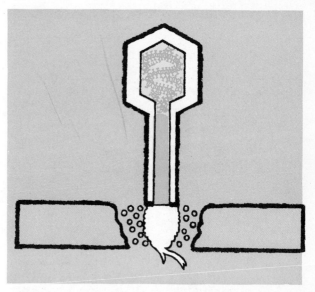

Closeup view of how bacteriophage attaches itself to the cell wall of a bacterium and, by chemical action of enzymes, "breaks a hole" in the defenses of the germ.

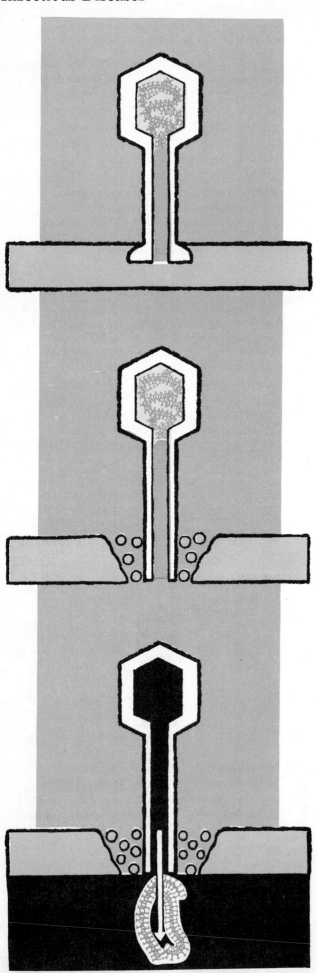

Steps by which a bacteriophage (virus) attacks a bacterium. TOP: The virus attaches to the cell wall of a bacterium. The hexagonal "head" contains infective molecules (nucleic acids). The "foot" contains specific enzymes. CENTER: Cell wall of bacterium is dissolved by enzymes. BOTTOM: Virus injects its infective nucleic acid into body of the bacterium.

life. New knowledge of what viruses are and how they work has shown that a pure molecule, containing chemical directions for life processes but not itself alive in the sense that a bacterium is, can cause infectious disease.

Viruses are composed, essentially, of a protein overcoat enclosing a core of nucleic acid. The latter is the same sort of chemical molecule that constitutes the heredity-dictating genes of living cells. But the hereditary material of viruses is inferior. It cannot "instruct" the virus to make its own enzymes and proteins or to transform raw materials into nutrients or to carry out complex chemical processes of life independently, as cells of bacteria and plants and animals and human beings can. Thus, viruses are absolute parasites. They can multiply only by raiding a living cell, commandeering the cell's chemical machinery, and forcing it to serve the virus's purposes.

How does a virus get into a cell? Its protein coat attaches itself to a small part of a cell membrane, a receptor patch, that fits it exactly. Not just any cell will suit a particular virus. Influenza viruses cannot cause paralytic polio, because they do not "fit" susceptible nerve cells. Many viruses which cause insect, plant, and animal diseases are harmless to man because human cells don't "fit," and it also works the other way around.

Once a virus is attached to a susceptible cell, rather astonishing events ensue. The virus dissolves a hole through the cell wall and its nucleic acid seeps into the cell and takes over its chemical machinery, "stealing" the cell's energy and forcing it to make virus protein and nucleic acid for the production of virus progeny. It is possible that we live peaceably with many viruses that do no detectable harm. But if enough virulent viruses invade enough vulnerable cells, we are sick in various ways.

There are no medicines that halt virus infections as antibiotics halt bacterial infections. The only exception is a drug that is useful in treating an inflammation of the eye caused by herpes simplex virus. Viruses within our cells are mischievously removed from non-toxic medicines harmless to the cell. Virus infections are self-limited. That is, if all goes well, they cure themselves. However, things don't always go well in severely ill, debilitated patients, and in patients with prior disease overlaid by virus infection. Supportive medical measures can be very important, sometimes life-saving, and viral infections may be complicated by bacterial infections for which there are specific drugs.

Fortunately, the general run of common minor virus infections — cold-like illnesses in winter, misnamed "intestinal flu" that hits suddenly and is gone in two or three days, and the like — are not terribly serious in healthy people, and the main problem is to make the patient as comfortable as possible and to keep him in bed. Common sense dictates that high fever or other severe symptoms be reported promptly to a doctor, for a number of diseases begin with symptoms that may be mistaken for an ordinary cold.

By far the best "treatment" for virus diseases of a serious nature is immunization. Vaccination of course has to be done prior to infection, since it takes days or weeks for vaccines to make the body produce immunizing antibodies. Oddly, antibody production is not stimulated by the nucleic acid part of viruses that cause disease, but by the protein overcoat.

The Common Cold (Coryza)

This is the most common and widespread infectious disease in populated areas. There is no need to describe sniffly symptoms well-known to the reader. The common cold or something indistinguishable from it is not produced by *a* virus but by one of a number of viral agents, including a group known as adenoviruses, of which a number have been isolated and studied.

Colds generally are very contagious, especially in young children. As one grows older the tendency to "catch cold"

decreases, possibly due to some developed immunity. Exposure to cold or wet has nothing to do with getting a cold. Contact with a cold virus, spread by somebody who has one, is what may produce a cold. Droplet infection (a sneeze can spray invisible particles across a room) is a major route of cold transmission. The least a cold sufferer can do to protect others is to muffle his coughs and use disposable paper tissues. There is no satisfactory immunizing agent to prevent colds, although there is evidence that immunity against limited kinds of "colds" caused by adenoviruses can be produced in limited situations.

At the first sign of a cold one should go to bed. This superb advice is generally ignored except by hypochondriacs and the indolent. Treatment is symptomatic, using aspirin, antihistamines, and steam inhalation to soothe stuffed-up passages. Infrequent complications generally result from secondary bacterial infections of the nasal sinuses.

Influenza (Grippe)

The "flu" comes on suddenly, with chills or chilliness, muscular aches, prostration, lethargy, loss of appetite, weakness. Onset may be so sudden (a matter of a few minutes) that it is hard to believe that a person could feel so bad so quickly.

Typical of influenza is its rapidity of spread and high degree of contagiousness under certain conditions. Older readers may remember the rapid spread of worldwide influenza in 1918-19, and all will remember the speed with which "Asian flu" spread in 1957.

Ordinarily, influenza is more annoying than serious, except in older people. But at times, for reasons unknown, it can produce changes in the lungs which make them much more susceptible to pneumonia caused by bacteria. This was what happened in the 1918-19 pandemic when people died by the millions all over the world from flu complications.

Bad weather, wetting and cold have nothing to do with catching influenza. The disease is produced by any one of three strains (A, B, C) of influenza viruses. Fairly effective A and B vaccines have been developed. However, "flu bugs" have a malicious ability to mutate, or change their character slightly, and each mutation requires its own vaccine. So-called Asian flu was such a mutation, and an effective component was promptly added to influenza vaccines. Immunization does not protect indefinitely and yearly booster doses are needed to maintain reasonable immunity. As a rule vaccination is recommended for elderly people, pregnant women, and in other circumstances best evaluated by one's doctor. The vaccine is prepared from fertilized eggs and this should be considered by persons who are allergic to egg protein.

Antibiotics may be given to prevent pneumonia in persons 50 years and older who have influenza. Otherwise, bed rest, aspirin, and plenty of fluids constitute the best treatment for most flu patients. Persistent fever or worsening symptoms may herald the onset of pneumonia. If pneumonia develops, antibiotic treatment should be instituted. Complications are uncommon except for pneumonia.

Yellow Fever

"Yellow Jack" once took its toll of thousands in American coastal cities. Today the focus of yellow fever exists largely in the jungles of certain South and Central American countries where a reservoir for the virus exists in monkeys. The disease is spread from man to man or monkey to man by the bite of certain mosquitoes. Onset is sudden, prostrating, fever is moderately high, and the pulse slow in relation to the fever. Vomiting of black blood may occur. Jaundice is present. There is no specific treatment, but there is a good vaccine which everyone who is going to be in the jungles of central or northern South America should take.

Cytomegalic inclusion disease is a not very well known viral disease that has no "popular" name. In most instances it is probably harmless and without symptoms, but on occasion may produce illness in newborn infants characterized by enlarged spleen and hemorrhages. No treatment of any value is known.

Cold Sores (Herpes Simplex)

Most people are hosts to *herpes simplex* viruses which produce "cold sores" or "fever blisters." Cold sores often develop with no apparent reason, but concomitant attacks are not uncommon in certain diseases such as lobar pneumonia, malaria, and meningococcal meningitis. Some women have an attack of herpes at each menstrual period. Between attacks the viruses apparently go underground and lurk there until lowered resistance or something else provokes them into action. Spirits of camphor or calamine lotion may help to dry the oozing pimply eruptions. Otherwise not much can be done except to grin and bear it. Grinning at times is uncomfortable.

Infants and children under two may have a feverish herpes infection that can be quite severe and sometimes requires vigorous supportive therapy. Probably this is a primary infection, after which the viruses remain latent in the body and the worst that happens is an occasional crop of cold sores. It is prudent not to let babies and small children come into intimate contact with people who have cold sores. Occasionally, herpes may infect the cornea of the eye and threaten vision. For this condition a drug called idoxuridine has recently proved effective.

Shingles (Herpes Zoster)

The term "shingles" comes from a Latin word meaning "belt," which defines the waist area typically affected by the disease doctors call *herpes zoster*. The responsible virus is similar to if not identical with that of chickenpox. Outbreaks of chickenpox have followed cases of shingles.

The virus affects certain nerve endings so selectively that, after characteristic skin eruptions appear, shingles is obvious to the experienced eye from the pattern of the lesions. Most often clusters of vesicles follow nerve pathways from the mid-back around to the abdomen, but nerves in the region of the eyeball may also be affected. Before the eruption appears, the patient has slight fever and some pain—often described as burning, itching, or stabbing—in the chest wall, lower back, or other affected area. Pain usually lessens after eruptions appear. These soon begin to dry and become encrusted, and disappear in two or three weeks. Generally there are no after effects, although some old people may have a severe neuralgia that persists for months before it fades away.

Shingles usually runs its course in a few weeks. Treatment is directed toward keeping the patient reasonably comfortable, easing pain, and preventing secondary bacterial infection.

"Parrot Fever" (Psittacosis, Ornithosis)

This disease is endemic in certain species of birds, especially parrots, parakeets, pigeons, and certain others. In most instances of this disease in human beings, it is acquired from contact with infected birds or their droppings or inhalation of microscopic particles of droppings disseminated in the air. However, the disease can be transmitted from person to person as the virus is present in the sputum of infected individuals. The infection produces an atypical type of pneumonia which may not be recognized for what it is.

Personally, the author has stood aghast in Atlantic City and other resorts where it is the custom for people to feed the pigeons. The risks of catching ornithosis are just too great. No protective vaccine has been developed. In the past the outlook for patients was not good, but proper antibiotics now give generally prompt recovery *if the nature of the illness is promptly recognized.* Unfortunately, physicians see many varieties of atypical pneumonia and are not likely to ask about exposure to birds, and patients and relatives are unlikely to mention or think about birds as causes of ornithosis, so treatment may not be started as early as it should be.

Lymphogranuloma Venereum

This is a generalized infection with acute and chronic involvement of lymph vessels and nodes of the rectum and genitals, transmitted by sexual contact. The infecting agent is a large virus similar to ornithosis viruses. The disease occurs all over the world and its fre-

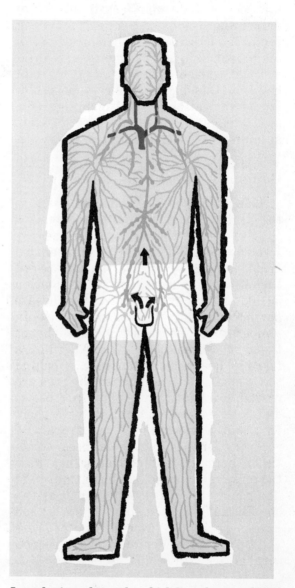

Lymphatic pathways by which *lymphogranuloma venereum* infection spreads from the genital area to regional lymph nodes and becomes generalized. The joints, eyes, nerves, and skin may be involved if the disease becomes systemic.

quency depends on the sexual promiscuity of the population.

A short-lasting, superficial genital lesion is an early manifestation. This is followed by inflammation of lymph nodes in the genital region. Eventually the nodes break down and discharge pus. If the disease becomes systemic, skin eruptions, arthritis-like signs and symptoms, involvement of the eyes, meningitis-like involvement of the nervous system, and rectal lesions producing pain and a pussy or bloody discharge may occur. Late manifestations include deforming lesions of the genital organs, rectal strictures, and hemorrhoids. A diagnostic skin test is accurate in about 90 per cent of persons who have or have had this disease. There is no specific treatment, although sulfonamides and antibiotics have some effect when administered over a fairly long period.

Dengue ("Breakbone Fever")

This viral disease does not exist in the United States, although an extensive epidemic recently occurred in nearby Puerto Rico. The virus is transmitted from persons by bites of mosquitoes of the *Aedes* genus. After an incubation period of five to eight days, the disease begins suddenly with a sharp rise in temperature, excruciating pain (hence the term "breakbone" fever), chills, a terrible headache, intense pain behind the eyeballs especially when the eyes are moved, backache, and pain in muscles and joints. Some patients have a rash. In about a week the fever drops and recovery ensues, but weakness sometimes persists and convalescence may take several weeks. Treatment is designed to make the patient as comfortable as possible. There is no known preventive vaccine, and as there are two types of dengue virus, a second viral attack may occur.

Colorado Tick Fever

This disease occurs in all the western states in which the woodtick *Dermacentor andersoni* is found. Although the disease has not been reported in the east, the virus has been found in dog ticks collected on Long Island. Symptoms begin four to six days after being bitten by an infected tick in spring or early summer. There is mild eye discomfort produced by light, chilly sensations, fever, generalized aching, especially in muscles and around joints, headache, nausea, and loss of appetite. This goes on for a couple of days, then everything clears up for a couple of days, then the symptoms recur and the second attack may last longer than the first. In rare instances a third attack may occur. Sometimes the attack may be single and last about a week. There is no specific treatment. Recovery almost always occurs and complications are rare. Recovery from the disease appears to give lifelong immunity.

Foot-and-Mouth Disease

This disease currently does not exist in the United States because it has been eradicated in animals. Even in countries where it occurs it is rare in man. It is characterized by fever and the appearance of small blisterlike lesions in the mouth and on the soles of the feet and palms of the hand. The disease is self-limited and non-fatal in man. Treatment is purely symptomatic.

Rabies (Hydrophobia)

This disease, always fatal, is produced by the bite of a rabid mammal (including bats). The virus, which is present in the saliva of an infected animal, does not pass through intact skin. The incubation period for rabies is from ten days to a year. The term "hydrophobia," or fear of water, derives from refusal of an infected animal or person to drink. This is not because water is not desired, but because efforts to swallow cause excruciating spasms.

In man, the farther from the head the bite of a rabid animal is inflicted, the better the results from so-called Pasteur treatment — that is, treatment-prevention. This consists of daily injections of graduated doses of rabies vaccine for two weeks.

The problem is what to do when one is attacked and bitten or comes in contact with saliva of a possibly rabid animal. The first thing to do is to try to apprehend the animal and place it under veterinary observation for rabies.

Failing this, or if the attack has been unprovoked and made on the neck or face, and the skin is lacerated, or the animal is pronounced rabid, immediate immunization with hyperimmune anti-serum should be undertaken, to be followed immediately by administration of anti-rabies vaccine. Of course the local lesions should be treated immediately by thorough cleansing with soap or detergent solution. *Get in touch with your doctor and your health department* as soon as possible if there is the slightest suspicion that the animal was rabid.

Coxsackie and ECHO Viral Infections

Coxsackie is a town on the west bank of the Hudson River below Albany. ECHO is not "echo," but stands for "enteric cytopathic human orphan" viruses — a striking example of a flight of fancy in scientific nomenclature.

ECHO translated into readable English means we have found a virus for which (at the time of discovery) we had no disease. So we have to look for one and attach it to the virus. The town of Coxsackie broke into the scientific literature when patients living there, who supposedly had infantile paralysis, turned out not to have polio but a disease caused by a new virus. There are more than a score of different Coxsackie viruses and heaven only knows how many types of ECHO viruses.

What diseases do they cause? Well, among others, *herpangina,* which is a very painful type of sore throat accompanied by fever. The area around the tonsils (or where the tonsils used to be) is fiery red, and oyster shell-white little blisters are seen. Herpangina frequently occurs in epidemics in summer camps for children. Treatment is purely symptomatic and recovery is prompt. Second or even third attacks have been reported, as there are many strains of the virus, and one does not immunize against another.

Epidemic pleurodynia or "Devil's Grip" is another disease produced by Coxsackie viruses. It begins with a sudden onset of pain in the chest or abdomen. The pain may be so dreadful that patients quickly come to the verge of collapse. Suddenly the pain may stop, only to reappear later. It scares the life out of patients so they take to their beds.

Relapses may occur over a period of a month. Involvement of the testicles, a type of pleurisy, and aseptic meningitis are possible complications. A fatal outcome is very rare. There is no specific treatment so all efforts should be directed toward relief of pain.

Aseptic types of *meningitis* are produced by Coxsackie and ECHO viruses, especially in children, and are frequently diagnosed as non-paralytic poliomyelitis. This type of meningitis is not fatal after the neo-natal period. Treament is purely symptomatic. The problem in this type of meningitis is to differentiate it from the early stages of poliomyelitis.

"Boston rash" and *rash with aseptic meningitis* are other ECHO virus diseases. Boston rash is a German measles or measle-like eruption accompanied by fever which clears up quickly. There is no specific treatment.

Rash with aseptic meningitis may occur in widespread epidemics. The symptoms are headache, stiff neck, feeling badly, and rash as described above. Treatment is symptomatic.

Poliomyelitis

The most important thing about this disease is that it can be eliminated if *everybody* is vaccinated, either with the Salk or Sabin vaccines, and then has booster doses when indicated.

The disease produced by the different types of virus is a brief, feverish illness accompanied by headache, sore throat, often vomiting and stiffness of the muscles of the neck and back. Usually the disease subsides and immunity is established. However, sometimes there is a lull in the infection and then a resurgence with paralysis. Rarely, the disease would progress rapidly to paralysis and death in a day or two. It may be presumed that most people who contracted this disease in the past never knew that they had poliomyelitis.

Encephalitis Lethargica

The cause of this illness, also called "sleeping sickness," is unknown, but it is suspected that it is a viral disease. It may start suddenly or gradually.

In its early stages, somnolence may be marked and there may be a paralysis of the eye muscles. In other cases the patient may be overactive with involuntary jerky muscle activity of the face and extremities. Mild or severe psychic disturbances may appear. In some cases death ensues in a few hours.

The illness may progress to a secondary phase with innumerable subjective complaints which may get the patient labeled "psychoneurotic." The patient may then recover, or progress to a third or chronic phase with symptoms of Parkinson's disease and emotional depression or deterioration. Parkinson's disease may occur years later after the patient recovered from a very mild attack of encephalitis. There is no specific treatment.

St. Louis Encephalitis

This disease, first recognized in this country as the result of an outbreak of a thousand cases in St. Louis in 1933, is produced by a small virus which is closely related to those of exotic-sounding viral diseases such as *Japanese B encephalitis, West Nile fever, Murray Valley fever,* and *Russian spring-summer encephalitis.* Certain species of mosquitoes transmit it.

Patients with this disease fall into three groups, the first being characterized by abrupt onset of illness with high fever, vomiting, headache, stiff neck, sleepiness, staggering, mental confusion, various tremors, and trouble in talking. Fever may last from four to six weeks.

The second group is comprised of patients who feel generally knocked out, have a bellyache, fever, and generalized pain in the muscles, which lasts from one to four days before symptoms of encephalitis (inflammation of the brain) develop. The third group consists of patients who have a mild form of the disease with headache and some fever. The case fatality rate increases with age. There is no specific medical treatment.

Post-Infection Encephalitis

This may follow measles, vaccination, mumps, influenza, chickenpox, smallpox, or German measles.

Two types of the disease occur. One, the *encephalitic* form, is characterized by rapid onset with fever, headache, vomiting and sleepiness. A transient weakness of the muscles may occur. Sometimes extensive paralyses are present. Light may hurt the patient's eyes.

In the other type, the *myelitic paralyses,* odd disturbances of sensation in the skin and a loss of control in holding the urine or stool may be noted. The case fatality rate is ten to 50 per cent. Those who recover rarely have any after effects. There is no specific treatment.

Equine Encephalomyelitis

As its name indicates, this is primarily a disease of horses, although birds such as pheasants and pigeons may contract it. Mosquitoes transmit the disease to human beings. There are two types of the virus, Western and Eastern. The latter produces a case fatality rate of 90 per cent; the Western variety is about one-third as lethal.

The onset of the disease is abrupt, fever may be quite high, convulsions may develop, coma may occur, and some patients have facial edema. A satisfactory vaccine has been produced for horses or mules, but it has not been used in man to any extent, except in laboratory personnel working with the disease. There is no specific medical treatment.

Viral Hepatitis
(Serum and Infectious Hepatitis)

There are two forms of the disease which have more or less identical symp-

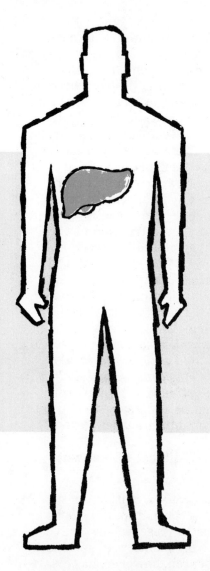

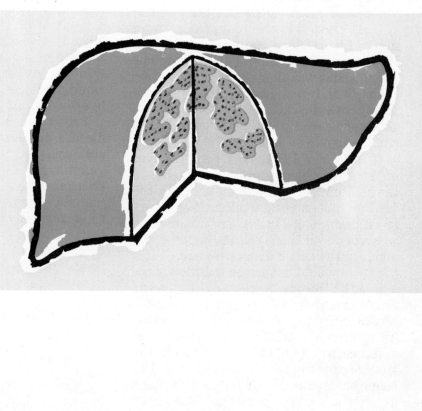

Infectious and serum hepatitis are caused by viruses. The target organ is the liver and a common manifestation is jaundice, although this symptom does not always occur. Most patients recover but convalescence may be prolonged. The most serious, but not common, complication is destruction of local areas of the liver, as shown.

toms but different incubation periods: *serum* (or long-incubation) *hepatitis* and *infectious* (or short-incubation) *hepatitis*. Serum hepatitis virus is found only in the blood or tissues of an infected person, while in infectious hepatitis the virus usually may be found early in the blood and also in the stools of persons who have the disease.

Serum hepatitis is generally produced by the transfusion of blood or plasma containing the virus. It occurs in about three per cent of patients receiving transfusions. *For this reason transfusions should be given only when really necessary.* It is generally agreed that if a patient is given only a single transfusion, he did not really need it.

Infectious hepatitis results from ingestion of food or water containing the

virus. There is also some evidence that an individual may directly transfer the virus to another, by hands contaminated with the infectious material. *It is a disease propagated by unsanitary conditions.* The viruses of infectious hepatitis are quite resistant to heat and standard chlorination procedures. It is likely that untreated sewage always contains some infectious hepatitis virus, so one should never eat shellfish from water into which untreated sewage flows. Small epidemics have been reported from camps where it was definitely shown that supposedly pure water was contaminated with the virus.

Carriers of both types of the virus have been detected. Those carrying serum hepatitis virus should never give blood for transfusions or for making plasma. Those who are carrying the virus in their stools should not work at food handling and should be very careful about disposal of their fecal material. Precautions as with typhoid carriers should be used.

Diseases produced by both these viruses were very much misunderstood until World War II. Previously, most instances of serum hepatitis occurred in clinics or hospitals where injections were given, for example, salvarsan for syphilis. Hence when these patients became jaundiced it was thought to be a reaction to the drug. Infectious hepatitis was commonly called "catarrhal jaundice" and was considered a mild although sometimes annoying disease.

It took World War II to open the eyes of American physicians and surgeons to the real nature of these diseases. In the Mediterranean theater alone there were more than 36,000 cases, and the disease was a problem in the China-Burma-India and Southwest Pacific theaters. Viral hepatitis would have been a major problem in the European theater had the war lasted another year; divisions transferred from the Mediterranean theater introduced it to the European theater. It is interesting that all major wars in the Mediterranean area have been marked by large outbreaks of serum or infectious hepatitis among western European troops introduced into that region, since Napoleon invaded Egypt in 1798.

Symptoms. Let's take a look at these two interesting diseases. The incubation period of serum hepatitis may be from seven to 180 days, that of infectious hepatitis, from 14 to 40 days. Patients may have infectious hepatitis in so mild a form that the correct diagnosis is never made.

In epidemic periods for either type of the disease, a considerable number of patients do not have jaundice.

In typical instances, onset of the disease is sudden; nausea, vomiting, loss of appetite, lethargy, and a mild sore throat are present. This seems to clear up after two or three days and then all of the symptoms described, except the sore throat, reappear in a much more severe form, jaundice becomes apparent, and there is abdominal discomfort due to the enlarging liver. Lethargy and weakness may become marked.

These signs and symptoms may clear up within a week, a month, or even three months. In some instances, rare to be sure, the disease progresses directly to cirrhosis of the liver. Relapses may occur, especially if the patient gets up too soon. Convalescence may be short or very prolonged — sometimes years go by before the patient feels really fit again. On occasion the progress of the disease is very rapid, and death from destruction of the liver occurs in three or four days.

Protection against the spread of the disease in a *closed institution* can be accomplished by injection of human gamma globulin. There is no specific treatment, but one thing seems to be true: *A person who has serum or infectious hepatitis should stay in bed until a test called the Bromsulfalein test indicates that liver function is within normal limits.* It will then be necessary to start a program to rehabilitate the patient physically.

Hepatitis is not a disease to fool with.

The search for causes. Although the diseases have long been thought to be caused by viruses, researchers have failed to isolate or identify a specific virus. Recent research, however, has disclosed a particle that occurs in the blood of most people who have had serum hepatitis. It was originally called *Au antigen*, since it was discovered in the blood of an Australian aborigine, but now is more commonly called *Hepatitis-Associated Antigen* (HAA). It is about one hundred times smaller than the smallest known virus. It is associated only with serum hepatitis. The antigen or an active part of it (called by some a *viroid*) may be the cause of serum hepatitis or a consequence of having had the disease.

The risk of acquiring serum hepatitis from transfusion of contaminated blood is measurably reduced by a screening test which detects HAA in donor blood. Such blood is rejected. Although present tests are not 100 per cent reliable, improvement of techniques and exclusion of commercial donors, who are much more likely to have HAA in their blood than the general population, should significantly increase the safety of blood transfusions. Another technique for preventing not only serum hepatitis but incompatible blood reactions is *auto transfusion*—use of one's own blood, withdrawn and stored prior to surgery.

A few persons with serum hepatitis have absolutely no history of blood transfusion, inoculation by contaminated hypodermic needles, or the like. Rarely, the disease may be transmitted in other ways. One of these is oral: there are always some loose blood cells in the human mouth. Inadvertent blood exchange may occur through cuts or abrasions.

Infectious Mononucleosis

This disease is considered to be of viral origin although it has not been proved to be so. It has a number of similarities to infectious hepatitis, and indeed it may "imitate" other diseases quite puzzlingly. It occurs generally in people in the first three decades of their lives and is most frequent in the 15 to 30-year age group. While sporadic cases are seen, infectious mononucleosis sometimes appears in epidemic form, and on occasion, in semiclosed populations such as private schools, a majority of the pupils will be affected. The route of transmission is not positively known, but an interesting hypothesis suggests that infectious mononucleosis is a "kissing disease" acquired by age groups most active in osculation. (The disease is unusual among people married for a long time).

The onset of the disease may be slow or sudden. The patient doesn't feel good; a sore throat — sometimes very severe — may or may not be present; fever is present but not very high. An important feature is enlargement of the lymph glands of both sides and the back of the neck ("swollen glands"). Other areas containing lymphoid tissue, such as the spleen, may also be enlarged. Some patients develop skin eruptions.

Generally the disease runs its course in a few days, occasionally a few weeks, and in some instances a few months.

Complications are rare, but a type of hepatitis with little or no jaundice may accompany the disease. Relapses do occur. In addition to the typical disease, a latent form has been described which has no signs or symptoms and is diagnosed only after white blood cell studies. (Mononuclear cells, from which the disease gets its name, are a class of white blood cell.)

In general, infectious mononucleosis is a relatively mild though often annoying and often alarming disease for which there is no specific treatment.

A blood test done in less than three minutes in a doctor's office can discriminate between "mono" and more serious illnesses such as hepatitis that have confusing similarities.

Strict, prolonged bed rest is not prescribed for the average "mono" patient as often as it used to be. The principal admonition is to avoid strenuous exercise, such as vigorous competitive and body contact sports, to avert the possibility of spleen damage.

Suspected Virus

There is persuasive but not absolutely conclusive evidence that "mono" is caused by EB virus, named for Epstein and Barr who discovered it in patients with Burkitt's lymphoma, a cancer of the lymphatic system that occurs in children in malarial parts of Africa. The EB agent is a herpes virus (different herpes viruses cause cold sores and shingles).

Evidence that EB virus is associated with and probably a cause of mononucleosis is supported by many findings. Mononucleosis patients develop protective EB antibodies. Such antibodies are found in about half the general population by four years of age. Several university studies have shown that large numbers of students have EB antibodies when they enter college, and do not get "mono." Those who do not have the antibodies are susceptible to infection, but for every two cases diagnosed in college there is one inapparent infection so mild that the patient is not aware of illness.

It is believed that EB virus is widespread; that most people are harmlessly infected by it early in life, often with mild or unnoticed symptoms, and build immunity; that some people reach early adulthood without immunity, and may acquire mononucleosis with overt or quite inapparent symptoms.

Infectious mononucleosis is a self-limited disease and the ultimate outcome is excellent. Serious complications, such as rupture of the spleen, are quite rare.

Cat Scratch Disease

This is presumed to be a viral disease and is more common than most people think. Following a scratch (occasionally a bite) by the family cat, a slowly healing, scabby ulcer develops at the site of the scratch. Then one finds a painless, benign swelling of regional lymph nodes, which may go on to suppurate or to heal spontaneously. It may take two weeks or two years for this to happen. Some physicians believe that administration of one of the tetracyclines shortens the course of the disease. If the lymph nodes suppurate, they must be incised and the pus drained.

Epidemic Hemorrhagic Fever

This disease occurs in northeastern Asia and was important to American forces in Korea. It is probably caused by a virus and is possibly spread by certain mites. The disease has a five per cent fatality rate under ideal conditions of treatment. There is no specific treatment, but symptomatic treatment designed to combat all deviations from normal physiological and biochemical states is very important to the patient.

Acute Infectious Non-Bacterial Gastroenteritis

These infections attack adults and children. They are characterized by abdominal cramps, nausea and vomiting, low fever or no fever, and diarrhea. The infection is associated with poor sanitation. Treatment, except in rare instances of debilitated or enfeebled persons, consists of fluid replacement.

RICKETTSIAL DISEASES

Rickettsiae are tiny micro-organisms named for their discoverer, H. T. Ricketts. They are larger than filtrable viruses and smaller than most bacteria, and have some of the characteristics of both — including the capacity to infect human beings and induce feverish diseases. Their normal habitat is the intestines of insects and various crawling and biting "bugs." From this reservoir, the

Rickettsiae, shown below, are intermediate in size between bacteria and small viruses. They cause various fever-diseases in human beings and are usually transmitted by lice, fleas, and ticks.

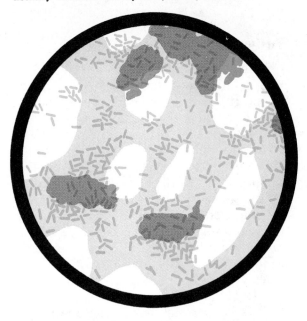

organisms may be transmitted to man. Since the customary vehicles of transmission are lice, fleas, ticks, mites, chiggers and infested rodents, control of vectors by sanitation and pesticides has reduced the incidence of rickettsial diseases in most parts of the world. Rickettsial diseases are quite rare in the United States, and some forms do not occur here, but in some parts of the country, as in tick-infested areas, there is some risk of rickettsial infection.

Rickettsial diseases are sometimes labeled "typhus," in a general way, with a subtitle indicating mode of transmission — for example, "louse borne" or "tick borne." *Typhus* (not to be confused with typhoid fever) comes from a Greek word meaning "stupor arising from fever." It is quite descriptive of fever with sudden onset, usually accompanied by skin eruptions and often, in severe forms, by involvement of the central nervous system. Antibiotics are so effective that these diseases no longer reach a threatening advanced stage if proper medical treatment is available.

Epidemic Louse-Borne Typhus Fever

This disease is transmitted from person to person by the bite of an infected louse. As Hans Zinsser said in his fascinating book, "Rats, Lice and History":

"The louse shares the misfortune of being prey to typhus ... If lice can dream, the nightmare of their lives is the fear of some day inhabiting an infected rat or human being. For the last may survive, but the ill-starred louse which sticks his loustellum through infected skin ... is doomed beyond succor. In eight days he sickens, in ten days he is *in extremis,* on the eleventh or twelfth his tiny body turns red ... and he gives up his little ghost ... To the louse, *we* are the dreaded emissaries of death."

Typhus fever has not existed in the United States for many years. During World War II, American forces in North Africa were faced by a major typhus epidemic (250,000 deaths), but it did not constitute a threat to our forces because all had been vaccinated with Cox vaccine for typhus. Infection therefore was rare and mild.

In the fall of 1943, soon after Naples was captured, epidemic typhus fever broke out in the Italian population. Due to the foresight of the then Col. William S. Stone, of the U. S. Army Medical Corps, adequate supplies of DDT were in the Mediterranean theater. Within a very short time most of the population of the city was dusted with DDT, and what would have been a fearsome epidemic was stopped dead in its tracks. Subsequently, in the late 1940's, it was found that chloramphenicol and the tetracyclines were highly effective drugs in the

treatment of epidemic typhus fever. So between vaccination and highly effective drugs, epidemic typhus fever holds no fears in this day and age.

Recrudescent Typhus (Brill-Zinsser Disease)

This is a rare but very interesting disease which still occurs in the United States among older immigrants from Poland or Russia. In 1934, Hans Zinsser isolated the typical rickettsial organism of epidemic typhus from three patients who had "Brill's disease." He theorized that the disease must be a recrudescence of a previous attack of typhus fever, because most of the patients he studied had had epidemic typhus fever many years before in Europe. Chloramphenicol or the tetracyclines cure this disease.

Murine Flea-Borne Typhus Fever

This disease occurs all over the world. The reservoir is in rats or mice. It is transmitted from these rodents to man by infected fleas, which, once infected, carry the causative rickettsiae the rest of their lives. The disease has been reported from most of the states in this country, particularly from the nine Southeastern states.

The disease is characterized by fever, headache, and muscular pains. A flat spotty rash appears on the trunk on the fifth or sixth day of the fever and then spreads to the extremities, face, palms and soles. Generally the patient tells a story of being in a flea-bitten area. Fatalities are rare even without treatment, but chloramphenicol or one of the tetracycline antibiotic agents is specific and brings about a rapid cure.

Rocky Mountain Spotted Fever

This rickettsial disease has occurred in the New England states (Martha's Vineyard), the middle Atlantic area, the Rocky Mountain area, in fact throughout the United States. It is carried by the woodtick in the West and the dogtick in the East. Once infected, the tick transmits the rickettsiae to its descendants ad infinitum. Before the introduction of specific antibiotic agents the fatality rate was around 20 per cent in the United States.

The disease occurs generally at times of year when ticks are abundant. It is characterized by chills, fever lasting about two weeks, severe pains in bones and muscles. A spotted eruption which becomes hemorrhagic appears after three to five days, first on the wrists, ankles, and back, and then spreading over the entire body. The tetracyclines or chloramphenicol are remarkably effective in treatment. If the disease is recognized when the rash appears, cure is almost certain. A vaccine is available for those whose risk of infection is high.

The important thing to remember is that all woodticks or dogticks are potential carriers of the disease. It is wise to inspect the body for ticks after being in a tick-infested area, or walking in the woods or tall grass. If a tick is found, remove it with a piece of tissue without touching it directly or crushing it. Parents examining children should remember that ticks crawl into the ear canals and may be missed on preliminary cursory examination.

Scrub Typhus

This disease occurs southward from Korea and Japan to New Guinea. Two species of mites transmit it to men from a reservoir in birds and mammals. If the disease is untreated, convalescence is protracted, often for a period of several months to a year. No satisfactory vaccine has been produced, but if the disease is recognized in its earlier stages and treated with one of the tetracyclines or chloramphenicol, recovery is prompt.

Q Fever

How did this disease, first discovered in Australia, get the odd name, Q fever? In early clinical studies it was called "Query fever" — that is, "doubt fever." No one knew what caused it. The disease is probably worldwide in distribution and man probably contracts it by inhaling dried Q-fever rickettsiae from various sources. Occasionally ticks are infected. Milk from infected goats, cows, and sheep may contain the organisms. Pasteurization is not entirely effective in getting rid of them. They may also be found in sheep's wool.

The disease has a sudden onset, irregular and often high fever, headache, and a patchy form of pneumonia like that seen in primary atypical pneumonia. Q fever is self-limited and very rarely causes death. As with several other rickettsial diseases, treatment with chloramphenicol or one of the tetracyclines seems to bring about a prompt cure. Most instances of Q fever are probably unrecognized.

Rickettsialpox

This apparently non-fatal disease is transmitted by mites from infected mice or other small rodents. It is a mild, brief disease characterized by fever, with an initial lesion at the site of the mite bite and a chickenpox-like rash. Most reports of the disease have come from New York City. Again, treatment with one of the tetracyclines or chloramphenicol brings about dramatic improvement in 48 hours.

Trench Fever

This is essentially a war disease which your author saw frequently in World War I and in World War II at the time of the capitulation of the Germans in Italy, when scores of patients with the disease were admitted to prison compounds. Trench fever is probably caused by a rickettsia, is transmitted by the louse, is essentially non-fatal, and where it keeps itself between wars is unknown. It is characterized by sudden onset, a discrete rash, fever, and pain in the bones, muscles, and joints. Treatment has always been symptomatic but the disease probably could be cured by antibiotics effective in other rickettsial infections. Infection is associated with conditions of trench warfare which has little place in today's military programs.

PARASITIC INFECTIONS

What purists call *metazoa* are more often called "worms," applicable to about anything that wiggles without legs. Another hightoned medical word for such disagreeable creatures is "helminths." All we need to know is that the organisms are multi-celled members of the animal kingdom and are very much alive. It has been estimated that two billion people in the world are or have been infected with roundworms or flatworms. We will not try to mention all the diseases produced by variants of such parasites, but will give attention to those that may affect people of the western world and travelers who visit countries where diseases they never heard or thought of are common in the population.

Flukes

These are types of parasitic flatworms that are almost never encountered in this country or Europe but which may be of concern to travelers in certain parts of the world.

Fasciolopsis. An intestinal disease of India and Southeast Asia, characterized by pain in the pit of the stomach and, at times, intestinal bleeding and anemia. A patient may harbor several thousand worms. Easily cured by hexylresorcinol.

Clonorchis (Liver Fluke). Common in Southeast Asia, especially in South Vietnam. Human beings get it by eating raw, smoked, or pickled fish. A chronic disease characterized at first by nondescript stomach complaints, later by liver enlargement, fluid in the belly, and nervous symptoms. Treatment is not satisfactory. Chloroquine has been recommended. Prevention: eat only well-cooked fresh-water fish.

Sheep Liver Fluke Disease ("Liver Rot"). Although the fluke which causes this disease is found in North American sheep, about one-third of reported cases are from Cuba. The fluke forms cysts and the disease is spread by eating contaminated watercress or drinking contaminated water. In endemic areas, don't eat watercress sandwiches or drink water of questionable safety. Treatment with emetine is effective.

Lung Fluke Disease. Most cases originate in Southeast Asia or Japan. Freshwater crabs and crayfish harbor this fluke. One gets it from eating them. Cook your freshwater crabs and crayfish thoroughly. The disease resembles tuberculosis in many respects. No specific treatment exists. One out of ten patients in one group was cured by long term treatment with chloroquine.

Schistosomiasis (Bilharzia)

Next to malaria, this is the most serious parasitic disease of man. Over 100,000,000 persons are infected. It occurs in the Middle East, parts of Africa, West Indies, northern South America, Central America, Japan, the Philippines, Southeast Asia, the Indonesian archipelago, and Portugal. There is an intestinal form and a urinary tract form caused by related but different organisms.

The *intestinal* form is ushered in by itching and a rash, hives, and sometimes asthmatic attacks. This is followed in a later stage by enlargement of the liver, not uncommonly seen in cities which have large Puerto Rican populations. The disease is contracted by being in fresh water — swimming, washing cars or clothes, wading — where the free-swimming form of the parasite hooks onto your skin and gets through it before you can say "Jack Henry." If you drink contaminated water the parasites go through the lining of your throat or esophagus quick as a wink.

There are several specific treatments. Your author considers tartar emetic the best drug, but patients often have a rough time with it. Stibophen is a good drug and is easier on the patient.

A relatively new drug, niridazole, has become the treatment of choice. It approaches 100 per cent effectiveness, is taken by mouth, is rather well tolerated, and often cures within a week.

A more heroic treatment which has been tried with some success employs the

Tapeworm eggs get into the body via the mouth, from consumption of infected raw or underdone meats. The adult tapeworm attaches itself to the intestines. The head at this point of attachment is very small compared to the rest of the worm. Segments of the worm may be passed in the stools but it is necessary to "get the head" to prevent regrowth.

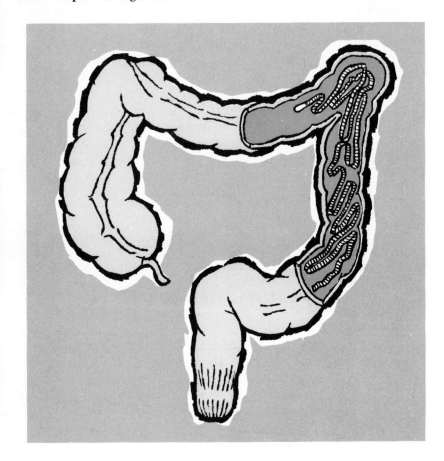

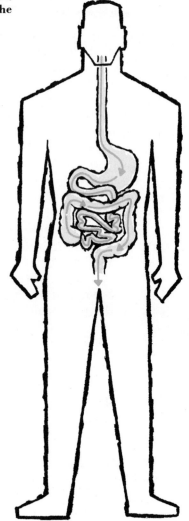

principle of a sieve. The patient's blood is circulated through filters which trap the worms and remove them from his bloodstream.

Freshwater snails are hosts to the parasite. Adult worms migrate to the bladder, intestine, and other organs. Diagnosis is confirmed by the presence of eggs in stool or urine specimens. Suspicion may be aroused by a history of a recent visit to the tropics.

The **urinary tract** form of this disease is of great antiquity, especially in the Nile valley where at one time practically every *fellahin* was infected. Many patients with this disease end up with cancer of the bladder. Treatment is essentially the same as for the intestinal form.

Prevention is simple but at times difficult. Keep out of contaminated fresh water—i.e., the Nile River, lakes in the Philippines, rice paddies in Korea or Vietnam. Swim in chlorinated fresh water swimming pools in the West Indies—or anywhere else in the tropics, for that matter.

There is a third form of Schistosomiasis which we have in the United States and which we should speak about. It is *"Summer Itch"* and is characterized by a prickling sensation a few minutes after the skin has been invaded. Then red spots develop, then little bumps, and next some of the bumps may turn into pimples. If you scratch too much you may infect them. Use agents such as calamine lotion with phenol to decrease itching.

Tapeworm

No, just because someone has a good appetite it does not mean that he is "feeding a tapeworm." With one exception, tapeworms do not produce serious disease. *Fish* tapeworms may produce an anemia which requires special care and at times is difficult to distinguish from pernicious anemia.

The two common tapeworms in the United States are the *beef* and *pork tapeworms*. People who harbor either of these two types may have nondescript abdominal complaints, but usually the diagnosis is made when they pass a part of the worm in a bowel movement. It is essential to "get the head" of the tapeworm when a deworming agent is given. The head attaches itself to the intestinal wall, and if the head is not passed the worm grows right out again.

Prevention consists of eating well-cooked meat (farewell to "steak tartare") and observance of ordinary sanitary practices.

Hydatid disease is relatively rare in this country. Sheep and goat herders, kennel-keepers and dog handlers seem most likely to contract it. The disease is caused by the larval stage of a variety of tapeworm, with formation of multiple fluid-filled cysts, particularly in the liver and lungs. There is no drug treatment; the involved area must be removed surgically if possible. Prevention in endemic areas consists in avoiding contact with dogs and taking care to prevent contamination of food, drink, and utensils with dogs' feces.

Whipworm infection occurs all over the world. A heavy infection is manifested by small, blood-streaked, semi-diarrheic stools, belly tenderness, pain, and at times a severe anemia. Treatment can be successfully carried out with dithiazanine. Prevention means observing ordinary sanitary precautions.

Hookworm

These small worms which attach themselves to the lining of the small intestine have been with us somewhere or other since time immemorial. The worms thrive between 30 and 36 degrees of latitude wherever people defecate on the ground and wear no shoes. Electric refrigerators and pasteurization practically did away with "cholera infantum" in babies; shoes and sanitary privies have done likewise with hookworm disease.

The larvae of the worms generally get through the skin of the feet and lower legs and produce a "ground itch." Then as they pass to other parts of the body they may produce bronchitis, big appetites, dirt-eating, constipation, headache, weakness, stupor, dropsy, and even death. Hookworm infection is easily cured with tetrachloroethylene.

Threadworms (*Strongyloides*) produce a chronic intestinal infection with manifestations similar to hookworm infection. In light infections there may be no symptoms, but in heavy infections there is usually abdominal pain, watery diarrhea, loss of appetite, anemia, nausea, vomiting, and emaciation. Dithiazanine is the drug of choice. Proper sanitary precautions prevent it. Don't be a barefoot boy in poorly sanitated areas.

Trichinosis

This infection is often mild and unrecognized but can be serious. It is caused

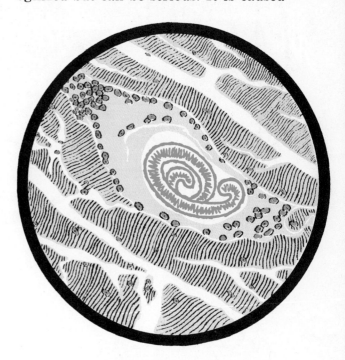

The coiled creature in the center of the drawing is an encysted form of the worm that causes trichinosis (*Trichinella spiralis*) embedded in strated muscle of its host.

by a worm called *Trichinella spiralis* which the victim almost always acquires by eating raw or partially cooked infected pork. Minute larvae burrow into voluntary muscles of the body, become encysted, and may survive in the muscles for years.

Symptoms during the invasion period may resemble "food poisoning," and be followed by muscular pains, weakness, fever, puffiness of tissues around the eyes and forehead, and sometimes odd signs and symptoms of nervous involvement. Thorough cooking of all products containing pork is a sure means of prevention.

Ascariasis (Roundworm Infections)

Three million of us have this occasionally very nasty infection. The large roundworm, *Ascaris lumbricoides*, is widely distributed but is more common in moist, warm climates. Its eggs usually reach the mouth by way of fingers that have been in contact with contaminated soil. The worm inhabits the small bowel. Larvae enter the bloodstream, reach the lungs, move up the throat to the pharynx and are swallowed, returning to the intestine where adult growth is completed.

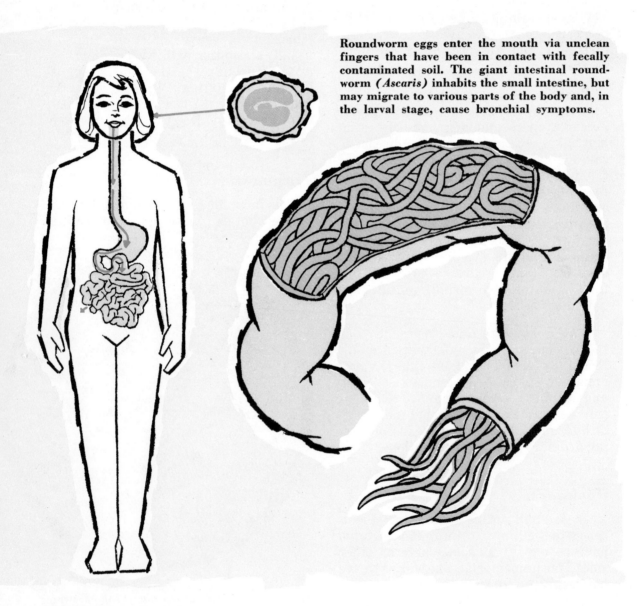

Roundworm eggs enter the mouth via unclean fingers that have been in contact with fecally contaminated soil. The giant intestinal roundworm (*Ascaris*) inhabits the small intestine, but may migrate to various parts of the body and, in the larval stage, cause bronchial symptoms.

Mild roundworm infection doesn't bother most people who have it. But migration of adult worms to various parts of the body may cause serious effects. To have a worm emerge from a baby's nostril or be found in a bed is shocking. Furthermore, if worms crawl into the esophagus they may produce symptoms of a perforated peptic ulcer and an unnecessary operation may result. Ordinarily, symptoms of infection with these worms are nondescript abdominal complaints and anemias.

Prevention is a matter of sanitation. Travelers may acquire the infection by eating uncooked salads in countries where human excreta is used as fertilizer. Roundworm infections can be safely and easily cured by piperazine compounds.

Leech infestation. Many people emerge from fresh water wading or bathing with a blood sucker on their foot. In this country bloodsuckers rarely cause any harm.

Filariasis. Threadlike worms produce this disease. Mosquitoes carry the larvae which are common in tropical and subtropical areas. Diethylcarbamazine kills the parasite in certain of its developmental stages. Arsenamide can be used against the adult forms. Prevention is a matter of mosquito control and precautions against being bitten in certain tropical areas.

Pinworm Infection (Enterobiasis)

It is said in medical books that infection with pinworms (also called seatworms) is not limited to poor people without sanitary facilities but is found even "in the seats of the mighty." Indeed it is. The characteristic symptom is itching around the anus.

The mature female pinworm, laden with as many as 10,000 eggs, comes out at night to deposit them on skin around the anus. This causes itching, which causes scratching, and transfer by the fingers is the usual mode of reinfection.

Piperazine or pyrvinium pamoate are very effective in eliminating pinworms. The main difficulty is to stop reinfection.

Eggs have been recovered from household dusts, bedding, clothing, and it is possible that viable eggs may be inhaled. If one member of the family is infected, others probably are, and it is important that everybody in the household be treated at the same time as the patient. A piece of Scotch tape patted down on skin around the anus will collect pinworm eggs, if any, and clinch the diagnosis under the microscope.

Good personal hygiene is important in preventing and interrupting the infection. Children should be taught to wash their hands after the toilet and before meals. Keep an infected child's fingernails clean and closely trimmed. During treatment and for a few days thereafter the child should wear cotton pants or a close-fitting garment to prevent dissemination of the eggs and contamination of the hands. This garment and night clothes should be boiled every day and bed sheets a couple of times a week.

The only bad effects of pinworm infection are itching, restlessness, and irritability, which are bad enough.

PROTOZOAN INFECTIONS

Protozoa are single-celled organisms, usually classified as belonging to the animal kingdom, though they hardly resemble what we think of as animals. The familiar bloblike ameba is an example. Most protozoa do not cause disease in human beings, but those that do are important. Malaria, for instance, is one of the world's most widely prevalent diseases. Some protozoan infections which sound rather exotic will be mentioned briefly since in these days of fast air travel some people may be exposed to infections not normally found at home.

Amebiasis (Amebic Dysentery)

This disease is caused by *Endamoeba histolytica*. It primarily affects the colon but may affect other organs, especially the liver.

Severe amebiasis is characterized by diarrhea with blood and/or pus and mucus in the watery discharges. Perforation of the bowel may occur. Infection generally takes place following the drinking of water contaminated with sewage containing amebae.

In nature, amebae exist in two forms. One is the active flowing organism which produces disease, the other is the *cyst* which represents a resting phase of the organism. Cysts are resistant to freezing and partial drying. However, boiling water effectively kills them. When cysts are swallowed and reach the colon, several active forms emerge and invade the lining of the colon.

It has been estimated that ten per cent of the people in the United States are infected — that is, carry cysts in their stools. The number who have symptoms is very small. But under some circumstances the amebae can give rise to severe and even fatal disease. The most famous epidemic in the United States, due to faulty plumbing in a hotel, occurred in Chicago in 1933.

Complications of amebic infection are hepatitis, abscess of the liver, abscess of the lung, and perforation of the bowel. Specific therapy with a tetracycline, emetine, di-iodohydroxyquinoline and carbasene, properly administered, will bring about a cure in severe disease. Mild disease can generally be cured by a single course of di-iodohydroxyquinoline.

Malaria

At one time, *malaria,* with worldwide distribution in tropical and temperate zones, produced more annual disability and probably more deaths than any other single disease. In the last half-century it has been gradually eliminated from many areas and deaths have decreased. Despite this achievement, malaria is still a scourge to many nations and it keeps some parts of the world uninhabitable. Indigenous malaria has virtually disappeared from the United States and Canada, but what with the speed of modern travel, persons who have acquired malarial infection elsewhere may present puzzling symptoms to a doctor who rarely sees a case of the disease.

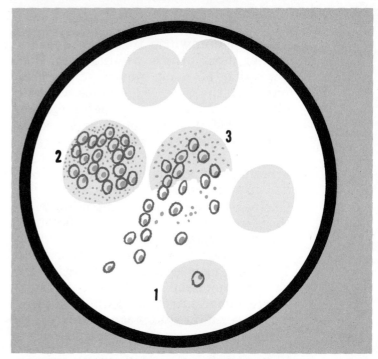

Drawing shows one phase in complex life cycle of malaria parasite; (1) individual parasite; (2) multiplication in human cells; (3) breakout from cells, with subsequent entry into red blood cells.

Malaria in man is produced by one of four specific parasites *(Plasmodia),* transmitted by *Anopheles* mosquitoes which exist all over the world. The mosquito is not a mere mechanical conveyor of the parasites. The latter go through a developmental cycle in the mosquito. Improperly sterilized hypodermic syringes may transmit malaria from one infected drug addict to another.

Malaria generally has a gradual onset accompanied by a sense of feeling ill, shaking chills and fever, or symptoms typical for the form of malaria the patient has. Delirium and coma (both bad signs) may develop early or late and death may occur. In one form of the disease, a diagnosis of dysentery may be made because of cramps, vomiting and bloody diarrhea. A serious complication is *blackwater fever,* in which the urine becomes dark or almost black in color.

Most people with untreated malaria get over it. Although they may have relapse after relapse, the malaria tends to "burn out." However, malignant tertian malaria which is produced by the *falciparum* type of parasite has a high death rate if not recognized and treated early.

Treatment of malaria by chemotherapeutic agents is now quite satisfactory, with proper administration of chloroquine and primaquine. Malaria may be suppressed over long periods of time, in persons residing in a highly malarial area, by giving one dose of choloroquine a week.

Trypanosomiasis

African sleeping sickness. This disease, African *trypanosomiasis,* is produced by the bite of an infected tsetse fly. It is generally fatal unless treated with arsenical compounds. Protection lasting at least two months can be obtained from a single injection of a compound called pentamidine.

Chagas' disease (American *trypanosomiasis*) is related to African sleeping sickness. It occurs in Central and South America. The bite of a specific insect, contaminated by the insect's feces, permits protozoa to enter the body. Victims are predominantly children. The disease may be mild or very severe, with symptoms of fever, edema of the face, and enlarged liver. No effective treatment is known; prevention is furthered by spraying houses to keep down the insect population.

Leishmaniasis

Kala-Azar, produced by a protozoan organism called *Leishmania donovani,* occurs in the Mediterranean basin, Middle East, India, China, North Central Africa and certain South American countries. It is transmitted by sandflies. In many parts of the world the dog appears to be the host of the parasite. As seen by the author in the Mediterranean theater, the disease has an onset resembling influenza. Recovery apparently takes place, then fever reappears, anemia is present, the spleen and frequently the liver are enlarged. With treatment with certain antimony compounds the outlook is good.

Cutaneous Leishmaniasis (oriental sore). This disease, characterized by single or multiple indolent ulcers, occurs in the Mediterranean area, Middle East, parts of Asia and Africa, and probably in Central and South America. Dogs, small rodents, and man appear to be the reservoir for *Leishmania tropica* which produce the disease. Sandflies transmit it. Treatment is the same as for kala-azar.

American Leishmaniasis is produced by organisms carried by sandflies. It occurs all over Central and South America and in southern Mexico. It resembles oriental sore, but in addition some patients have ulceration of the nose, mouth, and throat. Local treatment of mouth and throat lesions should be given in addition to treatment with antimony compounds.

Toxoplasmosis

This disease is a parasitic infection caused by *Toxoplasma gondii,* a minute animal (protozoan). About one-fourth of U. S. adults have antibodies indicating infection at some time, giving presumed immunity to further infection. The disease in adults generally runs a mild course, often with no noticeable symptoms, or discomfort resembling a cold. But if a pregnant woman acquires toxoplasmosis, there is grave threat of birth defects in her child: heart, brain, skull, eye damage, mental retardation.

The neonatal congenital form is acquired from the mother before birth, although the mother usually has no active symptoms. This form is characterized by severe congenital abnormalities, particularly of the nervous system. There is no satisfactory treatment and the outlook is not good. The other form is acquired after birth. In its acute stage, a red rash, fever, cough, pneumonitis, headache, muscle and joint pains, lymph node enlargement, inflammation of the heart muscle, and conjunctivitis may occur. Good results have been reported from the use of sulfonamides and pyrimethamine.

Many animals harbor the parasite in their tissues without harm to themselves. The principal mode of human transmission is thought to be raw red meat in which, after slaughter, the organism lives on unless killed by heat, drying, or prolonged freezing. Also, the infection may be transmitted by the feces of cats which, because of a peculiarity of the feline digestive system, may harbor the parasites at an infective stage. This discovery alarmed many cat lovers but it is not necessary to sacrifice kitty if sensible precautions are taken.

A blood test for toxoplasmosis is desirable if a pregnant woman eats raw meat or is in contact with cats. The test can tell whether or not she has protective antibodies, but not whether the infection was acquired prior to or during pregnancy. If she has no immunity, the following safeguards are presently recommended:

Home-cooked meats should be heated *throughout* to at least 140° F to kill toxoplasma organisms. This is the "rare" reading on home meat thermometers. But in restaurants or out-of-home dining it is safer to order meats well-done rather than on the rare side.

If there is a cat in the home, a veterinarian can test its feces to determine whether it is free of infection. If it is, the cat should be fed canned cat foods or commercial dry cat foods—no raw meat, no underdone table scraps, no hunting of mice or contact with other cats. Someone other than the expectant mother should empty the litterbox every day, wearing rubber gloves (it takes two to four days after excretion for feces to become infective). Litter should be incinerated or disposed of carefully. Don't dig in the garden if cat feces have been buried there. When visiting households where there are cats, do not pet or hold them. If there is a litter pan in the bathroom, there is no need for the pregnant woman to be concerned as long as it is undisturbed in her presence.

THE MYCOSES

Mycoses are infections caused by fungi. A mushroom is a fungus, but fungi of medical concern — except poisonous toadstools — are members of the vegetable kingdom, of which molds that grow on bread or cheese are representative. Fungi contain no chlorophyll. There are many varieties, including yeastlike forms and molds that produce penicillin. An antibiotic with "-mycin" in its name derives from some member of the mold family. Fungal infections of the skin are rather common and often quite stubborn (see Chapter 5).

Actinomycosis (Lumpy Jaw)

This is a rather uncommon chronic infection characterized by formation of abscesses which open and discharge pus. It appears to be more common in out-of-door workers. The most common portal of entry of the causative ray fungus is thought to be decayed teeth. Common sites of abscess formation are around the lower face and jaw, in the chest and lungs, and in the abdomen, especially in the area of the appendix. This latter type is life-threatening unless treated.

General supportive treatment plus adequate therapy with penicillin and/or sulfadiazine should be given and continued for about six months. Surgical drainage of areas containing pus is indicated. Dead tissue or bone should be removed surgically.

North American blastomycosis. This chronic granulomatous disease, caused by a yeastlike fungus, may occur only in the skin, only in the lungs, or it may be a systemic infection. The outlook for cure in the cutaneous form is good when skin lesions are treated by x-ray. Chances of recovery from systemic blastomycosis were greatly increased by the introduction of treatment with stilbamidine and hydroxystilbamidine by the author and his co-workers in the late 1940's. Amphotericin B is effective.

Cryptococcosis (Torulosis) is a subacute or chronic disease which may arise in any part of the body, especially in the brain and spinal cord and their membranes. It has a high fatality rate. The infecting organisms are apparently widespread in nature, having been found in fruit juices, milk from cows which had mastitis, and in pigeon dung. Your author never saw a patient recover from this disease until amphotericin B was developed. Now he knows of patients who have survived for at least four years after treatment.

Coccidioidomycosis

This disease is most frequently encountered in southern California but it appears to occur throughout the southwestern part of the United States. In some areas of California at least 80 per cent of the population has been affected at one time or another. Most persons with this disease, produced by *Coccidioides immitis,* have such mild infections that they are never recognized.

When severe enough to be recognized, the disease is characterized by headache, backache, fever, chills, night sweats, pleurisy, a general feeling of being ill. A *primary* form of the disease usually produces symptoms of an acute respiratory infection that is self-limited. There is a less frequent *progressive* form of the infection that can be serious. This may appear months or years after apparent recovery from an initial infection. The lungs may be involved, and other organs may be invaded as the disease progresses. There is evidence that amphotericin B is effective in early infections and useful in chronic cases.

Histoplasmosis

This systemic fungus infection has a harmless initial phase but in some instances progresses to a severe generalized infection. Thousands of persons have a benign form of the disease which causes no symptoms and is never recognized unless, by chance, chest x-rays taken for other reasons reveal calcified lesions in the lungs which may resemble healed tuberculosis lesions.

Histoplasmosis is most frequent in the Ohio and middle Mississippi valleys among persons living in humid rural regions. The causative organism, *Histoplasma capsulatum,* has been found in dogs, rats, skunks, and mice, and occurs in large numbers in droppings of bats, chickens and pigeons. Inhalation of dust containing spores may give rise to infections.

Histoplasmosis should be suspected in every infection in which there is an unexplained enlargement of the lymph nodes, with or without enlargement of the spleen and liver. Amphotericin B seems to be the best agent for treatment of this disease to date.

Candidiasis (Moniliasis). These infections of the skin or mucous membranes are produced by a yeast-like fungus, *Candida albicans.* Various forms of the disease include general eruptions, thrush, vaginal thrush, tongue inflammation, bronchitis, and lung involvement. The organism is universal. Debilitated persons seem to be especially susceptible to this infection. Amphotericin B should be used in severe or generalized infections.

Other Mycoses

A number of other deep-seated and quite rare fungus infections get their rather formidable names from the causative organism: *nocardiosis, maduromycosis, sporotrichosis, aspergillosis, chromomycosis, mucormycosis.* Early symptoms of many mycotic infections tend to be quite mild, and even well-established generalized symptoms may not be very intense, so there may be little sense of urgency in seeking medical help, but prompt diagnosis is important since, if untreated, such infections generally run a long chronic course and, if widely disseminated, may be fatal.

ON TAKING YOUR MEDICINE

Whether it is for an infectious disease or any other condition, the patient has no little responsibility for proper use of a drug prescribed by a physician. Directions for taking are stated clearly on the label. Strangely, not a few patients do not take the medicine as directed and some don't take it regularly or at all.

A doctor who writes a prescription considers the patient's condition, the drug, the dose, in giving directions for taking. It may make a difference whether you take your medicine at bedtime, or on getting up in the morning, or before or after meals, or at other specified times. Some drugs may irritate the stomach unless taken right after a meal. Others may be prescribed to relax the stomach before eating. Generally, drugs are absorbed more rapidly from an empty stomach, more slowly after eating. Drugs may be formulated to dissolve in the stomach, or in the small intestine, or large bowel, and some have built-in mechanisms for slow release over a period of hours.

Some drugs are excreted rapidly from the body and some slowly. Some tend to accumulate in the body after repeated doses, others do not. A physician takes account of duration of action in prescribing. Skipping a dose may dilute the effectiveness of a drug, and shortening the time between doses or taking an extra tablet "just to be sure" can have undesirable effects.

Sometimes a patient takes a prescribed drug to control, say, an infection, and after three or four doses feels so much better that he abandons his medicine. This can give germs, which are merely stunned but not put out of business if a drug is stopped too soon, a chance to regroup for a comeback. Take your medicine as long as the doctor says.

It is just as important to follow directions for use of "over the counter" drugs as for prescription drugs. Non-prescription medicines are not totally harmless if misused. They are considered safe for ordinary use if directions on the package are scrupulously observed.

Refills. A pharmacist may refill a prescription unless there are reasons why he should or must not. Narcotic prescriptions, by law, are not refillable. State or Federal laws require a new prescription for certain potent drugs.

There are many reasons why a doctor may limit the quantity of a drug despite the patient's hankering for a generous supply. He may want to observe reactions to a medicine. He may expect to shift the patient soon to a different drug. He may recognize, although the patient may not, that an ailment should respond rapidly to a particular drug and that if it doesn't, something different is needed.

THE HEART AND CIRCULATORY SYSTEM

by HOWARD B. SPRAGUE, M.D., ALBERT N. BREST, M.D., JOHN H. MOYER, M.D., and HOWARD C. BARON, M.D.

CORONARY ARTERY DISEASE

CORONARY THROMBOSIS

CONGENITAL HEART DISEASE

CONGESTIVE FAILURE

RHEUMATIC HEART DISEASE

IRREGULARITIES OF THE HEART BEAT

HIGH BLOOD PRESSURE

STROKES AND OTHER BLOOD VESSEL DISORDERS

OBLITERATIVE ARTERIAL DISEASE

ARTERIAL ANEURYSMS

VARICOSE VEINS

PHLEBOTHROMBOSIS

THROMBOPHLEBITIS

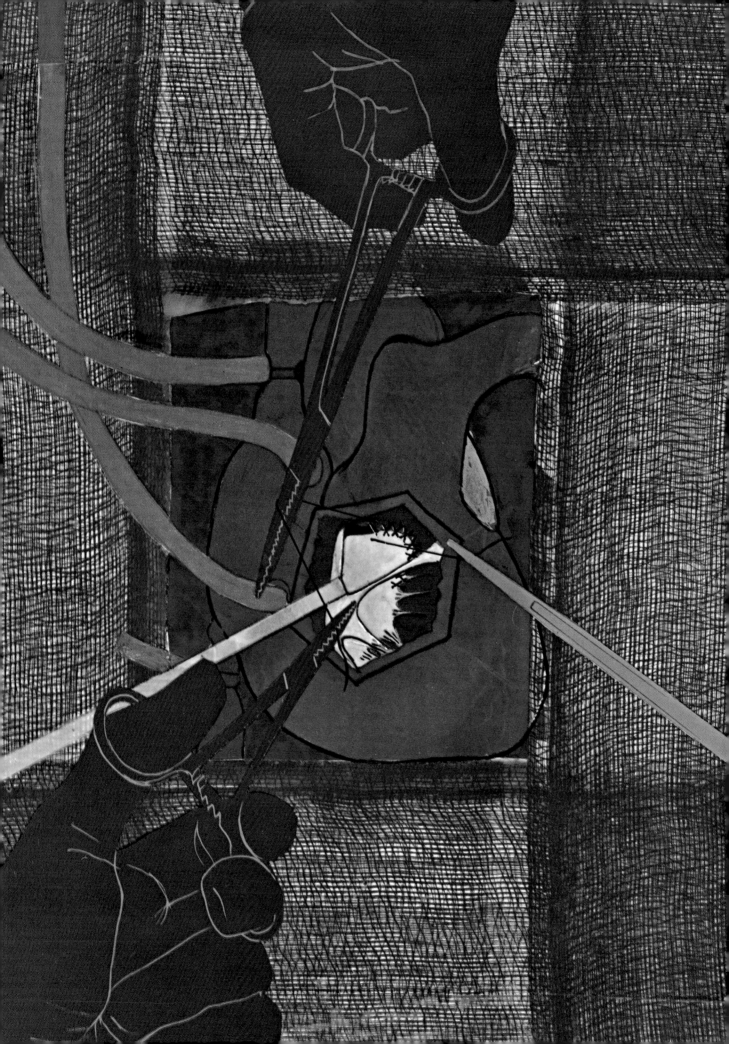

CHAPTER 3

THE HEART AND CIRCULATORY SYSTEM

by HOWARD B. SPRAGUE, M.D.

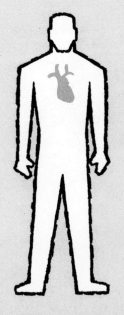

The figure above shows the position and relative size of a normal heart.

Heart-lung machines which bypass the heart and "breathe" and pump blood for the patient make open heart surgery possible. In such procedures the heart is drained, opened, and operated on under direct vision while the "mechanical stand-in" takes over.

The color plate shows a stage in repair of an interventricular septal defect — an abnormal opening in the wall that separates the right and left ventricles of the heart. Small defects of this sort may simply be stitched shut but larger defects, frequently the size of a quarter, require a patch.

In the drawing the surgeons are in the process of suturing the repairs.

The human heart is a remarkably tough hollow muscle about the size of your fist. It is relatively simple — nowhere near so complicated as the chemical-processing liver or the brain with its fantastic labyrinths of nerve pathways. In principle, the heart is an electrically-fired pumping machine which squeezes and relaxes at one point in a closed system of flexible pipes, to keep fluids within the pipes in constant circulation. All tissues depend on this circulation for their nutrition and disposal of wastes.

Perhaps because we can feel our hearts beat, and thump and pound dramatically in our ears when we exert ourselves extremely, and we know that when the heart stops, so do we, some people feel that the heart is a very delicate organ that needs coddling and babying. On the contrary, it is just about the sturdiest organ we possess, designed to do its vital work with a minimum of fuss or complaint.

The amount of work done by an uncomplaining heart — even though its owner merely lies in bed — is awesome. The heart beats about 70 times a minute, or more than two and a half billion beats in a lifespan of threescore years and ten. Less than one month after conception, the heart of a fetus begins to beat and continues for a lifetime. An adult heart pumps about 5 ounces of blood at each stroke, or 4,000 gallons a day. If compelled to, a stout heart can pump a volume of blood equal to the flow of water from a wide-open kitchen faucet. The work done by the heart in 12 hours could lift a 65-ton weight a foot into the air, or in a year lift its owner a hundred miles from the ground.

All this unceasing labor is accomplished one beat at a time without conscious effort on our part. Yet the heart is not an unresting organ. It rests between beats. It rests a little more than half the time. In a lifetime of 70 years, the heart rests about 40 years. It rests even when it is working its hardest, and gives an excellent lesson in the value of pacing exertion.

Externally, the heart bears little resemblance to a valentine or the pips of a playing card. It is roughly pear-shaped, with the apex or tapered part at the bottom. It lies almost centrally in the chest behind the breastbone in a diagonal position, its broad part directed up and to the right, and its apex or narrow end directed downward to the left. The apex is where the beat is felt, which is no doubt the reason for belief that the heart is a left-sided organ. Only a very little more of the mass of the heart ordinarily lies to the left of a midline through the chest.

The heart is well protected by the chest cage, and other defenses. It is almost impossible to injure a healthy heart by moderate periods of extreme physical exertion, partly because other muscles become exhausted before the heart muscle. And the heart has considerable "give" so that it can rebound from fairly severe blunt blows. It more or less hangs from blood vessels that give flexible support and allow a certain amount of movability.

Chambers and Valves

The phrase "two hearts that beat as one" usually suggests romantic harmony between two persons, but it applies equally well to the individual human heart. Functionally, we have two hearts which sustain separate circulations and indeed beat as one. The complete heart is divided into a right and a left heart by a solid muscular wall, the *septum*, which runs down the center and prevents blood in the two sides of the heart from mixing.

The right side of the heart receives "used" blood, returned from veins of the body, and pumps it to the lungs where it gets rid of carbon dioxide and picks up oxygen from inhaled air.

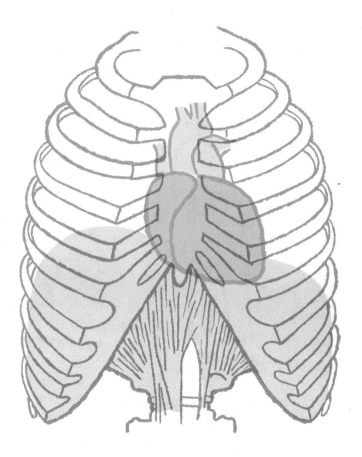

The fist-sized heart lies well protected within the rib cage, above the diaphragm. Its apex (where the beat is felt) tapers downward to the left, but the mass of the heart lies centrally in the chest rather than on the left side of the body.

The left side of the heart receives freshly oxygenated bright red blood from the lungs and pumps it to the body through a vast network of vessels.

This is quite simple in principle, although a cross-section view of the heart makes matters look rather complicated because of many "plumbing" connections and structures that in life are forever moving in little seas of blood.

Each side of the heart has two hollow chambers, an *auricle* (also called an *atrium*) and a *ventricle*. The auricle is mainly a receiving room and its walls are relatively thin since it does not do very hard pumping. The auricle has a trapdoor which opens into the ventricle below it. Ventricles do most of the pumping work and have thick muscular walls. The left ventricle which gives fresh blood its

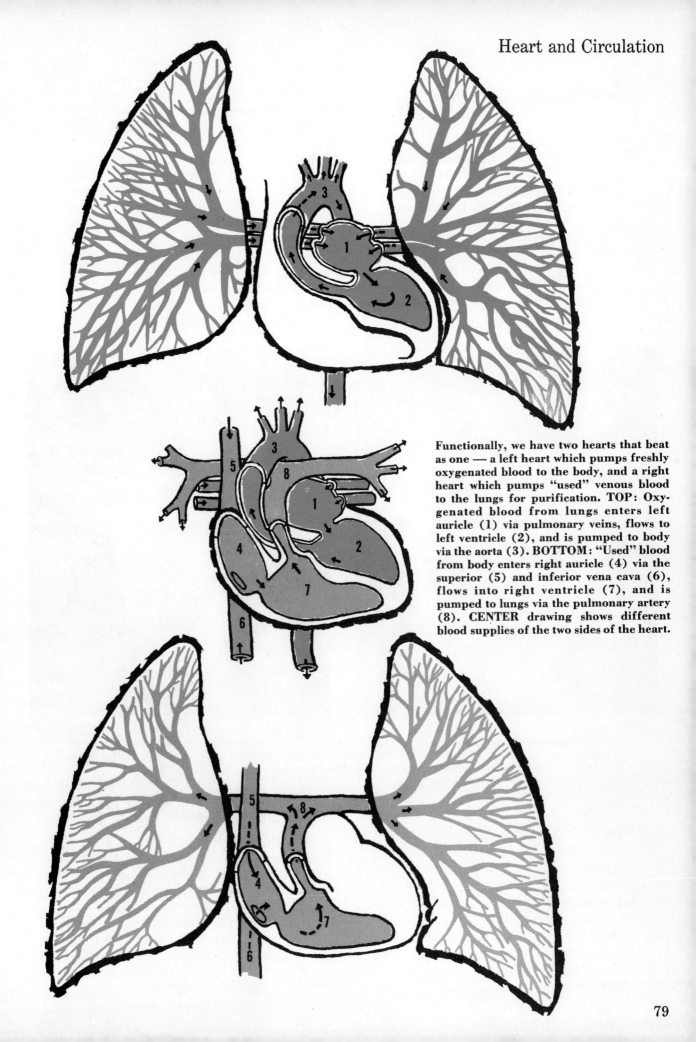

Functionally, we have two hearts that beat as one — a left heart which pumps freshly oxygenated blood to the body, and a right heart which pumps "used" venous blood to the lungs for purification. TOP: Oxygenated blood from lungs enters left auricle (1) via pulmonary veins, flows to left ventricle (2), and is pumped to body via the aorta (3). BOTTOM: "Used" blood from body enters right auricle (4) via the superior (5) and inferior vena cava (6), flows into right ventricle (7), and is pumped to lungs via the pulmonary artery (8). CENTER drawing shows different blood supplies of the two sides of the heart.

initial big push to all parts of the body is more muscular than the right which has only to pump spent blood to the nearby lungs.

As in an auto engine which has no power without compression, valves in the heart are necessary to seal pressure chambers tightly, so that contracting muscles have something to work against, and to provide an "exhaust" route. This is accomplished by four sets of heart valves which snap open and shut in precisely timed sequences, prevent backflow of blood, and keep it moving in one direction.

Simultaneously, the left side of the heart goes through the same cycle. Blood in the auricle goes to the ventricle through the *mitral valve,* so called because its two peaked flaps resemble a bishop's miter. The valve closes and the contracting ventricle moves the blood through another set of semilunar valves into a main artery, the aorta, for distribution to the body.

Under ordinary conditions these cycles are repeated 70 to 72 times a minute — or exactly at the rate of one's pulse. The rate of the heartbeat varies with bodily activity, rest, or excitement.

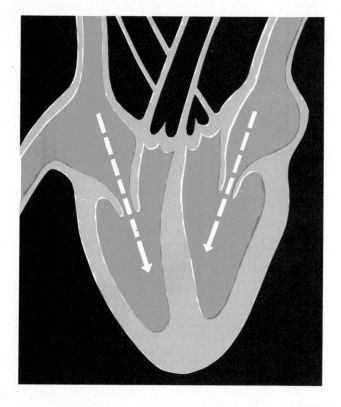 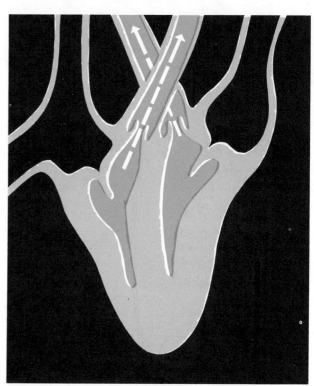

Mechanical pumping action of the heart. LEFT, in diastole, the ventricles are filling and the heart is relaxed or resting. RIGHT, in systole, the heart contracts and forces venous blood to the lungs and oxygenated blood to the body. Four sets of valves open and close appropriately.

In the right heart, blood moves from auricle to ventricle through the *tricuspid valve,* which has three triangular-shaped leaflets. Contraction of the ventricle moves blood through a *semilunar valve* (which has three cusps shaped like half-moons) into an artery that leads to the lungs. The semilunar valve opens at the same time that the tricuspid valve closes.

Heartbeat Regulators

Both sides of the heart beat in unison. The auricles beat first and then the ventricles. The part of the beat during which the heart relaxes and the ventricles are filling is called the *diastole.* The period of contraction is called *systole.* Thus, as well as a two-sided heart, we have two kinds of blood pressure—*systolic* and *diastolic.*

Diastolic pressure is the lower of two figures (such as 120/90) with which doctors express blood pressure readings. Here, 90 is the low pressure level in the arteries during the "runoff" period when the heart is resting. The figures record the number of millimeters a column of mercury is raised by the force of blood pressure.

Not all of the fine mechanisms and forces that trigger the heartbeat are known with precision. A small knot of tissue known as the *pacemaker* or *sinus node* is a vital spark plug. It is located in the upper part of the heart near where great veins enter the right auricle. It consists of specialized nerve and muscle cells which ignite a wave of muscle contraction in the heart. The wave spreads over auricular muscles and, although there is no direct connection, appears to travel from auricles to ventricles and

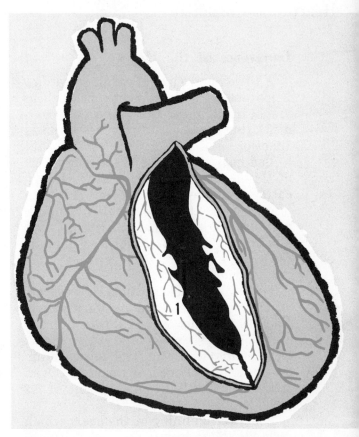

Cutaway section shows thick *myocardium* or heart muscle (1). The muscular wall of the left ventricle, which exerts greater pumping force, is somewhat thicker than the wall of the right ventricle.

The stimulus that triggers the heartbeat originates in the *pacemaker*, a specialized knot of nerve and muscle cells in the right auricle (1). Its impulse ignites a similar AV node that serves the ventricles (2) and (3).

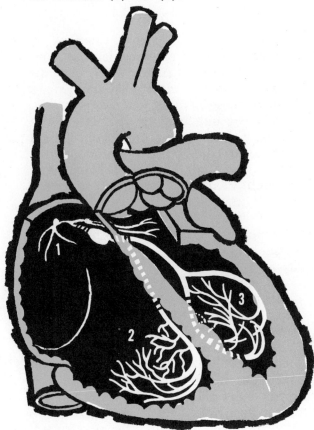

muscles of the valves over a bridge, the auricular-ventricular or *A-V node*. In some cases of disease or injury which interrupts communications between the sinus and A-V nodes, the ventricles may continue to beat independently but more or less erratically, under control of their own standby spark plugs, suggesting that there are complex safety factors which tend to protect the heart.

The electrical nature of impulses that spark the heartbeat is shown by the success of artificial pacemakers in triggering normal rhythms in some forms of heart disease. Artificial pacemakers are battery-powered devices, worn over the shoulder like a camera or implanted under the skin, which are connected to electrodes in heart tissue. The devices feed tiny jolts of electric current to a faulty heart, to spark its beat and keep it running rhythmically.

Various abnormalities of the heartbeat are called arrhythmias.

Heart and Circulation

Language of the Heart

A little knowledge of cardiac anatomy helps one to understand terms such as "myocardial infarction" and "endocarditis" that doctors use in discussing heart functions and disorders.

The heart is enclosed in a tough sack of tissue called the *pericardium*. Lubricating fluids beneath it permit free-slipping movements. Occasionally, the pericardium becomes inflamed, or adhesions may form, from causes such as rheumatic fever or extension of infections from neighboring parts.

The heart muscle is called the *myocardium*. It is a specialized and very powerful form of muscle, laid down in crisscrossed layers that give great strength, like laminated wood. The myocardium may become inflamed, or weakened, even starved to death, by impairment of its blood supply.

The internal lining of the heart which includes the valves is the *endocardium*. Bacteria may sometimes cause serious inflammation of the endocardium, especially in regions of the valves.

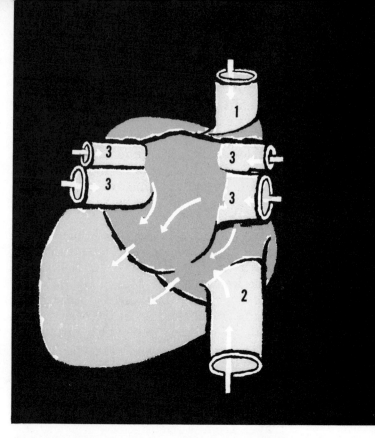

Rear view of heart showing great vessels which bring blood to the heart: superior vena cava (1) and inferior vena cava (2) bring "used" venous blood to right atrium (or auricle); pulmonary veins (3) bring freshly oxygenated blood to left atrium.

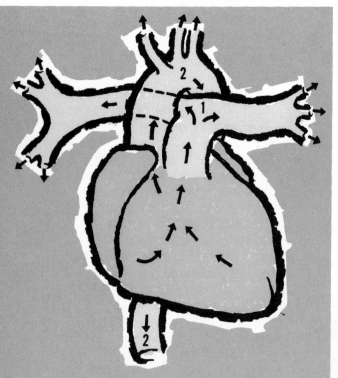

The great vessels which carry blood *from* the heart: (1) the pulmonary artery carries blood to the lungs for oxygenation; (2) the aorta carries blood to the rest of the body.

The broad upper part of the heart is entered by great vessels which arch and branch in quite confusing ways. Perhaps the easiest way to clarify the tangle is to think of these as input and outgo vessels. Two great outcarrying vessels emerge virtually side by side from the top central part of the heart. One is the *pulmonary artery* which carries "used" blood from the right heart to the lungs. It branches almost immediately into two divisions, one of which leads to the left and the other to the right lung. The other output vessel is a great artery, the *aorta*, which arches over the pulmonary artery. The aorta carries freshly oxygenated blood outward from the left side of the heart and distributes it through finer and finer vessels to all parts of the body.

Four vessels, two on each side, bring blood *to* the heart. These enter at the top and sides of the broadest part of the upper heart and discharge into their respective auricles. Two large veins, the superior (upper) and inferior (lower) *vena cavae* open into the right auricle and bring "used" blood that is returned to the heart for pumping to the purifying lungs. The upper vena cava brings blood from the head and arms, and the lower, from the legs and lower parts of the body. Two similar *pulmonary veins* opening into the left auricle bring oxygenated blood from the right and left lungs.

Blood inside the heart cannot nourish the heart muscle. Like other tissues, heart muscle must obtain its blood through circulatory channels. Heart muscle gets its blood through *coronary arteries* and the blood is returned by a collecting system of veins that discharge into the right auricle. Two sets of coronary arteries are quite conspicuous on the surface of the heart. The vessels follow a tortuous course and branch into finer and finer subdivisions. The name "coronary" was bestowed by early anatomists who fancied that the vessels resembled a crown encircling the heart.

The heart muscle or myocardium obtains its blood supply through the coronary arteries (1); the blood is returned via the coronary veins (2).

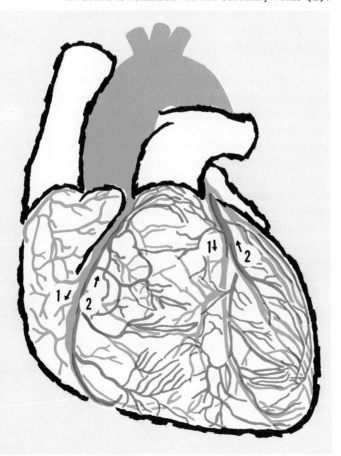

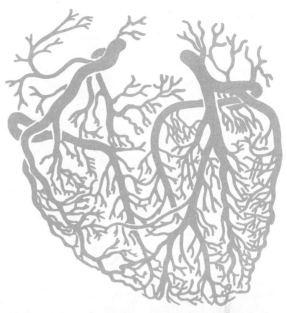

The coronary arterial "tree" branches from major vessels into finer and finer subdivisions that bring blood to local groups of muscle fibers.

Some Diagnostic Aids

Physical examination, a careful history of the patient, his complaints and symptoms, are of paramount importance in diagnosing heart troubles, as of other diseases. The physician's judgment is aided by tests and instruments which give important information about the heart's behavior. All tests require expert interpretation. Some are very sophisticated and others quite simple. For instance, a patient may be asked to do a measured amount of exercise, such as stepping up and down an abbreviated flight of stairs. The time needed for his pulse rate to return to normal gives some indication of his heart's reserve capacity.

Sounds and Murmurs. There is no such thing as a quiet heart. It is constantly clicking, lubbing, swishing, as its parts participate in variegated symphonies. The stethoscope, an instrument which when hung around the neck of a movie actor is a sign meaning "doctor at work," magnifies heart sounds for the physician's ears.

Heart sounds are better heard than described. Words are inadequate, but the typical heart sound is commonly approximated as "lubb-*dup*." The dull low

Heart and Circulation

"lubb" is caused by the closing of the valves between auricles and ventricles and is partly the sound of the ventricles' muscles contracting. The "dup" sound, shorter, higher pitched, almost clicking, is caused by closing of the semilunar valves in the exit-arteries. There is a fraction of a second pause between a dup and the next lubb. At that moment, the heart rests.

Other sounds from particular hearts are distinguishable by a trained ear. A rather soft swishing or hissing sound — a "murmur" — may indicate that blood is leaking back through an imperfectly closed valve. "Canned heartbeats," which are phonograph records of normal and abnormal heart sounds, are useful in teaching medical students what the heart is saying.

Electrocardiograms. A minute electrical impulse is set up whenever a muscle contracts. These impulses can be magnified by instruments and their strength and amplitude can be recorded on paper as squiggles with peaks and valleys. An instrument called the *electrocardiograph* detects tiny electrical changes in contracting heart muscles; its record is an *electrocardiogram.* Several leads from surfaces above different parts of the

Section of a normal electrocardiogram (EKG). The P wave (1) represents electrical changes occurring in auricles. The QRS (2) complex (downward, sharply upward, downward) measures the spread of electrical impulses through the ventricles; the T wave (3), subsidence of the impulse with relaxation of the muscle.

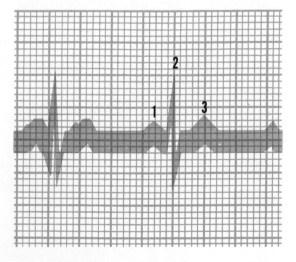

heart transmit impulses to the instrument for amplification. Normal hearts produce characteristic peak-and-valley tracings. Disordered hearts may produce tracings which differ in some particular and give clues to the nature of the trouble. The instrument is infallible, but interpretation of its findings requires a great deal of expert knowledge and experience.

X-rays. The shadowed heart imprints its outline on an X-ray photo of the chest. Comparison with standardized scales of healthy hearts gives information about enlargement, distortions, and abnormalities of the heart and its four chambers. With a fluoroscope, a physician may watch the living heart in action.

A number of highly refined procedures which must be carried out in hospitals by persons of special skills using special equipment are not used routinely and are not necessary very often. However, they are of value in assisting diagnosis of rare, puzzling, and complicated heart disorders, and some of them are useful tools in cardiac research.

By a technique called *angiocardiography,* the course of radio-opaque dyes through the heart valves and circulation can be followed, and defects visualized, by taking X-ray pictures at split-second intervals.

The heart has a "kick" which jolts the body imperceptibly. The kick, not unlike the recoil of a shotgun, is the recoil of a "discharged heart" when it contracts and squirts blood into the aorta. This slight nudge can be picked up by apparatus called the *ballistocardiograph,* which consists essentially of a delicately suspended cot on which the patient lies and instruments which amplify the minute heart-impelled quiverings of his body. The device gives information about the heart's energy output.

By a relatively new procedure, *cardiac catheterization,* blood can be withdrawn from the right and left heart through a tube inserted through a vessel of the arm. Analysis of the blood samples gives information that in some circumstances is of great value. Many delicate chemical tests are used in diseases of the heart.

The Nature of Heart Disease

It may seem inconsistent to discuss diseases of the heart as if these were detached from the blood vessels, that is, the arteries and veins through which the heart pumps the blood. The heart and the arteries are interdependent — the whole system is the "circulation."

In another sense, however, heart disease in its major forms is really *artery disease*. The common types of heart disease are *congenital, rheumatic, hypertensive,* and *coronary.* Other ailments also cause heart damage, such as infections, notably syphilis and virus diseases.

I say these disorders of the heart are chiefly vascular (that is, of blood vessel origin) for these reasons:

Congenital heart disease is the condition originating in the development of the infant before birth, from failure of the necessary twisting, joining, and division of two primitive arteries to take place in proper sequence, and with necessary completeness, as the heart is forming its four chambers, valves, and major inlets and outlets. For example, in one anomaly, *patent ductus arteriosus,* the artery which bypasses the lungs in the unborn child fails to close after birth and blood continues to flow through it. This can be cured by surgery.

In ***rheumatic heart disease*** the inflammation in the heart muscle is often "perivascular," that is, around the arteries in the heart muscle, and other blood vessels in the body may become inflamed in rheumatic fever.

In ***hypertensive heart disease*** the heart muscle becomes overworked because of spasm or narrowing of the arterioles or fine branches of the arterial system throughout the body, producing an increase in the resistance which prevents easy "run-off" of the blood into the organs. Thus the pressure in the arteries is raised and the heart is forced to pump out its blood against a high blood pressure.

In ***coronary heart disease*** we see the most obvious example of the primary role

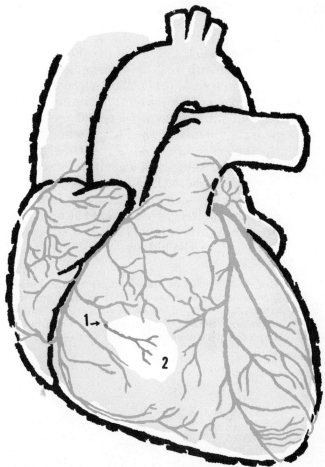

Obstruction of a branch of a coronary artery (1) cuts off the blood supply of the muscle fibers it serves, resulting in an area of *infarction* or death of tissues (2). This is a "heart attack."

of the arteries in producing the heart failure. "Coronary heart disease" is truly "coronary *artery* disease," because the heart muscle itself is normal except where the circulation to it has been reduced or cut off by narrowing or blocking of branches of the coronary arteries. English physicians call this "ischemic heart disease," which is a good term, because it describes the real damage to the heart from local reduction of blood supply to a portion of the muscular wall.

Thus in "coronary heart disease" we should always think of the constantly changing pattern of the circulation in the complex branching distribution of the coronary arteries. Some are becoming thickened and blocked with clots or fatty deposits narrowing the caliber. In some a clot in the artery is becoming partially dissolved and always nature is attempting to open up new channels to replace those which have degenerated.

Of course, the arteries in other organs are also subject to degeneration by arteriosclerosis or atherosclerosis. We recognize cramping pain in the calves of legs on walking as evidence of *ischemia* or local anemia of the leg muscles, when the arteries are obstructed to a point where the increased demand for blood flow cannot be satisfied. In general, however, people with aging changes in their arteries do pretty well unless the arteries predominantly affected are in the brain, the heart, or the kidney.

The drawing below shows stages of *atheroma* formation in blood vessels. TOP square, normal artery. CENTER, deposits developing in lining of artery. BOTTOM, arterial channel greatly narrowed by thickened wall; a clot may form.

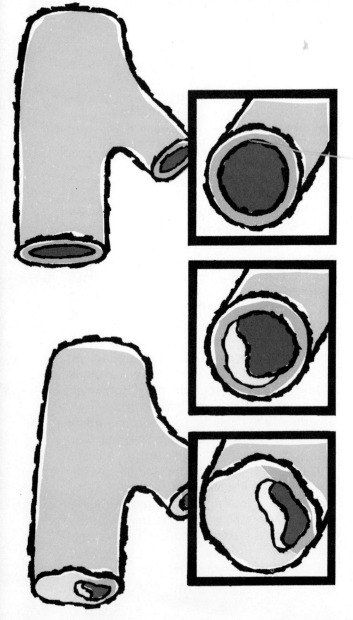

Heart Failure

The heart can fail in three major ways: by inability to pump out the blood adequately (*congestive* heart failure); by sending painful sensations to the chest (*anginal* failure); or by losing its normal, even beating and becoming irregular, or extremely slow or fast, or by having periods of complete stopping of the beat. The latter is called *heart block* and this refers to blocking of the electrical impulse which passes from atria to ventricles with each heart beat. It should not be confused with blocking of a coronary artery by a clot.

CORONARY ARTERY DISEASE

Atherosclerosis of the coronary arteries is the most common form of heart disease. It is in the nature of arteries to undergo thickening of their walls as they grow older. This occurs earlier and more severely in some individuals than in others, probably because of differences in heredity.

This is as "normal" a way as we know for a person to age and die. Dr. A. S. Warthin pointed out, many years ago, that this change in arteries and rapid senescence occurs in nine months in the human placenta and in about 75 years in the human male.

But this is not the whole, or even the major, mechanism of what goes on in coronary arteries when we have coronary disease and coronary "attacks." *Atherosclerosis,* as distinguished from *arteriosclerosis* ("hardening of the arteries"), seems to be a disease or at least a disturbance in the arteries themselves, or in the ability of the arteries to handle certain elements of the blood that circulates through them during years or decades.

Atheroma means porridge, or soft mush, and this is the type of fatty cholesterol deposit appearing in the lining and walls of affected arteries. Later there may be a deposit of calcium or lime salts in these diseased areas.

The major question in the control of this disease concerns whether or not the tendency to it is hereditary ("inborn error of metabolism"), or sufficiently dependent upon environmental influences so that something can be done about it on a preventive basis. There is little evidence that it can be reversed once it is well established.

Hereditary Aspects

The basis for assuming an hereditary origin is impressive. The outstanding fact is that in the early age period, especially under age 40, coronary atherosclerosis is almost entirely a male disease. Only after the menopause does its occurrence become equal in males and females. Women's glandular, or hormonal, arrangements before the menopause seem to provide a considerable degree of protection against coronary disease.

Another point is that young men suffering from premature coronary attacks are in general muscular and tend to put on weight after age 25. This body shape is that of the "mesomorph" with heavy muscles, whereas the slender, poorly muscled male is almost immune to coronary disease under the age of 40.

There are also families with a high incidence of coronary attacks and early death, and in some a family tendency to high levels of cholesterol in the blood, or a high level of uric acid. Recently a hidden tendency to diabetes has been demonstrated in some instances. Diabetes increases the susceptibility to coronary disease, even in the female, to a striking degree. High blood pressure also may be found with coronary disease, especially in women, and hypertension adds an important burden to the heart.

Incidence

There is a great deal of interest in heart attacks and in what seems to be an increase in heart disease as a cause of death. Sudden death is almost always a cardiac death. Coronary artery disease is by far the most common type of heart disease responsible for these events.

However, there are factors, aside from a true increase in the occurrence of coronary disease, that account for what has been called an "epidemic" of heart diseases. These are the increase in the average age of our population, the conquest of many infectious diseases previously fatal, the general improvement in the health of the population, and the greater accuracy in the diagnosis of coronary disease. There is also a tendency to label some deaths as "coronary" in origin when other fatal diseases are present.

It is the popular belief that coronary disease is something new, and indeed the recognition of acute coronary thrombosis is only about 50 years old. Heart deaths did not appear in the mortality figures of 150 years ago. But I have read Boston newspaper accounts of deaths occurring at that time and it is clearly evident that sudden coronary attacks were often the cause of unexpected demise.

In any event, this "epidemic" seems to have reached its peak and to be tapering off to some degree. But so long as more years are added to our life expectancy we may expect a high incidence of both coronary disease and cancer.

Environmental Factors

I have pointed out that the chemical and anatomical baggage that each man carries aboard the ship for his voyage of life is predetermined by his heredity. We should consider what are the buffetings of the voyage that may influence his coronary arteries to become obstructed at 40 or 80. What are the things he may do or that are done to him that will bring him to a coronary attack?

We actually know relatively little about what these influences may be in an individual case. We have some knowledge of differences in prevalence of coronary disease in different countries, but if these countries are medically primitive even this information is highly inaccurate.

In general, two factors seem to be involved — one is the effect of *atherosclerosis* and narrowing of the coronary vessels; the other is the tendency to *thrombosis* or clotting in these vessels. Not only are these two different things, but even the students of the pathology of

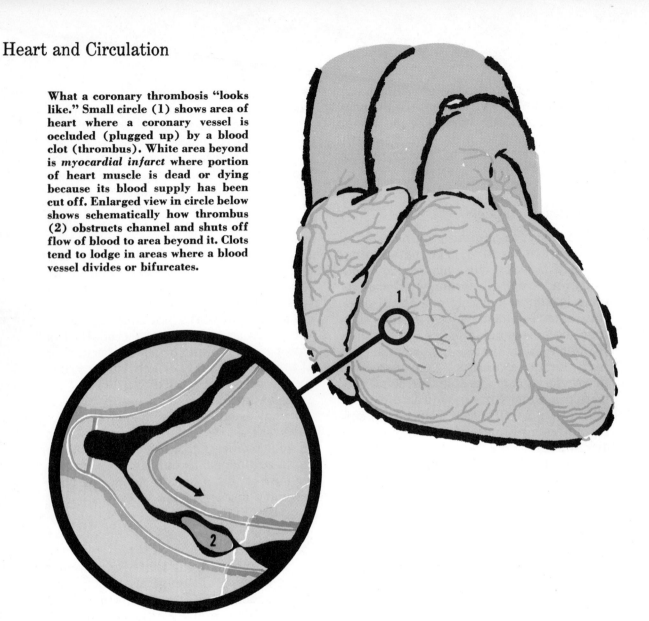

What a coronary thrombosis "looks like." Small circle (1) shows area of heart where a coronary vessel is occluded (plugged up) by a blood clot (thrombus). White area beyond is *myocardial infarct* where portion of heart muscle is dead or dying because its blood supply has been cut off. Enlarged view in circle below shows schematically how thrombus (2) obstructs channel and shuts off flow of blood to area beyond it. Clots tend to lodge in areas where a blood vessel divides or bifurcates.

the coronaries disagree on which comes first. One school contends that the lining of the vessels degenerates first and clots are formed on the affected areas; the other believes that we all form minor clots in our arteries and that the normal mechanism for dissolving them (*fibrinolysis*) is disturbed in the victim of coronary disease.

Whatever may be the genesis of this disease, it seems likely that prosperous nations have more atherosclerosis and a greater tendency to abnormal clotting than do the less favored ones.

The usual explanations for these differences are that the men in prosperous countries tend to be overweight, less physically active, consume richer diets, smoke more cigarettes, and live more competitive lives. It may be, as one study

suggests, that heavy users of coffee (over five cups a day) are in the group susceptible to coronary disease.

For each one of these factors there is some controversial evidence. It is impossible to submit much of this here, but I must emphasize a few points.

Exercise and Diet. Thin, active men living in the country and under the demands of daily physical chores tend to live long. I believe that it makes little difference what a man eats so long as he earns his calories by not gaining weight. Men who do not exceed their top weight at age 25 have a good life expectancy.

It is probably not a good thing for an automobile-riding, television-viewing, cigarette-smoking population to have a high fat or a high carbohydrate (sugar-starch) diet, but when it comes down to the individual it is very hard to prove that these sins of inertia are doing him in because we can never conduct a controlled experiment. The closest to it is now being carried out in several medical centers with men on special diets.

Studies on men in England (Morris) and in the United States (Paul), for example, show no correlation of the dietary intake with coronary disease, as compared to those who have not developed it.

A great deal of work has been done on the influence of the polyunsaturated fats (vegetable oils) as compared to animal fats and hardened fats (some of the margarines). It seems to me reasonable to reduce the total fat calories of our diets to 25-30 per cent and to consume half of this in vegetable oils (such as corn oil, safflower oil or cottonseed oil). The answers to some of these questions lie in the future, after the completion of predictive studies, and not in retrospective surveys in which the notoriously fallible memory of what we ate in the past is so important a datum.

Cholesterol. Much of the apprehension concerning diet centers about *cholesterol*, which has become a popular scare word, and the usual assumption of the transition from diet to coronary atherosclerosis is that fat or cholesterol in the food causes fat or cholesterol in the arteries.

This is too simple an explanation. Furthermore, a certain amount of fat and cholesterol is necessary in our food. Fat has a dozen virtues ranging from vitamin supply, to energy production, to lubrication and protection from atomic radiation. Cholesterol is needed in almost every tissue of the human body and, if not supplied in the diet, it will be produced by the liver. It is also essential to sex hormone production.

I think that the most that can be said at the moment is that flooding the digestive tract with large amounts of saturated fats and cholesterol is unwise and, in genetically susceptible and physically inactive men, will not only increase body weights but strain the mechanisms of fat utilization and excretion — which is only another plea for moderation.

The dietary research focus is shifting somewhat from a concentration on the effect of fats to the influence of carbohydrates, especially sugar. After all, the carbohydrates (starches and sugars) can be transformed to fat by the body. A hog is not fattened by feeding him fat but by giving him corn.

Professor Yudkin of London has pointed out that civilized man is a victim of the palatability of artificially produced sweets and that "the relative incidence of myocardial infarction in different countries is more closely related to the consumption of sugar than to the consumption of fat, or animal fat."

So active has been the investigation of dietary factors that almost everything has been incriminated, either from excess or deficiency in the diet — fats, proteins, carbohydrates, trace elements, vitamins, and soft water.

We had best not be dogmatic but realize, as Yudkin points out, that man has changed from an essentially protein- and fat-eating savage to a civilized creature enjoying palatable, calorie-rich carbohydrates and sugars in the past 10,000 years — which is too short a time for him to make a satisfactory adjustment. This dietary shift may well be a primary factor in the increase in obesity, dental caries, myocardial infarction, peptic ulcer, diabetes, and other diseases.

Susceptibility Prediction. The prediction of who is likely to suffer from coronary disease is best made by family history, weight gain after age 25 (from eating too much), presence or absence of high blood pressure, and roughly the level of cholesterol in the blood over 300 mg. per 100 cc. (in some studies over 260 mg.). We cannot really compare the latter test with the levels in other countries since the United States has no large groups with normally low cholesterol levels, i.e. under 200 mg., and our average is about 250 mg.

I would, however, caution against too much emphasis on cholesterol levels. Most doctors don't have their own blood cholesterol tested. I have had my own determined only once. Furthermore, there are wide fluctuations in the same person and all sorts of factors influence it. For example, emotion puts it up, but, to my way of thinking, this must be what nature intended and it is probably one of our defenses.

Tobacco and Stress. Of the many other mischiefs of a man's life that have been blamed for his development of coronary artery disease, I shall mention only two — tobacco and emotional stress.

The American Heart Association has published a statement opposing cigarette smoking in cardiac patients, and, in my experience, I know of no heart condition for which tobacco is useful. I regularly say to my patients "I don't know whether or not tobacco is a factor in your coronary disease. I only know that many men with angina are better if they don't smoke. You will have to find this out yourself, and this means complete stopping of cigarettes for at least three months, as a starter."

To those who have already had a heart attack, (coronary thrombosis) I say "those men who stop smoking and can hold their weight (or lose some if overweight) and can gradually increase physical exercise tend to do well. The crybabies who say, 'I can't stop smoking, I shall be a nervous wreck,' are generally not able to play the coronary game and win."

As for emotional stress the most popular and conscience-satisfying alibi for the coronary patient, or his wife, to explain the development of his heart disease, is the nervous strain he has been under.

The American public has no more wishfully-thought-out belief within its bosom than the desire to blame nervous tension for everything. We are supposed to be living in a peculiarly stressful era, a belief held by every generation since the world began. In 1895, for example, Max Nordau was impressed by the great increase in railway travel in Europe and by the increase in German book production and the number of letters handled by the English postal system as causes of "the vertigo and whirl of our frenzied life," and hazards to humanity's ability to adjust to stresses.

I can give supporting evidence, going back to Greek and Roman times, that every era had its belief in a Golden Age which was always before the current one. The Hindu religion favors the idea that each epoch in history is shorter and worse and the present one is the worst of all; but the interesting thing is that in the past half century the average age of Americans has increased by twenty years. Things may be tough but they are not destroying us yet.

Nervous Tension. The fact of the matter is that coronary disease is ubiquitous in civilized society because of the age of the population, and it is found in all economic levels and with all degrees of nervous stress. Studies in England show that regardless of occupational stress, the incidence of coronary disease is inversely related to the degree of physical efforts of the job—that is, the physically active have less of it regardless of whether they have jobs with much or little nervous tension.

Professor Arnott has stated this well:

"Psychological stress and strain has for long been popularly believed to play an important part in a wide variety of disease, including ischemic heart disease and essential hypertension. So far as I can see, this hypothesis has no scientifically credible basis whatsoever—in fact, most of the evidence adduced in its support is dubious and much of it absurd . . . The ready acceptance of this 'stress and strain' concept is very understandable. It nourishes the *amour propre* of the believer and it is readily acceptable to the unfortunate victim and his relatives. It places ischemic heart disease in being in the position of the unjust reward of virtue. How much nicer it is when stricken with a coronary thrombosis to be told that it is all due to hard work, laudable ambition, and selfless devotion to duty than to be told it is due to gluttony and physical indolence."

This is not to say that an emotional stimulus may not start an attack of angina; this is well known, but the nervous tension of life, I contend, is not the origin of the deposit of fatty substances in coronary arteries, except by its secondary influence leading to overeating, over-smoking and under-exercising. These are controllable by the individual.

The Pattern of Coronary Artery Disease

It may seem a pessimistic statement, but physicians today possess no method, test, or instrument for the early detection of coronary artery disease and are no

Nitroglycerine was first given for this disease in 1879; there is no better medicine for it yet. The character of the distress and its relationship to precipitating factors must be studied by the physician. It is not a good idea for the patient to diagnose his own ailment. A great many chest pains are harmless and related to organs other than the heart.

It is true that in some instances an electrocardiogram will reveal abnormal electrical waves in the heart to support a diagnosis of coronary disease, but when these are present the disease is well advanced. Indeed, by the time angina develops one or more branches of the coronary system have already been

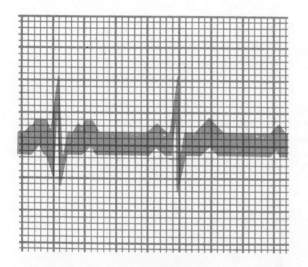 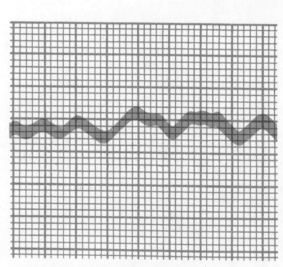

Example of how the electrocardiogram (EKG) assists in diagnosis of heart disease. At left, above, a normal EKG with characteristic peaks and valleys. At right, EKG of a patient with *ventricular fibrillation*, a condition in which ventricles quiver ineffectively and do not "squeeze" blood out to the body.

more capable of making the diagnosis of its clinical manifestations than they were in 1786 when the English physician, Heberden, described it in "Some Account of a Disorder of the Breast."

What I mean is that the earliest sign of coronary insufficiency is the sensation of pressure or strangling in the chest, or *angina pectoris*, and the diagnosis is made by the skilled assessment of what the patient tells the doctor and by whether or not a nitroglycerine tablet under the tongue relieves the patient of his distress.

blocked by gradual narrowing of the particular vessels that are involved.

Angina. By and large, angina shows itself by chest discomfort, often not called "pain" by the patient, brought on by situations demanding more work by the heart and greater blood flow through the coronary arteries. Such may be physical effort, emotional stress, the increased circulation required by the digestion of a meal, and particularly exertion in cold, windy weather.

Combinations of the factors are especially bad. I have often told a patient with angina that the worst thing he could do would be to eat a heavy meal, smoke several cigarettes, lose his temper, and rush out of the house carrying his suitcase up a hill against a cold wind.

Nitroglycerine is the sovereign remedy and should be used freely, and particularly before any effort or strain which is known by the patient to have brought on attacks in the past. These may include all sorts of stresses; from opening the garage door in the morning to giving an after-dinner speech, appearing in court, or sexual intercourse.

Living with angina. Development of angina pectoris does not mean an invalid's life. Often, simple alterations in routine living will reduce the symptoms considerably. Weight reduction, cutting out smoking, getting more vacations, rearranging business commitments, and getting more graded exercise will help.

Everyone with angina should realize that, while he has an obstructive process in his coronary arteries, so do 50 per cent of all men over age 45 in the United States; and furthermore, nature is always attempting compensation for this by opening up other arteries in the coronary system to produce a secondary or collateral circulation to help out. The patient's course depends upon the balance of these two factors in his heart.

Many attempts have been made to improve this collateral circulation by drugs having a dilating effect upon the arteries. The evidence for their effectiveness is colored by the influence of suggestion in relieving some patients with angina. However, they are worth a trial.

Recently, various surgical procedures have been attempted. These consist of trying to enhance the blood supply by transplanting nearby arteries into the heart muscle; through producing adhesions containing small blood vessels

A surgical effort to enhance coronary blood supply. Below, heart with diseased left coronary artery. At right, transplantation of nearby mammary artery into the heart muscle, in hope that new networks of vessels (collateral circulation) will develop to supply the threatened area.

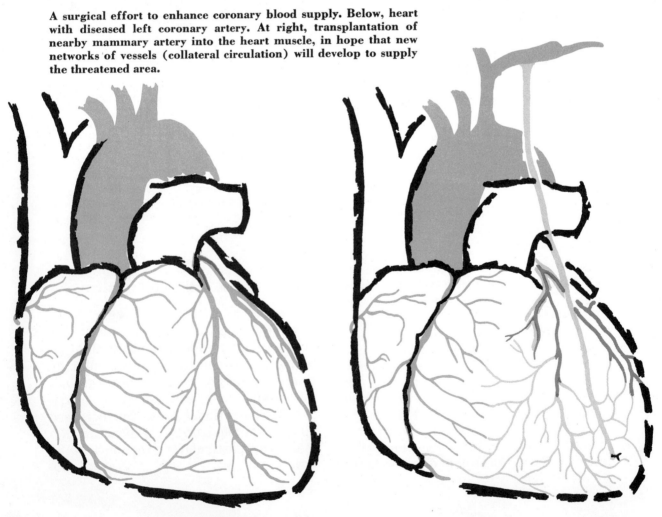

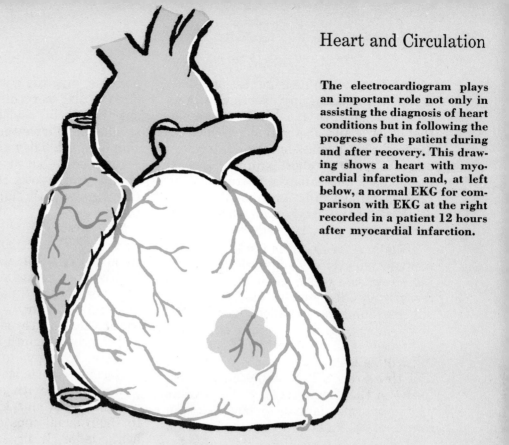

Heart and Circulation

The electrocardiogram plays an important role not only in assisting the diagnosis of heart conditions but in following the progress of the patient during and after recovery. This drawing shows a heart with myocardial infarction and, at left below, a normal EKG for comparison with EKG at the right recorded in a patient 12 hours after myocardial infarction.

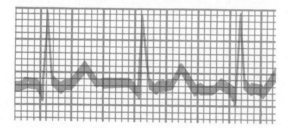

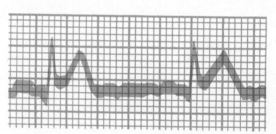

between the layers of the pericardium by introducing irritating substances into the pericardial sac; or by actual dissection or reaming out the deposits obstructing the coronary artery.

All of these procedures are in an experimental stage and I have not recommended them to my patients. Occasionally, angina may be reduced in special cases of thyroid overactivity by depressing the function of the thyroid gland by medical measures, including radioactive iodine.

One must face the fact that a person who has angina pectoris may die unexpectedly and coronary artery disease is not only the most common cause of sudden death, but in perhaps 15 per cent, sudden death is the first and only manifestation of the disease.

On the other hand, the average length of life after the diagnosis is made is well over ten years and many live much longer. Indeed, men who recover from the more severe forms of coronary blocking, namely acute coronary thrombosis, to the degree that they can return to work, die at a rate only about 15 per cent greater than unaffected persons with normal life expectancy.

CORONARY THROMBOSIS

What is commonly called a "heart attack" is one that kills its victim within a few minutes or causes a collapse which is survived long enough for him to be put to bed at home or in the hospital.

Usually the individual has a story of previous angina, but this new attack often comes when he is at rest or asleep or not involved in any exertion such as he has learned to avoid in the past. On the other hand, he may have had no earlier chest distress but is awakened by a severe crushing chest pain with sweating, nausea and collapse. Nitroglycerine fails to relieve him, and morphine and other sedatives, oxygen and heart supporting drugs may be needed.

Usually a fresh clot is found in a narrow coronary artery and in those surviving a few hours or days an area of heart muscle supplied by the blocked artery will be found to have died from loss of nourishment; that is, the structure of the muscle and its function of contracting will be lost *(myocardial infarction)*, and this area will be replaced by scar tissue in those who recover. The extent of the muscle damage determines the events of the next few days and weeks.

In general, survival for 24 hours introduces definite hope; survival for three days makes recovery from that attack likely; survival for a week is statistically very strongly optimistic, and at the end of three weeks most of the complications will have occurred.

The action of the heart rate and rhythm, the recovery of blood pressure, the disappearance of pain, the subsidence of fever, are all signs to be evaluated. There are more delicate indices also, certain blood enzyme tests, sedimentation rate, and so on, to guide the physician.

In this condition, the electrocardiograph has reached its highest function. It can not only make the diagnosis, but tell the area of involvement of the heart muscle, and something about the severity and extent of the damage and the speed of recovery.

Treatment. The treatment of each patient must be individualized but is always greatly aided by good nursing. Hospitalization is usually advisable because of the availability of emergency treatments. The use of oxygen, heart drugs, blood pressure stimulants, and anticoagulant medicines is the province of the physician. My own practice is to avoid the latter medication whenever possible, but this question of anticoagulants is still very disputatious throughout the world, and different statistical studies support either the use or omission of them. They are difficult and dangerous to use but may prevent some secondary thrombosis in the veins of very ill patients with sluggish blood flow in the legs.

The usual time interval for major recovery is three months, with a probationary period of six months and with improvement possible up to two years. The amount of time in bed and in the hospital will vary with the severity of the attack from three weeks to six weeks, but the third month is generally the one in which to return to full-time work.

Recent experience in industry shows that most men with good recovery and no residual heart muscle failure may return to their usual jobs even at moderately heavy labor. In my own experience, the exception is the operation of common carriers — trains, busses, street cars, airplanes. I never permit return to this work because of the increased liability of the company, even though the risk may be slight.

After recovery. As in the case of angina, coronary thrombosis need not lead to invalidism. The active life of President Eisenhower after his coronary attack has demonstrated this most forcibly to the American public. Most men after a coronary thrombosis go through a period of anxiety and depression, but as the years go on they realize that recovery usually means return to a comfortable, effective life.

I do not restrict my patients beyond the caution that they should avoid situations beyond their control — don't get caught in snow storms, don't swim way out to a raft when you have to swim back, don't drink so much that you lose your judgment, don't smoke, don't gain weight, exercise regularly, indulge in sexual relations when accomplishment is not merely a matter of masculine pride.

Losing one's temper is a luxury. This can be learned. I have one patient who used to become so incensed at his golfing errors that I have known him to break

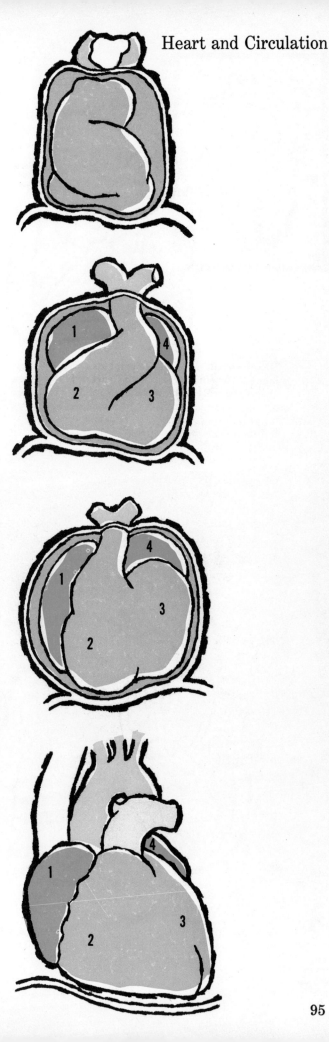

$50 worth of clubs in anger in a single round. He tells me that he now merely says "dear, dear" when he drives into the rough. His coronary attack came many years ago.

I have another patient who had three attacks of coronary thrombosis over 30 years ago and after retirement he married and is now living comfortably in his eighties in Florida.

Prevention. In view of the fact that many influences appear to be involved in the development of coronary artery atherosclerosis, it is indeed difficult to speak about prevention with any assurance. There is the feeling that it is one of the inevitabilities of civilized society, indeed a result of natural selection. It has been suggested that individuals who survived the terrible famines in Europe in the Middle Ages were those who inherently were efficient body "fat-storers", and this trait has become transmitted to an Age of Plenty when fat-storage has become dangerous rather than advantageous. We are putting in calories and not burning them up by daily chores. It may well be also that the greatest harm to the male is done in adolescence when overemphasis on rapid growth and large fat intakes in the form of milk are common. The adolescent female takes far less.

In any event, one must be impressed by such observations as that which indicates that the only way to make a male rat live as long as a female is to feed it only 70 per cent of what it would like to eat.

My own belief is that weight control, regular physical exercise, reduced fat and sweets, and no cigarettes constitute a formula for the young male in the United States that might have some protective influence on his coronary arteries. This prescription is unlikely to be filled so long as the automobile, television, the soda fountain, and cigarettes constitute so much of the horizon in daily living of our young.

In the embryo the heart develops from a simple tube which twists and divides in complex ways to form the multi-chambered mature heart. Developmental stages are shown at right with parts numbered: (1) right auricle; (2) right ventricle; (3) left ventricle; (4) left auricle.

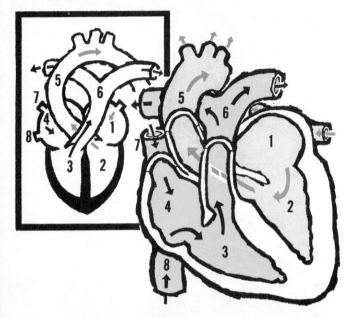

Blood circulation of a normal heart, with parts labeled for comparison with heart defects shown elsewhere. 1. left auricle; 2. left ventricle; 3. right ventricle; 4. right auricle; 5. aorta; 6. pulmonary artery; 7. superior vena cava; 8. inferior vena cava.

CONGENITAL HEART DISEASE

The development of the heart in the embryo is an enormously complex process. The human heart with its four chambers and valves originates as a tube which divides and twists in a fashion that permits a great variety of errors of construction if anything goes wrong.

Disturbances in oxygen supply to the mother, infections — chiefly viral — and deficiencies in nutrition, seem to be of major importance. Recently, we have seen the effect of certain drugs, notably thalidomide, in producing congenital defects of the limbs, and similar defects may appear in the heart.

The possibilities of combinations of cardiac defects are almost limitless, over 900 in one accounting that I made, but most of these are so severe that they lead to death of the infant before, or shortly after, birth.

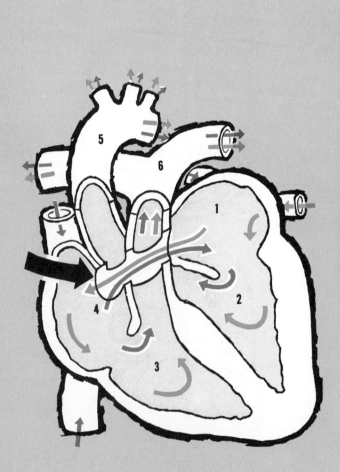

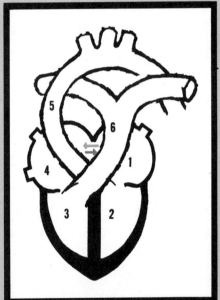

An inter-atrial septal defect allows blood to flow between the left atrium (1) and right atrium (4), with mixing of "blue" and "red" blood. This causes dilation of right ventricle (3) and right atrium (4), enlargement of pulmonary artery (6), and "blue baby" symptoms.

The errors of assembly consist chiefly of failure of development of *valves;* or of *septal defects,* that is, failure of holes in the partitions between heart chambers to close properly; or of persistence of the artery that by-passes the lungs *(ductus arteriosus)* which fails to close and cease its fetal function after birth.

arteries arise from the wrong ventricle; persistence of the improper aortic arches, which go back to the primitive gill slit stage of the embryo, resulting in rings of blood vessels surrounding and constricting the breathing (trachea) and swallowing (esophagus) tubes; and narrowing *(coarctation)* of the aorta.

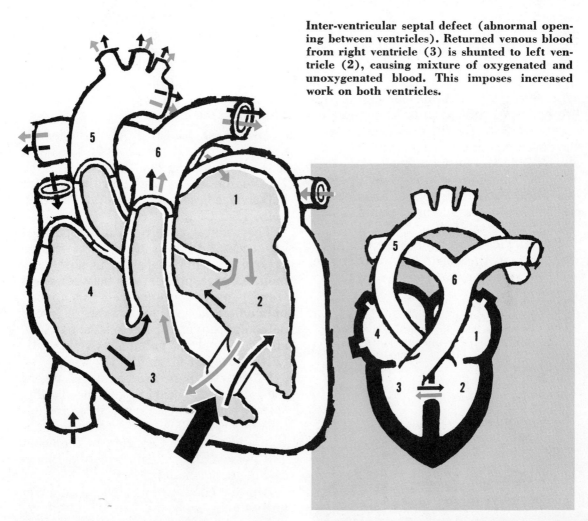

Inter-ventricular septal defect (abnormal opening between ventricles). Returned venous blood from right ventricle (3) is shunted to left ventricle (2), causing mixture of oxygenated and unoxygenated blood. This imposes increased work on both ventricles.

Many others of course occur, such as the emptying of veins from the lungs into the wrong atrium; origin of coronary arteries from the pulmonary artery, instead of the aorta, so that the heart muscle is being fed blue, unoxygenated blood, instead of red blood; lack of proper division of the heart into four chambers so that it may have only three, or even only two, chambers; incomplete rotation of the heart so that its main

The human heart, at first a simple tube, begins to be formed at about the third week of development of the embryo. The heart begins to twitch, and then to beat, somewhere around the fourth week of development. By the sixth week the four chambers are recognizable and complex changes are under way.

Diagnosis. Children with congenital heart disease are divided into two main groups — *cyanotic* (blue baby type) and *non-cyanotic* (with normal color). In some cases, the child may become blue in attacks.

The blueness of the cyanotic type is due to the mixing of venous blood, that has not gone through the lungs, with oxygenated blood. This may be caused by an abnormal communication or "septal defect" between the right and left heart chambers, or communication through an abnormal channel, such as a persistent ductus arteriosus, if there is a high enough pressure on the blue side of the circulation to force the blue blood over to mix with the red.

The tremendous growth of our knowledge of congenital heart defects during life has been built upon two advances of recent years — the cardiac catheter, and the development of cardiac surgery, with and without the "heart pump." The latter permits stopping of the patient's own heart and the carrying on of an effective circulation by a mechanical pump beside the operating table.

The *cardiac catheter* is a slender tube which can be threaded into a vein in the arm, or an artery, and pushed into the

Cardiac catheterization: A thin tube is threaded into a vein of the arm, through the right side of the heart, into the pulmonary artery (4), via the superior vena cava (1), right auricle (2), and right ventricle (3).

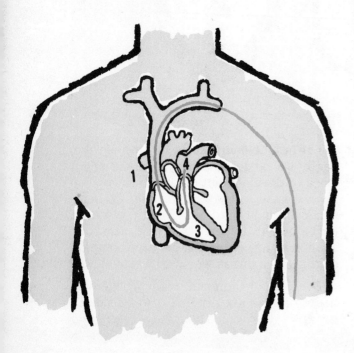

heart — most readily into the right atrium, right ventricle and lung vessels; special techniques are necessary for left heart catheter study.

The tube may be seen on the fluoroscopic screen of the x-ray and guided in the heart, it can be photographed by x-ray, it can be used to measure pressures in the heart and lungs and passed through septal defects. Through it can be drawn samples of blood from various areas in the heart for measurement of their oxygen content; radio-opaque material can be introduced through the catheter and its progress through normal or abnormal channels can be photographed by a rapid series of x-ray films or x-ray movies.

Treatment. Cardiac surgery is the major treatment for congenital heart disease. It has become possible even in the young infant and more and more defects are becoming correctable by surgery. (See Chapter 22.)

The earliest condition to be operated on successfully was the *patent ductus arteriosus*. This operation is now common. Later, septal defects between atria were repaired; narrowed *(stenosed)* pulmonic and aortic valves were freed; defects in the ventricular system patched, abnormally placed pulmonary veins resituated, vascular rings divided, and so on.

Of course there are instances where the defect in the heart is only one of widespread congenital abnormalities including the brain. This may be true in Mongolian idiocy where surgery of the heart will not correct the fundamental inherited germ plasm deficiency.

Another combined congenital anomaly is *Marfan's syndrome*. These individuals have a typical association of cardiac defect and dislocation of the lenses of the eyes. They are tall and slender with very long spider-like fingers and toes *(arachnodactyly)*. They are not usually suitable for cardiac surgery since the defect is a disturbance of the fundamental supporting structures of their tissues.

The "blue baby" is no longer a mere medical and nursing problem with only a hope of survival, but is a subject for intense study by modern methods because

Patent ductus arteriosus. In the fetus, the ductus arteriosus is a normal channel which short-circuits blood from the pulmonary artery (6) to the aorta (5), as shown in the small drawing. This channel normally is obliterated at birth; if not, the abnormal communication between the aorta and the pulmonary artery causes serious heart disease.

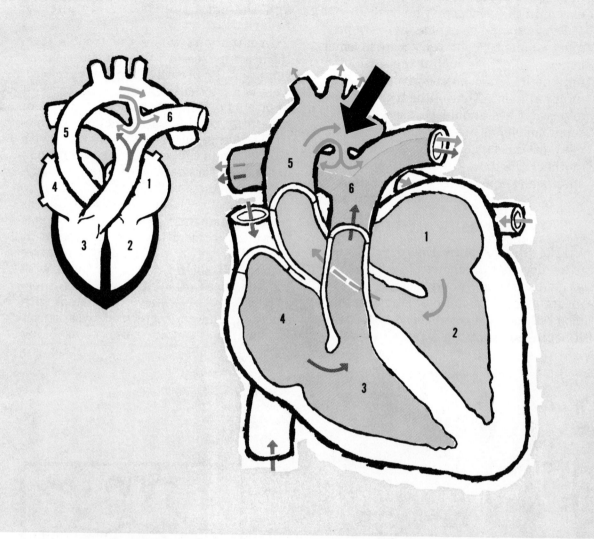

of the possibility of surgical relief. Still, by no means can all of these children be helped by surgery.

However, blue babies have survived to live useful lives even when constantly cyanotic. Dr. Paul White and I described in 1929 a famous musician and composer who lived to be 59 and who was severely cyanotic all his life.

Prevention. Present evidence favors the view that injury to the mother in early pregnancy is the major factor in congenital defects, although there may be a genetic or family tendency. This inherited tendency is not so strong as to advise a woman against having other children if she has given birth to an infant with a congenital heart defect.

It has been shown that German measles in the first three months of pregnancy results in cardiac anomalies in a high percentage of the babies. All girls should have their children's diseases in childhood and especially German measles and mumps. All virus diseases should be avoided if possible in pregnancy, particularly in the first three months.

Similarly, it is believed by some embryologists that any exposure to *anoxia* (low oxygen) can be dangerous to the fetus at this time — even airplane trips and high altitude travel. The latter view is supported by the high incidence of congenital heart disease in babies born in races living at high altitudes, as in the Andes Mountains of South America.

Errors in nutrition are not likely to be of great importance in the United States except in the very poorly nourished.

Drugs should be kept away from pregnant women except for accepted emergency medication, such as the antibiotics, but these should not be given for every minor ailment. None of the tranquillizers and sedatives should be used. There is some suspicion about cigarettes, but in view of the large numbers of smoking mothers the data are statistical and not specifically applicable to individuals.

CONGESTIVE FAILURE

Like other organs in the body, the heart often does not announce the early stages of its diseases. It is only when it has used up its reserve of muscular power, or of blood supply in its coronary arteries, that it begins to produce a warning signal.

In coronary disease this is usually the distress on effort called angina pectoris and the condition is called "anginal failure."

In situations where the trouble is in the heart muscle or valves, the presenting symptom is breathlessness *(dyspnea)*. This is a particular kind of shortness of breath or puffing, with increased rate of breathing, coming with exertion or sometimes waking the patient from sleep with oppression in the chest, desire to sit up in order to breathe better *(orthopnea)*, wheezing, and cough.

This latter disturbance is known as "cardiac asthma," and all of these breathing difficulties are a prominent part of what is known as "congestive failure." It should not be confused with the shortness of breath which is intermittent, not regularly associated with exertion, and characterized by a sensation which I usually refer to as being

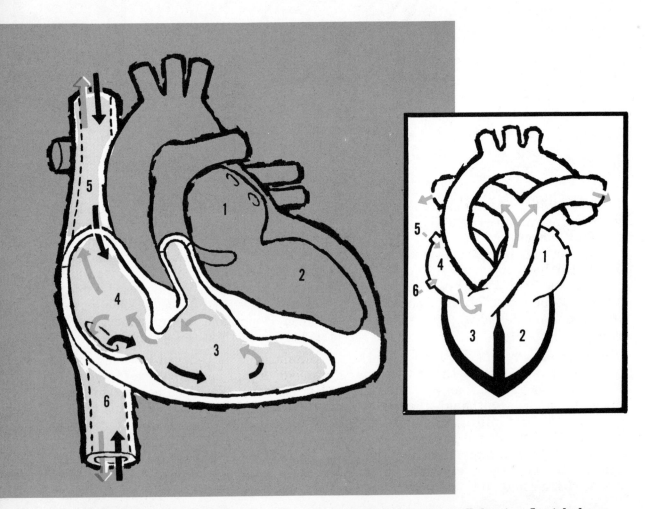

Congestive failure of right heart. Normal circulation shown in small drawing. In right heart failure, the right ventricle (3) has difficulty in delivering venous blood to lungs. Blood backs up in atrium (4) and superior (5) and inferior vena cava (6), causing dilation, with backup of blood, increased pressure in veins in upper and lower parts of the body and in the liver.

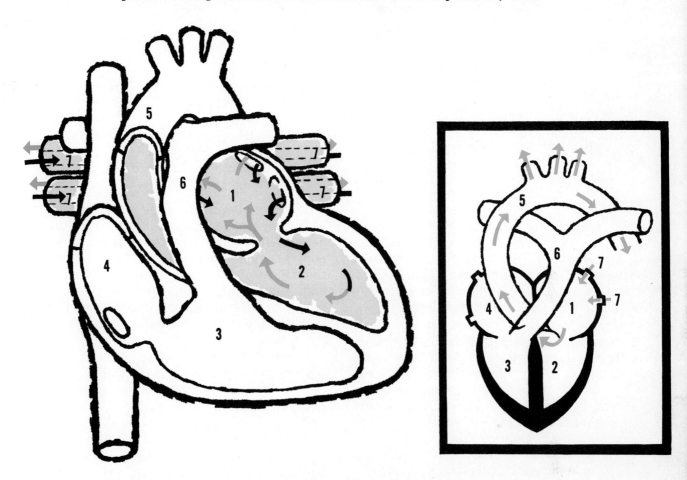

Congestive failure of left heart. In contrast to normal circulation (small drawing), ineffective discharge of the left ventricle (2) causes back-pressure in left atrium (1), enlargement of pulmonary veins (7), and increased pressure in lung vessels. Dotted lines show normal size of pulmonary veins.

"unable to take a deep breath," inability to get a satisfactory breath, or "get over the crest of the hill." This leads to deep sighing breathing and finally one of these breaths is effective. Then the symptom subsides, only to start again later.

This is an uncomfortable, but never serious, sensation and is found in all sorts of fatigue and anxiety conditions. It is usually more bothersome when the person is resting or working quietly rather than when he is asking the heart to do extra work.

True *congestive failure* occurs only with damaged hearts, but is often reversible with treatment and it may be kept under control for years with careful diet and medicine. It is of two kinds — right and left heart failure — but there may be a combination of these. The reason for differentiating the two types is partly to help in deciding the underlying cause of the heart disease.

In *right heart failure,* the right ventricle has difficulty in delivering the venous blood to the lungs and it backs up in the right atrium and then into the veins in both upper and lower parts of the body and in the liver.

This "venous stasis," or stoppage, with increase in pressure in the veins, results in leakage of fluid through the small vessel walls and collection of the fluid (edema) in the ankles, later the legs, or even most of the body in bedridden patients. Fortunately, this is not seen so commonly since the treatment has been better understood.

The old term for this was "dropsy," which is derived from the Greek word for water, and one may speak of a "water-logged" patient. Actually, in pure right heart failure the congestion is in the outer or peripheral parts of the body and the lungs are spared, but this is very rarely seen since both sides of the heart generally weaken together, especially if there is heart muscle disease, but the thinner right ventricle tends to fail first.

In *left heart failure*, the difficulty lies in the ineffective discharge of the left ventricle. This can arise from hypertension, obstruction of the aortic valve (stenosis), leakage of the aortic valve (regurgitation), leakage of the mitral valve, and other less common conditions. Mitral stenosis, on the other hand, spares the left ventricle and causes back pressure in the circulation behind it, that is, in the left atrium, and the blood vessels in the lungs. There is then "hypertension in the lesser circulation," namely, high blood pressure in the lung arteries and veins. The right ventricle, in trying to pump against this, will fail first.

Actually, when the left ventricle weakens and has trouble in emptying, this will result in much the same increase in pressure in the lung vessels, so that secondary failure of the right ventricle will occur. It is clear, therefore, that either mitral stenosis or left heart failure will reveal itself by causing the individual to become breathless with effort, because the effort calls for an increase in the amount of blood pumped by the heart which in turn will back up in the lungs.

Treatment. The most important advance in the treatment of congestive heart failure was made by a British physician, William Withering, in 1785. He discovered, after investigating various herbs used by an old woman in Shropshire to treat dropsy, that the foxglove, whose leaves produce the drug digitalis, was the active agent. He therefore used a decoction of the leaves and published a little book describing the effects. Digitalis is particularly effective when atrial fibrillation is associated with failure since it causes a blocking of many of the irregular useless signals from the atrium and slows the ventricles, as well as strengthening the heart muscle.

The proper use of this drug was forgotten after Withering's day and only in the present century have the ideal dosages and methods of administration in the individual patient been well established.

Another important step was the introduction of effective *diuretics*, that is, drugs stimulating kidney activity to eliminate the retained water. The most powerful have been the mercurial diuretics whose kidney stimulation was discovered by accident by Saxl in Germany in 1920 during the treatment of syphilis with a new organic mercury compound. These compounds have been improved and are still the most effective, but have to be given by injection.

A third advance was the re-emphasis of the importance of *sodium* in the diet of people subject to congestive failure. The body's congestion by water is fostered by the retention of sodium in the tissues and, indeed, the action of most diuretics seems to be the elimination of sodium through the kidneys and this takes the water with it.

Careful attention to the amount of sodium in the diet may make the use of diuretics unnecessary or, at least, permit smaller or less frequent doses. (See Low Sodium Diets, page 32).

The most common source of sodium in our food is table salt, sodium chloride, and this is readily controlled, but a person with a need for sodium restriction should be under careful medical control: first, to receive instructions about the sodium content of foods not obviously salty, and, second, to be sure that the sodium and other necessary salts, such as potassium, are not unduly depleted to a point where the chemistry of the body is so disturbed as to produce further complications.

The level of restriction is an individual prescription for each patient. It should be remembered that in certain areas of the country the drinking water is sufficiently rich in sodium to be a factor in the total sodium taken by the patient.

Chronologically speaking, the next step in treatment might be considered the ability to operate on the mitral valve and relieve stenosis. When this is the cause of heart failure, the direct attack on the mechanical obstruction is the most valuable treatment, but it is rarely the only treatment necessary.

In recent years, one more valuable drug has been added and that is the diuretic compound that does not contain mercury and may be taken by mouth. The basic drug is *chlorothiazide*, of which several modifications are available.

In describing these treatments, it is not my intent to disregard the common sense measures advisable for anyone

Rheumatic fever is apparently a sequel to a strepto-coccal infection, characteristically ushered in by a respiratory infection with sore throat. Involved cardiac areas may be the heart muscle (1), the pericardial sac around the heart (2), and most frequently the mitral (3) and aortic valves (4), rarely, the tricuspid valve (5).

hypertension and other ailments may trigger or perpetuate congestive failure.

Congestive failure is not necessarily a final stage of heart disease, that is to say, it may be a temporary situation responding to treatment, and after recovery the individual may lead a reasonably active, productive, comfortable life for years.

It might be compared to diabetes. If untreated the patient loses ground and

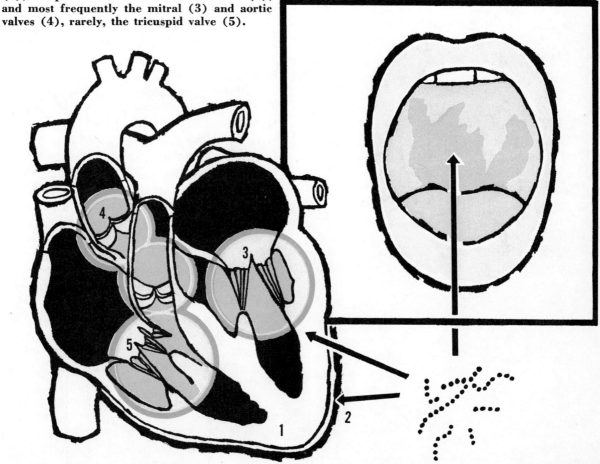

with heart disease. These include a routine of life within the limits of the individual's physical ability and one which does not produce symptoms; weight control; omission of tobacco (often a most important step in controlling cough); and the correction of any complicating disease. For example, anemia from the bleeding of stomach ulcer, infections of various sorts, diabetes,

may have a serious or fatal breakdown. With diet and insulin he is protected. Similarly, the cardiac learns to live with his disability and to cooperate with his physician faithfully.

RHEUMATIC HEART DISEASE

The most common cause of heart disease in children and young adults is ***rheu-***

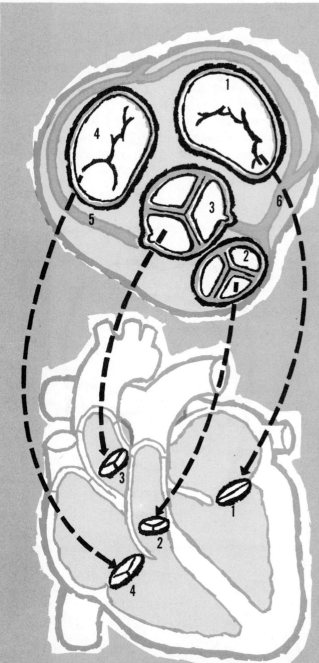

Upper part of drawing shows top view of heart with valves. Arrows lead to corresponding valves in sectional view below. Identification: 1. mitral (bicuspid) valve; 2. pulmonary (semilunar) valve; 3. aortic (semilunar) valve; 4. tricuspid; 5. right coronary artery; 6. left coronary artery.

matic fever. This disease is apparently a streptococcal infection which may appear also as scarlet fever or acute streptococcal nephritis (kidney inflammation). It has been decreasing in prevalence in the United States and Britain for over 30 years, but tends to occur in epidemic form wherever large groups of young men are brought together, as in military training camps.

It is more common in the colder months, especially the spring, and in temperate climates, but in recent years study has shown that rheumatic heart disease is found in the tropics, although the premonitory symptoms of sore throat and joint pains may be less obvious. I have seen it in American Samoa and Fiji and, except for tuberculosis, it is said to be the greatest cause for hospitalization of children in the Fiji Islands.

Symptoms. The characteristic stage of onset of rheumatic fever is a respiratory infection with sore throat. Culture of the bacteria from the throat shows a type of hemolytic streptococci.

Two or three weeks after this sore throat the child will show joint pains with swelling and redness of the larger joints of arms and legs, possibly nosebleeds, skin eruptions, a form of pneumonia, inflammation of the sac around the heart *(pericarditis)*, heart murmurs and changes in the electrocardiogram. Another sign may be *chorea* (St. Vitus Dance) and, in severe cases, small fibrous nodules may appear over bony prominences like knuckles, elbows, knees, ankles, and spine.

At the present time, the disease seems to be less severe than it was 40 years ago. The child may have only mild joint pains yet the heart valves and muscles may be affected.

The earliest sign of heart muscle inflammation may be the electrocardiographic evidence of a delay in the passage of the electrical impulse from atrium to ventricle. In rare cases this may lead to a degree of "blocking" of the impulse by inflammatory reaction, so that heart beats are dropped out, that is, the heart pauses momentarily. In only one case in my experience have these pauses been so long as to cause fainting.

The patient has fever and increased heart rate. The white blood cell count is elevated, and other delicate indicators, such as the sedimentation rate, show various signs of disturbance.

Valve damage. Murmurs and changes in the heart sounds occur. Some of these murmurs decrease and disappear with recovery, but loud murmurs produced at the mitral valve and those from the aortic valve mean true inflammation of the valve leaflets.

While the heart has four valves — *tricuspid, pulmonic, mitral,* and *aortic* — the latter two are commonly affected by rheumatic fever, the tricuspid rarely, and the pulmonic never.

With recovery from the acute stage, the inflamed valve becomes scarred and does not close properly, resulting in a leak *(regurgitation),* or it becomes narrowed by adhesion of the valve leaflets *(stenosis).* The effects of these mechanical disturbances in the valves are greatly influenced by the degree of injury to the heart muscle *(myocarditis)* which accompanies the valvular inflammation.

The heart enlarges by thickening of the muscle because of the greater work demanded by the leaking or obstructed valves, and stretches out by weakness brought on by the inflammation of the heart muscle.

Later it may develop irregularities in rhythm and finally atrial fibrillation with total and continuous irregularity.

We think of rheumatic heart disease as a malady of childhood and early life, but many individuals with "rheumatic hearts" live into the late adult years and even old age. It is believed that some cases of calcified aortic valve stenosis have their origins in childhood rheumatic infection, but this is notoriously an old man's type of heart disease and may be seen in the 70's and 80's.

Rheumatic infection is unlike most other diseases of childhood in that it does not characteristically run an acute course and then subside with a type of complete recovery that makes the child immune to other attacks. Quite the reverse, it may lead to a low grade, smoldering infection lasting for months or years. The tendency to recurrence is ever present, especially after colds and sore throats. This subacute state may be shown by vague joint pains (growing pains), skin rashes, nervous twitching of chorea, nosebleeds, poor appetite, weight loss, abdominal pain (sometimes mistaken for appendicitis), and the picture of a child chronically ill and "out of sorts."

Recurrent acute attacks may appear at intervals of a few months or, more often, ten to 12 months apart.

Rheumatic infection is to be suspected most commonly in our northeastern cities and in poorer economic conditions. There seems also to be some family tendency. The prevalence of this disease is shown by the fact that children who have rheumatic fever or have had it, as revealed by cardiac damage, comprise 0.75 per cent of the school population of New York City.

It has been thought that improved economic conditions are largely responsible for its decline. However, I have seen patients with acute rheumatic fever in families of a high economic level.

Wherever the streptococcus is prevalent, rheumatic fever is found—in Naval Training Stations at the Great Lakes, Air Force camps in Wyoming and Colorado, and in the cool climates of Mexico City and Britain. It may well occur throughout the world and its present decrease is probably only a phase in which it is waiting to appear like many pestilences that come out of hiding in times of war, crowding, and poor nutrition.

Clinical Course. The common cold with running nose and no fever is not the precursor of an attack of rheumatic fever. The "sore throat" is the potential danger signal, if accompanied by fever, and if a throat culture shows the typical streptococcus. This is the infection that should be treated early, and if this is done the incidence of rheumatic fever following it is strikingly reduced. Prompt treatment with penicillin is essential with moderately large doses (1 million units twice a day) continued for ten days.

If such treatment is not given, rheumatic infection may appear two or three weeks later, but it should be remembered that the number of children or young adults who develop this after a sore throat is really very small. Since, however, it is unpredictable, treatment should be given early and after throat culture has been taken. If the beta hemolytic streptococcus (group A streptococcus) is not found in this culture, no harm is done; but if it is, the full course of ten days of penicillin is advisable. Sulfa drugs were formerly found to be effective.

It may be very easy or very difficult to be sure of the diagnosis of rheumatic fever or even of the early stages of rheumatic heart disease. Some signs are unequivocal, such as pericardial inflammation or characteristic murmurs or electrocardiograms. Often a period of several weeks of bed rest may be necessary before the child can be judged free from active rheumatic infection. This is also why a child should be seen by his physician at intervals of a few months for at least three years after a bout of rheumatic fever, even if the heart appears to have escaped damage.

Generally, it is best for a rheumatic child to have daily preventive penicillin by mouth for several years after an attack, just how long is not really known. Some say "for life," but after a child grows up the treatment can be stopped if valvular disease is not clearly present and if he is alert to the knowledge that he should always have penicillin when he has a sore throat or other severe respiratory disease. This is the way I have treated my own son, who had severe rheumatic fever while serving in the Navy in World War II.

An attack of active rheumatism may subside in two or three weeks but usually we think of this as a disease lasting for six weeks, or longer.

Return to normal life may be permitted by the end of three months. Complications and daily symptomatic treatment in the acute phase should be in the physician's hands. Penicillin, aspirin, and the newer steroid hormones (cortisone derivatives) are the major drugs for this disease.

Chronic Rheumatic Heart Disease.

When the heart is permanently damaged by rheumatic fever, the course of the disease may be rapid and fatal in children in a matter of a few weeks or months, but the usual progression is slow and the most striking fact is that adults in their thirties to fifties, or even later, who can remember no episode of acute rheumatism in their earlier life, may be found to have valvular deformities due to rheumatic infection. There may be only a story of vague "growing pains" or frequent sore throats.

Individuals of this sort may be unaware of their heart disease until some severe strain is put upon the heart, such as infection, pregnancy, or competitive athletics; or when routine examination for life insurance or military service is encountered. Sometimes the arrival of sudden total irregularity of the heart, at a rapid rate (atrial fibrillation), will lead to heart failure and reveal underlying mitral stenosis.

The two valves commonly affected are the *mitral* and the *aortic*. Either one may develop a leak (regurgitation) or a narrowing from thickening and scarring (stenosis). The mitral valve is particularly liable to stenosis and the aortic to regurgitation. Furthermore, the stenosis of the mitral valve, putting a back pressure on the left atrium, is commonly associated with atrial fibrillation. Aortic regurgitation is a more serious condition, but there are gradations of stenosis and regurgitation as well as combined damage to either or both valves, that is, a valve may have some degree of both obstruction and leakage.

Surgery. It is in this area of rheumatic valvular disease that cardiac surgery has played one of its most dramatic roles.

The technique of cardiac catheterization permits study of the actual amount of blocking or leaking of the valves and a shrewd estimate of the actual size of the valve opening.

It is now readily possible to relieve the stenosis of the mitral valve; it is somewhat more difficult to remove the aortic valve obstruction; and it is still more difficult to repair the leaking valves. Rapid progress, however, is being made in fashioning artificial valves of human tissue or plastic materials. The ability to perform "open heart" surgery is aiding these advances, since the heart can be stopped while an artificial pump takes over the circulation during the operation.

Men and women with rheumatic heart disease usually live moderately active, useful lives under medical care, and now after cardiac surgery their life expectancy and work ability have been vastly improved. A certain number, perhaps 15 per cent, have to undergo second operations because of return of valve deformity from scarring. It is hoped that this percentage will decrease with improved surgical techniques.

IRREGULARITIES OF THE HEART BEAT
(The Arrhythmias)

Among the very early discoveries concerned with the action of the heart and circulation, the observation of the pulse beat and its disturbances was very important. In ancient days the wrist pulse bore many names from which the physician was supposed to make the diagnosis of different diseases.

It was described as slow or fast, hard or soft, full or weak, bounding, paradoxical (when it rose and fell in volume in an abnormal fashion during breathing), and so on. Many of these terms were originally Latin, such as "pulsus irregularis perpetuus" (in atrial fibrillation), or "pulsus caprizans," so-called by Herophilus of Alexandria around 300 B. C. because he thought it resembled the leap of a goat. This was probably a simple extra beat or "extra-systole."

The relationship between what went on in the heart and what could be felt by the finger on the artery at the wrist was not understood, but it is still true that

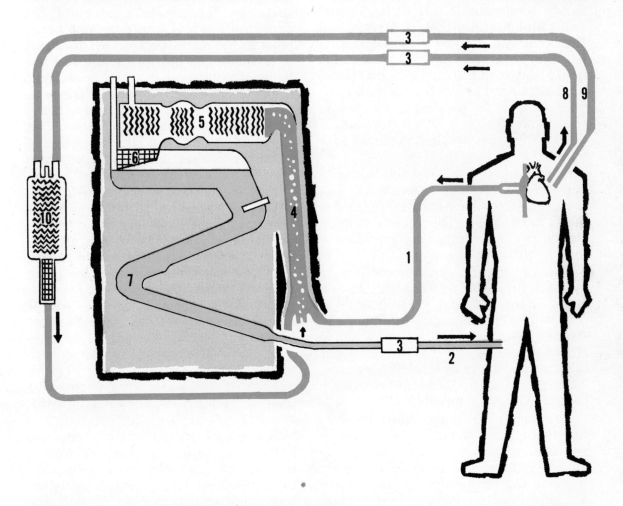

Schematic drawing of disposable bubble-type oxygenator, equipment for bypassing heart and lungs, in open heart sugery. Parts: 1. venous line; 2. arterial line; 3. pumps; 4. oxygenating column; 5. debubbling chamber; 6. filter; 7. reservoir; 8 and 9, cardiotomy return from surgical field; 10. cardiotomy reservoir.

careful observation of the character of the pulse can give a great deal of information about the heart and blood pressure.

Although much was learned in the last century by simple mechanical recording of the pulse with levers moving writing pens, the invention of the *electrocardiograph* by Einthoven in Holland in 1903 provided us with an instrument of extreme delicacy, capable of recording and explaining every kind of disorder of heart rate and rhythm. Indeed, the electrocardiograph was first used chiefly to study just these disturbances. It was not until about 40 years ago that its value in diagnosing heart muscle injury, as in coronary thrombosis and infarction, became recognized.

Rapid Heart. With exercise, emotion, or any stimulus asking the heart to speed up to provide more blood to the tissues, it will accelerate. It retains its normal sequential beating, that is atrium and then ventricle, but just goes faster. This is *sinus tachycardia,* or rapid heart beat under control of the sino-auricular node, or pacemaker. The rate may be quite fast. I remember once walking up the Washington Monument without stopping, a good many years ago, and my heart rate was 160 at the top.

Normal heart rate is variable throughout the day. It may average 72, but normal men can have daily resting rates of 35 to over 90. The rate is usually slower in the morning; it rises after a meal or with smoking.

There are great differences at different ages. An infant before birth may have a heart rate of 120, and when he is 80 it may be 60. The difference in animals is striking. The heart rate of an elephant is 46 per minute and that of an ostrich is 60, while that of a small bird, the bramble-finch, may be 900. The canary's heart beats 1000 times a minute.

A rapid heart from excitement or exertion is a normal response and is one of nature's reflexes to prepare the individual to fight or run away. The reason we have this *tachycardia* when we are anxious is often because we cannot decide which to do.

Normal Irregular Heart. Another normal alteration of the heart beat is called *sinus arrhythmia.* The heart speeds up when we breathe in, and slows down when we breathe out. This is more noticeable in children and young people and if any characteristic is to be applied to it, it should be considered a sign of a normal heart.

Other Disturbances. The most common disorder of heart rhythm is the *extrasystole* or *"premature beat."* This is a hesitation of the heart which, when felt in the pulse at the wrist, seems to be a skipping or dropping out of a heart beat.

Actually what happens is that a small area in the atrium, or ventricle, or even in the electrical network of heart nerves, becomes "irritable" and sends out a message before the next normal signal from the sinus node is due. This triggers off an early or "premature" beat and the expected normal one does not occur because, having just responded, the heart is refractory. What we usually feel is a temporary flutter in the chest or neck and a sort of "all gone" sensation that seems to call for a deep breath, and a heavy thump when the next beat comes. This thump is caused by a larger ejection of blood because the heart has paused and therefore has had more time to fill.

Few, if any, of us go through life without occasional or many premature beats. Often the individual does not even feel them at a time when we are actually recording them in the electrocardiogram. They are more common when we are at rest and sometimes make it difficult to get to sleep, especially for one who is apprehensive about them. They are never serious and occur in normal hearts probably more often than in those with disease. They may come singly or in groups, irregularly with periods of freedom, or be present for weeks, months, or years.

Most of us learn to live with premature beats and disregard them as merely bothersome, but they may mean that fatigue, coffee, tea, (or other caffeine-containing drinks), cigarettes, cocktails, late hours, or anxiety are nibbling at us.

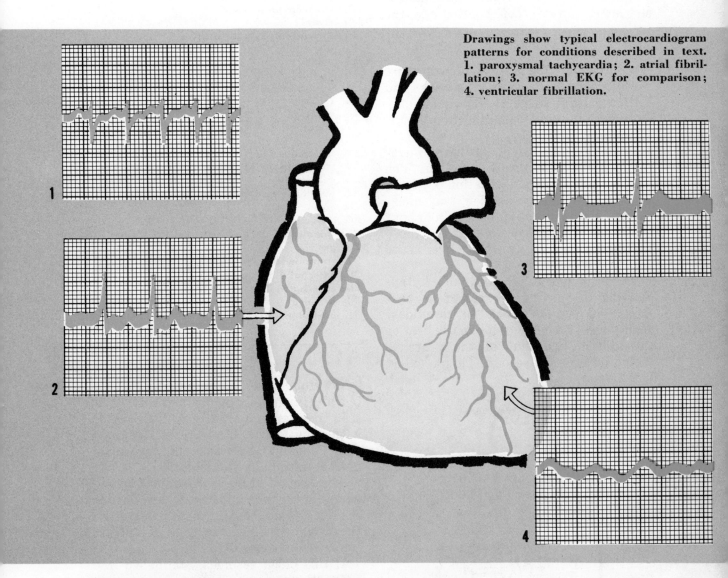

When a series of premature beats gets started all strung together at a rapid rate (like "beads on a string" as one of my patients called it), it is called *paroxysmal tachycardia*. Such attacks may show heart rates over 300, but mainly from 120-180. They start or stop abruptly and run for a few seconds up to several

usually more serious and harder to treat. Drugs are available that are generally helpful in preventing paroxysmal tachycardia. The most commonly used is some form of quinidine, a relative of quinine.

Various measures to stop an attack should of course be under the control of a physician.

Drawings show typical electrocardiogram patterns for conditions described in text. 1. paroxysmal tachycardia; 2. atrial fibrillation; 3. normal EKG for comparison; 4. ventricular fibrillation.

hours. Occasionally the attack may last for days or weeks and in one patient of Dr. Paul White's and mine a rather similar rhythm — "atrial flutter" — lasted for five years before spontaneously resuming normal rhythm.

Paroxysmal tachycardias may originate in the atrium or ventricle. The latter are

I have referred to the rapid, totally irregular rhythm of *"atrial fibrillation."* It is found most often with rheumatic valvular disease (chiefly mitral stenosis), thyroid overactivity, or coronary disease with congestive failure. However, it also can occur at intervals as short attacks for as long as 60 years in apparently normal hearts. Its occurrence should always lead to a careful medical survey because all organic causes should be ruled out before it can be considered innocuous or "functional." Digitalis is the drug of choice in treating an acute attack.

A far more serious and often fatal disturbance of rhythm is *ventricular fibrillation.* Since the ventricle is not pumping in this condition it is rapidly fatal unless the heart can be "defibrillated" by the new electrical machines that shock the heart out of its dangerous standstill.

Ventricular fibrillation occurs more commonly in acute coronary attacks and during cardiac surgery, although it may unexpectedly occur during other forms of surgery. The ability to terminate such attacks by defibrillating has been of dramatic service on many occasions. The onset of this form of fibrillation probably accounts for many sudden and unexpected deaths in individuals going about their daily tasks as well as in those in the serious stages of obvious acute coronary disease.

There is one other form of rhythm disorder of varying degrees of seriousness. This is *heart block.* In its mildest form there is a delay between the beat of the atrium and that of the ventricle which exceeds 0.2 second. This is called

ARTERIES ➡

1. carotid sinus
2. vertebral
3. thyrocervical
4. axillary
5. internal mammary
6. brachial
7. pancreaticoduodenal
8. superior mesenteric
9. radial
10. interosseous
11. ulnar
12. volar
13. digital
14. deep femoral
15. femoral
16. plantar
17. digital
18. external carotid
19. internal carotid
20. common carotid
21. subclavian
22. pulmonary arteries
23. aorta
24. celiac
25. splenic
26. gastric
27. common iliac
28. external iliac
29. anterior tibial
30. peroneal
31. posterior tibial

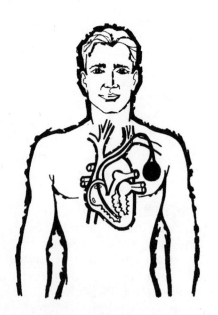

Implanted cardiac pacemaker, electrodes in right ventricle.

"first stage block" or prolonged P-R interval (in the electrocardiogram). It is seen in a few apparently normal people with slow hearts, but may be a sign of early rheumatic disease of the heart muscle, especially in children.

The second state is *"dropped beats"* when the block is sufficient to prevent the electrical impulse from passing from the atrium to the ventricle at certain intervals of time.

If this block becomes established in a proportional form, namely blocking at regular intervals, the atrium may beat twice as often as the ventricle (2:1 block) or three times to the ventricle's twice (3:2 block) or in some other relationship (3:1, 4:1, etc.).

Finally, in serious disease the impulse may be entirely blocked and we speak of *"complete heart block."* This is a somewhat confusing term because it sounds

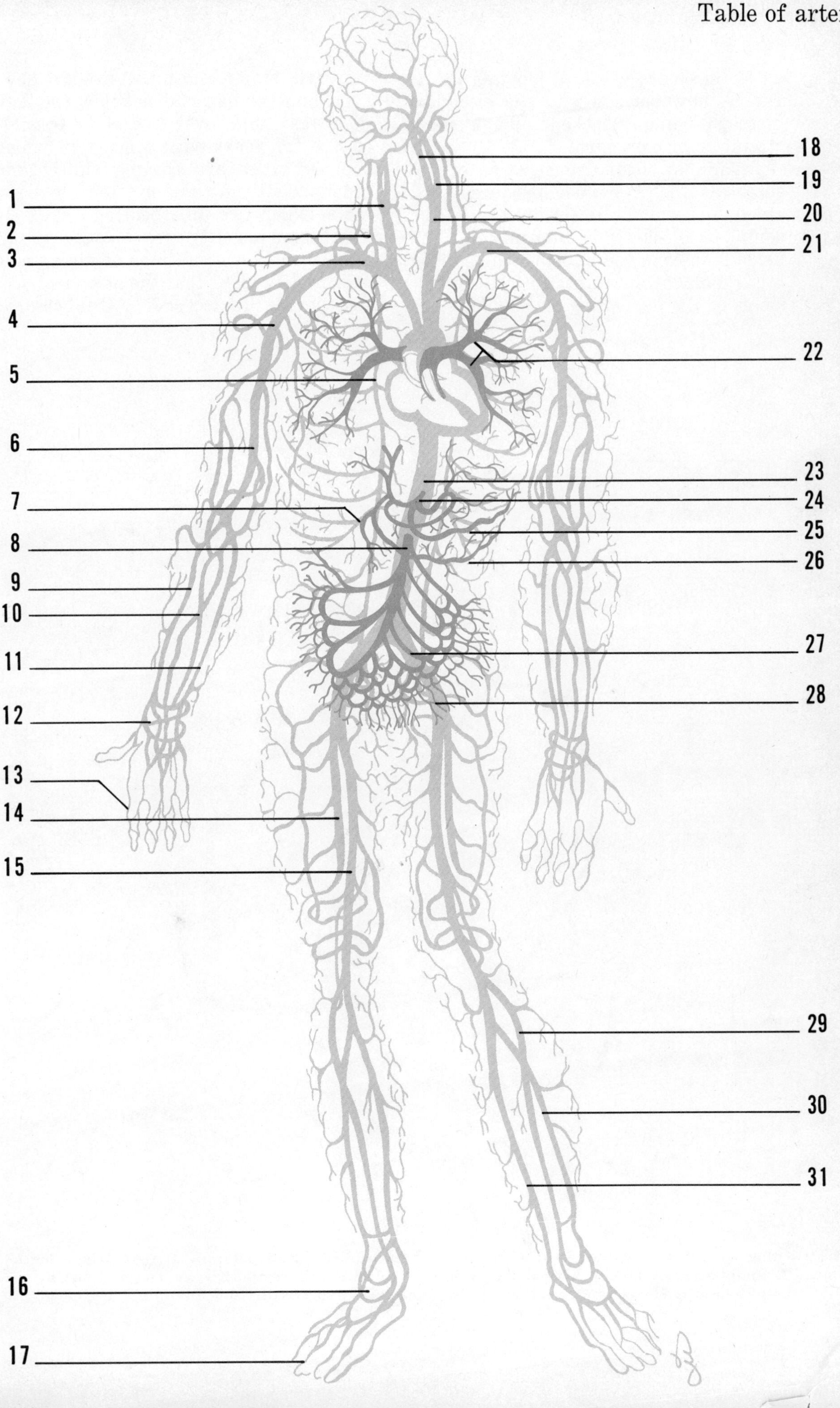

1 _____

2 _____

3 _____

4 _____

5 _____

6 _____

7 _____

8 _____

9 _____

10 _____

11 _____

12 _____

13 _____

14 _____

15 _____

16 _____

17 _____

18 _____

19 _____

20 _____

21 _____

22 _____

23 _____

24 _____

25 _____

26 _____

27 _____

28 _____

29 _____

30 _____

31 _____

as if the heart were all plugged up. It refers, however, only to the electrical message being "blocked" like a short circuit or broken wire.

Inflammation or degeneration of tissue near the A-V node produces this, chiefly in coronary artery disease. If this complete blocking is intermittent, the heart stops and the patient will be dizzy for a moment, or faint, go into convulsions, or die depending on how long the ventricle stops beating. Actually, however, another pacemaker below the A-V node may take over and it is possible to live for years with a heart in which the ventricles are beating slowly and independently, paying no attention to the atria which are also beating regularly at a faster normal rate.

It is in these conditions of high grade or complete block that the new *electrical pacemakers* are useful. One can be

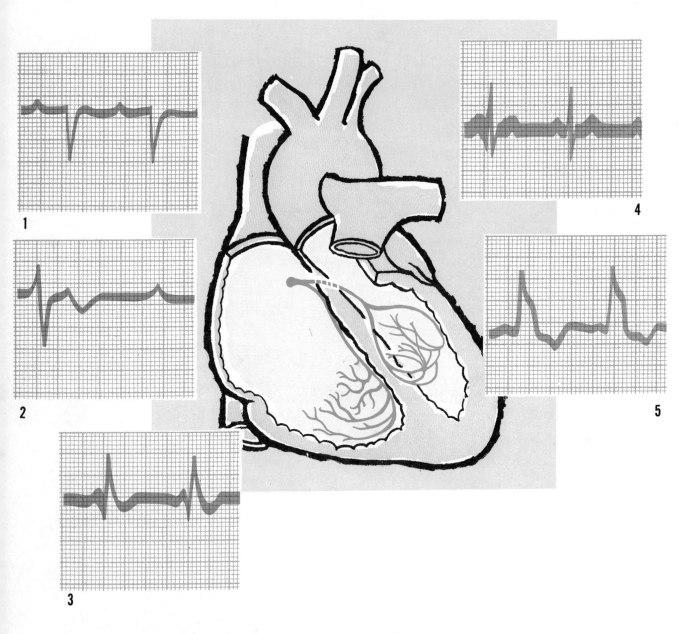

Other conditions described in text with typical electrocardiogram patterns. 1. first degree block; 2. complete heart block; 3. right bundle branch block; 4. normal EKG for comparison; 5. left bundle branch block. Interpretation of EKG's requires expert skills and training.

applied to the chest in an emergency, and later a small one can be implanted in the heart muscle with the battery pack under the skin.

These devices send a stimulating current to electrodes in contact with the heart muscle, thus triggering the "beat" and producing contractions at near the normal rate when the heart itself cannot do so reliably. Cardiac pacemakers have increased greatly in sophistication and reliability since the first ones, which were carried in an awkward and bulky package at the waist, with wires connected with electrodes in the heart.

Many patients need the permanent protection of a pacemaker implanted under the large muscle on the left side of the chest. The original installation of course requires surgery. Replacement of the mercury battery every couple of years or so also requires surgery but this is a relatively minor procedure since the pack is close to the surface and the heart itself is not invaded. It is possible that battery replacement may become unnecessary in improved pacemakers if tiny nuclear power plants that run on and on for many years, currently under development, prove practicable.

HIGH BLOOD PRESSURE (Hypertension)

by ALBERT N. BREST, M. D., and JOHN H. MOYER, M. D.

There is probably no bodily function which commands greater attention or has graver connotations, in the minds of the lay public, than does the blood pressure reading. On the other hand, there is probably no common function which is less well understood by the average layman.

Most persons recognize that a higher *(systolic)* blood pressure level exists, and to many, this is *"the"* blood pressure. Relatively few are aware that blood pressure varies with each heartbeat, giving rise to a lower *(diastolic)* pressure as well. The readings are commonly expressed as

140/90

in which 140 is the systolic and 90 the diastolic pressure.

Innumerable symptoms are often attributed to blood pressure elevation, but the condition is, in fact, frequently symptomless and insidious in its natural history. Often the word "hypertension" conjures up the picture of an anxious individual of the executive type, but this characterization need not exist at all. To the physician, hypertension denotes only an elevation in blood pressure. The hypertensive patient may be tense or relaxed, forceful or subservient, active or inactive.

The exact incidence of high blood pressure or hypertension is not known. Current estimates suggest that there are at least 10 million Americans with hypertension. It is noteworthy, however, that blood pressure elevation is a universal disease which is found among all societies.

Although most frequent after age 35, no age group is spared entirely.

The cause of blood pressure elevation remains disturbingly elusive in most instances. Nonetheless, sufficient scientific knowledge has been accumulated to provide a reasonable understanding of its significance. Furthermore, effective methods of therapy have evolved, especially during the past 15 years. These now make it possible to control high blood pressure in the overwhelming majority of cases and provide a current attitude of medical optimism.

Varieties of Hypertension. The arterial blood vessels consist of large-sized *arteries* and small-sized *arterioles*. The arterioles, by their elasticity, regulate the flow of blood from the arteries into the capillaries. The capillaries bear the responsibility for supplying nutritional requirements from the blood to the various tissues and organs of the body. "Blood pressure" refers to that pressure which is exerted by the blood against the walls of the arteries, as blood is propelled by the heart through the arterial blood vessels into the capillaries. The force of blood pressure is determined by several factors, including the pumping activity of the heart, the elasticity of the large arterial walls, and the degree of narrowing of the arterioles.

The blood pressure level fluctuates with each heart beat. The upper level, the *systolic* blood pressure, is the maximum pressure exerted within the artery when the heart is contracting actively and forcing blood out into the arterial blood vessels. The lower level, the *diastolic* blood pressure, is the pressure manifest within the arteries when the heart is relaxed and not contracting. The magnitude of the systolic blood pressure depends mainly on the pumping activity of the heart and the rigidity of the large arterial walls. On the other hand, the diastolic pressure is determined largely by the degree of constriction or narrowing of the arterioles.

The blood pressure is measured with an instrument called a *sphygmomanometer*. The levels are recorded in terms of millimeters of mercury. Normally, the blood pressure ranges between 100 and 150 (millimeters of mercury) systolic

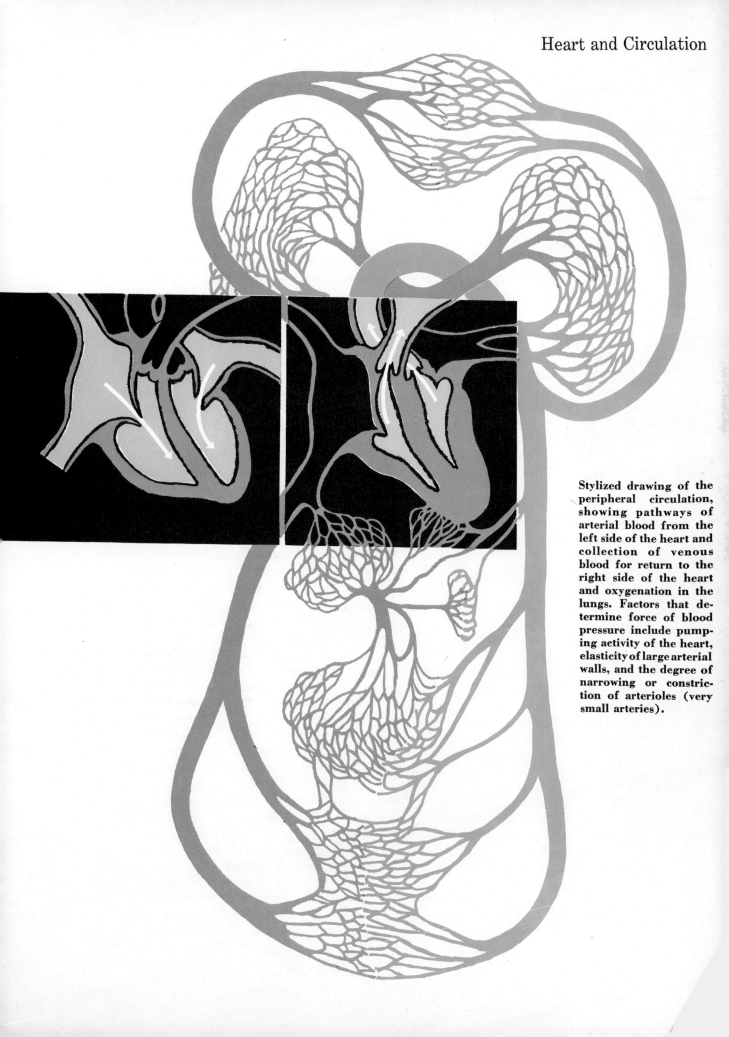

Stylized drawing of the peripheral circulation, showing pathways of arterial blood from the left side of the heart and collection of venous blood for return to the right side of the heart and oxygenation in the lungs. Factors that determine force of blood pressure include pumping activity of the heart, elasticity of large arterial walls, and the degree of narrowing or constriction of arterioles (very small arteries).

pressure, and 60 to 100 (millimeters of mercury) diastolic pressure. When the blood pressure (either systolic or diastolic) is elevated in excess of these figures, hypertension is said to exist. Blood pressure elevation may involve either the systolic blood pressure (systolic hypertension) or the diastolic blood pressure (diastolic hypertension) or both.

Systolic hypertension may be caused either by an increase in the amount of blood pumped by the heart or by loss of elasticity of the large arterial walls. The latter is the most common cause for systolic hypertension and is most often due to arteriosclerosis (hardening of the arteries). A mild degree of systolic hypertension, due to arteriosclerosis, is encountered not infrequently in many apparently healthy people as they grow older. At present there is no effective means to alter the cause or course of this type of blood pressure elevation. Less commonly, systolic hypertension is due to an increased output of blood by the heart; included among the causes for an increase in heart output are anemia and thyroid gland overactivity, both of which are potentially correctable.

Diastolic hypertension results from an excessive constriction or narrowing of the arterioles throughout the body. The greater the degree of arteriolar narrowing, the greater is the diastolic blood pressure elevation. Of the two types of blood pressure elevation, i.e., systolic and diastolic hypertension, the latter exerts the most injurious bodily effect when sustained over a long period of time. It is noteworthy that systolic blood pressure elevation usually accompanies diastolic hypertension. On the other hand, systolic hypertension occurs not infrequently in the absence of diastolic blood pressure elevation.

Since systolic hypertension is usually related to arteriosclerosis, a medical problem which is as yet insoluble, no further attention will be given in the ensuing discussion to this form of hypertension. All subsequent remarks dealing with the causes, effects, treatment, and prognosis (outlook) of hypertension refer specifically to the problem of diastolic blood pressure elevation.

Causes. Specific causes for diastolic blood pressure elevation (hereinafter referred to simply as high blood pressure or hypertension) can be found in 10 per cent of cases. The other 90 per cent of patients with high blood pressure are categorized as having "essential" or primary hypertension. Among the latter group, the causative factors responsible for hypertension remain obscure. "Essential" does not have the ordinary meaning of "necessary"; it means occurring without known cause.

Kidney disease is the most common known cause for hypertension. Patients with inflammatory diseases of the kidney such as glomerulonephritis (Bright's disease) and pyelonephritis (kidney infection) frequently manifest blood pressure elevation. Other kidney ailments, including polycystic disease and narrowing of the arteries which supply the kidneys, also may produce secondary hypertension. The exact mechanism whereby kidney diseases cause the blood pressure to rise is not clear. It seems most likely, however, that the kidney elaborates circulating biochemical substances which stimulate the arterioles to narrow.

Tumors of the adrenal glands also may cause secondary hypertension. Adrenal tumors may give rise to clinical disturbances such as Cushing's disease, pheochromocytoma, and aldosteronism, each of which is usually accompanied by hypertension. In these cases, it is clearly established that the tumor elaborates circulating hormones which sensitize the arterioles, causing them to constrict and thereby elevate the blood pressure.

The least common secondary type of hypertension is that caused by disorders of the nervous system, including infections of the brain (encephalitis) and brain tumors. In these instances, the mechanism for blood pressure elevation appears to be related to overactivity of the sympathetic nervous system. Since the elasticity of the arterioles is partly under the control of sympathetic nervous system activity, it seems likely that excessive stimulation of the latter is responsible for the accompanying blood pressure elevation.

When a physician finds that a patient has hypertension, his initial diagnostic survey is generally directed at the kidneys, adrenal glands and nervous system. That is, he attempts to discover the presence of any diseases involving these organs which might be responsible for the blood pressure elevation. Having proved that one of these diseases does exist, then the physician can direct his therapy at the specific underlying disorder. Having determined instead that no specific cause for the blood pressure elevation can be found, then the patient is categorized as having "essential" or primary hypertension. In the latter cases, therapy is necessarily supportive rather than specific.

Contributing factors. Although the fundamental cause for essential hypertension remains undefined, it is well recognized that several important factors contribute to the blood pressure elevation. Among these, hereditary predisposition is the most important. Other contributing factors include emotional stress, obesity, dietary salt, and excessive smoking.

Most patients with essential hypertension have a family history of this disease. Statistics indicate that if one parent has essential hypertension, there is a 50 per cent likelihood that the offspring from that marriage will develop hypertension sometime during their lives (usually initially manifest between ages 30 and 50). If both parents suffer from essential hypertension, the likelihood for the development of blood pressure elevation in the offspring increases to 90 per cent. These statistics emphasize the hereditary background of essential hypertension. However, essential hypertension may occur in the absence of a positive family history.

Specific causes of high blood pressure, involving the brain and nervous system (1), the kidneys (3), or adrenal glands (4), as shown in perspective drawing, may be found in ten per cent of cases. In the other 90 per cent the condition is called "essential hypertension," meaning of unknown cause. The heart (2) and large arteries (5) are "target organs" commonly damaged by hypertension.

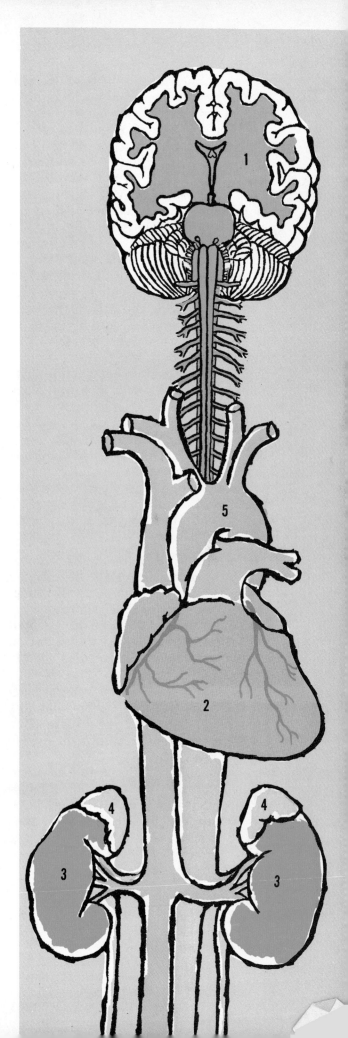

The classic prototype of the hypertensive subject is an individual who is tense, anxious, and excessively active; but the hypertensive patient often does not fit this characterization. Quite to the contrary, his personality may be docile and his activities sedentary. Regardless of the basic personality pattern, however, emotional tension does act usually as an aggravating factor to intensify the hypertensive process. Feelings of anger and frustration, in particular, tend to aggravate blood pressure elevation.

Patients with essential hypertension do not tolerate dietary salt in the same way as the normotensive individual. In the hypertensive patient, excessive dietary salt intake tends to increase the blood pressure level. In contrast, restriction of salt intake acts to lower blood pressure. Obesity and smoking are additional contributing factors in essential hypertension. Excessive weight probably adds to the hypertensive burden from a mechanical standpoint, whereas the nicotine content of cigarettes stimulates sympathetic nervous system activity and thereby aggravates blood pressure elevation.

Effects on bodily function. The importance of hypertension can be determined by surveying its effects on bodily function. Many such medical surveys have been conducted and it is well documented that sustained blood pressure elevation does inevitably cause serious bodily damage.

The natural history of hypertension is somewhat paradoxical in that the signs and symptoms of the disease often do not become apparent until the hypertension has been long-standing. Ultimately, however, the continuing accumulation of bodily damage does cause significant disturbances. The four "target" organs which bear the major burden of uncontrolled hypertension are the *heart, brain, kidneys* and the *large arterial blood vessels.*

The heart is the "target" organ which is most commonly damaged by hypertension. When the blood pressure is elevated, the heart must expend greater energy to circulate the blood. The heart muscle, like muscles elsewhere in the body, enlarges in response to excessive work. If the blood pressure elevation is uncontrolled and the excessive work load is sustained for a long period of time, the heart eventually is unable to meet the demands placed upon it and "heart failure" ensues. In the latter instance, the tissues of the body become congested with fluid.

In addition to heart enlargement, the blood supply to the heart (the coronary circulation) also suffers from long-standing hypertension. The cardiac burden often is so great that the heart cannot meet the increased requirements for circulation of blood through the coronary arteries to the heart muscle itself. As a result, coronary insufficiency develops with *angina pectoris* (chest pain) or even *myocardial infarction* (necrosis or death of a portion of heart muscle).

The brain is another "target" organ of hypertension. Long-standing or severe blood pressure elevation which is uncontrolled is apt to weaken the cerebral (brain) arteries giving rise, in turn, to cerebral hemorrhage. The occurrence of a cerebral hemorrhage or "stroke" reflects the severe stress which is imposed upon the large arteries by increased intra-arterial pressure.

Another prime target of hypertension is the *kidney*. The arterioles which supply this vital organ are particularly vulnerable. As a result of chronic renal arteriolar damage, the blood supply to the kidneys gradually diminishes and kidney function is reduced correspondingly. In a small number of patients, uremia or kidney failure results as the functional capacity of the kidneys is reduced to a level inadequate to meet the excretory needs of the body.

The fourth major area of insult involves the *large arteries*. The arterial walls, in particular, are severely burdened by long-standing blood pressure elevation. The eventual damage most commonly takes the form of hardening of the arteries (arteriosclerosis). Arteriosclerotic vessels lose their elasticity, their channels become narrowed, and blood flow to the tissues supplied by these vessels is compromised.

As general rule, the greater the hypertension, the more severe is the accompanying systemic damage. On the other hand, whereas severe hypertension may lead to serious and sometimes fatal complications within a few short years or sooner, mild to moderate hypertension exerts its effects much more slowly. The complications of mild hypertension often are not evident for 20 or more years.

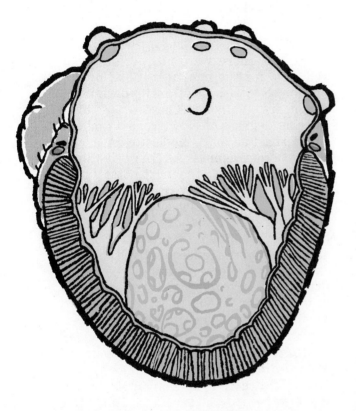

Cross-section of hypertrophied or enlarged heart, due to excessive work loads imposed by uncontrolled high blood pressure over long periods of time.

Statistical analyses indicate unequivocally that life span is eventually shortened as a result of uncontrolled hypertension. On the other hand, accumulating statistics also indicate that the outlook for the patient with hypertension can be normalized if the blood pressure elevation is reduced and subsequently maintained at normal levels.

Treatment. It has already been pointed out that the initial diagnostic approach in hypertension is to determine whether or not a causative lesion can be determined. If so, then specific treatment is directed at the causative factor. On the other hand, if the patient suffers from essential hypertension, then the blood pressure elevation is treated empirically.

It is fortunate indeed that effective antihypertensive drug therapy is now available which can control blood pressure elevation in most patients with essential hypertension, despite the fact that therapy in these cases is directed at the blood pressure level per se rather than the underlying disorder.

Overall management in patients with essential hypertension includes adjunctive therapeutic measures, specific antihypertensive drug therapy and, occasionally, sympathectomy or other surgical procedures. The adjunctive measures are directed at those factors which aggravate blood pressure elevation — emotional stress, obesity, dietary salt, and smoking. Surgery is reserved for the small group of patients who fail to respond to medical management.

Stress. Regardless of the basic personality pattern of the hypertensive patient, blood pressure elevation usually is aggravated by *emotional stress*. Thus it becomes imperative to minimize emotional excesses in hypertensive patients whenever possible. Recreational exercise suited to the age and condition of the patient is essential; conversely, periods of excessive physical exertion and mental fatigue should be avoided. Providing the patient with insight into the role of emotional tension also may be helpful in the control of the problem. Sedatives and tranquilizers may be useful therapeutic aids. They are, however, inadequate substitutes for an intelligent, well-planned way of life.

Diet. Appropriate dietary habit is likewise important in the patient with essential hypertension. Although it is often difficult for the obese hypertensive patient to reduce his weight to normal levels, he must appreciate that the loss of excessive weight may, by itself, significantly reduce blood pressure elevation. It is well established that reduction in salt intake also exerts a beneficial antihypertensive effect. The more severe the dietary salt restriction, the greater is the antihypertensive response.

Fortunately, since the introduction of effective drug therapy (especially potent diuretic drugs), it is no longer necessary to reduce the intake of salt so rigidly. With the use of the latter drugs, the patient is generally advised only to avoid the addition of table salt (although a modest amount of salt is allowed in cooking) and to refrain from eating excessively salty foods such as crackers, potato chips, and salty pork products. (See Low Sodium Foods, page 32). The reward for conscientious dietary effort is improved antihypertensive control.

Smoking. Elimination of smoking also is beneficial in the successful control of essential hypertension. It is acknowledged that discontinuation of smoking is a difficult chore. On the other hand, the benefit to be derived warrants the trial associated with withdrawal of the smoking habit. Even a reduction in cigarette smoking may be helpful.

In patients with mild hypertension, the various adjunctive therapeutic measures alone may control the blood pressure elevation. When the hypertension is more severe, the additional use of antihypertensive drug therapy is usually required. In most instances of hypertension, regardless of severity, the adjunctive measures plus specific antihypertensive drugs will provide adequate blood pressure control. However, in a small percentage (less than five per cent) of hypertensive subjects, it may be necessary to resort to surgical measures.

Surgery. Although various types of surgery have been utilized in the treatment of essential hypertension, the most successful procedure is *sympathectomy.* This consists of surgical removal of the sympathetic nerve fibers (within the abdomen) which are responsible for much, but not all, of the nervous regulation of the small arterioles. Unfortunately, the blood pressure reduction which follows sympathectomy is most evident when the patient assumes the standing position, whereas the supine blood pressure fall is usually less marked. Even when the blood pressure fall is incomplete, however, the response to antihypertensive drug therapy generally is improved following sympathectomy. Overall, surgery is usually reserved for those patients who cannot be controlled by the usual adjunctive and drug measures.

Antihypertensive drugs. Prior to 15 years ago, there were no specific drugs available for the management of hypertension. Now a host of antihypertensive drugs are available. These drugs have varying degrees of effectiveness and are categorized as mild, moderate, or excessively potent agents. Although it might seem logical to use the most potent antihypertensive drugs for all cases of hypertension, it is not practical to do so. Generally speaking, the less potent drugs have the advantage of producing fewer side reactions; consequently they are employed whenever possible. The use of drugs with greater potency is generally reserved for patients with the more severe degrees of blood pressure elevation.

The two major drug groups which possess *mild* antihypertensive potency are the *diuretic* and *rauwolfia* drugs. Diuretic drugs are compounds which deplete the body of excess stores of salt and water. Their salt-depleting effects provide obvious therapeutic benefit to the hypertensive patient. The rauwolfia compounds exert specific antihypertensive effects upon the arterioles, and they possess tranquilizing actions as well.

There are numerous diuretic compounds which can be taken by mouth, most of which belong to the chlorothiazide family. When used in equivalent dosage, all of these diuretic agents provide similar antihypertensive effects. Rauwolfia compounds also are available in various forms which exhibit similar antihypertensive effectiveness when used in equivalent doses.

In addition to their antihypertensive effects, the diuretic and rauwolfia drugs enhance the therapeutic effectiveness of the more potent antihypertensive compounds. Thus the diuretic and rauwolfia drugs can provide "background" therapy for the use of the more potent compounds. This "background" therapy decreases the untoward side reactions of the more potent agents and improves their overall effectiveness. Combination drug therapy with diuretics or rauwolfia makes it possible to use smaller doses of the more potent drugs, thereby achieving the same blood pressure-lowering effect, with substantially greater safety and comfort to the patient.

There are three major drug groups which possess *moderate* antihypertensive potency: hydralazine, veratrum, and methyl dopa. Although more potent than the diuretic and rauwolfia drugs, these agents possess a higher incidence of accompanying side reactions. They may be used alone in the control of hypertension, but more often these drugs are used in combination with the diuretic or rauwolfia compounds.

The most *potent* blood pressure-lowering agents currently available are the ganglion blocking drugs, guanethidine and pargyline. These various drugs have common therapeutic advantages and disadvantages. Because of their marked potency, it is necessary usually to begin treatment with small doses and then gradually increase the dosage until the desired degree of antihypertensive response is obtained.

The overall incidence of accompanying side reactions is greater than those with the less potent drugs. In addition, each of these potent drug groups exerts a greater antihypertensive action when the patient is standing than when he is in the supine position. In order to reduce their dosage requirement and to decrease the incidence of accompanying side reactions, these drugs are used most commonly in combination with milder antihypertensive agents.

The antihypertensive drug groups described above — diuretics, rauwolfia, veratrum, hydralazine, methyl dopa,

The sympathetic nervous system is responsible for much but not all of the nervous regulation of small arterioles. In closeup, removal of sympathetic nerve fibers within the abdomen, in *sympathectomy* procedure to control hypertension.

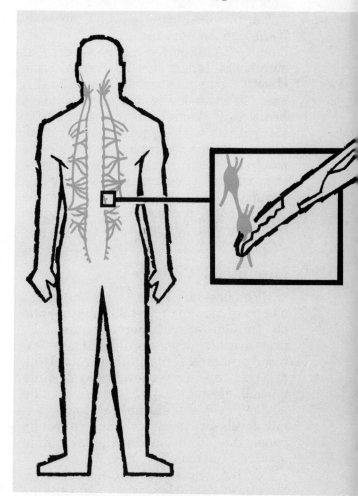

ganglion blocking drugs, guanethidine, and pargyline — are the most commonly employed blood pressure-lowering agents. However, other drugs are available and occasionally prescribed, according to individual needs. The current array of antihypertensive drugs is capable of controlling hypertension in the overwhelming majority of instances. At times, the patient must tolerate some annoying side reactions, but the benefits to be derived from blood pressure control invariably justify the means employed.

Outlook. It is evident from the preceding paragraphs that many questions about high blood pressure (especially essential hypertension) remain unanswered. Nonetheless, in spite of the many gaps in our knowledge, it has been possible to develop a logical and realistic attack on the problem. Particularly noteworthy is the fact that hypertension can now be controlled in most instances.

Uncontrolled hypertension leads inevitably to important "target organ" damage. It is comforting, however, that significant benefit can be derived from effective treatment, even when the disease is far advanced and organ damage has already occurred. It is important for the patient with hypertension to avail himself of the best treatment that science has to offer and to adhere rigorously to the medical program outlined by his physician. Only by this means can the patient hope to delay or prevent hypertensive complications.

Low Blood Pressure

Blood pressure levels around 90 (millimeters of mercury) systolic pressure and 60 (millimeters of mercury) diastolic pressure are often considered as "low blood pressure", but this figure is only an arbitrary one. Lower levels may be quite normal, depending on age, race, sex and environment. For example, we know that low levels are more common in young people than in old, and in oriental than in occidental persons.

Low blood pressures are, in most cases, harmless variations that warrant no treatment or concern. In fact, they may foretell good health and promise longevity. Recently, physicians have noticed that people with "low blood pressure" often escape arteriosclerotic cardiovascular disease. Recently, too, an insurance society, surveying blood pressures in four million applicants followed up for periods of 20 to 25 years, found that people with the lowest blood pressures live longer and stay healthier than those with normal or high blood pressures.

Although comparatively rare, some patients do have an underlying organic cause for low blood pressure. Organic causes include malnutrition, hormonal deficiences, and various cardiovascular disorders. However, in most cases, persistent low blood pressure is not harmful and so cannot be considered a disease.

Lay people often believe that many vague symptoms including easy fatiguability, lightheadedness, daytime drowsiness, and constipation stem from "low blood pressure". However, in this regard, it must be acknowledged that all of these symptoms are equally common in individuals with normal or high blood pressure; that treatment with blood pressure-elevating drugs generally fails to produce relief of symptoms; and, finally, that low blood pressure can be found in very energetic, strong, and obviously healthy people such as athletes, farmers, and laborers. Thus there is no correlation between blood pressure levels and the "typical" symptoms of low blood pressure.

Those patients with low blood pressure who are underweight or physically inactive may benefit by having their general health improved by diet, graduated exercises, and other supportive measures. Others may benefit from rest, because they may be fatigued from real overactivity. However, most have no physical problem at all.

STROKES and other Blood Vessel Disorders

by HOWARD C. BARON, M. D.

The patient who has suffered a stroke constitutes one of the major problems in medicine. The popular term "stroke," or sometimes "paralytic stroke," has about the same meaning as the medical word *apoplexy* — "to cripple by a stroke." All of these terms express the blowlike suddenness of symptoms. However, there is a great range of manifestations, from so-called "little strokes" which may cause a few minutes of confusion, passing dizziness, or slurring of speech, to major strokes which may be quickly fatal. A medical term that better describes the mechanisms of strokes is *cerebral vascular disease,* since the underlying cause is impairment of blood supply to the brain.

Although the stroke victim is usually middle-aged or older, younger men and women are by no means immune.

In bygone years, the care and treatment of a stroke victim was relatively simple. There was no preventive or curative treatment. All that could be done was to attempt to save the patient's life and reduce the ensuing paralysis as much as possible. Accurate localization of the cause of trouble was relatively unimportant, since there was no definitive treatment.

In the past decade, great advances in diagnosis and treatment of cardiovascular disease have been extended to include diagnosis and treatment of the patient who has sustained a stroke. One of the major advances has been the introduction of *angiography,* a method of visualizing blood vessels. In this technique, arteries supplying blood to a portion of the body or brain are visualized by means of a dye as x-ray films are taken of the affected areas.

Symptoms. A stroke may manifest itself in a variety of ways and produce many widely varying effects or symptoms, even though the underlying cause of the stroke is the same in most cases.

When a block occurs within one of the major arteries going to the brain, or within the brain itself, the blood supply to that portion of the brain is halted and the affected brain area stops functioning. If this situation is prolonged more than a few minutes, the brain cells in the affected area die. These effects are caused by an obstructing clot in an artery, or compression, spasm, or constriction of an artery sufficient in extent to interrupt the flow of blood.

The effect of this disruption of the brain's blood supply is prompt and in many instances overwheming to the body, because of the far-reaching role of the brain in maintaining normal body

Arterial blood supply to the brain: 1. vertebral artery; 2. internal carotid artery. In some cases, stroke results from interruption of blood supply to the brain from obstruction of the carotid artery, which is accessible to surgery, and may be correctable in suitable cases.

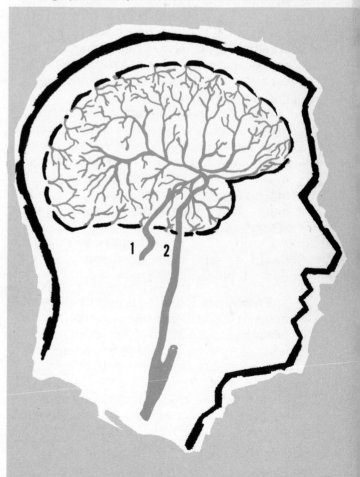

processes. For example, one small area of the brain largely governs the control of one arm or one leg. Should this area become damaged, the patient's control of that arm or leg is lost. The limb becomes weak or paralyzed. If the affected area is big enough, the paralysis affects one whole side of the body and *hemiplegia* (one-sided paralysis) ensues. The affected area is usually on the side of the body opposite to the affected side of the brain.

Various other areas of the brain control speech, sight, and complex activities. A vascular accident affecting one of these brain areas will be reflected in disturbance of function that the area controls. Persons who have suffered strokes often manifest difficulties of vision, speech, hearing and gait.

Causes. *Blockage of an artery* as the result of the formation of an arteriosclerotic clot or thrombus is the most common cause of strokes.

The next most important cause of stroke is *hemorrhage*. In this case, bleeding inside the brain case is brought about by a leak or rupture of an artery within the brain. This may be caused by a ruptured arterial *aneurysm* (a blood-filled sac formed by dilation of artery walls) or formation of an *angioma* (a tumor composed of blood vessels).

The third most common cause is blockage of an artery due to an *embolus* or clot that has broken off from a major clot elsewhere in the body, usually in the heart. This clot then travels through the arterial stream into the brain, where it lodges in a place narrow enough to hold it and block blood flow beyond that point.

Compression from tumors or swollen brain tissue may also impede the flow of blood.

Treatment. Despite major advances on many frontiers, treatment of the stroke patient continues to offer many problems. As recently as ten years ago we had no treatment worthy of consideration to offer. Today, therapy is offered under broad classifications such as surgery, anticoagulants, vasodilators, the cortisone drugs, and agents designed to dissolve clots.

The use of *vasodilators* (agents which dilate blood vessels) is designed to overcome the arterial spasm associated with certain forms of intracranial hemorrhage, to alleviate the spasm and to allow adjacent parts of the brain, unaffected by the hemorrhage, to receive an adequate supply of blood. The major disadvantage of vasodilators is that generalized vasodilation may actually reduce the blood supply to the affected area and further aggravate the cerebral difficulties that the physician wishes to overcome.

Another broad form of therapy is the use of *anticoagulants* to reduce the clotting tendency of the blood. The rationale for this form of therapy is that, with the reduction in the clotting tendency, further clot formation in the narrowed and diseased artery may be prevented.

However, the administration of anticoagulants is never free from risk, and the possibility of further spread of the intracranial hemorrhage which caused the original stroke is present. For obvious reasons, anticoagulants should not be given to a person who has suffered a hemorrhagic stroke. These drugs are potent and should be used only by physicians experienced in their use.

Surgery. Of all forms of available treatment, surgery in suitable cases represents the most hopeful approach to the crisis caused by stroke. In many instances, the obstruction to blood flow to a portion of the brain does not occur in the brain itself, but in a major artery of the neck, the *carotid artery*. Because of their location close to the surface at the sides of the neck, the carotid arteries are readily accessible to the surgeon. When this is the location of a thrombus or clot which obstructs blood flow to a part of the brain, its surgical removal may bring about a dramatic reversal of the patient's symptoms.

The substantial role played by obstruction of a major blood vessel outside the brain, in the production of stroke, can be appreciated from estimates that as many as 25 per cent of strokes are caused by a block in the carotid artery leading to the brain.

Obstruction of the carotid artery is mostly due to arteriosclerosis, but occasionally a blood clot from the heart may be the blocking agent. On occasion, kinking or buckling of the artery may be a cause. The site of obstruction is most frequently at the Y-shaped junction where the common carotid artery (the major artery of the neck) divides into the external carotid artery and the internal carotid artery which goes directly to the brain. The blockage usually begins with formation of an arteriosclerotic plaque (patchy deposit) just beyond the bifurcation. As the plaque grows in size, the channel of the artery is narrowed and blood flow to the brain reduced.

Symptoms and signs of carotid artery obstruction are variable, depending largely on whether the obstruction is partial or complete. When obstruction of the internal carotid artery is complete, the thrombus rapidly spreads into the brain. In cases of partial obstruction, the symptoms may be temporary loss of vision and bouts of fainting. The most frequent manifestation is intermittent impairment of function, either motor or sensory (e. g., impaired control of movements, or numbness) of a hand or foot, sometimes associated with a transient defect of speech or vision.

When a stroke has occurred due to a block of the internal carotid artery, the surgical procedure most frequently used is called *thrombo-endarterectomy* or *thrombectomy* of the artery. In this operation the artery is exposed, opened, and the offending clot removed. When the operation is performed by a trained vascular surgeon, complications and fatalities are rare. In most instances the patient is up and about the day after the operation, is home within a week, and returns to work within a month.

Operations designed to relieve the occurrence of transient strokes which have not left permanent neurological damage have a high percentage of good results. If the lesion in the carotid artery is extensive, the site of obstruction may be by-passed with one of the *vascular prostheses* now available. These are "artificial blood vessels" made of inert synthetic materials. Rapid advances in treatment of arterial occlusion outside of the brain itself have shown the importance of early diagnosis and early recognition of an impending stroke. Prompt surgery may prevent a major stroke.

Cerebral hemorrhage is a frequent cause of stroke. It is thought in these cases that the hemorrhage is due to rupture of a small blood vessel, generally in a patient with a long history of high blood pressure. This type of stroke can occur even in a patient with normal blood pressure. Usually the hemorrhage occurs deep within the brain, but in some instances it may occur in more superficial areas of the various lobes of the brain.

Distinguishing between a hemorrhage within the brain and a stroke due to blockage of one of the extra-cranial (outside the skull) blood vessels may often be extremely difficult. The importance of *arteriography*, or visualization of the blood vessels by injecting a dye into the blood vessel and x-raying it, is very great.

As a rule, patients sustaining intracranial hemorrhage are middle-aged persons with a long history of cardiovascular disease. Cerebral hemorrhages are not necessarily fatal as was once commonly believed, and attention is now being directed to methods of reducing stroke-producing effects of such hemorrhages by surgical evacuation of the blood clot.

A rather rare cause of stroke is *angioma* formation in a blood vessel of the brain. These weak vascular areas tend to bleed at a relatively early age, the peak incidence being at about 25 years. As a rule, hemorrhage from this type of lesion occurs at lower levels of blood pressure than primary intra-cerebral hemorrhage, and the natural mortality rate in this form of stroke is lower.

Another cause of stroke is development of an aneurysm of one of the arteries within the brain. *Aneurysms,* which frequently are congenital, are dilations of an artery wall, which may pouch out from the artery like a thin-walled balloon, or like an inflated weak spot of a tire inner tube. This weakened, dilated area of a cerebral artery is blood-filled, and if it bursts, blood seeps out, accumulates, presses upon delicate brain tissue, and produces a stroke or stroke-like symptoms with unconsciousness and one-sided paralysis.

Not infrequently, as a consequence of the aneurysm, spasm is produced in the arteries in the vicinity of the aneurysmal sac, making intracranial surgery particularly hazardous. Surgical treatment is generally a direct intracranial (within the skull) attack, with tying off

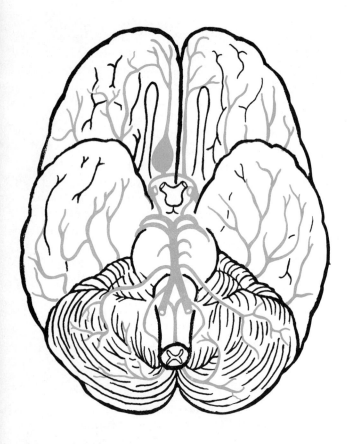

Base of the brain, showing vessels that supply blood to brain tissues. The balloon-like enlargement of a cerebral artery is an *aneurysm*, a weak-walled distended area that is susceptible to rupture and hemorrhage.

of the neck of the aneurysmal sac, or if there is no neck, enclosing the sac with gauze or with a plastic material which hardens and supports the area from the outside. The clot resulting from the hemorrhage is of course removed at the same time.

From a practical standpoint, when blockage of a carotid artery, or hemorrhage from angiomas is present, surgery has a great deal to offer the patient. However, in primary intracerebral hemorrhage due to aneurysm formation, surgery may have something to offer but not a very great deal.

Restoration of function. In restoration of function after occurrence of a stroke, *physiotherapy* plays an important part.

Certain deformities may occur after a stroke, which, if allowed to develop and progress, not only delay recovery but also impede the restoration of voluntary movements of affected parts. The most common deformities arise from *adhesions* of the joint, and *contractures* or shortening of the muscle or muscles of the paralyzed limb. These deformities occur most commonly in the patient who is paralyzed on one side of the body and who, either because of prolonged unconsciousness, threat of further complications, or further brain hemorrhage, must remain at prolonged bed rest.

One of the most important deformities that occurs and can be prevented is called "equinus foot deformity" with associated shortening of the Achilles tendon — the tough band of tissue that runs up the back of the heel. In this condition the paralyzed foot "drops" or assumes a drooping, downward-flopping attitude. Prevention or partial prevention can be achieved by using a bed cradle and a foot rest support (see Chapter 1) to maintain the foot at an angle of 90 degrees to the leg, and by daily stretching of the calf muscles when they begin to shorten or become spastic.

Another important maneuver is the placing of sandbags along the outside of the paralyzed leg to prevent an outward-rolling of the leg and foot. Equally important is the use of a splint to maintain the "bending muscles" of wrist and fingers in proper position, accompanied by movement of the affected parts at least twice a day.

Perhaps the most troublesome disability is "frozen shoulder," resulting from adhesions which form in and about the shoulder joint of the paralyzed limb. This condition generally occurs from immobilization of the joint. The newer cortisone drugs are quite commonly used in treatment of frozen shoulder. These compounds are injected into the joint and may give early relief of pain. However, their effects in improving the range of motion in the joint is not so consistent, and loss of joint function can take up to two years or more for restoration despite injection of steroids and diligent physiotherapy.

Physiotherapy is aimed at restoring voluntary power and is based on repetitive use of various forms of *active* rather than passive exercise. Exercises are started at the earliest possible stage of the illness and are based on simple principles. The most important of these is that *from the beginning it must be understood that it is the patient who has to make the major effort in moving the limb.*

Leg function is started first in an effort to make the patient ambulatory. Knee and hip exercises should be introduced as soon as the patient's general condition allows it. As soon as these exercises are accomplished, more complicated exercises are introduced and these again emphasize restoration of function.

Examples are: moving up and down the bed; rolling from side to side in bed, and then sitting on the edge of the bed. At this stage an attempt is made to restore sitting-balance control, and the patient is taught to resist attempts to unbalance him. It is important to re-establish balance awareness as early as possible. Once the patient has attained balance in sitting on the edge of the bed, he should be moved into a high-backed chair. With stable foot and ankle, preferably without a brace, he now requires only minimal power above the knee to stand or walk.

If the hemiplegic patient can raise his paralyzed leg only a few inches off the bed while lying on his back, there is sufficient muscle power in the thigh to permit walking maneuvers. Once he has assumed the standing position, exercises are first based on weight-bearing, marking time, and finally walking.

A set of parallel bars is of great help when early attempts at walking are being made. This may be followed by a "walking pulpit." When functional activity of the lower limb is achieved, mastery of the upper limb or restoration of its function may be more easily attained. Here the principle is simply a progression from passive movements to *active assisted movements* and then to unassisted voluntary movements.

It is best to follow a functional pattern of rehabilitation, with the accent on training those movements necessary for such activities as conveying food to the mouth, combing the hair, and other personal functions. The shoulder pulley for assisting shoulder movements is well known. It is important to concentrate on *outward* rotation of the shoulder, this being the most difficult movement for a hemiplegic to regain.

Flexion and extension of the forearm, and rotation of the arm inwardly and outwardly, are also difficult and must be practiced through all stages from passive movement to active movement and then to unassisted voluntary activity. Quite often, however, the fingers cannot be re-educated to any return of the real function the patient experienced before his stroke, except in mild cases. The fingers are often held tightly flexed and full extension is rarely possible.

Rehabilitation at home. Advantages of starting physiotherapy early in management of residual paralysis after a stroke, and realization that physiotherapy does not require elaborate or complicated apparatus, lead the way to early physiotherapy given in the home. Home physiotherapy has a great many advantages, not the least of which is that the economic burden is substantially lessened. The principal disadvantage of home physiotherapy is that the recovering stroke patient is deprived of association with others who are similarly affected, and thus does not have encouraging demonstrations of the heartening progress that can be made in overcoming disabilities.

There is no particular drug of value in helping the physiotherapy program to produce relaxation of spastic muscles. Best results are achieved when the patient's efforts are encouraged by a sympathetic family or physiotherapist, with understanding management of anxieties, lessened power of concentration, loss of memory and difficulties of communication the patient may have. It should be remembered that, in some cases of stroke, the patient may not be able to speak clearly or at all, but may understand what is said to him.

The long-term outlook. The best time to assess the patient's ultimate recovery of function, and of residual disabilities, is about three months after the time of the stroke. Realistic appraisal should be made of disabilities that remain, to relate these to the patient's social circumstances and a suitable rehabilitation program. Of particular relevance are evaluations of the patient's range of voluntary movement in sedentary and active situations, his abilities to feed himself and manage his toilet, and capacities to perform household duties or undertake forms of employment.

At about this stage a retraining program may also be necessary. For example, the left hand may be retrained to take over some of the functions of a paralyzed right hand. Aids in retraining, such as modifications of the clothing, perhaps replacement of buttons by zippers, may be instituted. Modifications of household fixtures may be desirable, such as handrails in the bathroom and possible elimination of stairclimbing.

Perhaps the single most important factor in rehabilitation of the stroke patient is *initiation at the earliest possible moment,* as soon as the patient's general condition warrants, a psysiotherapy program.

Once the maximum recovery of function is achieved, assessment of residual disabilities and retraining efforts should be instituted.

The defeatist attitude which used to surround the patient with a stroke is certainly no longer justified. Treatment of cerebral vascular disease is in a stage of rapid evolution and every patient with a stroke should be studied individually in an effort to apply the best possible treatment.

Accuracy in diagnosis of cerebral vascular disease has been dramatically extended by methods of visualizing arterial obstructions by x-ray techniques. Since strokes are commonly caused by blocks in the carotid artery within the neck and in certain of the arteries within the brain, surgical treatment in appropriate cases may be dramatically effective. While medical treatment of occlusive diseases of blood vessels has not progressed to a stage of rigid therapies, the use of vasodilators, anticoagulants, clot-dissolving enzymes, and steroids such as cortisone, all have their appropriate indications for use. An intelligent program of rehabilitation after assessment of the residual defects will often restore the stroke victim to society in a useful capacity.

OBLITERATIVE ARTERIAL DISEASE

As long as arteries function as tubes conveying blood, they can be said to be adequate. A major occurrence that can render an artery inadequate to convey blood is obstruction. The most common cause of obstruction to an artery is *arteriosclerosis obliterans* — closure of the arterial tube brought about by degenerative disease. Reduction in size of the *lumen* (the internal tube-like channel) of an artery often occurs as a result of arteriosclerosis ("hardening of the arteries"). But sufficient reduction of blood

flow to cause malfunction of tissues supplied by the artery does not occur unless the reduction is pronounced. It is obvious that considerable disease of the arterial wall must exist before tissue malfunction can occur.

Blockage within an artery develops from an *atheromatous plaque* or deposit of fatty material within the lining of the artery. This is a consequence of *atherosclerosis,* a form of arteriosclerosis with fatty degeneration of connective tissue of the arterial walls. Thrombosis of an

At left below, cross section of a normal artery. At right, partial closure of the arterial tube brought about by degenerative changes. Deposits of fatty material in the lining of an artery *(atheromatous plaque)* may lead to thrombosis and blockage of blood flow.

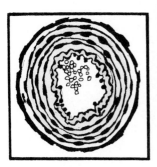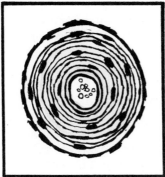

artery is the usual factor which precipitates the patient's symptoms. (A *thrombus* is a blood clot which remains at the point of its formation; an artery in which this occurs is said to be *thrombosed*). The artery, which at first was partially blocked, becomes completely occluded or thrombosed over a length varying from a half inch to six to 12 inches. Any artery in the body is susceptible of being blocked in this manner.

Arteriosclerosis is a rather broad category which includes diseases of the major arteries such as the aorta, iliac, and femoral arteries. Loss of elasticity and changes in the appearance and structure of lining coats of the arteries are brought about mainly by degenerative changes which increase in frequency with age and which affect the arterial system of such vital organs as the heart, brain, kidneys, and major blood vessels to the extremities. The term "generalized arteriosclerosis" is erroneous. Arteriosclerosis may be prevalent throughout the arterial system, but it is rarely generalized to the extent that all arteries of the body are affected equally or similarly.

Processes of thrombosis. When an artery "thromboses" due to atherosclerotic disease, a sequence of changes occurs. The thrombus, or clot, sets up severe inflammatory reaction which spreads to the covering (adventitia) of the artery and then into surrounding tissues. Frequently, collateral circulation (new networks of blood vessels) develops around the blockage. This may be sufficient to keep tissues alive, but not sufficient to supply adequate blood to muscles during exercise.

Once an artery has thrombosed and caused symptoms, there is danger that other arteries in the body will become blocked in a similar fashion. Atherosclerosis is a progressive and exasperating disease. Fortunately its course is not steadily downhill, but rather, after each thrombosis, there may be a period of improvement as collateral circulation develops. Intervals of improvement vary in different patients from a few weeks to 20 years or more between episodes.

This tendency to spontaneous improvement between episodes of thrombosis makes it very difficult to assess the disease process accurately. While patients with symptoms of atherosclerotic thrombosis have decreased life expectancy, it is important to stress that the course of the disease is highly variable. Some patients are markedly affected, but others lead long, active and useful lives with an interval of years between thrombotic episodes.

Absence of atherosclerosis is very rare in middle-aged and elderly persons. The disease is much more prevalent among men than women. Atheroma formation is uncommon in women before the menopause. However, in patients with diabetes the sex incidence of atherosclerotic symptoms is about equal, perhaps because diabetes is more prevalent in women.

Symptoms. Atherosclerotic disease rarely causes symptoms until an artery becomes completely or partially blocked. Thrombosis of the lower portion of the aorta and major vessels of the legs (a common area for atherosclerosis) causes three main types of symptoms.

Intermittent claudication, which means "intermittent limping," is the most common symptom. The patient, after walking a certain distance, develops pain in the calf muscles, due to inadequate flow of blood through these muscles. The blood flow is adequate when the patient rests, but inadequate to meet increased demands of muscles in a state of increased physical activity.

Patients with this symptom usually state that pain comes on after they have walked a definite distance — a city block, two city blocks, or a quarter of a mile. The pain may of course come sooner if the patient walks at a faster rate or walks uphill.

Another symptom is *pain at rest*. This is ominous evidence of severe blockage of arterial blood flow to the affected area. As a rule, these pains are worse at night, and may be eased by a hanging-down position of the leg or aggravated by elevating the leg.

Another distressing symptom may be *anesthesia,* or loss of sensation in the entire extremity or a portion of it. This frequently occurs after a major blockage of blood flow involving the entire foot, and may portend necessary amputation of the extremity.

Atherosclerosis of major vessels of the lower limbs rarely causes a patient to complain of symptoms other than intermittent claudication or rest pain. However, a frequent complaint is that the feet and toes are unduly sensitive to cold. Some patients may complain of numbness of the feet and toes without a feeling of coldness. These minor symptoms may manifest themselves before major symptoms of advanced arteriosclerosis of the major vessels of the lower limbs occur.

Treatment. Perhaps the best advice to give a patient with atherosclerotic obliterative arterial disease is to recommend some form of physical exercise every day, such as a walk of at least several blocks. In this manner a compensating circulation may be built up to improve blood flow to the affected limb.

A diet with a low content of fat which contains a predominance of unsaturated fatty acids is advisable. It is essential that tobacco be eliminated, as its blood vessel constricting tendencies contribute to development of symptoms associated with the disease. It is important that patients with evidence of recent thrombosis of a major artery stop smoking.

Alcohol is a vasodilator and useful in treatment of this disease when taken in moderate amounts, not only for its vasodilating role, but also for its mild sedative action, particularly in patients who have some pain associated with the thrombosis. *Anticoagulant* therapy should be instituted after thrombosis of a major artery under direction of a physician to prevent further spread of the thrombosis. Not infrequently it will be on a long term basis.

Prevention of infections of the extremities is most important. An infection may often precipitate gangrene in a patient with advanced atherosclerotic disease of an extremity. The feet should be kept clean and dry, the toe nails carefully cut, and corns or bunions treated by a competent practitioner. Shoes should be comfortable and well fitting, neither too tight nor too loose. At the slightest suspicion of an actual infection, inform your doctor immediately.

Posture in bed is of great importance for patients with thrombosis of a major vessel of the leg. The ideal position for the affected limb is slightly below the level of the heart. Raising the head of the bed about six inches achieves a satisfactory sleeping posture. On no account should an affected limb be raised above the level of the heart.

Exposure to cold should be assiduously avoided. Patients with advanced disease whose occupation exposes them to cold weather may have to change occupations. The feet should not be allowed to become wet and the patient should avoid chilling, since it will constrict blood vessels. *No hot objects should ever be placed in contact with the skin.* Hot water bottles and electric heating pads should never be used to warm the feet, no matter how cold they become.

Anything which may produce cuts or nicks in the skin, bruises, or crushing injury should be avoided. This means avoidance of crowded places where the patient's feet may be stepped on. Should a minor injury occur, the patient should go to bed and call his physician. The importance of proper care of the feet in all cases of arteriosclerosis obliterans cannot be over-stressed. Prevention of any mechanical, chemical, or heat injury to the skin of the feet and toes is very important. Many cases of gangrene which occur in patients with this disease can be traced to some supposedly minor and usually preventable injury to the feet.

Patients with atherosclerotic occlusive arterial disease may be benefited by surgical reconstruction of the affected artery after thrombosis, if the arterial patient. However, in patients who meet the necessary criteria for surgery, results are gratifying in about 90 per cent. In these successful instances, restoration of adequate flow to the blood-starved limb will be manifested by relief of symptoms.

Another form of surgery sometimes used is *sympathectomy*, in which an

Aneurysm of the abdominal aorta, the portion of the great artery from the heart that continues below the diaphragm and branches into the common iliac arteries that lead to the legs. Normal structures are shown at left below. At right, an aneurysm (1) or ballooned-out area displaces blood vessels (2) and kidneys (3). Most of these aneurysms, generally spindle-shaped, occur just below the area where renal arteries branch off to the kidneys.

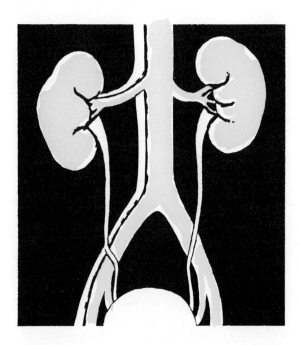 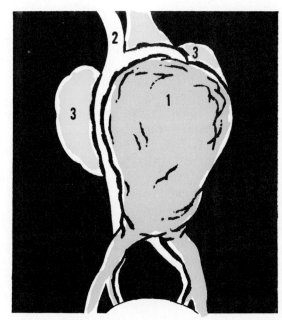

vessels beyond the thrombosis are open and adequate. In the patient who meets these requirements there is a good chance of restoring adequate circulation with relief of disabling symptoms. The involved artery may be opened and the thrombus removed. Another operation is a by-pass procedure, using an "artificial artery" of synthetic fabric to convey blood around the block.

The outcome of various arterial reconstructive procedures depends on many factors, such as the amount of collateral circulation, degree of blood insufficiency, and the age and general condition of the

attempt to overcome arterial spasm accompanying the disease is made by cutting certain of the sympathetic nerves to the involved arteries. At present it is the only procedure that can be offered to patients with extensive and irreparable arterial disease.

ARTERIAL ANEURYSMS

An *aneurysm* or ballooned-out weak spot of a major artery such as the aorta may occur at any point along its course.

The portions of the aorta that lie in the chest and in the abdomen are common sites of aneurysms.

The essential factor in aneurysm formation is damage to the middle layer of the artery wall. When only the thin lining and outer fibrous tissue layers remain to withstand repeated pulsing forces of blood flow, the artery begins to dilate or balloon out. Progressive dilation ensues in the weakened area, and as the aneurysm develops, pressure is exerted upon tissues that surround it.

Syphilis is a major cause of aneurysms of the *thoracic aorta*, which lies within the chest. Atherosclerosis may also lead to aneurysms in this region, but as a rule is more likely to produce diffuse dilation of the aorta than the characteristic sac-like aneurysm seen in syphilis.

In its early stages the aneurysm may cause no symptoms, or may be associated with only slight discomfort. Usually, symptoms result from pressure upon adjacent organs and tissues. Thus, the symptoms produced depend largely upon the location and size of the aneurysm.

Most aneurysms of the *abdominal aorta* occur just below the area where the renal arteries branch off to serve the kidneys, and the dilation usually extends downward to involve the common iliac arteries which lead to the legs. These aneurysms generally are spindle-shaped and result from atherosclerotic disease of the aorta.

The major symptom is generally pain in the upper abdomen or lower back, which may extend to the lower extremities. Presence of pain is an important symptom, for it often indicates a rapid and progressive enlargement of the aneurysm. The outlook in this disease, *if untreated,* is grave. The majority of patients may develop actual rupture of the aneurysm, with intense pain and death due to blood loss. The average period of survival after occurrence of symptoms from an aneurysm is from one to two years, with rupture of the aneurysm being the most common cause of death.

Recent advances in vascular surgery have greatly improved the outlook for patients with arterial aneurysms. The involved segment of the artery, including the aneurysm, is removed, and replaced, with a "synthetic artery" which restores normal blood flow within the arterial tree. Results of operative treatment for aneurysms have been increasingly gratifying and surgery has been a major factor in reducing the extremely high death toll of the past.

VARICOSE VEINS

When man assumed the upright position in his evolution, his new vertical posture subjected his venous system, at best relatively inefficient, to many new burdens.

Our network of veins serves to drain the capillary beds and body tissues of "used" blood and return this blood to the heart. The venous flow is assisted in its return to the heart by the rhythmic sucking action of breathing, muscular contraction in the extremities, and valves located in the veins of the legs. If the walls of the veins were rigid, the rhythmic respiratory movements of the chest wall might be sufficient to draw toward it all available blood in the venous system. Unfortunately, these walls are not rigid, nor are they even similar to the walls of the arteries which are strongly muscular and elastic.

Gravity assists venous blood from the head and neck to return to the heart. But venous flow from the legs is against the force of gravity, an "uphill" proposition, and valves which are present in both the deep and superficial veins give an indispensable "lift" to returning blood. Valves in our veins are arranged in such a way that blood flows past them toward the heart. They prevent backflow, and are located at irregular intervals along the main veins, but generally occur at sites of communication between the deep and superficial vein systems in the lower legs. The two set of veins (*deep* and *superficial*) in the leg lie, as their names imply, near the skin surface and deeply beneath it.

The superficial set of veins, the *saphenous system,* lies between the deep layers of the leg and the skin, surrounded by subcutaneous fat. The deep set, termed the *femoral veins,* lies between muscular compartments deep within the leg. These two systems connect in the area of the knee and in the groin. Important valves are located at these junctions. The two systems also connect by a number of communicating veins with valves. In this manner the flow can traverse many alternate routes.

"Varix formation" is a medical term for what is popularly known as "varicose veins." Obvious varicose veins are obvious indeed, as swollen, tortuous, unsightly bluish cords. Varicosed veins are permanently dilated and there is associated impairment of valves within the veins. The condition is mostly seen in superficial veins of the legs.

More women than men have varicose veins. Factors such as infection, injuries causing obstruction of venous flow, poorly oxygenated venous blood, and metabolic waste products, contribute to the occurrence of the condition.

How varicosities develop. The defect responsible for varicosities in the legs is failure of the valves to function in communicating veins between the deep and superficial venous systems. When the valves no longer prevent backflow of the column of venous blood, abnormal pressures dilate the superficial venous system, causing stagnation and pooling of blood.

Congenital factors are important. There appears to be an inborn defect presented as a weakness in the vein walls. Family tendencies to varicosities have been observed to manifest themselves earlier in the lives of those whose parents, one or both, have had the defect.

Statistical comparisons between people whose occupations require standing and walking and those in more sedentary professions, reveals no difference in the rate of incidence of varicosites. Prolonged standing may aggravate a pre-existing weakness or tendency toward the formation of varicose veins. Prolonged compression, or constriction of

Schematic drawing shows vein patterns in the leg. Superficial veins (1) have communicating channels (2) to deep veins (3). Valves in the veins (shown in insert) keep blood moving toward heart and prevent backflow. Impairment of valves permits stagnation and pooling of blood and leads to dilated or varicosed veins.

the leg by garters, contributes to the formation of varicose veins.

Varicose veins in pregnancy. The increased incidence of varicose veins during pregnancy is not always consistent with the thought that increased back pressure upon the veins of the legs causes this phenomenon. Dilated veins sometimes appear as early as the second or third month of pregnancy. Occasionally, the most severe symptoms of varicose veins occur in the early rather than late stages of pregnancy, leading to the speculation that factors other than pressure may produce dilation of the vein walls.

Varicose veins which are present or which develop during pregnancy, or are aggravated by pregnancy, must be carefully watched because of the danger of infection *(phlebitis)* of the vein. An elastic stocking from the toes to the knee will suffice in most instances. However, if the varices become severe or disabling, surgery may be required. As a rule the varices diminish in size following delivery.

Obesity is often cited as a contributing factor toward development or aggravation of existing varicose veins. Many middle-aged overweight persons with varicose veins also suffer from flat feet and other deformities of the feet. Sometimes, it is not easy to decide which of these conditions is causing discomfort. Here, a trial use of an elastic stocking may indicate the role of the varicosity in the production of the patient's complaints. If suitable relief is not obtained with an elastic stocking support, operative removal of the varicosities may be beneficial.

Symptoms. A great disparity often exists between the way varicose veins look and the symptoms they produce. Seldom is there any correlation between the extent of varicosity that is apparent upon inspection of the leg, and the symptoms produced. Not infrequently a leg with minimal varicosities may cause severe or excruciating symptoms, while on the other hand, some legs with severe varicose veins cause minimal or no symptoms.

As a rule, varicosities cause symptoms of tenseness, burning, or itching of the skin. Other early symptoms are heaviness, a drawing sensation, and a cramping feeling in the calf of the leg. Often, after long standing or walking, the legs feel heavy or have a "woody" sensation or feeling. Severe pain is absent except in the presence of an ulceration of the skin, or an infection of the vein. Then it is often of an intense burning character.

The external appearance of a leg with varicosities is variable. In the female with an abundant fat pad under the skin, comparatively little evidence of varicosities may show even though extensive varix formation may be present. In the thigh, with its thick fat pad, no veins may be visible; however, in the calf and lower leg, masses of veins may stand out, resembling tortuous blue cords. The presence of small dilated veins just underneath the surface of the skin is also indicative of the presence of varicosities.

VEIN CHART→

1. axillary
2. superior vena cava
3. right atrium (heart)
4. inferior vena cava
5. hepatic
6. portal
7. pancreaticoduodenal
8. superior mesenteric
9. hypogastric
10. femoral
11. anterior tibial
12. peroneal
13. superior sagittal sinus
14. external carotid
15. internal carotid
16. subclavian
17. innominate
18. pulmonary veins
19. gastric
20. splenic
21. ulnar
22. radial
23. inferior mesenteric
24. median
25. external iliac
26. great saphenous
27. popliteal
28. posterior tibial
29. marginal
30. cephalic
31. brachial
32. basilic

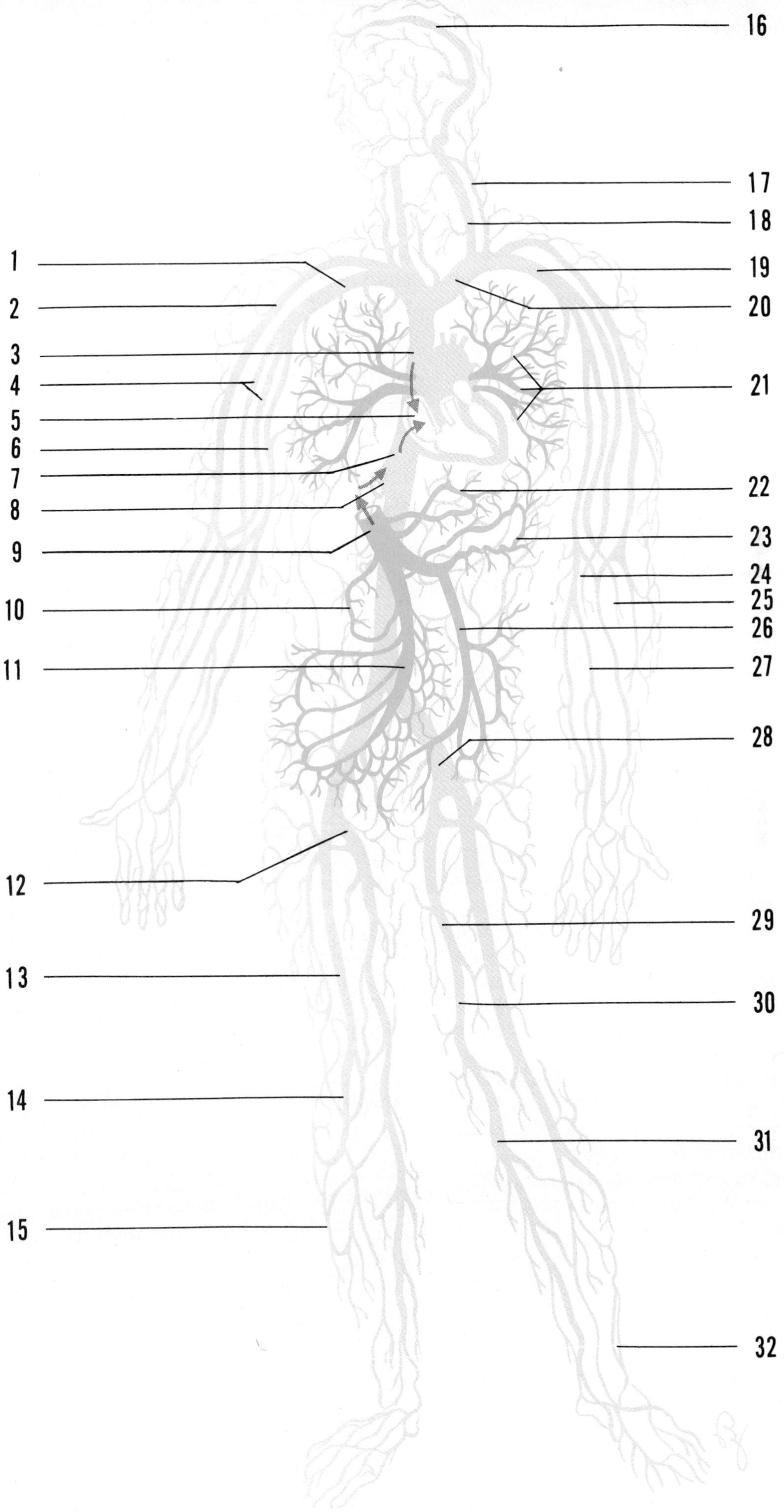

1

2

3

4

5

6

7

8

9

10

11

12

13

14

15

16

17

18

19

20

21

22

23

24

25

26

27

28

29

30

31

32

Complications. An area of pigmentation or brownish discoloration of the skin may be evidence of irritation and local malnutrition of the skin due to venous blood stagnation. Quite often, this occurs before the formation of an ulcer of the skin.

Another complication of varicosities may be rupture of one of the veins, with loss of a considerable amount of blood. This may occur in individuals who have varicosities just under the skin. In such instances, the veins have a deep blue color, covered only by a thinned-out layer of skin. A simple abrasion of the skin may result in considerable blood loss without associated pain. This type of bleeding is easily controlled by elevating the leg and applying a pressure bandage over the site of bleeding.

Another common complication of long-standing varicosities is varicose dermatitis or inflammation of the skin over the varicose vein. The skin appearance varies from a brownish, leathery discoloration to an acutely inflamed, reddish, burning aspect. The most common site is the skin over the lower third of the leg. This varicose dermatitis is frequently the forerunner of an ulcer of the skin, caused by a local malnutrition and irritation of the skin due to venous stagnation in the area. An accompanying bacterial or fungus infection in the affected region is not a most uncommon experience.

Treatment

Non-operative. Non-operative treatment of varicose veins of the legs includes the use of some form of well-fitted elastic stocking for support, and the injection of sclerosing (hardening) chemicals. The latter form of treatment is generally reserved for persons who for some reason cannot undergo surgery or whose varicosities are not very extensive or severe.

The principle of the elastic bandages or elastic stocking is very simple. Elastic pressure upon the dilated varicose veins forces blood into other venous channels which can more effectively carry it toward the heart. Elastic bandages or elastic stockings compress the superficial veins, shunt the venous blood through the deep vein, and more effectively aid its return to the heart.

The injection treatment consists of injecting a chemical solution directly into the varicose vein to obliterate the varicosity and aid in shunting the blood to the deep system of the veins.

Operative. Surgery for varicose veins is designed to remove swollen or dilated superficial veins along with the incompetent valve system. Thus, pooling and stagnation of the venous blood is prevented and the normal flow toward the heart is aided by shunting the blood from the remaining veins into the deep venous system of the leg. A number of satisfactory operations have been devised.

Perhaps the simplest is ligation (tying-off) and division of the superficial venous system at its junction with the deep venous system in the groin, and severance of all the small venous branches arising from this area.

The operation of choice consists of ligation and removal of the main *saphenous* vein (superficial vein system) and veins involved, and includes individual ligation and division of any incompetent communicating or perforating veins that might tend to compromise the results of operation. In addition, the great saphenous vein is stripped as described below and in this way the entire dilated or tortuous vein is removed.

Stripping

In the stripping procedure, an operative instrument is passed from the ankle to the groin through an incision on the inner side of the ankle at the level of the shoe top. The entire vein is then removed. The same ligation and stripping operation is followed in varicosities that involve the lesser saphenous vein, a portion of the superficial venous system. In this instance, the site is exposed through a small incision behind the knee. There is every reason to believe that with the removal of the varicose veins, the circulation is aided greatly and venous stagnation overcome.

As long as the cause of varicose veins is unknown, operative elimination of all varicosities provides the most realistic hope of complete cure in most cases. In some persons, varicosities may persist or may develop after surgery. These are generally new varicosities rather than recurrences. Here, the treatment need not necessarily entail additional surgery but rather simple office injection of a sclerosing solution.

Postoperative care. Results following adequate varicose vein ligation by one of the accepted operative procedures are usually excellent. The removal of the dilated, tortuous varicose veins aids in the return of venous blood to normal functioning channels, and prevents stagnation and increased back-pressure of blood from the veins within the leg.

After operation, the patient is generally allowed out of bed, instructed to walk for five minutes out of every hour on the first postoperative day, ten minutes out of every hour on the second postoperative day, and discharged from the hospital on the third or fourth postoperative day. An elastic stocking or an elastic bandage is generally used for additional support of the lower leg for the first several weeks postoperatively, as an aid to the shunting of blood through the healthy veins into the deep veins of the lower leg and then to the heart. In due time the stockings are discarded. Any remaining small varicosities may be treated in the postsurgical period by injection treatment.

Today, operative treatment for varicose veins is effective in reducing symptoms in approximately 95 per cent of patients suffering with varicose veins.

PHLEBOTHROMBOSIS

Spontaneous clot formation may occur in veins in any part of the body, but most commonly in the legs. Among the most common causes of this form of clotting, especially in the veins of the lower limbs, is slowing of the circulation with stagna-

tion of the blood or damage to the vein wall from outside injury.

When this combination of circumstances occurs, some persons will develop *phlebothrombosis.* Here, the clots may form in the veins, most frequently in those of the calf muscles. The clots are loosely attached to the walls of the vein and may break off and pass in the venous blood to the heart and thence to the lungs, causing dangerous *pulmonary embolism* or blood clot to the lung.

In this condition as opposed to phlebitis or thrombophlebitis in which a very tenacious clot is formed and adheres rigidly to the vein wall, inflammation is often completely absent, although in some cases, a secondary inflammatory reaction may occur purely from irritation by clots.

As a rule, the signs of phlebothrombosis are rather vague. A slight temperature elevation or a slight elevation of the pulse rate without any of the more usual causes, may be indicative of the condition. Tenderness in the calf of the leg is most important, and individuals may complain of aching or cramps in the leg but it is not a general rule.

Treatment of this condition may include anticoagulant therapy, in which drugs are given to reduce the coagulative ability or clotting of the blood. In certain individuals in which a "warning embolus" has occurred, the patient may be subjected to ligation of the veins above the suspected site of the phlebothrombosis as a preventive measure.

THROMBOPHLEBITIS

Large and small veins are subject to a variety of inflammatory processes, both bacterial and non-bacterial. The cause in many instances is poorly understood, especially in the non-bacterial group. Veins are commonly affected by being in close proximity to an infectious or bacterial process. In these instances, the vein wall becomes inflamed and a rigid or adherent clot develops.

This type of clot rarely if ever gives rise to the fatal "blood clot on the lung" or pulmonary embolus. The condition is usually confined to the area immediately around the vein. It is generally apparent to the patient as a painful, tender redness in the skin confined to the course of the vein.

Treatment generally consists of rest, elevation of the involved limb, and, on occasion, a course of an anticoagulant drug administered by a physician. After effects can be most annoying, in that they may result in the production of a second-ary varicosity in the area, as a result of obliteration of the valve within the vein, destruction of the vein wall, or loss of integrity of the vein wall with pooling of the blood in the area.

Milk leg and *phlegmasia alba dolens* are terms used for a kind of clot formation that occasionally occurs shortly after childbirth. Massive swelling of the affected leg gives a whitish "milky" appearance. There is little risk of embolism in this condition.

BLOOD-FORMING ORGANS AND THEIR DISORDERS

by CHARLES A. DOAN, M.D.

Composition of Blood • Formed
Elements • The Lymphatic System •
Characteristics of Blood Cell Formation
• Hereditary Backgrounds

BLOOD GROUPS

BLOOD TRANSFUSIONS

THE ANEMIC STATES

Iron Deficiency Anemia • Pernicious
Anemia • Other Macrocytic Anemias •
Polycythemia

SPLENIC DISEASE

The Hemolytic Anemias • Acquired
Hemolytic Anemia • Molecular Diseases
of Blood • Hemoglobinuria • Red Cell
Enzymes • Purpura • Other
"Bleeding Diseases" • Neutropenia •
Panhematopenia • Diagnostic Procedures

THE LEUKEMIC STATES

THE CHRONIC LEUKEMIAS

Chronic Myelogenous Leukemia •
Monocytic Leukemia

THE ACUTE LEUKEMIAS

THE LYMPHOMATA

Other Lymphomata • Plasma Cell
Diseases • Hypo-Aplastic Syndromes

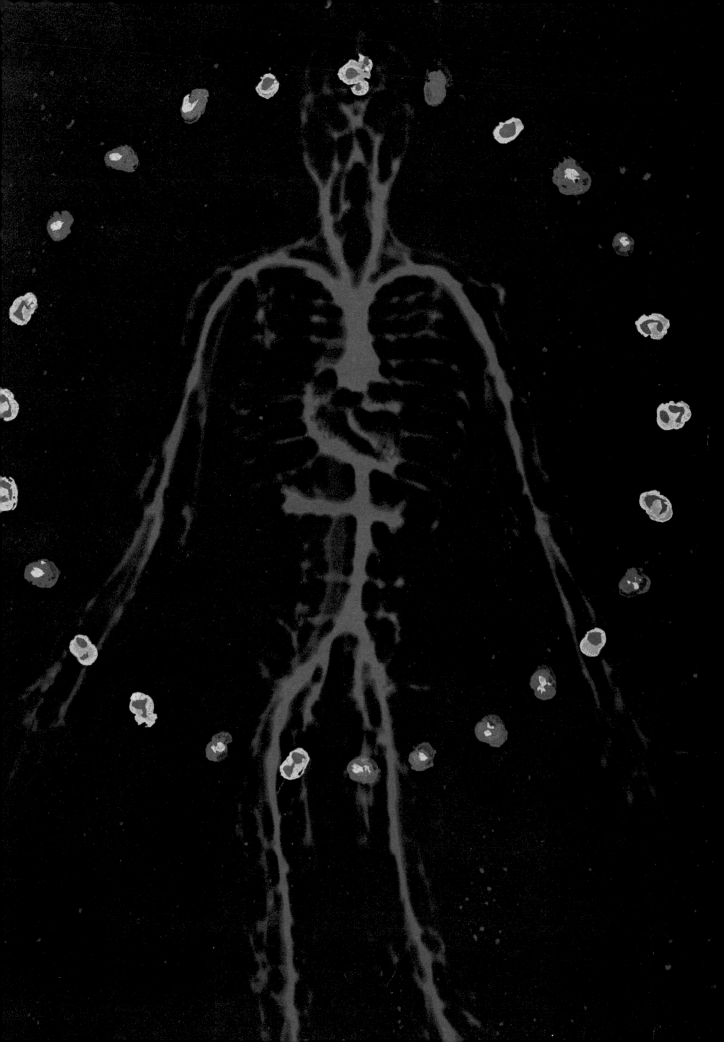

CHAPTER 4

BLOOD-FORMING ORGANS AND THEIR DISORDERS

by **CHARLES A. DOAN, M. D.**

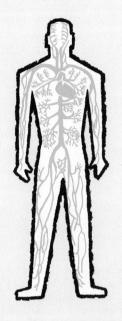

The formalized figure shows a circulatory pattern that is familiar to everybody — networks of vessels that carry blood to and from every cranny of the body.

This chapter concerns the *quality* of what is circulated.

Functions and disorders discussed here fall within the medical specialty of *hematology*, concerned with the composition of blood and lymph, the "second circulation" known as the lymphatic system, the prodigious activities of structures and blood-forming organs that incessantly manufacture, destroy, salvage and renew the hundreds of constituents that protect and sustain the body in myriad ways.

The functions discussed — formation of blood elements, "filter-trapping" of germs, removal of debris, and many other unceasing activities — are not performed by a single kind of cell or organ, but by a complex meshwork of internal defenses known as the *reticulo-endothelial system.*

Without oxygen, no living cell can survive. Without a specialized system of oxygen transport to cells, no complex multi-cellular organism such as man could exist. Thus, red blood cells which carry oxygen to and carbon dioxide away from the thirty trillion cells of the human body are basic requirements for health and life itself.

Perhaps the next most essential requirement for human survival in a hostile environment is our inborn, protective cellular and humoral defense forces — the police, army and ammunition — which automatically respond throughout life to countless threats of invading bacteria and many other challenges.

It is our so-called Reticulo-Endothelial System which performs these two basic functions: oxygen-carbon dioxide transport and internal defense.

The term *reticulo-endothelial,* especially if abbreviated to *R-E system,* may sound strange to the average lay reader. But anemia, "swollen glands," hemophilia, leukemia, enlarged tonsils, lymphoma, are much more familiar and meaningful to most persons. These and other similar conditions exist in the matrix of the R-E system. The concept of a pervasive, protective, versatile R-E system is important in considering disorders of the blood and blood-forming organs.

The system takes its name from its own characteristic cells. It comprises the basic *reticulum* cells (meaning "like a net") of the widespread, diffuse connective tissue framework of all organs, and the *endothelium* which lines blood and lymph vessels that permeate every cranny of the human body. The system is not a localized organ like the heart, but more like a gossamer meshwork woven through the body to perform many diverse activities such as blood and bile formation, the disposal and conservation of worn-out red cells, destruction of foreign invaders, debris removal and other far-flung operations.

In the bone marrow, spleen, lymph nodes and liver, these particular cells perform specific functions with which we shall be dealing in this chapter.

Fortunate is the person and the family who has inherited a strong and vigorous R-E system.

Formed Elements

Red blood cells (erythrocytes) are not as most cells, in that in mammals they extrude their nuclei when they become fully mature before entering the blood-stream. But they grow and multiply by nuclear division in their maturing youth, and survive for an average life of 120 days (4 months) within the circulating blood stream, as hard-working viable bags of hemoglobin.

Red cells are formed in the red marrow of bones. The process is called *erythro-poiesis.* Red cells are disk-shaped and slightly concave on both sides. Some 50

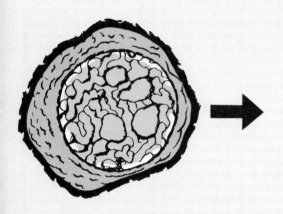

Mature red blood cells do not have nuclei, hence are more precisely called corpuscles. At left, immature nucleated cells developing in red marrow of bones. Arrow indicates an individual mature *erythrocyte* in the circulation. The concave disklike shape allows the cell to bend and squirm its way through close quarters, as in some capillaries so narrow that the red cells must move through in single file. It has been estimated that the bone marrow produces 5,000,000 red blood cells per second to replace an equal number that have worn out after a busy lifetime of about four months.

Composition of Blood

Blood is a liquid tissue, not much more liquid than some tissues which seem quite solid. If a blood specimen is allowed to stand in a test tube, solid and liquid portions separate. Moist solids constitute almost one-half (45 per cent) of blood volume. The rest is a clear, slightly yellowish fluid called *plasma.*

Plasma carries hundreds of different substances in solution or suspension. These substances include nutrients assimilated from the digestive tract, minerals, antibodies, hormones, gases, enzymes, blood-clotting proteins and breakdown products of metabolism. Watery plasma is also the fluid medium in which individual blood cells move through the body in enormous numbers.

red cells strung side by side could be covered by the period at the end of this sentence. However, red cells often vary from this "ideal" shape and size, both in health and disease. Some of these qualitative differences are important in diagnosing certain blood disorders.

Erythrocytes are soft, jelly-like, elastic, readily distorted units which turn corners and slip through extremely narrow capillary blood channels without damage or rupture.

Red cells get their color from an iron-containing pigment, *heme,* which combines with protein to form *hemoglobin.* This remarkable molecule has the ability to pick up oxygen and hold it very loosely, and to do the same with carbon dioxide, depending upon their relative environmental concentrations. Where oxygen is

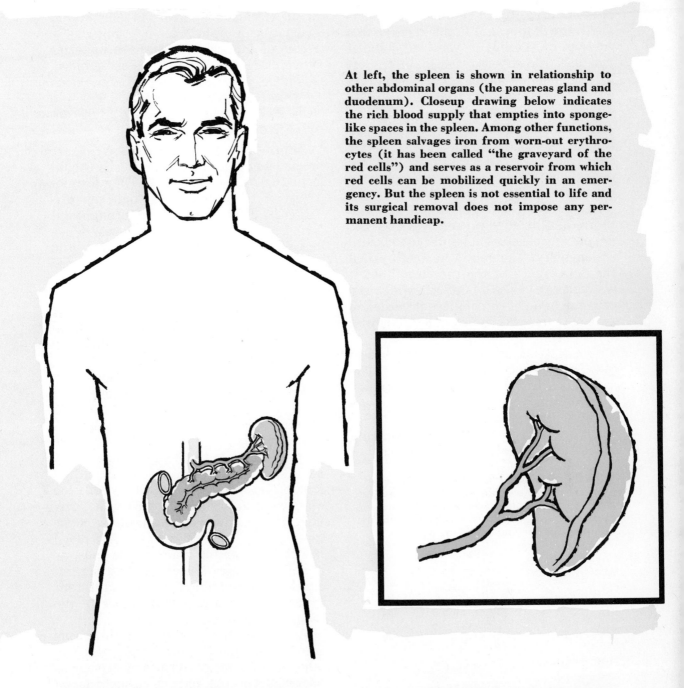

At left, the spleen is shown in relationship to other abdominal organs (the pancreas gland and duodenum). Closeup drawing below indicates the rich blood supply that empties into sponge-like spaces in the spleen. Among other functions, the spleen salvages iron from worn-out erythrocytes (it has been called "the graveyard of the red cells") and serves as a reservoir from which red cells can be mobilized quickly in an emergency. But the spleen is not essential to life and its surgical removal does not impose any permanent handicap.

abundant, as in the lungs, hemoglobin coming from the tissues picks up new oxygen and drops its load of carbon dioxide. Where the opposite condition exists, as in the vicinity of cells, hemoglobin drops its load of oxygen and in exchange picks up carbon dioxide, a waste gas of metabolism. Thus the function of red cells is to work like an endless belt containing trillions of gas buckets, bringing fuel-gas to cells and carrying exhaust-gas away.

The red cells lead a rough-and-tumble adult functional life that is relatively brief. Worn-out red cells are broken down and their constituent parts salvaged by the same R-E system which creates them. Particularly in the spleen, but also in the liver, R-E cells take out fragments of old erythrocytes, save the iron, and discard residues in the form of bile pigments excreted by the liver.

The normal adult *spleen* is a fairly plump pulpy organ weighing about 5 ounces and located in the abdomen, underneath the diaphragm in the general area covered by the flat of your left hand if you place it just below the ribs on the left side. Unlike any other organ, blood that enters the spleen empties into widely dilated vessels which form the spaces. This structure makes the spleen function like a sponge, which may become engorged and friable, and it may be and not infrequently is ruptured by external blows, falls, diving and other accidents. Fortunately, it is not an organ essential to life and its surgical removal does not impose any permanent handicap to health or longevity. The spleen has been called the "graveyard of the red cells," but it also serves as a reservoir from which red cells can be quickly mobilized if needed in an emergency, as for example during a severe hemorrhage.

The destruction and rebuilding of red cells balance out in healthy persons. The rate of death of the red cells is not known with absolute precision, but has been credibly estimated to be on the order of 5,000,000 per second, with an equal rate of creation. In health a complete turnover

White blood cells are larger and much less numerous than red blood cells. The two large cells shown below are *neutrophils*, one of the family of *granulocytes* which contain granules that become visible when dyed.

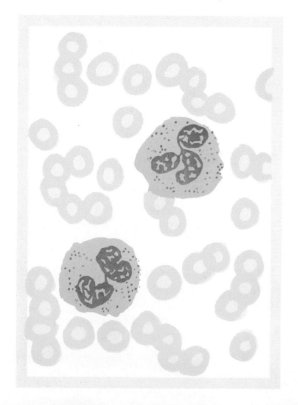

of all circulating red blood cells occurs every four months. This is prodigious in terms of numbers, but less so in terms of volume. A cubic millimeter of blood, about the volume of a fair-sized pinhead, contains approximately 5,000,000 red cells. The body of the average adult contains five to six quarts of blood.

White blood cells (leukocytes) are much less numerous than red cells (about 5 to 10,000 per cu. mm.). They are not truly white, but colorless, and their differential characteristics are brought out by various staining techniques. They have different shapes and sizes and motility and are usually larger than red cells. Pathologists and hematologists distinguish several varieties to which have been given technical and sometimes overlapping names, based on internal structure or a specialized avidity for accepting certain dyes.

One family, the *granulocytes*, have tiny granules which become conspicuous when dyed. These are manufactured in the red marrow (the yellow marrow is all fat). Another family, the *lymphocytes*, are manufactured in the lymph nodes, spleen and Peyer's Patches of the intestinal tract. The third type of white cell, the *monocyte*, arises in the diffuse connective tissues and the spleen and in some lymph nodes. If a given sample of blood has too few or too many white cells, or abnormalities in structure, or a significant disproportion between different types, these are important clues in the diagnosis of disease.

A primary function of the white cells is to ingest, digest, destroy and thus overwhelm invading bacteria and even nonbacterial foreign particles, such as an imbedded thorn. The process is called phagocytosis ("I eat") and obviously is a first line of defense against germ infections.

A representative granulocyte is not unlike an ameba. It moves like an ameba, swelling part of its structure in one direction and pulling the rest after it. When bacteria get into the body, white cells in the blood "gang up" on the invaders. The neutrophilic granulocytes, commonly known as "polys" from their multiple or

How a white blood cell ingests, digests, and destroys bacteria by the process known as *phagocytosis*. At left below, a neutrophilic granulocyte approaches a cluster of streptococci. In center, the white cell manipulates its shape to engulf the germs. At right, ingested bacteria undergoing destruction within the white cell. Red blood cells in background.

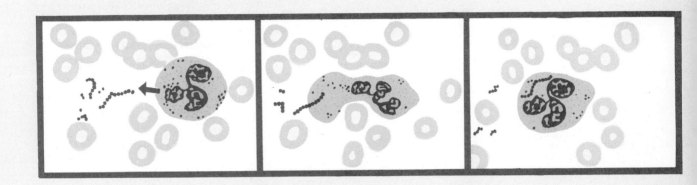

polylobed nuclei, move through the capillary walls, shrinking, expanding, tugging their jelly-like selves between seemingly impenetrable endothelial lining cells of the vessels. They travel unerringly to bacteria, engulf and digest them.

Everybody has seen the successful results in the form of a little collection of pus (white cells) that may have collected around some minor injury. The pus contains debris of demolished bacteria and white cells (some dead, some still surviving on the battlefront). As might be expected, when the R-E system mobilizes its forces to fight infection, the circulating white cell count goes up. The normal 5,000 to 10,000 white cells per cubic millimeter of blood is doubled, tripled or quadrupled according to the demands of the emergency. This finding often suggests or helps to confirm the presence, the type and the severity of an infection.

Blood platelets (thrombocytes) are tiny cytoplasmic blood elements, only about one-fourth the size of red cells and also without nuclei. They, too, are formed in the marrow. They help initiate blood clotting by triggering certain plasma constituents into a very complicated series of coagulative steps. Some forms of hemorrhagic disorders are associated with platelet deficiencies.

A *blood count* of the various cells is made from an accurately measured volume of freshly drawn blood appropriately diluted for the preservation of the specific type of cell desired. A specially prepared slide with a gridlike screen marked off in many squares facilitates accurate counting of the various types of cells under the compound microscope.

The Lymphatic System

Not uncommonly, children with upper respiratory or other infections develop tender "swollen glands" in the neck. These are enlarged lymph nodes, part of the lymphatic system which is part of the pervasive R-E system.

The *lymphatic system* is a sort of secondary circulation, inextricably intertwined with the vascular circulation of the blood. The tissue spaces surrounding cells are bathed in tissue fluids which filter out from circulating blood plasma through the capillary walls. Any excess fluids must be returned to the circulation promptly, lest tissues become hopelessly water-logged (edematous).

The return trip begins with diffusion of the tissue fluids into infinitesimally small *lymph capillaries* which have blind ends. The milky fluid in these capillaries is known as *lymph*. Countless of these finely branched lymphocyte-containing channels merge into larger channels of a drainage system that flows back toward the heart. All below the diaphragm unite in a collecting center in the abdomen, the *cisterna chyli*. Similar collections derive from the head and upper torso. Eventually, these large lymph vessels join in the thoracic duct which empties

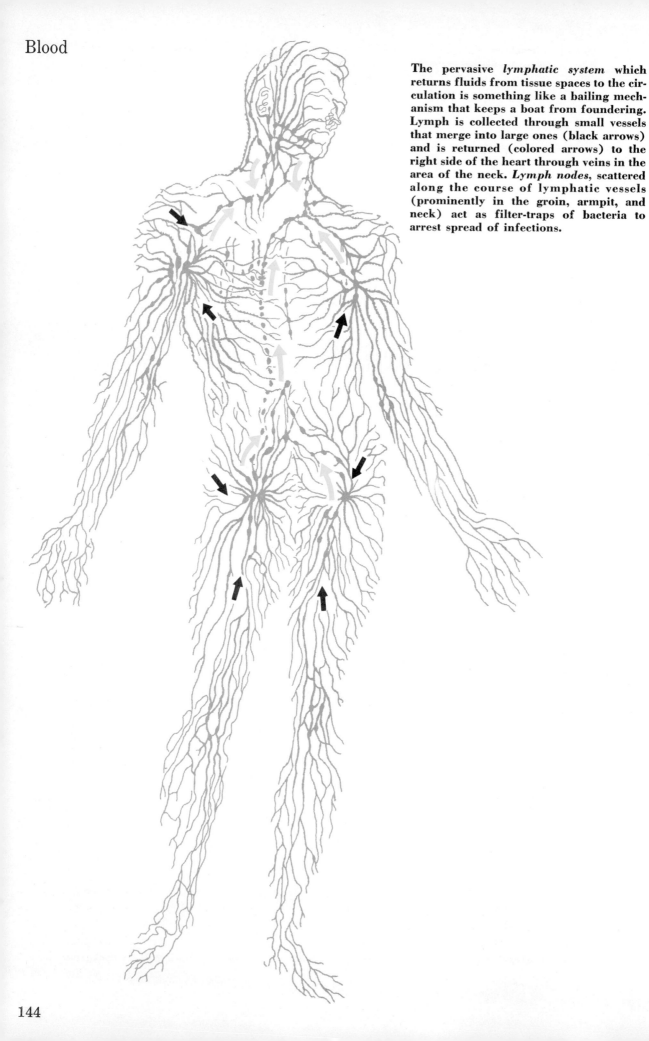

The pervasive *lymphatic system* which returns fluids from tissue spaces to the circulation is something like a bailing mechanism that keeps a boat from foundering. Lymph is collected through small vessels that merge into large ones (black arrows) and is returned (colored arrows) to the right side of the heart through veins in the area of the neck. *Lymph nodes,* scattered along the course of lymphatic vessels (prominently in the groin, armpit, and neck) act as filter-traps of bacteria to arrest spread of infections.

into a large neck vein, returning all venous blood once again to the right side of the heart.

Lymph is moved along by the massaging effects of the muscles, and squeezing, sucking actions of body movements such as breathing, assisted by a series of valves in the lymph vessels. Thus the fluids that leak from the blood into tissue spaces for nourishment of the cells are returned for re-circulation repeatedly, as are the red blood cells. In this aspect, the lymphatic system is something like a bailing mechanism that keeps a boat from foundering.

Lymph nodes are the small, lumpy enlargements along the course of the various lymphatic vessels.

These structures, also called lymph glands, have interspaces like baffles through which lymph is forced to flow. This filtering arrangement is an efficient trap for bacteria and minute foreign particles such as cell debris. The lymph nodes are also the chief sites of the origin and growth of the lymphocytes.

It is estimated that there are more than a hundred lymph nodes, or glands, scattered throughout the body along the line of the lymphatic vessels. Those most commonly involved in complaints of "swollen glands" are in the neck, armpits and groins. Each is a potential dam to arrest the spread of infection from an extremity to the main body organs, and these sentinel glands may swell and be painful when they put forth an heroic effort to defend the body. For instance, an infection of the hand may cause enlargement of lymph nodes in the armpit. There are, however, many other causes of enlarged nodes, and this "sign of trouble" should always be called to a physician's attention promptly.

Characteristics of Blood Cell Formation

Though broadly distributed over the body, nevertheless the reticuloendothelial system does represent a functional unit somewhat comparable to the cardiovascular renal and central nervous systems, with which there is complete integration. A unique feature of the R-E system is the retention throughout life of early embryonic characteristics for the continuous origin and differentiation of the blood and connective tissue cells.

In the earliest growth stages of the tiny human embryo, certain cells called *angioblasts* differentiate. From these, the first hemoglobin-making red blood cells, the first blood plasma, and the first *endothelial* cells that will later participate in the formation of blood vessels and blood cells are immediately derived. Shortly thereafter the so-called *reticulum* cells differentiate which help to form the non-skeletal connective tissue framework, and from them arise the first defensive white blood cells. In a sense, fixed reticulum cells in connective tissue, and endothelial cells which line blood vessels, are perpetually embryonically youthful, since capacities exhibited almost at life's beginning persist throughout life.

The heart and its large communicating vessels begin to develop early in embryonic life from the network of vessels

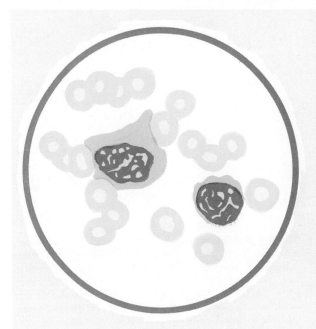

Lymphocytes are white blood cells with large nuclei and little cytoplasm. They are manufactured in the lymph nodes, the spleen, and certain structures in the intestinal tract (Peyer's Patches). Lymphocytes come in small, medium, and large sizes. Red blood cells in background.

formed from the small islands of angioblasts. The heart is a specialized pump which begins beating long before we are born. Protective mechanisms, develop very early, in addition to the granulocyte mechanisms which keep the blood fluid within its channels, but in times of emergency promptly solidify blood to plug a "hole in the dike" from which we might otherwise bleed to death. The blood platelets, important to prompt blood

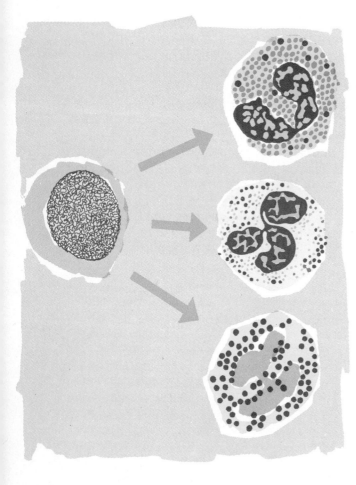

The *myeloblast* is the "mother cell" in the bone marrow from which the *myeloid* (bone marrow) family of granular white cells develops. At right, top: *eosinophil*; center, *neutrophil*; bottom, *basophil*. Technical names derive from stainability by acid, neutral, or basic dyes. In their circulating state the white blood cells are colorless.

coagulation, derive from other specially differentiated cells *(megakaryocytes)*, which appear in the embryo at about the same time as white blood cell differentiation.

In the last three months of intra-uterine fetal growth, formation of red and white blood cells and platelets occurs in the spleen, the immature skeleton being mostly cartilaginous tissue or gristle at that time. But after birth this function gradually changes location to the developing bone marrow. Thereafter the marrow produces red cells, the three types of white cells known as granulocytes *(neutrophils, eosinophils, and basophils)* and the blood platelets. But in certain pathologic states such as progressive fibrosis of the marrow, the spleen may resume the blood cell-producing activities that it performed in embryonic life.

Lymphocytes continue to be produced in the spleen and lymph nodes, tonsils and adenoid tissue in nose and throat, and a few other areas such as patches in the small intestines and the appendix. Large *mononuclear* or *monocytic* white cells come from the connective tissues everywhere, from the spleen whenever needed, and occasionally from peripheral lymph nodes, but never, normally, from the bone marrow. Large phagocytic or scavenger cells of connective tissues, spleen, bone marrow and liver arise in part from the endothelium and in part from the reticulum.

An important advantage of the R-E system in medical diagnosis is the relative ease with which a "sample" of its functioning status can be obtained. A drop of blood obtained from the finger or ear lobe is actually a biopsy specimen, more readily obtained than a comparable section of lymph node, kidney or liver tissue. It is now also easy to obtain a direct sample of bone marrow from sites such as the breastbone, crest of the hipbone, and accessible parts of the vertebrae, where there is relatively easy access to the marrow through cartilage. Direct observation of the efficiency of blood formation may be obtained from careful microscopic examination, preferably of the living cells.

Hereditary Backgrounds

It is well known that each of us inherits from our forebears a variety of gene characters which govern our height, weight, physiognomy, eye and hair color, and other attributes. Genetic studies show that the R-E systems of some families are more susceptible to related diseases than those of other families. This is not to say that the same blood diseases are inherited directly, but in some families there is a greater incidence of R-E disorders, such as low resistance to infections in general, a tendency to polycythemia (too many blood cells), various leukemic and lymphoma states, and certain types of anemia.

By the same mechanism, some families seem to inherit a superior R-E system which responds sensitively to the slightest pathogenic stimulus and functions at a high level of efficiency throughout many years of a long life. Thus, in addition to environmental factors, there are inborn susceptibilities and resistances which either handicap or aid the physician in treating specific disease that may occur in the individual person.

Fortunately, we are getting increasing knowledge, with the necessary wisdom, to discover and compensate for certain of the inherent defects involved in specific hematologic diseases. The discerning physician with insights which come from experience, adequate histories, complete physical and appropriate laboratory examinations, may hope more often than not to succeed in re-establishing desired balances of health.

There are, of course, no generalizations which can safely be made about an individual patient with any illness. Each patient has his particular inheritance and whatever environmental stresses that have beset him. Moreover, each disease has "degrees" of intensity which we usually speak of as chronic, subacute or acute. And today an ever-increasing variety of drugs and agents must be fitted to individual needs as precisely as a Yale lock requires its specific key to function. Every patient presents a new research problem to his physician, and diagnosis is only the first step of many which will either promote well-being or, failing, will allow disease to continue until the right answer can be found.

It is with this general background of fact and philosophy that we shall approach those diseases which, primarily or secondarily involve the reticulo-endothelial system. We shall point out dramatic advances in knowledge and control of these diseases that have been made over the past fifty years, and discuss diseases of which at the present time we have only partial knowledge and, therefore, only partial control.

BLOOD GROUPS

In thick preparations of blood cells, the red cells often tend to stick together and form a continuous overlapping chain such as happens when a deck of cards is spread out on a table to draw for the cut. This phenomenon is called *rouleau formation.* While studying this phenomenon microscopically in preparations of fresh blood, Dr. Karl Landsteiner, an Austrian investigator, in 1898 observed certain red cell incompatibilities. In mixtures of blood cells from one patient with plasma from another patient, he observed in some instances a true agglutination or tight clumping of the red cells which was different from the rouleau formation.

From these studies he divided the population into four groups — people having in their blood what he called Factor A, or Factor B, or both (AB), or in the fourth instance (O) no agglutinating factors at all. His first published account mentioned that this phenomenon might some day be important in human blood transfusions. Relatively little clinical attention was given to the matter until World War I when there was great need of supportive transfusions for wounded soldiers. At that time, Oswald Robertson and Peyton Rous of the Rockefeller Institute did extensive studies on the preservation and transportation of blood, but not until World War II did blood transfusion become widely and safely available on a large scale.

With great intensification of studies of lifesaving blood transfusions, it was inevitable that factors other than the original ABO groups would be discovered. Landsteiner, who in the meantime had come to the Rockefeller Institute from Vienna, discovered a further division of human red blood cells into those that produce specific antibodies in the macacus rhesus monkey and those that do not. This led to "Rh positive" and "Rh negative" classifications of red cells (see *Pregnancy* chapter).

Other factors, M and N, have been described, and much rarer incompatibilities have been found and named after the families (such as Lewis, Kell, and Duffy) in which they were first discovered. All of these findings (and other factors are discovered from time to time) mean that a well-equipped blood-typing laboratory with a specially trained staff is essential for the maximum promise of safe transfusion for every recipient.

BLOOD TRANSFUSIONS

Even with every caution with respect to compatibility of the red blood cells, post-transfusion reactions still occur. Feverish and allergic reactions without destruction of the red cells may be produced by transfused white blood cells and platelets in patients who have received multiple transfusions. Many of these reactions can be prevented by removal of the centrifuged "buffy coat," which is comprised largely of white cells and platelets, before transfusing "packed" or "washed" red blood cells, where only the red cells are needed.

Some five million transfusions of whole blood are given annually in the United States and the rate will increase in the future. It is necessary to be aware of certain hazards which may be associated with this important therapeutic procedure. One of the main contraindications for blood transfusion is myocardial failure or decompensation of the heart in the elderly. Under such circumstances, if blood transfusion is mandatory, it must be given very slowly, so there will not be an overload of blood to be handled by a heart already weakened.

When the circulation is competent and intact, the speed with which the blood volume readjusts to the added transfused blood is amazing. The plasma passes into the connective tissues almost as rapidly as the blood is given, and the patient ends up with his same original blood volume within an hour or two. The same thing works in reverse for the donor, with plasma from his tissues coming into the bloodstream almost as rapidly as the blood is taken out, to reestablish normal blood volume of the donor within a matter of minutes or hours.

The patient should have blood from a relaxed, rested donor, because fatigue products, which accumulate after eight hours of strenuous physical effort, for example, will be transmitted by the donor's blood to the recipient, and he will feel as tired (or as rested) as the donor was at the time the donation was given. Likewise, blood from allergic persons, such as those having hives or asthma, may transmit these symptoms to a recipient. If the donor has taken penicillin and the recipient is sensitive to this drug, a serious reaction could follow a transfusion from this source. Care is always taken, of course, not to transfuse blood with a positive Wassermann reaction indicating syphilis, or from a donor who has had viral hepatitis within the past year, or malaria.

In patients who require many transfusions over many months, there is danger of overloading the cells with iron (*hemosiderosis*). Methods of "unloading" iron under these circumstances will be invoked by the alert physician. Meticulous care in preparation of glassware or plastic bags used as containers in transfusion of blood will prevent so-called "pyrogenic" reactions which are due to bacterial products transmitted to the blood in transit. Since most transfusions are not direct from donor to patient, and the collected blood is rendered non-coagulable with sodium citrate, large numbers of transfusions in close succession raise the possibility that citrate intoxication of the recipient may occur.

Despite all of the possible difficulties that can happen, blood transfusions are truly lifesaving, and in actual practice serious reactions are exceedingly rare.

Blood donors. To healthy donors of blood for transfusion, may we say that, under ordinary circumstances, this is the best "tonic" you can possibly have for your own system. It was shown in World War II studies that the giving of blood stimulates the bone marrow as physical exercise stimulates the muscular system. A healthy man regenerates the first pint of blood he gives in approximately four weeks. If he then gives a second pint, he regenerates the same amount in three weeks, and if he then gives a third pint his bone marrow regenerates it in two weeks.

Every donor, therefore, is not only doing a priceless favor for an ill or injured patient, because in many cases there is no substitute for human blood, but he is doing himself a favor and actually strengthening his own blood-forming organs by "exercise."

THE ANEMIC STATES

It is probably safe to say that everyone is or will be anemic at some time during his or her life. *Anemia,* a lower than normal level of hemoglobin in the circulating blood, is the most common single objective finding in medical practice. Every physician must learn to identify the different mechanisms which cause anemia, and thereby be prepared to correct or eliminate the specific cause.

Iron Deficiency Anemia

The most commonly encountered anemia in the world today is iron deficiency anemia. It is a *hypochromic* anemia (red blood cells are paler than they should be).

There are two causative factors. First and most common is a nutritional deficiency of iron, most frequently encountered in the premature infant, the growing child and the pregnant woman. The second is chronic blood loss.

As the body grows in height and weight, or in pregnancy assumes the nurture of a parasitic fetus, an increasing volume of red blood cells is demanded, and need for additional iron and proper protein for the synthesis of hemoglobin increases. If sufficient iron is not available from food, or is not absorbed efficiently through the digestive tract, an iron deficiency occurs, with a decrease in the hemoglobin of each red blood cell. The cells may not be decreased in number, but the total volume of circulating hemoglobin—hence, of oxygen available to cells—is diminished. Under such circumstances, proper oral doses of medicinal iron of almost any type (the ferrous iron molecule is more effectively utilized) will correct the anemia very promptly.

Chronic blood loss may be quite unsuspected. A symptomless peptic ulcer, hemorrhoids which bleed only intermittently, excessive menstrual flow and other conditions may cause chronic blood loss and iron deficiency anemia. It is essential to detect and correct the cause of the blood loss, while providing iron supplements.

During the early years of life the normal hemoglobin values are identical for both sexes. But with the onset of menstruation in girls and until the menopause, hemoglobin levels of females average one to two grams lower than in males of the same age range (females, 12.6 grams; males, 13.6 to 14 grams). After the menopause there should be no significant difference. It is a medical axiom that in the adult male any hypochromic anemia must be due to chronic blood loss and the site of bleeding must be sought for until it is found.

Sometimes a patient cannot take oral iron because of distressing reactions such as gastric cramps or diarrhea. There are forms of iron that a physician may inject intravenously to bypass the gastrointestinal tract. This gets the iron directly to the bone marrow to furnish the intact blood-making machinery with material for restoring the normal hemoglobin level.

Recent intensive studies of iron metabolism in a number of laboratories have given quite complete knowledge of how iron is absorbed and utilized. The only excuse for iron deficiency anemia in our country today is the patient's unawareness of symptoms or failure to get proper treatment from a physician.

Symptoms. Any kind of anemia may be virtually symptomless or symptoms may be severe to the point of incapacitation. So insidious is the onset of anemia in many instances that the person may not be conscious of any significant change in strength or endurance; in others, symptoms appear early and increase.

Many persons who are not naturally rosy-cheeked, because they lack a rich network of capillaries near the skin surface, do not even recognize the characteristic pallor which is the commonest objective sign of anemia. And the universal use of cosmetics masks the developing pallor to the casual observer who ordinarily does not inspect the conjunctivae, gums and mucous membranes of the mouth where the physician makes his observations.

Many Spartan women adjust to a lowered hemoglobin level by sheer force of will and attribute their tiredness to excessive demands of home or job. They do not realize how much more they could do and how much better they would feel with more nearly normal hemoglobin levels to lift their energies.

Pallor and easy fatigability, then, are the commonest direct signs of anemia.

Indirectly, many vague aches and pains may derive from anemia. Excessive irritability and breath-holding episodes may mark the iron deficient infant. Sore skeletal muscles may arise from insufficient oxygen to meet the work load, and the heart muscle may protest with attacks of angina pectoris due to anemia rather than to coronary sclerosis and narrowing of vessels feeding the heart.

Only a discriminating physician can distinguish between simple iron deficiency anemia and the more serious and complicated anemias. A simple blood test may give the lead, and when indicated, a bone marrow examination with quantitative serum iron studies and indicated laboratory tests to rule out other possible complicating factors will confirm the diagnosis.

It pays to be *sure*. Do not accept a "therapeutic test" for iron deficiency anemia—that is, an iron-containing prescription or proprietary compound — before *proof* that all that is needed is iron. Precious days or weeks may be lost on self-medication by guesswork if anemia is due to one of many causes other than iron deficiency. Only the trained physician has the skill to recognize and treat these causes.

Caution. An overdose of iron, especially in children, is dangerous, even fatal. Keep all iron medications out of reach of children. Prolonged iron medication, or iron released from multiple long-continued blood transfusions, may lead to iron deposition *(hemosiderosis)* in the skin and some vital organs—heart, pancreas, liver, kidneys — with impairment of functions. This is known as *hemochromatosis*. The alert physician will recognize this tendency early and take steps to reverse it.

Pernicious Anemia

Giant red cells *(macrocytes)* are found in the blood in certain anemias. Each red cell appears to be overloaded with hemoglobin *(hyperchromic)* while the total red cell count is decreased. This is one of the characteristics of **pernicious anemia** — a name that once was all too descriptive, but now is retained only out of respect for tradition. As recently as 1925 this disease was invariably fatal; today the life expectancy of the properly treated "P. A." patient is about the same as that of the general population. However, it is simpler to continue to call the disease "pernicious anemia" than a "macrocytic, hyperchromic, megaloblastic anemia", and to leave these finer discriminations to the hematologists.

In sharp contrast to the small, pale, hemoglobin-deficient red blood cells of simple iron deficiency anemia, the few large cells in pernicious anemia are fully filled with hemoglobin and appear to be more highly colored *(hyperchromic)* than normal. Many bizarrely shaped red blood cells appear as the anemia becomes more severe, and there is an accompanying decrease in blood platelets and total white cells.

The life span of abnormal red cells in pernicious anemia is quite short. They are subject to easy dissolution and give up their hemoglobin (hemolysis) more readily. This breakdown results in an increase of pigments which frequently give a lemon yellow color to the skin. The urine also takes on a deeper coloration from excreted red cell breakdown products.

Basically, pernicious anemia results from failure of red blood cells to develop and mature normally. The disease occurs chiefly in later life, very rarely before the age of 30, and most commonly in the 50's and 60's. A direct study of the bone marrow usually confirms the diagnosis. Despite the scarcity of red cells in the blood, the bone marrow is packed with young so-called "megaloblastic" precursors of definitive red blood cells which fail to mature normally. These have many of the gross appearances of cancer cells; the yellow acellular fatty marrow of long bones is replaced by deep red, highly cellular tissue. In days when pernicious anemia was invariably fatal, pathologists mistakenly described the disease as a malignancy of the red cells of the bone marrow.

Symptoms. Pernicious anemia may first be present in three quite different symptom complexes.

(1) Most frequently there is an insidious increase of fatigue and weakness, with an anemic pallor which progresses to the typical lemon yellow color of the skin and mucous membranes. The tongue becomes smooth, red, and painful.

Or (2) the onset may be heralded first by gastrointestinal symptoms predominantly, more particularly, dyspepsia-like complaints of indigestion which reflect a beginning destruction of certain essential glands in the stomach wall.

Or (3) even before external signs of anemia appear, there may be evidences of early spinal cord degeneration. Deterioration of parts of the nervous system is manifested by incoordinated gait and gradual onset of numbness and tingling in the toes and fingers, spreading to the feet, hands, legs and arms. Impaired perception of pinpricks, light touch, heat and cold stimuli often develops in a "glove and stocking" distribution. Impotence occurs early and disturbances of bladder control are common. This is the most serious form of pernicious anemia. If the condition is recognized early and treated adequately, the neurological symptoms may be stopped and reversed.

Underlying mechanisms. What is wrong with the pernicious anemia patient's red blood cell producing centers? One of the great triumphs of modern medicine is knowledge of subtle chemical factors concerned with blood cell production and maturation and of treatments which have changed pernicious anemia from an invariably fatal disease to one that can be controlled with practically complete success.

Some 40 years ago, Dr. George Whipple was making pioneering studies of effects of various foods in stimulating hemoglobin production. His studies, done at the Hooper Institute in California, used dogs made anemic by chronic bleeding. Dr. Whipple found that liver was one of the best foods for stimulating hemoglobin regeneration in his anemic dogs.

In Boston, Dr. George Minot at the Peter Bent Brigham Hospital and Dr. Francis Peabody, Professor of Medicine at the Harvard Medical School's Thorndike Memorial Laboratory, were making intensive studies of human pernicious anemia, testing their patients with the dietary substances which Dr. Whipple's studies with dogs indicated might be helpful. Dr. Minot found that most of his patients would rather suffer from pernicious anemia than eat liver regularly in large daily amounts. Fortunately, there happened to be two patients who really liked liver well enough to consume the one-half pound prescribed daily, long enough to suggest that their pernicious anemia was being relieved.

By gradually ruling out other elements in the original liver-containing diets which might have caused the improvement, and by camouflaging the raw liver sufficiently to persuade other patients to ingest it, Dr. Minot with his medical hospital resident, Dr. Murphy, demonstrated that liver itself, and alone, could stimulate the stalled bone marrow blood factories in pernicious anemia patients to once again produce normal mature red cells in normal numbers. Harvard's famed biochemist, Edwin Cohn, was then called in and promptly isolated the "active fraction" from beef liver. Injectable and oral liver extracts soon freed pernicious anemia patients from the necessity of eating large unappetizing amounts of raw liver every day in order to live.

Meanwhile, Dr. William Castle, then a medical resident under Dr. Francis Peabody at the Thorndike Memorial Laboratory, Boston City Hospital, was studying the possible physiologic relationships of the stomach to pernicious anemia. Various symptoms of "indigestion," as we have indicated, are common in the disease. Typically, the pernicious anemia patient's stomach produces no free hydrochloric acid, and there are various degrees of atrophy and glandular inflammation in the stomach wall, as studied pathologically.

Dr. Castle found that ground beef digested by normal gastric juice, first in vivo and then in vitro, could also enable a pernicious anemia bone marrow to mature normal red cells. This *extrinsic factor,* obtained from an external source —(red muscle meat)—is now known to be Vitamin B_{12}, the most potent of all the known vitamins. Dr. Castle then hypothesized that an *intrinsic factor* is produced by normal stomachs, but insufficiently or not at all by the stomachs of pernicious anemia patients. The exact chemical formula of the "intrinsic factor" enzyme is still unknown, but its vital relationship to red blood cell production is perfectly clear.

Strictly speaking, a pernicious anemia patient does not suffer either from a lack of Vitamin B_{12} or from a primary blood cell disease. It is a gastrointestinal disease. An ordinary mixed diet normally provides ample amounts of the vitamin. Because of his atrophic gastritis, the pernicious anemia patient lacks enough of the "intrinsic factor" (digestive enzyme) to utilize the dietary Vitamin B_{12}, and the stores of the essential red cell "maturation factor" resulting from this interaction are gradually depleted from the liver. As the bone marrow becomes deprived of this stimulus, the symptoms and signs of pernicious anemia gradually appear.

Treatment. Injection of minute amounts of Vitamin B_{12} into a pernicious anemia patient brings one of the most immediate and dramatic responses in all medicine. The patient's subjective complaints change overnight. Gastric symptoms subside, the appetite returns, and a new sense of well-being is obvious within 24 hours. Objectively, the first laboratory sign is a sharp drop in circulating serum iron and within 12 hours arrested red cell elements in the bone marrow may be seen to have begun to mature. In seven to ten days, the bone marrow is changed from a congested and arrested "factory" to a normally productive one. Certain white cells which had been displaced by rapidly proliferating primitive red blood cells return to normal numbers and function. All minor neurological symptoms disappear, and major neurological manifestations will regress in direct proportion to their duration and severity.

An incredibly small amount of Vitamin B_{12} — one microgram, or about $1/28,000$ of an ounce a day — is often sufficient to keep a pernicious anemia patient in good health. In the average patient, injection of a readily determined maintenance dose of Vitamin B_{12} every four to eight weeks is sufficient to maintain normal red cell production, except under conditions of infection or unusual stress, when larger doses are needed. Much larger doses are required if the vitamin is given by mouth. Treatment must, of course, be continued for the rest of the patient's life, since Vitamin B_{12} does not "cure" the basic biochemical defect of insufficient intrinsic factor production, but effectively bypasses it.

Masking action of multi-vitamins. Folic acid, as part of the Vitamin B complex (see Chapter 14), has the same ability as Vitamin B_{12} to overcome the purely anemic symptoms of pernicious anemia.

Folic acid, however, is powerless to protect against the potentially serious effects of the disease on the central nervous system. Thus there is danger that if multiple vitamins including folic acid are taken without a physician's advice, as self-medication, the characteristic anemia may be masked and go unrecognized while neurologic degeneration progresses beyond a point of no return. Whenever the previously described neurologic symptoms appear, whether or not there are typical symptoms of anemia, it is very likely that pernicious anemia is in the background if not in the foreground, and immediate differential medical diagnosis is imperative.

Stomach cancer. There is a considerably higher incidence of stomach cancer in patients with pernicious anemia than in similar age groups in the general population. Evidently, atrophic degeneration of the stomach walls, characteristic of pernicious anemia, predisposes to the development of cancer. Once the diagnosis of pernicious anemia has been made, it is important that a barium x-ray study of the upper gastrointestinal tract be done at least every six months, symptoms or no symptoms. Stomach cancer may develop silently without early symptoms, and early detection is essential to surgical cure.

Other Macrocytic Anemias

Very rarely, a strict vegetarian or a person prevented by poverty or faddism from getting an adequate diet over a long period of time may develop an anemia resembling pernicious anemia but due solely to lack of extrinsic factor or Vitamin B_{12}. Such anemia is promptly corrected by providing the missing factor and instituting healthful eating habits.

A primary stomach cancer may so completely destroy or inhibit tissues which produce intrinsic factor that a macrocytic anemia will be the first sign of its presence.

Surgical removal of the stomach for peptic ulcer or cancer removes the major source of intrinsic factor, and if sooner or later a progressive macrocytic anemia develops, injections of Vitamin B_{12} are specific for its reversal.

Tropical sprue, or sprue in the temperate zone, are conditions of intestinal malabsorption which may imitate pernicious anemia but should be readily differentiated by the character of the stools and other characteristic symptoms.

A few years ago, *macrocytic megaloblastic anemia of infancy* was not uncommon in 9 to 12-month old infants fed on formulas lacking Vitamin C and B-complex vitamins. Vitamin B_{12} failed to correct this condition, which paralleled iron deficiency anemia in other babies of the same age raised on a milk formula without supplements. Folic acid plus Vitamin C proved to be specific for red cell maturation in this condition. This observation, together with the finding that an occasional pernicious anemia patient requires folic acid as well as Vitamin B_{12} for satisfactory red cell production, has proved that both vitamins are essential for the complete maturation of the red cells.

The outlook for patients with the above mentioned anemias, with the possible exception of gastric cancer, is now excellent. The group of macrocytic anemias has been discussed in some detail because relatively recent knowledge marks the first appreciation of the fact that a nutritional deficiency may simulate the cellular distortions of cancer, and may cause a progressively fatal disease not due to malignancy. These findings have initiated a new era in nutritional studies and a more hopeful approach to at least some others of the so-called malignant diseases.

Polycythemia

Polycythemia or erythrocytosis is a condition of too many red cells crowding the circulating blood. A *relative polycythemia* occurs when there is loss of plasma without comparable loss of blood cells, with a corresponding concentration of red cells.

Restricted fluid intake alone may lead in a few days to a decrease in plasma volume, or loss of water and electrolytes due to vomiting, diarrhea, excessive sweating, extensive burns or traumatic shock can lead to excessive plasma loss. Restoration of fluid balance with proper amounts of water and electrolytes promptly abolishes the relative polycythemia.

The red blood cell-forming mechanism in the bone marrow is very sensitive in its response to increased oxygen needs by the body. People who live at very high altitudes commonly have seven to eight million red cells per cu. mm. to compensate for the lowered oxygen saturation at those altitudes. There are also certain diseases (e.g., silicosis, emphysema, chronic fibrosing tuberculosis, some forms of congenital or acquired heart disease) that result in compensatory increases in red cells. Certain brain tumors and tumors of the kidney are regularly associated with polycythemia.

Primary polycythemia, or *polycythemia rubra vera* (too many red cells, true), is, we believe, an inherited chronic disease which involves an increase in all of the cellular elements of the bone marrow — red cells, granulocytes, and blood platelets. A careful family history and blood studies of blood relatives of patients with polycythemia vera will frequently show a familial pattern. In most of these patients the polycythemia does not follow the course of a malignant disease.

The *diagnosis* can usually be made just by looking at the patient, who characteristically shows marked redness of the skin, especially of the face and cheeks, with purplish lips (cyanosis) because of the high carbon dioxide content of the circulating blood, bluish nail beds, and purple coloring of the fingers.

The symptoms complained of are not different from those of extreme anemia. There is malaise, easy fatigability, often mental clouding with difficulty in thinking clearly, and it is a paradox that a patient with well-developed polycythemia rubra vera (PRV) may, in one and the same week, either suffer from a venous thrombosis or almost bleed to death. The thrombosis is understandable since many of these patients have four to five million circulating blood platelets instead of the normal 750,000 per cu. mm. It was not clear why such patients might bleed extensively from the gastrointestinal tract until the role of prothrombin or blood coagulation was discovered.

Prothrombin, a plasma factor essential for blood coagulation, is made from Vitamin K by the liver, and the vitamin must be absorbed through the gastrointestinal tract for liver processing. The characteristic cyanosis of mucous membrane of the lips and skin of PRV patients also exists throughout the intestinal tract and absorption of food substances is much less efficient. One of the first laboratory determinations to be made in a new patient with PRV is the plasma prothrombin level, and if this is low, an injection of Vitamin K (short-circuiting the gastrointestinal tract) will bring an increase in prothrombin in a few hours.

Treatment. Since we believe PRV to be an inborn trait and know of no acquired cause, treatment is approached from the standpoint of decreasing the number of circulating cells and slowing down their overproduction if possible. The obvious thing is to remove the surplus circulating red cell volume, and this can be done by venesection — "bloodletting." The absolute blood volume in PRV is often increased from the normal five quarts to seven or eight liters, and often as much as 75 per cent of the blood volume is comprised of cells, whereas the normal is around 45 per cent.

Combined with removal of blood is restriction of iron-containing foods, so that one may "starve" the bone marrow of iron necessary for the manufacture of hemoglobin. These measures, however, are only temporary and have no favorable influence on the elevated blood platelets and white cells.

In 1941, when *radioactive phosphorus* (P[32]) became available following the invention of the cyclotron by Ernest Lawrence, his physician brother, Dr. John Lawrence, and his medical associates, were able to show that P[32] is best for slowing down bone marrow over-activity in PRV. During the first year of artificial isotope production by the cyclotron, we in our clinic were permitted to share in early P^{32} studies and to begin treatment of PRV and other blood studies with radioactive phosphorus, which we have continued to the present day.

The half-life of P^{32} is approximately 14 days. It may be given intravenously or by mouth, and dosage can be controlled accurately without danger of depressive activity continuing too long, which was a disadvantage of longer-acting sources. The phosphorus is carried directly to participate in the calcium-phosphorus metabolism of the bones, where it very promptly and effectively suppresses all cell types to the extent controlled by the skilled physician. The only precaution is that one must not precipitate an anemia and a depression in the white cells beyond physiologic levels. Where radioactive isotopes are not available there are other chemotherapeutic suppressive agents that are effective. With our present understanding and methods, PRV is now almost as effectively and continuously controllable as pernicious anemia.

SPLENIC DISEASE

At birth the spleen, which previously had been almost the sole site of blood cell production, relinquishes this vital function to the bone marrow. If the bone marrow fails for one reason or another, the spleen may again become a blood-forming organ in later life.

The spleen has an abundant blood supply. It has a smooth muscle capsule and muscular bands which extend into the body of the organ and account for its contraction and relaxation. The unique vascular pattern of the spleen is conducive to reservoir-like containment of blood cells brought to it by the splenic artery. The organ is adapted to entrapment of old, senile red blood cells, preparatory to their dissolution with salvage of iron from hemoglobin for later resynthesis in the marrow. The human red cell has an average life span of 4 months,

which means that the entire red cell population of the body is completely renewed about three times a year.

A hormone secreting function has long been suspected but never proved for the spleen. There are no obvious ducts or groupings of secretory cells as in ductless endocrine glands (e. g., thyroid and pituitary), but there are large numbers of reticulo-endothelial *phagocytes* (engulfing, digesting cells) which conceivably might give rise to circulating hormones. These cells can avidly ingest damaged cells or foreign particles, and probably play a role, along with certain white cells, in formation and transport of antibodies important in mechanisms of immunity.

No function inherent in the spleen, however, is essential to either health or longevity. A person can live as healthily and as long without his spleen as with it. But it has been learned by costly experience that a disordered spleen may cause chronic invalidism or prove fatal in certain diseases if it is not removed.

Recently there has been new emphasis on the blood-forming role of the spleen. Animals exposed to otherwise lethal doses of total body irradiation survive longer if their spleens are shielded, apparently because of more rapid regeneration of blood-forming tissues in these marrows than in those animals whose spleens are not protected. The studies suggest that the spleen exerts some influence on blood formation and that life-saving repopulation of the bone marrow in emergencies may derive from it.

It is, then, to a clinically diverse but physiologically related group of diseases in which the spleen plays a major role that we shall now devote some attention.

The Hemolytic Anemias

Congenital hemolytic jaundice is an inherited condition resulting in production of small, globular, fragile red blood cells (microspherocytosis) by the bone marrow. Spherical red cells are less resistant to rupture and to normal wear and tear than normal red cells which are shaped like indented disks. This susceptibility to destruction with resultant escape of hemoglobin gives rise to the most prominent signs of the disease — jaundice and anemia.

From birth, the inherited trait results in a precarious balance of red cell production and destruction. The balance may be tipped toward destruction by the ordinary vicissitudes of life, or by mild stress such as a mild infection or simple fracture, which may precipitate a "hemolytic" crisis with an increase in jaundice and pallor. Under such circumstances, there is always a sharp increase in the percentage of young red cells recently delivered into the circulation.

The course of the disease may be (1) quiescent, symptomless, or (2) productive of chronic invalidism consonant with the degree of anemia, with or without pigment gallstones, or (3) an acute crisis may threaten life itself. Such spontaneous or secondarily precipitated crises are a constant threat to a person who has inherited this trait. For that reason, when the diagnosis is certain, it is advisable to elect to remove the spleen prophylactically during a time of quiescence rather than to undertake surgery during an acute crisis. The spleen is the principal site of red blood cell destruction in this disease, and its surgical removal *(splenectomy)* should cure. Through the years, splenectomy has been proved to be curative in a very real sense, and after more than 40 years of personal experience we have no hesitancy in urging it as the treatment of choice for congenital hemolytic anemia at any age when any degree of symptomatic activity has been demonstrated. Smaller accessory spleens are often found in these patients, and all splenic tissue must be discovered and removed by the surgeon if a relapse is to be avoided.

Chronic hemolytic anemia over a prolonged period will almost surely result in formation of pigment stones in the gallbladder. Thus, splenectomy not only controls the anemia but when performed early and promptly prevents the formation of this type of gallstone complication.

Acquired Hemolytic Anemia

Within the past decade, so-called *idiopathic acquired hemolytic anemia* has been shown to be closely associated with immunologic mechanisms. In many such cases, specific antibodies to the patient's red blood cells can be demonstrated. These *acquired* factors are in contrast to the inherited abnormalities of congenital hemolytic anemia. However, the two types of hemolytic anemia are not mutually exclusive. If the type of anemia is in doubt, blood relatives of the patient should be examined by appropriate laboratory tests. When there is no characteristic family history and there have been no recurrent episodes of hemolytic jaundice in the patient's history, the disease may be of the acquired type and immunologic studies are indicated.

Results of treatment show some degree of overlapping which may reflect incomplete differentiation of the two mechanisms or some superimposition of the acquired on the congenital type of hemolytic jaundice. Treatment with adrenal corticosteroids (cortisone et al.) is not recommended in the true congenital type, but may be of value in patients with the acquired type of the disease. The latter often, but not always, attain the same completely satisfying results from removal of the spleen as patients with the hereditary form of the disease virtually always do. When either splenectomy or steroid therapy alone fails, the other should be tried with hope of success.

Molecular Diseases of Blood (Hemoglobinopathies)

Hemoglobin is a marvelous molecule with a heart of iron. Its iron-containing part *(heme)* is smaller than the globin portion, which is a protein. Relatively simple chemical units known as amino acids (there are 22 different kinds) are linked together in precise sequences to form proteins. We can imagine a meaningful word spelled by a large number of letters. If a couple of letters are transposed, or a wrong letter used, the word is obviously misspelled. A similar seemingly trifling error in sequence of hundreds of amino acids does not produce a misspelled word but creates a unique molecule. It may closely resemble another molecule, but it will be subtly different. If the molecule is important to some body function, the seemingly trifling difference may be manifested as some form of disease. If so, it is truly a molecular disease, caused by a change in the structure of a molecule.

Just such hereditary "misspellings" of hemoglobin occur in some people. Linus Pauling, the Nobel prize-winning chemist, first demonstrated that such an error is responsible for a disease, sickle cell anemia. Many similar chemical errors, called *hemoglobinopathies*, have been identified. There have been more than 20 recognized at the present time. Most of them are designated by a letter of the alphabet, the current list extending from A through S inclusive. Only the usual A (adult) and F (fetal) hemoglobins are considered normal. Abnormal hemoglobins do not always cause frank disease. Sometimes they do, however, and the application of this modern knowledge has greatly enhanced our understanding of once mysterious blood disorders.

Sickle cell anemia occurs predominantly in the Negro race, although a few instances in Caucasians have been reported. Fortunately, only about two per cent of those who carry the trait develop a significant anemia.

The name of the disease reflects the tendency of these abnormal red blood cells to take sickle-shaped or oat-shaped forms, because of the distorting effect of the abnormal hemoglobin molecule. As the sickling increases, the blood becomes more viscous and the red cells more fragile, leading to hemolytic anemia, clogging of veins, and impairment of blood supply to many organs, including the lungs, central nervous system and long bones.

The course of the disease is punctuated by crises with fever and attacks of pain referred to the arms and legs, heart, or abdomen. Treatment of such crises must

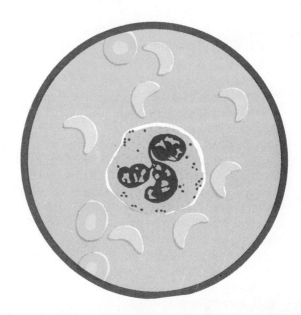

In sickle cell anemia, some of the red blood cells are sickle-shaped or oat-shaped instead of disk-shaped. This is due to distortion by an abnormal hemoglobin molecule that is hereditary. The white blood cell in the center contains no hemoglobin and is not affected.

be symptomatic, with or without oxygen administration or supportive fresh whole blood transfusions. It is important at times to recognize the underlying condition in these patients in order to avoid the implication that an emergency abdominal operation is necessary.

In childhood, there is often initial enlargement of the spleen in sickle cell anemia. This may be associated with a secondary hypersplenic syndrome in which splenectomy is definitely indicated. If the patient survives to adult life with repeated thromboses and fibrosis, the spleen shrinks greatly in size but crises nevertheless occur. These patients should avoid going to high altitudes or flying in airplanes without pressurized cabins.

Counseling and Screening for Sickle Cell Disease

Current public and private research efforts are under way to improve the treatment and recognition of sickle cell disease—a disease that is perfectly well understood but which is not presently curable because the inherited defect is hidden in the structure of hemoglobin molecules. About 2,500,000 black Americans carry the sickle cell *trait,* and can transmit it to offspring; only about one in 400 trait-carriers has frank sickle cell *anemia.*

Sickle cell disease is inherited recessively (see Chapter 25). That is, if only one parent has the trait, there is an even chance that each child born to them will or will not have the trait, but none will have anemia. If both parents carry the trait, for each child born to them, there is a 50 per cent chance that it will inherit only the trait, a 25 per cent chance that it will have sickle cell clinical anemia, and a 25 per cent chance that it will be entirely normal, with neither the trait nor the anemia.

Mass screening programs for sickle cell have been made feasible by several tests, especially of youngsters in school, with follow-up, if indicated, of blood relatives. Persons and families who have the trait but do not know it can be so informed. What to do about this knowledge is another matter. Affected persons can consult their own doctors, or seek genetic counseling, or do nothing. The predicament is the same as that posed by recessive genetic diseases such as cystic fibrosis: counselors can only explain the risks involved but cannot make or impose decisions.

Experimental treatments of painful sickle crises, not without potential hazards, give hope that better methods will become available. One treatment that has gained adherents, and raised questions, involves the intravenous infusion of a solution of urea in sugar, in the hope of breaking up log-jams of sickled cells that plug blood vessels. The treatment requires intensive care facilities, indwelling catheters, and skilled teams. In our own hands this treatment has not proved successful. The same precautions hold for a newly developed antisickling cyanate agent. Since crises generally abate with conservative supportive measures, benefits are hard to evaluate, and there is some doubt that medicines can actually reach the blocked sites. No known treatment can change the basic defect in the hemoglobin molecule. But in view of progress in "molecular engineering," who can say what effective treatments the future holds?

Thalassemia or *Mediterranean anemia,* or, as it is frequently called in this country, *Cooley's anemia,* derives its name from the fact that it occurs predominantly in the peoples bordering on the Mediterranean sea and their descendants elsewhere in the world. Like sickle cell anemia, it may occur either as a relatively symptomless trait, *Thalassemia minor,* or as a severe anemia, *Thalassemia major.*

In the major disorder, which is frequently fatal during childhood, the red cells are very small and very low in hemoglobin concentration. Usually both the spleen and liver are enlarged. Such patients may be benefited by splenectomy if a hypersplenic crisis is precipitated.

In general it may be said that splenectomy is beneficial, in theory and usually in practice, in all of the hemoglobinopathies whenever increased hemolytic action of the spleen is shown to exist.

Hemoglobinuria
(Hemoglobin in the Urine)

Paroxysmal nocturnal hemoglobinuria is a rare form of chronic hemolytic anemia. The patient's morning urine has a dark red appearance. The constant feature of the disorder is iron from the blood in the urine. The defect is in the red blood cell which is abnormally sensitive to a slight increase in acidity of its environment. Accumulation of dark red urine during the night is probably due to increased plasma acidity in areas of the circulation less active during sleep. Onset of the disorder is insidious and the course chronic. Splenectomy has not proved to be of any value.

Paroxysmal hemoglobinuria. The patient passes dark-colored urine transiently after exposure to cold during the winter months, or more rarely after strenuous exercise. The dark red or almost black urine contains hemoglobin, other substances, and sometimes intact red blood cells.

The paroxysmal attack comes on anywhere from a few minutes to 6 or 8 hours after the patient is chilled. The chilling may be surprisingly slight. There is headache, pain in the back and legs or abdomen, chills followed by fever of 104°F. or higher, blueness of the skin, and transient rise in blood pressure. A test shows that hemoglobin separates from the patient's blood when a sample is chilled in a test tube and subsequently warmed in a precise way. A history of syphilis and a positive Wassermann reaction point to the probable underlying cause. Specific anti-syphilis therapy has been reported to alleviate the symptoms.

In certain patients there is no history of syphilis and their blood does not hemolyze when tested as described above. At basis are auto-immune reactions, entirely unrelated to syphilis, which leave the red blood cells abnormally susceptible to physical or chemical injury.

Red Cell Enzymes

Manifestations of newly found hereditary deficiencies of the human red blood cell fall within the broad category of the hemolytic anemias. The red cell carries a quota of enzymes, which are protein molecules that catalyze farflung chemical processes of the body. Sometimes the red cell does not inherit a normal supply of enzymes. A few malaria patients develop hemolytic anemia after treatment with primaquine, an anti-malarial drug. They are said to be "primaquine sensitive."

The cause of this unusual reaction is now known. These patients have a deficiency of a specific red cell enzyme. No harm results unless primaquine or something else triggers a hemolytic anemia. Various other drugs — sulfonamides, some common pain relievers, and even the Fava bean, an ordinarily harmless food — have been shown to cause hemolytic reactions in persons who lack a protective enzyme because of their inherited constitutional makeup. In addition, infectious hepatitis, infectious mononucleosis, and certain bacterial pneumonias and viral infections of the upper respiratory tract seem to take advantage of the enzyme deficiency to produce an hemolytic anemia.

Certain other relations of specific enzyme deficiencies to various disorders are being elucidated. We may expect additional revelations in this field, which is a relatively new area of research. Only the alert physician trained to recognize the varied mechanisms which underlie the hemolytic anemias will be able to identify the several entities and prescribe appropriate treatment.

Purpura
(Purple Patches in Skin and Mucous Membranes)

Blood platelets or *thrombocytes* are essential for normal coagulation of blood, as when we cut or scratch ourselves. They are present in normal blood in numbers ranging from 700,000 to 1,000,000 per cubic millimeter. Platelets are small fragments of mother cells in the bone marrow known as *megakaryocytes*. If for any reason there are fewer than 50,000 platelets per cubic millimeter, evidence of bleeding from tiny blood vessels may appear in the skin and mucous membranes. A general term for such bleeding is *purpura.*

Small hemorrhages may occur spontaneously as well as after mild injury. Tiny pinpoint hemorrhages (*petechiae*), larger purplish patches in and beneath the skin, or "black and blue" spots are warnings to seek the cause of bleeding. If these painless signs are ignored, bleeding gums, prolonged nosebleeds, or severe urinary or gastrointestinal hemorrhages or prolonged menses may follow.

At the first appearance of these signs the patient should consult his physician. Blood studies should be made. If normal blood platelets are present in normal quantity, then other mechanisms of abnormal bleeding such as Vitamin C or K deficiency or toxic hemorrhagic infections may be identified and treated.

Our present chief concern, however, is with bleeding which does reflect a great reduction in numbers of circulating blood platelets. When this is the case, the next step is a careful study of the bone marrow (readily obtained by needle aspiration from the breastbone or backbone) to determine whether "mother" megakaryocytes in the marrow are capable of producing normal populations of platelets.

Idiopathic thrombocytopenic purpura is a formidable term which means bleedings occurring with deficiency of platelets from unknown causes. We shall considerately refer to it hereafter as ITP. Most times the causes can be discovered and corrected.

Many industrial chemicals and a number of important drugs may be toxic to the mother cells in the bone marrow of susceptible persons. Just as some people react differently to foods or pollens, so do some react differently to drugs and chemicals which most persons tolerate without difficulty. Effects of toxic influences which interfere with normal production of blood platelets can readily be seen by direct microscopic studies of living marrow cells. Usually the toxic agent can be identified by a physician who knows which substances are most likely to cause marrow damage and who by careful analysis of the patient's history and exposures can track down the probable offenders and eliminate them.

On the other hand, if the bone marrow shows an increase in numbers and activity of platelet-producing cells without parallel increase of platelets in the blood, but rather a continuing severe deficit, the possibility of abnormal screening-out and pathologic destruction of platelets by the spleen is immediately suggested. Platelets are so tiny that the spleen is not grossly enlarged by their excessive accumulation, so absence of an enlarged spleen does not exclude the incrimination of this organ in ITP.

One of the most dangerous crises to face any physician is uncontrolled and uncontrollable bleeding. Transfusions of fresh whole blood or platelet suspensions can only be temporarily effective. The precise mechanism underlying such a purpuric catastrophe must be established at the earliest possible moment, as only the specific remedy can be ultimately lifesaving.

ITP in childhood is often acute and self-limited. Bleeding from membranes of the mouth is common. History of a recent viral infection, in children especially, may point toward a toxic delayed-action depression of marrow cells, readily established by direct microscopic observation. This demands supportive whole blood transfusions while efforts to demonstrate an autoimmune basis—reaction of the body's own cells to foreign substances—are made. Corticosteroid drugs should also be started immediately and spontaneous recovery may be expected, beginning within a few hours to a few days, if it is a true autoimmune reaction. Should discontinuance of the drugs be followed by a return relapse with again a dangerous decrease in platelets, and the marrow still shows an increase of megakaryocytes, splenectomy is definitely indicated.

In our experience, ITP on the basis of autoimmune mechanisms is more likely to occur in children below teenage. In such instances it may be that there is an inborn instability of the spleen, so that spontaneously, or from some minor stress, the organ suddenly begins to withhold platelets from the circulation although platelets are being delivered from the marrow in abundance. Another theory is that hypothetical inhibiting substances from the spleen suppress the delivery of platelets from the marrow and that a failure of central delivery is responsible for symptoms.

Supporting the concept that the spleen plays a major role in the usual case of ITP is the amazing rapidity with which the platelets return to the circulation as soon as the surgeon interrupts the spleen's activity by tying off the splenic artery.

Expert bone marrow interpretation is the key to differential diagnosis and treatment of both chronic and acute thrombocytopenic purpuric crises. As soon as all relevant factors can be analyzed and the diagnosis confirmed, immediate emergency splenectomy is as necessary to survival as is an emergency appendectomy to avert a threatened rupture and peritonitis.

The term *hypersplenism* suggests an excessive increase in the destructive processes of the spleen. If the spleen is definitely enlarged in a case otherwise suggestive of ITP, the possibility of a *secondary* hypersplenic mechanism is to be suspected. If confirmed, splenectomy is desirable and even necessary in such patients, and the hematologic response will be as prompt and permanent as in a *primary* hypersplenic purpura. Not infrequently, when the spleen is removed for an apparent hypersplenic ITP, an unsuspected disease — splenic tuberculosis, sarcoidosis, Hodgkin's disease, and others—is discovered, and specific treatment can be begun for the underlying disease not previously recognized.

Will removal of the spleen endanger the patient's future health and longevity? A confident answer "no" can be given. British Lord Dawson of Penn made long-term studies of patients whose spleens had been removed for congenital hemolytic anemia and who fought through the trenches in World War I without less strength or greater susceptibility to infection or wound complications than their comrades. We have followed patients whose normal spleens have been removed after traumatic rupture, for ITP and other hypersplenic states since 1930, without finding any evidence of heightened susceptibility to infections or interference with normal health and longevity, or of any handicap to normal growth and development in children.

Other "Bleeding Diseases"

Hemophilia is the best known of the hereditary "bleeding" disorders. It is no longer so utterly hopeless a disease as it once was thought to be, although the defect in clotting ability of the blood is permanent and the patient must learn to live with it and adapt his activities to his inborn handicap.

Classic hemophilia is the result of varying degrees of deficiency of a constituent of blood plasma which has an essential role in the very complicated processes of blood coagulation. The substance is called *anti-hemophilic factor* or *AHF*. In the numbering system of blood clotting factors, it is Factor VIII. Inability to produce this factor, or not enough of it, is passed on by female carriers who themselves do not have symptoms but transmit the disease to male descendants.

There is remarkable variability in bleeding tendencies of hemophiliacs. In some patients the condition is only troublesome when a tooth must be extracted or some fairly severe wound is suffered. Other patients are so acutely sensitive that they cannot walk across the floor without getting joint hemorrhages. They may develop crippling joint deformities and be confined to a wheelchair.

Treatment is important and should be given in a hospital, however minor the cut or accident, since recurrent delayed bleeding is common and may be difficult to control. Appropriate coagulation tests evaluate the activity of AHF which not only varies from person to person but in the same person from time to time.

Only fresh whole blood, fresh plasma, freshly freeze-dried or freshly frozen plasma furnish the deficient anti-hemophilic factor. Intravenous administration must be continued every one to three days until healing is complete. Even in males with a minor inheritance of the defect, careful and prolonged administration of AHF is necessary in preparation for and after major surgery.

Many efforts have been and are being made to obtain potent AHF concentrates, for preventive as well as therapeutic uses, but none have been successful to date. This is because AHF potency begins to diminish as soon as blood which contains it is drawn from the circulation. Apparently the factor is not stored in the body and must be manufactured continuously by each of us for ourselves. It has not been possible to make the hemophiliac's body produce the deficient factor and the physician cannot build up a reserve for the future in the patient.

Care of hemophilic infants and children taxes the emotional and financial resources of parents and it is important that the family as well as the patient learn to live with the disease. Babies who inherit the trait gradually learn to avoid bumps and bruises as they grow up. A prolonged session or two in a hospital teaches the important lesson — *prevention!*

Parents should do all within reason to safeguard their small hemophilic boy. The sides of the child's bed, playpen, or high chair should be padded. Toys should be soft, without sharp edges or parts. Finger and toenails should be trimmed carefully. Be watchful to keep cutlery and objects the child might pull onto himself out of his reach.

There is reason to hope that a potent AHF concentrate may eventually be developed as the ultimate goal in treatment. In the meantime it is important to follow the advice of a specialist in handling unavoidable complications which hang over heads of these patients.

Christmas disease is named not for the season but after the family in which it was first discovered. It is also called Hemophilia B. Symptoms are indistinguishable from classic hemophilia, but are caused by hereditary deficiency of a different blood clotting element, Factor IX. It is unlike hemophilia in two important respects: (1) Some of the female carriers may themselves have a mild bleeding tendency. (2) Factor IX, unlike Factor VIII, is relatively stable in stored blood which therefore may be used effectively in treating bleeding episodes.

Pseudo-Hemophilia Type B is a rare familial bleeding disorder. In addition to deficient AHF, there is prolonged bleeding time not seen in hemophilia. This disease occurs as frequently in women as in men. Prolonged vaginal bleeding is the common complaint in women. Fresh whole blood is essential in treatment, since AHF will not correct the prolonged bleeding time.

Hypo-Afibrogenemia. Plasma factors essential for blood coagulation have been numbered from I to XII, and doubtless more will be added. Factor I is *fibrinogen,* which derives from the liver and forms the solid fibrin clot which seals the break in a damaged blood vessel. There are two kinds of Factor I deficiencies. *Congenital afibrogenemia* is a rare hereditary condition best treated with the specific plasma fraction I. *Acquired hypofibrinogenemia* may be precipitated by certain complications of pregnancy, incompatible transfusions, or by metastases of malignant disease. Treatment is by intravenous fibrinogen or fresh whole blood.

Another plasma constituent having an influence on blood coagulation is *plasminogen.* If this factor is high, fibrin dissolution may occur so rapidly that there is no apparent fibrin clot at all. Chemical inhibitors are available to decrease the plasminogen, and intravenous fibrinogen may restore this essential.

Neutropenia

Of the 5,000 to 10,000 white cells per cubic millimeter which normally circulate in the blood as mobile defense forces, about 70 per cent are so-called neutrophilic granulocytes.

In ***primary splenic neutropenia*** (-penia: poor, want), no other disease entity can be found. The bone marrow shows hyperactivity for granulopoiesis. Symptoms are those of chronic invalidism, chronic recurring infection, weakness and general feeling of illness. Removal of the enlarged spleen brings immediate recovery of the granulocytes to normal, chronic ulcerations heal, foci of infection clear up and a normal state of health returns.

Cyclic neutropenia is a periodic decrease of neutrophilic granulocytes in the circulating blood. There are more or less regular spontaneous recurring relapses and recoveries. During each relapse there develops a sore tongue and sore mouth, with flareups of chronic sinusitis, otitis, fever, and general malaise. These symptoms are relieved only when the granulocytes spontaneously return to normal, but recur again in a periodic cycle of approximately 20 to 30 days. Apparently this is a congenital condition reflecting some disturbed fundamental inherent regulatory mechanism of the individual. Splenectomy has not stopped the cyclic activity, but after removal of the spleen the cycling granulocytes do not fall to quite such critically low levels as before and the patient remains essentially free of symptoms.

So-called *Banti's syndrome* is associated with chronic liver damage resulting in cirrhosis. The secondarily congested enlarged spleen chiefly filters out the white blood cells and occasionally there is a mild hemolytic anemia. Removal of the spleen releases the granulocyte levels and tends to remove the danger of hemorrhage from the venous congestion in the stomach wall and along the esophagus. Early diagnosis and prompt operative interference are advisable because of the perisplenitis with dense adhesions which develops later and renders surgery dangerous if not impossible.

In *Felty's syndrome* there occurs chronic infectious arthritis, enlargement of the spleen, and a Banti-like decrease of granulocytes but without any liver damage. Removal of the enlarged spleen restores the granulocytes to normal. In approximately 50 per cent of the patients with this syndrome, symptoms of progressive and recurrent infectious arthritis are either ameliorated or completely eliminated, but it is not presently possible to predict which half. All experience better general health.

In none of the described neutropenic states has treatment with corticosteroid drugs been effective in eliminating the granulocyte deficit. Only splenectomy has been able to correct the underlying mechanisms and symptoms up to the present time.

Panhematopenia

One might suspect that if an unstable spleen can selectively screen out and destroy the specific types of formed elements of the blood, it might at times also attack and withhold all of the circulating bone marrow elements indiscriminately. Such a syndrome was first observed in an infant girl, resulting in chronic invalidism and diagnosis of hypoplastic anemia. Removal of the spleen after finding an intact, actively functioning bone marrow was followed by complete restoration of all normal circulating blood elements and complete clinical recovery. No other primary disease was found or developed in the patient in subsequent years.

Cases of secondary *hypersplenic panhematopenia* occur with a variety of diseases which involve the spleen and trigger a sieving mechanism which withholds all or practically all of the cells deriving from the bone marrow and brought to it. Splenectomy is curative insofar as the decreased cell count is concerned, while the primary disease is recognized and specific treatment instituted.

Diagnostic Procedures

The careful study of interreactions of spleen and bone marrow is vital in understanding the group of diseases involving either or both organs. At the same time, autoimmune reactions which may simulate the hypersplenic cell-withholding and destroying mechanisms must be differentiated.

The spleen lies in the abdominal cavity high up under the diaphragm on the left side behind the ribs and is in direct contact with the stomach and pancreas gland. While ordinarily not palpable, if the spleen becomes enlarged to twice or more its normal size (by weight, ten ounces plus), its tip frequently may be felt by the examiner, with characteristic notch and downward movement on deep respiration. In disease conditions the spleen may become enormously enlarged, filling the entire abdomen and weighing as much as 10 pounds or more.

If microscopic and laboratory studies of blood and bone marrow fail to give sufficient evidence, a direct sample of spleen tissue may be obtained by aspirating the organ with a hollow needle. This can be done safely because the enlarged spleen lies directly under the surface of the abdomen and the nearby stomach and intestines are displaced.

Blood vessel patterns may be studied

by injecting opaque substances directly into the body of the spleen and taking immediate x-rays. This is particularly useful in determining the position of any vascular obstructions, and the arrangement of splenic veins prior to certain operative procedures, especially if any "shunting" of the circulation is contemplated.

In progressive *myelofibrosis* of the bone marrow the blood cell-forming areas are gradually replaced by fibrous tissue. In most instances the spleen enlarges, and it is important to know whether the spleen itself is involved in the fibrotic process or whether it is resuming its embryonic function of blood cell production. In this disease it is often necessary to obtain a bone marrow sample by a surgical procedure when needle aspiration fails. This, with other indicated tests, helps the hematologist to decide the relative role of the spleen in any given patient and whether splenectomy will be beneficial. In properly selected patients, removal of the spleen will greatly relieve increasing discomfort from the enlarging tumor and increase the blood cell survival time, thus prolonging life more comfortably without weekly blood transfusions which otherwise might be required for many months and even years.

THE LEUKEMIC STATES

The word **leukemia** creates a picture of imminent physical disaster in the minds of many people, including doctors. It is true that leukemia, like many other diseased states, may progress to a fatal termination sooner or later. But, as is also true of so many other diseases now, there are increasing numbers of patients with this disturbance in the white cell equilibrium who live many years and die of unrelated superimposed diseases.

Just what is a "dangerous disease"? It is more and more impossible to generalize in this regard, because of the wide variation in resistance of human beings and their ability to respond to the variety of chemotherapeutic and antibiotic agents which we are finding to be more or less specific for different diseases. Any individual whose life is threatened with a fatal outcome has a "dangerous disease" for him. This is not necessarily true for other members of his family or community. Coronary heart disease, chronic nephritis, hepatic cirrhosis, diabetes, are all diseases with which some people live and from which others die prematurely. So it is with the leukemias. A physician who is an expert in the rapidly growing knowledge of the cause and control of these diseases may definitely influence favorably their otherwise progressive course.

Acute and chronic leukemias. It has been customary to divide the leukemic states into the *acute* and *chronic* leukemias. The terms were originally descriptive of the clinical course of the disease, the "acute" frequently having an onset similar to an acute infection (developing most frequently in children) with a fatal outcome in four to eight weeks. On the contrary, "chronic" leukemia characteristically has an insidious onset, occurs in middle and later life, and may remain quiescent or progress very slowly over a period of months and years before symptoms develop which interfere with the normal life of the individual.

While it is true that we do not yet know the basic causes of these widely varying disturbances in the normal equilibrium of the white cells, research is leading closer to those factors which either cause these changes or lower an individual's resistance to them. Fully as great progress has been made in the variety and specificity of drugs and other agents which may be used to alter, and in many cases, stop the progress of the leukemias, as in the control of any other group of diseases — notably, the yielding of bacterial infections to current chemotherapeutic and antibiotic agents.

Thus the term "leukemia" does not necessarily carry the same fatal connotation as formerly, any more than "pernicious anemia" any longer connotes an invariably fatal progressive red blood cell disease.

THE CHRONIC LEUKEMIAS

Any of the individual kinds of white blood and connective tissue cells may occur in pathologic excess without involving any of the others. The most commonly encountered leukemic disturbance involves the *lymphocytes* (50 per cent), and of these **lymphatic leukemias,** approximately 50 per cent are chronic and 50 per cent acute.

A relatively benign, chronic, symptomless *lymphocytosis* (excess of normal lymphocytes in the blood) is the most common finding in individuals, beginning in the late fifties and extending through the sixth and seventh decades of life. Fortunately, this is the easiest of all the leukemias to control for long periods of time. In the absence of symp-

toms and without any embarrassment of function of bone marrow or other nearby vital organs, no treatment may be necessary for months or years.

The physician who finds a mild elevation in the lymphocytes in circulating blood will know that sooner or later the tempo may increase. Watchful waiting and periodic blood and physical examinations of the patient are indicated, to determine if and when specific therapy may be needed. But in the absence of pathological manifestations, it is important not to label this stage "leukemia," but rather to describe it simply as "chronic lymphocytosis." It is important psychologically never to apply the term "leukemia" to a patient where there is no clear-cut evidence of progressive disease with objective symptoms.

In addition to a possible slowly developing anemia and decrease in blood platelets, when the bone marrow is invaded in chronic lymphatic leukemia, there may develop early or late enlargement

The most common leukemic disturbance, *lymphatic leukemia,* involves the lymphocytes. At left below, a smear of normal blood with a normal granulocyte (1) and a normal lymphocyte (2). At right, excess numbers of lymphocytes with large nuclei. A chronic *lymphocytosis* (excess of normal lymphocytes in the blood) is the easiest of all the leukemias to control for long periods of time.

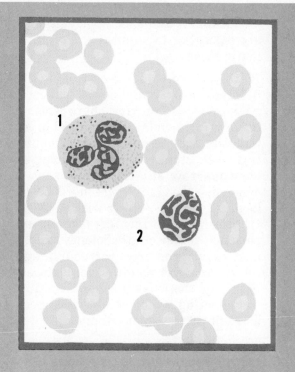
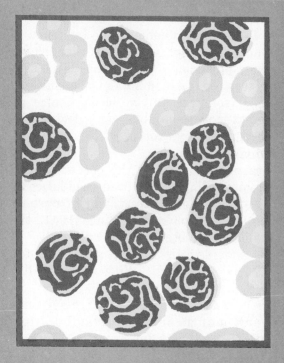

of the regional lymph nodes and/or spleen. These are the classical sites for development of the lymphocytes. Increase in lymphocyte production with swelling of lymph nodes may also occur without any change in the circulating blood cells.

More frequently, however, when a patient notices any peripheral lymph node swelling or discovers a solid mass in the upper left quadrant of his abdomen, a look at the peripheral blood will reveal an increase in the lymphocytes but they will still be small, qualitatively normal, mature lymphocytes. A bone marrow study by direct aspiration will reveal the degree, if any, of lymphocyte infiltration of the marrow with displacement of red cell and platelet formation.

In older men with benign enlargement of the *prostate gland,* who have a concomitant chronic lymphocytic leukemia, specific treatment for the leukemia should be instituted before considering urologic surgery. Asymptomatic infiltration of the prostate gland with lymphocytes in lymphatic leukemia is not uncommon. In such cases, specific treatment will generally reduce the size of the prostate gland and therefore the urinary symptoms.

Treatment. Whenever the tendency to abnormal lymphocytosis is recognized, many physicians prefer the patient to be seen by an hematologic consultant, who, from the fairly broad choice of agents now available, will decide the treatment program best fitted for the individual patient.

Since the turn of the century, deep x-ray irradiation has been used successfully in the initial treatment of chronic lymphocytic leukemia. Since 1941, the radioactive isotope of phosphorus, P^{32}, has provided an internal substitute for external radiation. With its half life of approximately 14 days, this *radioactive phosphorus* may be given once every month or two to ambulatory patients, without interruption of their daily routine.

With either x-ray or cobalt bomb therapy a course of daily treatments is necessary. This may require hospitalization, with more or less severe side reactions, with temporary interference of the patient's occupation. The oral nitrogen mustards may be given but this means taking pills daily, which may lead to forgetfulness or a state of fear and invalidism.

Complications. There are several complications to be kept in mind in chronic lymphatic leukemia:

1. Fifty per cent or slightly more of such patients show a lowering of the antibody globulins, and if the granulocytes are also reduced in absolute number, there may be increased susceptibility to infections. When acute infections develop they should not only be treated promptly with the indicated chemotherapeutic agent, but also with gamma globulin.

2. Herpes zoster *(shingles),* a painful virus disease of the sensory nerve sheaths, seems to have a higher incidence in chronic lymphatic leukemia patients. Shingles is a self-limited disease, but requires great patience on the part of both the patient and the physician. More specific treatments are emerging to supplement symptomatic measures.

3. If the spleen becomes prominently involved in the lymphocytic leukemia process, a secondary hypersplenic hemolytic anemia or depression of platelets may be precipitated, requiring splenectomy when confirmed by bone marrow studies. When such a syndrome develops there need be no hesitancy in proceeding with surgery. In some 35 such instances in our experience, the specific deficiency of cells has been promptly corrected, and there has never followed any exacerbation of the leukemia nor any later complication which might have been a result of the splenectomy.

4. There is always the potential danger of a "packed bone marrow" with infiltrative lymphocytes. Prevention is

worth many pounds of cure! At the very first sign of marrow embarrassment, P³² or an oral nitrogen mustard compound should be used. A course of deep x-ray to the flat bones, or intravenous nitrogen mustard, may be necessary in far advanced cases.

Chronic lymphocytic leukemia, then, is the type of leukemia to choose if you have the choice, and you will have better than a fifty-fifty chance of continuing to live a useful life with this disease and not to die from it.

Chronic Myelogenous Leukemia

The myeloid cells of the bone marrow may either be involved singly or the three types (neutrophils, basophils, and eosinophils) may be jointly involved, along with the megakaryocytes, in a chronic bone marrow hyperplasia (abnormal multiplication of cells). The lymph nodes are not usually involved in this condition, but the spleen becomes enlarged early — in some patients it fills the entire left side of the abdomen — and may be the first sign. A secondary anemia will arise if the developing red cells in the bone marrow are sufficiently displaced.

Characteristically, *in chronic myelogenous leukemia,* the cells are relatively mature, with only a small percentage of very young "blast" cells to be found in blood and bone marrow. The spleen, being a reservoir for bone marrow elements, tends to become engorged with excess white cells resulting from overproduction from the bone marrow.

Treatment. Once again, we have an increasing number of therapeutic agents which are helpful. X-ray irradiation is the time-honored method of reducing the enlarged spleen and in most cases is still the best initial treatment when the spleen is excessively enlarged. Along with reduction in size of the spleen there is a diminution in the production of cells from the bone marrow. At times, a remission may be induced by direct irradiation over the spleen which will last months and even as long as three years, without

further treatment. Once the spleen has been sufficiently reduced, we like to change to radioactive phosphorous P³², which with small oral doses every four to eight weeks will hold the hyperplastic tendency in check indefinitely.

New chemotherapeutic agents are finding a useful place in the treatment of this as in the other leukemic states. Some are more effective in one type of leukemia than in another, and at different times in the same patient. Several of the purines (for example, *6-mercaptopurine)* have been found effective, as well as *busulfan* (Myleran), an alkylating agent. There are other agents such as *ethyl carbamate* (urethane) and *demecolcin* (a colchicine derivative) which in special circumstances may be used effectively. Duration of control currently with the usual initial agents ranges from two to seven years, rarely longer.

It is, however, the continuing advice of the physician-hematologist which must be followed if maximum benefits are to be obtained for the individual patient during the prolonged course of this chronic disease.

Unlike chronic lymphocytic leukemia, which seldom if ever changes to more acute forms, chronic myelogenous leukemia characteristically evolves sooner or later into the subacute or acute *myeloblastic* phase (proliferation of cells from which the myelocytes develop). We are not certain why this basic change in the maturation of the cells occurs. But when this change does occur in the peripheral blood, reflecting a sudden bone marrow predominance of myeloblasts, there is usually a sharp change in the clinical condition of the patient. A reversal of the previously high platelet level allows bleeding manifestations to develop, secondary infections reflect the marked immaturity of the granulocytes, fever and malaise develop, and the patient for the first time feels ill.

The treatment of this phase demands a prompt change in medication, and we are just beginning to get new chemical agents which will handle this otherwise critical emergency. The purines, of which there are three different molecular structures available as this is written, are the most important of these newer agents now available. Another newer agent known as *vincoleucoblastine,* derived from the periwinkle plant, has proved effective in some instances.

This field of therapy is changing so rapidly that no published volume can keep up with the speed of development of new and hopefully better agents. The discerning family and the intelligent patient will seek the best possible current advice in centers of hematologic specialization. This will give the only assurance that every possible therapeutic measure will be made available to the patient as soon as it is approved for clinical use.

I have said that chronic myelogenous leukemia characteristically evolves into more acute phases. Approximately 85 per cent of patients developing this disturbance begin with *chronic* cellular changes, and therefore may be assured months and years of normal activity. Only some 15 per cent first present with the full-blown *acute* clinical picture which requires, at once, the best and latest highly specialized drugs. The cells in this phase are not unlike the megaloblasts in pernicious anemia, which can regularly be matured with Vitamin B_{12}. When we know as much about the maturation requirements of the myeloblast as we now do about the megaloblasts, it is to be hoped that maturation factors similar to Vitamins B_{12} may be found for the myeloblasts.

Other varieties. A relatively rare variety of myelogenous leukemia is *chloroma,* characterized by an invasive tumor-like greenish growth in various organs and tissues, including the marrow. The treatment is that of acute myelogenous leukemia.

There is a third myeloid abnormality, *acute myeloblast-sarcoma*—a true malignant change which must be studied as other neoplastic diseases are being studied with hope of ultimate control. It is this third form of myeloid leukemia which is hardest to control, but very recently new drugs (as Cytosar) which give real promise of controlling even this

phase of the disease have begun to emerge from the laboratory. All too brief remissions have been accomplished with some of these agents, but they have been remissions in which the patient has returned to normal health and activity. It is to learn how to prolong these remissions that the intensive research of many laboratories is being directed today.

Monocytic Leukemia

The large *mononuclear* or *monocyte* is the third of the major white cell groups represented in the peripheral blood. These cells are direct derivatives of the diffuse connective tissues throughout the body. They have no primary source in the bone marrow, with minimal generation in the lymph nodes and somewhat more often in the spleen.

These cells have a high phagocytic (ingesting) capacity. The monocyte can substitute defensively for the neutrophilic granulocytes when the latter for any reason become dangerously diminished. If the cause for depression of the granulocytes does not at the same time depress the basic origin of the monocytes, there is a compensatory increase in monocytes which may prevent overwhelming infection until the granulocytes can recover.

In *tuberculosis,* the prominent epithelioid cells making up the center of the typical tubercle are altered monocytes. The stimulated monocytes overflow into the blood at the expense of the lymphocytes. The normal circulation ratio of lymphocytes to monocytes is three to one. A ratio higher in lymphocytes means increased cellular resistance; the reverse reflects progressive tuberculous lesions.

Acute monocytic leukemia is more common than the chronic form. Usually the patient has minimal lymph node enlargement, and only rarely an enlarged spleen. A dentist may be the first to see these patients because of bleeding and hyperplastic gums, attributed by the patient to pyorrhea and neglected mouth hygiene. Immediate blood studies are indicated before any dental manipulation and before the underlying platelet deficiency results in more serious bleeding problems, including a not impossible cerebral hemorrhage.

The purines have been found to be helpful in a number of patients with the more acute monoblastic leukemias, but corticosteroids should be used with extreme care, if at all. In at least some instances these derivatives of the adrenal gland seem to accentuate the process. In all of the acute leukemias, supportive fresh whole blood transfusions and antibiotic therapy, to control hemorrhage and infection, are essential while "buying time" for the more specific drugs to work.

Fortunately, very few leukemias of any type are associated with pain. The critical level of the various cell types is fortunately very low, so that except for weakness from the anemia and occasional deep bone pain from pressure of invading cells, the leukemias are relatively asymptomatic. Radioactive phosphorus is dramatically effective in relieving the deep bone pain caused by endosteal pressures, and the radioactive agent should be used promptly to give comfort when the need indicates.

Chronic monocytic leukemia is as readily managed as chronic myelogenous or chronic lymphocytic anemia. It may follow a very benign course for months, even years, with few or no subjective symptoms. Here the physician's discriminating knowledge may be very reassuring to the patient, because the chronic phase of monocytic leukemia is not so likely to metamorphose into an acute phase as is the chronic myelogenous type. Treatment is symptomatic until and unless the monocytes impinge upon vital functions of other organs, particularly the bone marrow, in which case suppressive agents are usually effective.

At times, chronic monocytic leukemia may be confused with chronic Hodgkin's disease (see page 170). In some cases, chronic Hodgkin's disease, with lymph node pathology indistinguishable from chronic monocytic leukemia, may terminate as an acute monoblastic leukemia.

THE ACUTE LEUKEMIAS

In describing the chronic leukemias we have mentioned the circumstances under which certain of the acute leukemic phases develop. We have also mentioned that acute leukemia is encountered much more often in youth than in maturity or old age.

Fully 90 per cent of all the acute leukemias of childhood involve the *lymphocytic* cells, and almost all of them show a true neoplastic sarcomatous (malignant) change in the lymphocytes. The incidence rises rapidly after one year of age, reaches a peak during the third year of life, and drops sharply. The lowest incidence of both acute and chronic leukemia is from ten years of age through the teen age period.

Lymphosarcoma usually strikes suddenly in a previously healthy child. The symptoms are those of an acute infection, with or without hemorrhage, with or without generalized lymph node enlargement or enlarged spleen. There is fever, loss of appetite, sore throat, anemia, deep bone pain (often interpreted as rheumatic fever), with joint involvement or aching muscles.

Only the internal organs and tissues may be involved, with no evidence of lymphosarcoma cells in the circulating blood. In this instance, a bone marrow and/or lymph node biopsy must be obtained to make the diagnosis. More frequently than not, typical lymphosarcoma cells may be seen in the circulating blood. To see and to identify *one* typical lymphosarcoma cell is to make the diagnosis.

This is a disease which may start in any organ of the body, including any lymph node. The disease spreads from a single local focus to other areas of the body via blood or lymphatic channels. Symptoms vary widely, according to the organ or organs involved. When the bone marrow is primarily involved, progressive anemia with pallor and weakness develop as the sarcoma cells displace red blood cell formation. If the kidney is the site of origin, the initial clinical picture is one of nephritis.

Treatment. The story of the first breakthrough in chemotherapy for acute lymphosarcoma is fascinating. Folic acid vitamins (pteroyl-glutamic acid) had shown striking but not complete effects in stimulating the normal maturation of red blood cells in pernicious anemia. Analogues, or close structural relatives, of pteroyl-glutamic acid were synthesized. Biochemists hoped that an analogue would be a more effective blood cell maturation factor. But instead of being metabolically stimulating, as folic acid had been found to be, the newly synthesized compounds were extremely toxic for blood and tissue cells.

Dr. Sidney Farber of Children's Hospital in Boston, with the "prepared mind," undertook to see whether this highly toxic action might be put to use in restraining the overgrowth of leukemic cells. At that time, the average survival time of children with acute untreated leukemia was four to eight weeks. It was found that the drugs (Aminopterin and Amethopterin), though very toxic, could bring remissions in a considerable percentage of these patients.

To achieve a remission, a toxic level of tolerance has to be approached. But remissions when obtained are complete, the patients return to normal health, and circulating sarcoma cells disappear from the blood, marrow and other organs. The duration of effectiveness of these drugs in sustaining remissions was found to range from nine to 18 months.

At this point our ingenious biochemists synthesized *6-mercaptopurine,* as theoretically offering a means of interference with the synthesis of abnormal amino acids of lymphosarcoma cells. This chemical agent proved able in many instances to take up where Aminopterin left off, and in virgin cases to initiate remissions, and 6-mercaptopurine and several of its analogues have proved to be less toxic, and at the same time to be effective for much longer periods of time in selected individuals.

Youngsters have been carried in satisfactory remission for as long as five to eight years with maintenance doses of 6-mercaptopurine alone, or with small supplemental doses of corticosteroids. Always, however, relapses have recurred, usually secondary to bacterial or viral infection, showing the precarious equilibrium of these individuals in times of remission.

One asks why, if a disease with a life expectancy of eight weeks untreated can be given a remission lasting eight years with treatment, it is not possible to hold this tendency in check for 80 years. We are hopeful that the "next step" is just around the corner.

THE LYMPHOMATA

The *lymphomata* include all of the diseases which primarily involve the lymph nodes and lymphatic system. Chronic and acute *lymphatic leukemia, lymphosarcoma,* and *lympholeukosarcoma,* have already been discussed.

Hodgkin's disease is perhaps the next most common of the remaining lymphomata. The name derives from an English physician who in 1832 described a small group of patients with prominent lymph node swellings in the neck. Hodgkin's disease involves primarily the *reticulum cells* of the lymphoid tissue rather than the lymphocytes. It is the reticulum cell counterpart of lymphosarcoma, which is primarily a disease of the lymphocytes themselves, and, like lymphosarcoma, probably starts in one cell in one location of the body. It is thus very important to discover Hodgkin's disease early, in the hope that it may be stopped locally before it becomes disseminated.

Hodgkin's disease may start in any lymph node, but commonly is first discovered in nodes above the collarbone or lower nodes in the neck region.

Diagnosis. Any lymph node swelling in this area which cannot be explained by a condition such as infected tonsils, or which does not recede spontaneously in eight to 12 weeks, should be aspirated or removed surgically for study. If the study shows only a non-specific inflammatory reaction, attention is directed to local tissues which may be chronically infected.

If, however, a reticulum cell type of hyperplasia is found, with other typical changes, Hodgkin's disease is confirmed. Rarely, local surgical dissection of all lymphoid tissue in the area may be followed by a "cure." However, it is not possible to be certain that there is no insidious early spread of the process, and to be on the safe side a "tumor dose" of deep x-ray or cobalt bomb therapy should follow the surgery. If the diseased node is classifiable as stage one, the measures suggested may assure more than five-year survival in approximately 65 per cent of such patients, and ten per cent will survive beyond ten years.

Hodgkin's disease manifests itself most often in the second or third decade of life, more commonly in men than in women. Intermittent low grade fever is characteristic, itching of the skin is a common complaint, and lymph node enlargement may be discovered in any of the regional groups of nodes. The outlook is most grave when the disease starts in the abdomen. Not infrequently there is involvement of a bone. Often, a spontaneous fracture may be the first evidence of the disease.

Frequently, the reticulum cells in the lymph nodes have all of the characteristics of neoplasia (new abnormal growth), consistent with what is sometimes called a *reticulum cell sarcoma*. This does not differ materially from so-called Hodgkin's sarcoma, described originally by Ewing, a famous pathologist who devoted a lifetime to study of this disease.

Management. In its early and more benign states, Hodgkin's disease is not incompatible with normal life and activity. We do not know its true incidence, because undoubtedly there are many persons walking the streets today with asymptomatic lymph glands of this type who have never consulted a physician. The specific cause of the disease is a mystery, although many different organisms have been incriminated, and not the least of current suspicions implicates viruses as possible agents.

In absence of specific measures, treatments to suppress growth and extension of the particular cells involved are employed. As mentioned, x-ray and radioactive cobalt have been used successfully in selected cases, especially when the disease is discovered early and is apparently limited to one location. Unfortunately, many patients are seen only after diffuse dissemination of the disease has occurred, and spray irradiation to the whole body has not proved successful in our hands.

A number of chemotherapeutic agents can slow down and in some instances stop the progress of Hodgkin's disease for months and years. I have personally studied patients in New York City with Hodgkin's disease diagnosed by Dr. Ewing some 25 years earlier who lived all this time with occupational independence and without diminished physical strength. Occasional courses of deep x-ray therapy had proved quite effective.

With such evidence of inherent chronicity and longevity in many patients with Hodgkin's disease, the optimistic physician accepts every new case with the realistic hope that this patient too will be one of those who will be amenable to medical management. This optimism is increasingly justified by the variety of available therapeutic agents which favorably affect the progressive stages of the disease.

Alkylating agents, particularly the various oral nitrogen mustards, are proving to be very effective for maintenance therapy in many patients. When "shingles" (herpes zoster) complicates Hodgkin's disease, intravenous Pactamycin now appears to be helpful in controlling both this viral complication and the underlying Hodgkin's disease. Involvements of the liver, kidneys and lungs have been most difficult to control in the past. With the development of *vincoleucoblastine* (VLB), however, we now have a drug which is proving to be effective in reversing these manifestations. *Hexamethylmelamine* is another new drug which gives promise of "backing up" VLB, at least in selected patients, if the latter drug loses some of its potency.

Other new experimental drugs are under clinical study. Current medical literature cannot keep up with rapid developments in applied therapy, and efforts to find the basic cause of Hodgkin's disease give a fresh basis for optimism for future control of the disease. Patients in whom Hodgkin's disease is diagnosed, and their families, should look to an informed clinical research center for the latest month-to-month information in this field. There is constant interchange of information between medical centers where new drugs are being tested clinically.

It is becoming increasingly evident that when patients no longer respond to the usually effective chemotherapy, the R-E system is becoming ineffective in its defense mechanism. Mathé has suggested restimulation with an antigenic challenge, as for example, using BCG vaccination. Sokol and associates at Roswell Park Cancer Research Center in Buffalo have found that failure to respond with the development of a P.P.D. positive reaction, when it has been initially negative, is a serious prognostic sign. But if a reactive response can be elicited from the patient, the prognosis is greatly improved.

In the patients non-responsive to an antigenic challenge, it may be possible to give them a new supply of R-E cells by transplanting under the skin embryonic fetal thymus tissues. This is the newest and latest approach to prolonging the effectiveness of the usually dependable chemotherapeutic agents, and when successful, may extend the life expectancy indefinitely.

Other Lymphomata

Reticulum cell sarcoma may occur spontaneously, fullblown, without having first shown the tumorous characteristics of early Hodgkin's disease. The therapeutic approach is the same as in Hodgkin's sarcoma. There is the same hopeful optimism in this disease as in Hodgkin's disease.

Giant follicular lymphoblastoma is initially indistinguishable clinically from early Hodgkin's disease or lymphosar-coma, and only a node biopsy may reveal the differential diagnosis. The name is descriptive of great enlargement of individual lymph follicles, but without loss of normal structure of nodes or invasion of the capsule such as occurs in neoplastic malignancy. The clinical course usually is relatively benign and is influenced by radioactive phosphorus or other lymphotoxic agents when necessary.

The spleen becomes involved in a large percentage of these cases, and its surgical removal may be necessary as in other secondary hypersplenic syndromes. In our own series of patients, reviewed after ten years, only one in four progressed into lymphosarcoma, while 75 per cent have remained as the benign giant follicle lymphoma without progressive symptoms. We feel justified in giving optimistic reassurance to patients who present this picture, but we recommend observation at regular intervals to discover any incipient change.

Leukemic reticulo-endotheliosis. There are several related syndromes which involve the basic reticulo-endothelial system and its "stem cell." The latter lacks all of the differential characteristics of the definitive blood and connective tissue cells, and when it remains at this undifferentiated level and multiplies without maturation, a condition known as *leukemic reticulo-endotheliosis* develops. In a recent survey of 26 cases studied in our Clinic, the course was variable: 46 per cent followed a chronic pattern, 23 per cent showed a subacute picture, while 31 per cent had an acute and rapidly progressive course. Among the chronic group a "splenic form" of the disease developed, requiring deep x-ray therapy to the enlarged spleen, but an acute "crisis" required splenectomy in five patients. Selected alkylating nitrogen mustards with corticosteroids have been helpful in some instances.

Lipid endothelioses. The best known of the group of so-called lipid endothelioses is a "familial large-celled spleno-megaly" first described by Gaucher in 1882, often called *Gaucher's disease.*

Since more than a third of reported cases have occurred in multiple members of the same family, it is assumed that an hereditary factor is important.

Few complete genetic studies have been attempted, but it is hypothesized that Gaucher's disease represents a genetic mutation, transmitted as a simple dominant trait which gives rise to a disturbance in fat metabolism with deposition in the spleen of certain large cells (Gaucher's cells) which contain a lipoid (kerasin). The disease appears to be transmitted in increasingly severe form, with manifestations at an ever-earlier age, in succeeding generations, so that eventually the mutation may "extinguish" itself by permitting only unaffected offspring to survive.

There are few diseases in which the spleen becomes so large. In some of our patients, the spleen has assumed huge proportions, precipitating a deficiency of cellular elements in the blood; in these instances, splenectomy has given complete and permanent correction. Only in infancy is the course of the disease rapidly progressive and fulminant; this probably represents the final "extinguishment" of a mutation arising in previous generations. Any patient with this disease who survives the first few years of life has a good prognosis.

Another lipid dystrophy occurring only in children is known as **Letterer-Siwe's syndrome.** In this disease there is reticulum cell hyperplasia without storage of lipoid substances in cells. Fever, bleeding tendencies, middle ear angina, progressive anemia, enlargement of lymph nodes, spleen and liver, a focal destruction of bone suggest either an acute sepsis or acute leukemia. Antibacterial, anti-viral, and anti-leukemic agents have thus far failed to stop the progress of the disease.

Xanthomatoses. In addition to Gaucher's disease and Letterer-Siwe's syndrome, there are two other of the disturbances of reticulo-endothelial cell storage that are known collectively as the *xanthomatoses* (abnormalities of lipoid metabolism with formation of lipoid tumors).

Nieman-Pick's *lipid histocytosis* has a special predilection for infants of the Jewish race. These infants show gastrointestinal disturbances, general malnutrition, and iron deficiency anemia. They fail to gain in weight and mental development, display skeletal abnormalities, and show striking enlargement of the spleen, liver, and lymph nodes. Numerous complications during early life make survival beyond the second year very problematical.

Lipophagic granulomatosis *(Hand-Schuller-Christian disease)* usually develops insidiously during the first decade of life. The reticulo-endothelial cell hyperplasia in this condition is associated with disturbance of cholesterol metabolism, with deposits of cholesterol in subcutaneous tissues and bones. Irritability, excessive thirst and urinary output, bulging of the eyes, swelling of the gums, loosening of the teeth, and deep bone pain and tenderness may develop. Symptoms reflect the gradual encroachment of abnormal cells on surrounding tissues. Irregular punched-out areas are more frequently found in the skull than in the long bones. Small papular lesions with yellow centers known as *xanthoma* (the word means "yellow tumor"), which reflect disordered cholesterol metabolism, may appear over the face and trunk.

Premature extensive arteriosclerosis, usually found at autopsy in these patients, is perhaps associated with the disturbed cholesterol metabolism. Fatal lipid invasion of abnormally porous cranial bones occurs in an estimated 85 per cent of these patients. However, spontaneous regression of bone lesions has sometimes occurred and x-ray therapy has seemed to clear some of these skeletal lesions.

Plasma Cell Diseases

We have not heretofore mentioned the **plasma cell,** a "first cousin" to the lymphocyte. The plasma cell is normally found in the walls of the intestinal tract and in the healing phase of chronic infectious lesions, and is thought to play an important role in the defense mechanisms of the body. Probably any mutational disturbance of the plasma cell may take any of the three forms of disease described below.

Multiple myeloma is most commonly found localized in the bony skeleton, causing destructive lesions with scattered areas of abnormal porousness ("Swiss cheese appearance") and leading to spontaneous pathologic fractures. On microscopic examination the entire first stage maturation range of plasma cells can be found in localized nests eroding the surrounding bone. When this condition is suspected, x-rays of the skull and pelvis are taken. It is these areas that most frequently show the identifying lytic lesions.

Usually the rare appearance of plasma cells in the circulating blood is consistent with conditions of chronic infection. In other instances, however, an excess of plasma cells may pour into the blood, in which case we have the picture of *plasma cell leukemia.*

When "metastases" are found in upper respiratory passages, the cornea, pleura, and elsewhere, in addition to the bone lesions, the generalized dissemination and invasion of plasma cells is known as *plasmacytoma.*

Multiple myeloma is twice as common in males as females and almost all cases occur after the age of 40. As already stated, often the first evidence is a pathologic fracture of a rib or vertebral body. Deep bone pain, worst at night, is the most common symptom. This reflects the "boring in" of plasma cells eroding the bone and pressing on nerve endings.

The first sign may arise from kidney involvement, and examination of the urine will often reveal the presence of so-called "Bence-Jones protein." Usually there is an abnormally high amount of protein in the blood plasma. Bence-Jones protein precipitates out of solution at certain temperatures, and its ease of deposition in kidney collecting tubules will gradually reduce kidney function, with uremia as the terminal event. This is perhaps the most important criterion influencing the prognosis for the patient with multiple myeloma.

Periods of spontaneous remission and exacerbation are to be expected. Deep x-ray therapy over sites of spontaneous fracture or the thin shell of vertebral bodies sometimes results in recalcification in these areas, relief of pain, and lessened threat of vertebral body collapse. Ethylcarbamate (urethane) has been the drug of choice until recently. In approximately 50 per cent of cases, this drug will control fever, skeletal pain, and acute symptoms within two to four weeks, with concomitant slowing down of bone erosion. More recently, an alkylating agent, Cytoxan, has been used with benefit and perhaps less toxicity than urethane, which may damage the liver over the long pull. Other alkylating agents are being given clinical trial, and it is hoped that plasma cell disorders may be better understood and soon come under more consistent control.

Hypo-Aplastic Syndromes

Thus far we have discussed overproduction of cellular elements by the bone marrow. The other end of the spectrum —inadequate production — seems to be occurring with increasing frequency. These hypo-aplastic, pancellular, bone marrow syndromes differ only in degree of marrow paralysis.

Fanconi's syndrome bears the name of the Swiss investigator who first described it in 1929. Extra digits, double kidneys, cleft palate, imperforate anus, and other characteristics have been described, but the principal cause of fatality is progressive bone marrow *aplasia* (atrophy; without ability to develop new blood cells) which advances slowly until it becomes incompatible with life beyond the early teen age. There is an apparent genetic defect in which the congenital aplastic anemia is the most serious and usually fatal inheritance.

Toxic agents. Until the mid-1920's, approximately 90 per cent of the hypoaplastic anemias of identifiable cause were traced to industrial toxins that "poisoned" the cell-producing mechanisms of the marrow. It became recognized that the bone marrow may be susceptible to many volatile "inhalable" chemicals as well as to those that may enter through the skin or gastrointestinal tract. Industry itself now demands toxicologic studies on all new chemical compounds before introducing them into their processes, with the result that industrial-induced bone marrow depression now constitutes ten per cent or less of cases seen by today's physicians.

New drugs and chemotherapeutic agents have now largely supplanted industrial toxins as triggers of aplastic anemia. Many lifesaving drugs, well tolerated by the great majority of patients, may in an occasional rare individual incite an idiosyncratic reaction with the bone marrow as the chief target. Physicians have learned that the institution of any new drug should be preceded by physical and laboratory surveys of the patient, including always a blood study and bone marrow observations when indicated. An initial dosage considerably less than the anticipated therapeutic dose should be started and observed until there is assurance that the drug carries no immediate toxic side effects that outweigh its benefits. Cumulative drug toxemia as well as allergic sensitization after repeated courses of drug therapy must be considered.

Other instances of bone marrow aplasias of seemingly indeterminable cause are called *idiopathic aplastic anemias*. These probably can be reduced to the vanishing point by assiduous history-taking and probing of the patient's memory for possible precipitating factors. This statement is justified because of the inherent resiliency of the normal bone marrow in repairing transitory damage, if earliest signs of depression are recognized promptly and the inducing agents stopped forthwith. *Prevention* is the principal and only always successful treatment for aplastic anemia.

Bone marrow transplants. Intensive studies in transplantation of organs now being made include applications in hypo-

aplastic anemia. Bone marrow transplantation, now in its experimental phase, may well become an accomplished procedure tomorrow.

Some patients with hypoplastic marrows have taken as long as two to three years of supportive and stimulatory therapy before regeneration became adequate, so that such measures should be vigorously undertaken and continued with the hope that recovery of normal blood cell equilibrium will occur in time.

The Reticulo-Endothelial System is one of the most important pillars sustaining human health. The well-trained obstetrician, pediatrician, internist and hematologist, working as a team in cooperation with their patients, have a heretofore unparalleled opportunity to preserve the hematopoietic functional integrities so essential to sound mental and physical health.

Auto-Transfusion

Risks of blood-bank transfusions—hepatitis, mismatching, various immune reactions—would virtually vanish if the patient's own blood could be transfused when needed. "Auto-transfusion" is not exactly new. Banked autologous blood has been used occasionally for patients with rare blood types. But doctors have generally felt that patients could not replace the withdrawn red cells adequately and would come to surgery weakened from blood loss.

We found during World War II in the Red Cross Blood Program that healthy men could replace blood volume almost immediately and regenerate the red cells removed in the average 500-cc. blood donation within four weeks. A second similar donation of red cells was regenerated in three weeks, and a third consecutive donation in two weeks. In women, this sequence did not follow because of the regular 21-28 day menstrual blood loss which delayed the build back.

This information led to the acceptance of our soldiers on rest leave as blood donors for use by the Army. It was found after repeated blood donations—"exercise of the bone marrow"—our soldiers thus prepared could withstand much larger blood losses from battle wounds without shock.

This practice could be applied to patients anticipating elective surgery.

More recent experience at one institution indicates that many patients can give their own blood for their own use if an iron solution is injected immediately after drawing blood. Normal men treated with iron were able to regenerate red blood cells rapidly enough to permit a unit of blood to be drawn five times a week for as long as 22 weeks. Blood volume was restored within 12 hours after blood was drawn. If only one unit of blood was needed, it was drawn 48 to 72 hours before surgery. If several units were needed, a period of 48 hours was maintained between blood drawings. Auto-transfusion may be feasible, with obvious advantages as to safety and cost, in as many as half of elective operations. There is adequate testimony to the regenerative powers of healthy blood-forming organs.

CHAPTER 5

THE SKIN AND ITS DISORDERS

by SAMUEL M. BLUEFARB, M.D.

Layers of the Skin · Sweat Glands · Oil Glands · Hair and Nails

ACNE VULGARIS

Rosacea · Pruritus · Colloid Baths

ECZEMA

COSMETIC DERMATITIS

Drug Eruptions · Prickly Heat · Psoriasis · Pityriasis Rosea · Lichen Planus · Warts

BIRTHMARKS AND MOLES

Vascular Nevi · Moles

CANCER OF THE SKIN

DERMATOSES DUE TO THE SUN

BALDNESS

Common Baldness · Infections of the Skin · Pemphigus

RINGWORM OR FUNGUS INFECTIONS

Yeast Infections

PARASITIC INFECTIONS OF THE SKIN

Pediculosis · Scabies

COMMON SKIN CONDITIONS IN OLDER PEOPLE

MISCELLANEOUS SKIN CONDITIONS

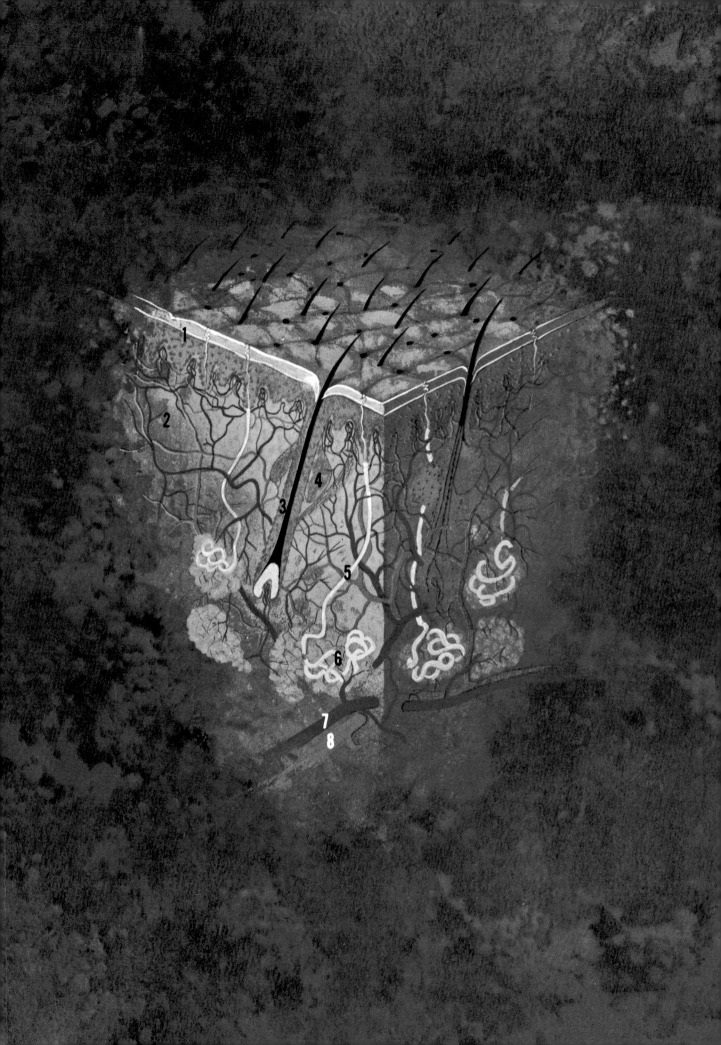

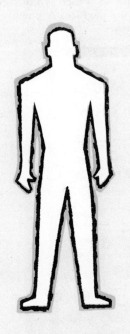

CHAPTER 5

THE SKIN AND ITS DISORDERS

by SAMUEL M. BLUEFARB, M.D.

The skin is the largest organ of the body and, with the exception of the brain, probably the most complex. It wraps the adult body in about 20 square feet of tissue, at once tough and delicate, weighing some seven pounds. Within this prosaic covering are millions upon millions of minute structures and mechanisms of surprising intricacy — microscopic oil wells and geysers, structures that waterproof and prevent entrance of bacteria and harmful materials from the outside world, nerve endings that whisk electrical messages of pain or cold or heat to the brain which "feels" them, chemicals that make Vitamin D with the assistance of sunshine, structures that excrete and others that participate in production of antibodies against foreign proteins.

The seemingly smooth skin of a baby or beauty contest winner may deceive the eye but not the microscope. Human skin is furrowed by ridges and valleys, pitted with tunnels from which hair tips project, moistened by salt water and lubricated by an invisible moving film of oils. And it is incredibly alive, continually renewing itself and casting off dead cells that worked incessantly and wore themselves out in service to their owner.

With profound truth, the skin has been called "the mirror of the body." If beauty is only skin deep, the skin's connections reach the innermost parts of the body. Some symptoms that are visible in the skin do not arise primarily in the skin but in other organs. Thus the skin is an "early warning system," and its examination, very important and informative in physical diagnosis, occasionally furnishes the first clue to identification of serious systemic diseases.

Some of the things the skin warns about are "false alarms" or at least have no connection with organic disease. Associations between the skin and the mind are very intimate and very complicated. There is, for instance, a kind of emotion that is expressed almost instantly by a blush — a rush of blood to the face — and

The skin enwraps the entire body, and with its modified structures such as hair and nails is virtually all the public sees of us, and thus is pre-eminent in personal appearance.

A section of the skin shown in the color plate reveals it to be a complex organ. The outer layer, or *epidermis* (1), is itself many-layered (see page 168). The *dermis* (2), also called the *corium* or "true skin," is a dense, elastic layer of fibrous tissue that contains and supports many important structures of the skin. An indefinite layer of cushiony subcutaneous tissue lies below it.

Hair follicles (3) have their roots in the dermis. *Sebaceous glands* (4) secrete their oil (sebum) into the hair follicles and thence to the surface of the skin. Coiled *sweat glands* (6) open directly to the surface of the skin via ducts (5). Blood supply is furnished by *arteries* (7) and *veins* (8).

absence of a blush under circumstances that theoretically should provoke it may suggest something else about emotions. Psychic influences on the skin are powerful indeed, and may even provoke some people to dig and scratch at it as a "bad" organ or one which they wrongly feel is punishing them for some sort of misbehavior.

Like other organs, the skin is subject to its own diseases. Dermatology is the branch of internal medicine concerned with diagnosis, interpretation, and treatment of diseases of the skin. Since the skin is a "two-faced" organ, with an internal and an external surface — and consisting, as it does, of many types of tissues—it is susceptible to a great variety of disorders. Some of the more common are infections, inflammations, new growths, degeneration, wasting, overgrowth, and congenital abnormalities.

Skin diseases are diagnosed by evaluating the patient's history and his objective and subjective symptoms. The latter are symptoms which are not visible but which are described feelingly by the patient: itching, heat, pain, burning, or "crawling" sensations. Objective symptoms are those which can be seen. These are the most important symptoms in dermatology because the chief instrument of the dermatologist is his eye. Fortunately, in most cases, visual examinations suffice for the diagnosis of skin troubles.

An obvious function of the skin is to mark the boundary between "us" and the world, and to enclose the internal seas in which we live so that we do not evaporate to death. Yet controlled evaporation from the skin is essential to life, lest we be heated to death by our own body fires. Countless highly specialized anatomical structures are intricately interlaced within an integument that varies in thickness from a thirty-second to an eighth of an inch.

Layers of the Skin

Anatomically, the skin is a layered organ, although as far as the owner is concerned it functions as a unit.

The outer skin, or *epidermis*, has several anatomical layers. The topmost horny

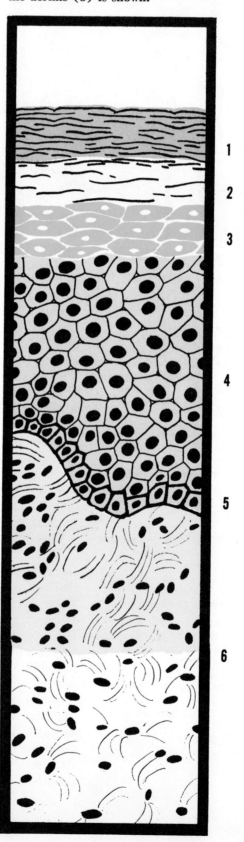

Layers of the epidermis: 1. Outermost horny layer, or stratum corneum; 2. stratum lucidum, a shiny ill-defined layer; 3. granular layer; 4. prickle-cell layer; 5. germinative layer, a single row of columnar cells in which young cells develop and move to the surface. A portion of the dermis (6) is shown.

layer *(stratum corneum)* is composed of dead cells that are always being worn off. We shed our skins continuously, not all at once, as some reptiles do. Brisk rubbing with a towel peels off little rolls of material composed of dead outer skin cells that never will be missed. This incessant shedding of flaky material goes mostly unnoticed, unless we complain of dandruff or peel off insensate skin patches after a sunburn.

New cells originate in the germinative layer at the bottom of the epidermis. These fresh young cells mature and move upward, changing gradually, until they in turn become dead horny cells that fall off our skins into oblivion. Layers of the epidermis are renewed from below. Pigment granules of material known as *melanin* are present in lower epithelial layers. These proliferate under stimulus of certain wavelengths of sunlight and become visible as suntan or freckles.

Beneath the epidermis is the *dermis*, also called the *corium* or "true skin." It contains connective tissue, is strong and elastic, and is the part of animal skins that makes leather when tanned. It is laced with blood vessels, nerve fibers, receptor organs for sensations of touch, pain, heat and cold, contains muscular elements, hair follicles and oil and sweat glands. The surface of the dermis is cobbled, ridged and valleyed, and is fitted to and impressed upon the under surface of the epidermis above it. (A blister, incidentally, is a collection of fluid between the epidermis and dermis).

Ridges are most conspicuous in the hands and feet and their digits, and their patterns, unique to the individual person, are the basis of fingerprint identification and the common footprint identification of newborn babies. However, these pressure ridges have a more fundamental function. They help to "slip-proof" the fingers and make it possible to pick up small objects and do delicate manipulations. Rarely, a person's fingertip ridges may be obliterated by acids or other causes, and the person has great difficulty in picking up a pin.

Beneath the dermis is an indefinite layer of subcutaneous tissue with fatty

and resilient elements that help to cushion the skin above it. This layer plays a part in complaints about wrinkles. Absorption of subcutaneous fat and softer parts of the skin removes "bouncy" supporting

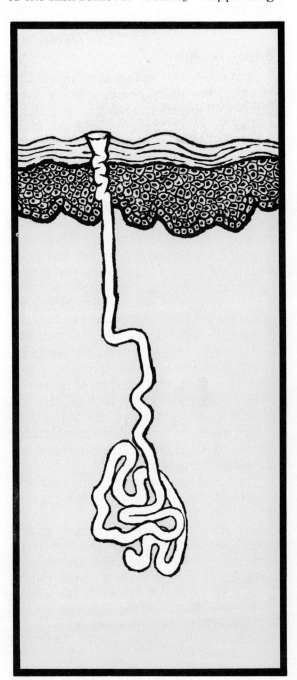

A sweat gland: the coiled lower portion which lies in the dermis or subcutaneous tissue is the secretory part. The upper end makes its way through the epidermis in a corkscrew manner and terminates in a trumpet-shaped opening. Eccrine glands of this sort produce a watery secretion that is very important in dissipating excessive body heat.

material, and since the external skin does not have the capability to shrink at the same rate, it tends to collapse and become enfolded in wrinkles. Subcutaneous layers of fat also have insulating properties.

Sweat Glands

Our skins are equipped with upward of two million tiny glands which excrete fluids well known as sweat, or more genteelly, as perspiration. The working or secreting parts of the glands are intricately coiled little tubules in the dermis. Ducts for discharge of sweat tunnel upward to the surface of the skin.

There are two kinds of sweat glands, producing different kinds of sweat. One kind, called *apocrine sweat,* is not very important physiologically but has some social significance. Apocrine sweat glands open into hair follicles and are limited to a few regions of the body, particularly the underarm and genital areas. They are inactive in infants, develop with puberty, and enlarge premenstrually. Apocrine sweat contains complex substances that give it a somewhat milky appearance. Freshly produced sweat is normally sterile and quite inoffensive. Its decomposition by bacteria gives rise to perspiration odor and to innumerable products designed to subvert it.

The other kind of sweat, called *eccrine,* is of towering importance to our comfort if not our lives. Multitudes of *eccrine sweat glands* are present almost everywhere in the skin, except the lips and a few other areas. They are crowded in largest numbers into skin of the palms, soles, and forehead. Ducts of the glands corkscrew their way through the epidermis directly to the skin surface.

Sebaceous glands are associated with hair follicles, except in a few non-hairy parts of the body. Cells in the small sac-shaped glands, which may have several lobes, form fat droplets which, mixed with cast-off cell materials and debris, is sebum or "skin oil." Sebum seeps through a duct into the hair follicle, lubricates the hair shaft, and works to the surface to lubricate the skin.

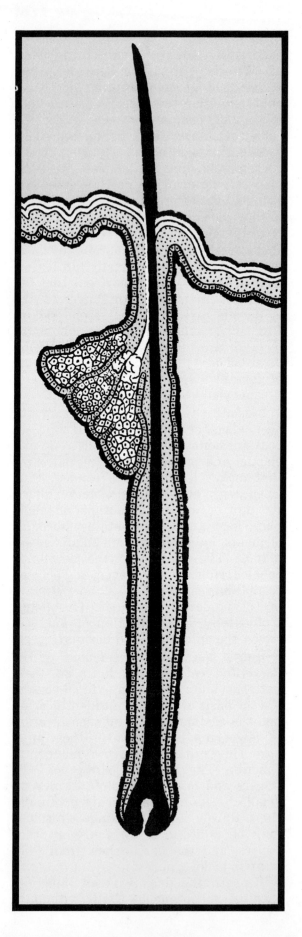

Eccrine sweat is little more than extremely dilute salt water, clear and watery in appearance. Its function is to help the body to dissipate excessive internal heat. The skin and its sweating mechanisms are parts of a vital heat-regulating system that keeps us from burning up alive. A thermostat-like center in the brain sends out flashing nerve-orders when we are too hot. The heart pumps more blood to the skin. One square inch of skin contains about 15 feet of minute blood vessels. These dilate to carry more blood when we need to lose heat, constrict when we need to conserve warmth. A little heat is radiated from skin surfaces. But by far the most efficient means of body-cooling is evaporation of water — sweat. This process goes on even though the skin may seem to be dry. "Insensible" perspiration is sweat that evaporates as soon as it is formed.

Sweat that rolls off the skin in rivulets without evaporating is not doing as efficient a cooling job as it should. Humidity on a hot day impedes evaporation and gives substance to the cliche, "it isn't the heat but the humidity." Sweat glands have a prodigious rate of output — two quarts or more a day — under some extreme circumstances.

Oil Glands

We have about as many oil-secreting or *sebaceous glands* in the skin as we have sweat glands. Most of these glands occur in or near hair follicles, and excrete their oils through the narrow pit of the follicle. Fatty materials in the flask-shaped glands are changed into a complex oily substance, called *sebum*, which seeps into the hair follicle and works its way to the surface where it spreads as a thin film.

The primary function of sebum, as is proper to oils, is lubrication — in this case, of the hairshaft and horny surface layers of the skin. A certain amount of natural skin-oil is necessary to keep skin and hair soft and pliable. In addition, chemicals in sebum play a part in maintaining the so-called "acid mantle" of the skin. The surface of normal healthy skin

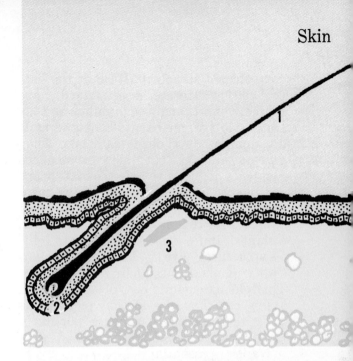

Growth of a hair (1) occurs at the root (2) where the bulbous lower end of the hair rests closely upon a cone-shaped structure, the *papilla*. Sudden contraction of erector muscles (3) attached to the hair follicle causes "gooseflesh."

is slightly acid in reaction; a tendency toward alkalinity is thought to increase the susceptibility of skin to fungal infections and other disorders or perhaps is a consequence.

Oil glands are distributed over almost the entire body, and are largest in regions of the forehead, face, neck, and chest — typically, the areas involved in common acne, a condition with which cell-clogged oil glands are associated. However, the palms of the hands and soles of the feet are poorly greased. That is a reason why skin of the inner hand becomes whitened, wrinkled, and soggy-looking if immersed for some time in water.

Hair and Nails

Hair is a modified form of skin cells, and so are fingernails and toenails. The major structural material is *keratin*, produced by the same processes that change living cells into dead, horny cells of the outermost skin layer. However, hair and nails are almost total keratin.

Hairs grow in almost the entire skin, though in many areas they are so inconspicuous or vestigial that they are never noticed. At the bottom of a *follicle*, which is a narrow skin-pit, lies a *papilla*, a tiny cone-shaped structure. Here at the hair root cells proliferate, move upward, shape the hair shaft, and lose viability as they cornify or become horny. Hair and nails are composed of dead materials. They give no pain when cut; there are no nerve filaments or blood vessels. The latter are confined to living cells from which hairs originate.

Most hair tips project from the skin at a slant. Minute muscles attached to follicle structures have the fascinating potentiality of making the hair stand on end. This phenomenon is best observed in an angry cat. The closest that most of us come to it is the experience popularly known as "goose pimples."

Nails are essentially the same in structure as hairs, except that nails are flat, hard plates. The living part of a nail lies in the matrix back of the half-moon or *lunula*. If the dead nail plate, which constitutes most of the visible part of the nail, is destroyed by injury, a new nail will grow if the matrix is intact.

ACNE VULGARIS

Common acne (blackheads and pimples; the common "bad complexion" of adolescence) is one of the most common skin diseases and, in its mild form, may be a normal accompaniment of puberty. Acne is due to the overactivity of the *pilosebaceous apparatus* (hair follicles and sebaceous glands) which results in oversecretion of oil by these glands, associated with thickening of the pores.

The onset of acne is associated with the physiologic increase of sex hormones at puberty in boys and girls. Acne never occurs in eunuchs.

The primary sites of acne lesions are the center of the face, the chest, upper back, and shoulders. There is usually an associated oiliness of the scalp with some degree of dandruff. The primary lesion of acne is the *comedone* (blackhead). The blackhead is darkened by air, not by dirt as parents usually assume.

Treatment. Topical measures (those applied locally to a surface) are designed to achieve a continuous mild drying and peeling of the skin, to remove excessive oil, and to prevent obstruction of the follicles which leads to blackhead formation. The most simple measure is the use of ordinary soap and water, twice daily if not oftener. Several special soaps which intensify the cleansing and "unplugging" action are available.

Topical preparations usually contain resorcin and sulfur, either singly or in combination. Sulfur is a valuable topical agent because of the peeling it produces.

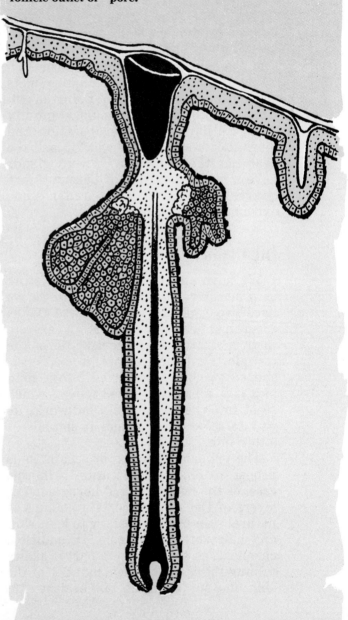

A blackhead or *comedone* is the earliest lesion of common acne, associated with oversecretion of oil and thickening of the hair follicle. Oil and cell debris, exposed to air, thickens and plugs the follicle outlet or "pore."

"Peeling" of the skin, actually a removal of superficial layers, may also be produced by application of "dry ice" (carbon dioxide). This is mixed with acetone and applied to the skin with a gauze-wrapped cotton applicator. Ultraviolet light treatments will also produce peeling of the skin.

Soap and water, cleanliness, topical preparations, and perhaps a covering agent to conceal a blemish or two, may be all that are needed in mild cases of acne. However, there is a tendency to pick and squeeze at lesions, and severe cases of acne with inflamed pimples and even pus-filled cysts may require special treatment.

When there is no appreciable improvement with other measures, x-ray therapy is indicated. This remains the most effective treatment, but it must be administered cautiously to selected patients by a dermatologist trained in this field of medicine who is qualified to administer it safely and effectively.

Proper care of the scalp is important because seborrhea is often present. The hair and scalp should be shampooed frequently. Cosmetic preparations having a greasy base, as well as hair pomades, should not be used.

Things to avoid. Certain foods and drugs are *acnegenic stimuli* — that is, they exacerbate the acne process, and it is of prime importance to avoid them.

Certain dietary restrictions are advisable because some foods apparently produce aggravation by causing follicle irritation. Nuts, chocolate, and sharp cheeses are principal offenders.

Foods and drugs containing iodides or bromides may produce acnelike eruptions as a result of follicular stimulation. Therefore, sea foods and shellfish should be avoided, and in severe cases a non-iodized table salt should be used. Certain cough mixtures and other medicines contain iodides, and bromides are present in some sedatives, "cold" tablets, and "nerve" medicines. Any of these which a patient happens to be taking will be recognized by a physician who can advise accordingly.

Infection and inflammation. Secondary pyogenic (pus-producing) infections may play a part in some cases of pustular or cystic acne. In such cases, antibiotics may be administered systemically. In my experience, systemic antibiotics have proved to be a most potent measure in the management of many patients having these forms of acne. Although antibiotics do not cure the basic condition, their use is justified in an attempt to bring the pustular and cystic elements under control and thus prevent scarring.

In some instances, emotional stimuli may contribute to a flareup of acne, since stress alters the production of sebum.

Acne pits and scarring. Much experience with *dermabrasion* has been gained in this country in the past ten years. Dermabrasion as performed by dermatologists is a highly technical procedure for treatment of skin pits and scars, to produce a smoother skin. It is also called "surgical planing" or "wire brush surgery." It is a relatively minor operation which ordinarily can be done in the dermatologist's office.

An instrument not unlike a dentist's drill, with a small rotating wire brush on its end, is used to plane off layers of skin by high speed abrasive action. A local refrigerative anesthetic is applied to the skin and the skilled operator planes the skin to remove defects. Expert knowledge of skin structures and mechanisms of planing is of course essential. Healing takes place beneath a crust in a week to ten days, and the new skin surface that forms is usually much smoother and presentable than the old.

The perfectionist who expects 100 per cent improvement will be disappointed. Not all pits and scars can be planed to a state of complete disappearance, but the improvement is usually most gratifying. Patients who expect planing to solve personality problems, or any problems other than cosmetic ones, will be disappointed.

Summary. Treatment of acne is individualized and many-sided, in view of the many factors that affect it. Efforts should be made to prevent or overcome the overactivity of the oil-producing glands.

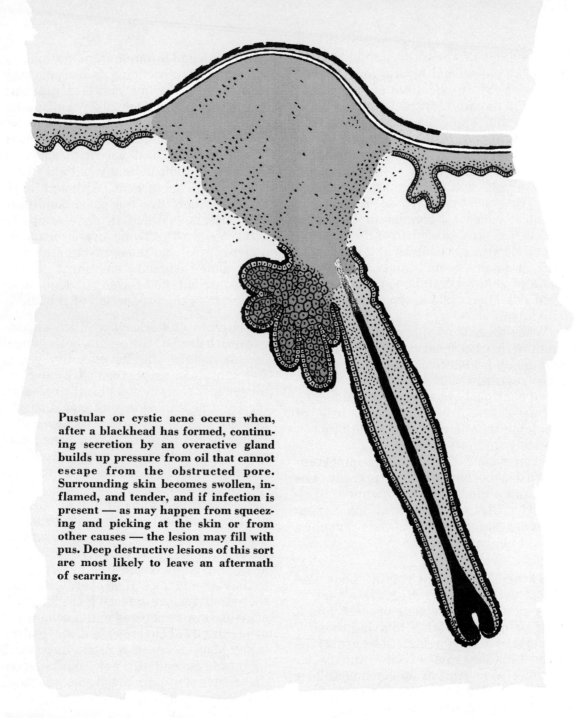

Pustular or cystic acne occurs when, after a blackhead has formed, continuing secretion by an overactive gland builds up pressure from oil that cannot escape from the obstructed pore. Surrounding skin becomes swollen, inflamed, and tender, and if infection is present — as may happen from squeezing and picking at the skin or from other causes — the lesion may fill with pus. Deep destructive lesions of this sort are most likely to leave an aftermath of scarring.

Measures include topical therapy, ultraviolet light, carbon dioxide "slush," x-rays, avoidance of certain foods and drugs, and antibiotic therapy.

Rosacea

Acne rosacea, not at all related to common acne, is a chronic disease which affects the skin of the middle third of the face. This "flush area" includes the nose and adjacent portions of the cheeks, the chin, and the center of the forehead. This area has a rich blood supply and the disease begins with intermittent dilation of superficial blood vessels.

The redness varies from a mild red to a deep bluish-red color. Eventually the dilation of the superficial blood vessels becomes permanent, and the skin constantly red. Dilation causes enlargement of the skin of the nose. The familiar "red nose" of alcoholics and dyspeptics, depicted by artists and cartoonists, is due to rosacea.

The disease occurs most frequently in middle age, and in women, in whom it is associated with gastrointestinal disturbances or pelvic disease. Many rosacea patients have concomitant focal infections. Infections of the gallbladder, appendix, teeth or tonsils can produce pus-forming lesions. In some instances there is absence of free hydrochloric acid in the stomach.

Persons with rosacea must avoid any food or drink that will cause flushing of the face. They must avoid hot and spicy foods and alcoholic beverages. All foci of infection must be eliminated and any disturbance in the gastrointestinal tract or pelvis must be corrected. Hydrochloric acid is administered when necessary. Vitamin B complex capsules may be helpful. Antibiotics and superficial x-rays are given for pustular lesions. Astringent lotions are prescribed for topical use.

Pruritus (Itching)

Everybody has experienced "normal" itching from, say, a mosquito bite or some other transient obvious cause. Prolonged, persistent, annoying and even maddening itching is another matter.

Pruritus is not a disease in its own right but a symptom which may occur as an initial or accompanying manifestation of many conditions, some of them minor and some serious. In addition to relief of itching, determination of the underlying cause is important. Most often, itching is an accompaniment of parasitic diseases such as scabies ("itch mite"), fungus infections, dermatologic diseases such as the eczemas, allergies, excessively dry skin, and the like. But it may arise from an obvious systemic disease such as chickenpox or a less obvious one such as diabetes or leukemia, described elsewhere in this book.

There are helpful topical medications for relief of itching, and some systemic drugs may be prescribed under certain circumstances, but many commonly used drugs that are taken orally may themselves be a cause of itching reactions, and a succession of different medications applied to the skin without a doctor's advice may make matters worse. Annoying itching may result from contact of wool or scratchy clothing with the skin, especially in a warm and dry environment, in which case a shift to non-irritating garments next to the skin gives relief. For extensive itching, colloid baths described below are helpful, and well tolerated by people with excessively dry and sensitive skin who are irritated by frequent ordinary baths, especially in the winter.

Colloid Baths

A colloid bath can be prepared by adding one pound of refined corn starch to a tubful of warm water. Stir the starch with cool water to make a thin paste before putting it in the tub. A similar amount of bran or oatmeal enclosed in a cheesecloth bag with a half pound of baking soda will serve the same purpose.

ECZEMA

Eczema, sometimes referred to as *dermatitis,* is not a disease but a symptom complex of many causes and clinical variations. The term "eczema" is derived from a Greek word meaning "to boil over," quite descriptive of inflamed and sometimes weepy skin.

The principal symptoms of the various eczemas, or dermatitis, are redness, swelling, sensations of heat and itching. The changes of dermatitis are reversible and the skin recovers, unmarked and intact, provided there is no underlying infection or that ulceration has not occurred from too vigorous scratching.

Since the skin is "two-faced" — that is, has an inner and an outer aspect — substances that irritate it may be of internal or external origin, and often there may be a combination of the two factors. The various types of eczema or dermatitis are described below.

Contact dermatitis is a reaction of the skin to material that comes in contact with it, as the name indicates. This substance may be a primary irritant, such as a strong acid or alkali, injurious to any skin, or it may act by sensitization induced by previous contact with it, as in *cosmetic dermatitis*. Contact dermatitis is the most frequent dermatosis seen by a dermatologist.

The skin disturbances that patients with contact dermatitis complain of are similar in all cases, but differ in degree of acuteness. The initial reaction occurs in the area of contact, and there is sharp delineation between the inflamed and normal skin. Clues to the cause of contact dermatitis can frequently be discovered by noting the location of the eruption, its configuration, by patch tests, and by careful taking of the patient's medical history.

Chemical agents are responsible for the greatest number of contact dermatoses. These agents in the home, industry, and in fact everywhere around us, are so numerous that it is impossible to mention them all. Some of the chemical agents most frequently responsible for contact reactions in various areas of the body are:

Head and neck: Ragweed, cosmetics, dusts, sprays, hair dyes, jewelry, furs, plastics, oral preparations and poison ivy. The common offenders in *cosmetic dermatitis* are nail lacquer, permanent wave solutions, hair dye and lipstick.

Hands and forearms: Occupational contactants, detergents, cleansers, plastics, and foods that are handled.

Trunk: Articles of clothing, metal clasps, rubber, cosmetics, and deodorants.

Legs and feet: Clothing, elastic garters, poison ivy, shoes, and topical medications.

Identification of the offending contactant is accomplished by patch testing. This is done by applying the suspected substance to an area of skin that is free of eruption and noting whether or not there is a reaction. Once the responsible substance is discovered, it must be removed from the patient's environment to effect a cure. Nothing can be done if the patient continues to come in contact with the substance.

The dermatitis tends to clear uneventfully if the process is not perpetuated by ill-advised treatment or if secondary bacterial infection does not occur.

Poison ivy dermatitis. This plant has probably spoiled more vacations than all other mischiefs of nature combined. The "poison" is an oily substance in the plant (urushiol) that is also present in poison oak and poison sumac. There is no reaction to poison ivy the very first time one is exposed to it. But a later exposure produces an acute, intensely itching, blisterlike eruption on an inflamed base. The blisters are usually grouped and often "streaked," because of tendency to spread along scratch lines. Spread to other parts of the body occurs by direct transfer of the oily substance, usually by the fingers from scratching. However, the fluid that oozes from blisters is not itself "contagious."

One attack of poison ivy does not give immunity to later attacks, but rather an increased susceptibility. Some people are so exquisitely sensitive to poison ivy that they react to such remote contact as the smoke from burning plants, contact with pets that have brushed against plants, or tools and clothing.

Avoidance of the plant is the best "treatment." Poison ivy is easy to recognize by its notch-edged leaves that grow in *clusters of three* — a pair of leaves opposite each other, with a third one that grows out between them at the tip of the stalk.

If exposure to poison ivy is suspected, prompt washing of the skin with soap and water may remove the plant oils before damage can be done. But this has to be done quite soon after exposure. Very mild cases of ivy poisoning, perhaps a few small blisters in a small area of skin, may be eased by applying cool wet compresses at intervals, or applying a paste of baking soda held in place by a soft gauze bandage.

Severe cases should have medical care. Patients with very severe, widespread involvement may be relieved dramatically and the duration of the dermatitis may be considerably shortened, by administration of systemic corticosteroid drugs. In selected patients who cannot avoid the plant, and who have severe repeated attacks of contact dermatitis, hyposensitization with one of the oral extracts may be advisable. Hyposensitization by injection of poison ivy extract is of no value.

Hand eczema (housewife's eczema). This dermatitis affects persons with a dry skin and is precipitated by the chemical action of soap and alkali. Most lesions begin with mild dryness, redness, and scaling. As the condition becomes more severe by continued use of soap and water, fissuring and crusting occur, with eventual blisters and, ultimately, thickening of the skin. Frequently the condition involves the left fourth finger under the rings. It is more prevalent during winter months.

Undoubtedly the increase in this condition is associated with the advent of potent detergents. The more efficient the detergent, the greater its solvent action on keratin or fats of the skin. It appears that a superior cleansing agent not only cleanses with great effectiveness but tends also to "dehydrate" the skin. Thus the skin tends to become harsh and fissured, with dry eczematous lesions on the fingers, wrists, or back of the hands, and inflammation of skin between the fingers and around the nails.

Even without irritative agents, constant immersion of the hands in water alone tends to produce deleterious and macerative changes. The tissues tend to become less resistant to hitherto innocuous chemicals. If, in addition, a fat solvent such as a detergent is used on an already dry skin, the "soil" is ready for the development of typical housewife's eczema.

Management of this dermatitis is tedious, painstaking, and at best palliative. However, patients may be greatly benefited by a few simple measures.

The first is ***reduction of the irritation.*** Cotton-lined rubber gloves, or cotton gloves under rubber gloves, should be worn, for periods of not more than 15 minutes. Since heat will penetrate these coverings, hot water should not be used.

Dishwashing should be done by soaking the dishes in hot soapy water for 30 minutes to emulsify the debris. At the end of this period the water will be sufficiently cool for washing with cotton-lined rubber gloves.

For ***bathing infants,*** a pair of cotton gloves should be worn over the cotton-lined rubber gloves to prevent slipping. Diapers should first be rinsed in clear water to remove the ammoniacal urine.

Because handling of fruit juices, fruits, vegetables, and raw meats is frequently irritating, the use of canned or frozen products is recommended. Patients with hand eczema should avoid contact with wool, as in knitting or making beds. Since ordinary handcleaning methods are not advisable, a tepid boric acid solution may be used for this purpose. If cotton gloves are worn at all times the hands will require little cleaning and the patient will not need to wash them too frequently.

Atopic dermatitis (generalized neurodermatitis) embraces allergic and infantile eczema. Although the lesions occur most frequently on the "bends" of the elbows and knees, they may involve any part of the body. In infants the eruption usually appears first on the scalp and face. These patients are prone to acquire hay fever or asthma later in life, and heredity plays an important role.

Atopic dermatitis usually occurs in three separate stages: infantile, childhood, and adolescent or young adult stage. The childhood phase may immediately follow that of infancy or it may occur several years after the infantile eczema has disappeared. In the adolescent stage the skin becomes thickened (lichenified), more dry, and of a darker color.

Itching is without question the predominant symptom of atopic dermatitis. Associated findings may be cataracts, intolerance to high temperatures and humidities, and precipitation of symptoms by emotional stress. While allergy (see Chapter 20) is present in more than 50 per cent of these patients, its exact role in the production of the skin lesions is not certain. In many cases, diet and environmental factors can be shown to provoke recurrences, but other factors such as cold, humidity, heat and stress do so equally.

Topical application of properly selected steroid drugs is probably the most successful therapy at present. A change of environment is frequently beneficial.

Although medical management is often successful, the results are usually symptomatic rather than specific in nature. For intractable atopic dermatitis, the systemic administration of corticosteroids remains the most effective therapy. But possible side-effects from this therapy make it essential that it be employed judiciously in conjunction with all known medications to give the patient maximum relief with minimum risk.

Seborrheic dermatitis (seborrheic eczema) usually involves areas of the skin in which the oil glands are most abundant, such as the scalp, sides of the nose, behind the ears, and the center of the chest. ("Seborrhea" means "flow of oil"). The lesions are covered by a greasy scale and have a yellowish-brown tinge so they appear and feel oily. On the scalp there may be some dry scaling, as in dandruff, or the scales may be profuse and greasy.

Dandruff — fine, whitish, slightly greasy scales — is often associated with a "dry" form of seborrhea without inflammation.

Seborrheic dermatitis probably has several underlying factors. These may be hormonal, infectious, or nutritional; patients are usually partial to diets rich in fats and sweets.

Treatment of seborrheic dermatitis is unsatisfactory because the condition can merely be controlled, not eradicated. Frequent washing and shampooing of excessively oily skin and scalp, with use of such medication as a doctor may advise, is helpful but not curative.

Nummular eczema is another dermatitis of unknown cause. It is always associated with dryness or dehydration of the skin and can appear at any age in either sex. The lesions ("nummular" means "coin-shaped") occur as plaques, usually on the back of the hands, outer surfaces of the arms, and outer aspects of the legs and thighs. It is most common in housewives, dishwashers, surgeons, and persons who are in constant contact with soap and water, continually dehydrating the skin. The eruption commonly recurs in the winter (with exposure to cold, chapping, rough clothing such as wool) and often clears in the summer.

Infectious eczematoid dermatitis occurs in proximity to discharging lesions or an external focus of infection. It may occur about infected wounds, from nasal secretions, infected secretions from the ear, or around the ear or cutaneous lesions. Treatment is directed to the underlying infection.

Lichen simplex chronicus (localized neurodermatitis). The first symptom is itching without visible skin lesions. Constant scratching of the affected area produces thickening of the skin.

Patches of lichenified (thickened) eczema may occur on the thighs, legs, or feet, and often appear on the nape of the neck in women after the menopause. These thickened, darkened lesions are of a leathery consistency. The itching can be controlled with appropriate therapy.

Stasis dermatitis. Eczema of the legs, sometimes called *varicose* or stasis dermatitis, is due to incompetency of the valves in the veins, leading to impaired circulation (see *varicose veins*, Index). Stasis dermatitis is common in elderly persons and the condition may become chronic. The patches of dermatitis may become pigmented, thickened, and may even ulcerate, leading to painful lesions. Treatment is rest in bed, elevation of the legs, and application of soothing medicaments.

COSMETIC DERMATITIS

This dermatitis is usually due to *sensitization* rather than to primary irritation. A sensitizing agent is one which does not cause demonstrable changes on first contact. However, subsequent contact with the same or other areas may cause specific changes in the skin or mucous membrances after five to seven days or more.

Cosmetic dermatitis is cured by removing the offending substance from any contact with the skin. The location of the dermatitis — e. g., lips, scalp, fingers — is one clue that helps to identify the cause. However, the detection of a particular sensitizing agent is not always easy, and the nature of the lesions, a painstaking check of preparations the patient uses, and knowledge of the chemical components of cosmetics, may be required to bring the culprit to bay.

The most common preparations which cause dermatitis are nail lacquers, scalp preparation, face creams, lipstick, and perfumes.

Creams. Among the widely used creams are bleaching, freckle, lubricating, emollient, cleansing, hormone, vanishing and foundation, and vitamin creams. Reactions are most likely to occur from freckle, bleaching, or cleansing creams.

In *freckle cream* the most likely irritants are acids, or oxidizing agents such as perborate, hydrogen peroxide, or zinc peroxide.

There are three types of *cleansing cream:* 1. A *liquefying* type containing mineral oil, paraffin, and white petrolatum. 2. A *cold cream* type containing mineral oil, beeswax, borax and water. 3. An *emollient* type containing mineral oil, yellow petrolatum, beeswax, borax, water, and lanolin or vegetable oils, or an absorption base or other emulsifying agents such as sulfonated oils. The most common irritants in such creams are the petroleum oils, detergents, and perfume.

Astringent creams are used to close large pores. They generally contain salts of zinc sulfate, aluminum sulfate, or bismuth subnitrate. They may also contain resorcinol or salicylic acid, both of which are likely to produce dermatitis.

Depilatories are used most frequently on the legs, but when used on the chin may cause a dermatitis of the face and eyelids. This action is usually that of a primary irritant. The chief irritating ingredients are sulfides or sulfhydrates of an alkali or alkaline earth. Others are mercaptan carboxylic acid or its salt, alkaline stannate solutions, and newer preparations containing calcium thioglycolate, which appear less likely to cause dermatitis.

By far the most common cause of cosmetic reactions affecting the *head and face* are the hair and scalp preparations. These include dyes, bleaches, lacquers, tonics, and waving lotions.

Hair dyes are of various types: vegetable, metallic, synthetic organic (amine or aniline), and sulfonated azo dyes. The amine and aniline dyes are the most effective and are used most extensively in beauty parlors. They contain paraphenylenediamine and paratolylenediamine and constitute the greatest health hazard. Numerous eye injuries have resulted from paraphenylenediamine and its use in eyebrow and eyelash preparations is now forbidden.

Before dyeing the hair, beauticians are required to apply the dye to a small area behind the ear. This is covered with collodion and the site examined 24 hours later for evidence of irritation. This test is not completely reliable, because sensitivity may not develop for several days, and the quantity of dye used for a patch test is minute compared to that used for the entire scalp. Dermatitis from hair dyes may involve the scalp, face, ears, and eyes, or it may become generalized.

Scalp lotions are also frequent causes of dermatitis. These contain ingredients such as resorcinol, arsenic, tar, sulfonamides, glycerine, and quinine, all of which are capable of causing dermatitis.

Permanent hair waving is now chiefly done by the "cold wave" process. This consists of applying solutions of chemicals to soften the hair so that it loses its elasticity and will take a curl. Oxidizing solutions are then applied to "set" the curl. Gums or resins may be added to "hold the curl." The reducing agents are generally inorganic sulfides or thioglycolates; the oxidizing agents are usually iodates or peroxides. "Home permanents" usually contain the same ingredients but in more dilute form.

Dermatitis may result from the reducing agents or the gums or resins. Often the dermatitis is *due to misuse* of the products, especially when using home permanents, from failure to follow directions carefully or from too much stretching of the hair.

Wave-setting solutions, used in setting hair after shampoos, rarely cause dermatitis. The chief ingredients are gums, such as acacia or karaya.

Hair lacquers, used to hold the hair in place, are solutions of gum resins or other colloidal material of an alkaline aqueous or alcoholic nature. In one "outbreak" of dermatitis among users of hair lacquer pads, a resin of maleic anhydride was found to be the offender.

Hair bleaching preparations may occasionally cause dermatitis, especially if the compounds used are from chlorine or oxalic acid. Hydrogen peroxide and ammonia are the most commonly used bleaches and, if properly used, do not produce irritation.

Hair "straighteners," used primarily by persons with kinky hair, consist of perfumed petroleum jelly or a gum solution such as tragacanth or benzoin. However, they may contain alkaline mixtures with sodium hydroxide or sodium carbonate which may cause a dermatitis.

Lipstick dermatitis is generally in the form of a cheilitis (inflammation of the lips and angles of the mouth). Bromofluorescein dyes are the most frequent offenders in lipsticks. Other dyes, perfumes, oils, waxes, fats or flavors may cause a dermatitis. The indelible lipsticks are the greatest offenders.

Eyelid dermatitis and dermatitis of the face, ears, and chest result largely from nail lacquers. These areas are frequently touched by the nails and the lacquer agent can be transferred. The cause is generally found to be the resins in lacquers; the dye or solvent is often not responsible.

Perfumes have long been known to cause cosmetic dermatitis. They may also lead to sinusitis and rhinitis. Perfume consists of alcohol, a natural or synthetic flower oil, and a fixative such as musk or ambergris. Because of their complex composition, it is very difficult to identify the ingredients in a perfume that causes a dermatitis.

Drug Eruptions

The drugs which most frequently cause skin eruptions are those which are most commonly used. Lesions which result from oral or injected drugs are numerous and varied. They may be generalized or limited to certain body areas, and vary in severity from simple redness of the skin to gangrene. They usually appear suddenly.

It should be stressed that *any* drug may produce any type of skin reaction. Drugs frequently associated with skin eruptions include barbiturates, sulfas, tranquillizers, salicylates (chiefly aspirin), opiates, biologicals, bromides, acetanilid, phenolphthalein laxatives, and the antibiotics.

Prickly Heat

Prickly heat (miliaria) results from obstruction of some of the sweat ducts, so that trapped sweat cannot reach the surface and escape. This condition is brought about by high temperatures due to fever or hot "perspiry" weather. The eruption typically consists of inflammatory pinhead-size lesions, accompanied by itching and burning sensations. Occasionally there is secondary infection and formation of tiny pustules. Treatment demands avoidance of excessive heat, application of a dusting powder or soothing lotion, and wearing of light loose garments. Prickly heat disappears quite promptly in a cool environment.

Psoriasis

Psoriasis is one of the most common skin diseases, in some form affecting an estimated six per cent of the population. The cause is unknown; faulty metabolism of fats and neurogenic disorders have been suspected. It is likely that the cause may be found to be an enzyme defect affecting keratinization (the process by which skin cells become horny).

The disease affects both sexes, adults more commonly than children. Psoriasis can occur in families and in about 25 per cent of cases the disease is hereditary.

Psoriasis rarely affects the general health. It has periods of remission and recurrence, usually abates during the summer and recurs in winter.

Initially there is a bright red, sharply defined, elevated lesion covered with a thick, dry, silvery scale. Removal of the scale reveals tiny bleeding points. The finding is characteristic of psoriasis. The lesions heal without scarring. They may coalesce to form patches of bizarre and spiral shapes. The affected sites are usually the elbows and knees, scalp, nails, and the lower back.

There is no single preferred method of treatment nor any drug that will cure psoriasis. The simplest forms of treatment are topical applications as the doctor advises. A well known treatment used in hospitals is the Goeckerman treatment. This consists of the application of crude coal tar ointment followed by ultraviolet light. Recently, for the "stubborn" type, the use of aminopterin

"Prickly heat" results from entrapment of sweat in layers of the skin close to the surface, from obstruction or disruption of sweat duct outlets. At left below, a normal gland delivering sweat to the surface of the skin. At right, rupture of a duct in the prickle-cell layer of the epidermis; sweat produced by the gland cannot escape and an intensely burning, itching, minute pimple forms. Relatively few of the 2,000,000 sweat glands are affected at one time.

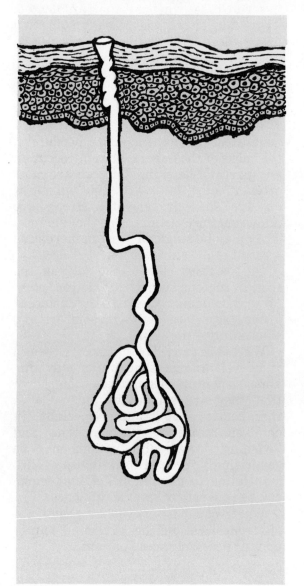

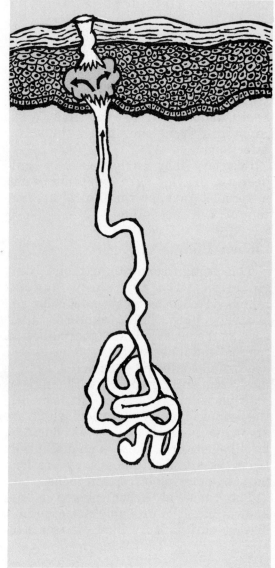

has been advocated, but this drug requires careful supervision by a physician since it can cause undesirable changes in the blood.

Corticosteroid drugs will control psoriasis but will not cure it, and continued use of these drugs would make the treatment potentially more harmful than the disease. Their use is usually restricted to patients whose handicap in society or employment is extremely severe.

Pityriasis Rosea

This is a common disease of young adults. It is self-limiting and terminates in six to eight weeks with complete recovery.

The first symptom is a solitary, rounded lesion, known as the "primary" or "mother" patch, which is usually mistaken for "ringworm." Similar but smaller oval-shaped lesions appear within four to ten days. These are usually on the trunk where their symmetrical distribution resembles a Christmas tree. The lesions usually do not occur on the face, seldom appear below the elbows or knees, and as a rule are not "itchy." The condition is neither contagious nor infectious.

Recovery may be hastened by mild peeling of the skin with sunlight, ultraviolet rays, or the topical application of a drying lotion.

Lichen Planus

This benign condition exhibits many variations. The dry, shiny, angular lesions have a somewhat violet color and are very itchy. "Thin skinned" areas such as the wrist surface, genitalia, lips, tongue, and inner surfaces of the cheeks are usually affected. The wrist area is most frequently involved, with single or multiple patches of lesions. In the mouth, the lesions occur as white dots which are arranged in circles or lines, producing a lacelike network. There is no discomfort from these lesions unless they are irritated by smoking or certain foods.

The cause of lichen planus is not known, but it is probably not a specific disease entity. More likely it is a syndrome resulting from various factors. In recent years emphasis has been placed on neurogenic factors or some type of infection, but a causative organism has not been isolated.

Lichen planus has been known to occur following the use of drugs (bismuth, gold, atabrine, arsenic, para-aminosalicylic acid, isoniazid). The role of emotional factors is uncertain. Onset may coincide with an emotional upset but this may be only a "trigger" factor in precipitating symptoms.

Treatment is merely palliative and cure depends upon spontaneous resolution of the disease process. Topical therapy consists of itch-relieving creams and superficial x-rays for localized lesions. Antimalarial drugs may be administered internally, and steroid drugs may be used in severe cases when not contraindicated. There may be considerable pigmentation of the skin after the lesions disappear, but this gradually fades.

Warts

The **common wart** ("seed wart") usually occurs on the hands, especially on the backs of the fingers, but may occur on any part of the skin. Children are most often affected, but warts may appear at any age. These dry, elevated lesions have numerous projections on the surface. They may be single or very numerous as a result of autoinoculation.

On the thick skin of the soles of the feet, in regions subject to friction, *plantar warts* appear as yellowish translucent lesions associated with discomfort and thickening of the skin.

Warts are caused by viruses. Although it is well known that warts may disappear spontaneously, it has been shown that they are sometimes amenable to therapeutic suggestion. Especially in children, impressive "hocus pocus" and "wishing away" ministrations may be surprisingly successful, giving some substantiation to popular belief that warts can be relieved by "magic influences."

Warts can be removed by chemicals, electrodesiccation, or excision, appropriate to the individual patient.

Molluscum Contagiosum. This is a viral infection of the skin in which there is an overgrowth consisting of single or multiple rounded pimples. It is of a pearly gray color with a central depression from which a "cheesy" plug, called the molluscum body, can be squeezed. Lesions usually occur on the trunk and buttocks but can involve any area of the skin.

on the skin or mucous membranes. The lesions are small raspberry-like vegetations of granulation tissue which are secondary to skin infections. They are usually soft, have a supporting stem, and occur singly. The scalp, lips, and fingers are the most common sites of involvement. The growths bleed easily due to their vascular matrix. Treatment

Xanthelasma is a not uncommon disease of the eyelids in persons past middle age, manifested by characteristic raised yellowish spots that usually begin at the nasal side of the eyelids. The drawing at the right shows a cross section of an eyelid with the lesion, which in most instances is associated with high levels of cholesterol in the blood. The plaques begin as yellowish spots of pinhead size and enlarge over a period of time.

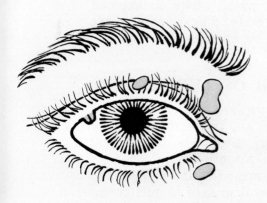

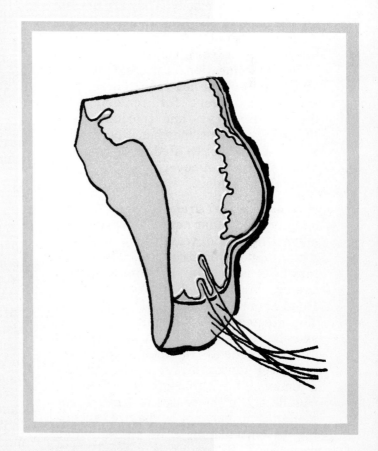

It is essential to remove all the lesions because the disease is contagious. Treatment consists of curetting the lesion or expressing the cheesy contents. A drop of liquid phenol or tincture of iodine may be applied to each lesion.

Granuloma Pyogenicum. This common type of rapidly growing tumor appears

may be either by excision, electrodesiccation, or cautery.

Xanthelasma is the most common form of *xanthoma* ("yellow tumor"). The condition occurs when there is a high level of cholesterol and cholesterol esters in the blood. The lesion occurs on the eyelids. They are flat, soft, yellow-colored plaques of varying size. This sign may be a forerunner of angina or high blood pressure. Treatment consists of a cholesterol-free diet and chemical or surgical removal of the lesions.

BIRTHMARKS AND MOLES

Vascular Nevi

Nevus flammeus (portwine stain). These pink to bluish-red lesions, usually with a smooth surface, most often occur on one side of the face or neck but they may be widespread and involve as much as one-half of the body. They are present on the nape of the neck in about 10 per cent of the population. The mucous membranes may also be involved.

The discoloration is present at birth and usually does not fade. There is no satisfactory agent for removing the lesion. Grenz rays and thorium-X will lighten the color somewhat. Radium and x-rays should not be used for this type of vascular nevus. A covering cosmetic will conceal the lesion.

Hemangioma (strawberry mark). This variety of vascular nevus affects only the superficial blood vessels and has very little supporting structure. The marks may be present at birth or appear later in life as pinhead-sized or larger growths, ranging in color from scarlet to purple. The affected sites commonly are the face, shoulders, scalp and neck, but they also appear frequently in other regions. Generally the mark grows slowly but there is a tendency for it to regress more or less completely in the course of time. Treatment may or may not be required according to circumstances in an individual case. This birthmark is susceptible to radiation, especially radium. Carbon dioxide snow may also be used.

Moles

The *common mole* or *nevus* is a frequent benign lesion which develops during the first few years of life. In the beginning they are flat and of various shades of brown or black. Moles enlarge slowly and most of them become elevated.

Some have hairs on the surface. At adolescence, and during pregnancy, all moles tend to darken and enlarge.

A person in his twenties has an average of 40 to 50 moles. These tend to disappear and by the age of 60 years the average is four per person. But it is possible for moles to appear at any time up to 30 years of age.

Moles that darken or increase in size, or appear after the age of 30, can be dangerous and should be removed. Moles which repeatedly become infected or are subject to irritation should be removed. When a suspicious mole is removed it should be sent to a laboratory for microscopic examination. Rarely, the pathologist's diagnosis may be *malignant melanoma* for which surgery is the usual therapy.

Moles are also removed for cosmetic reasons. These moles are usually elevated brown lesions which occur on exposed parts of the body. These lesions are considered to be harmless.

CANCER OF THE SKIN

This is the most frequently encountered form of cancer, and the form most likely to have a happy outcome with early and proper medical attention.

All of these growths are visible, and with the proper degree of suspicion and alertness on the part of patient and doctor, the diagnosis can be made early in the progress of the disease, and treatment can be instituted with extremely satisfactory results. As a rule, skin cancer is nearly always so characteristic in its appearance that a diagnosis can be made immediately. However, microscopic confirmation of the clinical diagnosis should always be made.

The two most common types of skin cancer are the basal cell and squamous cell types.

The *basal cell* variety originates as a small fleshy nodule, most often in parts of the face. The basal type usually progresses slowly and it takes many months to reach a diameter of one-half to one inch. After about a year the small nodular lesion ulcerates centrally and begins to bleed. This is usually the time when a patient consults his physician and gives a typical history of the lesion. It is a crusted lesion from which the crust is shed at intervals, leaving an ulcerated, bleeding surface. However, another crust then forms and the sequence is repeated.

Basal cell cancers do not metastasize or spread, but if neglected they may extend under surrounding normal skin and cause serious trouble. Basal cell cancer can be destroyed by local measures employed by a specialist.

Squamous cell cancer, in contrast to the basal cell type, usually appears on preexistent, precancerous lesions. They may appear on any area of the skin or mucous membrane. The lips, mouth, and genitalia are likely sites of development.

Treatment is essential since squamous lesions will increase in size and large fungoid masses may appear. Metastases usually occur late in the course of squamous cell cancer.

Predisposing factors in the development of squamous cell cancer are leukoplakia (white, thickened patches) of the lips and mouth, smoking, and excessive exposure to the sun's rays of blond and blue-eyed persons. Skin cancer is more frequent among people exposed to large amounts of intense sunlight over long periods of time. Keratotic (horny) growths in exposed areas of skin, most frequently present on the face, ears, neck, and scalp, may be premalignant forerunners of squamous cell cancer. The lesions are benign as long as the individual is not exposed to sunlight.

DERMATOSES DUE TO THE SUN

Skin eruptions may be caused by allergy to a physical agent such as light.

Berlock dermatitis is an eruption produced by the application of certain plant product substances, followed by exposure of the skin to sunlight. Oil of bergamot is a constituent of some perfumes and colognes. It will, in sensitive persons, result in an area of discoloration at the site of application, such as the sides of the neck and the flexor surfaces of the arms and wrists.

Light-sensitization by drugs. Increasing numbers of drugs sensitize the skin to sunlight. Many of these drugs may be taken for weeks or months without any adverse response, but when the patient is exposed to light of the proper wavelength for a sufficient period of time the dermatitis occurs. The eruption is usually limited to areas exposed to the sun and may vary from redness of the skin to hives and eczema. Drugs which are capable of producing such a reaction include the sulfas, tranquillizers, antibiotics, barbiturates, and salicylates, to mention only a few groups. Discontinuance of a specific drug, or avoidance of exposure to direct sunlight, brings a disappearance of the eruption.

Sensitivity to Sunlight

Lupus erythematosus. This disease occurs in two quite different forms, the discoid and systemic varieties.

Discoid lupus erythematosus is characterized by red, circular or discoid lesions. Their initial appearance is often preceded by exposure to sunlight. The center of the lesion is depressed and dilated pore openings plugged with a fine scale are found on close examination. This is a chronic disease of the skin. The patient should avoid exposure to sunlight and ultraviolet lamps. If this is not feasible, a sunscreen preparation may be used. Therapy with antimalarial drugs under close medical supervision may be beneficial.

Systemic lupus erythematosus is a deep-seated disease with symptoms only incidentally manifested in the skin. Reddened patches occur on exposed areas of the body. A "butterfly distribution" is sometimes present — patches on the cheeks and bridge of the nose somewhat resemble a butterfly with open wings. *Systemic* lupus is one of the so-called connective tissue or collagen diseases. For fuller discussion of this group of diseases, See Chapter 19.

Freckles usually appear in susceptible youngsters around the age of six years or so. Redheads and blue-eyed blonds most often have the type of skin that is sensitive to sunlight. Freckles occur as a result of exposure to light, and once they appear they are a lifetime acquisition. They do not become cancerous and are strictly cosmetic blemishes, or for that matter, rather attractive "beauty spots." Freckles are usually darker in summer and less pronounced in winter. This reflects the stimulating action of sunlight on pigmentation.

Prevention of exaggerated freckles is about the same in principle as prevention of sunburn. A wide-brimmed hat, a sunscreen preparation, cosmetics, or staying in the shade, lessen the incidence of freckle-darkening sunlight to some degree. Covering cosmetics can mask facial freckles very satisfactorily, if the owner is greatly disturbed by them. Bleaching preparations are of little benefit. Sometimes, "skin peeling" measures can lessen the conspicuousness of freckles, but such procedures should be in the hands of a dermatologist experienced in their use.

Sunburn is a burn in every sense of the word. Massive sunburn is not only excruciating but can make one very ill. Skins differ in the speed with which they build up defenses at the first seasonal exposure to hot sunlight, as at a beach. There is no warning of a bad burn at the time it is being inflicted; symptoms come later, perhaps after several hours. Graduated exposure to the sun builds up protection not so much from the increase in pigment known as "tanning," but from increased thickness of the skin.

The first exposure of unprotected skin to sunlight at a beach should be limited to about 15 minutes. Increase this exposure about five minutes a day for a week. By that time the skin should be reasonably well conditioned for bathing suit activities. However, some skins do not tan; they just burn or freckle.

Lotions and creams containing chemical agents that block the burning wavelengths of sunlight, called sunscreens, can prolong the period of safe exposure to the sun quite effectively. At the same time, the more effective of these agents delay the process of pigmentation or tanning, depending on the amount of tanning wavelengths that filter through. There are also complete sunblocking agents that not only prevent burning but tanning as well. Swimming may remove protective agents from the skin.

Babies and young children must be protected by adults who limit the youngsters' time in the sun or apply appropriate sunscreen agents.

Sunlight is most intense at high noon, when the sun is directly overhead, and for a couple of hours before and after noon. It may be wise to begin the first sunbathing exposures around 4 p.m. when the angle of the sun is lower. Water and sand, however, reflect sunlight and intensify its burning properties. Bad burns can also be inflicted through a hazy atmosphere. Ointments containing local anesthetics suffice for treatment of mild sunburn, but a severe case may require medical treatment.

Excessive, repeated, continued exposure of the skin to attain and maintain a deep tan has undesirable consequences over long periods of time. Physiologically, such skins tend to become prematurely aged, with an eventual unyouthful leatheriness and lack of suppleness that is irreversible.

BALDNESS

Physicians, particularly dermatologists, are frequently consulted by patients who complain of loss of scalp hair. Medical science has accumulated a good deal of knowledge concerning the physiology of hair growth. Some types of hair loss can be dealt with quite effectively, but other types cannot.

Alopecia areata (patchy baldness). In this condition, hair is usually lost from a single spot, generally in the scalp but sometimes in the bearded area. The bald spot is usually about the size of a dime or a quarter. The hair loss may occur suddenly, but this is not common.

Common male baldness follows a definite pattern. The hair recedes from the forehead, temple, and crown, as shown in drawing, and the bald areas tend to merge, but a fringe around the ears and back of the head always remains.

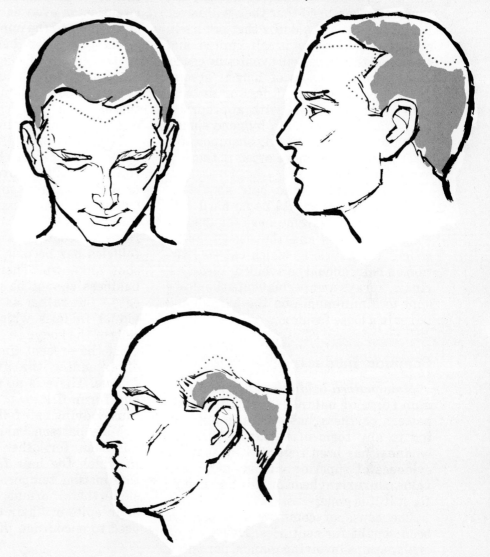

There is no inflammation or any obvious skin disorder or systemic disease. Baldness in the patches is complete. Almost invariably the hair returns spontaneously, in a few weeks or months, but sometimes the new growth lacks pigment and is lighter than surrounding hair. The condition may recur. Very rarely, loss of hair may involve the entire scalp (alopecia totalis), and if this occurs in childhood it is likely to persist for years.

Diffuse loss of scalp hair in women. The growth of hair on the scalp progresses in a cycle. A hair grows continuously for some years, then goes into a "resting" phase, and at the end of several months falls out. A new cycle then begins. The turnover rate is about 50 to 100 hairs per day.

An increasing number of young women under 40 years of age complain of diffuse loss of scalp hair. Whether this condition is actually increasing or whether more women happen to consult their doctors about it is not certain. The onset of hair loss is usually insidious and involves the top of the head, in a pattern of diffuse rather than patchy thinning common in older women but not in the young. After the fifth decade, such loss of hair is considered to be a consequence of aging.

The anxiety of younger women with diffuse hair loss is understandable, but they can be assured that they will never have the type of baldness that occurs in men. Their condition is self-limited, and even though severe, will eventually cease.

Occasionally a loss of hair is accompanied by excessive oiliness or dryness which can be treated with appropriate measures. General scalp hygiene should be maintained with weekly shampoos for most women, and more often if there is excessive oiliness.

Manipulation of the hair should be gentle and there should be no hard rubbing or use of extreme heat for drying. "Tight" hairdos and the use of brush rollers (or anything which causes traction on hair) should be avoided. Bleaches, rinses, sprays and permanents should be kept to a minimum and the hair should be set in a loose fashion.

Common Baldness

Male pattern baldness. The most common form of baldness, so-called male pattern baldness, has remained unyielding to any form of therapy. Although baldness has been regarded by some as evidence of superior virility, most men value a luxuriant head of hair and mourn for it if it is gone.

The cause of common baldness has been sought for centuries. However, all explanations involving glands, parasites, nutrition, nerves, and injury have been found to be inadequate, or at best to explain but a part of the process. It is well established that heredity is a factor in common male baldness. Genetic studies have been made of families in which it occurs. This type of baldness does not occur in men who fail to mature sexually.

The typical male "pattern" is not a general thinning of the hair but baldness of characteristic areas of the scalp. In its most extreme form there always remains a fringe of hair at the side of the head, running around the back of the head from ear to ear. (This classic pattern is shown in busts of Hippocrates, "the father of medicine".) The extent and rapidity with which hair is lost varies. Commonly, the hair begins to recede at a relatively early age, in the twenties or even earlier, from the area at the sides of the upper forehead in front of the temples. A bald spot may appear on the crown of the head, and balding areas may merge until only a side-fringe remains, but within this pattern area there are various degrees of denudation as the process continues or slows.

"Hair restorers" and treatments to reverse this process have been promoted for years but a cure for male pattern baldness remains unknown. It is quite evident that in this type of baldness the scalp is normal in every detectable respect except that the activity of the hair follicles has become suspended for reasons unknown. Therefore this form of baldness cannot be regarded as a "disease," but rather as a disability of individual follicles which die before other cells of the body.

At the present time no way is known of extending the lifespan of the hair follicle. There is no miraculous salve or any form of known treatment that will cause a dying hair follicle to produce hair.

Male pattern baldness should not be mistaken for other forms of alopecia in which the hair follicles have ceased to function temporarily, and often resume their normal function regardless or in spite of "hair tonics" that may be used to encourage them.

Infections of the Skin

Bacterial and viral infections with skin manifestations (e.g., shingles, boils, cold sores) are discussed elsewhere in this book. See *Index*.

Pemphigus

Pemphigus vulgaris is an uncommon but serious skin disease of unknown cause. It is characterized by the occurrence of crops of *bullae* (large blisters). These may be distributed on both sides of the body but have no definite geographical arrangement.

In many cases a moist, eczematous patch appears first, usually on the scalp, the umbilical region, or in the armpit. The so-called "primary" lesion of pemphigus is rarely recognized until other blisterlike lesions appear. These may vary from the size of a small pea to an egg and are single or grouped. The blisters often appear in mucous membranes of the mouth and throat as well as the skin.

When the bullae rupture a raw, red, moist surface remains. The lesions on the skin cause little discomfort other than tension or slight burning, and heal without scar formation. In the mouth, because of trauma and maceration from food particles, the bullae rupture early and leave raw surfaces which become covered by a loose, yellowish membrane. These lesions are tender and painful and interfere seriously with eating and nutrition.

Skilled treatment of pemphigus is essential. Administration of corticosteroids drugs with necessary precautions has greatly improved the outlook for patients with this disease.

RINGWORM OR FUNGUS INFECTIONS

Tinea capitis (ringworm of the scalp). This superficial fungus infection of the scalp occurs in children before puberty. It is characterized by loosening and partial loss of scalp hair in patches, breaking off of the infected hairs, and loss of luster. It is spread by direct contact with an infected person, a comb or headgear worn by an infected person, and by infected animals, usually pets. Children should be discouraged from "trying on" each other's caps or garments. The infection can be eliminated by oral griseofulvin tablets, one grain daily.

Tinea circinata (ringworm of smooth skin). This superficial fungus infection of the smooth skin may occur as a scalp lesion or as a round patch, a solid plaque, or a patch of eczema. It is often secondary to an infection of the scalp, feet, or nails. It may also be due to contact with an infected playmate or animal, and may

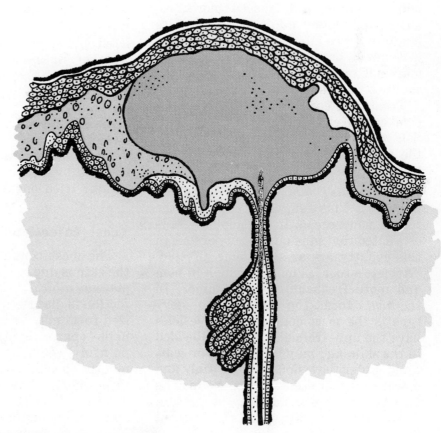

Cross section of a *pemphigus* lesion in a very early stage, in which there is intercellular edema (fluid accumulation) with formation of a small *bulla* or "blister."

occur in children in association with ringworm of the scalp.

The lesion is usually red-ringed and up to six inches in diameter. At times there may be minute blisters (vesicles) along its border. The surface is scaly and the central part of the lesion looks like normal skin. This infection responds to treatment and any fungicidal ointment, such as Whitfield's ointment, will cure it.

Tinea cruris (jockey strap itch). This superficial fungus infection is confined to the inner surface or upper parts of the thighs, where moisture, warmth, and friction are favorable for the growth of the fungus. The fungus infection is spread by infected articles of clothing or athletic suspensories. Itching is usually pronounced.

Treatment consist of keeping the area dry and the frequent application of fungizone lotion.

Tinea versicolor is a fungus infection of the skin manifested by scaly, dark brown to yellow spots and patches without inflammation. It is more evident in warm weather and is seen more frequently in young adults who perspire profusely. The affected areas are darker in summer but show no sign of inflammation. Examination with a Wood's light shows a fluorescence of the lesion.

Treatment consists of using a fungicidal cream such as Whitfield's ointment, Selsun shampoo to the affected areas, or the use of a 20 per cent sodium hyposulfate solution.

Tinea pedis ("athlete's foot," dermatophytosis). This fungus infection of the feet is widespread, if not popular. It is estimated that nine out of ten persons in this country are at some time affected. "Athlete's foot" is more common in men and more frequent in the summer. In the *acute* form, the vesicular (blister) type is the most common. The vesicles have the appearance of grain embedded in the skin, and may be grouped or scattered. Later the lesions become scaly and maceration is present. The scales may be branny, or large scales may be present due to the sodden skin. Crusts are present due to drying of the confluent vesicles.

In the *chronic* variety, the skin becomes thickened, and scaling and fissuring may be present. The toenails may also become involved.

Active treatment consists of the use of wet dressings in the acute phase and fungicidal ointments in the chronic phase. Excessive perspiration of the feet is a common predisposing factor. Dry skin with a normal "acid mantle" is not attacked by athlete's foot fungi with much success. Trapped sweat leads to macerated, sodden skin (at first, particularly between the toes of the little-toe side of the foot) and in an environment of steamy moisture and injured skin, the fungi may "dig in."

The causative fungi are ubiquitous and probably nobody can avoid them at all times. It is sensible not to walk barefoot on moist surfaces in crowded places, such as locker rooms and bathing pools, but the antiseptic foot baths provided in many of these places are of little or no value. Good foot hygiene is important in the prevention and treatment of athlete's foot. To cut down on excessive sweat and its entrapment, light shoes should be worn. Perforated or otherwise ventilated low shoes are preferable in warm weather. Special care should be taken to dry the feet thoroughly after bathing, especially between the toes. Frequent use of a dusting powder may be helpful. Socks should be clean. Exposure of the bare feet to open air is beneficial. Inflamed and macerated skin should not be insulted by a succession of potent medications tried one after the other.

Yeast Infections

The most common yeast infection of the skin is due to the yeastlike organism, *monilia albicans*. Systemic monilial infection is discussed elsewhere. The localized form may be in the skin around the nails (paronychia), beginning as red painful swellings; at the angles of the mouth (perleche); in the folds of the skin and the webs of the fingers; in the mouth (thrush); or around the anal and genital regions, in which case itching is a predominant symptom.

Moisture, in the form of increased sweating or prolonged immersion in water, favors the growth of the organism. Persons whose hands are frequently soaked in soap and water are prone to hand infections. Diabetics, debilitated and obese persons have decreased resistance to the organism, and the use of some antibiotics tends to set up conditions favorable to monilia.

For the local varieties of this yeast infection, gentian violet solutions or a topical fungizone lotion or cream may be used to advantage.

PARASITIC INFECTIONS OF THE SKIN

Pediculosis

Pediculosis means "lousiness." It is a term applied to skin diseases produced by lice, of which there are few varieties.

Pediculosis of the scalp is most often due to neglect and is seen most frequently in children. The head louse is readily transmitted by personal contact and such objects as combs and headgear. Impetigo is usually seen on the back of the neck because the lice, in feeding on the scalp, produce small wheals which itch intensely. The child then scratches, abrades the surface of the skin, and a secondary bacterial infection results. Examination of the infected scalp with a magnifying glass will reveal numerous *nits* or eggs firmly attached to the hair shafts. These mature into adult lice in a few days.

Pediculosis pubis is an infestation of the short hairs of the pubic region by the pubic louse. This creature is short and squat like a crab and the infection is commonly referred to in the vernacular as "the crabs." Rarely, the parasite may infest the armpits and even the eyebrows.

There is intense itching but very little dermatitis. When itching in the pubic and anal region is out of proportion to the amount of dermatitis present, examination with a magnifying glass to detect nits or pubic lice, which are comparatively large, should be done. The condition is seldom seen in women or in men with ordinary good hygienic habits and facilities for cleanliness. The lice may be transmitted through sexual intercourse, by wearing underclothes or bathing trunks of an infected person, or by sleeping in an infected bed.

Pediculosis corporis is due to the body louse. In contrast to the head and pubic louse, the nits are not present on the hair but in clothing, blankets, and bedding. The body louse mostly stays in the seams of clothing and comes out to attack the skin for nourishment in areas which are in constant contact with undergarments, such as the waist, shoulders, upper part of the back, and the extremities. In these areas there are linear, scratched pimple-like lesions, and because of intense itching and scratching there is usually some type of secondary infection such as boils. In long-standing cases, because of the constant scratching, the skin takes on a brown pigmentation. The infection is most common among elderly indigents, vagrants, and alcoholics, who seldom bathe or change clothing.

Treatment. Head and pubic lice are eradicated easily by specific proprietary preparations such as Topicide, Cuprex, or Kwell. Two applications about 20 minutes apart are usually sufficient but in some cases it may be necessary to repeat the treatment

For body lice, the body should be bathed in warm water and thoroughly soaked for ten or 15 minutes, then rinsed in clear water. A mild emollient or boric acid ointment is then applied.

Sources of louse infestation such as clothing, bedding, hairbrushes, etc., should be thoroughly laundered, dry-cleaned, or discarded.

Scabies

This is commonly called "the itch," for the very good reason that intense itching, most severe at night, is the outstanding symptom. The female *itch mite* burrows a tunnel in the top layer of the skin (stratum corneum) and lays eggs in it. The minute burrow looks like a fine

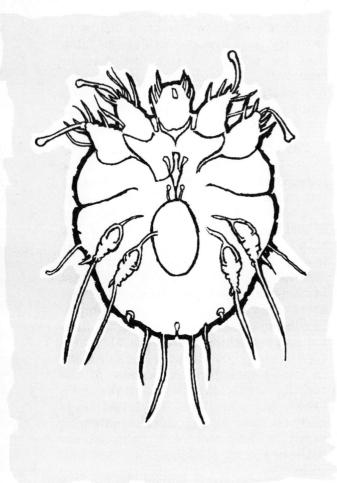

This exceptionally ugly creature in underside view is a horrendously magnified depiction of *Sarcoptes scabiei*, the itch mite, responsible for scabies. The fertilized female burrows into the horny layer of the skin, never deeper, and lays her eggs. Severe itching is due to sensitization of the host.

wavy line with a tiny pimple at one end, but it may be difficult to see because of overlying excoriations and redness caused by scratching. The skin areas most commonly affected are the waistline region, the buttocks, finger webs, and elbow and underarm regions.

Once diagnosed, proper treatment cures scabies promptly. A prolonged hot bath is taken and a scabicide ointment is applied to the entire body from the neck down. This may be repeated the next morning. Newer scabicides are somewhat easier to apply and less objectionable than traditional sulfur-containing preparations.

Scabies is very easily transmitted

and persons of quite fastidious habits may sometimes be affected.

COMMON SKIN CONDITIONS IN OLDER PEOPLE

For obvious reasons, women recognize the approach of senescence earlier than men. They note with apprehension the first facial wrinkles, the first gray hairs, the "fading complexion," and changes of bodily contours.

In elderly persons the surface of the skin may appear wrinkled, furrowed, and slightly more shiny than in younger persons. There is a tendency toward dryness and cracking of the horny layer, and the color may be yellowish with a sallow grayish hue. There may be areas of discoloration, "spots," scaling, and scattered redness.

When senile skin is pinched into a fold it usually feels thinner, lacks elasticity and turgor, and is slow to spring back to its flattened state. This is one of the simplest indicators of biological aging and reflects a lessened resilience of connective tissues of the body generally.

This loss of elasticity is frequently combined with loss of fat under the skin, with coarse folding of superfluous skin over areas deprived of "support from below." This occurs particularly over flexor (bending) areas and in relation to certain facial muscles concerned with "expression." These factors may be partly responsible for changes in the facial contours of older persons, and often are more dependable than lines and wrinkles in estimating the age of an individual. In addition, there are innumerable very fine wrinkles which result from atrophy of the dermal papillae (tiny nipple-shaped elevations) and flattening of the epithelium. These wrinkles increase steadily with age.

Hair. Although a tendency to lose body and scalp hair occurs with aging, there may be an increase of *coarse* hairs on exposed areas of the skin. While men are concerned with the loss of scalp hair at this age, women may note the appearance of coarse hairs on the upper lip and chin. The downy hairs within the ears and nose may become thicker and more conspicuous and the eyebrows may become bushy.

Although *gray hair* is popularly associated with aging, its time of onset is so greatly dependent on hereditary factors, and so variable, that it can never be used as an index of age. Some people "turn gray" at a very youthful age but their bodies do not necessarily or usually age prematurely.

Nails are also affected by age. The rate of growth of the nails diminishes and they may become either coarse and thick or thin and brittle.

Evaluating "skin age." In evaluating aging skin it is important to distinguish between changes resulting from the aging process and changes which result from chronic exposure to sunlight and weather. A truly senile skin can only be detected by thorough examination of unexposed areas of the body.

Premature "aging" of the skin noted on the face and hands of farmers — or of sailors or outdoors workers or indeed anyone continually exposed to sun and weather for many years — is readily recognizable. Wrinkling, atrophy, splotchy distribution of pigment, and keratoses (horny growths) are usually seen, and not uncommonly, skin cancer. However, the unexposed skin of people with "old" facial and hand skin is often completely free of any degenerative changes.

After determining the degree of skin degeneration that is due solely to exposure, and the degree due solely to aging, hereditary factors must be considered. The texture and depth of color of the skin, with consideration of racial groups, are of great importance in determining the resistance of the skin to the damaging influences of environment.

"Rejuvenation" of the skin. Our multi-million dollar cosmetic industry is conclusive proof of the universal interest in preserving a youthful appearance. Unfortunately, neither cosmetic products nor the medical specialty of dermatology can rejuvenate an aging skin and there is no remedy (other than superficial embellishment) for the changes which occur with advancing age.

The use of hormone creams has been widely publicized in recent years. Extensive studies have disclosed that they are neither harmful nor beneficial, except for some evidence of local tissue hydration— a slight swelling from water retention. Most dermatologists discourage the use of such creams and probably will continue to do so until their absorption through the skin is proved to be negligible even with exorbitant use. There appears to be no danger from average or recommended use, but effects of quantities that might be absorbed by massive use, much greater than recommended, by a woman zealously intent upon achieving a rapid return to youth, are more difficult to determine.

Special skin conditions of the elderly. Older persons are subject to the same skin diseases as young adults. Recognition and treatment of these conditions is much the same, regardless of the age of the patient. Nevertheless, a few conditions which occur frequently in "aging" skin merit special attention.

Pruritus. Itching is one of the most frequent and annoying infirmities of the aged. A recent survey in a home for the aged disclosed that 42 per cent of the residents complained of itching.

The typical patient is an elderly man who complains of generalized itching, without apparent skin lesions. The skin is dry but not necessarily extremely so. There is the usual thinning and atrophy of old age and some scattered excoriations. Because this picture is so common it is often dismissed lightly as "senile pruritus." Actually, it is doubtful whether senility of the skin *per se* ever results in pruritis. Most frequently the itching follows *external irritations* or *internal disease*.

External irritation may result from an acquired dryness of the skin, usually associated with cold weather, since the sebum or skin oil does not spread properly at low temperatures. Too frequent bathing and contact with itch-provoking garments such as wool are other external irritants.

Numerous internal diseases without obvious lesions may induce itching. Arteriosclerosis is perhaps the most common. The patient should be examined with particular reference to diseases of the blood, lymph nodes, liver and kidneys. Generalized itching may be the first sign of hepatitis, diabetes, nephritis, and tuberculosis, as well as leukemia, carcinoma, or lymphoblastomatous diseases. To add to the confusion, early symptoms of mental deterioration are frequently accompanied by itching.

Generally, itching which occurs during the winter months is associated with dryness of the skin and contact with woolen clothing, and responds well to simple treatment. This includes less frequent bathing, avoiding temperature changes, discontinuance of woolen clothing, and the local application of bland creams. If the pruritus has not abated after two weeks with these methods, search for an underlying disease process should be done with laboratory studies.

Senile purpura. This condition is more dependent upon old age than environmental exposure. Although it is relatively common and was first described over a hundred years ago, it seems to receive little attention at present.

Most commonly the characteristic hemorrhages of this condition occur on the extremities, but they may occur in other areas, even on the conjunctivae. The purpuric color gradually fades and leaves diffusely mottled areas of yellowish-brown pigmentation. Generally the skin is almost always extremely thin, fragile, and transparent.

Stasis dermatitis. Acute and chronic eczematous dermatitis of the leg is common in elderly persons. Most often it is associated with edema-producing conditions, especially varicose veins and chronic episodic phlebitis. The dermatitis may exist in varying degrees of severity for years, with or without ulceration. Contrarily, leg ulcers with edema may occur and continue for years without eczematization of the surrounding skin.

However, ulceration and eczema generally occur together.

Cancer of the skin is more frequent in elderly people. This condition has previously been discussed.

Removal of Wrinkles

Among the surgical procedures for correction of skin scarring, *dermabrasion* or "planing" is employed most frequently. This is a relatively simple office procedure which consists of local anesthesia sprayed on the involved area, after which the upper layers of the skin are abraded by a motor-driven wire brush or diamond head.

The operation is best performed in one session and the patient may go home immediately. Usually no after-pain medication is required. The treated and adjacent areas of skin may become quite swollen but this will subside within a few days. The scab formation will separate in a week to ten days. The reddish-pink discoloration disappears in three to four weeks but cosmetics may be used during this time. The patient may resume normal activities after the second week. Because the new skin is sensitive to sunlight, unnecessary exposure should be avoided. For optimum results the operation may be repeated in four to six months.

The age of the patient does not appear to be a factor in the success of this procedure, and all selected cases derive some benefit. Although dermabrasion is an office procedure, special equipment and assistance are required and the operation is not inexpensive.

Dermabrasion is used primarily to correct scars from acne and for superficial wrinkles, but may be used to remove superficial skin blemishes, moles, tattoo marks, or scars from injuries. It also has corrective and preventive value in management of aging skin. By removing the upper layers of the skin, wrinkles and minor blemishes are made less conspicuous.

Results from this procedure will depend on the shape and depth of the scars

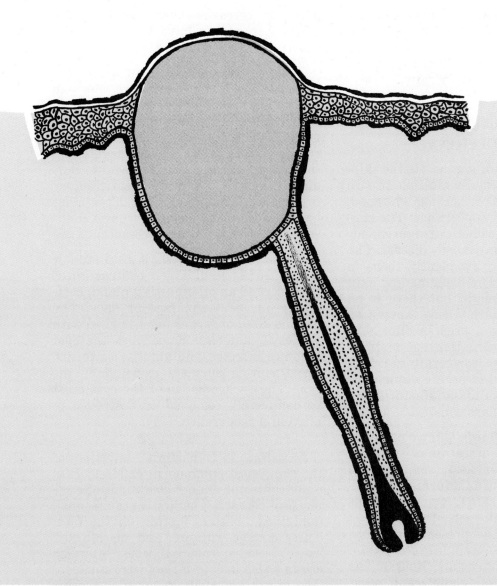

Sebaceous cysts or wens are fluctuant tense swellings of the skin, ranging up to marble size and larger. The cyst occupies the expanded end of a sebaceous gland duct that has become obstructed. The drawing shows an infected sebaceous cyst with pus formation following rupture of an obstructed duct.

or wrinkles. Facial scars respond to dermabrasion better than scars of the neck, shoulders, back, or chest. Miraculous results should never be anticipated, particularly when the scarring is deep, narrow, or of long duration.

Dermabrasion is not the treatment of choice for malignant lesions of the skin since far superior methods are available. Persons who have such lesions are prone to have subsequent ones. Proper therapy will eradicate the particular growth but will not prevent the occurrence of other lesions in untreated areas. However,

such lesions occur less frequently, or at a later time, on "new" skin produced by dermabrasion. The procedure thus has some prophylactic value for aging skin.

There are other methods for improving the appearance of wrinkled or scarred skin. One is *cryotherapy* — freezing the skin with carbon dioxide. If sufficient peeling is induced, there is improvement in small flat scars of acne and shallow wrinkles.

Another procedure consists of the application of cauterizing chemicals which are neutralized when the desired action has been obtained. This procedure is quite successful when properly employed, but should be administered only by physicians who have had experience in this exacting form of therapy.

MISCELLANEOUS SKIN CONDITIONS

Vitiligo is a loss of pigment in the skin. Patches of skin, usually multiple in size and shape, lose color, become whitened, and give a piebald appearance. The condition is purely a cosmetic disfigurement, not associated with systemic disease. The cause is unknown; frequently there is a family history. The depigmented skin is sensitive to sunlight but there is no change in its texture. Drugs known as *psoralens* have been used in efforts to encourage re-pigmentation but restoration of normal color is generally not complete. Depigmented areas, if conspicuous, may be masked quite satisfactorily by tinted opaque preparations.

Ichthyosis ("fish skin") is a congenital abnormality of cornification of the skin, associated with dryness, scaling, and warty growths. The mild form, known as *xeroderma* (dry skin), usually begins during the second year of life and is characterized by the presence of dirty, greasy, dry, rough, or slightly scaly skin, frequently broken up by fine fissures. The secretions of the oil glands, and occasionally the sweat glands, are deficient. There is no specific treatment. Emollients, ultraviolet light, and colloid baths are helpful. The skin is sensitive and does not tolerate irritants, particularly those which "defat" the skin, such as deter-gents or kerosene. Ordinary soap and water baths may have to be reduced, especially in the winter.

Keloids occasionally form after skin injury. Keloids are like dense, elevated scars. They usually occur after burns, scalds, cuts or surgical wounds, anywhere on the skin, frequently in the breastbone region. There is no way of foretelling their appearance after an injury. Surgical removal is not very satisfactory because keloids tend to recur. Treatment by irradiation or local injection of cortisone may give satisfactory results.

A *wen (sebaceous cyst)* is a skin tumor which usually results from obstruction of the outlet of an oil-secreting gland, commonly on the scalp, face or back. The marble-sized or larger mass is filled with "cheesy" material. Sometimes the cyst becomes infected and an abscess forms. Treatment is surgical excision of the cyst. The enclosing sac of the cyst must be completely removed or destroyed to prevent a recurrence.

Impetigo is a bacterial infection of the skin, most common in children. It is quite contagious under conditions of close physical contact. The first signs are small fluid-filled "blisters," often on the face. These enlarge, rupture, and the affected areas become covered with brownish crusts which look as if they were stuck on. The crusts are easily removed, exposing moist red skin underneath, which quickly crusts over again. Impetigo is easily cured by adequate treatment with an antiseptic ointment prescribed by a doctor, applied after removal of the crusts by thorough washing with soap and water.

CHAPTER 6

THE LUNGS AND CHEST IN HEALTH AND DISEASE

by J. A. MYERS, M.D.

The Lungs • Why Don't Lungs Collapse?
• Inside the Lungs • Vital Exchanges of
Gases • How We Breathe • Vital
Capacities

TUBERCULOSIS

Tuberculosis Eradication • Bronchitis
• Bronchiectasis • Lung Abscess •
A Word About Coughs • Pleurisy •
Empyema • "Devil's Grip" •
Pneumothorax • Emphysema •
Pneumoconiosis • Sarcoidosis • Lipoid
Pneumonia • Hyperventilation •
Hiccup • Cancer of the Respiratory Tract

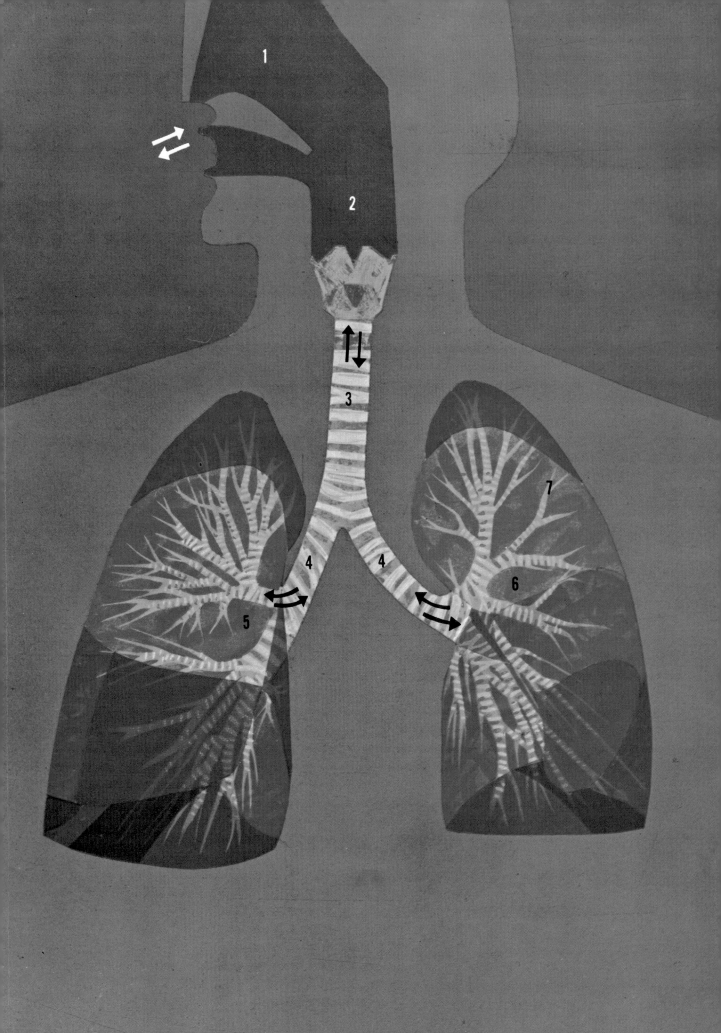

THE LUNGS AND CHEST IN HEALTH AND DISEASE

by **J. A. MYERS, M. D.**

Hemoglobin of red blood cells picks up oxygen and "lets go" of carbon dioxide in the oxygen-rich environment of the lungs. Carbon dioxide is a waste product of metabolism which must be removed.

Air is inhaled through *nasal cavity* (1), *nasopharynx* (2), and *trachea* (3). The main *bronchi* (4) go to the *right* (5) and *left* lungs (6). The bronchi divide into finer and finer tubes called *bronchioles* (7). The right lung has three lobes, the left lung two, and each has segments (shown in different colors) supplied by branches from the main bronchi.

Exchange of gases takes place in millions of tiny air cells *(alveoli)* located at the ends of bronchioles like clusters of grapes. Here, a thin film of blood is separated from the air in the lungs by the very thin surfaces of the alveoli. Venous blood diffuses its waste-load of carbon dioxide through these surfaces into the air cells, and oxygen from inhaled air diffuses through the walls into the blood. Carbon dioxide is expelled with exhaled air. Pathways of inhalation and exhalation are shown by arrows.

An average adult breathes more than 12,000 quarts of air a day. This is not only the body's largest intake of any substance, but the most immediately important to life. We can go without food for many days and water for many hours without fatal results. But life without air terminates in a very few minutes.

The lifegiving component of air is oxygen, which constitutes a little less than one-fifth of its volume. Almost all of the rest of air is nitrogen, with minute amounts of several other inert gases. More than half of our body weight is oxygen (water is eight-ninths oxygen). Ordinary combustion is a rather violent combination of oxygen with fuels such as coal, wood, or gasoline, producing flame and heat. A similar but marvelously controlled process called *respiration* goes on incessantly in every one of our trillions of body cells.

We need oxygen to burn food and release energy. Cells use oxygen and produce carbon dioxide in their vital activities. The one must be supplied continuously, the other removed, else living machinery comes to a halt in a very short time. "Respiration" is a common synonym for breathing. However, cells do not inhale or exhale or breathe in the ordinary sense. Physiologists think of respiration as a basic process of cells, the interchange of gases. What goes on in our lungs is vital, but only a way-station to what goes on in our cells.

Many small organisms obtain oxygen by diffusion from their environment. In man and higher animals the problem is more complicated. Billions of internal cells are shut off from direct contact with an oxygen-rich atmosphere. An efficient means of bringing oxygen

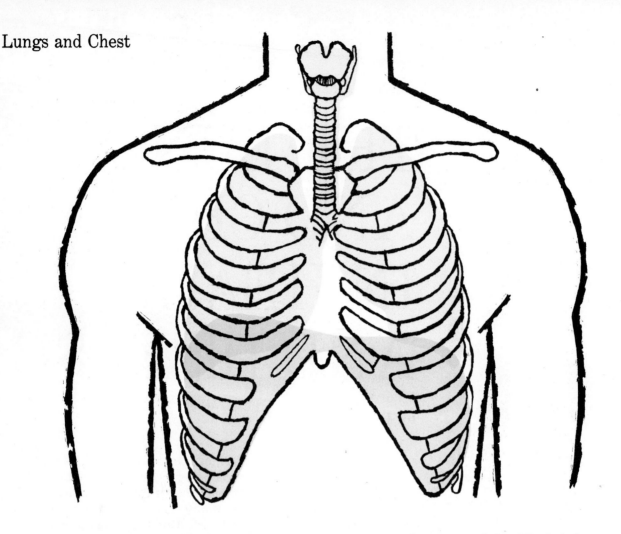

The lungs lie within the flexible rib cage, normally have but one fixed attachment (at the windpipe), and thus have considerable range of movement. The bases of the lungs rest above the diaphragm, the principal muscle of breathing.

from the outside world to every cell, and of removing carbon dioxide, is vitally essential. This transport system is provided by the blood in conjunction with specialized organs, the lungs.

The Lungs

Our two lungs lie on either side of the chest cavity. In gross appearance they are cone-shaped, grayish in color, verging toward black in city-dwellers (infant lungs are pink). Their bases rest on a dome-shaped transverse muscle, the *diaphragm,* and their top-parts (apices) are in the root of the neck. The lungs normally have but one attachment, in the region where the bronchi join the windpipe, and thus are quite freely movable.

A deep fissure divides each lung into a lower and an upper *lobe.* The left lung, slightly smaller than the right, has two lobes. In the right lung another horizontal fissure somewhat below the middle produces a third or middle lobe. It is now known that each lobe is divided into segments, each of which can readily be separated from the others. Before this was known, surgical removal of a small area of diseased lung tissue required removal of an entire lobe *(lobectomy)* or even a whole lung *(pneumonectomy).* Today, if a condition is limited to a lung segment, only the involved segment is removed, leaving the remainder of the lobe for normal function.

Each lung is completely surrounded by a thin, glistening membrane, the *pleura,* inseparably attached to its outer surface. The inner surface of the chest wall has the same pleural lining. Normally, there is no space between the lung and chest wall membranes, although the area is called the *pleural cavity.* It can become an actual cavity in certain circumstances of disease or accident.

Normally, the opposed fluid-lubricated surfaces of the pleura glide and slide easily over each other as the lung expands and contracts during respiration. Otherwise, breathing would be very painful.

The lung pleura contains no pain-transmitting fibers. Thus, like the lung itself, the pulmonary pleura may be involved in any abnormality without causing pain. However, the pleural lining of the chest wall is richly supplied with pain fibers, so that when it is involved in disease, "pleurisy pains" are experienced. It is involvement of this chest-wall layer of pleura which may cause excruciating pain in conditions such as pneumonia, tuberculosis, and cancer.

At birth the lungs are solid and contain no air. The baby's first breath establishes pressure within the lungs essentially the same as atmospheric pressure. As the infant's chest-cage enlarges faster than the lungs, this internal pressure forces the lungs to expand to fill all of the available space within the baby's chest.

Why Don't Lungs Collapse?

Lung tissue is extremely elastic. The natural tendency of a lung is to "pull itself together" — to shrink like a rubber sponge that has been overextended. The urge to collapse is counteracted by a pull in the opposite direction. The lung surface clings tenaciously to the chest wall, not by physical bonds, but from negative pressure — vacuum — of the pleural cavity. Normally, this negative pressure acts somewhat like a suction cup to pull the lung against the chest wall and keep it expanded. If the air-seal or vacuum of the pleural cavity is broken, the lung may collapse. This may occur

The right lung has three *lobes*, indicated by solid lines in the drawing; the left lung, two lobes. Dotted lines indicate *segments* which can be separated independently. The *bronchi* are shown cut off, for clarification of the drawing.

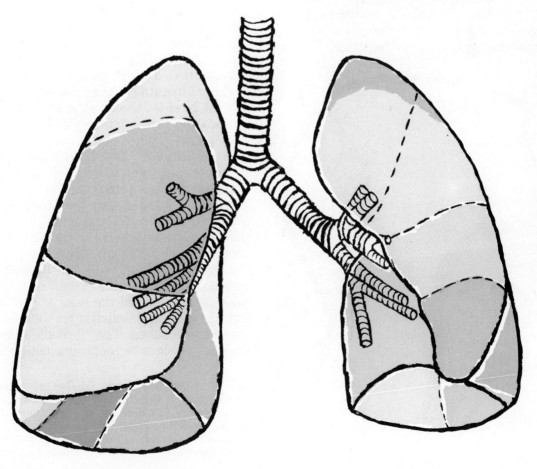

from a stab or gunshot wound that leaves an opening from the chest wall into the pleural cavity so outside air rushes in. Or disease in a lung may erode through the inner layer of pleura, allow air from the lung to enter the pleural space, and cause collapse.

Advantage is taken of this mechanism in treatment of certain lung conditions. Introduction of measured amounts of air through a needle into the pleural cavity collapses a lung partially or completely, to a degree controllable by the physician. The procedure, known as *artificial pneumothorax*, has been used extensively to rest a lung, as part of the treatment of tuberculosis. It may also stop bleeding in instances when severe pulmonary hemorrhages occur.

Fortunately, pleural cavities of each lung are independent of each other. Collapse of one lung does not have any effect on functions of the opposite lung.

Inside the Lungs

Air that is drawn in through the nose and the upper throat is warmed and moistened on its trip to the lungs.

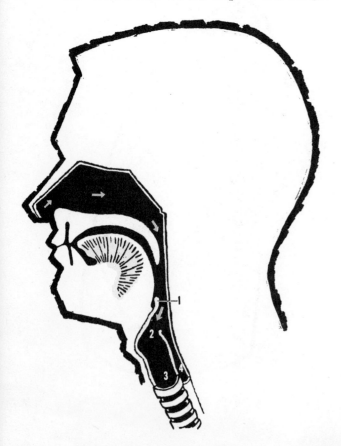

Both food and air follow the same throat passageway for a short distance. At about the level of the Adam's apple the passage becomes continuous with the *esophagus* or gullet toward the back, and the *larynx* (voice box) toward the front. The larynx is a tubular air passage about two inches long in women, somewhat longer in men. Its upper opening is guarded by an ingenious trapdoor, the *epiglottis*, which permits the passage to keep open for the passage of air, but closes it when food or liquids are swallowed. A simple attempt to swallow and inhale at the same time demonstrates that it cannot be done. Occasionally, if the opening is closed imperfectly or not in time, we experience a spasmodic choking reaction commonly called "swallowing the wrong way."

The lower part of the larynx is continuous with the *trachea* or *windpipe*, an air-tube between four and five inches long. The trachea is kept from collapsing by numerous C-shaped rings of cartilage, which can be felt by running a finger up and down over the lowest part of the front of the neck, just above where the bone begins. Here the trachea is very close to the skin surface and readily accessible to a surgeon who can make an artificial opening *(tracheotomy)* to permit air to enter the trachea and bypass a suffocating obstruction of the larynx above it.

Approximately at a level with the top of the heart, which lies behind it, the trachea divides into two *bronchi,* one going to the right and the other to the left lung. The right bronchus is a more direct continuation of the trachea, and a more common site of lodgment of foreign particles inhaled or "swallowed the wrong way." The main trunk of a bronchus passes toward the base of the lung, but divides and subdivides into eversmaller air tubes. The "bronchial tree" does resemble tree roots, branching into

Arrows show pathway of inhaled air warmed and moistened in nasal passage. A "trapdoor," the *epiglottis* (1) opens to permit intake of air through *voice box* (2) and *windpipe* (3). The epiglottis closes to confine swallowed food to the *esophagus* (4) and prevent it from entering lungs.

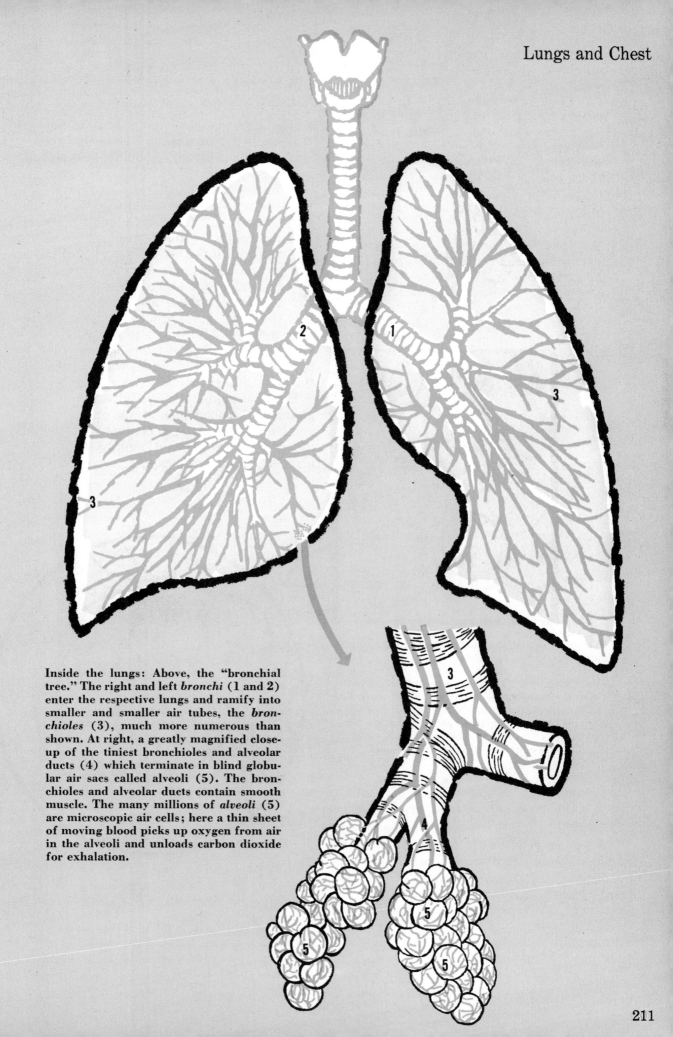

Inside the lungs: Above, the "bronchial tree." The right and left *bronchi* (1 and 2) enter the respective lungs and ramify into smaller and smaller air tubes, the *bronchioles* (3), much more numerous than shown. At right, a greatly magnified close-up of the tiniest bronchioles and alveolar ducts (4) which terminate in blind globular air sacs called alveoli (5). The bronchioles and alveolar ducts contain smooth muscle. The many millions of *alveoli* (5) are microscopic air cells; here a thin sheet of moving blood picks up oxygen from air in the alveoli and unloads carbon dioxide for exhalation.

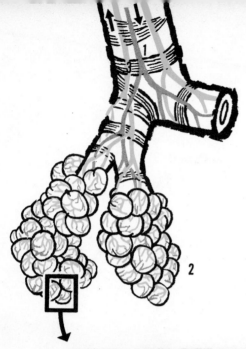

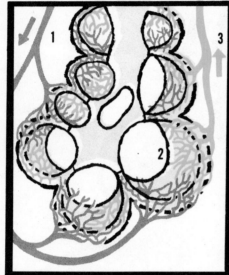

Vital Exchanges of Gases

The largest surface of the body in contact with the outside world is not the skin, which, if flattened out, would cover perhaps a bit less than two square yards. The inner surfaces of the alveoli, continuous with the bronchioles, bronchi, and trachea, are technically outside the body, in contact with the atmosphere. If the walls of all the air cells were spread out as one continuous area they would cover a surface the size of a tennis court. Yet this immense surface is compacted into the small space of our two lungs. It is incredibly thin. It has to be, to effect absorption of oxygen from air and dispersal of carbon dioxide waste gases through unimaginably delicate surfaces.

Let us consider a single alveolus as a globular chamber open at one end. Oxygen-containing air is in contact with the inner wall. The blood supply of the alveolus, laced with capillaries, is very

Exchange of gases in lungs. Top drawing: a pulmonary artery (1) brings venous blood with carbon dioxide load to alveoli (2); pulmonary vein (3) carries oxygen-enriched blood back to heart. In square immediately above, microscopic section shows blood vessels in thin walls of air-containing alveoli. In an air cell at right, oxygen molecules (4) diffuse into blood and carbon dioxide molecules (5) diffuse out of blood.

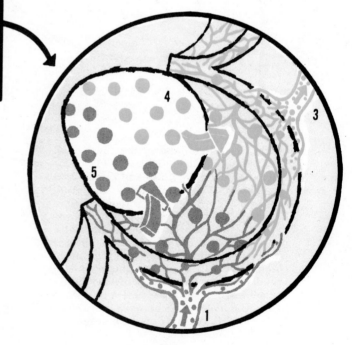

tinier and tinier rootlets. The tiniest lung tubes, the *bronchioles*, after many divisions terminate in blind globular air sacs. These outpouchings, called *alveoli*, resemble microscopic clusters of grapes. We have some 400,000,000 alveoli, each of which is an infinitesimal respiratory chamber. It is here that remote body cells maintain essential lines of communication with the outside world.

rich. The capillary wall is only one cell thick, and so is the air-sac wall. Gas molecules can move across these surfaces in accordance with laws of diffusion of gases. A key substance is the hemoglobin of red blood cells, which has a remarkable capacity to pick up and transport oxygen and carbon dioxide.

Bright red arterial blood pumped out of the heart is rich in oxygen obtained in the lungs. The deoxygenated, duskier blood returns through veins to the heart.

This vital exchange of gases transpires through gossamer surfaces of air cells which, in effect, continually expose a vast, thin, moving sheet of blood to the external world.

In this way, every cell of the body is in constant indirect contact with the air around us, and waste gases are disseminated into the atmosphere.

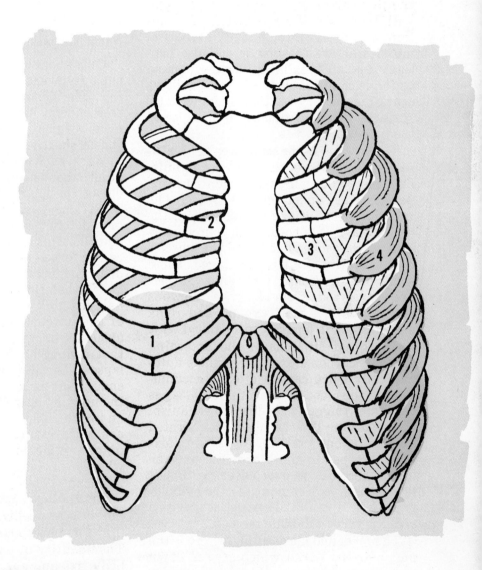

Accessory structures of respiration. Contraction of the *diaphragm* muscle (1) causes the chest cage (2) to expand, and the lungs, held to the inner surface of the chest cavity, also expand. *Intercostal* muscles (3) between the ribs and *serratus* muscles (4) arising from ribs assist contraction and expansion of the chest cavity, but most of the work is done by the diaphragm.

Hemoglobin serves as both a dump-cart and pickup truck in this incessant transport system. In our arteries, hemoglobin carries oxygen to cells, "dumps it," picks up carbon dioxide, and in the lungs reverses the procedure. Every breath we exhale contains about 100 times more carbon dioxide than the atmosphere around us.

How We Breathe

Air tubes within the lungs have muscle fibers. But lungs per se have no muscles. They are passive organs, expanded and contracted by movements of ribs and diaphragm which force air to flow in and out, much like a bellows.

The lungs are enclosed in a flexible

"box," the *thoracic cavity*. The chest cage boxes in the lungs, except at the bottom, which is enclosed by the diaphragm. Contraction of the diaphragm causes it to pull downward and expand the chest cavity, assisted by *intercostal* (between-the-ribs) *muscles* which elevate the ribs. The lung surfaces, clinging to the sides of the box through vacuum-like pull of the pleural cavity, necessarily expand with the box and air rushes in. Relaxation of the diaphragm and intercostal muscles allows the box to collapse partially, and air is exhaled. The mechanical action is comparable to that of a bellows containing a very elastic sponge with its surfaces securely attached to the sides of the bellows.

Nerve centers. The sequences of breathing — about 18 respirations per minute, or some 25,000 diaphragm contractions per day—are under nervous control. The breathing center is in the medulla at the top of the spinal cord. This center coordinates the movements of all the muscles of respiration. If it is damaged, as in some polio patients, breathing muscles are paralyzed from lack of nervous orders. "Iron lungs" expand and relax the chestbox in a purely mechanical way.

The great stimulus of the breathing center is carbon dioxide. We inhale automatically when carbon dioxide accumulates in the blood to a certain level — gas molecules trigger a feedback mechanism to the brain. This can be demonstrated by holding one's breath. As carbon dioxide increases in the blood, the urge to inhale becomes so overpowering that it is not possible to commit suicide by holding one's breath. Intake of oxygen reduces carbon dioxide tension.

The principal nerve of breathing is the long *phrenic nerve* which passes down the sides of the neck through the chest cavity to the diaphragm. The nerve lies close to the surface of the body in the lower part of the neck just above the collarbone. When a lung, particularly one with tuberculous involvement, could not otherwise be put to rest, surgeons have gently crushed and interrupted fibers of the phrenic nerve, which regenerate and regain communication with the diaphragm in two or three months during which the lung is at rest.

Complex nervous pathways may give rise to sensations of pain in body areas remote from the site of trouble. It is not unusual for pain originating in the chest wall pleura to be felt in the region of the appendix, and pain from the diaphragm may be felt in the shoulder region.

Vital Capacities

Only about one-eighth of our total lung capacity is exercised in ordinary breathing. The body's respiratory reserve is tremendous. An entire lung may collapse, or be surgically removed, without resulting in shortness of breath.

With each quiet breath-cycle of an adult, about a pint of air flows into and out of the lungs. This is known as *tidal air*. If one continues to inhale at the end of quiet inspiration, a bit less than an additional half-pint of *complemental air* can be forced into the lungs. Similarly, if one continues to exhale at the end of ordinary exhalation, as much as a pint and a half of *supplemental air* can be forced out of the lungs. However, there remains about a pint and a half of *residual air* that cannot be forced out. A lung collapses when removed from the body, but enough air is always entrapped so that the lung floats if placed in water. Before an infant takes its first breath, the lungs are solid, contain no air, and sink if placed in water. This test determines whether or not a baby was stillborn.

Vital lung capacity is measured by inhaling as deeply as possible and blowing as much as possible into a spirometer. The quantity of expelled air varies with body size and age. A medium-sized man may have a vital capacity of 4,000 to 4,500 cubic centimeters between the ages of 20 to 40 years. However, as the elasticity of tissues decreases with age, the vital capacity diminishes and may be as much as 20 per cent less at age 60 and 40 per cent less at age 75. It is important to allow for this natural decrease with age, since otherwise diminished vital lung

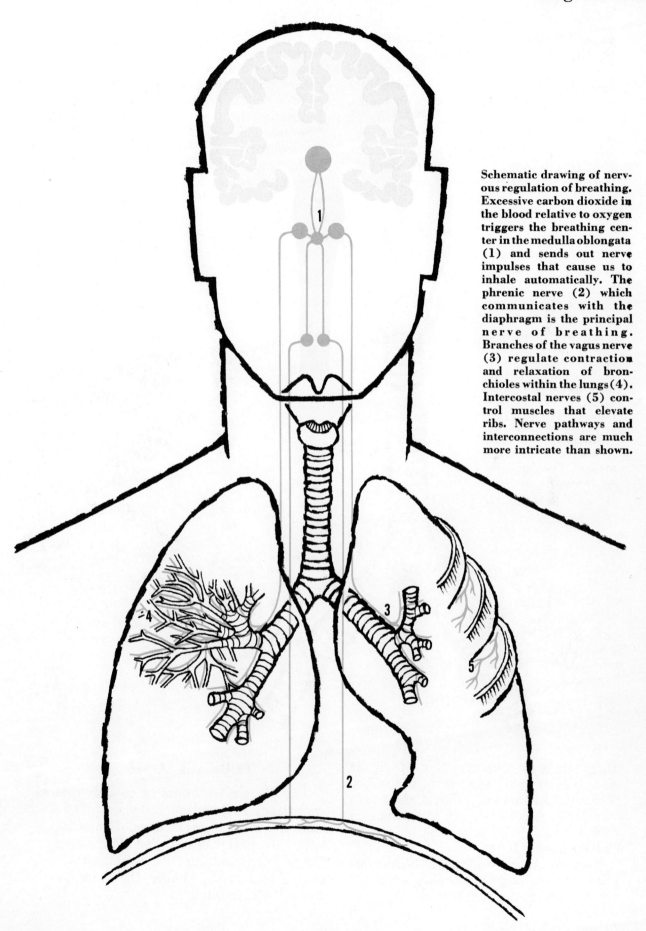

Schematic drawing of nervous regulation of breathing. Excessive carbon dioxide in the blood relative to oxygen triggers the breathing center in the medulla oblongata (1) and sends out nerve impulses that cause us to inhale automatically. The phrenic nerve (2) which communicates with the diaphragm is the principal nerve of breathing. Branches of the vagus nerve (3) regulate contraction and relaxation of bronchioles within the lungs (4). Intercostal nerves (5) control muscles that elevate ribs. Nerve pathways and interconnections are much more intricate than shown.

capacity may be attributed erroneously to other factors.

The respiratory tract has efficient self-cleansing mechanisms. From the entrance of the larynx to the tiniest bronchioles, the air passages are lined with *ciliated epithelium*. Millions of specialized cells with microscopic hair-like projections beat in rhythmic, sweeping movements that propel a thin film of mucus over

tective mechanism beginning with *vibrissae* (filtering hairs) of the nose, and extending to microscopic respiratory chambers, prevents about 99 per cent of dust and other foreign materials from entering or remaining in the lungs. The one per cent that is not eliminated is promptly engulfed by phagocytic cells and deposited in small masses of lymph tissue.

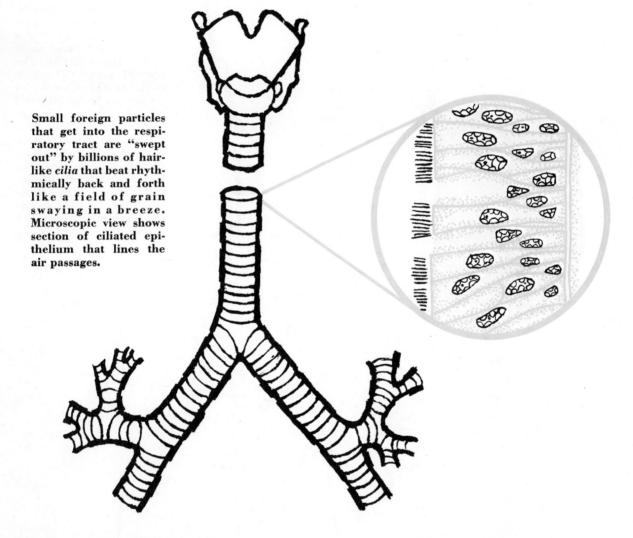

Small foreign particles that get into the respiratory tract are "swept out" by billions of hair-like *cilia* that beat rhythmically back and forth like a field of grain swaying in a breeze. Microscopic view shows section of ciliated epithelium that lines the air passages.

their surfaces. The direction of mucus flow is always outward from the lungs. The inner surfaces of millions of air sacs (alveoli) are covered with a moving film of fluid which joins uninterruptedly with that of the air tubes.

Foreign particles entrapped on mucous currents are constantly carried away from the lungs. An extraordinary pro-

TUBERCULOSIS

The disease we know as tuberculosis was attacking people on the plains of the Ganges in prehistoric days. Centuries before Christ it was called *phthisis*, a Greek word meaning "to consume slowly or waste away" — hence the familiar word, "consumption."

There are disseminated forms of tuberculosis which affect far-flung parts of the body. Tuberculosis may affect membranes of the brain, the bones, structures of the urinary tract, and other organs. However, about 90 percent of cases are tuberculosis of the lungs, or *pulmonary tuberculosis*. It is this serious and too common disease that we shall mainly discuss.

Tuberculosis deaths in the U.S. have diminished greatly since the beginning of the century. Tremendous advances in prevention, detection, and treatment by drugs, surgery, and other measures have tended to give the public the impression that tuberculosis is no longer a common health threat. Unfortunately, this is not the case. About 10,000 Americans a year die from tuberculosis. In 1962 nearly 55,000 new active cases were reported and about 43,000 of these were in an advanced stage.

From 40,000,000 to 50,000,000 persons in this country harbor the germs that can cause active tuberculosis. This does not by any means suggest that large numbers of these persons will "come down" with the disease — only that any one of them, at any time, may be stricken by an "explosion" of germs which have been carried like a hidden land mine in the body. The world over, tuberculosis today causes more incapacity and kills more people than all of the other communicable diseases combined.

Symptoms. Primary infection with tuberculosis does not immediately cause any overt symptoms. By the time symptoms are noticeable, perhaps many years after primary infection, the disease is well advanced. Unbearable fatigue may be the first sign that something is wrong. The patient may cough and seem to have bronchitis. There may be fever in the afternoon but not in the morning. The physician may hear abnormal sounds in the lungs. Blood may be coughed up.

Long before any of these symptoms appear, however, tuberculous infection can be detected by a very simple skin test. This is commonly done by the family physician, who is the most important figure of all in efforts to wipe out tuberculosis.

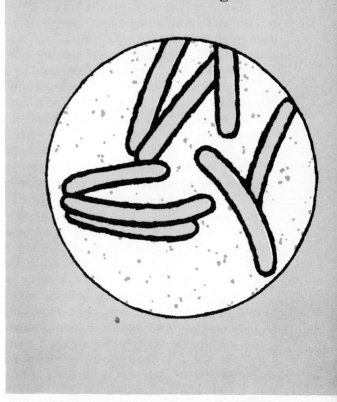

Tubercle bacilli are long, straight, or slightly bent organisms that are killed by exposure to direct sunlight, but which can survive outside the body for long periods in moist, cool surroundings.

To understand how the skin test works, we need to know something about the nature of tuberculosis and how it spreads.

The causative germ. The "something" that causes tuberculosis was unknown until less than a century ago. The great destroyer had been thought by some doctors to be a contagious disease and by others to be inherited. In 1882 the great German bacteriologist, Robert Koch, announced to the world that tuberculosis was caused by a long-shaped bacterium, the *tubercle bacillus* (Mycobacterium tuberculosis), which infects man and animals.

Soon this great discovery led to knowledge of how tuberculosis spreads. The germs are present in droplets of material sprayed into the air from the lungs of a person with active tuberculosis during coughing spells, and are also present in the sputum. Practically all persons with contagious tuberculosis swallow germs which are eliminated via the intestines. Other affected organs which communicate directly or indirectly with the outside may also discharge tuberculosis germs. For example, if tuberculosis affects the kidneys, germs are eliminated in the urine. Infections of lymph nodes or bones and joints may burrow through the skin and discharge material containing tubercle bacilli.

The two main routes by which tuberculosis germs get into the body are via the digestive tract (swallowed) and the respiratory tract (inhaled). Less frequent portals of entry are the eyes, and occasionally the genital organs.

Direct sunlight kills tuberculosis germs within a few minutes. However, if the germs are protected by materials such as sputum and pus they may live much longer, and in dark, cool places may survive for several months.

Body defenses. When tubercle bacilli enter the body they are met by millions of defensive white blood cells *(neutrophils)*. These cells ingest the bacilli, and, carrying germ particles within them, enter the blood and lymph streams and circulate through the body. Some of

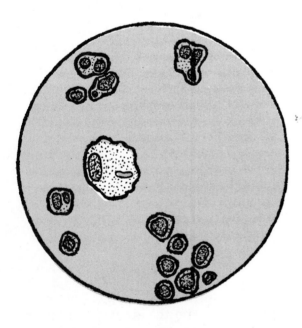

White blood cells *(neutrophils)* come to the defense of the body by ingesting hostile germs. Here a tuberculosis germ has been ingested by a protective white cell.

these white blood cells with their tubercle bacillus content may be deposited in various organs such as bones, brain, joints and kidneys. More are deposited in the lungs than in any other organ. This is a very rapid process. It occurs within an hour after bacilli enter the body.

Now a remarkable process gets into action. Defense elements begin promptly to build tiny cages around the germs and wall them off. The first walls consist of white blood cells, then scar tissue forms, and finally, in many cases, the germs are imprisoned in limestone and even bone encasements.

At this stage the person has a *primary* tuberculosis infection. Affected areas are nearly always microscopic in size and cause no illness. However, tissues of the body including the skin become sensitized to the protein part of tubercle bacilli — very much as an allergic person with hay fever is sensitive to the protein of ragweed pollen. As we shall see, this is the basis of skin tests for tuberculosis, and the mechanism involved if active tuberculosis develops later. It takes six or seven weeks for this sensitization to the tubercle bacillus to develop.

Reinfection by liberated germs. The walling-off of areas containing tubercle bacilli is exceedingly effective. Occasionally some of the germs escape and reach other parts of the body. More often, after nature has gone to the trouble of building walls around the germs, she treats these structures as foreign bodies by resorbing the scar tissue, calcium, or bone of the walls. Thus the germs are liberated on tissue that is highly allergic or sensitized to their protein. This is called *endogenous reinfection* (from within). It is responsible for practically all of the incapacity and death from tuberculosis.

Tissues upon which endogenous reinfections are implanted are so highly sensitized that the protein of the germs acts like a deadly poison which kills cells and tissues on contact. The result is a disease as different from that caused by the primary infection as if they were produced by two different kinds of germs. The primary infection sets the stage for all the destruction the tubercle bacillus is capable of producing. It only remains for them to escape and lodge on sensitized tissue to set a progressive and destructive disease in operation.

Lifelong infection. After the body becomes invaded by tubercle bacilli the encapsulated germs are likely to remain alive and virulent for the rest of the person's life. An infant infected with the germs may die at the age of 90 from some other disease, although he has harbored living tuberculosis germs throughout a long lifetime. However, the fact is that anyone who becomes invaded with germs of tuberculosis has microscopic areas of disease from which destructive disease may evolve at any time. It is encouraging that many such persons live long lives without ever developing incapacitating tuberculosis. Another heartening fact is that methods of detecting destructive forms of tuberculosis soon after they start are available. When found in early stages, nearly all cases can be treated successfully.

Detection in apparently well persons. Before the first years of our century there was no way of recognizing tuberculosis infections unless the disease was so far advanced as to cast shadows on x-ray film or produce symptoms such as germs in the sputum. The tragic result was that tuberculosis was rarely detected until it was approaching or in the consumptive stage and was contagious to others; thus the disease perpetuated itself.

In 1890 Koch produced *tuberculin* (a sterile liquid containing substances extracted from tuberculosis germs). At first it was hoped that tuberculin might cure tuberculosis, but it proved to have different and very important uses. Skin tests with tuberculin afford a safe and accurate method of determining the presence of tuberculous infection. The test is so sensitive that entirely symptomless primary infections in apparently well persons can be recognized.

How tuberculin tests work. As we have seen, the skin (as well as other tissues)
of a person who has been invaded by tuberculosis germs is sensitized to the specific protein of the tubercle bacillus, *tuberculoprotein.* This is present in tuberculin and purified protein derivatives. Introduction of tuberculin into deeper layers of the skin brings tuberculoprotein into contact with tissues. If the tissues have been sensitized by the presence of tuberculosis germs in the body, there is a characteristic allergic reaction. There is an area of hardness or swelling or both at the site of administration. This is a *positive* tuberculin reaction.

Various methods have been used to introduce tuberculin into the skin. In 1903, Clement Pirquet of Austria introduced a method of applying tuberculin to a scratch in superficial layers of the skin. The "Mantoux test" gets its name from a French physician who in 1908 introduced a technique of introducing measured amounts of diluted tuberculin into the skin through a needle.

The "puncture method" has been in wide use for about 30 years. This consists of placing a drop of tuberculin solution on the skin and passing a needle through it into deeper layers. The most recent modification is known as the *"tine test."* This employs an instrument with tinelike needles which make four skin punctures. The needles are covered with dried tuberculin which enters layers of the skin along with the needle points.

A properly administered tuberculin test tells with great accuracy whether or not tuberculosis germs are present in a person's body. There are a few exceptions. The test may be falsely negative if tubercle bacilli have not had time to sensitize tissues sufficiently to react to tuberculin. This takes up to seven weeks after bacilli enter the body. If an individual does not react positively, the test should be repeated in about two months. If a person in a family, office or school is found to have contagious tuberculosis, immediate testing of his associates may miss many whom he has infected. It is better to test associates about two months after the contagious case is discovered, or to repeat the test about two months later in those who did not react at first.

A large number of bacilli closely resemble the tubercle bacillus under the microscope and some of these may cause their hosts to react to tuberculin. However, non-tubercular bacilli can be differentiated by laboratory procedures. The tuberculin test is the master key to tuberculosis eradication since it detects the presence of tuberculosis germs earlier than any other method of examination. It not only identifies infected persons, but by examining associates of those who react to the test it may be possible to locate contagious cases that are unsuspectedly spreading the disease.

Chest x-rays. A positive tuberculin reaction practically always means that the person is infected with tuberculosis, but there is no immediate way of telling when if ever the infection may "explode" in destructive disease. Consequently it is important that the family physician keep watch and give periodic checkups to positive reactors. X-ray films of the chest are valuable though not infallible diagnostic aids. Diseased areas of the lungs tend to cast shadows on the sensitized film.

Periodic x-ray films of the chests of children under 12 years of age are not recommended, although an initial film of the chest of a child who becomes infected under the age of 12 is indicated because other abnormalities may be brought to light. However, periodic x-ray film inspection of the chests of adults who react

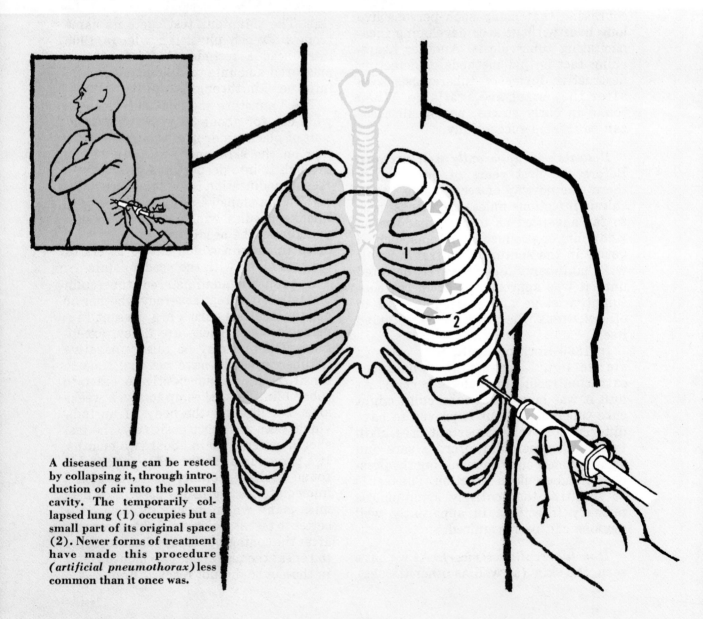

A diseased lung can be rested by collapsing it, through introduction of air into the pleural cavity. The temporarily collapsed lung (1) occupies but a small part of its original space (2). Newer forms of treatment have made this procedure (*artificial pneumothorax*) less common than it once was.

positively to tuberculin is an important part of followup examinations although it does not constitute a complete examination. X-rays may reveal lung shadows two or three years before symptoms and physical signs of disease are manifested. Yet a clear or negative x-ray film may be deceptive, and annual x-ray study of the chest of adult reactors to tuberculin is prudent.

Shadows of the heart and diaphragm obscure about one-fourth of the lung area from view on the usual single x-ray film, and there is no opportunity to focus on different areas. Special techniques have been devised to bring to view areas not ordinarily visualized. For example, a series of films can be made, each focused at a different angle through the entire chest. Such films are known as *planigrams* (stratigrams, tomograms). These often disclose areas of disease which cast no shadow on the ordinary single film.

Treatment of tuberculosis. From the days of the Babylonians down to the discovery of the tubercle bacillus, every medicine known to man, and hundreds best left unknown, were fruitlessly tried in efforts to find a treatment that would cure consumption. Useless nostrums and quackery thrived in partnerships that did no good for the patient. There were enthusiasts for diet fads, change of climate, long sea voyages, horseback riding, walking, woodchopping and the like. The most helpful measures were hospitalization and bed rest, begun in Germany in the latter half of the past century. There was a great surge in sanatorium building during the first decades of our century. Sanatoriums have been enormously important to the patient and the community, by offering the best treatments known and by isolating contagious cases, thus stopping the spread of tubercle bacilli in families and communities.

Collapse of the diseased lung by introducing air into the pleural cavity *(artificial pneumothorax)* was tried in the 1880's and became the most commonly used and important method of treatment until 1947. The effect of collapse is to rest the lung, inhibit multiplication of tubercle bacilli, and stimulate formation

of scar tissue to seal off the germs. This also helps to make contagious disease non-contagious. Adhesions may prevent a lung from being collapsed by usual methods. The same result can be attained by surgical removal of rib segments so that the chest wall collapses with the diseased lung. Many thousands of people now living and working were treated successfully by lung collapse procedures. The lung does not remain permanently collapsed, but gradually reinflates itself.

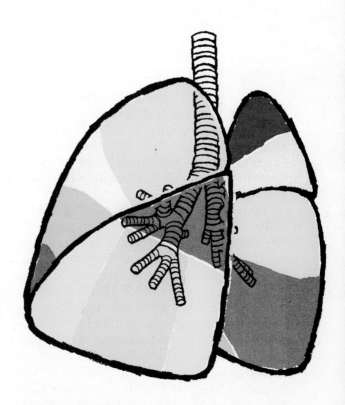

Segmented structure of the lungs enables segments containing local areas of tuberculosis to be individually removed by surgery. Surgeons cannot remove all areas of tuberculous disease.

Something new was added to tuberculosis therapy when streptomycin, discovered in 1944, was found to break through the defenses of tuberculosis germs. This antibiotic is a potent anti-tuberculosis drug, but has an unfortunate weakness. Tubercle bacilli tend to become streptomycin "resistant." That is, when the drug is given alone over a substantial period of time, strains of tubercle bacilli which are not affected by streptomycin tend to emerge. Another drug, PAS (para-aminosalicylic acid) also restrains the growth of tuberculosis germs, but less potently than streptomycin, and PAS-resistant strains also emerge. It was soon found that if smaller doses of streptomycin are given in combination with PAS, emergence of resistant germ families is quite effectively suppressed over longer periods. In 1951 another very potent anti-tuberculosis drug, isoniazid, came into extensive use. Present chemotherapeutic treatments now employ drug combinations, commonly, either streptomycin or isoniazid combined with PAS and, more recently, either of these drugs combined with rifampin.

Surgery. For years the chest was a citadel no surgeon dared to invade in depth. Antimicrobial drugs, advances in anesthesia, supportive measures, surgical techniques and knowledge of lung anatomy, have made it possible to eliminate small areas of tuberculosis by removing lung segments containing them.

Treatment of course is individualized. Generally the antituberculosis drugs are continued on prescribed daily doses for at least a year and usually much longer, after removal of as much of the diseased areas as possible when this is indicated. Drugs and surgery have aided in restoring many tuberculous persons to substantially normal working lives. However, it is not possible to exterminate *all* of the patient's tubercle bacilli. Surgeons cannot remove all areas of disease nor can any drug or combination of current drugs wipe out all the patient's germs. Therefore every patient who has made a good recovery should have the watchful care of his physician for the rest of his life.

Facts and fallacies. Many false beliefs about tuberculosis grew up during centuries when basic facts about the disease were unknown. Many of these beliefs persist despite the growth of knowledge which underlies modern tuberculosis control programs.

Infection is not inevitable. A belief that all adults are infected with tubercle bacilli and cannot hope to escape them stems from the fact that, in places where tuberculin testing was first used, almost all adults reacted positively. It was felt that tubercle bacilli are present everywhere and cannot be avoided. Tuberculosis germs are spread by people and animals with contagious disease. Excreted germs may remain alive for some time but they do not multiply except in the tissues of people and animals, whence they may escape to infect others. Tuberculosis germs are present only where contagious individuals are present. In some parts of the world contagious patients are few and pre-contagious patients (tuberculin reactors) are readily found and watched for possible onset of disease. In such places there are many people who do not come in contact with tubercle bacilli and who do not react to tuberculin tests.

Race and tuberculosis. Among American Indians, Negroes, and some other population groups, the incidence of tuberculosis has been high. However, this does not mean that some peoples have naturally low resistance to tuberculosis and others naturally high resistance. The facts are rather that people living in crowded and economically deprived circumstances are somewhat more exposed to cases of contagious tuberculosis in the community. Often there is greater tendency of the patient to continue work and usual activities in spite of symptoms of disease, so that tuberculosis tends to be farther advanced when it is finally discovered, and the mortality rate correspondingly high.

The opposite belief that some people have an innate resistance to tuberculosis is as ill-founded. Jews are often thought to have such resistance, since in general they have not suffered so much from tuberculosis as some other peoples. However, this is largely due to hygienic practices such as washing hands before eating, prohibition of meat from animals suffering from consumption, avoidance of exposure to contagion, seeking medical help on appearance of symptoms and submitting to treatment promptly.

There is no well documented evidence that defensive forces of the human body with respect to tuberculosis differ with race or nationality.

Mental illness and tuberculosis. High mortality from tuberculosis among patients in hospitals for the mentally ill in the past century led to the belief that mental disorder predisposes to tuberculosis. But in those days patients were admitted to mental hospitals without examination to detect tuberculosis, a contagious disease. In those closed communities, tuberculous infection spread, as it does not under modern conditions of tuberculosis control.

Age susceptibilities. The tuberculosis death rate of infants at the end of the past century was indeed high, but not because of extreme vulnerability to the disease. The true cause for high incidence of infection and mortality was intimate contact with contagious cases, including parents, grandparents, elderly neighbors, etc. Infants were helpless to defend themselves against fondling and kissing by such persons. Unpasteurized dairy products consumed by infants were often teeming with the living bovine type of tubercle bacilli.

Teenage boys and girls do not have peculiarly low resistance to tuberculosis, although many cases are discovered at this age. This is mating time when boys and girls associate in groups and enlarge social contacts outside the home, and intimate contacts are numerous. As tuberculosis develops and becomes contagious it usually causes no symptoms, and teenage boys and girls with unsuspected contagious tuberculosis can transmit it to their associates. Today this is less common since fewer children enter the teenage period with primary tuberculous infection.

Heredity. Tuberculosis is not inherited in the same sense that eye color is inherited. Very rarely, congenital tuberculosis may be acquired before birth from an infected mother whose tubercle bacilli cause disease of the placenta and fetus. Practically all infants are born free of tuberculosis and acquire the disease, if they do, from invasion by tubercle bacilli after birth.

Tuberculosis Eradication

For more than a third of a century we have known how to eradicate tuberculosis. Yet some 50,000,000 people in the U.S. harbor tubercle bacilli. No improvement can be expected until every person who reacts positively to tuberculin is recognized as a case of tuberculosis. These are the persons, together with those whom they infect, who will provide contagion, incapacity, and death from tuberculosis in the future. The microscopic areas of disease they carry are like machine gun nests or concealed weapons.

Eradication programs must start during the prenatal period. Great care must be taken to be sure that there is no person with contagious tuberculosis in the home, in the hospital where the infant will be born, and that no such case comes in contact with the infant thereafter.

This means adequate examination of the mother, father, relatives and neighbors who may frequent the home, as well as nurses, physicians and orderlies if the child is to be born in a hospital. Before starting school the child should be tested with tuberculin periodically to detect an infection that might have occurred. Tuberculosis is rarely transmitted from one gradeschool child to another. It is high school students and personnel such as teachers, bus drivers, janitors and cooks who offer a possible threat. Tuberculosis outbreaks in schools are usually traced to such persons who were not adequately examined for the disease.

Some years ago the Committee on Tuberculosis of the American School Health Association, working closely with state tuberculosis associations, devised a method by which schools can be made safe for children and personnel. This project consists of giving tuberculin tests to 95 per cent of children of all grades and to 100 per cent of school personnel, with appropriate followup of positive reactors. Schools which meet these qualifications are awarded certificates which, to remain valid, must be renewed each year. Eradication of tuberculosis in any community depends on protection of generations of children against tuberculosis germs as they go through life and replace the older generations now so extensively infected.

Bronchitis

The condition commonly called bronchitis is usually more extensive than the name indicates. It is often an acute infection of the air passages beginning with the nose and extending through the bronchioles. It may "act like" a common cold which "settles" in the nose or chest. Raw or burning sensations are felt in the back of the throat, then in the larynx, and later a burning, tight sensation may extend down the windpipe and the bronchial tubes. Occasionally the first manifestation is hoarseness.

Acute bronchitis may result from inhaled irritants such as fog, smoke, chemicals. It may be part of such conditions as chickenpox, influenza, measles and whooping cough. It may be due to allergy.

Usually there is mild fever for a day or so and after a few days pus-containing sputum is abundant. Usually, symptoms gradually disappear without after effects. However, in elderly people with emphysema acute bronchitis can be serious. Among children an acute condition known as laryngotracheobronchitis occurs, causing severe illness. The main problem is one of keeping airways open.

Chronic bronchitis usually develops slowly and appears in people past life's midway point. It occurs about four times more often in men than women, and more often among city dwellers than rural residents. In Great Britain about one-fourth of deaths of men of this age period are caused by chronic bronchitis. In that country the disease causes about 30,000 deaths annually. It usually begins with tracheobronchitis, with recovery, but repeated attacks occur until finally the condition persists continuously, usually with more severe symptoms during winter months.

The most significant symptom is cough, which may be constant or intermittent. Nearly always mucus is coughed up which may be clear, or may contain pus, or streaks of blood. In many cases no

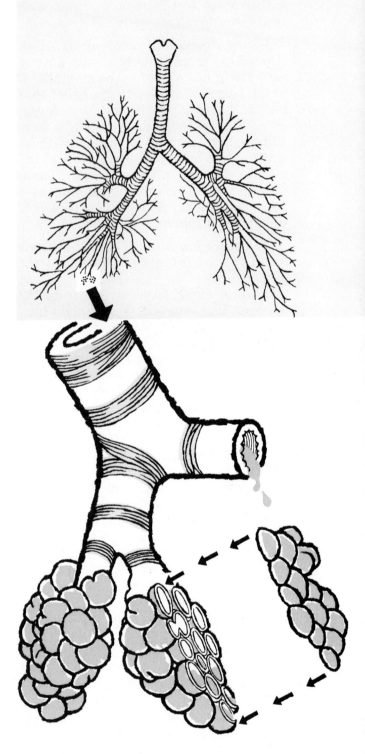

Cough and expectoration are characteristic of *bronchitis.* Closeup view of a section of the bronchial tree shows exudate dripping from a cut-off bronchiole. At right, directly above, exploded view of alveoli shows exudates in air cells that should contain only air.

medical help is sought since the patient is not severely ill or incapacitated. If a physician is consulted, his thorough examination usually reveals an essentially normal chest. Nevertheless, cough and expectoration persist.

Symptoms of chronic bronchitis may be caused by other more serious conditions, for example, tuberculosis. In all cases the

be so severe as to break one or more ribs or rupture a bleb on the surface of the lung, causing spontaneous lung collapse. Severe coughing may precipitate inguinal hernia, cause hemorrhages of the eyes or brain coverings, rupture blood vessels and impair "sweeping" cells (cilia) which remove foreign particles from the lungs. Large amounts of mucus

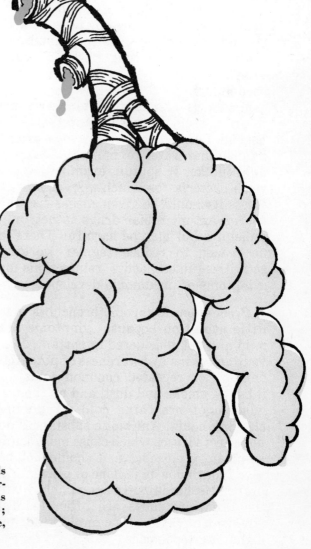

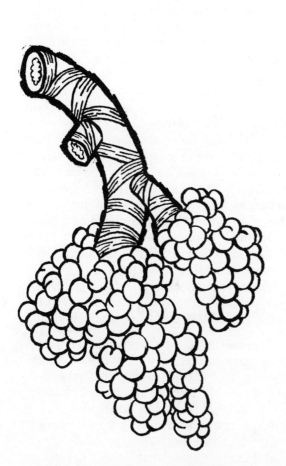

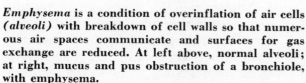

Emphysema is a condition of overinflation of air cells *(alveoli)* with breakdown of cell walls so that numerous air spaces communicate and surfaces for gas exchange are reduced. At left above, normal alveoli; at right, mucus and pus obstruction of a bronchiole, with emphysema.

sputum should be examined from time to time not only for tuberculosis germs but for other infecting organisms for which there may be specific drugs.

The outlook is good in chronic tracheobronchitis per se. However, there can be unpleasant complications. Coughing may

and pus may obstruct the bronchioles, with resulting emphysema.

Treatment begins with removal of any discoverable cause of irritation such as dust or smoke. Inhalation of cold air should be avoided. Room temperatures should be kept at 65 to 70° F. with relative humidity of about 40 per cent. Air should circulate gently—not in cold gusty drafts. Air should be filtered if possible.

There should be effort by the individual to suppress coughing except as necessary to raise secretions. In some persons coughing becomes a useless habit which perpetuates the bronchitis. No drug which completely suppresses the cough reflex should be taken. Cough should be controlled, but it is essential to clean the air passages. Sleeping pills and sedative drugs should be avoided by persons with chronic bronchitis, since they numb the sensibilities so the cough reflex does not operate normally and secretions accumulate.

Medicines intended to soften secretions in air passages (expectorants) may be helpful. This may be aided to some extent by drinking water to maintain adequate fluid intake. If sputum examination reveals bacteria for which a specific drug exists it should be given. Otherwise the use of antimicrobial drugs is not only unhelpful but may be harmful. There is no reason to reduce regular working activities unless acute reinfections or symptoms of pneumonia develop.

Prevention of chronic bronchitis gets little attention because symptoms are mild and not considered important. Prevention begins by awareness of potential dangers of repeated common colds, of inhaling smoke and dust, and by the unwisdom of breathing cold air during sleeping hours. Antibiotic substances do not affect viruses which cause most acute respiratory episodes and should not be given continuously in hope of preventing bronchitis flareups. Drugs which dilate the bronchial tubes are often helpful when bronchitis is complicated by asthmatic tendencies.

Bronchiectasis

The term *bronchiectasis* means dilation of the bronchial tubes. Dilations may be uniform or may appear as outpouchings on the outer walls of the bronchi. This abnormal condition may be present at birth but more often is acquired. It most frequently has its origin in children and young adults. Usually it is recognized some time after an attack of pneumonia such as occurs with influenza, measles, chickenpox and other illnesses. Generally infections are present which produce abscesses and large amounts of bad-smelling pus. Cough and expectoration of large amounts of sputum are characteristic symptoms.

Foreign bodies which obstruct the bronchial tubes may also cause bronchiectasis. One of the most common is peanuts which small children may "inhale." The peanut enters the larynx and passes as far into the bronchi as size permits. The object together with inflammation and swelling block the bronchi. Air trapped in that part of the lung absorbs and a condition known as *atelectasis* results. This dilates and damages the walls of the tubes and provides ideal conditions for multiplication of pus-forming bacteria. The foreign body may be removed through a bronchoscope, or destruction in surrounding bronchial walls may release it.

True bronchiectasis is an irreversible condition. Occasionally there is a "dry" form with little cough or expectoration.

Diagnosis of well-established bronchiectasis can usually be made on a basis of a history of having an attack of pneumonia or having aspirated a foreign body. Cough is not as continuous as in chronic bronchitis and is more likely to occur on changing position of the body. For example, stooping over to pick up an object from the floor is likely to cause severe coughing with expectoration of a large quantity of pus. If the disease is in the upper fourth of the lung, accumulations occur mainly while in the reclining position. A frequent symptom of bronchiectasis is bleeding which may range from streaks in the sputum to profuse hemorrhage.

A procedure known as *bronchography* enables one to determine the location and extent of bronchiectasis with great accuracy. It consists of introducing a tube through which a solution that is opaque

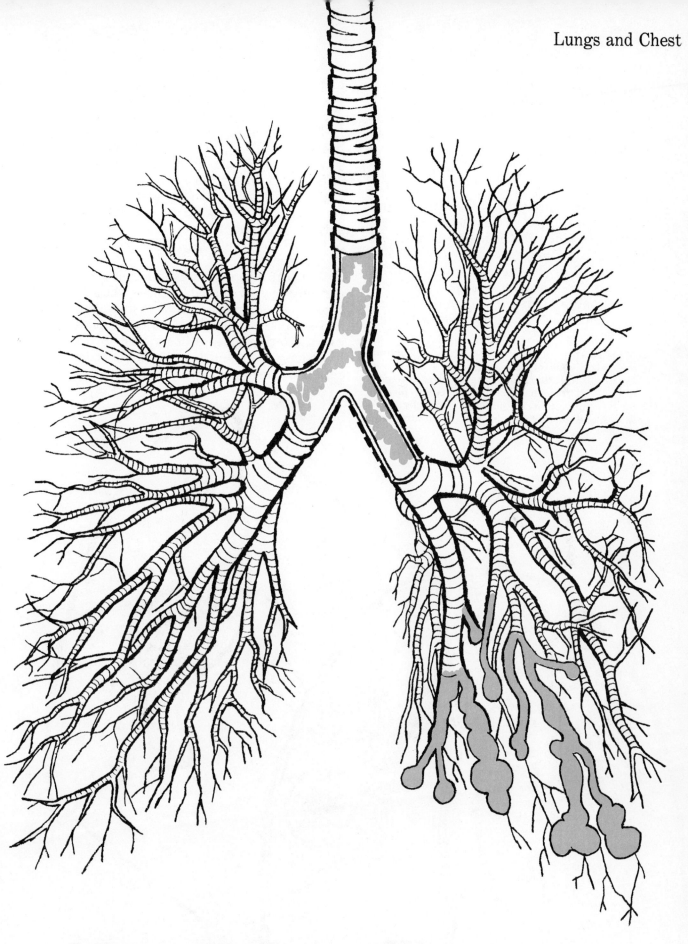

Bronchiectasis is a condition of dilation of the bronchial tubes that may result from obstructive foreign bodies and infections that produce abscesses and large amounts of pus. Cutaway view shows dilated pus-filled outpouchings for comparison with normal bronchial tree. Prompt treatment of pneumonia, especially in children, is important in preventing bronchiectasis.

to x-rays is poured into the windpipe. The opaque solution can then be made to flow into desired parts of the lung by tilting the patient's body, and x-ray films show the size, shape, and location of dilated bronchi.

Treatment of bronchiectasis is palliative unless surgery is indicated. Postural drainage—lowering the head and chest over the side of a bed, for instance, so that gravity helps to drain secretions — is helpful in preventing large quantities of pus from accumulating in the bronchial tubes. This reduces putrefaction and helps to decrease the unpleasant odor

A *lung abscess* is a local area of pus formation. Exploded view of left lung shows abscess in bronchioles infiltrating lung tissue. Abscesses may result from bronchial obstruction, foreign bodies, inhalation of material normally swallowed, and pus-forming bacteria from abscessed teeth or elsewhere.

of the sputum. Antibiotics may be used if susceptible organisms are present.

Surgical removal of the diseased area is the only definitive treatment for bronchiectasis. If the disease is localized so it can be removed a complete cure is effected. If too extensive for complete removal, the more involved areas may be removed with reduction of symptoms. If surgical treatment is refused or contraindicated, treatment is limited to palliative measures.

Value of surgery in established cases can only be appreciated by those who saw bronchiectasis when it was so prevalent and so untreatable. There was no more incapacitating disease. Its victims often lived long lives and were invalids from childhood until death. Many, in addition

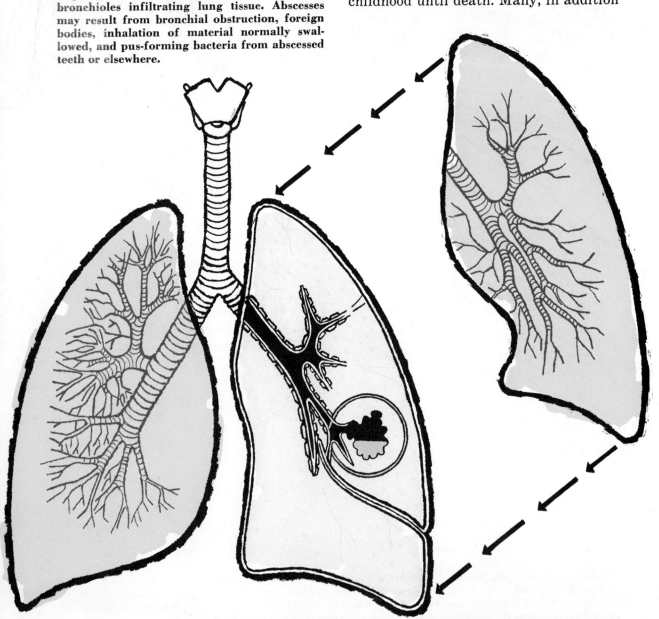

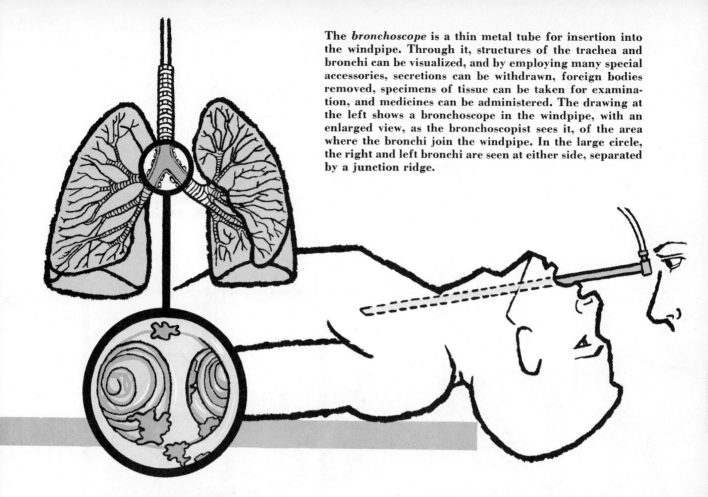

The *bronchoscope* is a thin metal tube for insertion into the windpipe. Through it, structures of the trachea and bronchi can be visualized, and by employing many special accessories, secretions can be withdrawn, foreign bodies removed, specimens of tissue can be taken for examination, and medicines can be administered. The drawing at the left shows a bronchoscope in the windpipe, with an enlarged view, as the bronchoscopist sees it, of the area where the bronchi join the windpipe. In the large circle, the right and left bronchi are seen at either side, separated by a junction ridge.

to being totally incapacitated, were miserable with pleurisy pain, pulmonary hemorrhages, repeated respiratory infections and extreme shortness of breath. They had paroxysms of coughing, often with sputum so fetid they were ostracized socially.

Chief factors in prevention of bronchiectasis are prompt treatment of pneumonia, especially in children, and making certain of complete recovery, using bronchoscopy if necessary to remove plugs which may obstruct bronchi. Bronchoscopy should be employed at the slightest intimation that foreign bodies have been aspirated by children or persons of any age.

Lung Abscess

Any area of local pus formation involving lung tissue is known as lung abscess. As we have seen, abscesses may be caused by bronchial obstruction and foreign bodies. Another cause is aspiration — inhalation — of materials into the lung which normally are swallowed and pass harmlessly through the digestive tract.

This may happen if the person is in an unconscious or semi-conscious condition or if normal reflexes are depressed. Material containing pus-forming bacteria may originate from the mouth if pyorrhea or abscessed teeth are present. Campaigns for good mouth hygiene have probably played a large role in reducing the incidence of pulmonary abscess.

Occasionally lung abscess from pus-forming bacteria accompanies pneumonia and fungus diseases of the lung. Abscesses in neighboring structures may burrow through and cause lung abscess.

Symptoms. Chill followed by fever may be the first manifestation of lung abscess. Usually there is not much cough or expectoration in early stages. Sudden coughing up of half a cup or more of pus occurs when an abscess ruptures into a bronchus. Bloodspitting varying in amount from streaks in the sputum to fatal hemorrhage may occur.

Abscesses usually cast shadows on x-ray film, but not always. Microscopic studies of sputum often determine the cause of lung abscess.

229

Treatment. In single abscess ten or more days usually pass before spontaneous rupture of pus occurs. During this time bed rest is needed with mild sedatives, but no drugs to control cough. As soon as sputum is available it is studied to identify responsible organisms, so that proper drugs specific for the organisms can be administered.

as long as there is drainage of pus. If postural drainage is not adequate, removal of secretions and pus with a bronchoscope may be necessary. If there is no great improvement within two or three weeks, surgical consultation is advisable. A surgeon may carry out procedures such as open drainage through the chest wall that will markedly hasten recovery. With-

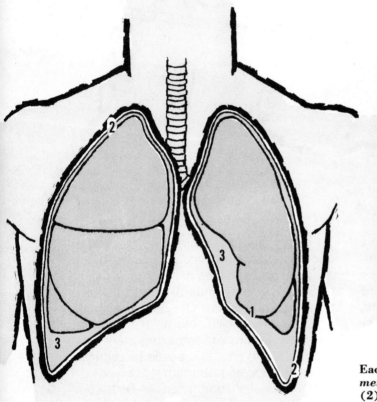

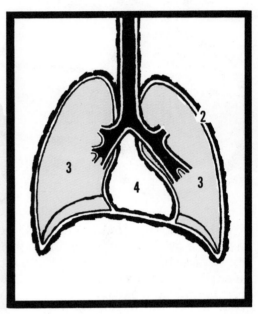

Each lung is surrounded by a glistening *pleural membrane* (1) and the inner surface of the chest (2) has a similar pleural lining *(parietal)*. The *pleural cavity* (3) between these sliding opposing surfaces is normally not a cavity at all, but entry of bacteria, penetrating wounds, erosion of disease areas of lungs, chest, abdomen, etc., can cause an actual cavity. In square, relationship of heart space (4) to pleural spaces is shown.

After an abscess ruptures and the patient's condition is satisfactory, *postural drainage* often helps to keep the area of disease reasonably free from pus. Posture which assists gravity to drain the pus depends upon the location of the abscess in the lung. For practical purposes, the position which produces the most coughing and eliminates the most pus suffices. This posture should be taken several times a day, continued each time

out such surgical consultation the patient may be jeopardized by complications resulting in long periods of invalidism.

A Word About Coughs

It must always be kept in mind that cough is an important protective mechanism. Foreign material which enters the larynx and passes along the lower respiratory tract normally triggers the cough reflex. Foreign material moved up the windpipe by beating cilia causes cough and clearing of the throat. Therefore it is never good to take drugs which completely inhibit the cough reflex. When cough is severe, prolonged, and "brings nothing up," a mild cough sedative is justified but not a drug which completely stops cough.

Conditions which depress cough and gag reflexes include unconsciousness, overindulgence in alcohol, cerebral accidents, diabetic coma, injuries to the head, anesthesia, and others. Persons in such defenseless states require body posture to prevent foreign material from entering the lower respiratory tract.

Deep sleep, particularly among elderly persons, and drugs taken to promote sleep, may depress reflexes enough to prevent cough from keeping the windpipe and bronchi clear. Foci of infection in tonsils, sinuses, gums and teeth provide rich sources of pus-forming germs if materials enter the lower respiratory tract when persons in such states are unable to defend themselves. Such foci should be removed or treated. Unexplained, severe attacks of coughing, in children and others, should be investigated by a physician.

Excessive, prolonged or useless coughing may often be eased by quite simple methods. Dry air in heated homes can irritate sensitive membranes. A source of moisture may minimize dry, hacking coughs. A vaporizer or steam tent helps to liquefy secretions of patients with congested nose and throat membranes. Chewing and swallowing a cracker or cookie may help to move "tickling" accumulations down the throat.

Pleurisy

Practically any disease that causes inflammation of the lungs may result in *pleurisy*. The first symptoms may be sharp, knifelike pain, a "stitch in the side," followed by fever. The thin, glistening layer of pleura which is inseparably bound to the lung has no pain fibers, but the opposing pleura is richly supplied. Normally the pleural layers glide over each other on a thin film of lubricating fluid. Disease may cause the pleura to become inflamed and adherent, or fluids may accumulate in the interspace, separating the layers, and pain subsides.

Normally there is no communication between the lungs and the pleural spaces. However, lymph channels draining from the head, neck, chest wall and abdomen may transport disease agents to the pleura. Disease areas in the lungs, chest wall and abdomen may erode into the pleural spaces. Thus, the cause of a particular case of pleurisy is always sought. Presence of pleural fluid is detected by examination including fluoroscopic and x-ray film inspection.

Tuberculous pleurisy results from invasion of the pleura by tubercle bacilli which have established disease areas elsewhere, commonly in the lungs. This sets up an inflammatory process with outpouring of fluid. Treatment of tuberculous pleurisy consists of repeated removal of as much fluid as possible through a needle, and anti-tuberculosis drugs, much the same as in pulmonary tuberculosis. If fluid is allowed to remain, its fibrin content may be deposited so thickly on the pulmonary pleura that the lung cannot re-expand, when the fluid is absorbed, to occupy the space which contained the fluid. Then a surgical procedure known as *decortication* becomes necessary to remove the peel of fibrin so the lung can expand.

Dry pleurisy may follow pneumonia and subside with the underlying disease, while measures to relieve pain are taken.

Wet pleurisy with large accumulation of fluid usually requires removal of fluid by needle aspiration. Pleural fluid often appears in persons with congestive heart failure or rheumatic fever. Patients with brucellosis, tularemia, fungus infections, chest malignancy, and cirrhosis of the liver may have pleurisy with fluid secondary to the disease.

There is a condition known as "simple pleurisy" of unknown cause. Attacks of pleural pain occur and may persist for a few hours or several days or weeks. No abnormality can be found. It is believed

Tuberculous pleurisy, resulting from invasion of pleura by tuberculosis germs, results in profuse outpouring of fluid. In contrast to normal lungs, above, the pleural space of the affected lung contains trapped fluid, shown being removed through a hollow needle.

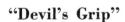

that disease is present near the periphery of the lung and is too small to be located with present methods of examination. These cases usually respond to treatment consisting of a tight binder around the chest to reduce breathing movements of the chest wall, mild sedatives, and rest as complete as possible until the symptoms diminish and disappear.

Empyema

When pus accumulates in the pleural space the condition is known as *empyema*. Formerly, empyema developed in some five per cent of persons after attacks of lobar pneumonia and rather frequently after pneumonia caused by hemolytic streptococci. It was the latter organism which caused such destruction during the influenza pandemic of 1918. Lessons learned during World War I led to the practice of aspirating pus through a needle while keeping close watch on the patient's vital capacity, and instituting open surgical drainage when the patient can withstand it. Empyema has become relatively rare since the advent of antibiotics for treatment of pneumonia and diseases associated with pus formation.

"Devil's Grip"

Sudden, knifelike chest pain which may radiate over the appendix heralds the onset of *epidemic pleurodynia*, sometimes called the "Devil's Grip." Initial symptoms resemble those of pneumonia, tuberculous pleurisy, and collapsed lung. There is fever for a few hours or a few days. The disease runs its course in about ten days. It is caused by a virus. There is no specific treatment. The patient is kept as comfortable as possible and isolated to prevent infecting others, since the disease is communicable and, as the name implies, tends to occur in epidemics.

Pneumothorax
(Collapsed Lung)

A young man walking in the street, or lying in bed, or watching television from an easy chair, is suddenly stabbed by excruciating pain in the side of the chest below the armpit. The pain is intensified each time he takes a breath. This is the typical acute symptom of *spontaneous pneumothorax* — collapse of a lung.

What has happened? Somehow, air has entered the normally airless space between the pleural membranes of the inner chest wall and the lung surface. The airless pleural space normally exerts negative pressure—i.e., a vacuum, a pull — so that the elastic lung which is filled with air at atmospheric pressure expands to fill all available space. When this vacuum-seal is broken, the elastic lung pulls itself together and shrinks in size— something like a stretched rubber band released from tension. The degree of collapse depends upon how much air comes into the pleural space.

Symptoms. Pain in this event is often felt under the armpit but it may occur over the heart, under the breastbone, in the shoulder area or down the arm. If collapse is extensive, shortness of breath usually follows the pain. In some persons the onset is mild and the first symptom may be slight shoulder ache, mild chest pain on respiration, or a feeling of slight pressure in the side of the chest. It is likely that many persons who have partial spontaneous pneumothorax do not consult a doctor and that the condition is more common than is supposed. Severe symptoms usually begin to subside within a few hours.

The most common form of spontaneous pneumothorax results from rupture of a bleb on the surface of the lung. The bleb is like a blister filled with air under pressure. It may be congenital or possibly is formed by coalescence of overdistended air sacs in the lungs. Its rupture permits air from the lung to enter the pleural space. This rupture may occur during sleep and has nothing to do with the patient's preceding activities; the lungs are constantly expanding and deflating.

There are other forms of pneumothorax. A penetrating wound or a splinter of bone from a broken rib may cause *traumatic pneumothorax.* A number of diseases which involve the lung may burrow through the pulmonary pleura and allow air to escape into the pleural space. Artificial pneumothorax is employed to collapse the lung deliberately in treatment of tuberculosis. But spontaneous pneumothorax occurs in absence of any demonstrable disease or injury, and is not necessarily associated with tuberculosis as it was once thought to be. It may occur at any age, but is most frequent in young men 20 to 25 years old and less common in women.

Treatment of simple spontaneous pneumothorax depends upon the extent of collapse, complications, and rate of re-expansion of the lung. If the lung is not more than 50 per cent collapsed, and initial symptoms subside, hospitalization and bed rest are usually not necessary. The patient is advised to reduce physical activity to a minimum until the lung is completely re-expanded. With a greater degree of collapse, particularly if the lung does not start to re-expand rather promptly, a period of a few days to a week in bed may be recommended. If the lung is then re-expanded, normal living may be resumed.

During the re-expansion period the patient should report promptly any symptom such as pain, shortness of breath or pressure. Fluoroscopic or x-ray film inspections enable the doctor to assess the progress of re-expansion. A collapsed lung may be re-expanded in a couple of days by withdrawing air from the pleural cavity through a needle or catheter. This is not advisable in simple uncomplicated cases but may be desirable if the lung is not re-expanding satisfactorily.

Occasional complications of spontaneous pneumothorax require treatment. Rarely, fluid accumulates in the pleural cavity and sometimes this should be withdrawn. In some cases, blood from a ruptured vessel appears in the pleural cavity and should be withdrawn. The most serious complication is *tension pneumothorax.* This is caused by a flap of the pleural rupture which allows air to enter the cavity but prevents if from going out, like a one-way check valve. Extreme pressures can build up, as in an overinflated tire, displacing adjacent organs. In such emergency it is imperative that air be released through a needle or catheter, and surgical repair of the tear may be necessary.

Occasionally, simple spontaneous pneumothorax appears on both sides almost simultaneously, or first on one side and on the opposite side at a later time. About a third of persons who have an initial attack of spontaneous pneumothorax have a recurrence subsequently. If there have been more than two recurrences, the best procedure is performed by a surgeon who expands the lung and roughens the pleural layers so they become adherent. This obliterates the pleural cavity and makes subsequent attacks of spontaneous pneumothorax impossible.

Persons who have or have had pneumothorax should avoid high altitudes or unpressurized airplane cabins. This is because the volume of air in the pleural cavity increases with altitude.

Emphysema

The term *emphysema* derives from Greek words meaning "overinflated." The overinflated structures are microscopic air sacs of the lungs (alveoli). Tiny bronchioles through which air flows to and from the air sacs have muscle fibers in their walls. These structures may become hypertrophied and lose elasticity. Then air flows into the air sacs easily but cannot flow out easily because of the narrowed diameter of bronchioles. The patient can breathe in but cannot breathe out efficiently. There is too much stale air in his lungs. As pressure builds up in the air cells their thin walls are stretched to the point of rupture, so several air spaces communicate and the area of surfaces where gas exchange takes place is decreased. The ultimate result is shortness of breath, overwork of the heart, and sometimes death.

Several types of emphysema have been described, but the one of great import-ance is known as chronic hypertrophic pulmonary emphysema. The condition is probably as old as the human race and has long been the bane of physicians everywhere. In some persons emphysema never reaches a stage where it causes inconvenience or incapacity. Persons whose symptoms, particularly shortness of breath, are quite severe usually have the disease in an advanced stage. In recent years emphysema has been extensively publicized and many believe that it is becoming more common. How much of this is due to more extensive reporting of cases is not known. The disease is not communicable or reportable to health departments, and many more people are living to older ages when emphysema is most prevalent. Symptomatic emphysema is most frequently recognized in persons between 50 and 70 years of age.

Of suggested basic causes, obstruction of the bronchioles is most plausible. Many emphysematous patients give histories of repeated colds and respiratory infections which come closer and closer together. Some studies associate emphysema with smog and heavy cigarette smoking. Smog, smoke, and inhaled irritants may increase mucus secretion in the air passages and cause obstruction of bronchioles with entrapment of air beyond the obstruction. Diseases such as tuberculosis and silicosis may involve such large areas as to cause overwork and expansion (hypertrophy) of remaining normal lung tissue.

The lungs contain much elastic tissue essential to their function. A general decrease in elasticity of body tissues begins around the age of 40 (first noticed by many people when bifocal lenses are needed for reading). Because of the large reserve of lung capacity, decreased elasticity may not be apparent until 60 to 65 years of age when shortness of breath may become noticeable. Excessive abdominal fat tends to lift the diaphragm, reducing lung space and making shortness of breath more noticeable. Age and weight should be considered when presence of emphysema is suspected.

Chronic pulmonary emphysema is irreversible. Broken-down walls of air cells never regenerate. There is no specific treatment. However, one may hope to stop the progress of the disease. A heavy smoker should give it up. Those living in smog-smitten areas should seek escape. The patient who has bronchial asthma should avoid allergens. Abdominal supports in the form of tight or elastic belts may be worn to decrease the abdominal space and push the diaphragm upward. In chronic emphysema the chest becomes enlarged and the over-distended lungs depress the diaphragm and restrict its respiratory movements. Special breathing exercises appear to be helpful.

Pneumoconiosis ("Dusty Lungs")

The term *pneumoconiosis* indicates a lung condition due to inhalation of minute particles, usually fine mineral dusts. There is no specific treatment for this group of diseases, but they are rapidly disappearing because of very effective preventive measures.

Normal chest, at left below, tends to become "barrel-chested" in chronic emphysema, at right. Loss of elasticity and narrowed diameter of tiny bronchioles makes it difficult for air to escape from air cells (*alveoli*) and too much "stale air" tends to accumulate.

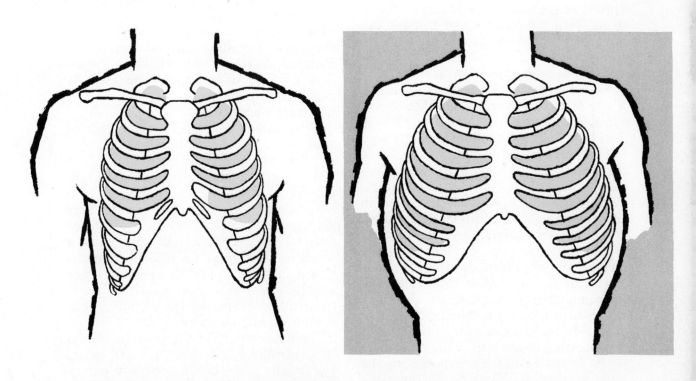

Antimicrobial drugs may be used when they are effective against specific organisms associated with excessive secretions causing obstruction of bronchioles. Obstructions may be partially eliminated by drugs which tend to liquefy thick secretions or dilate bronchial walls. For large air-containing pockets on lung surfaces, which become so distended under pressure as to compress the lung, surgical removal may give considerable relief. Appropriate measures will be prescribed by a well-informed physician according to individual needs.

The most ubiquitous mineral dust is silicon dioxide. About 60 per cent of the earth's crust is composed of silicon-containing material, of which about one-fifth is free silicon dioxide. Silica enters the body through food, drink and air. It is present in bones, skin, nails, connective tissue, blood and the lungs, and is often considered a normal constituent of the body.

Exposure to high concentrations of silica dust for a long period of time, 20 years or more, may cause a condition known as *silicosis*, in which fibrous tissue is built around clusters of fine silica particles in the lungs. Excluding and extruding mechanisms of the respiratory tract protect most persons against severe silicosis even when high concentrations of dust are inhaled. In a strict sense, all adults have silicosis. The condition varies through a wide range, from persons who have microscopic nodules to those with extensive fibrosis of both lungs.

Diagnosis. Mostly, only very tiny particles, 10 microns or less in diameter (a micron is a millionth of a meter), reach the air sacs of the lungs. Some are entrapped in lymph nodules and nodes. Where particles of silica are deposited, fibrous or scar tissue is laid down around them. Before a diagnosis of silicosis can be considered, there must be accurate information about the length of time the patient has been exposed to air containing certain quantities of fine silica particles. X-ray films show three general stages of silicosis, ranging from small nodules in the lungs to larger confluent shadows.

There are no significant symptoms in the first and second stages, and often these are lacking in the third stage. Usually the only symptoms that occur in silicosis are due to complications which develop in some third-stage cases.

Tuberculosis, once thought to be a serious complication, appears to be a matter of the amount of tuberculosis in the community rather than the extent of silicosis. In the past much emphasis was placed on right-sided heart failure as a complication of silicosis. This may come about from the burden imposed on the right side of the heart by compression and obliteration of pulmonary vessels by fibrous tissue surrounding them. Some instances of right-sided heart failure occur in extremely advanced cases of silicosis, among persons over 50 years old, an age at which cardiovascular disease is common. There is no evidence that cancer of the lung is more common in silicosis patients than in the general population. Silicosis per se causes no significant disability, regardless of its stage.

Silicosis is rapidly being eradicated by preventive methods which include reduction of dust counts, good industrial housekeeping, masks, and mixtures of substances with silica dust which form aggregates too large to pass through the bronchioles to the lungs.

Of other dusts that may cause significant pneumoconiosis, asbestos is most important. Processed asbestos is broken down to fibers and particles so long and large that they lodge in terminal bronchioles and do not reach air cells of the lungs. Fibrous tissue develops around particles in walls of the bronchioles, and walls of terminal air cells become thickened and their capacity is reduced.

Long, continuous exposure to asbestos dust with more than 5,000,000 particles per cubic foot of air is a prerequisite to diagnosis of *asbestosis.* In early stages there are no symptoms or abnormal x-ray findings. As more fibrous tissue is deposited it begins to cast x-ray shadows. As time passes, shortness of breath may begin and increase.

The outlook depends on the extent of the condition and complications that may develop. Progressive cases may result in bronchiectasis and failure of the right side of the heart.

Inhalation of beryllium by persons working in or near beryllium plants or with broken neon light bulbs may cause a condition known as *berylliosis.* Progressive shortness of breath and cough are usually the first symptoms of the acute respiratory form. In the chronic form symptoms appear more slowly.

Cortisone and ACTH may be useful in controlling the condition. In acute pneumonic cases death occurs in one to eight per cent. The remainder recover in about four months. Use of beryllium in the fluorescent light industry was discontinued in 1949. However, care should be taken in destroying old fluorescent bulbs made prior to 1949.

Sarcoidosis

A score or more of names have been applied to the condition known as *sarcoidosis.* The characteristic feature is nodules which appear in various parts of the body. The cause is unknown. When

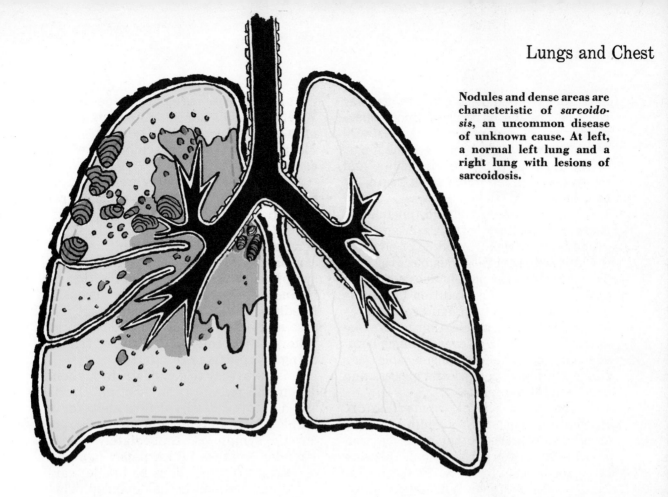

Nodules and dense areas are characteristic of *sarcoidosis*, an uncommon disease of unknown cause. At left, a normal left lung and a right lung with lesions of sarcoidosis.

sarcoidosis appears in the lungs the areas of disease range from small nodules to large dense areas throughout the lungs. Areas of sarcoidosis strongly resemble those of several other diseases and can only be differentiated by microscopic examination. If sarcoidosis involves the lungs extensively and tends to progress with deposition of scar tissue and cavity formation, the outlook usually is not good.

Most patients with sarcoidosis are in reasonably good health when first seen by a doctor, but now and then an individual appears chronically ill. Observations of sarcoidosis are relatively recent, and the natural course of the disease in many patients over long periods of time is uncertain. The longer persons with this condition have been followed, the more apparent has become the seriousness of the disease, with recurrences and late complications. Sarcoidosis is a disease of remissions and exacerbations. One area of disease may be clearing while others are evolving in different parts of the body.

A considerable number of persons with sarcoidosis have later been found to have tuberculosis, but no definite relationship between the two conditions has been established. To date no specific means of treatment of sarcoidosis has been found.

Lipoid Pneumonia

Oils that are harmless in the digestive tract may be very dangerous if they trickle down the windpipe into the lungs. This misdirection is never intentional. It may happen in infants and debilitated persons and even in normal persons. If certain oils are "inhaled," or trickle down from nose and throat into the larynx and thence to the lungs, *lipoid pneumonia* may result. This condition is caused by inability of the lungs to break down and get rid of oily substances which thus remain in lung tissues.

Cod liver oil, lard, cream and animal fats cause greater irritation in the respiratory tract and are more likely to be removed by cough than mineral oil (liquid petrolatum), castor oil, olive oil or poppyseed oil. Some of these substances, particularly mineral oil, cause so little irritation that they scarcely stimulate the cough reflex at all. Oily nose sprays are not so common as they were before the hazards of lipoid pneumonia were recognized. Yet oils still reach the nose, and sometimes the lungs, in the form of drops or ointments, and many people take mineral oil regularly as a laxative.

In some cases of lipoid pneumonia there is shortness of breath and low grade fever. If small amounts of oil enter the lungs at short intervals but over long periods of time the patient does not notice any symptoms. The condition usually is of long duration, and if oil aspiration is stopped and no complication occurs the patient recovers. However, if much damage has been caused, considerable scar tissue may be deposited and abscess and cysts may develop.

There is no specific medication. *Prevention* consists of avoiding the use of oily substances in the nose, as well as mineral oil for constipation. Oils and fatty foods should not be forced on infants who resist them. When lipoid pneumonia occurs in infants, it is often learned that they struggled and coughed when they were given cod liver oil, milk, and other fat-containing food.

When persons are ill, unconscious, enfeebled, their senses dulled, great care must be taken in giving oils and fats, as the cough reflex may be severely impaired. During vomiting periods they should be placed in such position that vomitus does not drain into the windpipe.

Hyperventilation (Overbreathing)

There are people who have attacks of air hunger, a feeling that they can't get a satisfying breath, accompanied by dizziness, faintness, numbness, tingling, pounding of the heart, and spasmodic muscle cramps. Their trouble is not that they get too little air, but too much, a condition known as *hyperventilation*.

Overbreathing or forced breathing triggers a strange chain of events. Our impulse to take in a breath of air is sparked by carbon dioxide which accumulates in the blood and acts on respiratory centers. When we inhale, the oxygen in air reduces carbon dioxide levels. When too much carbon dioxide is blown off there is increased alkalinity of the blood. This results in symptoms which can mimic disease.

Why does a person overbreathe in the first place? Usually there is some degree of anxiety, tension, and emotional distress. Overbreathing begins without the person's being aware of it, until enough carbon dioxide is washed out to cause symptoms which are so alarming that he begins to breathe even more vigorously. Needless apprehension about heart disease and other serious afflictions can be relieved if the innocuous cause of frightening symptoms is recognized.

It is quite easy to demonstrate the condition and reassure the "victim." He is asked to overbreathe deliberately for a couple of minutes to reproduce characteristic symptoms. Immediately thereafter he breathes into a paper bag and rebreathes from it. Thus he inhales carbon dioxide which he has exhaled. This restores carbon dioxide to its normal level and symptoms disappear. "Heart disease," panic, muscle spasms, will be no more if the reassured patient can learn to breathe properly.

Hiccup

Since we have mentioned breathing into a paper bag, this is a good place to mention *hiccup*, also spelled hiccough. Everybody has had hiccups. The cause is a spasm of the diaphragm resulting from some irritation of the nerves that control it. The result is a spasmodic intake of a little air which makes a peculiar noise as the glottis closes down.

Almost everybody has a favorite remedy for mild hiccups, and most of them work. Some people say to hold one's breath as long as possible, or to breathe into a paper bag, or to take nine consecutive sips of water from a cup without pausing. The basic principle of these and similar methods is the same. All of them decrease the intake of oxygen from air and thus increase the carbon dioxide level of the blood in a way that soothes the twitchy diaphragm.

Severe cases of hiccups that persist for days and exhaust the patient require medical or surgical intervention.

Cancer of the Respiratory Tract

Tumors are abnormal growths or swellings that may be benign or malignant. Malignant means cancerous and implies a tendency for the tumor, in time, to *metastasize* or spread to other parts of the body from the primary site of origin. A benign tumor remains localized, but is not necessarily harmless. It may cause serious or fatal interference with body functions. The respiratory tract has its share of both kinds of tumors.

Malignant tumors occur in the nose and throat, and the larynx is a common site. Benign tumors of the larynx occur most often in earlier years of life when use of the voice is greatest. Cancer of the larynx is about ten times more common in men than women. Prolonged hoarseness is one of the symptoms. Early surgical removal of the localized cancer often saves the patient's life, but at cost of loss of the vocal cords. However, most patients learn how to speak very satisfactorily by acquiring the knack of bringing up air, in a sort of controlled eructation, so that word sounds can be formed.

Cancer of the lung is the most frequent malignancy of the respiratory tract. Cancer in the bronchi and lungs evolves through a "silent stage" when lesions are microscopic in size and cause no symptoms. The conventional physical examination, including fluoroscopic and x-ray examination of the chest, is usually unavailing during early stages of lung cancer. Only after the condition is fairly extensive or productive of complications may abnormal physical signs be elicited.

The earliest symptoms are likely to be cough, expectoration, wheezing and *hemoptysis* (blood spitting). Symptoms of lung cancer become more severe as the disease progresses and often include shortness of breath, pulmonary hemorrhage and loss of body weight. If cancer is located near the surface of the lung the only symptom may be pain.

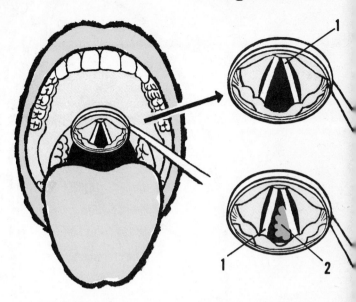

At left above, a normal larynx or voice box as it looks in the examiner's mirror. View at top right shows normal vocal cords (1) and surrounding structures, and below it, a malignant tumor (2) of the larynx.

As cancer grows in a bronchus it may partially obstruct passage of air coming from the part of the lung the bronchus supplies, so that air does not escape normally and the lung area is overdistended (localized emphysema). As the growth becomes larger it may completely prevent air from entering a part of the lung. Trapped air is absorbed and the airless part of the lung is in a condition of atelectasis.

Signs of emphysema first, and atelectasis later, may be identified in x-ray films, suggesting that the channel of a bronchus is blocked but not necessarily that the cause of obstruction is cancer. Again, a tumor near the lung surface may cause fluid to accumulate in the pleural space, casting a shadow on x-ray film.

However, there is no symptom or x-ray finding that is specific for lung cancer since there are other causes of localized emphysema, atelectasis, and pleurisy with effusion. But these findings point to the need for other examinations, one of the most important of which is bronchoscopy. With the bronchoscope the specialist may be able to see the affected area and remove a piece of the tumor for microscopic examination. He may also take a bronchial washing by introducing and withdrawing a saline solution which

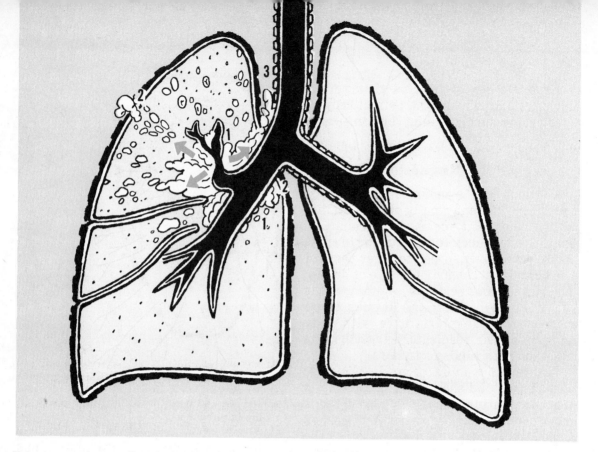

Primary carcinoma (cancer) of a main bronchus, with infiltration into lung tissue (1), extension through the pleura (2), and invasion to neighboring lymph nodes (3) and further extension. Cancer originating in other organs (stomach, uterus, breast, prostate gland, pancreas, and thyroid gland) often migrates or *metastasizes* to the lungs.

is studied for presence of cancer cells. Many bronchial ramifications are too small to permit visualization, but substances which are opaque to x-rays can be introduced. In this manner an obstruction of a bronchus may be located. The sputum can also be examined for cancer cells.

Tissue taken from a ridge at the bottom of the windpipe where the main bronchi diverge sometimes gives evidence of cancer that has spread from its original site in one of the bronchial passages. Another accessible area is just above the collarbone where small lymph nodes lie just under the skin. If malignant cells are found in the nodes it is evidence that cancer of the lung has metastasized — been transferred from its original site to a distant one by conveyance of cells through blood and lymph vessels.

Tests have been described at some length because it is important that permission be given the physician to do what he thinks necessary. However, in many cases the diagnosis is made with one or two diagnostic tests.

Physicians generally feel that most tumors of the chest, even benign ones, should be removed. Surgeons can enter the chest wall, locate the involved lung area, and remove a tissue section which a pathologist examines immediately while the chest wall is still open. The pathologist's verdict determines whether the surgeon will close the chest or first remove a lobe or even a whole lung.

Metastatic malignancies transferred from other sites are more common than primary cancer of the respiratory tract. In fact, about half of cancers of the breast metastasize to the lungs if untreated. Primary cancers of the stomach, uterus, prostate gland, pancreas, and thyroid gland often metastasize to the lungs. It is not unusual for cancer to appear in the lungs without the distant primary site at which the malignancy originated having been diagnosed, because of absence of symptoms. In fact, the primary lesion may be so small that it is neither suspected or located until an autopsy is performed.

THE NERVOUS SYSTEM

**by LEWIS J. DOSHAY, M.D., and
MADISON H. THOMAS, M.D.**

The Nerve Unit • The Nerve Impulse • Input and Output Pathways • Traffic Switches • The Central Nervous System • Peripheral Nerves • "Automatic" Regulators • The Human Brain • Clues to Disorder

NEUROLOGIC TESTS

PARKINSON'S DISEASE

BRAIN INJURIES

Brain Tumor

DEMYELINATING DISEASES

INFECTIONS OF THE NERVOUS SYSTEM

Neuritis • Neuralgias • Headache • Dizziness and Vertigo

SPASMS, CRAMPS AND TICS

Cerebral Palsy • Muscular Dystrophy

CONGENITAL MALFORMATIONS

EPILEPSY

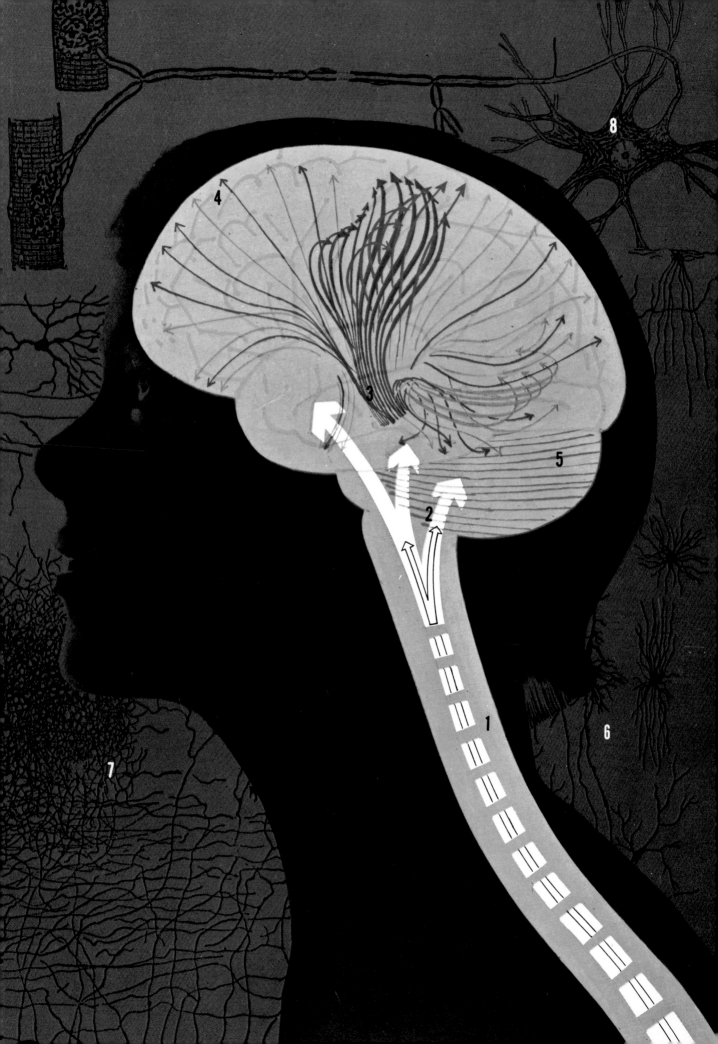

CHAPTER 7

THE NERVOUS SYSTEM

by **LEWIS J. DOSHAY, M.D.**

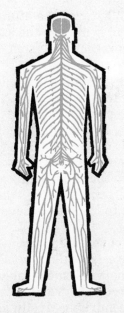

Without a nervous system, man would be doomed to a senseless, motionless, thoughtless vegetative existence, like a plant. The small figure above suggests the pervasiveness of the nervous system; the brain and spinal cord are in solid color.

The color plate shows, in a highly simplified way, some nervous structures and mechanisms that in the living body are incredibly intricate. Arrows suggest pathways of nerve impulses ascending the *spinal cord* (1). There are junctions in the *midbrain* (2) which includes the *medulla oblongata* and *pons,* and the *thalamus* (3); nearby is the *cerebellum* (5); and other fibers fan out to the *cerebrum* (4). Descending pathways are not shown.

Background structures are typical nerve cells of the *cerebral cortex* (6), the networks of fibers conducting toward the cortex (7), and a typical motor neuron of the peripheral nervous system (8) with its *axon* (the long fiber running across the top of the drawing) terminating in an "end plate" in striated muscle.

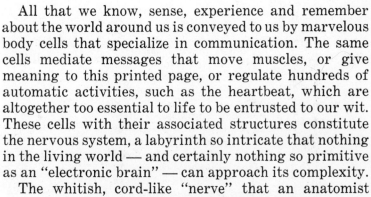

All that we know, sense, experience and remember about the world around us is conveyed to us by marvelous body cells that specialize in communication. The same cells mediate messages that move muscles, or give meaning to this printed page, or regulate hundreds of automatic activities, such as the heartbeat, which are altogether too essential to life to be entrusted to our wit. These cells with their associated structures constitute the nervous system, a labyrinth so intricate that nothing in the living world — and certainly nothing so primitive as an "electronic brain" — can approach its complexity.

The whitish, cord-like "nerve" that an anatomist sees is actually a bundle of hundreds or thousands of individual nerve fibers. Despite the complaints of some patients, nerves never become "tied in knots," nor do they jump, twitch, or jangle. Indeed, in their living surroundings, intact nerves are so deceptively placid that it is quite impossible for an expert with the best of microscopes to tell by mere inspection whether a nerve is working or not. Their messages are as invisible as a conversation in a telephone wire. But everything that sustains the highest processes of life, as well as humble vegetative processes, hangs upon the integration of billions of nerve impulses every minute that we live.

The Nerve Unit

The shape of a nerve cell resembles that of a drop of liquid which has splashed on a hard surface and flung out tentacles in various directions. The cell *body* is the central blob. Spraying out from it are short branched fibers which, from their resemblance to tree roots, are called *dendrites.* There is another long single fiber called

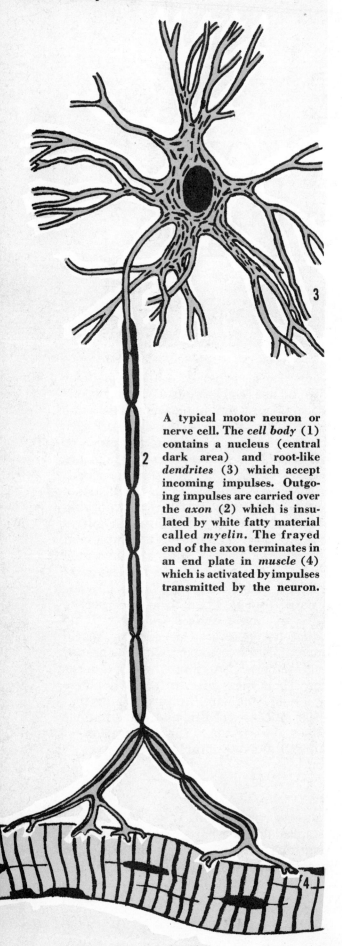

A typical motor neuron or nerve cell. The *cell body* (1) contains a nucleus (central dark area) and root-like *dendrites* (3) which accept incoming impulses. Outgoing impulses are carried over the *axon* (2) which is insulated by white fatty material called *myelin*. The frayed end of the axon terminates in an end plate in *muscle* (4) which is activated by impulses transmitted by the neuron.

an *axon* which ends in a brush-like tip. The complete unit is called a *neuron*.

This is the functioning unit that makes a baby cry when he is hungry or is pricked by a pin, or makes a man dodge out of the path of a car, or frown when he gets a tax bill. Whatever the stimuli, the job of the neuron is always the same — to transmit a nerve impulse from one part of its structure to another.

Dendrites accept incoming impulses and carry them toward the cell body. The axon carries impulses away from the cell body. "Nerves" vary in diameter according to how many axon fibers are bundled together like cables. Each fiber is an extension of a cell body that may lie a great distance away. The sciatic nerve which runs from the back to the toes is several feet long.

Most axons are covered by a sheath of white fatty material called *myelin*. "White matter" of nerve tissue is largely myelin-covered fibers, and "gray matter" the cell bodies and dendrites. Myelin acts very much in the nature of rubber that insulates electric wire and may serve other purposes. It is at least essential to healthy nerve function. Breaks or wasting away of the myelin sheath are characteristic of some disorders known as demyelinating diseases (see page 263).

We have billions of neurons — some 12 billion in the brain alone. This is fortunate, for we cannot regenerate nerve cells. The number we now have is the most we will ever have. Some are bound to be lost to the wear and tear of living. An elderly person has many fewer neurons than he did in his youth, but the original supply of billions of neurons was so generous that thousands can be lost without much impairment of function, if the losses are scattered and not concentrated into a particular nerve center or tract.

A limited amount of nerve repair is possible. All the metabolic processes of a neuron are directed by the cell body, and as long as this vital part is intact, the neuron functions. If a nerve fiber is cut or injured, the part attached to the cell body remains alive, but the part beyond the injury gradually withers away.

Sometimes the live part can extend itself through the withered component to reach its original destination and restore function. In favorable situations severed nerves can be rejoined by a surgeon. This can only be done with nerve tracts that are accessible to the surgeon. Many unfortunately are not.

The Nerve Impulse

A nerve is not like a wire and what travels over it is not ordinary electricity. Neurons do not make direct contact with each other. There are countless "breaks" along pathways that nerve messages travel. Electricity, on the other hand, travels over a continuous wire, at a speed of 186,000 miles a second. The greatest speed at which nerve impulses travel in the human body is somewhat more than 200 miles an hour. This is quite fast, but far from instantaneous, so we cannot safely or always rely on quick reflexes to get us out of trouble, such as might arise if we "tailgate" or follow too close to a car ahead of us. If the car ahead suddenly slows, it takes about a tenth of a second for nerve impulses to warn us, and another split second to act upon the information. There is always a slight lag in what the nervous system tells us.

Nerve impulses travel in chain reactions. One neuron triggers the next, like a train of gunpowder that ignites point by point as flame reaches it. This is an electrochemical process which is now quite well understood. It depends on movements of molecules back and forth across membranes of a nerve fiber.

The inside of a resting fiber is negatively charged, the outside, positively charged. This is caused by the relative abundance of potassium ions in the interior and sodium ions in the exterior. "Firing" of a neuron changes the permeability of the membranes, with an inward flow of sodium and an outward flow of potassium. This reverses the electric charge. Almost instantly, sodium-potassium movements are reversed and so is the electric charge. These alternating movements of molecules across membranes produce currents that propagate a nerve impulse. Reversals occur as frequently as 1,000 times a second.

Thus a nerve impulse is a series of tiny electrical leaks which travel over fibers and are boosted from one point to the next by chains of electrochemical relay stations which give local reinforcement of power.

A given stimulus either causes a single neuron to discharge or "fire" or it does not. Messages fired over nerve trunks are cooperative efforts of many neurons. Possible communications between individual neurons are virtually infinite in number, since the cells are not physically attached to each other. "Loose" connections permit uncountable numbers of different switching arrangements.

The junction where fine terminal branches of an axon come close to the dendrites of another neuron is called a *synapse*. There is no direct contact. A

A *synapse* is a region where terminal branches of an axon come close to dendrites of another neuron. Since there is no direct contact, nerve impulses must jump a "spark gap." This permits a great deal of selectivity.

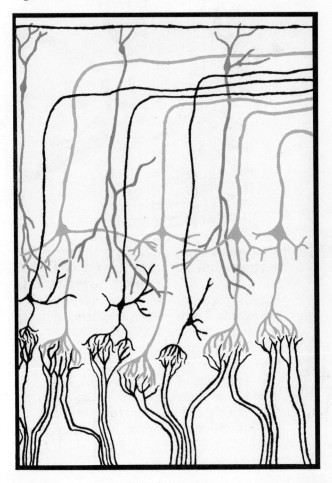

synapse is like a spark gap which a nerve impulse must jump across. The jump is facilitated by a body chemical, *acetylcholine,* which is essential for nerve impulse transmission. However, excessive accumulations of the chemical would cause a disastrous flood of impulses compelling various organs and tissues to run wild. This is indeed the effect of paralyzing "nerve gases" which cause a toxic build-up of acetylcholine. Our natural defenses include an antagonistic enzyme,

rerouting of nerve pathways should occur, we would perhaps be able to hear a flavor or smell a sunset. Something of this nature occasionally arises from growths in nervous tissues which may cause "unreal" but vividly perceived sensations, and there are hallucinations of taste, vision, and indeed all the senses which have no detectable physical basis.

The end results of torrents of nerve impulses—it has been estimated that we are bombarded by some three billion

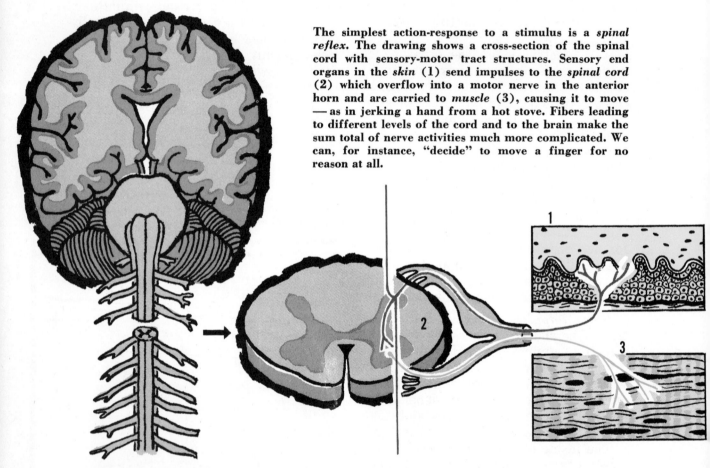

The simplest action-response to a stimulus is a *spinal reflex.* The drawing shows a cross-section of the spinal cord with sensory-motor tract structures. Sensory end organs in the *skin* (1) send impulses to the *spinal cord* (2) which overflow into a motor nerve in the anterior horn and are carried to *muscle* (3), causing it to move — as in jerking a hand from a hot stove. Fibers leading to different levels of the cord and to the brain make the sum total of nerve activities much more complicated. We can, for instance, "decide" to move a finger for no reason at all.

cholinesterase, which breaks down acetylcholine as fast as it is formed. Thus a fantastically rapid, never-ending buildup and breakdown of opposing chemicals keeps nerve impulses flowing in good order across synapses.

There is no difference whatever between nerve impulses except in frequencies per second. There is not a special kind of nerve impulse for seeing, another for hearing, another for smelling or tasting. If some incredibly mischievous

every second — depend on the pathways traversed by electrical leaks and the targets they reach.

Input and Output Pathways

Different neurons have certain differences in structure which need not concern us. A major distinction is between *sensory* and *motor* nerve tracts. Sensory nerves carry impulses *to* the central nervous system and motor nerves carry impulses *away from* it to effect action. Thus, a sensory nerve tract warns that a finger is resting on a hot stove, and motor nerves direct muscles to contract and jerk the finger from jeopardy.

Some nerve tracts are composed entirely of motor or sensory fibers, but others contain both kinds. Cell bodies of sensory nerves lie just outside the spinal cord, and those of motor nerves lie within it. From these areas, fibers run out to connect with distant body tissues, muscles, organs, glands, blood vessels, skin, eyes, ears, etc. The finely branched end of a motor neuron fiber which connects with muscle fibers is called an *end-plate*. Similar end-plates of sensory neurons connect with a variety of receptor organs, such as pain receivers in the skin or the light converters in the eye.

Communications between sensory and motor nerve tracts may reverberate through labyrinths of unfathomable intricacy to complete a stimulus-response circuit. A red light at a street corner does not excite an invariable and inbuilt mechanism of the body to step on the brakes. We have learned that a red light means "stop." A visual impression of color must be interpreted by the brain before impulses are channeled to motor nerve tracts which activate leg and foot muscles that push down on the brakes. The sequence involves thousands of neurons which steer impulses in effective directions.

The simplest stimulus-response circuit is a *spinal reflex*. This is an action which by-passes the brain. A familiar example is the knee-jerk reflex which everyone has experienced. A tap just below the kneecap of one leg hanging loosely over the other sends a stimulus over sensory nerve tracts to the spinal cord where motor nerves produce an irresistible jerk of the leg. The pupil reflex of the eye brings about an automatic constriction of the pupil to protect the retina when a light is shined on it. There are also more complicated ingrained stimulus-response reactions, as when an object flies toward the face, and the arm automatically rises to protect the eyes. Tests of various reflexes give physicians valuable information about the nature and localization of neurological disorders.

Traffic Switches

Few reflexes of the human nervous system are as simple as the reflexes of lower organisms which do a great deal of the organism's "thinking" for it. There are, for instance, important reflexes concerned with human bowel activity, but emotions, training, social taboos and conditioning can modify pure reflex actions. The nervous system is equipped with countless switches, junctions, and evaluation centers which channel ceaseless torrents of nerve impulses toward the proper decision and action with incomparable skill.

It should be obvious, therefore, that drawings of the nervous system which present a schema of the pathways of major nerve tracts are, in a sense, deceptive. It is nevertheless good to know where our sciatic nerve is located, especially if we have "sciatica," and perhaps to look up the radial or ulnar nerve or some other tract that particularly concerns us. The ulnar nerve, incidentally, can be felt where it passes over bone at the inward side of the elbow, and it is the source of tingling sensations when we bump the "funnybone." A drawing of the eye nerve and eyeball, showing the lens in the front part of the eye, makes it easier to understand why a cataract, which is a solidified form of the normally transparent lens, prevents vision from reaching the eye nerve and the brain.

However, drawings of the brain and spinal cord and their nerve connections to the body can show little more than a master plan of nervous organization. We must remember that infinite ramifications of finely branched nerve fibers permeate the entire body and modulate actions as exquisite as the expansion or constriction of tiny blood vessels, so fine that red cells must squeeze through them single file.

It would be a mistake to think of the nervous system as an entirely independent electrical switchboard. The central nervous system and the endocrine (hormone-producing) systems are intimately associated. For instance, nerves stimulate the adrenal glands to pour adrenaline into the blood and prepare the muscles for fight or flight upon order from the brain when danger threatens. But some special nerve cells also secrete neurohormones that in some respects act like adrenaline. We may think of the nervous system as a rapid-acting electrical system, and hormones as a more deliberate-acting chemical system, not independent but complementary, working in intricate co-ordination for our welfare.

The Central Nervous System

The central nervous system is headed by the brain, as is appropriate, and includes the spinal cord. The brain, the incredibly complex organ that makes man human, is so important that we shall later discuss it separately.

The spinal cord is a soft, fluted column of nerve tissue continuous with the lower part of the brain and enclosed in the bony vertebral column. Except for the 12 pairs of cranial nerves which connect directly with the brain, all the nerves of the body (spinal nerves) enter or leave the spinal cord through openings in the vertebrae. The cord is a slightly flattened cylinder, a little wider from side to side, about three-fourths of an inch thick and 17 inches long. All functions of the body depend upon the integrity of this intricate mass of cord tissue which weighs only an ounce and a half.

A cross section of the spinal cord reveals white tissue on the outside and a gray H-shaped mass in the center. The tips of the H, which is composed of nerve cell bodies, are called *horns*. Paralysis and wasting (atrophy) of muscles result if nerve cells of the horns are attacked or destroyed by disease, such as poliomyelitis. Sensory impulses of many kinds enter the outside white matter of the spinal cord, travel upward to the brain, or travel up far enough to trigger spinal reflexes at various levels. Motor impulses travel downward from the brain in the outside white matter to

reach spinal nerves which relay messages to various muscles, organs, glands and blood vessels.

Peripheral Nerves

There are 31 pairs of *spinal nerves* which emerge from the cord and are generally named for the vertebrae which they traverse. They are part of the *peripheral nervous system*, which also includes the *cranial* nerves and the *autonomic nervous system*. The division is somewhat arbitrary, since the nervous system works as an integrated unit, but there are certain specializations of duties and communications.

Each spinal nerve divides into two roots which enter the cord at different points. The "incoming" or sensory nerve fibers bulge into a *ganglion* (cluster of nerve cell bodies), enter the back of the cord and connect with gray matter of one of the horns of the H. "Outgoing" or motor fibers connect with the opposite horn at the front of the cord. The spinal nerve, before it divides into two roots, contains both sensory and motor fibers. The root arrangement permits complex relay systems to shunt impulses to the brain for analysis, or to complete a simple reflex.

Spinal nerves at different levels of the cord regulate activities of different parts of the body. If a specific part of the cord is injured, there will be characteristic abnormal reactions to neurological tests, which will indicate where the diseased part of the cord is located. If an arm is weak and atrophic, it points to disease in the cervical or neck part of the cord. If the leg is so involved, it will indicate a focus of disease in the lumbo-sacral or lower part of the cord.

The 12 pairs of *cranial nerves* arise in the lower part of the brain and their tracts branch out to innervate muscles of the face and eyeballs and to provide pathways for sensations of hearing, smell, taste, and vision. One of the cranial nerves, the *vagus* ("wanderer"), extends down the neck into the abdomen and sends ramifications to many organs in the chest and abdomen. The vagus nerve

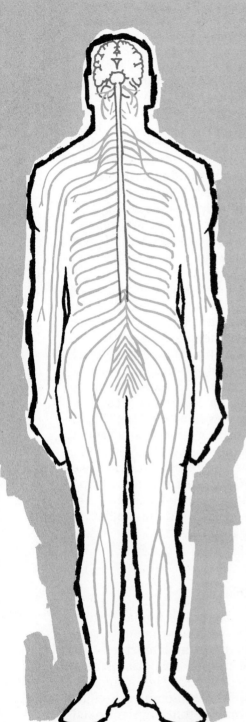

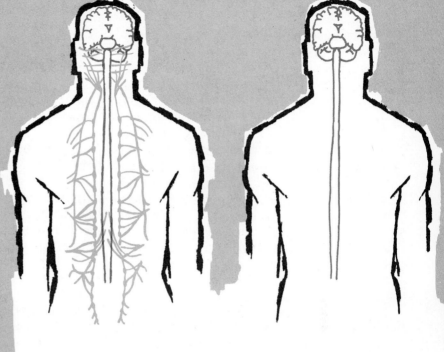

These drawings show different parts of the nervous system, on a basis of anatomy and division of labor, but it must be remembered that all parts are interdependent and that communication lines are marvelously intertwined.

The PERIPHERAL NERVOUS SYSTEM, at left, connects the central nervous system with the various tissues of the body. Pairs of *spinal nerves* at different levels of the spinal cord have "input" (sensory) and "output" (motor) connections, and messages can be relayed to and from the brain via the cord. Nerves leave the spinal cord through openings in the vertebrae and fibers fan out for relatively great distances to the tissues they serve. The peripheral system includes the *cranial* nerves that arise in the lower part of the brain, and the *autonomic* nervous system.

The AUTONOMIC NERVOUS SYSTEM (center) regulates "automatic" activities of breathing, heart action, peristaltic movement in the intestines, etc. It has two operating divisions *(sympathetic* and *parasympathetic)* which in general produce opposite and counterbalancing effects as the needs of the organism demand.

The CENTRAL NERVOUS SYSTEM (at right) includes the *brain* and *spinal cord*, a soft column of nerve tissue enclosed within the bony spine.

is concerned with regulation of breathing, rate of heartbeat, and the motility and gland secretion of the digestive tract.

Sometimes, by a surgical procedure known as *vagotomy,* certain branches of the vagus nerve may be interrupted deliberately, to diminish the flow of impulses. The objective, for instance, may be to reduce excessive acid secretion and hypermotility of the stomach in patients with peptic ulcers.

"Automatic" Regulators

We cannot be trusted to make our hearts beat by conscious effort in the same way that we flex voluntary muscles. Many functions continue while we sleep and require continuous adjustment to fedback information. These duties are delegated to the *autonomic nervous system,* which is a governor of involuntary functions that normally we give no conscious attention to.

The system is divided into the *sympathetic* and *parasympathetic* systems, which sounds quite complicated and has nothing to do with the ordinary meaning of the word "sympathy." However, the operating principle is quite simple: the two divisions have generally opposite effects and counterbalance each other.

Sympathetic nerve trunks lie on either side of the bony spinal column, connect with spinal nerves, and extend fibers to various organs of the chest and abdomen. Parasympathetic trunk lines (which include the vagus nerve) originate in the brain and the sacral part of the spinal cord. In general, both divisions reach and control the same organs — lungs, heart, liver, spleen, stomach, pancreas, adrenals, kidneys, colon, intestines, sex glands, bladder — but induce opposite effects.

For example, sympathetic impulses speed the heart and slow digestion.

Parasympathetic impulses do just the opposite. One set of impulses causes the muscle coat of blood vessels to constrict; the other, to dilate. Interplay between the two systems normally keeps body processes at a steady rate of activity, like stepping on the gas to climb a hill and applying brakes on the downhill side to maintain even speed. The parasympathetic system is chiefly concerned with digestion and repair of wear and tear to the body, whereas the sympathetic system is concerned with rapid adjustments in emergencies.

For instance, it is more important that the heart pump lots of blood into the muscles when we have to run away from danger than for the blood to go to the viscera for peaceful, normal digestion of food. Autonomic adjustments in such a situation speed the heart and suppress digestion which can later be resumed comfortably after we have escaped from a grizzly bear, or any threat requiring a flight-or-fight response. A simple example of penalties to be paid when we cross nature's purpose is the cramps suffered by an athlete who fills his stomach with food and immediately after starts running.

The Human Brain

And so we come to the human brain, and pause with awe and wonder to contemplate the marvels and mysteries of three pounds of pinkish-gray tissue contained within our heads. The brain contains upward of 12 billion nerve cells, each of which may potentially be linked to countless others. Possible "telephone connections" in switchboards of the brain are so numerous as to be incomprehensible. A credible estimate sets the figure at 10 followed by 23 zeros. The brain integrates torrents of nerve impulses into behavior. Its captaincy is indisputable, its finest workings, tantalizing enigmatic.

The brain and spinal cord are covered by membranes collectively called *meninges* (hence, "meningitis," inflammation of the membranes). The outer membrane

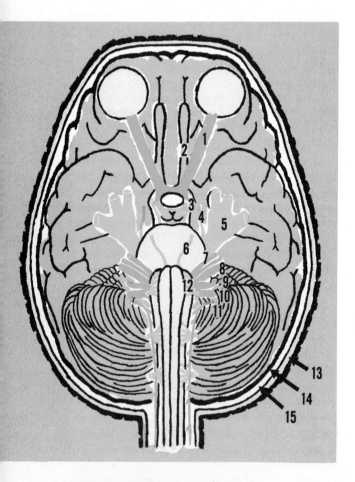

Functions of the 12 pairs of *cranial nerves*: (1) optic; (2) smell; (3), (4), (6) eye muscles; (5) trigeminal; (7) face muscles; (8) hearing; (9) tongue and throat; (10) vagus; (11) neck and back; (12) tongue. Brain coverings are *dura* (13), pia-arachnoid (14); spinal fluid, (15).

of tough connective tissue, the *dura mater,* is underlaid by a spidery web of *arachnoid* blood vessels. The inner membrane, the *pia mater,* closely follows the convolutions of the brain.

Grossly, the brain somewhat resembles a cauliflower with part of the stem attached. The most conspicuous part, the massive *cerebrum,* comprises all that lies above the level of the eyes. Its outer rind, the cerebral *cortex,* is a grayish layer of nerve cells about an eighth of an inch thick. Beneath is white tissue, at the base of which is an extra small center of gray substance called the *basal ganglion.* "Gray matter" is not necessarily superior to white, or vice versa. Gray matter is concerned with *distribution* of impulses across selected synapses; white matter, with their *conduction* along fibers.

Fissures, infoldings and convolutions of the cerebrum give it the aspect of a wrinkled walnut. These infoldings greatly increase the surface area of the cortex. Although the "wrinkles" may seem haphazard, they are quite uniform in normal brains and serve as useful landmarks in determining specific functional areas of the brain, such as speech, vision and hearing. A deep vertical fissure divides the cerebrum into two halves, a right and a left hemisphere. Other fissures divide each hemisphere into lobes.

"Phrenology charts" of sideshow barkers, which purport to show the location of "acquisitiveness," "amativeness," and other traits in relation to regions of the skull, have doubtless given some people quite fantastic and distorted notions of what goes on in their heads. Phrenology has no relation to actual localization of brain functions. Scientific "maps" of the brain are as yet quite incomplete, and there are many mysterious overlappings, but some specific functions are known to be centered in general areas.

The "seeing center" is located in the back part of the brain called the *occipital* lobe. Areas for hearing and smell are located in the *temporal* lobe at the side of the head. The sensory and motor centers are separated by a transverse fissure about in the middle of the top of the head. Other centers have become recognized through symptoms of disorders which affect them, and this special knowledge is helpful in diagnosing obscure neurological complaints and affords landmarks to the neurosurgeon in locating and removing brain tumors, an abscess, a bullet, or a clot in the brain.

Several "sub-brains" lie under the cerebrum and within its lower portions and are integrally connected with the cortex. These complex parts are "old" brains of animals that evolved long before man's cortex flowered so magnificently, and are principally concerned with life-sustaining functions rather than higher intellectual processes of reading and writing and intricate adjustments to environment for offense and defense. The brain has a large number of "parts," to which physiologists have given a bewildering variety of names.

Thalamus, hypothalamus and basal ganglia. These areas are concerned with regulation of sleep, heartbeat, appetite, metabolism, sexual drive, and other nonintellectual functions. The *brain stem* — the stalk of a cauliflower model — contains some important centers and continues downward as a continuation of the spinal cord. The *medulla oblongata* is a relay and reflex center and connects with higher brain centers via the *pons* (bridge). Deep in the brain stem, a pencil-sized mass of tissue called the reticular formation is thought to censor millions of clashing incoming impulses and to monitor information that excites and awakens the brain in some essential role to the conscious state. The *cerebellum,* an orange-size mass of ribbed tissue, lies at the back of the head behind the brain stem. It is concerned with body equilibrium, muscular co-ordination and the automatic execution of fine movements, such as catching a baseball without tipping over.

Pictures of the brain, and sections of the brain itself, are dismally static and cannot begin to express the wonder of the invisible switching, shuttling and electrifying nerve-impulse traffic that races about in us at all times.

Clues to Disorder

From knowledge of nerve structures and functions, physicians are often able to judge quite accurately the location where trouble lies.

Nerves from one side of the body eventually connect with the opposite side of the brain. Thus, a person whose right arm is paralyzed after a stroke is known to have suffered damage to the left side of the brain.

An abnormal reflex points to trouble along pathways of nerves that activate the reflex. Spastic (stiff) paralysis and flaccid paralysis result from damage at different points of nerve pathways. Inability to speak, or to recognize written words although spoken words are understood, and other strange disturbances, may indicate damage in brain areas concerned with specific functions.

All spaces around the central nervous system, including the four ventricles (cavities) of the brain, are filled with *cerebrospinal fluid*. This is very similar to other tissue fluids, but some diseases may cause certain chemical changes in its composition. In the lower back there is room for a hypodermic needle to be inserted between vertebrae to withdraw a sample of fluid. Chemical examination of the fluid is often helpful in diagnosing obscure diseases.

NEUROLOGIC TESTS

Other than special tests such as *electromyography* for muscle nerve disease, *electroencephalography* for epilepsy and other disturbances of the brain, *x-rays of the skull* for injury or brain tumor, and *spinal fluid studies* for possible brain hemorrhage or infection, there are few *laboratory-type* studies required for the diagnosis and treatment of neurologic diseases.

Standard tests performed by a neurologist in the office, clinic, or hospital include the following:

He will test the patient's steadiness in *body balance* by having him stand with his eyes shut and feet close together (Romber test). He will test the *gait* to note if the body and limbs move freely, if there is a limp in one leg, scuffing with the foot, an absent swing in one arm, a list of the body to one side, a droop of the head, involuntary hastening in gait, a falling forward or backward in walking, a twist in the spine.

He will note if there is a spontaneous *tremor* as in Parkinson's disease, or will ask the patient to bring his finger to his nose to exclude "effort tremor" or ataxia such as is found in multiple sclerosis, familial tremor and senile tremor. Handwriting samples are also taken to determine the nature and severity of the tremor.

Reflexes. He will test the state of the *muscle tendon reflexes* by tapping the muscle cord or tendon at the knee with a rubber hammer to bring forth the well known knee jerk or knee reflex. He will do the same at the elbow, wrist, and ankle.

An absent reflex in one arm or leg may suggest polio to the examiner. Absent reflexes on both sides may likewise indicate polio, or a past or present meningitis, or nerves damaged by diabetes or deficient in vitamins. Overactive reflexes on one side of the body may signify hemiplegia or paralysis; on both sides, it may signify a highly sensitive nervous system or an emotionally high-strung individual.

There are also skin reflexes to test, the most important of which is the *plantar scratch test* produced by stroking the bottom of the foot with a stick or finger. If the large toe rises while the other toes move downward, the response is a "positive Babinski sign" and signifies a past or current hemiplegia (one-sided paralysis).

Sensory tests. Loss or presence of sensations of touch, pain, heat, and cold in the skin of the face, body, and limbs is tested by means of a piece of cotton, a pin, and tubes of hot and cold water. A tuning fork applied to bones determines if there is a loss of *vibratory sense* and also determines if there is a loss of hearing when applied to the ears.

A look deep into the eyeball (fundus examination) with an ophthalmoscope can help to establish if there is an increase of pressure in the brain from a brain tumor, if there have been past or recent hemorrhages, if there is hardening of the brain arteries, or if glaucoma or a cataract is present. A light shined on the pupil by a lamp or flashlight gives information about the size, shape, and reflex activity of the pupil. An irregular pupil that is smaller than the pupil on the other side and is unresponsive to a flash of light suggests possible syphilis of the brain and the need for special blood and spinal fluid studies to exclude it. Examination of the pupils gives still other information.

The mouth and throat are examined to see if the muscles move equally on the two sides, and the tongue, to determine if it moves forward or to one side of the midline; these tests afford clues to weakness or paralysis of the tested muscles. Tests of heart action and measurements of blood pressure and weight loss or gain are made to record abnormalities that may bear on the patient's illness, or for future comparison.

PARKINSON'S DISEASE

Parkinson's disease is becoming one of the most common illnesses to afflict mankind. The last survey taken by the author, at the American Medical Association meeting in New York in June, 1961, showed a prevalence in this country alone of 1,200,000 Parkinson cases. Their numbers are increasing, first, because people live longer and Parkinson's disease is an illness of the middle and late years of life; second, because there is no cure for the disease; and third, because Parkinson patients live on for many, many years, so that their numbers accumulate.

Definition. Parkinson's disease is a slowly progressive disease of the *basal ganglia,* which is a small center or nucleus at the base of the brain. The disease does not affect the brain proper—that is the massive cortex and its nerve bundles —hence *there is no loss of speech, intelligence is unaffected, and there is never*

paralysis. Although the disease is progressive, in many Parkinson patients there are stationary periods of five to ten or more years when there is little if any worsening of symptoms.

Signs and Symptoms. The chief symptoms of this illness are shaking *(tremor),* stiffness *(rigidity),* and slow-

Nuclei of the *basal ganglia* at the base of the brain are shown in color below for orientation. Parkinson's disease is a progressive disease of small centers in this area. Since the brain proper is not affected, there is no impairment of intelligence, loss of speech, or paralysis.

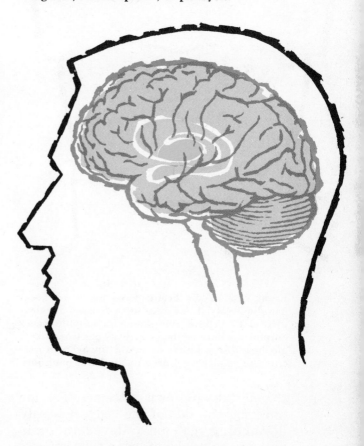

ness of movement *(akinesia).* A mild form of tremor, though at times embarrassing and annoying, does no harm except as it may interfere with employment in such vocations as a barber, tailor or waiter. Tremor of severe form affecting both sides of the body can impair health by interfering with eating and by producing a pronounced loss of weight, marked sweating, and insomnia. However, there are medications which, if tolerated by the patient, can control even

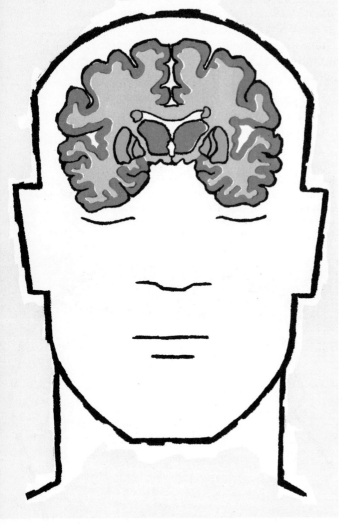

Front view of the brain shows nuclei of basal ganglia involved in Parkinson's disease. Surgical efforts to relieve symptoms in suitable cases employ various methods such as electrocautery, alcohol, a tiny knife, or liquid nitrogen to destroy the small target area in the basal ganglion.

the most severe form of tremor. Tremor affecting one side of the body, if highly disturbing, can be relieved in some patients by means of brain surgery.

Rigidity is the major problem in this disease. While tremor usually affects one or both arms and but rarely the head or legs, rigidity can involve the face muscles, the neck, shoulder, body, arms and the legs. If rigidity remains limited to one side of the body, it is not too severe a problem, except that free swing in the arm is absent, the arm tends to be held close to the body, and there is some scuffing and dragging of the foot. But speech

remains unimpaired, the mind is sharp, and the patient can work and take care of his family.

However, when rigidity spreads across the face, neck, and body and into the arm and leg of the other side, many problems can arise, especially under conditions of neglect. Rigid or frozen face muscles produce a fixed or masklike appearance of the face and eyes. Because the lips do not move too freely, the speech tends to become nasal, monotone, and indistinct in quality, even though actual verbalization is never lost. The neck muscles in front are stronger than the back muscles so that as they tighten, they tend to draw the head downward and cause the upper back to become rounded and hunched (*kyphos*).

With the head drawn downward and forward, the body tends to pitch forward into a propulsive form of walking. Under the added impact of gravity, this often leads to running or hurried short steps (*festination*), in the effort to prevent falling and sometimes they do fall unless they can stop against a wall or door. The frozen shoulders make it difficult to dress and put on a coat. The stiff and frozen fingers impair the skillful acts of everyday living such as cutting food, buttoning clothes, writing, typing and knitting. Stiffness of the back muscles makes it difficult for the body to shift its position in bed, or to get in and out of bed, chair or car.

Through neglect of treatment and insufficient use of rigid muscles, some of the muscle tissue wastes away through disuse and is replaced by connective scar tissue, which shrinks and shortens the muscle (*contracture*). Shortened and contractured calf muscles tend to pull the heels off the ground, forcing the patient to walk on his toes and pitching the body still further forward into propulsion and the greater hazard of falling. An occasional patient, to keep from falling forward, will arch the spine backward into a retropulsive posture as he walks and he is likely to fall backward if he gets off balance.

After falling once or more, and with body coordination slow and uncertain, such patients become very tense when faced with other hazards of falling, as when turning, entering an elevator, or crossing a threshold, so that the legs freeze or "glue" to the ground, which of itself leads to more falling. In time they become partially or fully dependent on others for safe navigation.

The droop of the head interferes with reflex swallowing of saliva, which accumulates in front of the mouth and with the pull of gravity leads to constant dribbling or drooling of saliva. It also leads to difficulties in swallowing food and liquids, so that weight is lost even under good nursing care.

Deformities develop in the hand, where the flexor muscles are stronger than those on the back of the hand (extensors), and as the flexor muscles stiffen and shorten, they tend to close the hand and twist the fingers out of shape. Similarly, the flexor or front muscles of the body, being stronger than the extensor or back muscles, tend to pull the body downward, which, added to the factor of gravity, can drop the body in extreme cases to almost a right angle to the legs.

The flexor muscles of the toes, being stronger than the extensor muscles on the back of the toes, often undergo contracture, draw the toes downward and produce painful cramps. In long-standing cases with advanced rigidity in body and limbs, contractures, poor balance, frequent falling and risk that the patient may severely injure himself, the family may for safety reasons confine the patient to a chair or bed. In this case, through lack of exercise, further wasting sets into the muscles, with progressive contractures and permanent invalidism.

The third common symptom of Parkinson's disease, the *slowness of movement* (akinesia), is not nearly as severe an impediment to the patient as tremor and rigidity, although in pronounced form it may hamper him in everyday activities such as dressing, getting in and out of a chair, getting out of bed and shaving, and it may lessen the capacity of the patient for rapid body adjustment to protect against falling.

Other symptoms sometimes mentioned are of little or no consequence. Autonomic symptoms are mentioned by some authorities, but actually the Parkinson patient suffers no greater autonomic disturbances than any other person. If he trembles a great deal, he will feel warm and will perspire. If he is sluggish, akinetic and motionless, his pulse will be slow and the blood pressure low. If the circulation to his feet and hands is poor, he will feel cold and chilly, just as any other person under similar circumstances who does not have the disease.

Types of Parkinson's disease. Three types of Parkinson's disease are often described in medical literature: the *post-encephalitic, idiopathic,* and the *arteriosclerotic* type. Actually there is only one type of true Parkinson's disease; that is the *idiopathic type.* "Idiopathic" means we do not know the cause.

The *arteriosclerotic type* has exactly the same type of symptoms and is part and parcel of the idiopathic type, except that the so-called arteriosclerotic form usually occurs in older people, so that their symptoms are more massive and usually set in with stiffness and heaviness of both legs, whereas in the younger idiopathic type, it usually sets in on one side of the body and commences with just a slight tremor in the hand which gradually progresses to involve the arm and the leg on that side with tremor and rigidity.

The *post-encephalitic form* is not true Parkinson's disease, since it is not a degenerative disease, but is caused by an infection that involves not only the basal ganglia but the entire nervous system. It was caused by a special virus during worldwide influenza epidemics of 1917 to 1927. This unusual variety of virus produced an encephalitis, which in addition to Parkinson symptoms left other symptoms such as drowsiness throughout the day, double vision, oculogyria (sudden attacks of the eyes drawn upward), and mental changes, such as are never seen in true Parkinson's disease. We have had no new cases of the sleepy lethargic form of encephalitis with Parkinson symptoms since the epidemics of 1927, and most of the cases from the original epidemics have since disappeared.

We have had many small epidemics of encephalitis due to other kinds of virus since 1927, but none of these produced Parkinson symptoms. Thus, the so-called lethargic encephalitis type of Parkinson's disease is of little current concern. Today the great challenge is the steadily growing number of cases of idiopathic Parkinson's disease, which can affect anyone from 30 to 80 years of age.

Diagnosis. Unlike diseases which are hidden from the surface and require intensive laboratory studies and investigations to reach a diagnosis, the symptoms of Parkinson's disease are on the surface and readily recognized even by a lay person. The *slow shuffling gait, the absent swing in one arm, the tremor in the fingers* and *the rigid bent posture* of the body are highly characteristic. In the very earliest stage there may be some difficulty in diagnosis, but once the symptoms are manifest there is no such problem.

Parkinson's disease must not be confused with *pre-senile, senile,* or *familial tremor,* which present symptoms of an entirely opposite nature, with no rigidity, no slowness of motion, and the tremor, instead of being spontaneous when the patient is at rest, appears *only* under the effort of doing something, as in lifting a spoon to the mouth. Multiple sclerosis is likewise characterized by an "effort tremor", but in addition presents many symptoms which are entirely different from Parkinson's disease.

Causes. Although the cause of idiopathic Parkinson's disease is presently unknown, research is shedding some light on its mechanisms. It has been found that certain drugs or chemicals, if administered to normal people, will within two weeks produce in them all the symptoms of Parkinson's disease. The fact that chemical substances can produce Parkinson symptoms in normal people indicates that the immediate cause of true Parkinson's disease must be toxic chemical substances, as yet unidentified, that accumulate in the basal ganglia, slowly damage or destroy cells in this brain area, and gradually produce tremor, rigidity, and slowness of movement.

It is also possible that poor blood circulation to the basal ganglia may be a contributing cause, since this could be responsible for a steady accumulation of toxic substances. However, it is clear that arteriosclerosis or hardening of the brain arteries *per se* is not directly responsible, since millions of people have advanced cerebral arteriosclerosis but never suffer from Parkinson's disease.

Perhaps a faulty liver may be responsible for the accumulation of toxic substances, or there may be a genetic predisposition to the disease. Much research will be needed to solve the problem. Even so, the fact that Parkinson symptoms can be produced with chemical substances unfolds the hope that through research or serendipity, some brilliant chemist may discover a chemical substance that will act as an antidote to prevent or arrest the progress of symptoms.

Favorable and Unfavorable Factors. The *unfavorable factors* are fully known to the patient and in most instances are exaggerated, hence they need not be expanded upon here. Some patients even dread to hear the word "Parkinson" and some families fear to inform the patient that he is suffering from Parkinson's disease, by masking the illness under the cloak of "bursitis", or "stiffness of muscles". This merely deprives the patient of knowing the true nature of his illness and keeps him from applying himself to intensive treatment at the earliest moment.

Still other patients mistakenly regard Parkinson's disease as an inevitably crippling disease, but this is not true. The only symptom that can cause deformities in the late progression of the disease is rigidity, for which we have good treatment, if applied early and intensively through the years. The greatest hazard to the patient is not the rigidity but the contractures which come from disuse and inadequate exercise of the affected muscles, so that in time they become replaced by connective scar tissue, shorten, and twist the body out of shape.

Favorable aspects of Parkinson's disease are often unknown to the patients and their families :

Parkinson's disease is not contagious and is not known to be inherited.

It does not shorten life; most Parkinson patients live for many, many years and some outlive their families and their doctors.

There is no pain unless treatment is neglected and contractures develop, or the disease is complicated by arthritis, sciatica, bursitis, or a muscle sprain.

There is no numbness and no paralysis.

There is never any loss of speech, even though speech may become muffled due to faulty use of lip muscles.

Since the brain proper is not affected by Parkinson's disease, there is no impairment of intellect, although some impairment of memory may occur in the elderly due to arteriosclerosis.

There is no blindness or deafness in this disease.

It does not produce headaches, convulsions, or vomiting.

For reasons unknown, Parkinson's disease tends to protect the patient against ailments such as cancer, tuberculosis, multiple sclerosis, etc. This must not be interpreted to mean that a Parkinson patient cannot possibly develop cancer, but clinical experience over 35 years proves that Parkinson patients rarely develop cancer although they are in the age range of 40 to 80 years when cancer is frequent.

Course and outcome. Families often inquire, "How long will my father live with his condition?" This is a difficult question to answer since it varies from patient to patient. Those who are fortunate enough to receive loving care can live on to 75, 80 or 85 years of age, when major arteries close and the patients go into a coma from which they do not arouse. Some patients, even after total disability and bed confinement, can under conditions of good nursing care live another five or more years.

Colds seem to have little effect on them and cancer stays away from their door, for reasons yet unclear. Should they develop infection, antibiotics spare them for a long time. The slowness of movement tends to preserve the heart and blood pressure and insulates the body against wear and tear, unless a patient happens to be agitated and depressed, or is severely tremulous. The usual duration of the illness is ten to 20 or more years, depending upon the age of onset and severity of the symptoms.

Treatment. Since we as yet have no means of cure or prevention of the disease, treatment must rest upon control of the symptoms and supportive psychotherapy. The latter does not imply that the Parkinson patient is mentally abnormal or that he requires special psychiatric treatment. Psychotherapy here is used in a broad sense to include proper orientation of the patient as to the nature of his illness and sympathetic encouragement and guidance on matters of exercise, hours of work, retirement, types of recreation, trips, vacations, personal, economic and family problems. The psychotherapy required by 98 per cent of Parkinson patients can be adequately provided by the family physician, who is most familiar with the patient's family life, his background and his problems.

The patient should be fully oriented with regard to his illness and its needs, so that he may not have to rely on stray bits of information derived from the neighbors, newspapers or magazines. To achieve the best results the patient should visit his doctor once a month because changes in medication have to be made from time to time as the remedies lose some of their original efficacy. Also, there are side-reactions that require attention of the doctor and some reactions, especially in the elderly, can prove more disturbing than the disease symptoms.

Some patients undergo a constant shift from doctor to doctor and medication to medication in a desperate drive to find a "cure". This is foolhardy. Most doctors are fully informed about the latest methods of treatment for the illness. It will serve the patient's best interest to select a doctor he can trust and cooperate with him to the fullest.

The treatment of the symptoms of Parkinson's disease consists of three phases, *medication, physiotherapy* and *exercise* by the patient. The surgical approach to symptom control is advisable only in cases where the above measures have been fully tried and failed.

Medication: The description of medication here provided aims to afford a better understanding of the drugs, their actions, and limitations, in order that the patient may more intelligently cooperate with his physician.

There are countless drugs to choose from and no single drug works effectively in all patients. Even aspirin is helpful to many people and yet others are made worse by it. Medication has to be tailored to the individual patient. Only the doctor knows which drug or combination of drugs is likely to prove best for each patient, and can make the required changes and adjustments as they become necessary from time to time.

Several drugs may be used as a single remedy for the treatment of all the symptoms found in some patients. Other drugs are useful chiefly for the specific action against a particular symptom and are added as they are needed. Some patients have to use as many as four or five drugs at one time.

The eight drugs most commonly employed against the Parkinson symptoms have been proved through the years to be entirely safe, if used within the therapeutic doses prescribed by the doctor. There may be an occasional complaint of dryness of the mouth, or blurring of vision, or nausea, drowsiness, or dizziness, but these do not constitute dangerous reactions and they usually subside when the amount of drug is reduced or another drug is substituted. The patient must not become alarmed by occurrence of minor side reactions.

Artane is the drug most widely used for this illness and it serves to control mild forms of tremor, stiffness and sluggishness. It also tends to provide extra

NERVE CHART →

1. facial
2. great auricular
3. spinal cord
4. dorsal scapular
5. suprascapular
6. axillary
7. subscapular
8. medial antibrachial cutaneous
9. ulnar
10. median
11. radial
12. lateral cutaneous femoral
13. sciatic plexus
14. femoral
15. sciatic
16. superficial peroneal
17. deep peroneal
18. cerebrum
19. cerebellum
20. great occipital
21. vagus
22. supraclavicular
23. phrenic
24. anterior thoracic
25. musculocutaneous
26. long thoracic
27. sixth intercostal
28. ilio-inguinal
29. genitofemoral
30. obturator
31. lumbosacral
32. lumbo-inguinal
33. external spermatic
34. common peroneal
35. tibial

energy to the patient, longer endurance at work, and mild stimulation. If used in very large doses, Artane may overstimulate and excite the brain, so that the patient may become somewhat delirious, confused and over-talkative, and may imagine he sees bugs crawling on the walls and on himself. These hallucinations disappear as soon as the drug is discontinued for 24 hours.

Pagitane is a drug with action fairly similar to Artane, as is Kemadrin. Akineton is still another drug that is fairly similar in action to Artane.

Cogentin is a drug with a potent specific action against *rigidity*, contractures and muscle cramps and spasm. It may be

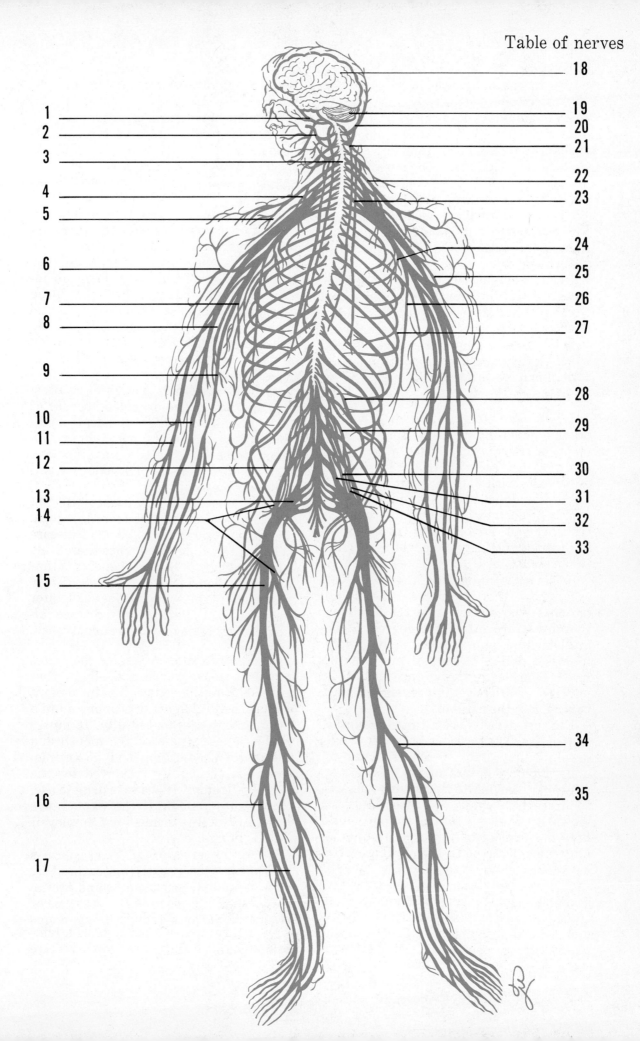

1

2

3

4

5

6

7

8

9

10

11

12

13

14

15

16

17

18

19

20

21

22

23

24

25

26

27

28

29

30

31

32

33

34

35

added to one of the above drugs, when the latter fail to adequately control these severe symptoms. It is rarely used alone. Patients with glaucoma and bladder disturbances should be particularly careful to avoid large doses of Cogentin.

Parsidol is a drug that is specifically useful against *tremor*. Patients who can tolerate it obtain good results. If not for the reactions of drowsiness and dizziness, huge doses would check the most violent tremor.

Phenoxene exerts a specific action as a stimulant. It is a gentle drug and never causes any disturbing cardiac side-effects. It tends to lose its original efficacy in the course of months, and Disipal, which has a fairly similar stimulating action, may be substituted.

Levodopa (L-dopa) is a drug which became generally available for management of Parkinson's disease in 1970, after extensive clinical trials. The brains of patients with Parkinsonism tend to be somewhat deficient in dopamine, a natural body chemical concerned with nerve transmission. Levodopa is transformed in the body into dopamine which reaches the brain.

Experience in many thousands of cases shows that symptoms in nearly all patients who are suitable for levodopa therapy improve to some degree. Some are benefited quite spectacularly, others to lesser but still worthwhile extent. Even when objective improvement is minimal, subjective improvement may be a boon to the patient.

Earliest benefits seem to be loosening of rigidity. The face is more expressive, drooling may stop, speech is easier to understand. As treatment progresses, movement begins to speed up; the patient seems to shake less often and less violently. Ability to control simple voluntary movements of muscles, limbs and fingers improves so that such simple acts as walking, rising from a chair, tying a shoelace, swallowing, are more readily accomplished. Muscular rigidity and tremor decrease. It is not possible to predict which patients will benefit most greatly or scarcely at all. Occasionally,

levodopa gives a sort of euphoria so the patient feels fine although objective improvement may not be measurable.

There is another side to levodopa. It does not cure; if discontinued, symptoms return. Large doses are necessary; side effects, usually several, are to be expected in all patients. When dosage is first begun, nausea, vomiting, and loss of appetite are common but tend to disappear when the maximum tolerated dose is attained. A few of the very numerous potential side effects are: abnormal involuntary movements; drop in blood pressure; dizziness; sedation; mental changes; abdominal distress; palpitations. Side effects may require reduction of dosage, with some loss of effectiveness. Some patients cannot tolerate levodopa at dosages high enough to be effective, and others are excluded because of heart disease or other physical conditions. Close medical supervision is obviously essential. Several months may elapse before benefits of levodopa treatment become apparent.

About one-third of patients will not experience much benefit from levodopa. It is imperative that Parkinson's disease be accurately diagnosed since there is no evidence that levodopa benefits other forms of neurological disease. Early treatment with levodopa does not alter the course of Parkinson's disease although symptoms may be well controlled.

Other medications. Besides the drugs described above there are others that prove helpful. Hyoscine is a natural plant product, helpful against tremor and to a lesser extent against rigidity. It causes considerable dryness of the mouth and blurring of vision. Benadryl, an antihistamine, is frequently employed for the control of tremor. It is a safe drug to use, except that patients who experience marked drowsiness must not employ it while driving a car.

Since the tremor of Parkinson's disease becomes greatly aggravated by embarrassment, nervousness and excitement, especially when in the presence of strangers, various tranquilizing drugs prove helpful to some patients as a temporary alleviant. They are more effective when not used too often and preferably in small doses, since they can cause mental fogginess and drowsiness. Alcohol if used in small amount helps to alleviate excitement and tremor in some patients, hence should not be prohibited where it proves useful.

For patients that suffer from insomnia, there is a wide assortment of remedies. The doctor will usually find the remedy that will best serve the patient.

Managing Side Reactions

Swelling of the ankles is a frequent occurrence among the very rigid and frozen Parkinson patients, especially those who spend many hours of the day sitting, which leads water to gravitate down to the ankles. A number of very effective drugs are available for swelling or edema of the legs and ankles.

For patients who suffer from marked slowness of movement, sluggishness, fatigue, depression, inactivity and drowsiness by day, and who fail to respond to previously mentioned drugs, there is a wide assortment of stimulants available. Various amphetamine stimulants prove helpful to some patients, and yet in other patients they tend to produce cardiac excitation, palpitations, and shortness of breath and have to be discontinued or used in very small amount. Thyroid in small dosage two or three times a day provides the extra energy that some patients require, although in some it tends to aggravate tremor and leads to over-excitement.

Vitamins are needed for patients who are undernourished or have difficulty in swallowing, hence live on erratic diets. Sometimes injections of B-12 prove helpful, also liver injections. However, people should not be gullible about reports of "miracle injections" or "miracle cures." Some patients, desperate for something new and different, turn to exotic drugs and treatments, not realizing that the most effective medications are well known to doctors.

The most common **side reactions** from the use of drugs for Parkinson's disease are *dryness of the mouth and throat,* *blurring of vision, nausea and indigestion,* and *constipation.* Mild forms of dryness of the mouth can be counteracted by sips of water, or the use of hard candies or chewing gum. However, instances of dryness that are severe enough to interfere with swallowing of food and with speech should be called to the attention of the doctor for changes in medication. Blurred vision is corrected by changes in the lens of the glasses to render reading easier, since Parkinson remedies blur *only close vision.*

Indigestion and nausea caused by pills can often be prevented by swallowing them with milk or buttermilk instead of water. Patients who gag and have difficulty in swallowing large pills and capsules will find it easier to do so if the capsule is pressed into the bottom of a teaspoon of applesauce or Jello. Vomiting is never caused by the standard drugs for Parkinson's disease and should it occur, all drugs are to be stopped and the doctor called. Parkinson remedies do not cause bladder retention, but they may slow the urinary stream among the male patients who have enlarged and obstructing prostate glands. Constipation can be aggravated by the above remedies, but rarely constitutes a serious problem.

Physiotherapy. For patients with rigidity, contractures, and frozen muscles and joints, and patients who have difficulty in performing their every day activities of life, *physiotherapy* is just as important and sometimes even more important than medication. Patients who suffer with tremor only or who have very minimal states of rigidity do not require physiotherapy, but it does no harm and often makes them more comfortable.

Physiotherapy should consist of *massage* to soften the muscles, and *stretching* to loosen the muscles and joints, so that the patient will gain greater freedom for exercise, work and his daily activities. Massage should be of the deep and vigorous type. Some physiotherapists fear to apply vigorous treatment because the Parkinson patients may look weak and frail, but actually most of the patients, though sluggish and frozen, are well preserved in body and can tolerate and need vigorous loosening of the muscles and joints, except in instances of cardiac disease.

Baking lamps, vibrators and whirlpool baths are of comparatively little advantage, but may be employed by the patient and family at their own leisure. The therapy visit should last an hour, since the hurried treatment of 15 minutes affords little benefit to the muscles. Most patients require physiotherapy treatment once or twice a week. In addition to massage and manipulation the physiotherapist can drill the patient in proper walking, in maintaining an erect posture, in getting in and out of the chair and bed with safety and in dressing.

The therapist is also equipped to advise the patient on matters of procurement and the use of various gadgets for preventive and corrective exercises. The patient must understand that he will need physiotherapy as long as he has rigid muscles, unless a cure is found. Some patients, who are not properly prepared by the doctor, expect miraculous results from one or two treatments and failing this, they stop all physiotherapy, which is a great loss to them and the doctor in terms of the later outcome.

Exercise. Every form of activity helps to maintain the health of *rigid muscles*, whether it be a walk in the park, a game of golf, a work-out in the gymnasium, or just playing checkers or cards. Patients should continue to work as long as possible and should not retire except under conditions beyond their control or on direction of the doctor.

Besides the exercises to be described, others can be improvised by the patient or family for the correction of specific difficulties in movement and performance. A wide variety of appliances are available that help to improve the range and effectiveness of exercise, among them dumb-bells, wall-pulleys, over-head pulleys, neck traction devices, vibrators, a stationary bicycle, electric power exercycle, a rowing machine, whirlpool bath and punching bag.

A *broom handle* can prove very effective for the exercise of bringing the arms across the head and back for five minutes two or three times a day, in order to loosen the shoulders and neck and correct a drooping head.

For *frozen fingers*, a rubber ball, sponge ball or tennis ball can be squeezed repeatedly, while watching television or reading a newspaper.

When there is difficulty in *finger coordination*, as in buttoning clothes or removing objects from the pocket, a simple exercise is to dump a jarful of large and small buttons, pennies and coins on the table and to replace the coins and buttons into the container.

Patients whose legs become frozen or "glued" to the ground, so that they fear to move and often fall, should practice walking a short distance and turning *with feet wide apart*, walking a short distance back and repeating the process 15 minutes several times a day, until the problem is corrected.

For the frozen mask-like expression of the face, the muscles of the forehead, cheeks and lips should be rubbed and loosened each day when washing, and the eyes should be shut tight a few minutes several times a day to strengthen and mobilize the lids. Frequent *smiling* greatly helps the expression and everyone else.

For tight and bent knees, the legs should be suspended on a chair or hassock half an hour each night.

Patients who tend to walk on the toes and scuff should practice goose-stepping and lifting the toes with each step they make.

When there is difficulty in putting on a coat, the patient should practice doing so 20 times a day, and will find the twenty-first time poses no problem. Every act that is difficult to perform should be repeated as a practice and exercise many times a day.

If getting out of a chair is a difficult problem, the patient should practice rising with *lightning speed* to overcome the pull of gravity and early drills should be rising from a hard chair, since soft chairs constitute a still greater challenge. In sitting down the patient must not fall into the chair. He should take ample time, since he is moving in line with gravity, should grip the arms of the chair and bend the body *sharply forward* as he lowers himself to the seat of the chair and then sits back. Problems of inability to turn in bed and inability to get in and out of bed can be counteracted by drills on a *floor mat* with the patient pulling on a knotted rope attached to a radiator, first by turning the body to the right and later shifting the body and turning to the left.

Difficulties in *speech* are most always due to freezing of the lips and can be corrected by talking into a mirror with forceful use of the lips in order to create clear sounds, or by reading aloud to the family from a newspaper 15 minutes each day.

Writing difficulties can be corrected by setting aside an hour each week, half of which is spent making circles to the right and left, zig-zag lines, large and small letters, figures and words, and the other half hour writing large and small words and figures on a scratch pad.

Exercises and corrective drills should be performed as faithfully as possible and with regularity, but not as an obsession or with compulsion. Parkinson's disease is not like a ruptured appendix, where a matter of minutes can be of serious consequence. Rather the aim should be to play with the muscles and keep them moving as comfortably and as often as possible.

Surgical Treatment. Brain surgery is employed to alleviate certain symptoms of Parkinson's disease. It finds its best use for the control of tremor, (a) if the tremor exists on one side only and (b) if the patient is young and a suitable subject for surgery. In some instances it may loosen a rigid arm on the side opposite to the operation, but not the leg. Surgery is not suited to patients with sluggishness, bilateral rigidity or stiffness of both sides of the body, bilateral tremor, advanced cerebral arteriosclerosis with memory impairment, confusion and mental changes, or to patients past 60 or 65 years of age. Some patients who have been operated on one side of the

brain may, after a lapse of a year or more, be operated upon the other side, but surgeons dislike operating on the two sides of the brain because speech may be impaired, mental sharpness may be lost, and there may be other complications.

Neurosurgery for Parkinson's disease is still experimental and exploratory. No single type of operation is universally employed by brain surgeons in this country. Some use electrocautery to destroy the target area in the basal ganglion; others use radioactive isotopes; others use a tiny knife; others use alcohol for the purpose; and still others the liquid nitrogen freezing method. Added to these are surgeons who are not happy with any of the above procedures and are exploring the ultrasonic method of destroying the target area, others the atomic "beam", etc. The operative procedure does not explain why some patients with tremor and rigidity are helped, why some are not helped, and why the rigidity and tremor eventually return to some who have been helped.

Brain surgery as a means of therapy should *only* be considered after all conservative efforts with medication, physiotherapy and exercise have been tried. Where tremor is the dominant symptom, among patients who are greatly disturbed by it and are hypersensitive to all forms of medication, brain surgery should be given serious consideration, since if the target area is successfully destroyed, there is a *dramatic* disappearance of the tremor.

The drawbacks to surgery are that the tremor may return to the same side that has been remedied, within a variable period of time; that tremor may suddenly appear and become very severe on the good side of the body; that the disease is *progressive by nature,* hence cutting out a tiny piece of the brain cannot serve as a total "cure" for Parkinson's disease.

Future outlook. The outlook for the Parkinson sufferer has materially improved over what it was ten years ago.

The nature of the disease is better understood and better medical remedies have been developed. Brain surgery, although still exploratory in nature, has been improved in safety to the patient and greater effectiveness against tremor in suitable cases. Much research is in progress and there are four Parkinson foundations dedicated to its support. The recent discovery that chemical substances can produce symptoms of Parkinson's disease in normal people opens the prospect that an "antidote" chemical capable of averting the onset of symptoms or arresting the progress of the disease may be found.

BRAIN INJURIES

Injuries to the head and brain constitute a seriously increasing problem.

Mild brain injuries that merely stun or daze or cause momentary unconsciousness (concussion) as a rule leave no permanent or lasting damage to the brain, although some patients may experience dizziness, nervousness, restlessness and headache as an aftermath for weeks or months. An x-ray of the skull is generally made to exclude fracture.

Unconsciousness that lasts several minutes or more following a head injury requires the close care of a neurologist. Some brain injuries, with or without fracture of the skull, can cause lasting damage to the brain tissue and leave residuals of severe headache, dizziness, and even paralysis or convulsions. *Very severe brain injuries* with hemorrhage and swelling of the brain substance (compression) can lead to death. The vast majority of head injuries, however, unless complicated by compensation situations, or by contusion or compression of the brain, leave no permanent ill effects, especially those occurring among youngsters at play.

Brain Tumor

Because the brain closely fills the tight compartment of the rigid skull, any added substance inside the skull cavity, be it a hemorrhage, an infection of the brain (encephalitis), or the covers of the brain (meningitis), or increase in blood circulation, or swelling of the brain (edema) due to an allergy or brain injury, or a new growth in the brain (brain tumor), will cause severe and constant headache until the *increase in intracranial (intra-skull) pressure* is relieved by spinal puncture (which removes fluid from the brain), by brain surgery, by drugs, or by the natural course of events.

Because of the *important centers located in the brain* and because of the fixed space inside the skull, any tumor or growth in the brain, whether benign or malignant, has to be considered malignant, since prolonged continuation of the increased intracranial pressure can produce blindness, or paralysis of one side of the body, convulsions, severe headache and vomiting.

It is therefore important that any sudden and persistent headache should obtain the early study and attention of a neurologist. Of course, some common sense has to be employed in such decisions, since every headache does not warrant an urgent rush to a neurologist, any more than every pimple or spot on the skin means cancer and a rush for a biopsy. When in doubt, however, it is wisest to consult a responsible authority on the subject.

There are many types of *brain tumor.* Some are easy to reach, especially if they are located near the skull, and may be removed completely. Others are deep seated in the brain and invade large areas of its substance, so that complete removal could only be accomplished at the risk of causing further damaging symptoms, paralysis, or even death. In such situations, a small portion of the brain tumor is removed to allow for the release of the increased intracranial pressure and the temporary easing of the symptoms, with the full understanding that the unremoved parts will continue to grow and lead to paralysis, numbness, blindness, vomiting, wasting of the body and ultimate death. Deep x-ray treatment into the brain can sometimes retard the speed of growth of special types of tumor.

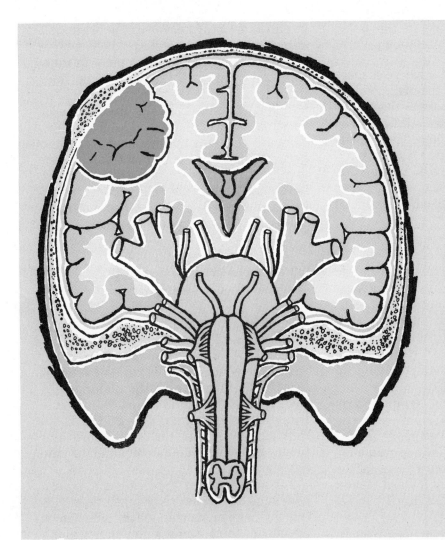

The brain is encased in a rigid skull and has virtually no room to expand. Hence any tumor, whether malignant or not, or any swelling or hemorrhage that exerts pressure on delicate brain tissues, is serious, and can produce blindness, convulsions, paralysis, headache and vomiting, and other symptoms if not relieved. The drawing shows a meningioma that has arisen from the dural layer and is infiltrating the cortex. Tumors located near the skull may be removed completely but deep-seated tumors that invade large areas of brain substance cannot be completely removed, although symptoms may be temporarily and partially improved by relieving intracranial pressure.

Certain tumors such as a *glioma* grow very slowly and, if situated in a so-called "silent area" of the brain, may not disable the patient severely for many years. When I was 15 years of age, an older brother of a friend had a glioma removed from the cerebellum part of the brain and continued to conduct his small business. When I was 25 years of age, he had a second operation for the removal of a remnant of the same tumor, which in the course of years had grown to large size. When I was 35, he had the third operation for the same regrown tumor, following which he became totally disabled. Research is continuing in many medical centers of the country for better methods of destroying brain tumors without injury to the patient.

DEMYELINATING DISEASES

These include a group of diseases of unknown cause that lead to a degeneration or disappearance of the *myelin* (insulation) around nerves, with an effect similar to stripping away the rubber insulation from an electric wire.

Demyelinated nerve fibers lose the power to conduct messages or impulses from the brain to the muscles, as well as messages of touch, pain, vision and hearing to the brain. In consequence, there may be paralysis or numbness in an arm or leg, or unsteady (ataxic) gait, blindness, loss of bladder and bowel control. Although some authorities speculate that an hereditary predisposition is responsible for the demyelination of the nerves, and others attribute the illness to some abnormal chemistry in the body, the actual cause remains unknown.

Multiple sclerosis is a strange disease that attacks any part of the brain, spinal cord and nerves with spots of degeneration, and is characterized clinically by paralysis, numbness, blindness, deafness, unsteady gait (ataxia), impairment of speech and mental changes. It usually begins during the early years of life, most often between 20 and 30 years of age.

The first sign of illness may be the sudden paralysis of a leg, or half of the body, or the sudden loss of vision in one eye. This could persist and slowly progress to add other symptoms, but usually the first symptoms disappear within weeks or months, to be replaced in the course of a year or years with a succession of the same or other symptoms, in various parts of the body.

The disappearance of symptoms is referred to as a "remission" and the re-appearance as a "relapse." These remissions and relapses may spread over a period of five, ten or more years, after which there is a tendency toward steady progression of the disease, until partial or total invalidism ensues.

There is no specific treatment as yet, nor any means of prevention of the disease. However, considerable research is under way in hope of reaching better understanding of the cause and the means to combat the illness. There is a Multiple Sclerosis Foundation that may be contacted for information as to the latest developments and prospects. Any person who develops sudden paralysis, numbness, blindness, or deafness, must obtain immediate study by a neurologist.

Amyotrophic lateral sclerosis. Because this medical term is so difficult to remember, it has come to be known in popular language as "Lou Gehrig's Disease", after the famous ballplayer who became afflicted with it. This illness differs sharply from multiple sclerosis, in that the patches of degeneration are not as diffusely spread out through the *entire* nervous system, but tend to localize on bundles of motor nerves in the brain and spinal cord, causing a slowly progressive paralysis and wasting (atrophy) of muscles on both sides of the body, sometimes more on one side than on the other. The hands often manifest the first signs of wasting and weakness, and later the legs. There is never numbness or blindness here. No specific treatment is, as yet, available for this disease, just as there is none for multiple sclerosis, although injections of B-12 and other vitamins (B-6) prove of some ameliorating value.

INFECTIONS OF THE NERVOUS SYSTEM

Infection may involve the brain, or the spinal cord, or the nerves and roots that emanate from the brain and spinal cord. Infection of the brain is called *encephalitis*, while infection of the meninges or covers of the brain is called *meningitis*. Infection or inflammation of the roots that emanate from the spinal cord and brain is called *radiculitis*, and of the nerves, *neuritis*.

Inflammation of the brain may cause headache, fever, nausea, vomiting, clouding of consciousness with sometimes coma or total unconsciousness, along with paralysis and numbness in parts of the body, blindness, or deafness, depending upon the brain areas involved.

Great influenza epidemics of 1917 to 1927 caused millions of cases of encephalitis due to a virus with a special characteristic of causing drowsiness and sleepiness, and Parkinson symptoms sooner or later. Hence the term "lethargic" was applied to this type of encephalitis. Most of the Parkinson cases produced by the lethargic encephalitis have since disappeared.

An occasional by-product of the lethargic encephalitis was a symptom called *narcolepsy*. This was characterized by a sudden attack of irresistible sleep during the day and many times a day, accompanied sometimes by sudden weakness and collapse to the floor, under stress of a surprising emotional stimulus such as fear or explosive laughter. In some attacks, the head would suddenly droop to the table during a business session or while attending classes. Narcolepsy is rarely seen these days. Amphetamine drugs are almost specific remedies for the problem.

Meningitis produces headache, vomiting, nausea, stiffness of the back, loss of reflexes, along with fever and other signs easily recognized by the neurologist. The newer antibiotics have proved of great help in combating the various germ infections that cause meningitis.

Neuritis

Neuritis takes in a wide group of disturbances affecting the peripheral nerves and roots after they leave the brain or spinal cord. Some are due to infection, others to compression of the nerves as they pass through narrow canals in the vertebrae and skull, and the cause of still other disturbances is unknown.

Shingles (herpes zoster) is due to an infection of a ganglion, or group of nerve cells perched on the root, by a virus. It

The layered membranes covering the brain and spinal cord are collectively known as the *meninges*. The drawing shows the *dura mater* (1), the outermost fibrous membrane; the middle *arachnoid* membrane (2), a very fine and delicate structure; and the *pia mater* (3), a membrane with a rich network of blood vessels. The arachnoid and pia are sometimes considered to be a single structure, the *pia-arachnoid*.

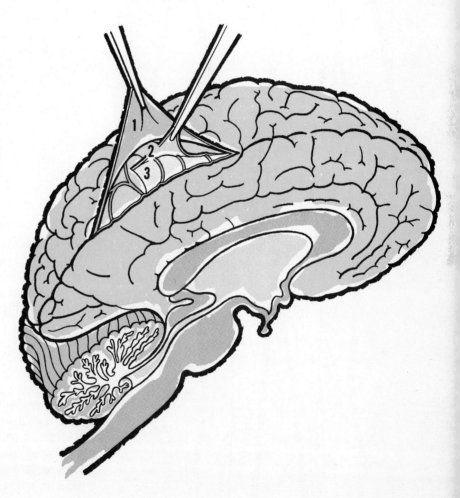

Among infections of the spinal cord, probably the very worst and most crippling form was that caused by the virus of poliomyelitis. This is rapidly and successfully being eliminated as a menace to the human race, through the development of oral and injectable vaccines within the past few years.

leads to excruciating itching and burning pain in a rash of blebs situated in a fixed zone of the body, usually the chest or upper face, on one side. There are measures of relief available, but no cure as yet. It tends to subside and disappear with the passage of weeks, but the itching in the area may remain for months.

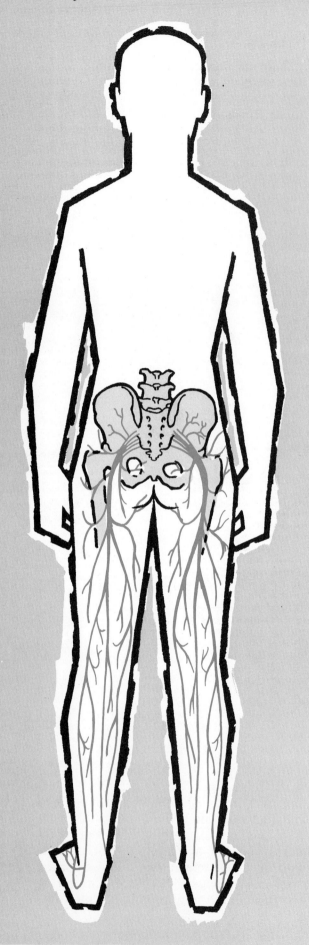

The *sciatic* (meaning "hip joint") nerve is the longest nerve pathway of the body. The drawing shows its distribution in the thighs and legs. A "nerve" dissected by an anatomist is actually a cable-like bundle of hundreds or thousands of individual fibers, each connected to its nerve cell body which may be a long distance away.

Sciatica, or sciatic neuritis may be due to infection of the nerve as it passes through the huge muscles of the buttock in its long course down to the foot, or it may be compressed by arthritic spurs at its exit from the vertebrae. There is severe pain down the leg, areas of numbness, loss of reflexes and sometimes weakness in the foot. Medication, baking, and stretching of the nerve help. Sometimes there is a recurrence of sciatica a year or years later.

Writer's cramp is not a true palsy, but occurs among people who have to write continuously under great pressure. What happens is that the muscles of the hand tire, tighten up, and fail to move temporarily. The situation is a physiologic rather than a true organic disorder and it clears completely under rest, a trip, or a change of work and pressure.

Polyneuritis is a disturbance that affects the peripheral nerves on both sides of the body at one time, sometimes of both arms and legs, along with some of the cranial nerves affecting the face, jaws, tongue and eyes. Motor as well as sensory nerves are involved, so that there is weakness, loss of muscle tissue (atrophy), numbness and loss of reflexes. It may be caused by infection, or by toxic substances as in uncontrolled diabetes, or by avitaminosis (lack of vitamins). It tends to subside with treatment, but may leave permanent minor residuals. Polyneuritis is, however, of rare occurrence, when compared to sciatica. "Lead polyneuritis" of painters is hardly ever seen these days.

Pressure Neuropathies (crossed leg palsies) are of comparatively rare occurrence. "Neuro" refers to nerve and "pathy" to pathology or organic abnormality, as distinguished from a physiological abnormality, such as writer's cramp, or a psychological abnormality, such as insomnia. The pressure neuropathy in crossed-leg palsy is entirely different from the direct compression of a nerve as it passes through the narrow canal of the spinal vetebrae, as in sciatica. In crossed-leg palsy the nerve is not compressed, but rather, poorly functioning or arteriosclerotic arteries fail to supply sufficient blood to the nerve, as a consequence of which there is tingling, numbness, and temporary loss of power in that leg. The condition often clears up under benefit of vasodilator drugs which bring more blood to the area, iodine compounds, massage, and the avoidance of crossing one leg *tightly* over the other. The problem is comparatively rare and occurs chiefly among elderly people with impoverished circulation or poor arteries.

Bell's palsy is a neuritis of the facial nerve. It is caused by infection and compression of the swollen nerve as it passes through a tiny opening in the skull below the ear, in its course to the muscles of the face. It is often caused by a draft of cold air during sleep that strikes the exposed side of the face near the ear. It also quite frequently occurs among chauffeurs who drive with an open window and are exposed to raw elements. The palsy is usually preceded the day before by a vague pain below the ear. The following day the patient cannot close the eye on that side, and in the space of hours there is complete paralysis of that side of the face, with a droop of the corner of the mouth, the mouth pulled over to the other side, and inability to raise the forehead.

In most cases the condition clears up within a month or several months and more rapidly with electric treatment and massage. The sudden appearance of paralysis of the face may prove alarming and embarrassing to the patient, but actually it tends to clear up without serious complication. However, during the time when the lid cannot be closed, a patch must be worn to prevent dust or rough particles from injuring the delicate cornea of the eye. In patients with severe injury to the facial nerve, there may be a residual slight weakness in the closing of the affected eye and a slight droop of the corner of the mouth for many years.

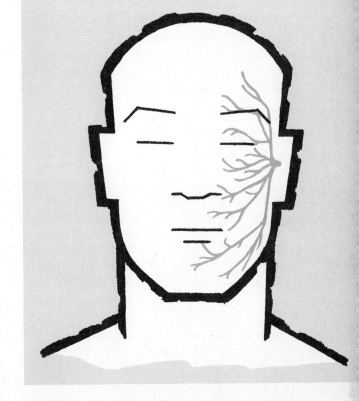

Distribution of the facial nerve which emerges from a tiny opening in the skull. The area controlled by the nerve is graphically evident in a person with Bell's palsy who is temporarily paralyzed in one side of the face and cannot control the muscles of the mouth, eye, and forehead regions on that side.

Neuralgias

Neuralgia is a painful condition in a nerve due to some unknown irritation or inflammation. Some authorities believe that *sciatica* (already described) is a neuralgia, while others regard it as a neuritis because there is weakness and a loss of reflexes in some patients.

Trigeminal neuralgia or ***"Tic douloureux"*** is the most common form of neuralgia and is characterized by repeated attacks of excruciating pain in one side of the face, usually involving the lips and nose most severely, sometimes also the gums and tongue.

The attack is often brought on by the mere touch of a trigger zone or area in the upper or lower lip, or the gum or nose, on the affected side. Speech is rendered difficult, because as the lip moves the trigger zone can set off the reflex neuralgic attack. Eating is also interfered with, because any contact of food with the sensitive zone of the lip or tongue may start the "tic douloureux" attack, leading the face to be sharply drawn up in reaction to the severe pain. Similarly, washing the face becomes a problem since touching the nose may start the attack.

The cause is not definitely known, but it is believed that operations and procedures about the teeth and gums may have something to do with setting up the trigger area through scarring that later leads to reflex irritation of some branch of the trigeminal nerve with the resultant tic douloureux attacks. A siege of attacks may last weeks or months, with each attack lasting seconds to a half minute and recurring countless times in a day. Another siege may recur a year or years later.

There is no specific remedy for the problem. Some patients use aspirin tablets but these fail to relieve the excruciating pain and spasm. Injections into the trigeminal nerve have been tried but have produced only temporary relief and sometimes worse complications. Various brain operations have evolved, but none of these have yet proved very satisfactory.

Headache

Next to pain, *headache* is probably the most common symptom to affect mankind. There is hardly a grown person who at one time or another has not experienced mild or severe headaches, for which most people take aspirin or a similar compound because it is often effective and does not require a doctor's prescription.

People of especially tense and nervous temperament may experience frequent or daily bouts of severe headache that is usually localized in the front or top part of the head. Those with rheumatism of the vertebrae and muscles of the neck will complain of headache in the back part of the head. This is actually not a true headache and may often be relieved by massage of the neck muscles and an ordinary aspirin tablet.

Nervous people are continually harrassed by real and anticipated problems and fears of dire things to come, so that through over-excitability the brain becomes overworked and filled with an excess of blood, which leads to headache. Such high-strung individuals may experience headaches for many years and be none the worse for it, and at times they obtain temporary relief from one or another medication. Some severe attacks may not respond to any medication. *Any severe and persistent headache should obtain careful study,* since headaches may also be caused by allergy, sinuses, colds, eyestrain, head injury, meningitis, a brain abscess, or brain tumor. Severe headache can produce

Repeated attacks of excruciating facial pain are characteristic of trigeminal neuralgia. The *trigeminal* ("three parts") nerve, one of the 12 pairs of cranial nerves, innervates the facial areas shown below.

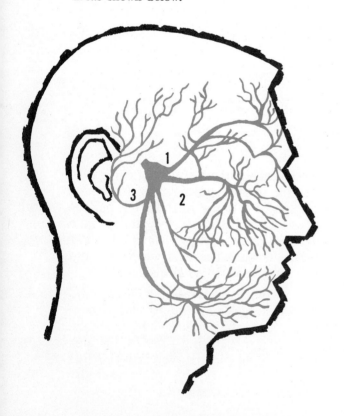

nausea and vomiting and impair the efficiency of work and daily activities.

Migraine is a special variety of intense headache that sets in with suddenness on one side of the head, lasts a day or two and disappears just as suddenly as it came, only to recur every few weeks or months with strange regularity. In women, it seems to come with the menstrual periods and disappears entirely when they reach the menopause. The sudden migraine attack may be accompanied by vomiting and temporary disturbances of vision. Many remedies are employed for migraine, including steroid compounds and ergot and caffeine preparations which may ameliorate some of the attacks when taken as a doctor directs, but they do not have any curative effect on the underlying condition.

Dizziness and Vertigo

Dizziness is almost as common a complaint, especially among older people, as headache. Dizziness is the lay equivalent of the medical term, *vertigo*. Dizziness is often loosely applied to include giddiness. *Giddiness* refers to a mild form of dizziness frequently seen among elderly people in which there is a *momentary* sensation of clouding of the mind and reeling or unsteadiness when they suddenly change position, as from a reclining to a sitting or standing position, or when they suddenly bend to pick up an object. It is believed to be due to hardening of the brain arteries, in which a sharp change in posture leads to a momentary flooding of the brain with blood, or the emptying of blood from the brain. Giddiness may prove frightening to some patients, but does not lead to any serious consequences and most patients learn to avoid making sudden postural changes.

Dizziness refers to a slightly more disturbing situation than giddiness that may last a few minutes to a half hour, during which there is some unsteadiness in walking and a slight reeling sensation, perhaps nausea, but rarely vomiting. It is usually due to a temporary impoverishment of brain circulation, caused by hardening of the brain arteries, by poor heart function, or by a drug that suddenly lowers the blood pressure. The patient will generally seek a sitting position for a few minutes until the unpleasant sensation passes.

Meniere's disease or syndrome is characterized by attacks that commence suddenly with violent dizziness, ringing in the ear, vomiting, a reeling sensation and unsteadiness of body equilibrium so severe that if the person does not lie down, he would fall to the floor. During the course of a severe attack, the patient is confined to bed and cannot move his head from one side to the other without experiencing disturbing sensations that the floor, bed, and chairs are turning around him. Such a bout may last several weeks before there is complete recovery.

Milder attacks may last a half hour to several hours. The attacks may recur at irregular intervals of weeks, months, or even a year or several years, but usually tend to disappear with the passing of time. Meniere's disease is due to a pressure change or circulatory disturbance in one of the tiny semi-circular canals of the ear, that have to do with body balance and equilibrium in space. It may be caused by an infection, an allergic condition, spasm of an artery, or a tiny hemorrhage in the ear canal.

SPASMS, CRAMPS AND TICS

Cramps are often noted among elderly people who suffer with poor circulation in the legs and are aroused from sleep, particularly during winter months, with painful cramps in one or both legs. The reclining position and cold weather tend to lessen the blood supply to the legs, so that by rising out of bed, moving about and rubbing the legs, the circulation is restored and the pain is relieved. Vasodilator drugs taken at bedtime afford relief to some patients and others obtain better sleep in special adjustable couches that permit the legs to be at a lower level than the rest of the body. *Spasm* is the technical name for "cramps".

Spasms can occur not only in peripheral muscles, such as the legs, but in many parts of the body and do not necessarily have to be caused by circulatory disturbances, but may be due to a variety of causes. Thus, we have spasm of the colon or spastic colitis in compulsive and highly tense people, spasm of the gall bladder due to gallstones, spasm of a tiny blood vessel in the semicircular canal of the ear that produces Meniere's disease, spasm of the ureter due to a stone from the kidney lodging there, and spasm of the throat that occurs among hysterical and highly nervous people ("globus hystericus"), which creates sudden choking sensations and difficulties in swallowing food.

There is also a fair consensus that spasm of the muscle wall of small arteries of the brain can lead to the so-called *minor strokes,* with dizziness, faintness, momentary unconsciousness and numbness, weakness or paralysis of one side of the body which lasts for a short period. The symptoms of these minor attacks disappear fairly quickly or gradually in the course of several hours, or a day or several days, but similar or sometimes worse spasms may recur in weeks, months, or even years later. (For discussion of *strokes,* see Chapter 3).

Torticollis or "Wry Neck" is a condition in which the muscles of one side of the neck are in a state of more or less continuous spasm and draw the head to the opposite side of the body. The patient will wrangle with the problem and repeatedly bring the face forward to the mid-line, but the spasm regularly recurs and pulls the head to the opposite side, to the great annoyance and discomfort of the patient.

The cause is not clearly understood, but it is believed to be due to a reflex spasm of the muscles, brought about by irritation or compression of the neck nerve roots, as they make their exit from the spinal cord through the narrow canals of the vertebrae. Injury to the neck may be a contributing factor in some of the patients, arthritis in others, nervous spasms possibly in others. The condition may disappear spontaneously with the passage of time, but in some patients it may remain for a lifetime. There is no specific medicinal remedy. Surgical procedures may be resorted to.

Tics. There is a wide variety of "tics" — nervous movements, such as the repeated shrugging of a shoulder, or the repeated pulling up of one corner of the mouth, engaged in, consciously or unconsciously, to achieve release of some inner emotional tension. These tics occur chiefly among young people, especially adolescents, but in some individuals they may continue through life. These belong in the realm of the psychiatrist, rather than the neurologist, except "tic douloureux" previously described. Tics can be annoying and exasperating but they seldom bode any physical injury.

Cerebral Palsy

"Cerebral" means brain-centered, and "palsy," paralysis. This is a condition present in children after birth, and affects brain centers having to do with muscular control. There is a considerable range in severity and nature of symptoms. Some afflicted persons walk with scissoring, floundering movements, awkward armflinging and head tossing and speak with difficult guttural sounds if at all. Some who are mildly afflicted do not appear to be conspicuously strange.

The cause or causes of cerebral palsy are not too clearly established. Some cases are due to brain injury during difficult childbirth, but many babies born with difficulty do not have cerebral palsy. Some cases are thought to be due to infections suffered by the mother or to toxic substances in her blood that reach and damage the brain of the fetus during its early developmental stages. Rh-factor incompatibilities are sometimes implicated.

The afflicted person may show chiefly one or a combination of symptoms such as *chorea* (involuntary jerking movements of different muscle groups), *athetosis* (a slow, writhing type of constant movement, chiefly in the fingers), poor sense of balance, tremor, and spastic muscles. Frequently, though by no means always, there is mild to severe impairment of intelligence; sometimes a normal intellect may be hidden behind difficulties of communication.

There is no positive prevention of cerebral palsy, other than careful prenatal and obstetrical care which may correct recognized abnormalities. Physical and speech therapy may overcome

Hydrocephalus (sometimes called "water on the brain") is a condition of increased volume of cerebrospinal fluid within the skull. *Ventricles* are cavities in the brain filled with watery cerebrospinal fluid that normally flows out of small openings, flows over the brain and spinal cord, and is absorbed into the bloodstream. If escape of fluid from the ventricles is blocked or if fluid cannot be absorbed, the ventricles become greatly distended and the head enlarges, as shown below in comparison of a normal child (left) with a hydrocephalic child (right).

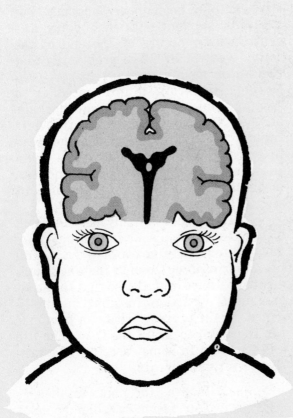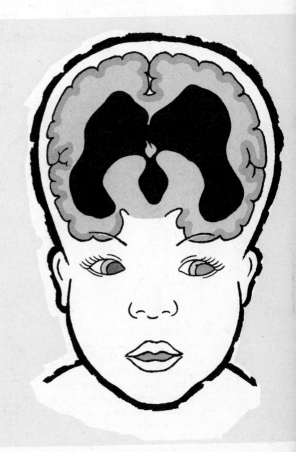

handicaps to some degree, and braces and other supportive measures may be helpful in individual cases.

Muscular Dystrophy

Although regularly described in textbooks on neurological disorders, *muscular dystrophy* is not a disease of the nervous system, but an intrinsic disease of the muscles due to an unknown cause. The fact that it affects several

members in a family would make it seem that some abnormal chemistry is inherited, which progressively destroys the muscle tissue so that in the course of several years there is barely anything left but skin and bones in the limbs, with weakness, total helplessness, and eventual wasting of the entire body.

While in many families the illness makes its appearance when the children are young, there are different forms of the disease that occur sporadically in

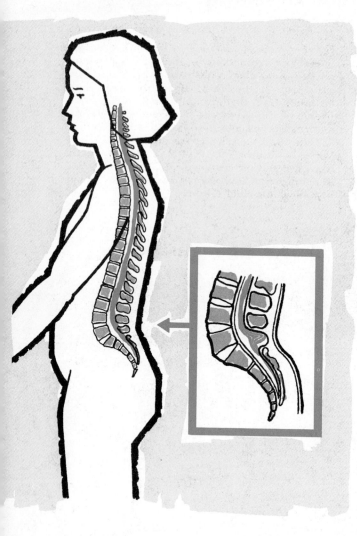

Spina bifida is a congenital malformation of the spine in which some of the vertebrae fail to fuse. The figure at the left shows a child with normal spine; in insert, spina bifida defect of the lumbar spine. In some cases, a sac containing fluid and parts of the spinal cord protrudes between the split vertebrae and appears under the skin, but more commonly there is no sac on the surface of the spine.

only one member of a family during adolescence or adulthood, which may remain in an arrested stage for many years or for life. There is as yet no specific treatment for this illness, but there is a Foundation that may be contacted for information on the latest developments.

CONGENITAL MALFORMATIONS

There is a wide variety of malformations of the brain, but the most common of these, *hydrocephalus* and *spina bifida*, are of most concern because many of the former and most of the latter survive to a full life, whereas bizarre malformations or "monsters" with half the brain missing do not survive birth, and the extremely rare instance of "Siamese twins" is an odd curiosity.

Hydrocephalus is a term that expresses the true state of the problem, "hydro" meaning water and "cephalus," brain, that is "a brain filled with water." It is usually due to some malformation or infection of the brain while the fetus is still in its intrauterine existence. At birth the head may not appear abnormal, but it rapidly expands with each month and death usually occurs by the end of the second year of life. The problem is that the water usually present in the cavities of the brain is prevented from escaping, due to an abnormal blockage of the exit avenues, so that the fluid rapidly accumulates, expands the head to extreme size and destroys the brain substance, causing paralysis, blindness, feeble-mindedness, lack or absence of speech, and often convulsions.

Sometimes there is only partial block of fluid escape and such individuals may survive for many years or even to full life, and in an occasional instance sufficient substance remains, so that the adult is almost normal or normal in intelligence. Brain surgery creates a new exit for the trapped brain fluid, so that life and function in some cases may be preserved for many years.

Spina Bifida, as the name implies, is a spinal malformation in which some of the vertebrae fail to fuse, so that a sac containing the covers of the spinal cord, the fluid, and even the spinal cord itself may protrude between the split vertebrae and appear under the skin. When present it indicates that the malformation occurred before the fetus, in its intra-uterine existence, was three months old, since after that the vertebrae normally close and seal in the spinal cord and its covers. The abnormality usually appears in the lumbar or low part of the back.

The sac-protruding type fortunately occurs rarely. The more common type is called "occulta", because there is no sac on the surface of the spine, but there is a slight separation in the lumbar vertebrae that shows up on x-ray examination. In such malformations there may be a tuft of hair on the surface, and because of some underlying defect in the spinal cord there may be slight ataxia or unsteadiness in gait, some abnormalities in the reflexes of the legs and sometimes bladder and bowel incontinence. The sac type requires surgery, but for the occulta type no specific treatment is available nor usually indicated.

EPILEPSY

by MADISON H. THOMAS, M.D.

Epilepsy has been known from antiquity, but our understanding of it has developed only in the past century. When it appears, the family may not only be perplexed by the illness but confused by contradictory information about it. An understanding of what it is, what its problems are, and what can and should be done about it will provide the best basis for intelligent cooperation in an appropriate program of medical care. Answers to some of the more common questions about epilepsy are presented here, but only the person's own physician can solve individual problems.

What is epilepsy?

Epilepsy is a tendency to have seizures, or more technically, it is a tendency to recurrent episodes of alteration of consciousness or control, associated with indications of abnormal overactivity of at least some part of the brain at the time of an attack.

How is the brain involved?

The brain is a complex organ, more complicated than the largest electronic computer. It is delicately balanced to control or modify everything a person does. Even the simplest sensations are registered in the brain and this information is used as the basis for actions ranging from the simplest of responses to highly complex activities such as using a typewriter or playing an instrument. The whole brain appears to be used for abstract thinking and planning, but various parts of the brain specialize for particular activities such as speaking or moving a particular part. Normally, these parts all work in smooth harmony together, but if even a small group of cells become abnormally active, this may result in a seizure. If the overactivity remains in one area, the result is a *localized* or special kind of seizure. If it spreads throughout the brain, a more *generalized* seizure may result. After the attack is over, the brain cells return to their normal state. Thus, except for the brief time of a seizure, the person with epilepsy is usually able to function as normally as anyone else.

What are some of the names for seizures?

These include convulsions, "spells," blackouts, "fits," paroxysmal cerebral dysrhythmia, falling-out spells, fainting spells. Not everything called by one of these names is an epileptic seizure. For example, a person may lose consciousness, or faint, from inadequate blood flowing to the head as a result of a temporary heart irregularity or from lowering of blood pressure because of an emotional shock. Consciousness returns when blood flow is restored.

There are several characteristic kinds of epileptic seizures, depending partly upon the group of brain cells that become overactive and partly upon the person's age and other factors.

What is the most common type of epileptic seizure?

Convulsions or *grand mal seizures* are the most common form and may occur at any age. In these, the attack may begin with a warning feeling or *aura*, after which a brief, unnatural cry may be heard. The person loses consciousness and his body stiffens and jerks, and his color becomes dusky because the muscles used in breathing are involved in the muscular spasms. This change in color is not serious, because breathing is restored when the muscles relax again within a very few minutes.

Is such a convulsion harmful?

No, not ordinarily, unless the person injures himself in falling, though he may injure his tongue or lips. If the bladder is full when the attack begins, the convulsive seizure may cause it to empty; or he may rarely soil himself, which may add greatly to the embarrassment of an epileptic attack.

What should be done by a person who witnesses the beginning of an attack?

Really, very little need be done, as the attack will come to an end by itself. The person having an attack should be eased to the ground and protected from injuring himself, but it is no longer thought necessary to attempt to insert anything between the jaws. Turning the person on his side toward the end of the seizure will help get rid of any saliva and eliminate risk of choking if there should be vomiting after the attack. A report of careful observation of the attack may greatly help the physician in understanding the problem.

Many persons can resume their regular activities almost immediately after a seizure, but others will need a short period of rest and reassurance. Since the person has no memory for what goes on during the seizure, he will be helped if the person who is with him avoids excitement and explains to him that nothing very serious has happened.

What should be done if the person seems to go into another attack before he is fully recovered from the previous one?

A series of attacks such as this is called *"epileptic status"* and is a medical emergency. The person's physician should be notified *immediately* and his instructions followed explicitly. Most commonly, it is wise for the person to be treated for status at the doctor's office or hospital, as injections of medication are usually needed.

Are all epileptic seizures as dramatic as grand mal attacks?

No. Epilepsy is a medical term covering a wide variety of episodic disturbances and most of them are less noticeable than the convulsive form.

What are some of these forms of epilepsy?

Petit mal epilepsy, or "little sickness", is seen most in children and usually disappears after adolescence. Petit mal seizures consist of brief, sudden losses of consciousness, lasting only a few seconds. In these spells, the child simply seems to daydream or stare briefly, and there is usually no falling and only a slight movement of mouth, face or arms.

Psychomotor seizures may be highly variable, but there is always loss of memory for the attack. There is a clouding of consciousness accompanied by automatic performance of movements that often seem quite purposeful and have a varying degree of complexity. There may be restless, repetitive movements, automatic movements such as walking, chewing, or moving about the room, etc., so that at first glance it is possible to confuse these episodes with emotionally disturbed behavior.

Focal or localized seizures are so called because the disturbance underlying the attack seems to remain limited to one area of the brain, and hence the manifestations are limited to an area of the body, such as in the jerking of an arm or of a leg.

Peculiar feelings in one of the extremities may also represent a focal seizure. Any of these manifestations, as well as some of those applying to the special senses such as vision, hearing, taste, or smell may be followed by spreading to other areas of the brain and hence more widespread seizure manifestations.

If such a peculiar disturbed feeling or warning comes before a more general attack, it is called an aura, and often permits the person to take some kind of action to protect himself, such as lying down on a bed before the seizure starts.

There are other less common kinds of seizures which include muscle jerking, alteration of function of some of the internal organs, or peculiar feelings, and some of these require very special study to determine their exact nature.

What causes seizures?

There are two categories of causes of seizures: First, the response of the brain cells to specific and discoverable injury or disturbance by an outside factor; second, the intrinsic susceptibility of the person to seizures.

What outside causes can produce seizures?

Many things can happen to the brain to make it susceptible to seizures. A direct injury to the brain, as by the force of impact in an automobile accident or injury at birth, may cause some of the brain cells to become intermittently overactive and set off a chain of events that produces a seizure. An infection of the brain, such as encephalitis, may cause irritation at the time of the infection and convulsions may occur during the acute illness, or long after the acute infection has passed.

Anything that seriously interferes with the blood flow to an area of the brain may also cause a seizure, and this is the reason that epileptic attacks are sometimes a complication in persons who have had strokes. In a few cases, the effect of a brain tumor may similarly produce interference with brain cell function.

Use of alcohol, especially in excess, may provoke seizures. Inborn defects of brain structure or brain metabolism may also produce abnormality, one of whose symptoms may be seizures. Changes in the metabolism of the body, such as disturbance of blood sugar supply to the brain, may produce seizures, as may interference with the circulatory system.

It is because of this variety of possible causes that the physician may require use of extensive diagnostic studies. Since some of these causes can be corrected by direct action, their elimination naturally represents the best means of treatment. A specific correctible cause may not be found and reliance must then be put on preventing seizures by the use of medications and other measures.

What if no definite cause for the seizures is found?

In this circumstance, two conclusions are possible. First, the specific cause may have been relatively minor or obscure. For example, the occurrence of a specific injury to the head may not be known in the history of the individual, or the neurologic changes may be too obscure to appear as part of the findings in the examination. Secondly, there may be a varying susceptibility to seizures in different individuals, especially in the case of petit mal spells in childhood.

Can a person with epilepsy marry?

An increased susceptibility may occur in some families, although this familial tendency is not great enough in most cases to cause any real concern about a person with epilepsy having children. However, if two persons having epilepsy marry, the chance of their children having seizures is naturally greater than if only one of the parents has them. In general, it is believed that there is no valid reason for persons with epilepsy not to marry and have children, but the individual circumstances should be thoroughly reviewed by the person's own physician or sources of special help that may be suggested by him.

How is a diagnosis of epilepsy made?

In the case of typical grand mal convulsions, the diagnosis may be readily apparent to the most casual observer, but the observation of this symptom would still have uncertainty as to the cause of the attack. With the other types of seizures, a diagnosis may be made only after a very careful evaluation as it is possible for other conditions to resemble seizures enough to produce some degree of uncertainty. The family physician may use a variety of special helps or consultation with other physicians to assist him in the diagnosis. The basic study rests on a careful evaluation of the history in a particular case, supplemented by physical and neurological examinations and special studies.

Why is the patient's history important?

A careful review of the history given by the patient as well as by observers who have witnessed an attack is the basis for establishing the diagnosis.

Since the person may not be able to report anything except warning feelings or after effects, it is extremely important that someone who has seen an attack should give the physician an accurate description of what takes place during the period of unconsciousness. The history will also reveal clues to other kinds of illnesses that may contribute to an understanding of the cause of the attacks.

How does the physical and neurological examination help in diagnosis?

These examinations do not help in determining if a person has seizures, but they may lead to an understanding of the cause of the seizure. For example, evidence of abnormality of heart function may lead to understanding that the seizures are in reality being triggered by changes in the blood supply to the brain. The finding of localized weakness or changes in the reflexes may point to some localized disturbance of the brain as the cause of the seizures.

What special examinations are used?

One of the most important special tests in a case of suspected epilepsy is the *electroencephalogram* ("brain wave" or EEG). By placing tiny metal disks over the scalp and connecting them by wires to the electroencephalograph, it is possible for the tiny electrical waves given off by brain cells to produce a record of the brain activity by activating pens moving across the surface of a moving sheet of paper.

The electroencephalograph or EEG machine is built on the same principle as a radio or TV set, using amplifying circuits to build up the tiny brain potentials some 50 million times or so in order to produce a written record. These patterns show the nature of the brain activity and may reveal evidence of localized disturbance in almost any area of the brain. The results of this study offer a valuable guide in both diagnosis and treatment of epilepsy.

X-rays of the skull are commonly taken to discover evidence of injury or other disturbance of the skull or its contents. Special injection techniques permit the introduction of a dye substance into the arteries that supply the brain with blood *(arteriogram or angiogram)*, or air into the cavities within the brain *(pneumoencephalogram)*, to provide special information about possible causes for the epileptic seizures, but these tests are less frequently needed.

Spinal fluid examination is often considered wise in the presence of suspected epilepsy, since the fluid which is easily secured from the lower end of the spine originates in the spaces within the brain and may give evidence of infection or other disturbance of the brain. The pressure is measured at the time of the test and a small sample of the fluid is sent to the laboratory for additional study. Other special tests include examination of the blood, urine, and chemical constituents of the blood, such as the level of blood sugar.

Since some cases of epilepsy are the result of serious injury to the brain, it is not unusual for psychologic testing to be done in particular cases, as a means of further appraisal of the patient's resources in meeting day-to-day challenges.

What can be done to control seizures?

Medication is the backbone of the management of epilepsy, but other general health and psychological considerations are important, too. With proper use and regularity of medications, 85 per cent or more of persons with seizures can be satisfactorily controlled, with over half of them being made completely free of any seizure recurrences.

How are the medications used?

To be effective, the medications must be taken with great regularity. The physician will usually prescribe a regular daily dose to be taken once or twice a day or on occasion several times a day for control of the seizures. It may be that the initial dosage will be inadequate for control, and subsequently increased amounts of the same medication or additional types of medication will be required. A growing child often requires adjustment of dosage of the medications to keep pace with growth.

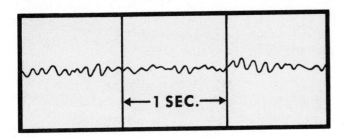

Normal EEG.

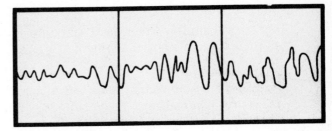

Petit mal shows fast and slow pulse with large voltage changes.

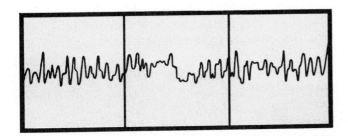

Grand mal seizures show rapid changes in voltage.

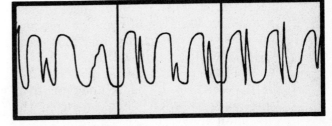

Jumpy, irregular waves are associated with psychomotor epilepsy.

An *electroencephalograph* is a machine that amplifies electrical activity of the brain ("brain waves") and records activity of various parts of the brain as peaks and valleys on a strip of paper. This written record is an *electroencephalogram* or EEG. Expertly interpreted, the EEG is helpful in diagnosis of seizures and related disorders. The drawing shows EEG's fairly representative of certain conditions. The EEG record of an individual patient covers many feet of paper on which impulses are recorded through electrodes applied to different parts of the scalp.

It is possible that some of the side effects of the medications will be troublesome enough that a particular medication will have to be replaced by another, but with perseverance and cooperation between the patient and his physician, a satisfactory balance of medications can usually be worked out.

Why is regularity in taking medication important?

Absolute regularity of taking a medication is important for two reasons. First, since control of the seizures depends on having an adequate saturation of the body tissues with the proper medication, a seizure may recur if this level is allowed to drop. Secondly, it has been observed that abrupt reduction of medication will accentuate the likelihood of seizures. Hence, it is of extreme importance that the patient and his family understand that regularity of schedule is essential to a successful program.

A variety of means have been used to help insure that no dose is missed, including marking a calendar, taking the medication in association with some other fixed function each day, such as with meals, or by counting out the medication each time. Many families have been helped by the device of securing seven small vials from their druggist, labelling each one with a day of the week, and then at the beginning of the week putting the proper dosage for each day into a separate vial. This permits the person who should use the medication to check on himself to see that the vial is empty at the end of each day, and in turn some other member of his family can unobtrusively check the vial.

If a dose is inadvertently missed, the physician will usually give instructions for making up the missed medication. If a particular schedule is difficult to maintain, the physician will often help by trying to simplify the dosage schedule so as to avoid having to take medications at school or at work.

Are there any serious complications from the medications?

It used to be thought that medications produced some mental dulling, but with modern drugs this is no longer considered true, except perhaps for a temporary effect if larger than optimum doses are being used, with the effect clearing when the medication is reduced. Some medications will produce unsteadiness in walking, blurring of vision, or nausea, but these are temporary and disappear when the dosage is adjusted. A few medications can produce skin reaction or disturbances of blood, kidney or liver functions, so when these are used the physician may request periodic laboratory tests. However, regardless of the medication, the patient should be alert to report any apparent untoward effects.

How much do epilepsy medicines cost?

For a large proportion of persons with epilepsy, complete control of their seizures can be attained with the use of medications that cost from a few cents up to perhaps ten cents a day. In other cases, where more than one medication is needed, or where some are more expensive, the cost may run to a dollar or more a day. In each case, the physician will usually try to use the medication that is safest and least expensive, provided it will accomplish the desired result of complete seizure control. Especially after the preliminary diagnostic studies are completed, the cost of medical supervision will usually be easily within the reach of most persons, as follow-up visits can be rather widely spaced after a person becomes stabilized on his medication.

How long must medicines be continued?

The physician usually recommends continuation of medications for one or more years after the last observed attack. For the convulsive seizures, this is usually at least two or three years, but it may be longer, depending upon the appearance of the person's EEG and other considerations. The medication should never be discontinued except on the advice of one's physician.

Are there special dietary needs for the person with epilepsy?

No, not as a general rule. The patient should simply have a well-balanced nutritious diet, but this need not be different from the other members of the family. Occasionally, the physician may prescribe a special ketogenic diet to augment the effectiveness of medications, but even this special diet is being used less frequently as new and more effective medications are developed.

Will a brain operation help the person with epilepsy?

If the diagnostic study reveals that the cause of the seizure is a blood clot or tumor or similar condition that can be helped by surgery, the physician will recommend this. In other carefully selected cases that have been found not to respond adequately to medications, an attempt may be made to remove by surgery the limited area of cells causing the seizure discharges. This is not always possible to do, so that this kind of surgery is approached only after very careful study of the total problem.

Does epilepsy affect intelligence?

Persons with epilepsy may have emotional problems the same as everyone else, but epilepsy is not considered a form of mental illness. In general, the intelligence of persons with epilepsy parallels that of the general population, with about as many having above normal as below normal intelligence. Famous persons who had epilepsy include Lord Byron, Dostoevski, Julius Caesar, Handel, Alexander the Great, William Pitt and others.

In the limited number of individuals whose seizures are the result of extensive damage to or disturbance of the brain, naturally their capabilities will be limited by this underlying impairment, so that special schooling and other care may sometimes be necessary, even though the seizures themselves may be readily controlled by effective medication.

What social and psychological factors affect the person with epilepsy?

Although most persons with epilepsy are basically stable, emotionally healthy, and productive, there are social and psychological problems which may make life more difficult for them. Ancient superstitions about the illness may occasionally result in exclusion from social groups. The attitude of parents or teachers may vacillate between overprotection and at times outright rejection of the child with the seizures, and either of these may bring to the surface symptoms of emotional maladjustment. It has been said that this illness is unusual because the attitudes of the persons around the individual may create more of a handicap than the actual illness itself. Continuing public information and education programs are doing much to eliminate the unfortunate attitudes that may add to the person's burden.

The person with epilepsy has realistic problems to deal with, including the uncertainty he feels about the possibility of recurring attacks, the uneasiness he may feel from isolation, the uncertainty of a self-image because of appearing to be entirely well and yet having to take a medication, and finally, by a lack of adequate understanding of his own illness. Many a person with epilepsy has been able to avoid the pitfalls of self-pity, anxiety and feelings of rejection by seeking a clearer understanding of the illness from his physician and others who can advise and counsel him. In so doing, he reaches a new level of emotional maturity coupled with a compassion for others with any kind of medical problem.

Are there legal restrictions on persons with epilepsy?

In only a few states are there remaining any of the outmoded restrictions on marriage and sterilization for persons with epilepsy, there having been a recognition of the lack of medical basis for these statutes in recent years. In some states, employment for persons with epilepsy is encouraged by workmen's compensation laws that provide financial protection to employers. Drivers' licensing laws are variable in the different states, and in some states physicians are required to report all cases of epilepsy in an effort to prevent them from driving. Since use of motor vehicles for transportation may be an important part of a man's way of living, such laws may keep him from securing medical care or may encourage him to secure a license under false pretenses. Many states grant licenses after a demonstrated period of control, subject to continuation as long as the control remains good, and the experience in these states has been excellent.

Are there problems of education for persons with epilepsy?

This is a variable picture. Since most patients with epilepsy have normal intelligence and the seizures are reasonably well controlled, children can and should be enrolled in regular school classes. There are a few children with serious damage to the brain, or other causes of mental deficiency, who also have seizures, who should be placed in special classes because of the mental deficiency rather than because of the seizure problem. If seizures are too frequent to be tolerated in the classroom, special arrangements should be made temporarily until satisfactory seizure control can be established.

At the college level, in the past there have been quite restrictive rules pertaining to the acceptance of persons with epilepsy, but this is fortunately improving, so that a person whose spells are reasonably well controlled with medication may be accepted in an increasing number of educational institutions.

What kinds of employment are suitable for persons with epilepsy?

A person with even moderately well controlled attacks can perform well in an extremely wide range of employment situations, as long as he is not required to operate high-speed or dangerous equipment such as motor vehicles, airplanes, hoists, or other things by which he or others might be injured in the event of an unexpected seizure. With proper placement and adequate training, a person with seizures proves to be an excellent worker, and many highly skilled professional people are found among the ranks of persons with epilepsy.

The United States Department of Labor, in 1961, published for the guidance of all United States Employment Service offices the following: "The physical abilities of a person with epilepsy are impaired only during the seizures and the usually short period of recovery following them ... Persons who have become seizure-free or those having only minor or very infrequent seizures are capable of physical and mental activity of a normal person ..."

Where can one secure further information about epilepsy?

Several of the states and larger cities have voluntary health organizations devoted to the problems of epilepsy. National organizations that will supply further information are the American Epilepsy Federation, 77 Reservoir Road, Quincy, Mass.; United Epilepsy Association, 111 West 57th St., New York 19, N. Y.; National Epilepsy League, 208 No. Wells St., Chicago, Ill.; and the Epilepsy Foundation, 1729 F St., Washington, D. C. The American Epilepsy Federation Film Library, 2201 Grand Ave., Merchandise Mart Bldg., Kansas City, Missouri, has educational films about epilepsy that are available for showing to health organizations interested in them. The Public Health Service of the U. S. Department of Health, Education and Welfare also has information available about epilepsy. "Employment of Epileptics in the Federal Service" is available from the U. S. Civil Service Commission, Washington 25, D. C.

KIDNEYS AND GENITO-URINARY TRACT

by R. H. FLOCKS, M.D.

The Secreting Kidney • The Filtering Unit • The Collecting System

INSTRUMENTS AND TESTS

STONES

Kidney Stones • Congenital Malformations • Injuries • Infections • Nephritis • Albumin in the Urine • Childhood Nephrosis • Tumors of the Kidney • Renal Insufficiency • Artificial Kidneys

URINARY TRACT

Obstructions • Ureters • The Bladder • Cancer of the Bladder

THE URETHRA

The Male Urethra • Injuries • Tumors • Strictures • Infections • The Female Urethra

THE PROSTATE GLAND

Examining Methods • Prostatitis • Benign Enlargement • Cancer of the Prostate • Other Disorders of the Male Sexual Apparatus • The Testes

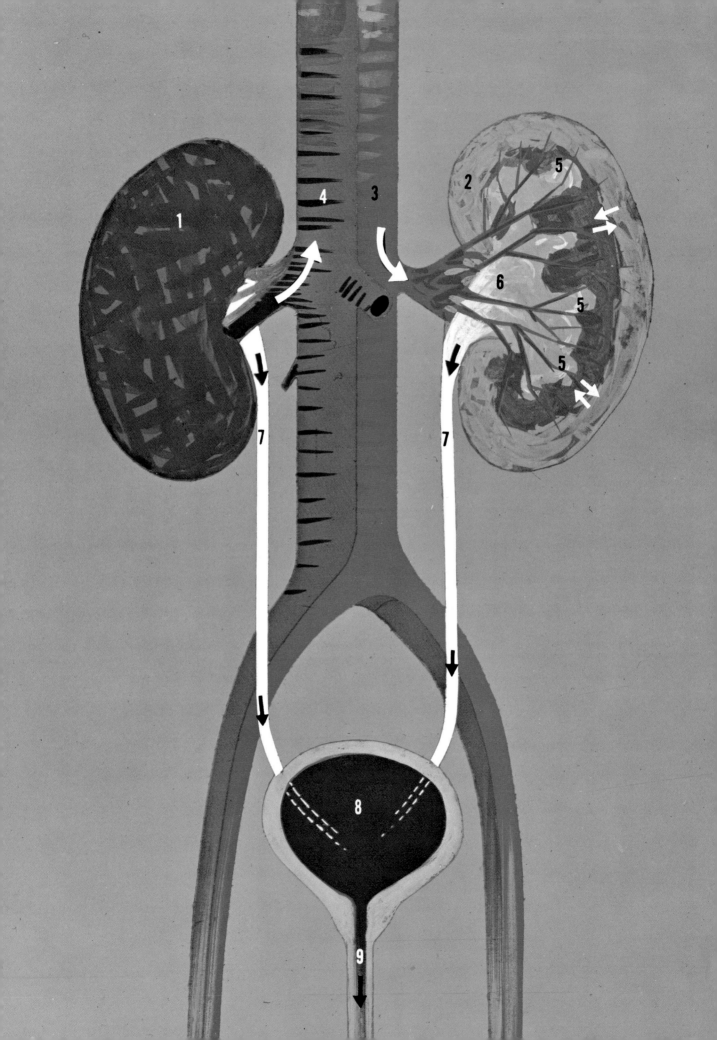

CHAPTER 8

KIDNEYS AND GENITO-URINARY TRACT

by R. H. FLOCKS, M.D.

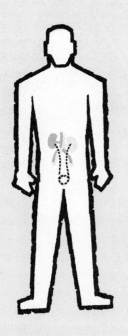

The kidneys form urine, filter many materials from the blood, and return materials to the body to maintain proper concentration of electrolytes and fluids.

The color plate shows the solid right kidney (1) and cross section of the left kidney (2). Each kidney receives blood from the *renal artery* (3) and blood is returned to general circulation through the *renal vein* (4). The vessels divide into tiny branches which permeate the kidney tissue. The white arrows show the direction of blood flow.

Microscopic urine-forming units(*nephrons*)are packed tightly into the curved outer part of the kidney. Here, urine is concentrated and collected into cuplike chambers called *calyces* (5) which open into the kidney cavity or *pelvis* (6). The black arrows show the direction of flow of urine.

The pelvis merges with the *ureter* (7), a tube which carries urine into the *bladder* (8). The bladder is a distensible storage chamber from which, at convenient times, accumulations of urine are disposed of via the *urethra* (9).

We live in an "internal sea" of fluids. The heart and circulatory system move blood to and from all parts of the body. Our kidneys incessantly filter various substances from the blood, reabsorb some of them, and concentrate wastes created by the chemical processes of living into urine which passes from the body through these mechanisms. The kidneys regulate the volume and composition of body fluids. The heart is a mighty organ that pumps blood, in a sense, blindly; the kidneys monitor the quality of what the heart pumps, so that an organism is not fatally poisoned by accumulation of harmful end-products of its own metabolism.

The labors of our kidneys are prodigious, but silent, and far less dramatic than the throbbing of the restless heart. About one-fourth of the blood pumped by each stroke of the heart passes through the kidneys. Our entire internal environment passes through the kidneys about 15 times a day. Approximately 1,700 quarts of blood flow through the kidneys every day, but only about one-thousandth is converted into urine.

The kidneys and urinary tract function as a unit, with a certain division of labor. The primary function of the kidneys is to form urine; of the urinary passageways, to dispose of it. Physicians who specialize in the treatment of kidney and urinary tract disorders are called urologists.

The Secreting Kidney

Most people have seen kidneys in meat markets and are familiar with the shape and deep-maroon color of the organs. The human kidney is a bean-shaped organ weighing about half a pound. We have two kidneys,

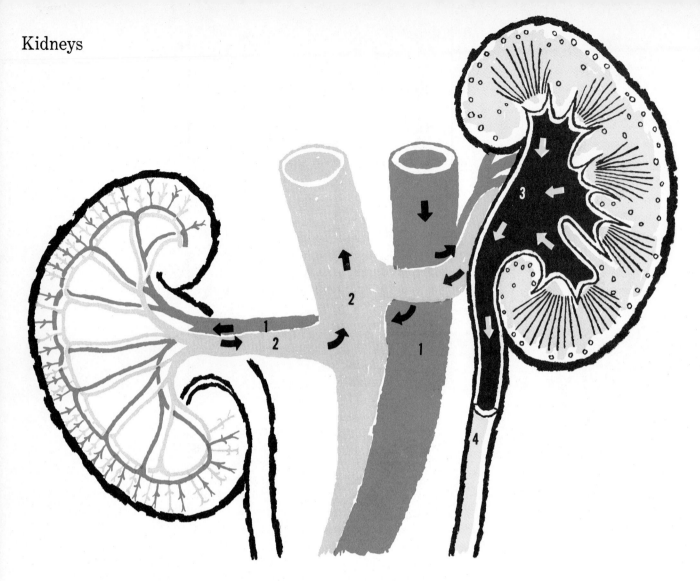

About 1,700 quarts of blood flow through the kidneys each day. This rich blood supply arrives via the *renal artery (1)* and returns via the *renal vein (2)*. Black arrows show blood pathways. The kidneys filter materials from the blood in highly selective ways and concentrate about 1½ quarts of urine per day. Urine is collected in the *kidney pelvis (3)* and flows down the *ureter (4)* to the bladder.

located behind the abdominal cavity (not in it) and protected at the rear by the spinal column and big muscles of the back. The tops of the kidneys are just underneath the chest cage. The right kidney, above which lies the liver, is usually a little lower than the left. Fat-cushions and somewhat flexible supports permit some protective range of movement, and minor variations of position which are not necessarily abnormal or a threat to health.

A half-section of the kidney, cut vertically, shows a mass of functioning tissue curved around a concave area, the *hilus.* The kidney receives its blood supply from the *renal artery,* usually a single large artery (there may be two or three moderate sized arteries) which divides into smaller and smaller branches which course through kidney tissue and filtering units. The blood is then collected by an intricate system of confluent vessels which flow into the renal vein to return blood to the general circulation.

Kidney cells have certain functions like glands of internal secretion. Local anemia of the kidneys causes pressor (pressure-elevating) substances to be secreted in amounts larger than are normally necessary to maintain the blood pressure, and hypertension may ensue. The kidneys also have other metabolic functions that are not clearly understood. But the primary urine-forming function of the kidney is accomplished during the passage of blood through tiny filtration chambers of marvelous delicacy.

The Filtering Unit

The urine-forming unit of the kidney is called a *nephron*. It is a microscopic filtration plant of exquisite design, consisting of several intricate structures. These units are packed tightly into the thick, curved, outer part of the kidney. They are largely what we see when we look at a cut section of this area of the kidney — except that the naked eye cannot distinguish an individual nephron, but only vague striations which point toward the central cavity.

A round-headed pin that bends back upon itself about halfway down its length in a hairpin turn is a very rough approximation of the shape of a nephron. The top is a cup-shaped structure known as *Bowman's capsule*. If you push your fist deeply into a soft rubber ball, the shape of the ball is roughly like that of Bowman's capsule—cup-shaped with a double wall. Nested in the capsule is the *glomerulus* ("little ball"), a tufted network of intricately laced capillaries. Practically all the constituents of blood, except blood cells and most proteins, can pass from the capillaries into the space between the double walls of the capsule. The resulting fluid, or filtrate, contains many dissolved materials, some of which are indispensable for the body's welfare, and some of which are harmful.

The filtering process of the glomeruli is physical, not chemical. Blood in the capillaries is under much higher pressure than fluids around them. The filtrate is "pushed" through the walls. If blood pressure drops sufficiently, the urine-forming process ceases. Filter surface areas compacted into a kidney the size of a small fist are astonishingly great. The filtering surface of glomeruli of a single kidney is as large as the surface of the entire body, and the glomerular capillaries of both kidneys would stretch more than 35 miles if laid end to end.

The filtrate is very dilute, and is mostly water. Out of some 180 quarts of filtrate a day, an average adult concentrates about 1½ quarts of urine. If all the filtrate were lost from the body, we would be in a perpetual state of unbearable thirst, and loss

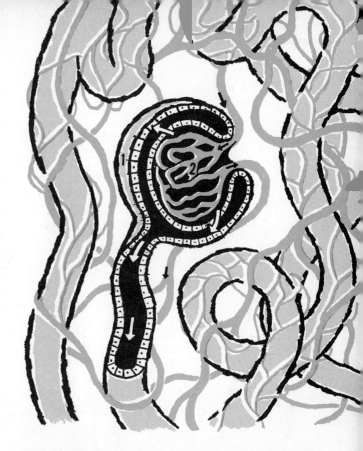

The double-walled cup-shaped chamber (1) is a *Bowman's capsule* of the kidney. The tufted network of capillaries within it is a *glomerulus* (2). Blood constituents pass into the space between the double walls as a dilute filtrate (colored arrows) which enters the kidney tubules, where most of the water and some other materials are reabsorbed and the remainder concentrated as urine.

of essential dissolved materials would in a short time be fatal. Obviously, it is essential to our lives that most of the filtrate and many of its dissolved materials be reabsorbed, while harmful materials are excluded. This is a function of the kidney *tubules*, in which residues are gradually concentrated into urine.

The capsule forms the head of a tubule, into which the filtrate flows freely. The tubule descends, bends upon itself in a hairpin turn (Henle's loop), and takes an ascending course. This meandering, convoluted course, full of complicated twists and turns, increases the length of the tubule acceptable within a small space, as one might fit a 10-foot length of garden hose into a narrow 5-foot pipe by bending the hose in the middle and doubling it back upon itself. Large amounts of water and selected dissolved materials are reabsorbed and returned to the body as fluids traverse the tubules. The concentrate at the "delivery end" of the tubules is ready for collection as urine.

Kidneys

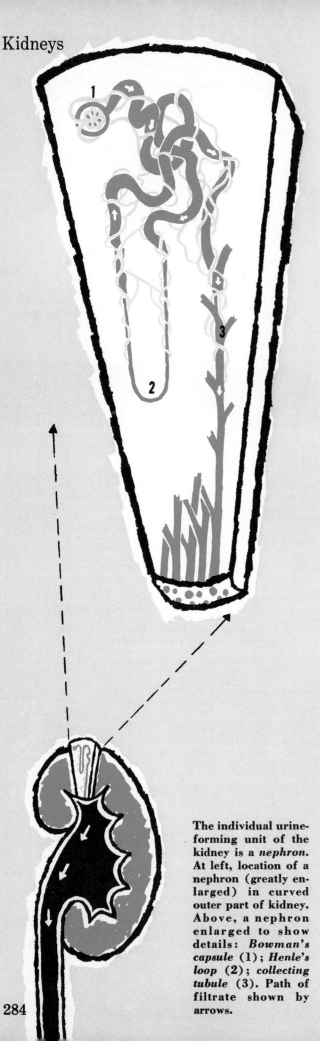

The individual urine-forming unit of the kidney is a *nephron*. At left, location of a nephron (greatly enlarged) in curved outer part of kidney. Above, a nephron enlarged to show details: *Bowman's capsule* (1); *Henle's loop* (2); *collecting tubule* (3). Path of filtrate shown by arrows.

This system of filtration, selective reabsorption, and excretion, is carried out by upward of 1,000,000 nephrons in each kidney. The nephrons of both kidneys put end to end would stretch well over 50 miles, affording such ample reserve capacity that one-half of one kidney is quite capable of sustaining life.

The kidneys regulate vital acid-base and fluid and electrolyte balances that must be kept within extremely narrow limits compatible with life. In the biological sense, electrolytes are dissolved salts or ions that participate in countless occult chemical processes of the body. Perhaps the most familiar electrolyte is sodium, an element of common salt. About 2½ pounds of salt passes through the tubules daily, but only a bit less than a third of an ounce is excreted in urine.

If salt intake is excessive, or ability of the kidneys to excrete it impaired, a condition of *edema* — fluid retention and water-logged tissues — results. On the other hand, salt depletion may cause dehydration and severe symptoms, such as the painful "heat cramps" of normally healthy persons who sweat profusely from continuous strenuous exertion in hot surroundings, drink vast amounts of water, and lose excessive quantities of salt in perspiration. The kidneys safeguard the balance of many other electrolytes which are of ceaseless and profound consequence to health.

Some kidney disorders primarily affect the glomerular filtration units, and others the tubular reabsorption units. Many rashly self-diagnosed complaints of "kidney trouble", such as legendary pain in the flank, or excessive or uncomfortable urination, have little or nothing to do with the kidneys as such, and only a physician, after examination, can determine the true nature of the condition.

The Collecting System

The collection and disposal of urine is a function of the urinary passages, distinct from the manufacturing functions of the kidneys. Urine from the ends of the tubules flows into several small cuplike chambers called *calyces* (Greek for "cup"), which merge into two or three major calyces that open into a single cavity, the *kidney pelvis*. This is a funnel-shaped sac which extends partly outside the kidney and merges at its lower end with the *ureter*, a narrow tube through which urine from the kidneys passes into the bladder.

Urine passes steadily, drop by drop, out of the kidneys. If urine had to be disposed of as steadily as it is produced, we would be seriously inconvenienced, not to mention the structure of society. The bladder is a storage organ which retains urine until disposal is convenient. Ordinarily, when the bladder collects half a pint or more of fluid, complex nerve signals notify the owner and the organ is emptied. However, the bladder is very elastic, and under some abnormal conditions may retain several quarts of fluid and greatly distend the lower abdomen.

The *urethra*, a passageway which extends from the bladder outlet to the outside, is relatively short in females but considerably longer, 8 to 9 inches, in males. The lower urinary tract of males is closely associated with reproductive organs, and is more properly called the genito-urinary tract, described on page 300. The urethra is a conduit surrounded by sphincter muscles, somewhat like purse-strings, which constrict the outlet until the owner voluntarily releases muscles to empty the bladder.

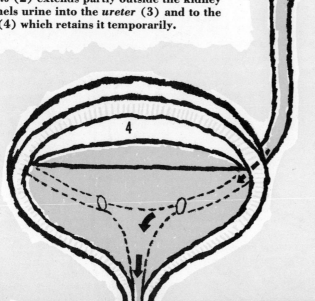

Collecting system of urine shown in cross section. The cuplike *calyces* (1) receive urine from nephrons (suggested by small black arrows). The *pelvis* (2) extends partly outside the kidney and funnels urine into the *ureter* (3) and to the *bladder* (4) which retains it temporarily.

INSTRUMENTS AND TESTS

Techniques for studying the functions of the kidney and visualizing the structures and processes of the urinary tract have been highly developed in recent years. Very exact knowledge of urological conditions can be obtained with the assistance of highly refined instruments, chemical analyses, x-ray visualization, and tests of function.

Urinalysis. Diagnosis of disease by inspection of the urine is an ancient and honorable practice, pursued centuries ago by Babylonian magi and Chinese, Hindu, Greek and Roman physicians of the time. In medieval days, the flask of urine was held in high esteem by patients and by practitioners who made diagnoses merely by looking at the portentous fluid.

Today, a properly analyzed urine specimen can tell many precise tales about conditions of the body. A complete urinalysis is not always necessary; it depends on what the doctor wants to learn about a particular patient's condition. The mere volume of urine passed in 24 hours may, for instance, be significant. Odor and color are gross qualities, and frightening color does not always have frightening significance, as when reddish urine is traced to eating too many beets. Tests for sugar, albumin, specific gravity and acid-alkaline reaction are more or less routine, but more sophisticated tests may be ordered to determine the presence of specific kinds of inorganic crystals, bile, pus, blood cells, bacteria, proteins and other elements. Cultures may be necessary to identify the particular germs

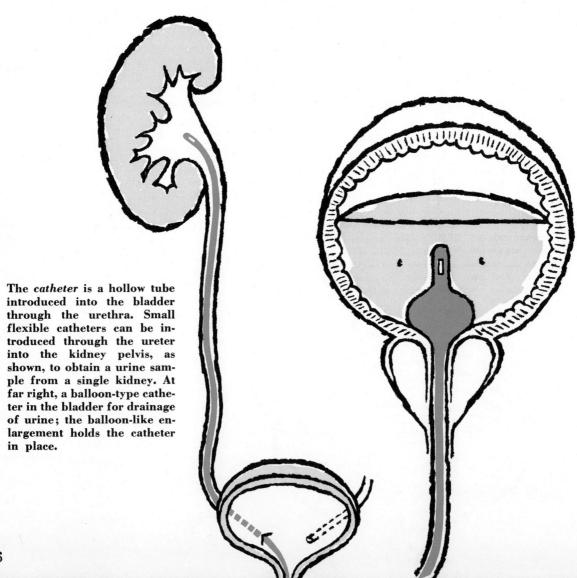

The *catheter* is a hollow tube introduced into the bladder through the urethra. Small flexible catheters can be introduced through the ureter into the kidney pelvis, as shown, to obtain a urine sample from a single kidney. At far right, a balloon-type catheter in the bladder for drainage of urine; the balloon-like enlargement holds the catheter in place.

responsible for a urinary tract infection, so that effective antimicrobial drugs may be used against them. Urine tests alone of course do not tell the whole story about a patient's condition.

Catheters. Greeks and Romans used catheters before the time of Christ. Specimens have been found in Ephesus and Pompeii. A catheter is a hollow tube for introduction into a cavity through a narrow canal, such as the urethra. Catheters of antiquity were made of bronze, copper, and silver, and later pewter, wood, and processed leather were used. Flexible catheters came into existence about the middle of the eighteenth century. In 1752, Benjamin Franklin described a flexible catheter in a letter written to his brother, and at about the same time the Surgeon General to Frederick the Great introduced an elastic catheter covered with India rubber.

Anciently, the catheter was primarily introduced into the bladder (more easily in women than in men, because of the shorter female urethra) to drain abnormal retentions of urine, and it still serves that purpose. However, development of smaller, more flexible catheters has enabled more delicate procedures to be carried out. An example is catheterization of the ureters. This small instrument makes it possible for urine to be collected separately from each kidney, a matter of importance in assessing the relative efficiency of the paired kidneys.

Cystoscopy. From the catheter, the beginning of instrumentation of the urinary tract, it was a tremendous leap to the modern *cystoscope*. This remarkable instrument consists essentially of a hollow tube with a tiny electric light bulb at its tip, which can be passed into the bladder. Various systems of viewing lenses are then introduced. Thus the interior of the bladder, the tubes leading into it, and the urethra can be inspected visually.

Modern cystoscopes embodying refined improvements are exceedingly versatile instruments. Forms of the cystoscope can be used as operating instruments for destruction of tumors and removal of stones and foreign bodies from the bladder. Recent improvements in the light systems have made it possible to see in the ureter and kidney pelvis, and it is likely that excellent instruments for inspecting the urine-collecting chambers of the kidney's interior will be developed.

X-Rays. Developments in x-ray apparatus have tremendously improved the study of the urinary tract and kidney function. Plain films can now be made which show the outlines of urinary tract structures. Other details can be visualized by injecting radio-opaque substances and making an x-ray film — an *excretory pyelogram*. This enables the entire urinary tract to be visualized and shows any distortions or disturbances associated with disease processes. It is also possible to introduce such substances into particular regions through cystoscopes and catheters. Recent developments in *cinefluorography* make it possible to take motion pictures of the urinary tract in action, following the introduction of opaque media.

Since the main function of the kidney is to clear certain substances from the blood, its ability to do so is a measure of kidney function. Highly specialized studies of the chemical constituents of the blood and ability of the kidneys to clear dyes or other substances give important information about how well the organs are doing their job.

STONES (Calculi; Lithiasis)

Kidney Stones

One of the oldest surgical operations is "cutting for stone." Samuel Pepys describes his own operation (on March 26, 1658) quite vividly, and notes in his diary that he spent 24 shillings for "a case for to keep my stone, that I was cut of." Benjamin Franklin has written eloquently of the symptoms of stone in the bladder which he and many of his contemporaries had. The specialty of cutting for stone was known in the time of Hippocrates, and was quite a restricted specialty. Hippocrates admonishes fellow

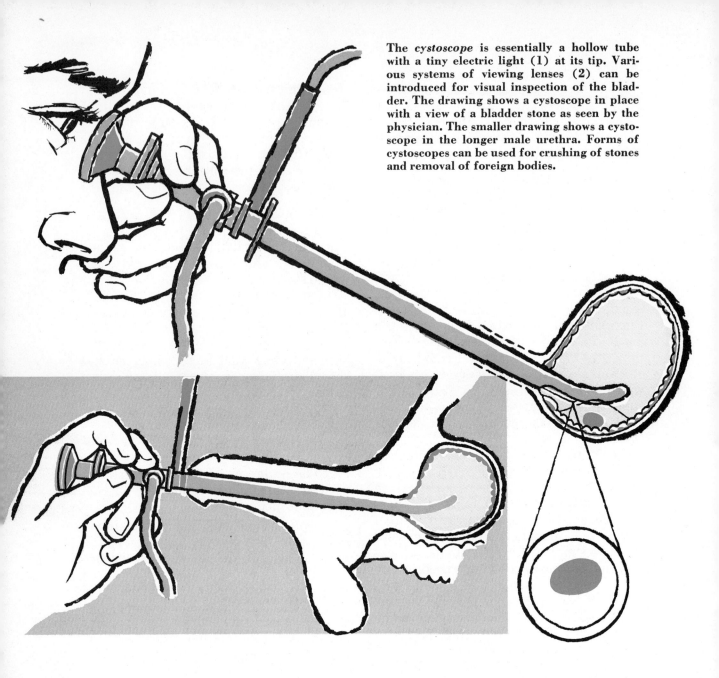

The *cystoscope* is essentially a hollow tube with a tiny electric light (1) at its tip. Various systems of viewing lenses (2) can be introduced for visual inspection of the bladder. The drawing shows a cystoscope in place with a view of a bladder stone as seen by the physician. The smaller drawing shows a cystoscope in the longer male urethra. Forms of cystoscopes can be used for crushing of stones and removal of foreign bodies.

physicians not to cut for stone, but to leave this condition to the specialist. Many operative procedures for removal of stones were developed in the seventeenth and eighteenth centuries.

Stones in the kidney and urinary tract are quite common, and still a major problem of urology. How kidney stones form is reasonably well understood. Urine is a complex supersaturated solution of many substances, including mineral salts. Under the right conditions, certain of these substances may precipitate out, condense upon some microscopic nucleus — perhaps a bacterium or a speck of mucus — and grow larger and larger.

Stones, then, are formed of dissolved substances brought to the kidney. *Why* they form in some people but not in others is not at all well understood. Prevalence of stone varies geographically; in some areas it is endemic. For example, the southeastern part of the U. S. is an area with high incidence of kidney stones. The location of stones in different parts of the urinary tract has varied historically. At present, in certain areas of the Near East most stones are present in the bladder and are found in children.

Despite these subtle mysteries, a great deal of practical medical and surgical knowledge is available to the troubled patient. Stones come in many shapes, sizes, and differences in structural material. If a stone can be obtained from a patient, analysis of its chemical makeup gives valuable information. Calcium phosphate stones are very common; among other kinds are urate and cystine stones. The latter are primarily due to an error of metabolism in the body's handling of an amino acid of protein foods. Sometimes a tumor in certain areas, such as the parathyroid glands, increases the excretion of calcium and phosphorus in the urine and predisposes to calcium phosphate stones.

Other factors that may encourage stone formation are obstructions anywhere in the urinary tract which may cause urine to "back up" and not drain freely from the kidney; prolonged recumbency; infection; and abnormally concentrated urine which may result from insufficient intake of water. It is obviously important to correct any abnormalities in the urinary tract which may predispose to the formation of new stones, and to correct changes in the urinary tract which may have been brought about by the presence of stones.

Some stones thrive in acid urine, others in alkaline. Medicines and special diets, such as an acid-ash diet, may help to maintain desired balances and deter future stone formation. There are other medical measures which a doctor can institute from his special knowledge of the patient's body chemistry and physical condition. It is of immediate importance to remove stones that are causing serious trouble, and this generally requires surgery (see Chapter 22). Sometimes it is desirable to remove the entire kidney, if its function has been markedly impaired by a large stone or stones, and if the remaining kidney is healthy and quite capable of continuing the labors that it has shouldered anyhow. Naturally, it is far more desirable for a person who is susceptible to stone formation to co-operate with his doctor in regular checkups, with x-rays and other measures, which may keep trouble from progressing and do everything possible to avert eventual surgical removal of a kidney.

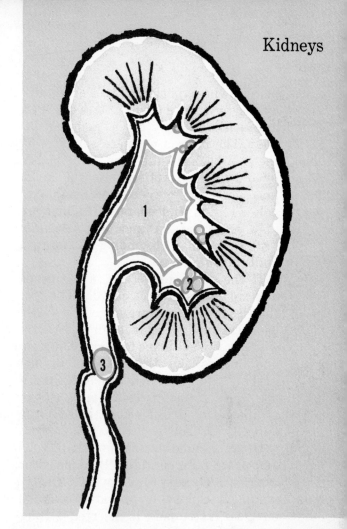

Kidney stones range in size from tiny crystals to *staghorn* stones which occupy practically all of the space of the pelvis (1) and take on the antlered shape of the cavity. Small stones (2) may be passed without incident. A stone that moves down and blocks the ureter (3) causes excruciating pain.

Some stones cause no symptoms, at least for a long time. Fine crystals, no larger than grains of sand, may pass down the ureter and to the outside world without the patient's being aware of it. Some "silent" stones are too large to enter or obstruct the ureter, but they may move about in the kidney and do quiet injury to delicate tissues. Some stones may practically fill the kidney pelvis and take on the irregular shape of the cavity, like a cast. These are called *"staghorn" calculi* from their antler-like appearance.

Many stones, however, do cause acute attacks of excruciating pain. A bout of "kidney colic" is never forgotten by the person who experiences it. The agony is caused by a stone which enters the ureter and works its way down, gouging as it goes. The pain is not necessarily felt in the mid-back, in the area memorialized by old-time advertisements for kidney nostrums, but may be referred to the pelvic region. Indeed, pain is not invariably excruciating, and the immediate symptoms may be nausea, vomiting, chills and fever.

If the stone gets stuck in the ureter, and medical measures can do little more than relieve pain, surgery will probably be necessary to remove an obstruction which can cause urine to back up, distend, and injure the tract above it most gravely. Stone-harried kidneys generally are more prone to infections; modern antibacterial drugs afford potent measures of control.

Often a stone passes into the bladder and acute pain subsides. Bladder stones are relatively easy to remove with instruments which leave no operative scar. The surgical instrument is inserted through the urethra, the stone grasped and crushed, and the particles withdrawn. Occasionally, a stone will lodge in the urethra and prevent urination. Its removal is comparatively easy and always an immense relief to the patient.

Congenital Malformations

Some malformations of the kidney do not significantly interfere with function and ordinarily will cause no difficulty to the person who has them. Other malformations do impair functions, sooner or later, and in varying degrees. Malformed kidneys which have been functioning quite well may be pushed beyond their capacity by injury or disease which overburdens them. Whether or not symptoms are evident, it is important to know that congenital abnormalities are present in an individual person, what they are doing, and how well the kidneys are performing their duties. Studies of function and anatomy previously described elsewhere give such information.

Before birth, the kidneys arise in the pelvic region and, in the course of prenatal development, migrate upward, rotate on their long axes, and settle down in their normal positions in the upper lumbar region. This complicated, twisting ascent is subject to aberrations which result in malformations.

Ectopic kidneys are "out of normal place." A kidney may fail to ascend to its normal level. Or it may cross to the opposite side of the body from which it originated. Then, the two kidneys may lie separately but close together on the same side of the body, or they may be fused together to form a single mass of kidney tissue which may be mistaken for an abdominal tumor. Such malformations may function well, but are prone to infection and obstructed outflow which causes collections of urine to distend the pelvis of the kidney (*hydronephrosis*).

Solitary kidney. Very rarely, a person is born with only one kidney. Or fused kidneys, described above, may in effect be a single kidney. We can do very well with only one kidney, but not with none at all. A solitary kidney may impose no particular difficulty, but the person does not have a "spare." Ordinarily, a severely injured or diseased kidney is simply removed if the other kidney is normal. This cannot be done if there is only one kidney since death would result.

Horseshoe kidney. As the name of this anomaly indicates, the paired kidneys, instead of being separate, are linked at their lower ends by a band of thin or thick tissue, giving a shape resembling a horseshoe. The bridge may or may not contain functioning tissue.

Polycystic kidneys are congenital and have a tendency to "run in the family." Usually, both kidneys are studded with bubble-like cysts which fill the interior with sponge-like cavities and, on the surface, resemble blisters. Polycystic disease recognized in infancy has a serious prognosis, but in adults the disease usually progresses slowly and is consistent with an active life.

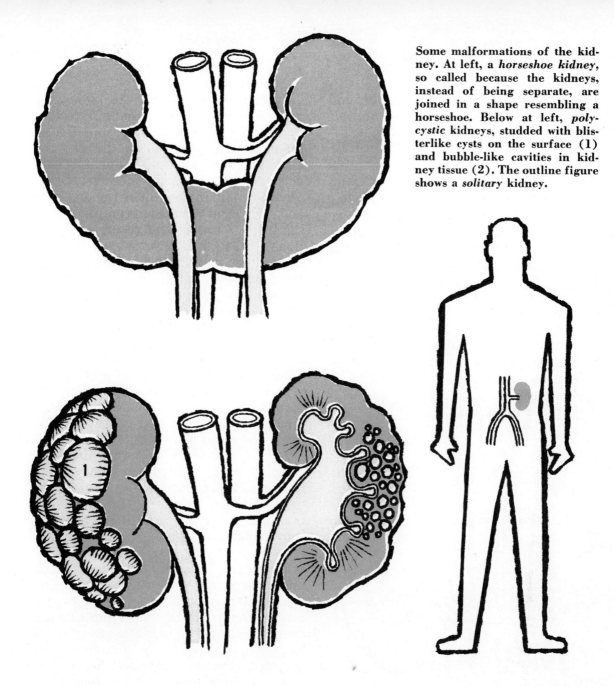

Some malformations of the kidney. At left, a *horseshoe kidney*, so called because the kidneys, instead of being separate, are joined in a shape resembling a horseshoe. Below at left, *polycystic* kidneys, studded with blisterlike cysts on the surface (1) and bubble-like cavities in kidney tissue (2). The outline figure shows a *solitary* kidney.

Injuries

The kidneys are quite resiliently moored and well protected, and injuries are relatively rare. However, crushing and penetrating injuries do occur sometimes, and the immediate problem ordinarily is one of bleeding from a very vascular organ. It may be possible to repair the injured structures, or a kidney may have to be sacrificed, depending upon the nature and extent of injuries.

Hematuria (blood in the urine) is always a symptom requiring immediate investigation by a physician to determine its cause. Sometimes, the startling discovery of blood in the urine is followed the next day, or for days thereafter, by clear urine, and the person may be lulled into feeling that nothing serious is amiss. There may not be, but intermittent hematuria may be of serious import and its first appearance is a warning to consult a physician. There are many possible causes of hematuria, some exceedingly grave, others trivial. Of the trivial variety, microscopic hematuria—presence of inconspicuous blood cells in a urine specimen—resulting from violent sports activity or exercise is perhaps the most common. The condition is not uncommon in boxers, basketball players, wrestlers and others subject to body blows and multiple episodes of forced forward crouching.

Infections

Infections of the kidney and its pelvis (*pyelonephritis*) are quite common. They are of extreme importance because chronic and recurring infections tend to induce changes which in time may interfere seriously with kidney function. In many ways the conditions seem to be related to high blood pressure. Some cases, particularly if untreated or neglected, progress to *renal insufficiency*— incapacity of the kidneys to filter toxins adequately from the blood. Retention of these infectious wastes leads to *uremia* or "uremic poisoning."

Infections can reach the kidney by various routes: direct ascent of infecting organisms from the bladder; spread from infections in surrounding tissues; and via the bloodstream and lymphatic channels. Acute infections manifest themselves by pain in the kidney region, fever and chills, and changes in composition of the urine. Chronic and recurrent infections tend to manifest themselves more insidiously in symptoms such as headache, nausea or vomiting.

The urine may contain pus (*pyuria*), colonies of micro-organisms, many white blood cells, and other products of inflammation. Identification of the infecting organisms enables effective antibiotics or other drugs to be given to destroy the organisms. Many acute and chronic infections respond to proper chemotherapy, rest, and general care in the form of fluids and other measures.

However, many kidney infections are complicated by obstructions and conditions which prevent free drainage of the urinary tract. Infected teeth and other foci may introduce infecting organisms into the bloodstream and thence the kidneys, in continuous supply. Extra-renal sources of infection must be recognized and cleared up, and there is need for urological investigation to recognize and correct abnormalities which impede good drainage and perpetuate low-grade infectious organisms. Early diagnosis and treatment is important and neglect may lead to kidney damage that is difficult if not impossible to reverse.

Nephritis ("Bright's Disease")

In 1827, Richard Bright of London described a disease which thenceforward bore his name and is probably the best known of medical eponyms (diseases named for the discoverer). Bright's disease is not a single entity. Several varieties are now recognized, and there is some confusion about definitions. In a very broad way, the group of diseases may be called *nephritis* — inflammation of the kidney not resulting from infection in the kidney. Fine blood vessels of the *glomeruli*, the filtering units of the

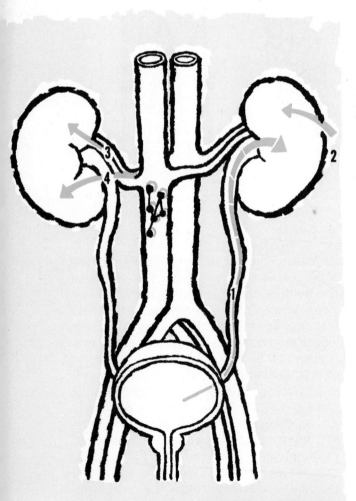

Infections may reach the kidneys by various routes: 1. ascending infection from the bladder and ureter; 2. from adjacent tissues; 3. from the bloodstream; 4. from lymphatics.

nephron, are commonly affected; hence the awkward term, *glomerulonephritis*.

Although germs are not a direct cause of nephritis, recent research has incriminated certain strains of germs as probable indirect causes. Acute glomerulonephritis may occur several days after a patient has suffered an infection caused by group A hemolytic streptococci, of the sort that often cause "strep throat" and scarlet fever. Delayed-action toxins produced by the germs are thought to be responsible.

Salts of mercury and some other metals can cause nephritis. The kidneys, guardians of the blood's purity, filter and excrete innumerable kinds of harmful substances day and night. Metabolic diseases may produce scarring in the kidney and inflammatory reactions. And the very vascular kidneys are subject to sclerotic or artery-hardening processes. This form of nephritis is called *nephrosclerosis*.

Acute glomerulonephritis usually affects young people, but no age is exempt. Symptoms include loss of appetite, headaches, nausea, vomiting, and scanty urine. There is puffy waterlogging of tissues. The urine contains much albumin (protein), evidence of kidney damage. Blood pressure usually rises. The patient is kept in bed and his diet carefully regulated with respect to intake of fluids, sodium, and other food elements. The great majority of patients recover completely and rarely have a second attack.

Chronic glomerulonephritis has a more serious outlook, though it is by no means to be regarded hopelessly. The condition may be latent for many years during which no active treatment is required. Dropsy is not quite so common a symptom of active disease as in acute glomerulonephritis. There is often anemia and a sallow complexion, and wastes tend to accumulate in the blood from diminished capacity of the kidneys to excrete them. There is albumin in the urine. Blood pressure rises. Although kidney impairment increases slowly, there may be a latent period, even of many years, during which the patient may feel quite well and be able to carry on an active life. Inflammatory

reactions tend eventually to cause renal insufficiency, uremia, and there may be accompanying congestive heart failure. The chronic condition has many aspects of generalized vascular disease in which the kidneys are conspicuously involved.

The relationship between high blood pressure and vascular kidney disease is of great interest because of the general high incidence of hypertension. Special tests to uncover these relationships are now available, such as *renal arteriography*—x-ray films of kidney vessels. When high blood pressure is present, these special tests should be carried out by a team of urologists and internists to rule out or confirm renal causes of hypertensive disease. When renal artery obstruction is demonstrated, surgical correction is frequently possible, as by constructing a bypass of the affected artery.

Albumin in the Urine

Albumin is a protein, like egg white, which is present in the urine of some persons, and probably at some time or other in the urine of almost everybody. Albumin is a useful substance and healthy kidneys normally do not excrete it wastefully. Therefore *albuminuria* (albumin in the urine) suggests damage to the filtering apparatus of the kidneys. However, some infectious diseases and even such things as violent exercise and other stresses are frequently associated with transient and harmless albuminuria. Some people have albumin in their urine "naturally" without any evidence of kidney disease. The symptom of albumin in the urine has no great significance until its meaning is interpreted by a doctor who studies the whole patient.

Childhood Nephrosis

Any degeneration of the kidney without signs of inflammation is called *nephrosis*. The term is most often applied to a cruel disease of children, childhood nephrosis. Most of the patients are between one and a half and four years of age when the disorder is recognized. The outstanding symptom is massive edema, distorting the small body with swollen accumulations of fluids. The first signs may be a slight puffiness about the eyes or difficulty in putting the child's shoes on.

The cause is not known. A preceding streptococcal infection apparently plays no part, as it does in acute glomerulonephritis. A great deal of research is devoted to determining the mechanisms of the disease, which involves the kidneys and may progress to kidney failure, but also appears to involve metabolic processes outside the kidneys.

Treatment has been greatly improved by use of steroid drugs (of the cortisone family) and antibiotics to prevent severe infections to which the nephrotic child is peculiarly liable. Judicious administration of steroids commonly reduces the massive edema and brings about remissions. Treatment is of course adjusted to

the individual patient. Refractory cases usually require prolonged hospital treatment and the financial burden upon the family is great. The hopeful aspect is that many of the patients do not develop kidney failure, the threat of severe infections is held at bay with antibiotics, and heartening numbers of children reach a state of good health without any permanent kidney damage from the disease.

Tumors of the Kidney

Tumors of the kidney are not uncommon. They may be benign, or they may be malignant — that is, cancerous, with ability to spread to other parts of the body (metastasize). The benign tumors are essentially cysts of the kidney, fluid-filled sacs. These may occur in one kidney or both, and may produce a large mass in the abdomen of the patient.

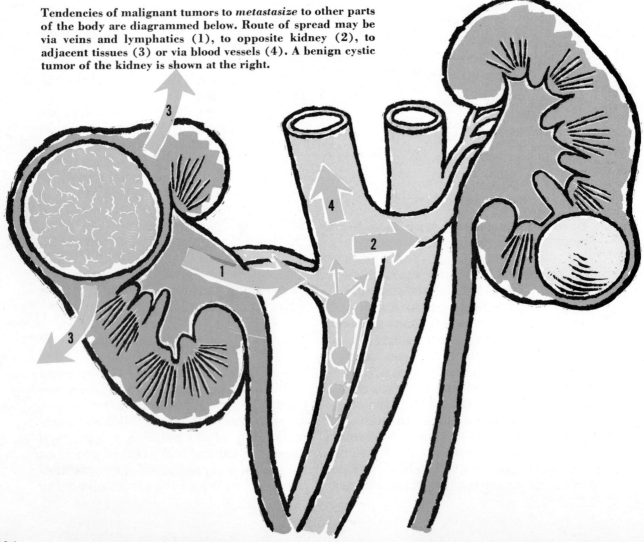

Tendencies of malignant tumors to *metastasize* to other parts of the body are diagrammed below. Route of spread may be via veins and lymphatics (1), to opposite kidney (2), to adjacent tissues (3) or via blood vessels (4). A benign cystic tumor of the kidney is shown at the right.

Malignant tumors practically always affect only one kidney. They arise in functioning tissue of the kidney. In general, kidney malignancies occur in two periods of life, in infancy, and in mid-adult life. Broadly speaking, there are two types: the so-called *Wilms' tumor* of childhood, and the malignancy of the adult, the so-called *hypernephroma*, which occurs primarily in persons over the age of 40. There are other malignant tumors which need not be discussed, because they are extremely rare and their effects are quite similar to those of Wilms' and hypernephroma tumors.

Symptoms. Evidences of such kidney tumors are primarily pain in one side or the other, bloody urine, or appearance of a mass in the abdomen in the region of the kidney. The symptom of bloody urine may not be accompanied by pain. There may be periods when there is no blood in the urine, and precious time may be lost in hope that the symptom will "go away." It is always a symptom that calls for immediate investigation, although it may originate from quite another cause than cancer. As with all cancers, the best hope of cure lies in early treatment.

A mother is often the first to discover a Wilms' tumor, as an abdominal mass, in the course of caring for her baby. The tumor usually occurs before the age of seven. A mass that can be felt in the abdomen is not necessarily a Wilms' tumor. A very large hydronephrosis, which we will discuss later, can also produce a mass and is much more common than Wilms' tumor. Congenital cysts of the kidney also may produce a large abdominal mass. Every child who has a palpable mass in the abdomen should be investigated promptly.

The treatment for Wilms' tumor and hypernephroma is removal.

Renal Insufficiency

We have mentioned "renal insufficiency" in the above discussions. The term is quite simple. It means that the kidneys are unable to filter all the wastes and poisons from the blood. Thus, various amounts of toxic materials remain harmfully in the body. If the kidneys fail completely, death results in a few days, from *uremia* or "uremic poisoning." This is a damming-up of toxins which is fatal unless corrected.

There are degrees of uremia. Early symptoms are headache, loginess, itching, muscle discomfort, with or followed by nausea and vomiting. The patient becomes drowsy, perhaps has convulsions, and lapses into coma and death.

Insufficiency is relative to the capabilities of a particular pair of kidneys. Insufficiency may result from some acute, repairable condition, or from gradual and irreversible damage and destruction of kidney tissue over a period of years. A major purpose of good urological care is to prevent insidious kidney injury and whenever possible to eradicate causes of insufficiency by such measures as clearing up infections and removing or bypassing obstructions.

Great advances in treatment of renal insufficiency have been made in recent years. One of the mechanisms artfully employed by the kidneys is *dialysis*. This is the separation of substances in solution, having different diffusibilities, by passing them through a porous membrane, such as membranes of the kidney filters. Similar filtration can be achieved by techniques of *peritoneal dialysis,* in which membranes of the abdominal cavity do the work of the diseased kidneys temporarily. Blood passed through peritoneal membranes is cleansed and returned to the body. The technique has proved very successful in treatment. Absorptive resins placed in the gastrointestinal tract are useful adjuncts.

Artificial Kidneys

Almost everybody has heard something about so-called "artificial kidneys." These are indeed artificial and mechanical, but they do the work of human kidneys quite remarkably for short periods of time. There are several variants of the artificial kidney, but all rely on pretty much the same principle as the living kidney itself: diffusion of blood through a membrane to extract wastes and return cleared blood

Kidneys

General principles of an artificial kidney which clears wastes from the blood are shown diagrammatically. Impure blood from the patient (1) is pumped (2) through coiled membranes surrounded by fluid (3). Substances diffuse through the membranes in the fluid *(dialysis)*. Cleared blood is returned to patient (4). Flowmeters and traps to remove bubbles from blood are part of the apparatus.

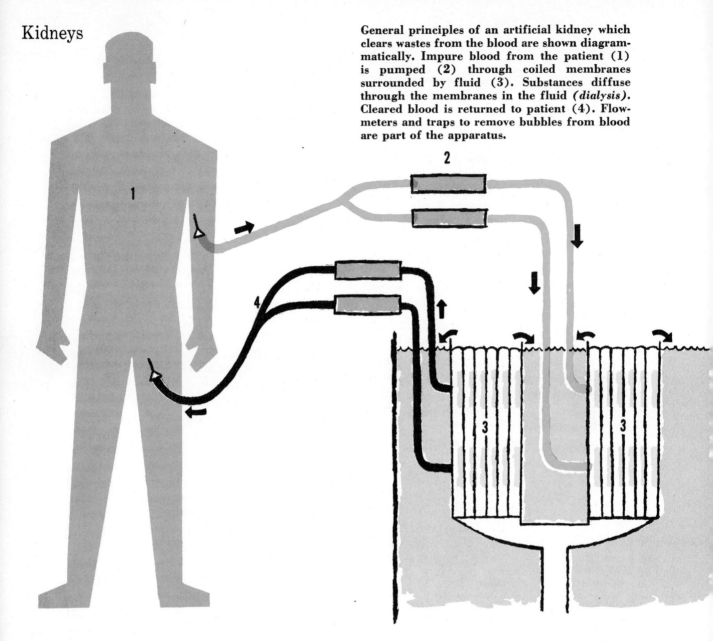

to the body. Artificial kidneys perform this function, called *hemodialysis*, outside of the body.

In essence, blood from an artery in the patient's arm passes through coiled membranes (commonly of cellophane), dialyzable materials are filtered into surrounding fluid, and the cleared blood is returned via one of the patient's veins. Pumps, flow meters, clot and bubble traps keep the blood moving safely. Hemodialysis is a hospital procedure requiring dependable apparatus and the skills of a team of specialists.

Kidney substitutes can only be used for a relatively short time to aid the body until the renal disease has been overcome and the kidneys can resume their normal function. Excellent results are attained in reversible kidney disease, for which the body needs only a relatively short period of outside support while the kidneys marshal their defenses. Transfusion reactions, poisoning, acute renal failure due to postpartum hemorrhage, are examples of conditions in which the artificial kidney may be lifesaving.

For the patient whose kidneys are irreversibly scarred, degenerated, and hopelessly inadequate, the machines are less practical because artificial hemodialysis must be permanent and frequently and regularly repeated. Unfortunately, present artificial kidneys are not suited for simple use in the home. A few patients have had permanent tubes inserted into an artery and vein of the wrist, for easy connection to an artificial kidney, and

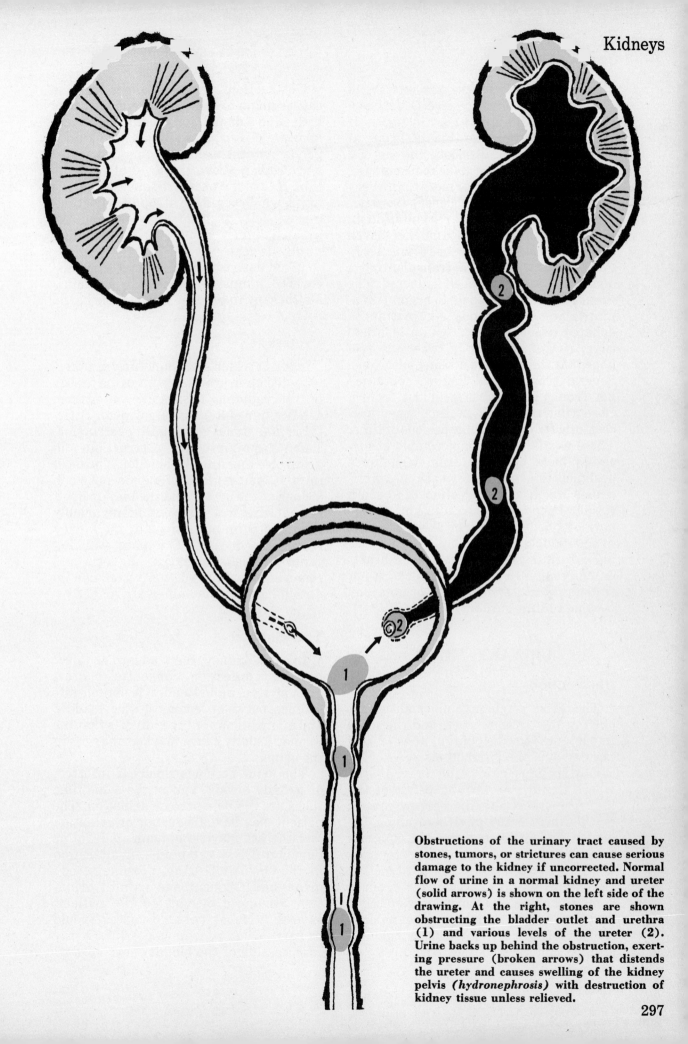

Obstructions of the urinary tract caused by stones, tumors, or strictures can cause serious damage to the kidney if uncorrected. Normal flow of urine in a normal kidney and ureter (solid arrows) is shown on the left side of the drawing. At the right, stones are shown obstructing the bladder outlet and urethra (1) and various levels of the ureter (2). Urine backs up behind the obstruction, exerting pressure (broken arrows) that distends the ureter and causes swelling of the kidney pelvis (hydronephrosis) with destruction of kidney tissue unless relieved.

once a week or so these patients spend a day in a hospital to have their blood cleared. But the great cost in terms of the patient's time, the time of teams of specialists, hospitalization and special apparatus, presently makes unremitting treatment impossible for more than a very few of those who might benefit from it.

Successful kidney transplantation in identical twins has focused much research upon this possibility for the future. Technical surgical details of transplanting a donated kidney have been mastered. The great remaining obstacle to organ transplantation is the body's rejection of donated tissue, except from an identical twin, as a foreign body. There is real hope that this obstacle is being overcome. Several transplanted kidneys, obtained not from an identical twin but from a close relative, have now functioned successfully for considerable periods of time. These partial, or perhaps complete, successes have benefited from techniques designed to suppress formation of antibodies involved in rejection of foreign tissue. Preparatory irradiation of the patient's body and use of antimetabolite drugs which controllably depress the blood-forming organs have given heartening results. In the future, perhaps not so distant, transplantation of organs may become routine surgery.

URINARY TRACT

Obstructions

The most common abnormalities involving the urinary tract, and the most important from the point of view of kidney damage, are obstructions.

Obstructions can occur in the area where the urine-collecting pelvis of the kidney merges with the narrow ureter, or they may occur anywhere along the ureter. For example, a stone or congenital stricture may obstruct the ureter anywhere along its course. Or obstruction can occur within the bladder from a tumor which blocks the openings of both ureters into the bladder, or it can occur at the bladder neck from congenital lesions, tumors, stones, or strictures.

Obstruction anywhere along the line causes urine to back up, as a river backs up behind a dam. Back pressure produces *hydronephrosis*, a swelling of the kidney pelvis, and the ureter becomes distended and swollen above the level of obstruction. Hydraulic pressure squeezes kidney tissue which begins to atrophy. Functioning capacity is gradually lost and the inflated kidney is at risk of becoming totally useless.

When destruction of any nature is discovered, it must be removed by appropriate therapy to prevent irreparable harm.

Ureters

Injuries which tear, puncture, or otherwise disrupt a ureter permit urine to seep into surrounding tissues like water from a burst pipe. Repair is surgical. Strictures and stones may cause obstruction. Tumors may produce obstruction and gross bleeding into the bladder. The most important single difference between lesions of the ureter and the kidney itself is that ureteral obstruction invariably produces pain, but lesions of the kidney frequently do not. The pain warning generally leads to early diagnosis and removal of an obstruction which can do untold harm to the kidney above it.

The Bladder

Like the kidney, the bladder is subject to injury, infection, congenital malformation, stones and tumors. A notable difference between lesions of the bladder and many lesions of the kidney is that the former usually cause marked changes in the urine.

The urine becomes cloudy if infected, or grossly bloody, and at the same time there are disturbances of urination. The patient may have frequency of urination and the act may be difficult, painful or burning. These symptoms of alteration in the clarity of urine, possible bloody urine, and frequent and painful urination are quite evident to the patient. Investigation of possible causes should be carried out as soon as possible. X-ray examination of the bladder *(cystogram)*

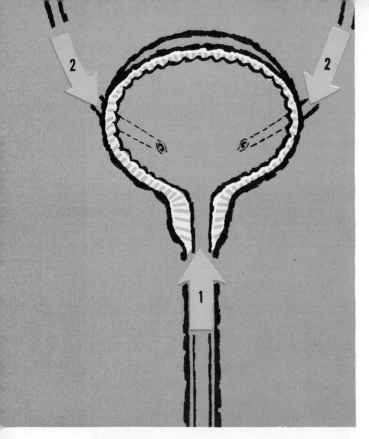

Infections causing *cystitis* most commonly reach the bladder via the *urethra* (1) from an outside source, especially in females. Infections can also descend from the upper urinary tract via the *ureters* (2).

or direct observation of the interior of the bladder by means of a cystoscope may be necessary.

Cystitis (inflammation of the bladder) is especially common in women. The short female urethra is a pathway to invasion by infecting organisms. Occasionally infection may descend from the kidneys to the bladder but the opposite route is much more common. The urethra is often infected and inflamed *(urethritis)* and the site of the most distressing symptoms. A physician's diagnosis of simple acute cystitis is usually not difficult. Symptoms are pain on voiding, frequency, perhaps backache, not much fever unless the upper urinary tract is involved, which is not often the case. Ordinarily an acute infection is cleared by antimicrobial drugs. It may or may not be necessary to identify the specific causative organisms to determine the treatment most effective against them. Chronic or recurring cystitis may require examination with a cystoscope and other

measures to detect abnormalities that may perpetuate the condition.

Congenital malformations of the bladder primarily involve failure of the bladder to close into a sac with a normal outlet. The anomaly is called *exstrophy* of the bladder. The malformed bladder has only a back wall and no abdominal covering. Urine from the ureters comes out to the surface of the body and the patient leaks urine constantly.

Correction is by surgery, and very difficult. In some cases, plastic surgery suffices. Other cases require diversion of the urinary stream into "unnatural" channels which direct the flow from the outside to the interior of the body. The stream may be diverted into the rectum. Or an isolated section of the bowel may be employed as an artificial bladder *(ileal bladder)*. This delivers urine to the skin surface in a localized area where it can be collected in a suitable container. There are of course no sphincter ("pursestring") muscles and the patient cannot start or stop the flow.

Bladder function may also be interfered with by neurological disease. Inability to empty the bladder may be due to damage to motor nerves, or injury to sensory functions may prevent sensations of bladder enlargement which normally trigger the urge to void.

Enuresis (involuntary discharge of urine) is normal in children up to about the age of three or four. "Automatic" control of urination is a complicated nervous function which takes time to develop. Bed-wetting problems in older children often involve psychic factors. Nocturnal enuresis is common in certain neurological conditions, for instance, the "uninhibited neurogenic bladder." When enuresis persists after the age of four, a search should be made for some local lesion involving the bladder or some neurological lesion.

Incontinence of urine occurs frequently in elderly people. It is usually associated with hardening of the arteries in parts of the brain, or with blood vessel injury associated with strokes, and is part of the general arteriosclerotic processes of advancing age. The resulting enuresis is similar to that which normally occurs in children under the age of four.

Cancer of the Bladder

It is extremely important that persons who have any difficulty or abnormality of urination be carefully examined to ascertain whether any lesions are present in the bladder.

Cancer of the bladder is one of the most common in this country. It is almost as common as cancer of the lungs, although it has not received as much publicity. At the University Hospitals in Iowa City, more than 75 new patients with cancer of the bladder are seen yearly.

The most common evidence of cancer of the bladder is grossly bloody urine, but frequency of urination and cloudy urine may also be important symptoms. When detected early, the outlook is good, when late, poor. Treatment consists of destruction of the tumor by a combination of surgical removal and irradiation therapy. Small tumors may be removed through the urethra with an instrument called the resectoscope. Larger lesions require more radical surgery with x-ray therapy.

THE URETHRA

The male and female urethras are different. The female urethra is simply a conduit to carry urine from the bladder to the outside. The male urethra performs the same service, and, in addition, is the passageway through which reproductive materials from the sex glands and associated structures are transported to the outside.

A number of conditions involve the urethra without prejudice as to sex, but we will discuss the male and female urethras separately because of different susceptibilities to some disorders.

The Male Urethra

The *meatus* is the external opening of the urethra, the terminus of the urinary system which begins with the kidneys. The male urethra is about nine inches long, and is divided — not physically, since it is continuous, but for purposes of description — into two portions. The portion which begins at the bladder outlet and runs through the prostate gland is the *posterior or prostatic* urethra. The rest of the structure is the *anterior urethra*, primarily located in the shaft of the penis.

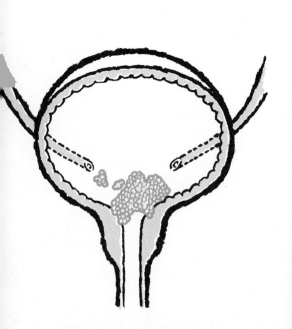
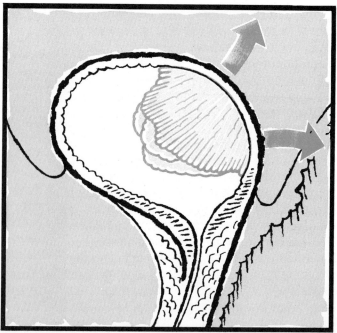

Symptoms of grossly bloody or cloudy urine or frequency of urination do not necessarily indicate cancer of the bladder, but should always be investigated immediately to determine the cause. At left, a papilloma (tumor) blocks the entrance to the urethra. At right, a malignant tumor of the rear wall of the bladder does not completely obstruct urinary outflow. Unless detected and removed early, malignant tumors may spread (arrows) via the lymphatic system to nearby tissues.

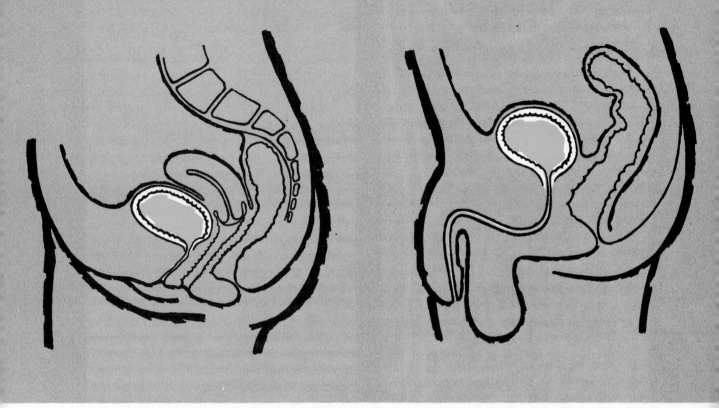

The female urethra, above, is short (about 1½ inches) and is a relatively simple channel from the bladder. The male urethra, at right, is not only longer (about 9 inches) but is more complex because it passes through the prostate gland and receives materials from the sex glands and associated structures.

The posterior urethra contains openings through which the surrounding prostate gland empties its secretions which are carried away in the act of urination. Here, too, are openings of the ejaculatory ducts which carry spermatozoa from the testicle where they are formed to the urethra, to be carried to the outside.

Certain small glands in the anterior urethra (glands of Littre) are important in keeping the urethra lubricated, particularly during sexual intercourse. Cowper's glands, situated in the perineum, also secrete a lubricating fluid and empty into the anterior urethra. It will be seen that the anterior urethra directs two quite different forms of traffic, carrying urine, and materials for reproduction, to the outside.

Because there are marked differences in symptoms and consequences of lesions involving the posterior as compared to the anterior urethra in the male, it is desirable to distinguish them. This knowledge is extremely important because of tremendous differences in effects of lesions in the two areas.

Malformations. Occasionally, a stricture — abnormal narrowing — of the posterior urethra is present at birth or may occur later in life. But for all practical purposes, no congenital anomalies of the posterior urethra exist unless they are associated with exstrophy of the bladder which has previously been described. Congenital anomalies of the urethra are, essentially, defects in construction of the tube itself, and are primarily related to the anterior urethra.

Hypospadias is failure of the urethra to close on the underside, so that instead of a tube it is more like an open trough. Ordinarily, this is a situation which does not extend into the posterior urethra, so that sphincter muscles which control urination function normally and the patient is not incontinent of urine. However, the trough-like external opening on the underside of the penis interferes with

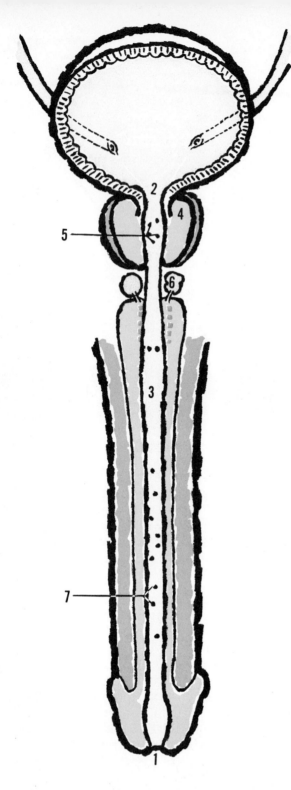

The male urethra from its beginning at the bladder to its termination at the *meatus* (1). The *prostatic* or *posterior urethra* (2) runs through the prostate gland; the rest is the *anterior urethra* (3). The encircling *prostate gland* (4) and the ejaculatory ducts have openings (5) into the prostatic urethra. *Cowper's glands* (6) secrete lubricating fluid into the anterior urethra, as do the *glands of Littre* which have small openings (7) into the forward portion of the urethra.

normal delivery of the urinary stream and with the transport of semen into the female reproductive tract. Plastic reconstruction is indicated if hypospadias is present to any marked degree.

Epispadias is a comparable but less common malformation, in which the upper side of the urethra remains open. The defect may be a slit or roofless channel running for a short distance from the end of the penis on the upper surface, or it may traverse the shaft of the penis more extensively, or the opening may begin and end at the base of the penis. In the latter case, normal sexual intercourse is not possible. Occasionally the posterior urethra is involved, with malformation of bladder sphincters so that the patient cannot control urination, much as would be the case with an exstrophied bladder except that in this case the bladder surface is normally formed. The problem is to restore urinary control and then to form a new tube by plastic surgery, from the re-formed sphincteric area to the outside. Usually the prostate gland, testes, and scrotum are not involved in this abnormality.

Injuries

Injuries to the urethra are serious for two reasons. In the first place, the urethra is a very vascular organ, subject to recurrent engorgement of erectile tissue and alterations in size consequent upon sexual function. Injury to an organ so richly supplied with blood can cause severe hemorrhage, pocketing of blood under the surface and extensive blood loss. In addition, since the urethra is a conduit for urine, an injury which "breaks the pipeline" permits urine to seep into surrounding tissues where it can do nothing but harm.

If the injury is in the posterior urethral region, urine will seep into the perineum and tissues around the bladder and its presence will not be obvious on external examination. It is more difficult to recognize, and more dangerous, than urinary seepage which may occur from "forward" parts of the urethra, and it will create a serious situation very rapidly unless satisfactory drainage and repair of the injury is carried out.

Seepage of urine through tears of the anterior urethra is usually recognized very quickly since there are no sphincters in this area to hold back the evidence. Bleeding is almost constant and, with no sphincter muscle to restrain it, blood drips from the external opening of the urethra. Furthermore, when the patient voids, an alarming swelling of the penis and scrotum is bound to be noticed and called immediately to a physician's attention. Early repair of the tear, and either sidetracking the urine to bypass the injury or satisfactory reconstruction of the conduit, is necessary if severe disability and even more serious consequences are to be avoided.

Strictures

Following injury or infection, stricture of the urethra is not uncommon. A stricture is any abnormal narrowing of the channel which impedes the free flow of urine or in extreme cases shuts it off. Symptoms are slowing of the flow, desire to urinate frequently, and dribbling at the end of the act.

Among the underlying causes of urethral strictures are physical or chemical injuries, congenital malformation and inflammations.

The three most common areas of stricture are: the bladder neck, following operative procedures near the area where the posterior urethra merges with the bladder; the bulbous urethra in the general area where the interior urethra begins; and the meatus or external open-

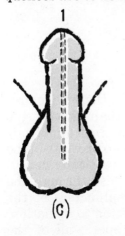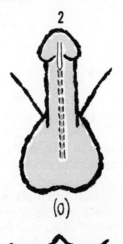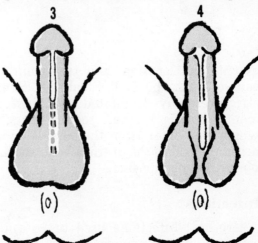

Hypospadias is a congenital malformation in which the male urethra fails to fuse completely on the underside, so there is a trough-like opening of various length instead of a closed tube. 1. Dotted lines show normal urethra. 2. Open defect of terminal portion of the urethra. 3. Imperfect closure of half of the urethra. 4. Urethra open its entire length.

Tumors

Malignant tumors of the posterior urethra are rare unless they arise in the prostate gland (see page 308). Malignant tumors of the anterior urethra are also extremely rare. Blood in the urine and constriction of the urethra with difficulties of urination are symptoms to be investigated without delay. Early radical removal of the tumor combined with irradiation is the treatment of choice.

ing. Strictures of the meatus and contractures of the bladder neck may be congenital in origin and cause difficulty in urination in children. In fact, bladder neck contracture is more common than once was thought, particularly in little girls, and is the precursor of urinary tract infections and serious upper urinary tract difficulties. These can be corrected surgically, once they are recognized by means of x-ray and cystoscopic studies. Strictures vary in their nature,

Strictures or abnormal narrowing of the urinary outlet are not uncommon; congenital contractures of the bladder neck may cause difficulties of urination in children. Below, an abnormal urethral growth causes constriction; at right, stricture of the urethra resulting from infection.

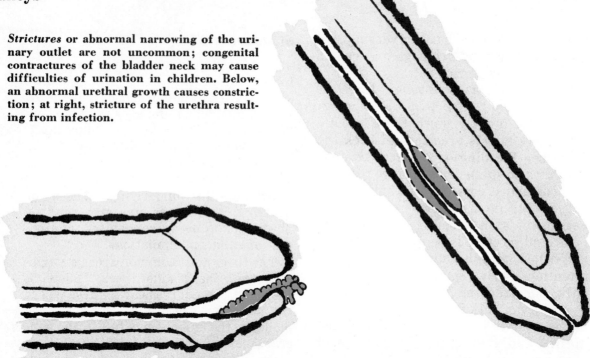

extent, and location, and treatment of course must be individualized. Some strictures may be dilated with instruments (bougies), others require surgery which may enter from the outside or be accomplished in the urethra with special operative instruments.

Infections

Urethral infections used to be quite common, with gonorrhea as the most common precipitator in the young male. In the age group of 45-and-up, infections of the posterior urethra associated primarily with non-specific infections of the prostate are not uncommon. Usual symptoms of an infected urethra are burning sensations when urinating and a frequent urge to do so.

Urethral infections are treated as infections anywhere in the urinary tract, by establishment of adequate drainage, removal of any dead tissue or scar tissue, general care to improve the patient's health, and use of antibiotic or other appropriate drugs, which may require bacteriological identification of the causative organisms from studies of urine and secretions.

The Female Urethra

As already mentioned, the female urethra is much shorter than that of the male, averaging about an inch and a half in length. Since there is no prostate in the female, the urethra is practically devoid of glands, but it does pass through the internal and external sphincters of the bladder which give volition to urination. It runs close to the upper wall of the vagina and its function is purely to transport urine from the bladder to the outside. There is no participation in reproductive function as in the male.

Infection of the bladder neck and urethra is common, and because of the urethra's short length, location, and contiguity to a contaminated environment, infecting organisms are readily transmitted to the bladder to cause infection there. Such an infection needs to be treated carefully so that it does not go on to form a stricture of the urethra and cause a vicious cycle of obstruction, infection, more scar tissue, more obstruction and still more infection. Such a situation may be the precursor of infection ascending up the ureters to the kidney pelvis and the kidneys themselves, producing acute or chronic pyelonephritis which has been shown to be related to hypertension. Therapy for such infection is adequate dilation of the urethra, removal of scar tissue if necessary, and removal of congenital bladder neck contractures if present.

Rarely, cancer occurs in the female urethra. Radical removal with adequate diversion of the urinary stream and possibly associated irradiation therapy is the treatment of choice.

THE PROSTATE GLAND

Accessory sex glands of the male and structures intimately associated with the lower urinary tract traditionally fall within the scope of urology.

The *posterior* or *prostatic urethra* runs through the *prostate gland* and contains muscles that hold urine in the bladder until it is ready to be expelled. Most of the *anterior* (frontal) *urethra* is in the shaft of the penis. The prostate is a mucus-secreting gland with three major lobes, continuous with each other, completely encircling the posterior urethra. The gland has openings through which its own secretions are emptied into the urethra and carried away in the process of urination.

The prostate is a sex gland which develops under the influence of male hormones; it is rudimentary in infants. Ejaculatory ducts which carry male germ cells (spermatozoa) from the testicles enter the prostate and open into the urethra. The scrotal sac contains the *testicles* (testes). Spermatozoa mature in enormous numbers in certain tissues of the testis, while other cells produce male sex hormone which enters the blood stream. Spermatozoa travel through the seminal ducts from the testes to the region of the ejaculatory ducts where there is a reservoir-like structure called the *seminal vesicle*. The latter empties at the time of ejaculation into the posterior urethra through the two openings of the ejaculatory ducts. Simultaneously, the prostate gland contracts and similarly empties its materials. The combined substance, called semen, is then ejaculated by

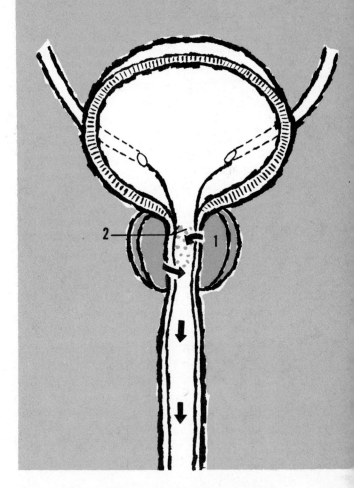

The prostate gland (1) is is an accessory sex organ that encircles the urethra at the bladder outlet and discharges its secretions through prostatic ducts that have tiny openings (2) into the prostatic urethra. Spermatozoa from the seminal vesicles are also discharged into this portion of the urethra.

a wave-like motion in which the frontal part of the urethral sphincter opens and the rearward aspect closes to prevent secretions from entering the bladder.

The prostatic secretion is important in supplying substances for maintenance of spermatozoa in their perilous course in the female genital tract. The secretions maintain delicate acid-base balances and supply substances needed by spermatozoa to carry out their metabolic activities during this period.

Diseases of the prostate gland which surrounds the posterior urethra are very common and very important. Congenital anomalies of the prostate are so extremely rare, unless they are associated with exstrophy of the bladder, that we may disregard them. The two major conditions to which the prostate is prone are infections and tumors. The latter may be benign or malignant.

Examining Methods

First, a word about procedures and purposes of examination of the prostate. With the patient bending over, the doctor inserts a lubricated gloved finger into the rectum. His educated finger tells him a good deal about the condition of the gland, with which it is in contact. His sense of touch tells him that the prostate is firm, or soft and boggy, or stony hard, or hard in a few areas. He massages the gland with a few gentle strokes to expel secretions which will be studied later. The expressed secretions may be found to contain pus, indicating infection, or other elements which assist diagnosis. Prostatic massage is also a useful therapeutic measure to empty the prostate and relieve congestion. The examining procedure takes only a couple of minutes or so and is not attended by any real discomfort.

Urine specimens are also taken, commonly three of them. If the first specimen contains pus or organisms, but the other two, taken after the first passage of urine cleansed the urethra, are clear, infection is probably limited to the urethra. If all three urine specimens are contaminated, infection is more widespread, probably involving the prostate, urethra, bladder, and perhaps upper parts of the urinary tract.

Prostatitis

Infections of the prostate *(prostatitis)* are quite common. Prostatitis in younger men is more likely to be specific — that is, to be caused by particular organisms, such as gonorrhea germs — and to be a spread of infection which moves up the urethra to the prostate or beyond. In mid-life or later, prostatitis is essentially non-specific, non-gonorrheal, and may be associated with a non-specific urethritis which has spread upward to the prostate. Also, the infection may be blood-borne from a focus of infection elsewhere in the body, such as the sinuses, tonsils, teeth.

Acute prostatitis is encountered less frequently since the advent of antibiotics. Symptoms usually are acute indeed: fever, urgency, frequency—compulsions to urinate coming altogether too close. Occasionally there is blood in the urine at the beginning and end of urination. Sitting may be very uncomfortable at times because of pain.

Chronic prostatitis usually is not accompanied by fever. There is a good deal of frequency of urination both day and night. The urine will be cloudy and may or may not have some blood in it at the

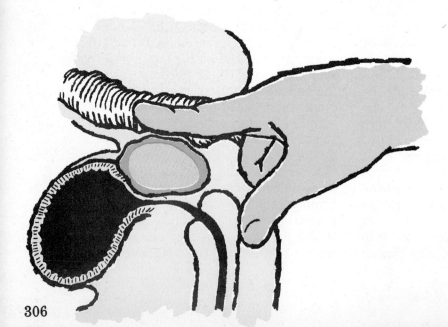

Side view of pelvis showing examination of prostate by finger in rectum. Firmness, bogginess, or hardness of areas of the gland are findings useful in diagnosis. In this instance, an abscess in the prostate has caused enlargement with constriction of the bladder outlet.

beginning or end of urination. Usually there is no history of prior acute prostatitis. Respiratory infections, abscessed teeth, and the like may be contributing factors. Not infrequently there are few or no significant symptoms.

But some patients have a variety of complaints such as diminished sexual drive, incomplete erection or premature ejaculation. It is easier for the physician than the elderly patient to remember that age erodes many virtuosities and that not everything may fairly be blamed on a misbehaving prostate.

Management of prostatitis is essentially the management of infection anywhere: establishment of good drainage, removal of the source of infection, and destruction of the infecting organisms. Since prostatitis is almost always associated with cystitis, the primary cause may be in the bladder itself, such as a stone or necrotic tumor which has predisposed to bladder infection. Prostatitis may be the first evidence of such a lesion in the bladder.

Benign Enlargement

A benign tumor, in medical language, is one which is not cancerous and does not invade other parts of the body. Symptoms of a benign tumor may, however, be anything but benign in the patient's estimation. This is certainly true of benign tumors of the prostate — the so-called *adenomatous hyperplasia* of the prostate. The condition is an overgrowth (hypertrophy) associated with aging. It is rare before 40. Incidence increases with age until, it is estimated, two-thirds of men between the ages of 60 and 70 have some degree of prostatic enlargement. Many have enlargement of such a degree and location that emptying of the bladder is interfered with.

The outstanding symptom of prostatic enlargement from whatever cause is urinary obstruction. All but a small proportion of lesions which obstruct the neck of the male bladder are in the prostate. Obstruction varies in degree and location, but the range of symptoms produced is characteristic. There is increased frequency of urination, especially at night, and the act may require more effort, or take several efforts to complete it. The stream may be slow to start, less forceful, decreased in caliber, and tends to end in terminal dribbling.

Surgery. Factors such as the extent of enlargement, state of kidney function and hazards to the upper urinary tract are considered in deciding whether or not surgery is advisable. A slight enlargement will be detected early in a prudent man who has regular examinations by his doctor, and can be watched. Bladder neck obstruction requires surgical care. Unrelieved obstruction dilates and weakens the bladder, and dammed-back urine can inflate the upper urinary tract and inflict serious damage, even to the extent of kidney failure and uremia. The patient is also very susceptible to superimposed infections which may add appreciably to the complications.

There have been tremendous advances in surgical care of bladder neck obstruction, including improvements in early diagnosis and recognition of changes in the urinary tract and kidneys resulting from prostatism or bladder neck obstruction due to enlargement of the prostate. An "emptying test" of the bladder is of value. This determines how much residual urine remains after the bladder should have emptied completely.

Relief of obstruction must be carried out slowly, with gradual decompression of a chronically overdistended bladder. Results of the obstruction, which are essentially infection and damage to kidneys, ureters, and bladder must be corrected if possible. Surgery for the condition is almost never an emergency and there is ample time to get the patient into the best possible condition.

There are four standard techniques of prostatectomy, three of which are "open" —the area is entered through an outside incision — and one of which employs the urethra as a route of entry. (See Chapter 22). Certain types of enlargements, and certain individuals, lend themselves best to one or another technique.

Benign enlargement of the prostate gland *(adenomatous hyperplasia)* can cause serious damage to the upper urinary tract by obstruction. Below, normal bladder and prostate with unobstructed urine flow (arrows). At right, enlarged prostate (1) compresses bladder outlet. If obstruction is unrelieved, the bladder (2) dilates and weakens; urine backs up (arrows) and enlarges and weakens the ureters (3), and dilates the kidney pelvis (4). Continued pressure can damage kidney tissue very seriously and the patient is susceptible to superimposed infections.

Cancer of the Prostate

Prostatic cancer is the most common cancer to afflict the American male. It is not uncommon in 40 to 50-year-old men, and the incidence increases steadily with age and is very high in men of 70 and over. It is estimated that about 20 per cent of all men over 60 have prostatic cancer. The estimate results from careful post-mortem studies of men of this age group who may have died from some

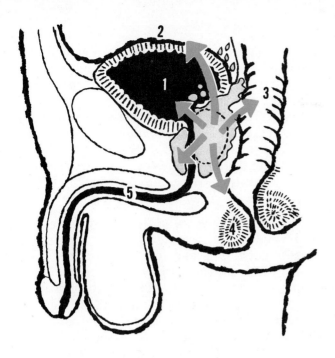

Routes of spread of cancer of the prostate to adjacent tissues: 1. bladder; 2. abdominal cavity; 3. rectum; 4. anal sphincters; 5. urethra. Early cancer of the prostate does not usually cause symptoms of bladder obstruction and the best hope of early discovery is rectal examination at intervals advised by a physician.

other cause without ever knowing that they had cancer of the prostate.

In contrast to benign prostatic hypertrophy, which very early begins to produce obvious evidences of urinary obstruction, prostatic cancer which starts in the outer region of the gland does not immediately involve the bladder outlet and therefore does not produce early impediment of the urinary flow or consequences of obstruction such as infection and renal insufficiency.

Prostatic cancer in early stages may be diagnosed by a routine rectal examination with palpation of the outer surface of the prostate by a finger in the rectum. Presence of a stony-hard area rouses suspicion of prostatic cancer. There are certain conditions — stones in the prostate, and certain chronic infections — which are sometimes difficult to differentiate from cancer by touch alone.

It is therefore necessary to take a biopsy (remove a small piece of tissue) from the suspicious area for study under a microscope to confirm or rule out the presence of cancer. This is a simple procedure requiring not more than 24 to 48 hours in a hospital. It is wise indeed for every man over the age of 50 to have a routine rectal examination every six months, so that if cancer is arising in his prostate it can be recognized early.

When prostate cancer is recognized early and treated by surgery and irradiation, the cure rate is very high. Adjunctive radiation therapy by interstitial insertion of radioactive isotopes of gold has proved of value in early cases. On the other hand, if the cancer is discovered late and has spread outside the confines of the prostate itself, the cure rate is very low. Too often, prostate cancer is discovered too late because it causes no early symptoms and the patient has not taken advantage of regular routine examinations of a simple nature which could have uncovered the condition when chances of cure were excellent.

Hormones. Prostate cancer is the first to be shown, by Dr. Charles Huggins, to be susceptible to the influence of hormones which modify its natural course. It is one of a few malignancies, including female breast cancer, that are "hormone dependent." Male sex hormones have an accelerating effect on prostate cancer; female hormones have an opposite and antagonistic action. The hormonal environment of prostate cancer can be altered beneficially by administration of female sex hormones and/or by castration which removes a natural source of male hormones. Alteration of the secreting powers of the anterior pituitary gland has also been shown to have a beneficial effect.

Hormone therapy does not cure cancer of the prostate, but temporary benefits may last for many months or even two or three years in cases of disseminated prostatic cancer which has spread to organs such as the bone marrow. Although prostatic cancer management has advanced strikingly in the past quarter century, its silent onset and insidious growth lead to late discovery and high incidence which can only be diminished by awareness of every man in his fifties

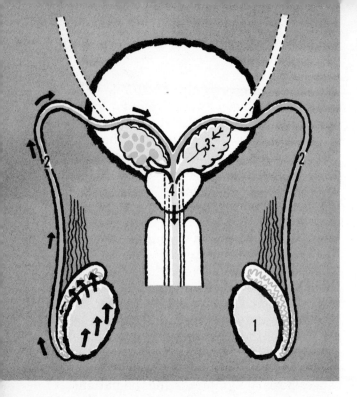

Rear view of male reproductive organs; arrows show route of delivery of spermatozoa to the prostatic urethra. 1. *testis*; 2. *vas deferens*, the excretory duct of the testis; 3. *seminal vesicles*; 4. *prostate gland*. Bladder in background.

or beyond that routine rectal examinations are superb safeguards against future trouble of a most serious nature.

Other Disorders of the Male Sexual Apparatus

Pouches of the *seminal vesicles* which contain seminal fluid are continuous with the prostate. Associated organs are the *vas deferens*, the excretory duct of the testis, and the *epididymis*, a portion of the seminal duct. Infections are the principal disorders of these organs, aside from rare congenital anomalies which may interfere with the conducting system of spermatozoa. Infection usually is secondary to infection of the prostate. Treatment is drainage and proper chemotherapeutic agents, with supportive measures such as hot sitz baths or hot compresses which give comfort.

The Testes

Hormone-producing interstitial cells of the testes are independent of the organ's spermatozoa-producing department (see Chapter 9). Tumors of the interstitial cells are extremely rare. Changes in the portion of the testes which forms the spermatozoa are relatively rare and are usually associated with various forms of intersex. These are congenital anomalies of considerable variety, mixture, and complexity in which the person's "true" sex is ambiguous.

Intersex. Rarely, a patient may have both male and female gonads which secrete both male and female hormones. The opposing organs may "cancel out" and prevent the production of spermatozoa. In some genetic anomalies the patient may appear to be male anatomically and yet be genetically female (as in so-called Klinefelter's syndrome). Determination of the sex of an infant would appear to be simple, and indeed usually is. But at times the external organs may vary in some way from the usual or normal and yet appear to be unmistakably of one sex or the other, and the internal arrangement is not inspectable. Major distortions will be recognized but lesser ones may not be. If a genetic male is brought up as a female, or vice versa, adult life may be anything but wonderful for the patient.

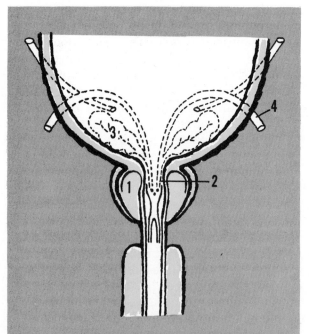

Front view of bladder, prostate and associated structures. 1. *prostate gland*; 2. *ejaculatory duct*; dotted lines indicate structures behind bladder: 3. *seminal vesicles*; 4. *vas deferens from testis*.

Some intersex conditions are correctible or reconstructible to a satisfactory if not total extent by timely surgery. There are many gradations and puzzling anatomical variations and elucidation frequently requires exploratory surgery.

In recent years there have been tremendous advances in understanding of genetic mechanisms involved in sex differentiation. Certain of the heredity-transmitting chromosomes may be duplicated, missing, or combined in abnormal ways to produce various degrees of male-female elements and even infertile "super females" with an excess of X chromosomes. Methods of determining the true sex by studying the nuclei of body cells are now quite practical.

Undescended testis or *cryptorchidism* is a condition in which one or both testes fails to descend from the abdomen, where the organs arise during fetal development, into the scrotum. The situation may be genetic and congenital, or mechanical or endocrine factors may interfere with migration of the testicle relatively late in individual development. If only one testis is involved the defect is probably mechanical in origin, but if it is bilateral the underlying mechanism may be hormonal, such as a poorly functioning

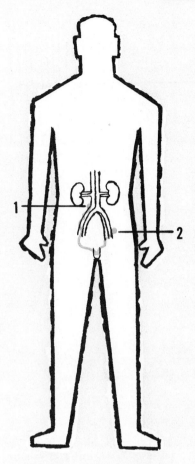

Undescended testes (one or both) remain in some part of the abdominal cavity, through some fault of development, instead of descending into the scrotum before birth. Drawing shows undescended right testis in kidney area (1); left testis in pelvic area (2). At internal body temperatures the testes are incapable of producing spermatozoa.

pituitary gland. Sometimes, improving function by administering pituitary extracts, or marking time until puberty, will ease the testicle into its proper position. However, surgical correction may be necessary. If such is the case, it is generally agreed that the operation should be done at an early age — before the age of five, and certainly before the onset of puberty.

A fully functioning testicle capable of producing spermatozoa requires an environmental temperature lower than that of the internal body. The dependent scrotum, with relaxing and contracting "thermostatic" muscle response, adjusts

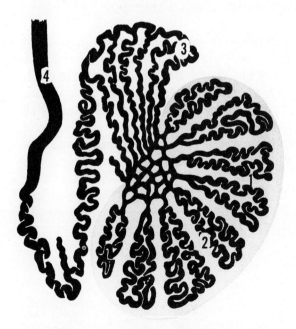

Cross section of testis showing 1. *spermatic tubules*; 2. *interstitial* (hormone-producing) area; 3. conducting tubules of the *epididymis*, a portion of the seminal duct lying upon and behind the testis; 4. *vas deferens* leading to urethra. Pathways of spermatozoa indicated by arrows.

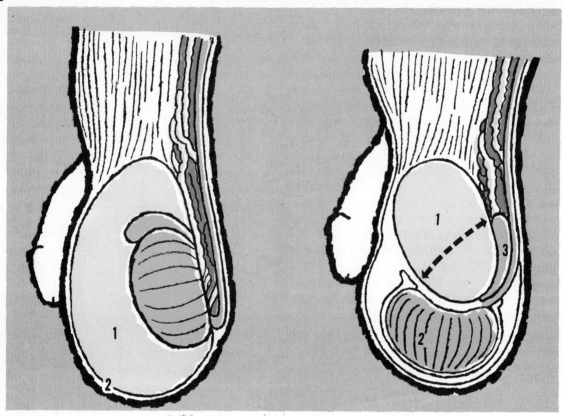

A *hydrocele*, above, is an accumulation of fluid (1) in the sac of the membrane that covers the testis (2), resulting in swelling of the scrotum. A *spermatocele* (right) is a similar cystic dilation (1) of sperm-conducting tubules, causing displacement of the testis (2) and the epididymis (3) that normally rests upon it.

this environment. The reason why sperm-producing tissues cannot function normally in the internal heat of the body is not clear but is one of the facts that nature appears to have ordained.

Tumors of the testicle are not unusual. They are highly malignant and may occur at any age, but are most common in the early teens and twenties. Any mass in the testicle, especially if it is not associated with fever, should be suspected of being the seat of a malignant tumor. Treatment is extensive surgical excision and, depending on the type of tumor, irradiation therapy.

Hydrocele is an accumulation of fluid in the scrotum, cystic dilation of the coverings of the testis. The swelling is obvious, varies in size, and may be painful. Hydrocele is frequently associated with hernias. *Spermatocele* is a similar cyst involving the sperm-conducting apparatus. Treatment is by excision.

THE ENDOCRINE GLANDS

by ROBERT B. GREENBLATT, M.D., and CHARLES WELLER, M.D.

Location of Endocrine Glands • Glands, Physique and Behavior • Hypothalamus • The Pituitary Gland • Acromegaly • Giantism • Dwarfism • Sexual Precocity • Sexual Infantilism • Panhypopituitarism • Persistent Lactation • Diabetes Insipidus

THE THYROID GLAND

Hyperthyroidism • Forms of Treatment • Hypothyroidism • Cretinism • Colloid Goiter • Nodular or Adenomatous Goiters • Thyroiditis • Tests of Thyroid Function

THE PARATHYROID GLANDS

Hyperparathyroidism • Hypoparathyroidism

THE ADRENAL GLANDS

Hypercorticoidism • Excessive Sex Hormone Secretion • Pheochromocytoma

THE TESTES

THE OVARY

The Amenorrheas • Excessive Uterine Bleeding • Ovarian Virilsm

INFERTILITY

THE MENOPAUSE

MISCELLANEOUS CONDITIONS

DIABETES

MANAGEMENT OF THE DIABETIC PATIENT

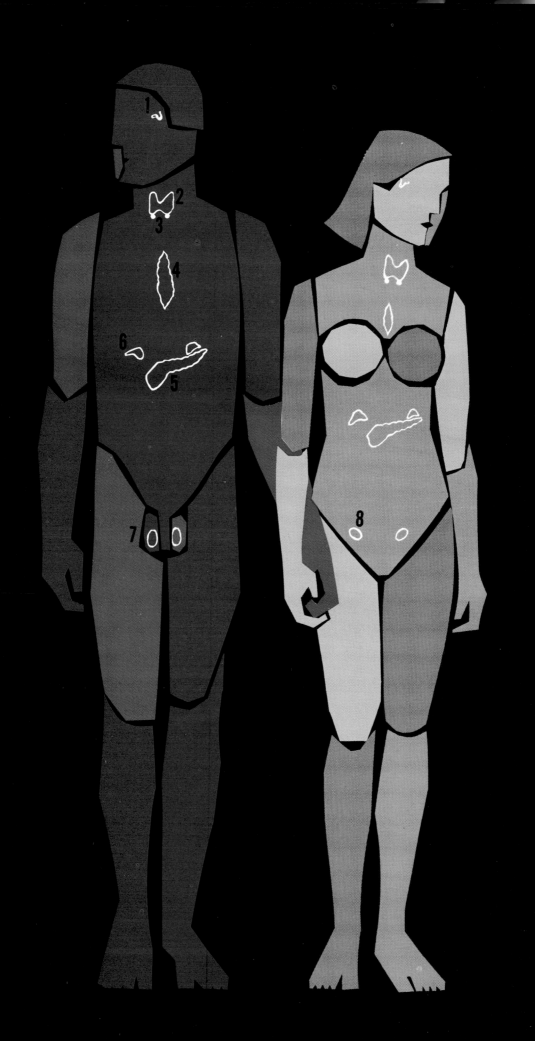

THE ENDOCRINE GLANDS

by ROBERT B. GREENBLATT, M.D.

A chemical system of communication between cells collaborates with the nervous system in adjusting the body to constant internal and external buffetings of environment. Chemical messengers or *hormones* are secreted into the bloodstream by endocrine glands located in various parts of the body, indicated in the small figure above.

The endocrine glands are the same in men and women, except for the *gonads*, the testes and ovaries of the respective sexes. The color plate shows the endocrine glands "in location" in a male and female figure: 1. The *pituitary* gland at the base of the brain; 2. the *thyroid* gland in the neck; 3. the *parathyroid* glands, imbedded on the surface of the thyroid; 4. the *thymus* gland, relatively large in infants but small in size in adults; 5. the *pancreas* gland which secretes insulin hormone as well as digestive enzymes; 6. the *adrenal* glands astride the kidneys; 7. the *testes*; 8. the *ovaries*.

Hormones are carried all over the body to reach the various organs and tissues they are destined to affect in delicate interrelationships.

Have you ever wondered, what is man, and what is woman? About the secrets of sex and the miracle of reproduction? Why some individuals are tall, others small; some fat, others lean; some slow, others quick; some strong, some weak? Or wondered how man copes with the daily hustle and bustle of a competitive world and faces rage, hate, and fear, yet finds time for love and laughter?

If you marvel at man's complex design and chemistry that enables him to adjust to his changing environment, heat and cold, food excesses and deprivations, the stresses of injury, infection and emotional strain, then you are interested in man's "endocrines". It is the function of the glands of internal secretion such as the pituitary, the thyroid, the adrenals, the gonads and others to maintain the constancy of the internal environment, i.e., the chemistry of the body.

"You are what you are because of your glands" is a somewhat trite statement but there is considerable truth in it. Nonetheless, the precept has been advanced that the individual is the product of his environment. This theme was so pithily expressed by Tennyson in epitomizing the exploits and adventures of Ulysses with, "I am a part of all that I have met." Fascinating as these postulates are, it is impossible to discount the very important place heredity and nutrition play in the molding of man, of nations, of civilizations.

Neither may the role of the endocrine glands be minimized, for in every individual they significantly affect the activity of every cell in the body, influence mental acuity, physical agility, build and stature, bodily hair growth, voice pitch, sexual urge, and behavior. In fact, the endocrine system tempers every waking and sleeping moment of life, and constantly modifies the way we feel, think, behave, and react to all sorts of stimuli.

Endocrinology is a science which concerns itself with the function of those glands which secrete into the blood stream one or more specific chemical compounds known as *hormones* or *endocrines*. Hormones are chemical messengers which arouse or set into motion certain functions necessary for the health of the body as a whole.

The ability of man to respond and adapt successfully to his changing environment is made possible mainly by the successful coordination of two great systems. One of these is the *nervous* system, the other is the system of *chemical* messengers.

The hormones are carried all over the body and reach the various organs and tissues which each of them will respectively affect. In the normal body, there is harmonious interrelationship between the endocrine glands. Under rare circumstances too much or too little of these specific compounds may be manufactured, resulting in certain disease states.

Location of Endocrine Glands

Various parts of the body harbor the endocrine glands, as shown in the drawings that introduce this chapter. The *pituitary* gland, the size of an acorn, is situated at the base of the brain and is protected by the skull. The *thyroid* and *parathyroid* glands lie in the neck; the *pancreas, adrenals,* and *ovaries* are in the abdomen, and the *testicles* are in the scrotum. *Gonad* is a general term for the ovary and testis.

The *thymus* gland which lies high in the chest is relatively large in infants but greatly diminished in size in adults. It is thought that the thymus plays a part in inciting immunological processes that give resistance to disease and infections. The pancreas gland has two "departments" — one, an endocrine department, with "islet" cells that produce *insulin,* a hormone; and another department which produces digestive enzymes that enter the upper intestinal tract. Little is known of the function, if any, of the *pineal* gland (meaning "shaped like a pine cone") which is situated at the base of the brain.

The pineal body appears to be a vestigial organ that probably once served a purpose in the course of human evolution.

There are other organs and tissues, not primarily thought of as endocrine glands, which secrete hormones as part of their functions. Acid-laden food in the stomach triggers the production of *secretin,* a hormone which stimulates pancreatic cells to turn out digestive juices at the right time. The kidneys also secrete hormone-like substances.

Glands, Physique and Behavior

Although endocrinology is a relatively new science, observations and experiments of an endocrinological nature are very ancient. The gelding of the stallion and the castration of male calves to make steers have been practiced for centuries. It has long been known that castration induces certain changes in the physical makeup and behavior response of both man and domestic animals. The castration of cocks changes them from crowing, fighting birds to fat, docile capons. It is evident that the "male sex hormone" is not only responsible for certain physical characteristics but also personality traits. It is indeed remarkable that the clinical entity which we recognize today as eunuchoidism was recognized as long as 2000 years ago. Matthew (19:12) records in his Gospel "For there are some eunuchs which were so born from their mother's womb".

Today, the young man so deprived of his heritage may be given solace and comfort, for he may be restored to physical fitness by substitutional therapy with testosterone, the so-called "male sex hormone". So, too, the young woman robbed of her birthright of the full-bloom of maturity because of poor or absent ovarian function may seek and receive aid.

A brief description of some disorders resulting from aberrations in endocrine function will give an insight into the manner by which the endocrine glands radically affect the structure and function of the body as a whole, as well as the workings of the mind.

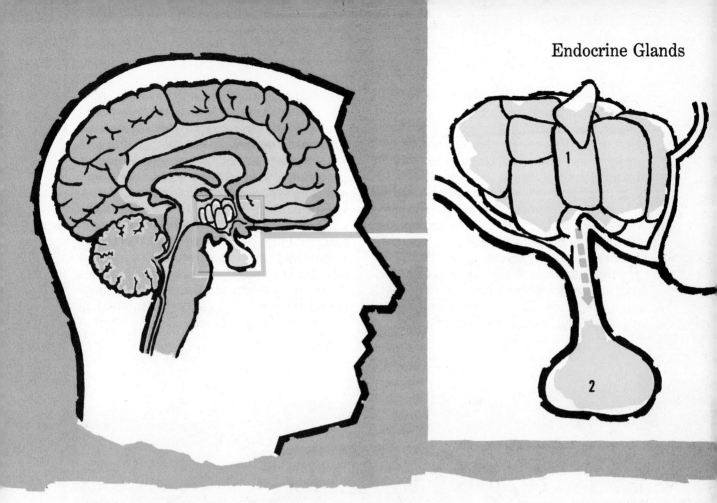

The *hypothalamus* is a small area of the brain that provides a link between the cerebral cortex or "thinking" part of the brain and the pituitary gland. At left above, orientation of the hypothalamus with the pituitary below it. Enlarged cross section shows nuclei that make up the *hypothalamus* (1) and the *pituitary gland* (2). Stimulatory and inhibitory agents originating in the hypothalamus play a part in directing pituitary function, suggested by arrow.

Let us take the thyroid gland as an example. Normal thyroid hormone production is necessary to maintain normal metabolism, and mental and physical activity. When too much is manufactured by the thyroid gland a state of hyperthyroidism supervenes. The mind, the heart and the oxygen consumption of the tissues are "pepped up" like a racing engine. Too little thyroid function, on the other hand, leads to mental sluggishness and physical inertia.

Let us consider other far-flung effects of endocrine function and disorder, with respect to particular glands.

Hypothalamus

The *hypothalamus* is part of the midbrain, the *diencephalon*. It is the "old brain" and the seat of those primitive instincts necessary to preserve the species, such as procreation, fight for self preservation, and flight from danger. Before man evolved to his present station, it is believed that the original brain was not covered by the outer brain or cortex. With the acquisition of a cortex man acquired intellect, memory, thought processes and rationalization.

The hypothalamus provides a connecting link between the cerebral cortex and the pituitary gland. Certain metabolic functions under the control of the hypothalamus are of considerable importance in endocrinology. Though the pituitary gland is considered the "master gland," nevertheless, there are stimulatory and inhibitory agents originating in the hypothalamus which direct pituitary function. This ancient area in our brain is also intimately concerned with regulation of energy balance through the control of appetite, sleep, body temperature, regulation of sexual function and control of water balance.

Lesions or disturbances in the hypothalamus may cause such endocrine disorders as *sexual precocity* or sexual infantilism; absence of appetite with extreme loss of weight, or insatiable appetite with enormous obesity; *diabetes insipidus* with its increased thirst and uncontrollable output of large amounts of urine; disorganization of the sleep rhythm and *narcolepsy*, as well as hibernating (low) temperatures and extremely high ones, too. Emotional disturbances, anxiety, and worry, and aberrations in "thinking" functions of the brain may upset hypothalamic-pituitary mechanisms. The young woman overanxious for pregnancy may cease to menstruate and will display many of the symptoms of pregnancy, such as nausea and abdominal swelling, yet not be pregnant.

Subject to re-interpretation in the light of this concept are the obesities in certain maladjusted individuals, forms of goiter in persons subjected to repeated psychic trauma, menstrual disturbances in women experiencing distressing emotional episodes, and endocrine imbalance in the neurotic, tormented young woman

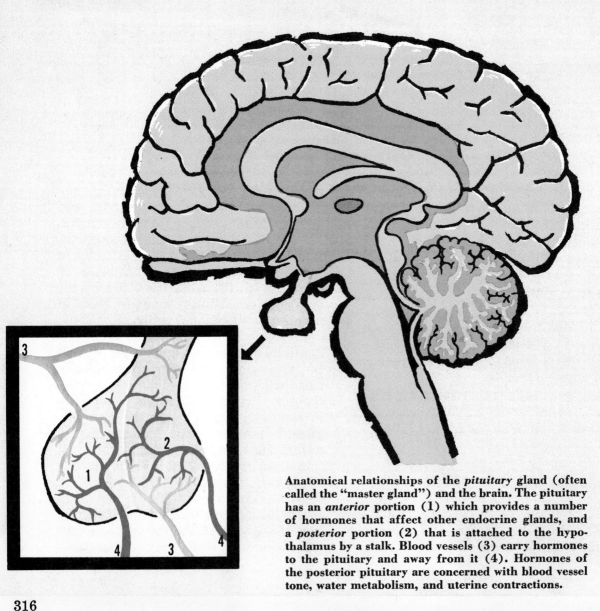

Anatomical relationships of the *pituitary* gland (often called the "master gland") and the brain. The pituitary has an *anterior* portion (1) which provides a number of hormones that affect other endocrine glands, and a *posterior* portion (2) that is attached to the hypothalamus by a stalk. Blood vessels (3) carry hormones to the pituitary and away from it (4). Hormones of the posterior pituitary are concerned with blood vessel tone, water metabolism, and uterine contractions.

with loss of appetite *(anorexia nervosa).* None too obvious mental hurts are reflected in disturbances of bodily function, just as illness and disorders of the body condition and shade every thought and action.

Indeed, the hypothalamus and the pituitary gland are both functionally and anatomically related. Our thoughts, our hopes and joys, our worries and our sorrows, our very nervous constitution—all profoundly influence the hypothalamus-pituitary partnership.

The Pituitary Gland

The *pituitary gland,* frequently referred to as the "master gland," is situated in a special protected cavity at the base of the brain known as the *sella turcica* ("Turk's saddle"). Its removal is followed by signs of thyroid failure, atrophy of sex glands and adrenal insufficiency. In the young, growth is arrested and weight loss is a frequent accompaniment.

The pituitary gland is divided into an *anterior* or forward part composed of glandular tissue and a *posterior* part composed of nerve-like tissue. The gland is connected with the brain by a thin stalk.

The anterior portion produces several hormones which stimulate distant structures or targets: *somatotrophin* (growth stimulating hormone); *adreno-corti-cotrophin* (ACTH) which stimulates the adrenal cortex; *thyroid stimulating* hormone (TSH); and *gonadotrophic* hormones which stimulate the ovaries and testicles. In the female the gonadotrophins are a follicle stimulating hormone, (FSH) and luteinizing hormone (LH). In the male these same hormones are known as FSH and ICSH (interstitial cell-stimulating hormone). The interstitial cells of the testis are the ones that produce so-called male hormones.

Other hormones of the pituitary gland are *prolactin,* which stimulates breast-milk production, and *melano-stimulating* hormone (MSH), which influences pigment production by certain cells of the skin, the melanophores.

The *posterior* part of the gland is an extension of the hypothalamus, that portion of the brain to which the pituitary stalk is attached. The posterior pituitary stores and secretes two hormones; one is *vasopressin,* which has to do with blood vessel tone and is the antidiuretic hormone influencing water metabolism; the other is *oxytocin,* which promotes uterine contractions and has the property of "letting down" milk in the lactating breast.

Altogether, the pituitary gland produces a number of hormones of diverse effects. Disorders of the pituitary gland are those of too much or too little hormone production. These will be discussed according to the particular hormone or hormones involved.

Syndrome	Hormone Involved	
Acromegaly		too much
Giantism	Growth stimulating hormone (Somatotrophin)	too much too early
Dwarfism		too little
Thyrotoxicosis	Thyroid stimulating hormone (TSH)	too much
Masked myxedema		too little
Cushing's Disease (of Pituitary origin)	Adrenal cortex stimulating hormone (ACTH)	too much
Adrenal insufficiency (of Pituitary origin)		too little
Sexual precocity	Ovary and testes stimulating hormones (Gonadotrophins)	too much too early
Sexual infantilism		too little
Panhypopituitarism	All pituitary hormones	too little
Syndrome of persistent lactation	Prolactin	too much
Diabetes insipidus	Antidiuretic hormone	too little

A brief description of each disorder follows. Disorders involving TSH and ACTH will be discussed in the sections devoted to the thyroid and adrenals.

Acromegaly

Acromegaly is a chronic progressive disease due to hypersecretion of the growth-stimulating hormone. In most instances, a benign tumor is the seat of the trouble.

The disorder is characterized by enlargement of the hands and feet, cartilaginous part of bones, soft tissues of the body, and such structures as the heart, spleen and liver. The frontal bones and jaw become prominent, the nose widens, the teeth become spaced, the lower eyelids are baggy, the tongue markedly enlarged. The thickened features of the face impart a bulldog look.

The diagnosis is readily made by the appearance of the spade-like hands and the coarse facial features. X-rays reveal many bony protrusions (exostoses), tufting of the bones at the tip of the fingers and toes, and general thickening of the long bones. The bony cavity at the base of the skull which houses the pituitary gland usually is enlarged. Frequently there is a concomitant diabetes mellitus which may persist even after the disease plays itself out. During the active phase, headaches are frequent, sexual drive wanes, and excessive strength gives way to progressive weakness. Lactation may be present in both men and women.

If the pituitary tumor is large enough to threaten or interfere severely with vision, due to pressure on the adjacent optic nerves, surgical interference is mandatory. Otherwise, deep x-ray therapy directed at the pituitary gland is often effective. In many milder cases, the female hormones have been used successfully to inhibit pituitary growth hormone in the female, and large doses of androgens have been similarly employed in the management of the disorder in the male, before the smoldering fires of activity are extinguished.

Giantism

The excessive secretion of growth hormone before the closure of the growing ends of bone has taken place results in abnormal tallness. Height is considered excessive when boys reach a height greater than six feet six inches and girls above six feet tall.

Not all cases of giantism are due to a hyperactive pituitary gland or adenoma. Excessive height may occur in eunuchoid males and in girls with primary loss of ovarian function, since in such persons there is insufficient sex hormone to inhibit the growth hormone or to hasten closure of the growing ends of bone (the epiphyses). Then, too, there are cases of genetic giantism which run in families and in certain races.

If uncomplicated by other endocrine disturbances, rapid growth due to pituitary hyperactivity or adenoma may be slowed in some instances by radiation to the pituitary gland. The administration of estrogens continuously for a period of a year or more in adequate dosage will hasten the closure of bone growth and will restrain further growth to one, two, or three inches if administered to girls with a trend toward abnormal height. Therapy should be started, if the growing ends of bones still remain open, when a height of 65 to 67 inches is reached.

One of the complications of treatment is excessive menstrual bleeding. This may be readily avoided by the administration of an oral progestin for five days in each month. In this manner regular menstrual-like bleeding may be induced. The progestogen must be continued for at least 12-18 months after discontinuing estrogen therapy to help regulate the menstrual cycle and avoid excessive bouts of uterine bleeding.

In males, it is more difficult to arrest linear growth but it may be accomplished by large doses of testosterone. However, on such medication one must expect a spurt of 3-4" of growth the first year.

Dwarfism

Lack of growth hormone production leads to a condition known as *pituitary dwarfism.* Pituitary dwarfs have the aspect of frail, fragile, miniature persons, reminiscent of a china doll.

However, these are rare. More frequent is dwarfism due either to constitutional illness, nutritional disturbance, parasitic disease, bone dystrophy, childhood thyroid deficiency, juvenile diabetes, and certain types of primary sex gland failure. Genetic dwarfism occasionally occurs in normal families, but as a rule is confined to racial groups such as the Pygmies of Africa.

There is also the boy and girl with a slow "growth clock," who present a problem in diagnosis and need for treatment. Such children have a retarded "bone age." This is, the rate of maturation of the growing ends of bones is less than is expected for a child of given chronological age. "Bone age" may be determined readily by x-ray studies of the hand. For psychologic reasons it may be worthwhile to help such patients attain their predestined growth earlier. The administration of anabolic agents — steroid drugs which have a constructive or "building up" action — along with a high protein diet has proved quite successful.

Dwarfism associated with *myxedema* (thyroid insufficiency) readily responds to thyroid medication. Constitutional illness can retard growth, and so can nutritional deficiencies and parasitic infections. Correction of the underlying cause usually proves helpful.

Achondroplastic dwarfs are not primarily endocrine problems and their status cannot be changed. Such dwarfs are characterized by short legs and arms, big head and face, and square nose with a depressed bridge. They are active, strong and usually intelligent. These are the usual "circus dwarfs." Attila the Hun was said to be an achondroplastic dwarf.

Sexual Precocity

Premature sexual development is termed precocious when both the secondary sex characteristics and maturation of the primary sex glands occur before the age of nine. When only the secondary sex characteristics show early maturation, without concomitant gonadal development, the condition is known as *pseudoprecocity*.

In the former, the inhibitory effects of the hypothalamus on the pituitary gland are lacking, and the ovary and testis-stimulating gonadotrophins (FSH and LH) are released prematurely. The ovaries are thus stimulated to precocious activity and breast development, growth of pubic hair, and menstruation occur. Immediate body growth is rapid, but so is the rate of bone maturation, resulting ultimately in reduced stature.

In boys, the voice changes, and the increased muscle mass, strength, and adult proportions of the genitals are striking. Hypothalamic lesions occur quite frequently in the male, accounting for the disturbed control over the pituitary. Pseudoprecocity may also be produced by feminizing tumors of the ovary and in boys, by congenital abnormal multiplication of cells of the adrenal gland *(adrenal hyperplasia)* as well as virilizing tumors of the testes.

Sexual precocity may be confined to one or two "targets," and may not represent excessive hormonal production but increased sensitivity of certain target structures to minimal amounts of hormones. Examples are precocious breast growth known as *thelarche*, and pubic hair growth known as *pubarche*.

Heterosexual pseudoprecocity occurs in females with virilizing adrenal tumors or with congenital adrenal hyperplasia. In such instances, pubic hair, enlargement of the clitoris, advanced bone age on x-ray, and high urinary *androgens* (substances which have masculinizing activity), aid in the diagnosis. Enlargement of the clitoris, with and without other manifestations, may occur in a female child as a result of hormone administration to the mother, during pregnancy, of androgens or certain progestins with mild androgenic activity.

Sexual Infantilism

Failure of development of secondary sexual characteristics does not become evident until the period of pubescence has passed. Such individuals retain the appearance of arrested childhood.

The infantile genitals, the scantiness or absence of pubic and underarm hair, the persistence of childlike features, may be indicative of a lack of gonad stimulating secretion by the pituitary gland. When only this gonadotrophic hormone is lacking, it is a selective form of pituitary failure. When some or all of the other pituitary hormones are absent, the condition is known as *panhypopituitarism*. Of course, the sexual infantilism may be not of pituitary origin but due to failure of the ovary or testis, and in such instances height may be normal or excessive. The bone age in either case is markedly delayed.

The eunuchoid male or the girl with sexual infantilism due to selective pituitary failure is best treated by replacement therapy with gonadal hormones, rather than by pituitary hormones. Growth and development of secondary sexual characteristics may be expected. Medication must be continued indefinitely.

In both the affected adult male and female, infertility is present, but with recent medical advances in making human gonadotrophins available there is the possibility of overcoming the failure of ovulation in the female and sperm production in the male. Such unfortunates, robbed of their heritage, may now hope and not in vain.

Panhypopituitarism

Destruction of the anterior pituitary gland with a loss of its secretory function is followed by a functional failure of the target organs under pituitary control, such as the thyroid, the adrenals, and the gonads. Loss of pituitary function may result from a tumor, cyst, necrosis, or calcification of the gland. Tumors in areas close to the pituitary will yield the same symptoms. Space-filling lesions are more common in men. The syndrome varies in severity and in the degree to which any one target gland is affected, and at what time of life the damage occurs. When severe, the syndrome is known as *Simmonds' disease*.

Panhypopituitarism is more common in females. When the syndrome follows post-childbirth hemorrhage it is known as *Sheehan's disease*. The sensitized pituitary gland of pregnancy suffers from temporary local deficiency of blood because of severe post partum hemorrhage.

Sexual infantilism and dwarfism occur in persons affected by loss of anterior pituitary function before puberty. In the postpuberal group, there is loss of sexual hair, unexplained anemia, weakness and fatigue, and in many there is loss of weight. If the hypothalamus is involved, obesity may be present. Low blood pressure, slow pulse, lethargy, poor tolerance of infections, intolerance of cold, atrophy of the genitals, absence of menstruation in the female, loss of sexual potency in the male, and premature aging characterize the disorder. The affliction pursues a prolonged course of chronic invalidism that may last 20 or more years, but the slow, inexorable sapping of vitality reduces the patient to a twilight existence, more vegetable than human.

The treatment is directed toward replacement of "missing" hormones, such as estrogens and androgens, adrenal cortical hormones when necessary, and thyroid medication. Menstruation may be induced by cyclic estrogen-progesterone therapy. Restitution toward semi-normalcy is not beyond the hope of every such individual. Where expanding pituitary tumors or other lesions are present, surgery and radiation therapy along with hormonal therapy are in order.

Persistent Lactation

Persistent lactation in non-menstruating women who are not nursing infants also occurs and is frequently associated with a pituitary tumor which apparently secretes the hormone, *prolactin*, which stimulates breast-milk production. Persistent lactation may occur in other circumstances, such as subsequent to chest and neck surgery or pelvic surgery. It has followed the use of certain tranquilizing drugs that influence hypothalamic function. Lactation may follow resection of the stalk of the pituitary gland, by severing the hypothalamic control of pituitary prolactin secretion. Lactation may be seen in patients with acromegaly. Persistent amenorrhea and lactation occasionally follow normal parturition; it is known as Chari-Frommel syndrome. Several women with the syndrome have been seen following several years on birth control pills.

Diabetes Insipidus

Diabetes insipidus (not to be confused with *diabetes mellitus,* or "sugar diabetes") is sometimes referred to as "water diabetes" because of the constant insatiable thirst and the tremendous output of clear-colored urine. It is as a rule a disorder which originates in the hypothalamus and involves the posterior pituitary gland. Hypothalamic centers secrete the *antidiuretic hormone* which checks urine secretion, and this hormone is stored in the posterior pituitary gland. Any lesion along the tract between the secretory hypothalamic centers and the storehouse will result in diabetes insipidus, provided the adrenal glands are functioning adequately.

The disorder is a failure of the kidneys to reabsorb water, due to an ineffective circulating level of antidiuretic hormone (ADH). There is another type of diabetes insipidus — the renal or nephrogenic type — in which there is adequate supply of antidiuretic hormone, but the renal tubules are insensitive to its action. In either case, as the disease progresses, constipation, dry skin, and loss of weight and appetite become pronounced. The person's life is confined between the water jug and the lavatory.

Thirst and excessive urine may occur with other conditions, such as diabetes mellitus, hyperparathyroidism, certain cases of renal disease, and sometimes have an underlying psychogenic origin.

The best test to help differentiate between true diabetes insipidus, nephrogenic diabetes insipidus, and psychogenic cases, is by the "water loading" test, followed by hypertonic saline infusion. Diuresis will cease in the normal and psychogenic cases, but continue in true diabetes insipidus. If a posterior pituitary hormone with antidiuretic properties (Pitressin) is then administered, diuresis will be arrested in true diabetes insipidus but not in the nephrogenic type.

Treatment is either the administration of Pitressin by injection, or posterior powder snuffed into the nostrils. Paradoxically, the chlorothiazide diuretics which enhance urine secretion have been found most useful, particularly in nephrogenic diabetes insipidus. Many patients with true diabetes insipidus also respond well, though not completely. Recently an anti-hyperglycemic agent, chlorpromazine, has proved effective in controlling diabetes insipidus, and holds much promise in use except in patients who already have low blood sugars.

THE THYROID GLAND

The *thyroid gland,* which weighs about an ounce or less, is located in the neck and is composed of two lobes joined by an isthmus or constricted part. It lies in front of and on either side of the windpipe and just beneath the larynx or voice-box. The thyroid gland is the central organ in a system that incorporates iodine into compounds of great hormonal activity, and makes them available for action in the tissues.

Iodine. The function of the gland is dependent upon a proper supply of iodine. Iodides are present in foodstuffs and enter the circulation following digestion. Inorganic iodine, i.e., the iodides, is taken up from the circulation and incorporated within the thyroid gland. The iodine combines with certain amino acids (tyrosine), and the hormone that results is stored as *thyroglobulin* in the acini or glands that make up the individual units of the thyroid gland. The hormone is released from the thyroid in the form of *thyroxine.*

Today, two pure thyroid hormone preparations are clinically available, the slowly acting *thyroxine* and the potent, rapidly acting *triiodothyronine.* Thyroid extracts are widely used and commonly are composed mostly of thyroglobulin and thyroxine.

The activity of the thyroid gland, its trapping, organification, storage, and release is under control of the pituitary's thyroid-stimulating hormone.

Thyroid hormone affects the metabolism of practically all the tissues of the body. The principal function of the hormone is to regulate the rate of oxygen

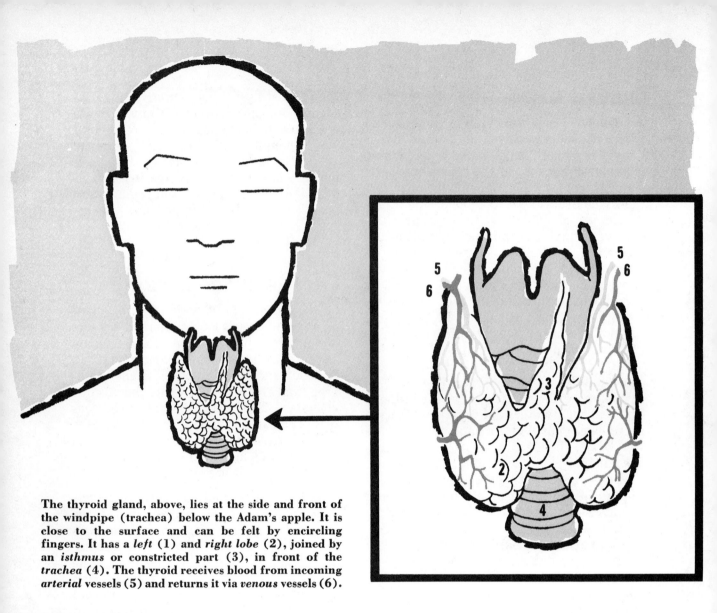

The thyroid gland, above, lies at the side and front of the windpipe (trachea) below the Adam's apple. It is close to the surface and can be felt by encircling fingers. It has a *left* (1) and *right lobe* (2), joined by an *isthmus* or *constricted* part (3), in front of the *trachea* (4). The thyroid receives blood from incoming *arterial* vessels (5) and returns it via *venous* vessels (6).

consumption, that is, the metabolic rate of tissues, which can be thought of as one's "rate of living." The hormone is required for normal growth and development of the brain and of muscle and bones. It indirectly affects the activity of other glands of internal secretion.

Too little thyroid hormone produces a low metabolic rate and slows down all the biologic processes. Even production of adrenalin by the adrenal glands is slowed down, and when too much thyroid hormone is produced, the heart muscle becomes sensitized to the circulating adrenalin, resulting in rapid heart action.

For good thyroid function, there must be normal pituitary function, normal iodine intake from food and water, and normal synthesis and release of thyroid hormone by the gland. Inadequate iodine supplies and excessive intake of iodides and certain drugs that impede hormone synthesis may result in thyroid enlargement and goiter development. There are several disorders of the thyroid gland and each of these will be discussed briefly.

Hyperthyroidism

Hyperthyroidism is known by a variety of names: *thyrotoxicosis, toxic goiter,* Graves' disease. There are two principal types of the disorder, one in which the thyroid gland is too active because of constant stimulation from the hypothalamus via the pituitary gland—a concept not completely substantiated since elevated levels of TSH cannot be demonstrated. In recent years, the presence of LATS—a long-acting thyroid stimulating substance—has been confirmed and believed to be responsible for accentuation of thyroid activity leading to thyrotoxicosis. The other type, frequently referred to as a toxic adenoma, functions independently of pituitary control. It is an autonomous tumor. The symptoms are similar except that in Graves' disease, bulging of the eyeballs (*exophthalmos*) is a frequent accompaniment. The symptoms are marked apprehension and alertness, nervousness, loss of weight, increased thirst, frequent urination, profuse perspiration, intolerance of heat, insomnia, frequent stools, rapid heart beat and palpitations. The skin is soft, smooth, warm and moist. The appetite may be ravenous but body weight cannot be maintained.

Advantages and disadvantages must be weighed in the selection of each of the three major methods of treatment now available to the patient. These are (1) *antithyroid drugs*, (2) *surgical interference* by removal of the tumor, or partial removal of the thyroid in cases of diffuse increase in size, and (3) the use of *radioactive iodine* or "the cocktail".

Forms of Treatment

Antithyroid Drugs. In young people with diffuse goiter of moderate size, there is much in favor of a long-term trial of antithyroid drug therapy. If successful, normal health and normal thyroid function may be restored. About 50 per cent may expect a long-lasting remission. If the response is satisfactory the treatment should be adequate and long enough, from one to two years or longer. A favorable response may be indicated in most instances by reduced pulse rate, increase in weight, and return of well-being feelings.

Treatment should be stopped in those patients who experience adverse reactions to antithyroid drugs, such as skin wheals, (urticaria), loss of head hair (alopecia), or marked drop in the white blood cell count (agranulocytosis). Blood counts should be performed regularly at monthly intervals and a drop to less than 50 per cent of the initial white blood cell count should serve as a warning. Only a few patients are adversely sensitive to propylthiouracil or methimazole, the antithyroid drugs of choice.

Surgery. It is the considered opinion of the author that surgery should be reserved for those patients who are unable to cooperate on a program of long-term therapy or for whom it is economically unsound; it should be reserved for patients with very large goiters and particularly those with adenomatous goiters.

The operation is an elective procedure to be undertaken only in patients who have been adequately prepared by drug treatment. The toxic patient must be restored to a more normal state prior to surgery by antithyroid drugs, and then two or three weeks of treatment with potassium iodide before the operation is added to the program. With such preparation, the operation is attended by few risks and the possibility of thyroid "storm" or crisis is avoided.

Radioactive Iodine has become the treatment of choice of most physicians for the elderly patient. Children and pregnant women are not suitable candidates for this form of therapy.

In the pregnant woman, radioactive iodine may damage the thyroid gland of the unborn child. In children, radioactive iodine therapy is proscribed because infants and children are quite susceptible to carcinogenic effects of radiation.

The greatest problem in treatment is selection of a dose of radioactive iodine, contained in water and drunk as a "cocktail", which will destroy enough but not all of the gland, and restore to normal the amount of hormone produced and released. In treatment, several small doses of two to three millicuries of radioactive iodine are administered two to four months apart, depending on need. In this manner excessive amounts are avoided.

General Considerations. The patient with a thyrotoxic condition needs rest, a quiet environment, good dietary intake, vitamin supplements, and some sedation before surgery and after. Reserpine may be employed to great advantage to help relax the over-anxious patient and slow the pulse rate.

Exophthalmos, or bulging eyes, may be a prominent sign in Graves' disease.

This may disappear or be reduced considerably with adequate management of the thyrotoxicosis. In some individuals the exophthalmos worsens in spite of treatment, and others who had minimal signs may develop severe exophthalmos following surgery. Treatment is difficult once severe or malignant exophthalmos has developed. Radiation of the pituitary gland has been used successfully in a few instances. Decompression operations which remove the posterior part of the bony eyeball socket are sometimes necessary to save vision. In the milder forms, diuretics, sleeping in a semi-recumbent position, tranquilizers, or cortisone-like hormones have been employed with some degree of success.

Hypothyroidism

Hypothyroidism (deficiency of thyroid hormone) leads to a slowing of both mental and physical processes. The skin becomes dry and puffy, hair is lost, and sensitivity to cold is a common complaint. Constipation, lethargy, fatigue, and a myriad of minor symptoms may be attributed to poor thyroid function.

Several types of hypothyroidism are recognized. One is due to the fact that the pituitary gland fails to stimulate the thyroid gland because of a lack of thyroid stimulating hormone. This type is known as *hypopituitary* or *masked hypothyroidism*.

The most common type, however, results from failure of the gland to produce adequate amounts of thyroxine. This happens when there is partial or more or less complete destruction of the gland by infection, auto-immunization, or radiation (x-rays or radioactive iodine). But most often it is due to an intrinsic biochemical defect, and the gland is either unable to take up or trap iodine, or unable to synthesize the trapped iodine properly to form the end product, thyroxine.

When thyroid deficiency occurs in an infant before birth, *cretinism* with retarded growth, mental, and sexual development is the result. When it occurs in childhood, the rate of growth is poor and sexual development markedly slowed, while mental faculties may not be too greatly affected. When it occurs in the adult, the disorder is known as *myxedema*. However, thyroid deficiency may be borderline and the diagnosis is frequently overlooked.

It is interesting that myxedema in adults is sometimes accompanied by oddities of behavior that may be attributed to a mental rather than a physical cause.

The diagnosis may be made by a persistently low basal metabolic rate (BMR), a low serum-bound iodine (PBI). (Details of tests of thyroid function will be discussed later.) Other tests employed are radioactive iodine uptake by the thyroid, and measurement of capacity of the red blood cells to take up radioactive triiodothyronine. The thyroid therapeutic test is frequently employed. This entails giving small amounts of thyroid medication and noting the response. The response must occur following the administration of small doses of thyroid medication. Thyroid deficiency states are very satisfactorily treated orally with dried thyroid extract, pure thyroid hormone (thyroxine), or triiodothyronine.

Cretinism
(Congenital Hypothyroidism)

A *cretin* is a child born with impaired or absent thyroid function. It is believed that the term is derived from the Old French and was meant to connote "little Christian" because these children were so gentle and well-behaved. Several types are recognizable:

A. *Endemic* goitrous cretinism is found in certain areas of the world, more so in some than in others. Poor iodine in the soil and water, as well as bacterially contaminated water supplies, have been incriminated. In these iodine-poor areas a goitrous mother gives birth to a goitrous child whose thyroid is permanently functionless. All tests for thyroid function will reveal extremely low values.

B. *Sporadic cretinism* may be divided into two types:

Anatomic abnormality in which there is actual absence of the thyroid gland (athyrotic cretinism).

Those with a *palpable thyroid* or even a goitrous one. In these an inborn error of iodine metabolism is present. One or more of the thyroidal enzymes is lacking, resulting in the improper synthesis of thyroxine. Pre-thyroid hormones may be produced in large amounts, but these are totally inadequate for the metabolic needs of the child. In such instances the serum bound iodine may be very high and so will the radioactive iodine uptake. The basal metabolism rate will be low (this test is difficult in infants).

The diagnosis is seldom made before the third month after birth. The mother first notices that the baby is a lazy feeder, but is impressed with his or her good behavior, for the baby cries and fusses little. Later, failure to gain weight, dryness of the skin, and constipation become noticeable. The apathy, the lethargy, the inability to sit up and the mental retardation arouse suspicion. The earlier the diagnosis, the more successful the treatment, for permanent mental damage with loss of intelligence occurs if thyroid hormone therapy is delayed.

The aspect of the full-blown cretin is one of dwarfism, sparse hair, dry thickened yellowish skin. The abdomen is distended (pot belly), the face is puffy, the tongue large, the lips thick, the bridge of the nose depressed. In the absence of a goiter, the condition may not be suspected, but failure to thrive, puffiness around the eyes, later tooth eruption, and constipation are early signs of hypothyroidism. Frequently an umbilical hernia is present and serves to alert the physician to the possibility of congenital thyroid deficiency.

The diagnosis is best confirmed by: (1) Radioactive iodine uptake (completely zero in the athyrotic cretin, but may be very high in the goitrous cretin). (2) Serum-bound iodine, extremely low but may be elevated in certain enzyme defects wherein incomplete forms of thyroid hormone are produced. (3) High serum cholesterol levels are usually present. (4) X-ray of the bones of the hand shows delay in appearance of centers of ossification, that is, delayed bone age.

Differential Diagnosis. Pregnant women receiving antithyroid drugs may in rare instances give birth to a baby with a goiter. The goiter, however, is transient, and the history of treatment during pregnancy helps with the diagnosis.

The main problem of diagnosis lies in separation of mongoloidism from cretinism. The slanting eyes, excessive flexibility of the joints, the short curved little fingers, the increased markings of the palms and soles of the feet, as well as the straightness of the upper crease of the hand and, not infrequently, a geographic (excessive furrous) tongue, are features distinctive of the mongolian idiot. Furthermore, the cretin is slow and lethargic, the mongol is active, cheerful, but at times unmanageable. Both, however, have defects in intelligence.

The treatment of cretinism is substitutional thyroid therapy. Treatment should be started as soon as diagnosis is made, to prevent mental retardation and to promote normal growth and development. Medication should be continuous and under the constant supervision of the physician. Some of the older cretins when treated with thyroid may become irritable and unmanageable, and as a rule their intelligence is not benefited by it.

Sporadic cretinism with goiter is treated in the same manner as sporadic cretinism without goiter, except that the child with a very large goiter may require surgery. Iodine prophylaxis (iodized salt and iodine in drinking water) has served to eradicate endemic cretinism in those areas where endemic goiter is prevalent.

Colloid Goiter

Colloid goiter, sometimes referred to as *endemic goiter,* is characterized by a

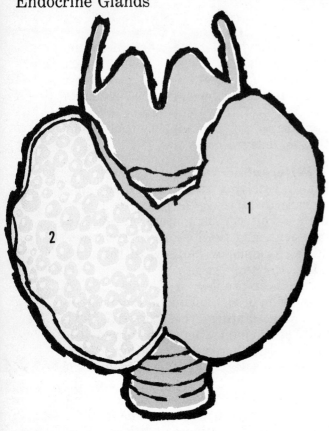

Colloid goiter (frequently called "simple goiter") is a soft, diffuse, symmetrical enlargement of the thyroid gland due to large deposits of thyroid hormone of poor quality, as may be caused by deficiency of iodine in the diet. The drawing shows an external view of the *left lobe* (1) and a cross section of the *right lobe* (2) of a thyroid with colloid goiter.

diffuse symmetrical enlargement of the gland without hyperthyroidism. Although usually there are no symptoms other than pressure that may result from enlargement, there are patients who show signs of depressed thyroid function.

The gland is enlarged because of large stores of hormones of poor quality. This excess storage is compensatory in an effort to supply adequate thyroid hormone. The disorder is called endemic goiter because of its frequency in areas in which the soil and water are deficient in iodine.

The introduction of iodized salt into the diet was followed by a dramatic decrease in the incidence of this type of goiter. Not all cases are caused by lack of iodine. Some are due to an inherent enzyme defect which is genetic. Others are due to excessive intake of *goitrogens* (goiter-inducing substances) in certain vegetables, such as cabbage. Sometimes the

thyroid enlarges in the female to goitrous proportions during puberty and pregnancy, presumably when the body's demand for iodine is increased.

Colloid goiter is a soft, symmetrical, smooth, glandular enlargement. The basal metabolism rate is usually normal, radioactive iodine uptake may be normal or elevated, and the serum-bound iodine is usually low. Treatment is surgical only when enlargement is so great as to cause pressure symptoms, or when surgery is desirable for cosmetic reasons. Iodine therapy for several weeks to months may produce excellent results. Iodine, of course, is most valuable as a guardian against the disease, and iodized salt should be used especially in those areas where this disease is endemic.

Nodular or Adenomatous Goiters

Nodular or *Adenomatous goiters* are the most common form of thyroid enlargements. Although symptoms of deranged thyroid activity are often lacking,

Nodular or *adenomatous goiter*, below, is so called for masses that may distort the surface (1) and interior (2) of the thyroid gland. Often there are no constitutional symptoms and only mild disfigurement, but it is possible for some adenomas to become toxic and produce symptoms of hyperthyroidism.

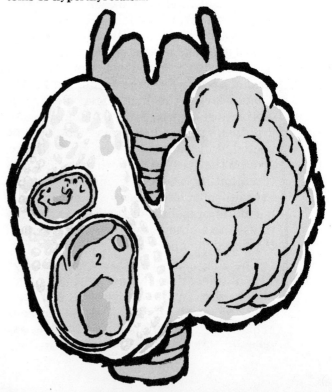

attention must be given to such goiters, because of the possibility of malignancy. The single nodule proves to be malignant more often than multiple nodules.

Surgery should be undertaken whenever a nodule is hard or fixed or causes pressure symptoms. If there is no absolute indication for immediate surgical intervention, suppressive doses of thyroid may reduce the nodule. Medication must be continued indefinitely.

Thyroiditis

There are several forms of *thyroiditis* (inflammation of the thyroid gland) to consider. The acute or subacute inflammatory form may be infectious in origin but more often part of a autoimmune process. The onset is sudden. Fever and malaise are associated with a tender swelling of the thyroid. Spontaneous recovery is the rule.

Chronic thyroiditis is seen more frequently than the acute types. Two kinds are recognized. Chronic *lymphadenoid thyroiditis* (Hashimoto's type) is usually found in middle-aged women. The gland is diffusely enlarged. In the early phase there may be some symptoms of thyrotoxicosis, but depressed thyroid function invariably appears in the later stage.

The second type is known as "woody thyroiditis" or Riedel's struma. The gland is enlarged, stony hard, and adherent to adjacent structures. The patient complains of a harsh, vibrating sound produced when exhaling and of difficulty in swallowing, with a constant feeling of pressure in the neck.

Tests of Thyroid Function

There is no one supreme test for thyroid function, but rather a battery of tests which give discriminating information about thyroid abnormalities. Fifteen years ago it was widely believed that all we needed was a basal metabolic rate (BMR) and perhaps a blood cholesterol test. Today we appreciate the fact that no single laboratory test can make a diagnosis without supporting clinical evidence. At times, continuing observation, more laboratory data, and therapeutic tests are necessary.

Most important of all is the interpretation of what appear to be inconsistent results. For instance, a patient on triiodothyronine (t_3) will show a very low protein-bound iodine (PBI) on testing. The low PBI might be unwarily interpreted as indicating a need for more thyroid medication. Actually, t_3 suppresses PBI and the reading is thus misleading. Another example is the child born with a large goiter. In spite of all the clinical signs of hypothyroidism, the radioactive iodine uptake may be very high because of the avidity of the goiter for iodine. The underlying defect, however, is inability of the gland to utilize the iodine, because of an inborn error of metabolism which results in hypothyroidism.

The following clinical tests are used to evaluate thyroid function.

Basal metabolic rate (BMR). The test measures the gross energy exchange when the body is in a state of rest. What is measured is the minimal rate of energy expenditure necessary to maintain the heartbeat, respiration and heat production — hence, "basal." Actually, oxygen consumption is measured, and computations based on age and skin surface are made. Normal values have a range of 20 plus or minus. The basal rate is governed to a great extent by the influence of the thyroid upon all the cells of the body.

In fever, leukemia, and a number of other circumstances, the BMR is elevated. The test is susceptible to many technical pitfalls. Nevertheless, the BMR is a useful test and should be employed in instances where diagnosis may be facilitated by its use, particularly when normal values are obtained in suspected hyperthyroid patients.

Protein-bound iodine of serum (PBI). This blood test, which measures the levels of protein-bound iodine in the serum, is today the most widely used of thyroid tests. The normal range is four to eight micrograms per 100 cc. of serum.

About three per cent of the patients with exophthalmic goiter (Graves' disease), and ten per cent with nodular (toxic) goiter with hyperthyroidism, have a PBI within the normal range, and so may about four per cent of patients with hypothyroidism. The test may also be below the normal range in patients with nephrosis, some types of liver disease, in patients receiving cortisone-like

cretinism in which too much iodine containing hormonally ineffective thyroid material or hormone is secreted. Also, PBI above normal range is seen in patients in whom organic iodine compounds have been administered for the purpose of performing gall bladder visualization tests, or outlining the Fallopian tubes in the study of the infertile woman, or outlining the bronchial tree in patients with bronchiectasis, or after pyelography. When allowances are made for error and interpretation, the PBI provides considerable information about thyroid function in the patient.

Radioiodine uptake. This test measures with great accuracy the uptake of a tracer dose of labelled iodine such as I^{131} by the thyroid gland. It does not measure, however, release of hormone by the gland. The test gives a clinical accuracy of 70 to 95 per cent. Normal values are between an uptake of 15 to 40 per cent in 24 hours.

However, patients receiving thyroid hormones, or iodides in abundance, will take up little radioiodine, and values are disturbed following iodine deprivation, antithyroid hormones in the treatment of thyrotoxicosis, and after a number of drugs such as perchlorate and cobalt. The test is an excellent one.

Another radioiodine test currently employed measures the avidity with which a patient's red cells bind triiodothyronine (t_3). A blood sample is incubated with labelled t_3 for a period of two hours. Then the red cells are washed repeatedly and the radioactivity which remains is estimated. The test is useful in patients who have received iodine compounds, since results are not affected by such therapy. The test has certain conveniences since no radioactive substance is administered.

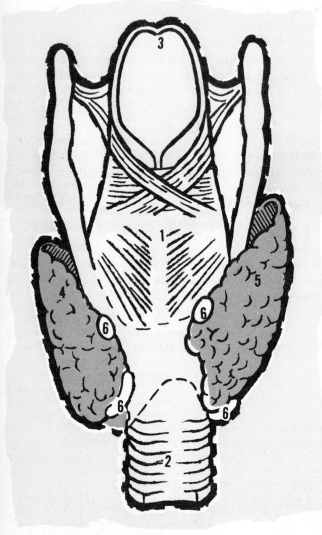

The *parathyroid glands* produce hormones concerned with maintaining a stable concentration of calcium in the blood. The drawing shows a rear view of the *larynx* (1), *trachea* (2), and *epiglottis* (3), with the bead-sized *parathyroid glands* (6) superficially imbedded in *lobes* (4, 5) of the thyroid gland. The parathyroids have an endocrine function entirely different from the thyroid gland.

THE PARATHYROID GLANDS

The *parathyroid glands,* four in number, are superficially imbedded on the back and side surfaces of each lobe of the thyroid gland. Each parathyroid is only slightly larger than a small bead, and

hormones and triiodothyronine (t_3), and after certain mercurial drugs are used.

It may be above the normal range in pregnancy, in patients receiving large doses of estrogens, and in some cases of occasionally one or more is "out of place" and lies behind the breast bone in the chest.

There are two parathyroid hormones — *parathormone* and *calcitonin*. Their function is to maintain a stable concentration of calcium in the blood. Parathormone is released whenever blood calcium levels are low. The hormone activates the transfer of calcium from bone to blood until the levels return to normal. Calcitonin, a newly discovered hormone produced by the parathyroids, is released during periods when there is excess calcium in the blood.

Removal of the parathyroids results in a sharp fall in serum calcium and a rise in serum phosphorus. The outstanding resultant symptom is *tetany* — excessive neuromuscular excitability. Tetany in mild form manifests itself as twitching and wrist and foot spasms, and in the severe form as convulsions which may be mistaken for epileptic attacks.

There are two main disturbances associated with parathyroid disease: *hyperparathyroidism* and *hypoparathyroidism*.

Hyperparathyroidism

Hyperparathyroidism in its primary form is as a rule due to a tumor of one or more of the glands, but occasionally results from an increased number of cells (hyperplasia) of the parathyroids. When this occurs, calcium is removed from bone. In the severe form, decalcification occurs, and bone cysts, benign giant cell tumors of the bone, spontaneous fractures, and skeletal deformities may result. The disease is then known either as *osteitis fibrosa cystica* or as von Recklinghausen's disease.

In the United States where calcium intake in the diet is usually adequate, this form of bone disease rarely occurs. The more common manifestation is kidney stones. Whenever a kidney stone is found to be a calcium stone, hyperparathyroidism should be suspected. In many cases, neither bone cysts nor kidney stones are found, but muscular weakness, loss of appetite, nausea, constipation, and excessive thirst and urination may be the only presenting symptoms. In prolonged cases, kidney damage due to deposits of calcium salts develops, and death may ensue from renal insufficiency.

The diagnosis is made by determining blood levels of calcium and phosphorus. In the typical case, serum calcium is high and phosphorus is low. However, in the presence of renal disease, the calcium and phosphorus may be normal.

Many cases, however, are borderline, in that the serum calcium levels are normal or only slightly above normal values. In such cases, repeated studies and observations are necessary, and special low calcium diets are administered to see if the urinary output of calcium remains low or elevated. If abnormally elevated, then hyperparathyroidism is suggested. Where the suspicion is strong, exploratory surgery is undertaken.

Secondary hyperparathyroidism is merely a compensatory increase in cells of the glands that occurs in certain disease states where there is a disturbance in calcium and phosphorus metabolism.

Hypoparathyroidism

Hypoparathyroidism results from parathyroid hormone deficiency. This may be an individual peculiarity, which is rare, or it may be a result of surgical removal of the parathyroid glands or damage to them during thyroid surgery. Serum calcium levels fall to low values and serum phosphorus levels are elevated.

In milder cases, signs of increased neuromuscular excitability may be elicited. A tourniquet around the arm will bring out spasms of the hand. When the condition is active, tingling, crawling, or burning sensations around the mouth may be the first symptom. Signs of tetany, confusion, and convulsions occur not infrequently. Cataracts and monilial (fungus) infections are common complications. X-ray study shows increased density of bone, and urine studies show absence of calcium.

The treatment for an acute attack of tonic convulsions or hand-or-foot spasms is intravenous calcium gluconate. Patients may be maintained in fairly good health by oral calcium, Vitamin D, and other compounds where necessary. Care should be taken to avoid overtreatment. Large doses of calcium carbonate have been recommended for treatment. Patients should remain under the constant watch of the physician.

A rare form of hypoparathyroidism is called Seabright-Bantam syndrome. It is a congenital disorder wherein hormone production is adequate, but hormonal action on peripheral tissues is ineffective.

THE ADRENAL GLANDS

One of the first diseases of an endocrine nature to be recognized was described over 100 years ago by a British doctor, Thomas Addison. In 1855 he described a disease caused by destruction of the adrenal glands, and to this day adrenal insufficiency is known as *Addison's disease*.

The adrenal glands are two small, triangular-shaped bodies lying immediately in front and above each kidney. The adrenal consists of two parts with distinct functions.

The outer part is called the *cortex*. This portion produces three important "sets" of hormones, such as:

Glucocorticoids, which are cortisone-like substances that influence carbohydrate, protein, and fat metabolism.

Mineralocorticoids, such as aldosterone, that regulate water and salt balances.

Sex steroids that act as an auxiliary source of male and female sex hormones.

The inner portion of the adrenal gland is known as the *medulla*. It is intimately connected with the sympathetic nervous system. Its hormones are *epinephrine* (adrenalin) and *norepinephrine* (noradrenalin).

Total destruction of the adrenal gland cortex leads to rapid death. In fact, in days gone by a diagnosis of Addison's disease was tantamount to a death warrant. An idea of progress made in the field of endocrinology may be gained from the fact that persons in whom both adrenal glands have been removed (and this is sometimes necessary) have now been kept alive in moderately good health for over 20 years.

Each of the two parts of the adrenal plays important roles in health and disease. One of the hormones secreted by the medulla, for instance, is *epinephrine* that is vital in enabling an individual to meet sudden dangers and emergencies. For instance, imminent danger — perhaps a car racing recklessly upon you — triggers an "alarm reaction" and prepares the way for emergency action. Epinephrine pours into the circulation, alertness is galvanized, carbohydrate reserves of the body are mobilized for quick energy, muscular strength is increased, pupils dilate for better sight and peripheral blood vessels contract. Thus endangered man can summon reserve strength for flight or fight, and minimize blood loss, if wounded, through constriction of blood vessels and faster clotting.

Energy stores are quickly used up and must be replenished to deal with further or continued stress situations. Epinephrine stimulates the pituitary gland to produce more ACTH hormone that stimulates the adrenal cortex. When this happens, cortisone-like hormones are released, to induce conversion of glucose from proteins and replenish the sugar stores in the liver and muscle that were used up in the alarm reaction.

Our ability to withstand prolonged stresses depends on the ability of the pituitary gland to respond to such situations by adequate secretion of ACTH to stimulate the adrenal gland.

Adrenal insufficiency. Acute adrenal insufficiency is also called "adrenal crisis." It occurs in acute. fulminating infections which rapidly destroy the adrenal glands; in massive hemorrhagic destruction of both adrenals, sometimes seen in the newborn; or when the glands are removed at surgery without proper substitutional therapy. This state also occurs in persons with chronic adrenal insufficiency who have been subjected to severe stress, such as infection, trauma, starvation, and overwork.

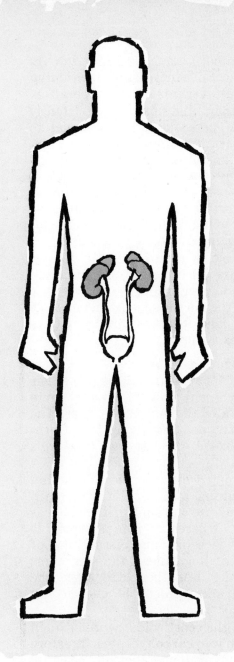

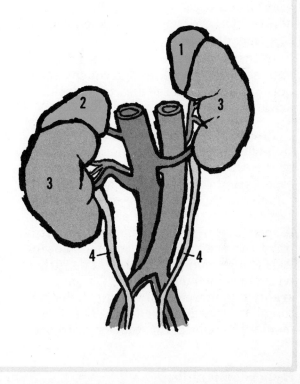

The *adrenal* glands (also called *suprarenal*, "above a kidney") are located as the name suggests and as shown in the figure at the left. The adrenal glands are small triangular bits of tissue with something of a "cocked hat" shape. The more detailed drawing shows the *left* (1) and *right* (2) *adrenal glands*, the *kidneys* (3), and *ureters* (4). Each adrenal gland has an outer "rind" or cortex, and an inner layer, the medulla, producing different hormones. The adrenal cortex is essential to life, but the medulla is not.

The symptoms are those of acute shock. Treatment is carried out by adequate replacement of adrenal cortical hormones such as hydrocortisone and desoxycorticosterone, salt and sugar replacement by infusions or by blood transfusions, and noradrenalin hormones to maintain blood pressure. In the presence of infection, heroic doses of antibiotics are given to supplement the above measures.

Chronic adrenal insufficiency (Addison's disease). The degree and severity of symptoms will depend on the extent of failure of the adrenal cortex. The signs and symptoms, in order of frequency, are weakness and fatigability, weight loss, mild pigmentation to marked bronzing of the skin, loss of appetite, vomiting, nausea, abdominal pain, intestinal disorders, and salt craving. Along with this there is low blood pressure, low blood sugar, emotional instability, loss of sexual hair in the female.

Acute prostration associated with relatively minor infections or gastrointestinal upset may be the first indication of underlying adrenal disease. Sometimes, loss of consciousness from acute hypoglycemia (low blood sugar) may be the presenting symptom.

In most cases, diagnosis is readily established by various tests. The most accurate test is determination of the ability of the adrenals to respond to an injection of ACTH.

With the aid of cortisone-like substances, salt intake, and frequent feedings of a well balanced diet, most patients are kept in moderately good health.

Pituitary hypoadrenalism is a condition which is rarely seen, but gives many of the same symptoms as Addison's disease, except that there is none of the skin pigmentation that is observed in most cases of primary chronic adrenal failure. A special test (Metapirone test) for pituitary reserve will reveal poor or absent ACTH production. Treatment is either with continued doses of ACTH, or preferably and more satisfactorily, substitutional corticoid medication. The treatment is the same as for Addison's disease.

Hypercorticoidism (Excesses of Adrenal Cortex Hormones)

Various disorders are associated with excesses and imbalances of the various hormones produced by the adrenal gland cortex. These are best considered with respect to the particular hormone "families" involved.

Excess mineralocorticoid production. Aldosterone is the most potent salt-retaining hormone or mineralocorticoid. Its excess production results in *primary aldosteronism,* a syndrome marked by loss of potassium and augmented alkalinity of the blood (alkalosis).

The patient is extremely weak, even paralyzed or afflicted with painful, jerky muscle spasms. Frequent urination, night urination, high blood pressure and headaches are some of the other symptoms.

Usually the condition is due to a small benign tumor or adenoma of the adrenal cortex. Occasionally, tumors occur in both of the adrenal glands, and in a few instances, excessive increase of functioning cells (hyperplasia) is found at operation.

Laboratory findings of persistently low serum potassium, high normal to elevated serum sodium, neutral or alkaline urine, and blood alkalosis in the presence of unexplained hypertension, lead one to expect primary aldosteronism. Confirmatory evidence is provided by assays for urinary aldosterone, a difficult and not readily available procedure.

Treatment is removal of the tumor. Results are dramatic. The so-called malignant hypertension, the weakness or paralysis, the muscle spasms and urinary frequency, disappear within a few days or weeks as a rule.

Excess glucocorticoid production (cortisone-like hormones) may be due either to a tumor (benign or malignant) or to hyperplasia of the adrenal cortices. The former is frequently referred to as *Cushing's syndrome,* the latter as *Cushing's disease.*

In Cushing's disease, the interacting hypothalamus and pituitary are involved, and the adrenal disturbance is secondary, whereas when a tumor is present, it is a primary disturbance of the adrenal. Regardless, the symptoms are more or less the same since the underlying mechanism is one of too much glucocorticoids.

Excess glucocorticoids cause protein breakdown into carbohydrates, interfere with carbohydrate metabolism and cause storage of fat in certain depots.

Thus, Cushing's syndrome is characterized by muscle-wasting of the extremities, but with large trunk and moon face and fat on the back just below the neck, giving a buffalo-hump appearance. The skin is thin and bruises easily. The bones, especially the vertebrae and ribs, are demineralized and brittle; there is a tendency to diabetes mellitus. The face is ruddy. There are usually purplish *striae* (stretch marks) on the protuberant abdomen.

Along with a "humpty-dumpty" appearance there is marked weakness and mild to moderate hairiness of the face.

High blood pressure is invariably a concomitant of the disease. In advanced cases, spontaneous fractures and collapsed vertebrae are not infrequently seen. Loss of sexual drive is the rule and mental aberrations are quite common.

Diagnosis is made by the demonstration of an adrenal mass which may displace one of the kidneys, as revealed by x-ray studies; the findings of increased glucocorticoids in the blood or urine; the poor utilization of carbohydrates when subjected to a loading test of sugar. The blood count will as a rule show an elevated red blood and white blood cell count, but low in eosinophils and lymphocytes. On occasion the pituitary gland is enlarged by an adenoma, since the disturbance often originates in the pituitary gland. In many, the pituitary tumor is so small as to remain undetectable until several years after the adrenal glands have been removed by surgery.

Treatment in the past has been removal of both adrenal glands with substitutional therapy by small maintenance amounts of corticoid hormones. The treatment after adrenalectomy is the same as for Addison's disease. In cases where the disease is caused by an adrenal tumor, the tumor or the involved adrenal is removed. In such instances, the opposite adrenal is usually atrophic and will remain so for periods varying from a few weeks to a year. In the meantime, maintenance therapy is administered to prevent an adrenal crisis.

In recent years there is a trend to direct treatment to the pituitary by radiation therapy in cases where an adrenal tumor has been ruled out. Some cases of adrenal hyperplasia are not due to a pituitary factor, but are caused by certain lung cancers producing excess amounts of ACTH-like hormone which stimulate the adrenal cortices.

Excessive Sex Hormone Secretion

Excessive sex hormone secretion by the adrenals may be due to tumor or hyperplasia. The main sex steroids produced in cases of hyperplasia are androgens, producing *virilism* in the female and *precocious puberty* in the male. A tumor, on the other hand, produces either androgens or estrogens in a paradoxical manner. As a result, the female is virilized while the male is feminized by the excess sex steroid secretion.

Abnormal sexual development. When hyperplasia of the adrenal cortex occurs with excess androgen production, it is in the main due to a congenital failure of the adrenal to synthesize its hormones properly because of a lack of certain enzymes. The result is that even in fetal life the adrenals produce abnormal amounts of steroids such as androgens.

When this happens, the female infant, in most but not all instances, will display signs of abnormal sexual development, i.e., external genitals that are partially male and female. This is known as *female pseudohermaphroditism*. In the male infant, the excess androgen production leads to premature development of the external genitals but this is not manifest until about the fourth or fifth year of life.

Diagnosis may be made in the female pseudohermaphrodite soon after birth by the presence of an enlarged clitoris, often mistaken for a penis, and a rudimentary vaginal canal which may resemble a common opening for the urethra and vaginal canal. Laboratory studies of sex chromosome materials can determine whether the infant is genetically male or female. As the child grows, pubic hair begins to appear about the age of five years. About age eight to 12, acne and facial hairs appear. Untreated, the female pseudohermaphrodite grows into a mannish individual: broad-shouldered, without breast development, and hirsute. In a few instances, menstrual periods have occurred for a few years.

In the male pseudohermaphrodite, the penis is usually normal at birth and early infancy, but within a few years enlarges gradually to adult size, while the testes remain small. Pubic hair appears by age four or five and body build and muscle mass increase rapidly, so that these children, like those with true precocious puberty, have been referred to as the "Infant Hercules". Though early growth is rapid, the ultimate height is far less than average because of premature closure of the growing ends of bone.

Because androgens are being produced at the expense of glucocorticoids, signs of adrenal insufficiency may develop and such individuals from infancy onwards may suffer adrenal crises due to excessive salt loss, or attacks of faintness because of low blood sugar. In a few cases there is salt retention with high blood pressure.

The diagnosis of congenital adrenal hyperplasia is readily made by urinary hormone determinations. X-ray of the hand for bone age in children will show a marked advance in the appearance of ossification centers and, as a rule, closure of the growing ends of bone, the epiphyses, takes place by the twelfth year.

Treatment of the child is by cortisone-like hormones in an amount sufficient to lower the abnormal production of androgenic hormones but not to induce a Cushing-like appearance. Medication in the female, if continued, will result in normal feminization, i.e., menstruation, ovulation and breast development; in the male there will be a greater tendency to normalization.

Plastic surgery of the genitals is performed when feasible in the female patient. The clitoris may be excised early, sometimes before the fifth year, and the narrowed vaginal canal enlarged at the same time or at puberty.

Adrenogenital syndrome. The adrenal cortex secretes sex steroids more or less similar to those of the gonads. The adrenal cortex is responsible for the greater part of the androgens (substances with masculinizing activity) that every female produces. In males, both the adrenals and testes contribute to the androgenic pool.

The adrenal cortex when functioning normally secretes some estrogen in both males and females. In the presence of tumor, the output of sex steroids is tremendously increased. Adrenal tumors with a predominant secretion of estrogen have been observed in boys and men. Clinically, the atrophy of the testes, loss of facial hair, and breast enlargement lead one to suspect that there is a feminizing adrenal tumor.

In the female, at any age, the tumor causes marked virilization. In the adult, voice changes, excessive hairiness, enlarging clitoris, and cessation of menstruation are usually but not always present. Diagnosis is made by the finding of large amounts of androgenic hormones in the urine which cannot be suppressed by glucocorticoid hormones. The treatment is surgical.

Pheochromocytoma (Tumor of the Adrenal Medulla)

Tumors that secrete excess amounts of epinephrine or norepinephrine or both arise in the *medulla* of one or both adrenal glands. Occasionally, the tumor arises from nests of cells of the sympathetic nervous system lying beside the great artery in the abdomen, the aorta.

Symptoms depend on which of the two hormones is predominant. The symptoms may be similar to what happens after the injection of a large dose of epinephrine: sweating, apprehension, tremor, palpitations, headache, abdominal cramp, nausea and vomiting. On the other hand, the symptoms may be similar to those caused by an injection of norepinephrine: a marked and sustained rise in blood pressure. In fact, the most striking symptom is paroxysmal attacks of high blood pressure which later may remain constantly elevated.

In most cases the signs and symptoms are due to a mixture of epinephrine and norepinephrine. An attack may be brought on by emotional stress, exercise, or massage of the loins. The diagnosis may be made by testing the urine during an attack for by-products of epinephrine and norepinephrine known as *catecholamines*. Another useful test is the administration of histamine to provoke an attack of high blood pressure. In those whose blood pressure is elevated, an adrenolytic agent such as phentolamine will cause a marked fall in blood pressure.

Treatment is surgical removal. Great care is taken during surgery to limit excessive elevation of blood pressure through manipulation of the tumor, and afterwards to prevent shock after removal. Phentolamine is administered during surgery and norepinephrine after surgery until the blood pressure becomes satisfactorily stabilized.

THE TESTES

The male gonads or *testes* lie in the scrotal sac and the normal size varies from that of a walnut to that of a pigeon egg. There are two parts to the testes, the *tubules* or excretory part which produces sperm, and the incretory part, the *Leydig cells* which produce the principal masculinizing hormone, *testosterone*. Leydig cells also produce small amounts of estrogens, the so-called female sex hormones.

The *testis* and associated structures, shown in detail below and in orientation figure at left. The *testis* (1) is the site of sperm and hormone production. Male germ cells originating in tubules of the testis pass into the *epididymis* (2) and the seminal duct or *vas deferens* (3). *Hormone-producing tissue* (4) produces the principal masculinizing hormone, *testosterone*, which enters the bloodstream. Sperm and seminal fluids are transported into the posterior *urethra* (5).

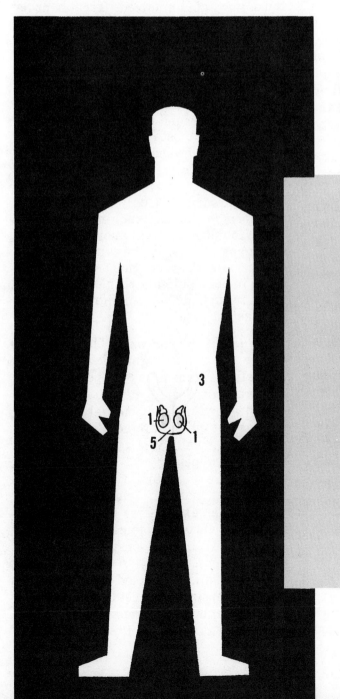

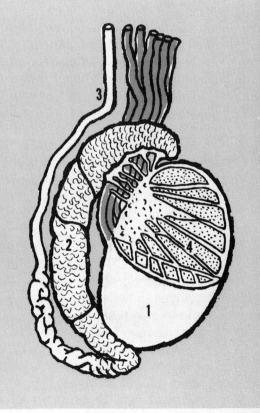

The testicle is under control of the gonad-stimulating hormones or gonadotrophins. Just before the onset of puberty, gonadotrophins are released, causing the testes to enlarge and to secrete increasing amounts of testosterone. This induces maturation of the secondary sex characteristics such as development of the penis, pubic and axillary hair growth, increased muscle mass, voice changes, eventually beard growth and all the signs of manliness in vigor, deportment and behavior.

With adequate gonadotrophins and androgen production, the tubular germ cells ripen into sperm cells. As these mature they are stored in little pouches (the seminal vesicles) on either side of the prostate gland. The prostate gland, supported by testosterone, provides fluid to nurture and sustain the vitality of the sperm. The seminal fluid is discharged toward the climax of the sexual act.

Disorders of the Testes

Eunuchoidism. When hypogonadism is due to primary failure of testicular development, it is known as *congenital eunuchoidism*. When the hypogonadism is due to selective failure of the pituitary, it is known as *hypogonadotrophic hypogonadism*.

Eunuchoid individuals frequently grow quite tall, lack beard growth, have small genitals and feminine distribution of pubic hair. The voice remains high pitched. Muscle mass is poor. Sex drive is absent. Not all are tall; some may be normal or even of small stature. Languor and lack of muscular strength are the rule. The bone age is markedly delayed. The emotional and psychologic stresses intensified by poor androgen function become deep-rooted.

Substitutional therapy with androgens yields most satisfactory results if treatment is not delayed beyond 15 to 16 years of age. Emotional and social stability, increased physical strength, and deepening of the voice may be achieved. Marriage may be undertaken and prove successful provided treatment is continued indefinitely. Of course, fatherhood is most improbable although an occasional fertile eunuch has been described following therapy.

Testicular tumors. Androgen-producing tumors of the testes, when they occur in prepubertal boys, cause marked maturation of all secondary sex characteristics: increased strength, voice changes, sexual hair growth, penile enlargement, advanced bone age. The unaffected testicle is usually atrophic. When they occur in adult men the symptoms may go unnoticed. Treatment is surgical.

Feminizing testicular tumors give rise to breast growth (gynecomastia) and recession of male characteristics. In a few instances these have occurred in childhood, but more commonly in adults. However, estrogen-producing tumors of the testes are most rare.

Another functional tumor of the testes is the *choriocarcinoma.* Occasionally, breast enlargement results because these tumors produce not only large amounts of chorionic gonadotrophin, similar to that found in pregnancy, but also estrogens. A positive pregnancy test is obtained with even markedly diluted urine in male patients with such tumors. They are usually very malignant tumors and metastasize early.

Klinefelter's syndrome. This is a syndrome that is diagnosed only after puberty. There is as a rule only a moderate degree of eunuchoidism, but breast growth, though not always present, may be quite extreme. The testes are unusually small. When sex chromatin studies are performed, most of these patients are found to have a pattern similar to that seen in females. Actually, they have an extra X sex chromosome so that their chromosome complex is composed of 47 instead of the normal 46 chromosomes.

Diagnosis is confirmed by absence of sperm, biopsy of the testes reveals complete hyalinization (from a Greek word meaning "glassy") of the seminiferous tubules. Treatment consists of plastic surgery of the enlarged breasts and androgen therapy to bolster poor androgen production. Such persons are infertile, though sexual relations may be quite adequate and normal.

Breast enlargement seen sometimes in boys with normal testes at puberty is usually temporary, although occasionally the breast enlargement may persist. Such boys are normal as to sperm production and the chromosomal pattern is similar to that of a normal male.

Undescended Testicles (Cryptorchidism). Failure of one or both testicles to descend from the abdomen to the normal position is not rare. In many instances the testes will descend spontaneously at puberty. However, it is probably unwise to wait on nature. A therapeutic trial with chorionic gonadotrophin or testosterone may cause earlier descent of the testis that probably would have descended at a later date. If medication fails, surgical measures should be undertaken before the eighth or ninth year. Not infrequently such undescended testes are poorly formed and nonfunctional, but at other times they are salvageable.

Disorders of sperm production. Semen analysis in the study of infertility or in a routine endocrine survey may reveal a very poor sperm count, or sperm of unusually poor quality and motility, or complete absence of sperm. In cases of poor sperm counts without other endocrine stigmata, the administration of small doses of testosterone, and at times large doses of chorionic gonadotrophin, have proved helpful. A history of high fever, mumps or some virus disease, is frequently obtained in such cases.

Male Climacteric. Unlike women, men rarely have abrupt slackening of gonadal function. Hence the counterpart of the menopause or female "change of life" is only occasionally encountered in men. The symptoms of loss of self confidence, asocial behavior, poor memory, insomnia, loss of libido, apprehension and nervousness, may respond to testosterone therapy and a trial course may be warranted.

THE OVARY

The ovaries, like the testes, have two functions: one, to provide ova or eggcells; and two, to secrete hormones. The hormones of the ovary are estrogens and progesterone, but under unusual conditions androgens may be produced.

The ovaries are awakened to activity when a young girl reaches 11 to 13 years of age. The "female hormones" serve to develop the secondary feminine sex characteristics of breast growth, pubic and axillary hair, maturation of the genital tract, and also the graceful contours of the female figure as well as the psychological development of ambitions and interests characteristic of the woman.

During the reproductive years there is a cyclic production of estrogen followed by estrogen and progesterone. When these hormones are withdrawn toward the end of each cycle, hormonal support to the lining of the uterus (endometrium) is withdrawn. Shedding of the lining takes place with passage of blood, hence monthly periods or menstruation. If fertilization of an ovum takes place and it implants itself favorably in the prepared endometrium, then a baby or fetus will grow.

A special structure, the *placenta*, develops from the implanted embryo and the placenta (which later becomes the afterbirth) produces hormones to support and maintain the pregnancy. Increasing amounts of estrogen and progesterone are produced until an abrupt cessation of hormonal production takes place coincident with the birth of the baby. About four days after childbirth, the breasts begin to lactate and milk is "let down", particularly when stimulated by the suckling of the baby.

Inadequate or absent ovarian stimulation by the pituitary gonadotrophic hormones, failure of the ovary to respond, or an abnormal response to the stimulation, results in many disorders ranging from complete failure to menstruate; irregular, infrequent menstrual cycles; excessive menstruation; secondary cessation of menses; and virilization in association with menstrual disorders.

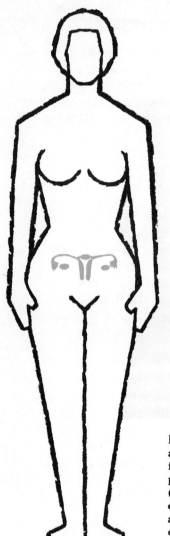

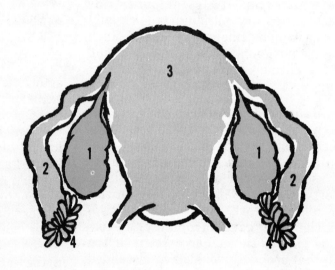

Principal organs of the female reproductive system, in orientation figure and in closeup. Ova (egg cells) mature and are released periodically from the *ovary* (1). The *oviducts* or *Fallopian tubes* (2) from the upper part of the *uterus* (3) terminate in open ends with fringelike processes *(fimbriae)* near the ovary. The tubes convey ripened ova to the cavity of the uterus. The oviduct is the usual site where fertilization takes place as an ovum encounters male germ cells that have traveled up the interior of the uterus. The many events of these processes are regulated by hormones, described on page 339.

The Amenorrheas
(Absence of Menstruation)

Amenorrhea is a symptom and not a disease. Amenorrhea may be primary, meaning that menstruation has never occurred. It may be secondary, in that menses may have occurred more or less regularly but have ceased to occur. The amenorrhea is said to be functional if menstruation occurs at irregular intervals, for instance every three to nine months or so. The amenorrhea is said to be physiologic when it occurs during pregnancy or for two to six months after childbirth or at the menopause.

Hypoovarianism: (inadequate function of ovaries). The young girl who has not menstruated by the end of the sixteenth year should be considered as having either delayed pubescence or endocrine disturbance. The delayed puberty may be a family characteristic, or be due to invalidism, a nutritional disturbance, or just a "delayed time clock." If it is endocrine in origin, the possibility of primary ovarian failure due to incomplete development, or secondarily due to pituitary failure, must be considered. The persistence of amenorrhea, neuter body contours, and infantile genital tract, together with the absence of breast development and scanty or absent pubic and axillary hair, characterize the young woman with sexual infantilism due to *hypoovarianism.*

Presence of chronic illness or malnutrition is apparent clinically. Short stature, with or without webbing of the neck,

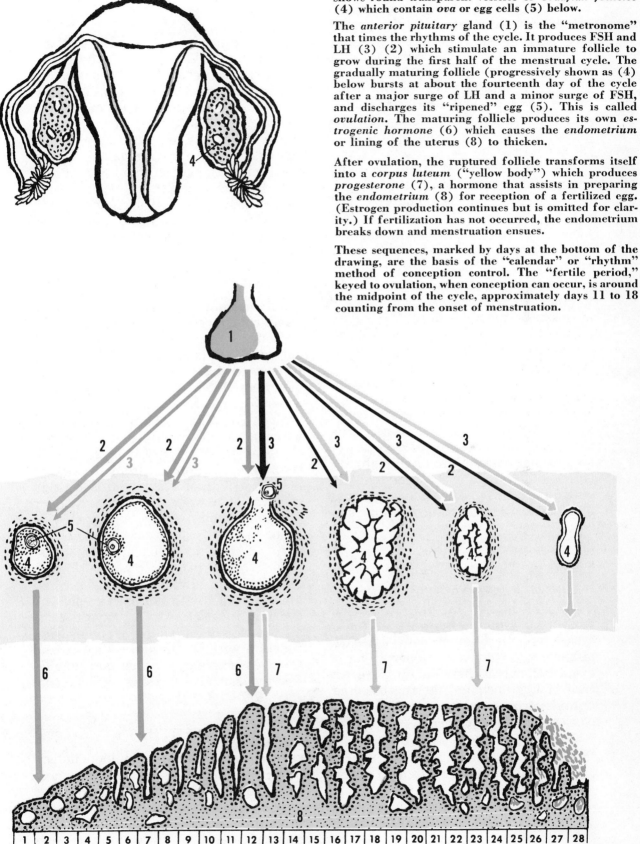

EVENTS OF THE MENSTRUAL CYCLE

Complex hormonal surges arise, subside, and intermingle during the repeated rhythmic events of normal menstrual cycles. At left, cross section of the ovaries shows round transparent vesicles or *Graafian follicles* (4) which contain *ova* or egg cells (5) below.

The *anterior pituitary* gland (1) is the "metronome" that times the rhythms of the cycle. It produces FSH and LH (3) (2) which stimulate an immature follicle to grow during the first half of the menstrual cycle. The gradually maturing follicle (progressively shown as (4) below bursts at about the fourteenth day of the cycle after a major surge of LH and a minor surge of FSH, and discharges its "ripened" egg (5). This is called *ovulation*. The maturing follicle produces its own *estrogenic hormone* (6) which causes the *endometrium* or lining of the uterus (8) to thicken.

After ovulation, the ruptured follicle transforms itself into a *corpus luteum* ("yellow body") which produces *progesterone* (7), a hormone that assists in preparing the *endometrium* (8) for reception of a fertilized egg. (Estrogen production continues but is omitted for clarity.) If fertilization has not occurred, the endometrium breaks down and menstruation ensues.

These sequences, marked by days at the bottom of the drawing, are the basis of the "calendar" or "rhythm" method of conception control. The "fertile period," keyed to ovulation, when conception can occur, is around the midpoint of the cycle, approximately days 11 to 18 counting from the onset of menstruation.

is a common accompaniment of ovarian agenesis and is known as *Turner's syndrome*. Hypothyroidism and juvenile diabetes mellitus can also be present with delayed sexual development.

In diagnosis, hormone assays for pituitary gonadotrophins help to ascertain whether the pituitary is at fault. Normal to high urinary and serum gonadotrophins are present in primary ovarian arrest, absence of gonadotrophins in pituitary failure. Those of pituitary origin may be caused by a cyst, tumor, or simply selective failure to secrete the hormone of the pituitary which stimulates ovarian function. X-rays of the pituitary gland and of the hand for bone age (delayed in sexual infantilism) are necessary in **arriving at an accurate diagnosis.**

Treatment. Replacement therapy with the female hormones, estrogen followed by progesterone, is indicated in sexual infantilism. Secondary sex characteristics will develop and withdrawal menstrual periods can be induced. It is essential to carry on with replacement therapy for at least a period of time equal to what may have been expected with normal ovarian function. Treatment is necessary to avoid demineralization of bone as well as for emotional stability and maturity. In cases of pituitary disorders causing sexual infantilism, some androgens may be added to permit growth of sexual hair.

Excessive Uterine Bleeding

Excessive uterine bleeding may occur with each menstrual period. This is known as *hypermenorrhea*. When it occurs irregularly for prolonged periods of time, it is known as *menorrhagia* or dysfunctional uterine bleeding. In every case of dysfunctional uterine bleeding, organic causes, particularly tumor or cancer, must be considered.

When the condition is due to endocrine imbalance, the bleeding can be arrested by potent estrogen-progesterone agents given in combination for five, ten or 30 days. The bleeding is usually arrested within 24 to 72 hours, and a withdrawal menstrual bleeding almost invariably follows within a few days after termination of medication and lasts four to six days.

When excessive bleeding is due to iron deficiencies, iron preparations are administered. When thyroid deficiency is present, thyroid medication proves effective. Hypermenorrhea is sometimes difficult to manage. If iron medication and agents that help clotting do not lessen the excessive flow, then inhibition of ovulation with an estrogen-progesterone compound may be administered each month from day five to day 25 for a period of six months. Correction of malnutrition, obesity, and psychosexual disorders will prove helpful in management.

Ovarian Virilism

The normal ovary does not secrete a significant amount of androgen. In the presence of enzyme defects in the ovary, considerable amounts of androgens may be secreted causing not only menstrual disorders but also varying degrees of *hirsutism,* i.e., hairiness.

When a masculinizing tumor is present, extirpation, of course, is the answer. When an enzyme defect is present, as in the Stein-Leventhal syndrome, treatment is by reduction of ovarian mass through removal of a wedge of tissue. Regular ovulatory menses may be expected to ensue in over 60 per cent of cases.

In all cases of virilism, adrenal disorders, of course, must be considered. Some types of hirsutism are genetic and are associated with normal adrenal and ovarian function. Under expert care, suppression of both adrenal and ovarian function with the newer corticoids and estrogens may prove beneficial if depilation by electrolysis first is undertaken.

INFERTILITY

In a world where 50 million human beings are added yearly to the population, the term "infertility" takes on two meanings. One refers to "involuntary infertility" which compels many barren couples to seek medical aid; the other denotes "voluntary infertility" sought by many to circumvent conception and limit offspring.

Involuntary infertility may be defined as the failure of conception to take place after two or more years of sufficiently frequent and normal coitus. The stigma of sterility should not be borne by the woman alone. The study of sterility should be the study of the barren couple. After physical examination of both male and female for general illness or abnormalities, specialized tests are undertaken.

The Study of the Male. A semen sample, after two or three days of abstinence, is obtained from the male in a clean bottle. A condom specimen is to be avoided. The specimen is kept at room temperature and transported to the physician's office within a few hours, but no longer than six or seven hours. A normal sperm count contains 40 to 100 million sperm per cubic centimeter, and two to four cc. is considered normal.

When there is complete absence of sperm the situation is usually hopeless. In those instances in which the sperm are of poor motility or the count is low, further studies are indicated and the possibility of improvement through a variety of treatments exists. The outlook, however, is uncertain unless a varicocele (varicose veins in the scrotal sac) is present. Tying of the internal spermatic vein or removal of the varices frequently corrects the infertility.

Study of the Female. It is important to establish whether ovulation occurs at regular or even irregular intervals. This may be determined by *basal body temperature records.*

During the preovulatory or estrogenic phase of the menstrual cycle, the basal temperature taken on awakening in the morning is much below normal, varying from 97 to 97.8° F. After ovulation occurs, the basal temperature rises by one-half to one degree and remains elevated for about 14 days.

In some women, this simple procedure, for some reason or other, yields inconclusive information. Ovulation may also be determined by the study of the vaginal

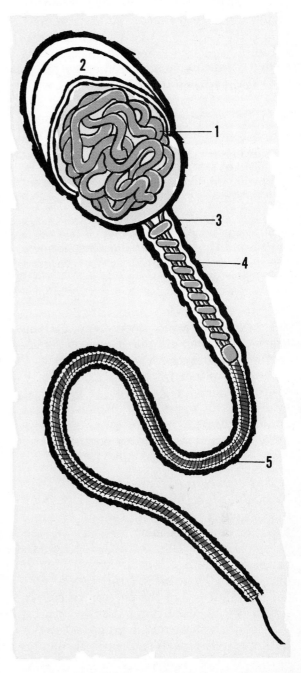

Electron microscopes disclose intricate details of the infinitesimal human spermatozoon (male germ cell). The nucleus (1) containing genetic material fits inside the headcap (2) like an acorn in its cup. The neck (3) contains two thick bundles of fibers which continue through the body or midpiece (4) and the tail (5). Spiral structures like binding threads coil around midpiece and tail.

mucosa and the cervical mucus every few days. The change from an estrogenic type of activity prior to ovulation, to a luteal type concurrent with ovulation, and from a clear watery cervical mucus (which forms a fern-like pattern on drying, readily observed under the microscope) to a thick tenacious one (which has lost its ability to fern) are indications that ovulation probably occurred.

It is then important to establish that the Fallopian tubes are open. These are tube-like structures which are attached on each side to the topmost part of the uterus and are the line of communication between ovary and uterus. The ovum that is discharged from the ovary is taken up by the fimbriated (fringed) end of the Fallopian tube for transport to the uterus.

It is in the Fallopian tube that *fertilization* of the ovum by the sperm takes place. Sperm deposited in the vaginal canal are attracted to the clear, watery mucus of the cervical canal. The sperm migrate through the mucus of the cervical canal and work their way up the uterus, into the Fallopian tubes. If fertilization occurs, then the fertilized egg descends further into the uterine cavity to find a nest for itself in the prepared lining of the womb (the progestational endometrium).

There are two tests to establish the "openness" of the Fallopian tubes:

The Rubin test. This is accomplished by *insufflation* (blowing a gas or powder into a body cavity) with carbon dioxide, to determine whether the gas in the uterus travels through the Fallopian tubes into the peritoneal cavity. This is determined by a measuring device and the fact that gas in the peritoneal cavity irritates the diaphragm, the breathing muscle at the base of the lungs, after the patient sits up. Referred pain in one or both shoulders is an accepted sign that the Fallopian tubes are patent or open.

Uterosalpingography. This is the injection of iodized oil into the uterus, after which x-rays are taken. The uterus and tubes are outlined and free oil is dispersed into the abdominal cavity. This test yields more information than the Rubin test.

To establish, for a certainty, that ovulation occurred and that the endometrium has properly prepared for "nesting" of the fertilized ovum, an *endometrial biopsy* is performed during the last week of the cycle. The tissue sample from the lining of the uterus may be obtained by the physician as an office procedure, or as a hospital procedure by performing a dilatation and curettage (D & C) under anesthesia (see Chapter 22). A healthy secretory or progestational endometrium signifies that ovulation occurred and the endometrium was prepared for gestation.

Having established all these facts, it is necessary to learn whether there is any incompatibility between the partners with respect to sperm reception by the cervical mucus. A *Sims-Huhner test* is performed as follows: the couple is advised to have marital relations the night before the examination (after two or three days' abstinence). The semen deposited in the vaginal canal is examined the next morning by the physician. As a rule, the sperm found in the vaginal secretions are immobile when examined under the microscope, but the sperm found in the aspirated cervical mucus should show good motility and progressive motion. The compatibility test is best performed just about or before the expected time of ovulation.

Treatment of the infertile female depends on what is found on examination. Closed or blocked tubes may be amenable to surgical repair. About ten percent of the cases are benefited. Cervical mucus infection which traps sperm and prevents migration requires local treatment to clear the infection. Failure of ovulation may be due to some psychophysical or glandular disturbance, and when corrected ovulation may readily occur or again be resumed.

Failure of ovulation sometimes is difficult to correct. However, recent progress in this field holds much hope. Human pituitary gland extracts, rich in follicle-stimulating hormone (FSH), are capable of stimulating the ovary but are available only in limited amounts for experimental use. Urinary extracts with similar properties, obtained from postmenopausal women, are proving of value in correcting ovulation although presently unavailable in the USA.

After a course of treatment with the FSH preparation, another hormonal agent, human chorionic gonadotrophin, is then employed to bring on ovulation. This latter substance has been marketed for many years and is derived from human pregnancy urine. These agents are proving a boon to those women who are fortunate enough to be able to obtain treatment with FSH of human origin. That of animal origin (sheep pituitary glands) is valueless in human beings but good for sheep.

However, a new chemical agent, clomiphene citrate, has been found to be capable of stimulating ovulation in non-ovulatory women. This agent is now generally available. The incidence of pregnancies that have followed its use suggests a most important breakthrough in the field of reproductive physiology.

CONTRACEPTION

Ever since man became aware of the relationship between sexual intercourse and conception, he has searched for some method—mechanical, medicinal, magical—which would prevent pregnancy or limit the number of progeny. The limitation of offspring for whatever reasons— ill health, economics, planned spacing of childbirth, or personal reasons—should be the mutual decision of the partners concerned. Several methods are available:

Coitus interruptus: The almost self-evident method of birth control (withdrawal before ejaculation), now known as Onanism, remains the most widely used method to this day. It is a practice that hinders emotional fulfillment and contributes to sexual dissatisfactions, especially of women. Moreover, it is an undependable method of birth control.

Barriers to cervical insemination: A. *Impediments:* The ancient Egyptians used medicated vaginal tampons composed of lint soaked in a mixture of acacia and honey as a barrier to semen deposited in the vagina. For many years, a variety of spermicidal agents have been incorporated into vaginal jellies, sup-

positories, creams, and foams. The chief advantage of their use is the simplicity of application, while the disadvantages are messiness and excessive lubrication. Effectiveness is reduced by an inadequate waiting period prior to coitus. Failures are said to range from 10 to 15 percent.

B. *The Condom, or Sheath:* First introduced in Europe during the sixteenth century, the condom became a popular contraceptive device only after the discovery of a method for vulcanization of rubber in the mid-nineteenth century. It is highly effective if properly used and if applied before too much sex play has taken place. The escape of a small amount of semen into the vagina before application of the condom may result in pregnancy. Failures may be caused by a tear or break in the condom; the risk is in the neighborhood of one percent.

C. *The Diaphragm:* A forerunner of the diaphragm, consisting of half a shelled-out lemon used as a cervical cap, was described by Casanova in the eighteenth century. It is interesting to note that citric acid (lemon juice) is in itself a good spermicidal agent. The advantage of the modern diaphragm which is inserted in the upper vagina to cover the cervix is that it is virtually without side effects. However, the failure rate ranges from three to ten pregnancies per 100 women exposed for a year, depending to some extent on motivation and intelligence of the user. If the diaphragm is improperly inserted, or used without a spermicidal vaginal cream, the failure rate increases considerably.

Rhythm method: In the 1920s, Ogino of Japan and Knaus of Austria advanced evidence that conception might be avoided by abstinence from sexual intercourse during the fertile period of a woman's cycle, i.e., between the eleventh and eighteenth days of the cycle. Actually the "safe" period varies widely, since ovulation may occur earlier than expected or may be delayed by such factors as illness, worry, fear, or other stresses. The advantage of this method is that there are no side effects, but watching the calendar is tantamount to love "according to plan." The method is wholly unreliable in women with irregular menstrual cycles and the failure rate may approach 20 to 25 percent.

Surgical sterilization. Voluntary surgical sterilization of both men and women has increased considerably in recent years. The procedures afford a virtually certain way of avoiding accidental pregnancies. Although in some cases the effects of sterilization have been reversed to restore fertility, sterilization should be considered to be permanent by those who contemplate the operation. For this reason, doctors usually require the consent of both partners. Voluntary sterilization is legal in every state; in Utah its use is limited by statute to reasons of "medical necessity."

Vasectomy, the male operation, gets its name from the tiny tubes through which the sperm (male germ cells) enter the semen. The doctor closes these tubes so that sperm cannot enter the man's sexual discharge and thus cannot cause pregnancy. The relatively minor operation takes about half an hour. It is usually performed under a local anesthetic in the doctor's office or clinic and a man can often return to his job the same day. Vasectomy in no way interferes with a man's potency, performance or sexual satisfaction—the only difference is that his seminal fluid does not contain sperm and hence it is not possible for him to impregnate a woman.

Tubal ligation, the female operation, is common and safe but somewhat more complicated and usually requires a brief stay in a hospital. The doctor makes a small incision in the abdomen and cuts and ties the tiny tubes (oviducts) through which a "ripe" egg cell travels to the womb each month. Pregnancy is not possible because no egg can reach the womb or entrance duct to be fertilized by sperm it might encounter there. As with the male operation, tubal ligation does not impair a woman's sexual interest and enjoyment in any way. She is just as feminine as before; menstruation continues as usual; the ovaries and womb are unchanged and female hormones continue to be produced.

Fees for surgical sterilization vary, but the average cost of a vasectomy is somewhere in the neighborhood of $150. The cost of tubal ligation is more variable, in part because of hospitalization for a few days. Frequently, tubal ligation is done shortly after a woman has given birth to a baby and is conveniently present in the hospital.

The national voluntary agency in sterilization information is the Association for Voluntary Sterilization, 14 West 40th Street, New York, N.Y. 10018.

The intrauterine contraceptive device (IUD): The IUD must be inserted by a physician or personnel trained in the technique. Grafenberg, in 1928, used an intrauterine ring made of fine spun silver. The method fell into disrepute because of corrosion of the metal, irritations, and infections. With the advent of plastic material, the idea has been revived and now some half-dozen forms of non-irritating devices are available. The IUD is best suited for women who have borne children, though it may be satisfactorily employed by those who have not, if inserted on the first or second day of menstruation.

Pregnancy rates have been estimated about 1.5 to 6 per 100 women years. The failures in some instances are due to loss of the device without the user's awareness; however, pregnancies do occur with the device in place. Among the side effects of IUDs currently in use are irregular, excessive bleeding, pelvic cramping, and pelvic infection. Acute infection, or perforation of the uterus, complicated at times by intestinal obstruction, has been encountered and several deaths have been reported. In a few instances, severe shock has followed insertion of the device.

"The pill": Dr. John Rock and the late Dr. Gregory Pincus reported in 1956 that a formulation of combined estrogen (mestranol) and a progestogen (norethynodrel), given in adequate doses and administered daily from day 5 to day 25 of the cycle, would prevent ovulation.

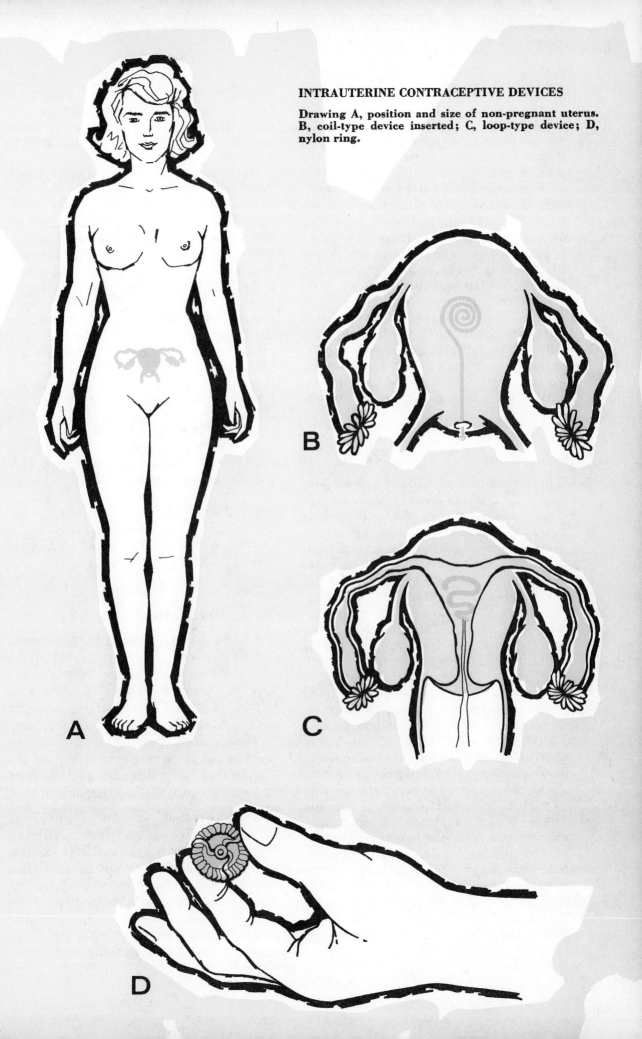

INTRAUTERINE CONTRACEPTIVE DEVICES

Drawing A, position and size of non-pregnant uterus. B, coil-type device inserted; C, loop-type device; D, nylon ring.

It had been recognized for a number of years prior to the discovery of the birth control pill that estrogens alone were capable of inhibiting ovulation, and it was felt by some researchers that the combination of estrogen with a progestogen for the 21 days was unnecessary. A preparation consisting of a potent estrogen, followed by 5 days of a progestogen, was shown by Greenblatt in 1961 to be an effective oral contraceptive and believed to be more physiologic. In 1963, Goldzieher was able to report on a significant series of cases using a sequential estrogen-progestogen to block fertility. Thus the "second generation pill" was established, and these two regimens are in extensive use throughout the world today. Physician and patient now have a choice in selecting an oral contraceptive regimen.

Side Effects

Since millions of women are now on the "pill," there is bound to be a significant incidence of coincidental illness, as well as side effects from the drug.

Many side effects have been attributed to the pill. Some are trivial, others quite dangerous. Nausea, vomiting, breast engorgement, breakthrough bleeding, weight gain, headaches, brownish discoloration of the face, visual disturbances, loss of sex drive, are side effects which may cause some women to abandon the pill. The more serious condition with which the pill has been associated is *thromboembolic disease,* through an increased tendency to blood clotting.

Prolonged use of the pill has led to aberrations in *carbohydrate metabolism, liver function,* and *blood pressure* levels. These changes are temporary, reverting to normal on discontinuance of the pill. There is an incidence of secondary amenorrhea, sometimes complicated by persistent lactation, which occurs on discontinuance of the pill, but this incidence is probably no greater than that which follows normal pregnancy. There is no evidence at this time that these drug-induced alterations pose any serious hazards to health.

Objections to the pill have been raised because of fear of thromboembolic disease, the possibility of cerebrovascular accidents, and possible relationship to cancer.

As to the first, there appears to be a legitimate basis for concern, and any woman with a history of phlebitis or varicosities should not be placed on the pill. Should signs of phlebitis develop, the pill should be discontinued and precautionary measures taken until the condition subsides. As to cerebrovascular accidents, a cause and effect relationship has not been established, but women who develop headaches or visual disturbances on the pill should go on to some other contraceptive method. As to cancer, there is no evidence to support the assumption that the pill will cause cancer. Indeed, clinicians with the greatest experience in the field of oral contraception feel that there may be a decrease in the incidence of cervical and endometrial cancer. This writer earnestly believes this to be the case, for after more than a decade of extensive use of the pill, he has not encountered a single case of cervical, endometrial, or mammary cancer that could be attributed to the drug.

THE MENOPAUSE

The menopause literally means "cessation of menses," and refers to that period in a woman's life when reproductive function has come to an end. Coincident with this loss of reproductive capacity there is a decline in hormonal secretion by the ovary. A better name for the menopause is "change of life", or the "climacteric", for it marks another rung in woman's progression through life.

Symptoms of the menopause are brought on by an estrogen deficiency which upsets the hypothalamic control of the autonomic nervous system. Hot flashes, sweats, depression, apprehension, nervousness, insomnia, headaches, crawling sensation of the skin, itching or pruritus of the external genitals, spasms, choking sensations, and heart

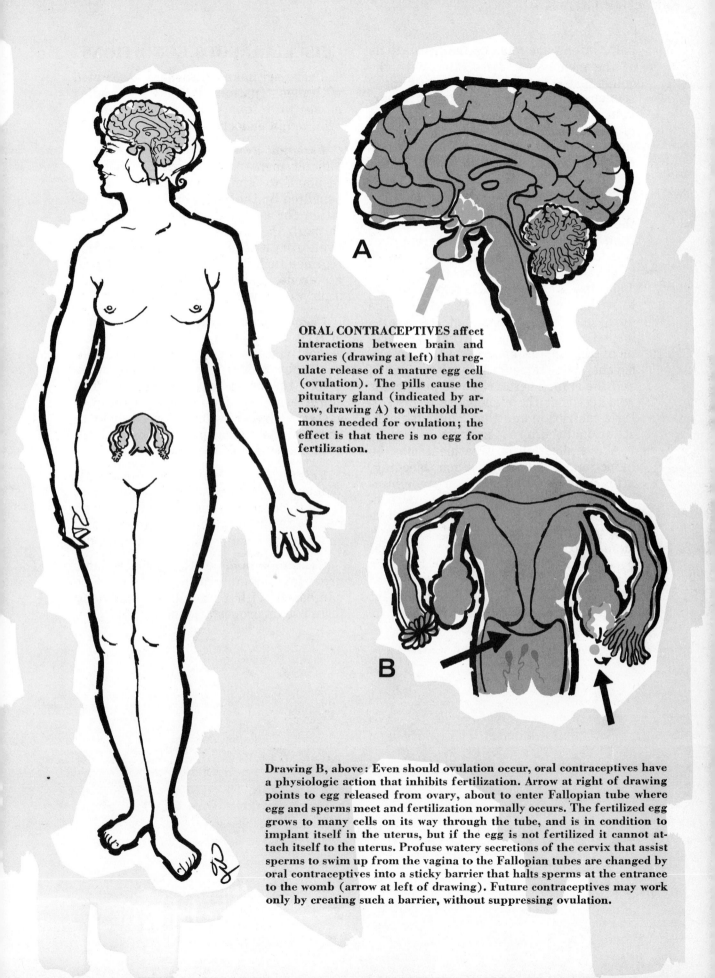

ORAL CONTRACEPTIVES affect interactions between brain and ovaries (drawing at left) that regulate release of a mature egg cell (ovulation). The pills cause the pituitary gland (indicated by arrow, drawing A) to withhold hormones needed for ovulation; the effect is that there is no egg for fertilization.

Drawing B, above: Even should ovulation occur, oral contraceptives have a physiologic action that inhibits fertilization. Arrow at right of drawing points to egg released from ovary, about to enter Fallopian tube where egg and sperms meet and fertilization normally occurs. The fertilized egg grows to many cells on its way through the tube, and is in condition to implant itself in the uterus, but if the egg is not fertilized it cannot attach itself to the uterus. Profuse watery secretions of the cervix that assist sperms to swim up from the vagina to the Fallopian tubes are changed by oral contraceptives into a sticky barrier that halts sperms at the entrance to the womb (arrow at left of drawing). Future contraceptives may work only by creating such a barrier, without suppressing ovulation.

palpitations are various manifestations of the menopause. Associated with the subjective symptoms there may appear sooner or later objective evidence of hormonal lack such as senile vaginitis, loss of mineralization of bone, with bone and joint aches, bladder irritation, and urinary incontinence.

Management. The administration of estrogenic hormones will readily arrest the symptoms of the menopause. At one time many physicians felt that treatment was unnecessary since the menopause is a physiologic and natural occurrence. This view is changing. There is no reason to withhold treatment, not only for the duration of symptoms, but for a prolonged period of time. Estrogen replacement therapy is of great value to the psyche, bone strength, healthy joints, and the skin. There are some physicians who feel that the menopause is physiologic castration and that continued substitutional therapy is in order.

A complication of treatment may be induction of bleeding. Such bleeding, after proper investigation, may be minimized by lessening the dosage or permitting bleeding to occur by adding five days of an oral progestational agent each month to induce a short withdrawal period. In this way, the fear that the bleeding might be due to cancer will be eliminated and the intelligent patient will know when to expect it.

MISCELLANEOUS CONDITIONS

There are many disorders associated with menstruation that may be handled more judiciously by the physician oriented in endocrinology.

Essential dysmenorrhea (painful and difficult menstruation) which does not respond to simple measures may be benefited by the cyclic inhibition of ovulation for a period of six to 12 months through the use of estrogens from day five through 25. The last five days of this regimen includes a small amount of progesterone. Painless menses at regular intervals may be so induced.

Premenstrual tension is the syndrome of irritability, depression in some, restless activity in others, bloating and swelling, that occurs for about one week before the onset of menstruation. The administration of diuretics and/or progestational agents for the week prior to onset of menses has proved most helpful in management of the syndrome.

Frigidity is a common complaint. Women who have known libido and lost it are the ones in whom sex drive may be readily restored by the administration of small non-virilizing doses of testosterone.

Nymphomania, i.e., the uncontrollable urge for sexual gratification, may be dampened with tranquilizers and long term use of progestational agents.

DIABETES

by CHARLES WELLER, M.D.

Diabetes mellitus is an inherited disease which occurs when the body cannot make full use of some of the foods we eat — mainly the carbohydrates or sugars and starches. The pancreas, a large gland lying beneath the stomach, does not make available enough insulin to burn these foods as energy or store them for future use. Starches and sugars increase the blood sugar content until the sugar passes through the kidneys and into the urine. This loss of carbohydrate energy causes the symptoms of diabetes and can lead to an illness which can be fatal if it is not properly controlled.

It is estimated that there are more than 2,750,000 known diabetics in the United States. In addition, there are about 1,250,000 people who are unaware of having diabetes, and more than 3.5 per cent of the total population who are presently destined to become diabetic.

The exact cause of the disease is not known. There are probably many factors involved. With some individuals it may be due solely to a lack of insulin production in the pancreas as a result of inflammatory or other changes in that organ. In other cases, certain ductless glands concealed in the brain and other parts of the body may be at fault. For reasons unknown at present there may develop an inability on the part of the tissues to utilize insulin.

There is no doubt that the great majority of people who have diabetes get

Anatomical location and details of the *pancreas gland* and surrounding structures. The *pancreas* (1) produces digestive enzymes which drain from collecting channels into the *duodenum* (2), in proximity to the *bile duct* outlets (3) from the *gallbladder* (4). The pancreas also produces a hormone, *insulin*, in islet cells that are independent of the enzyme producing structures. Insulin enters directly into the bloodstream.

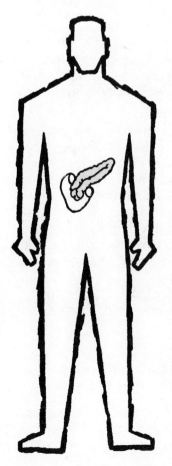

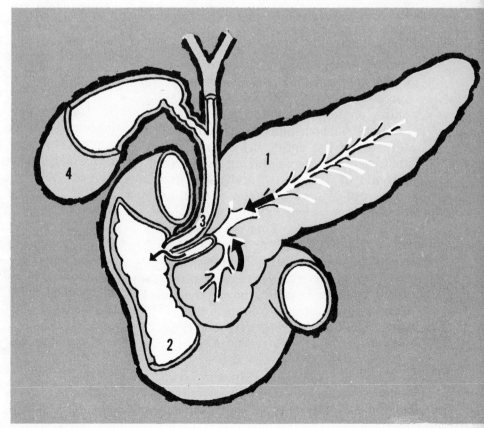

it on an inherited basis. That is, diabetes is inherited according to the Mendelian laws of heredity, with the diabetes being a recessive trait.

If a diabetic mother marries a diabetic father, the chances are that all their children will eventually develop diabetes at some time in their lives. If a diabetic mother marries a non-diabetic father, some of the children may not develop diabetes, but may be carriers of the disease. The diabetes may skip one or more generations and eventually become apparent later on.

Anybody is susceptible to diabetes from shortly after birth to over 90 years of age. Statistics show that men apparently reach their greatest susceptibility at about 51 years of age, whereas women reach it at about 55. Unmarried men appear to be more prone to develop diabetes than those that are married, and married women seem to be more likely to develop the disease than unmarried women. A mother seems to be more likely to develop the disease than one who has never borne children. However, it is not known why this is so.

There are some important clues to suspect the development of diabetes before overt symptoms appear. Diabetes may be strongly anticipated in individuals with a family history of diabetes or with an obstetrical history of overweight babies (nine pounds or over), repeated stillbirths or miscarriages, severe congenital defects in the child, infections of the bladder or kidneys during pregnancy, toxemia of pregnancy, and rapid development of overweight after pregnancy.

Sometimes sugar is found in the urine during pregnancy. This may not prove to be true diabetes, but may be what is termed "gestational diabetes." That is, the individuals just have sugar in the urine until their pregnancy is over and do not develop the symptom again until some time later on in life. However, a certain percentage of these will develop true diabetes some years after the pregnancy.

There are some individuals who have what is termed "renal glycosuria." This means that even though they spill sugar in the urine, their blood sugars always remain normal. This is not true diabetes mellitus. However, a percentage of people with renal glycosuria may eventually develop diabetes later on in life.

Sometimes some individuals develop what is called *spontaneous hypoglycemia*. That is the direct opposite of diabetes. They have too little sugar in the blood and they develop symptoms of weakness, marked perspiration, and fainting, symptoms of an *insulin reaction*. Eventually, after many months, these individuals may develop true diabetes.

Diagnosis. How do we diagnose diabetes? The simplest way is to test the urine for sugar two hours after a high starch meal. If it is positive, then we take a blood sugar two hours after a high carbohydrate feeding, such as candy or a lot of starches. If the blood sugar is abnormal, the individual is considered to have diabetes.

However, there are some cases which are borderline, and in those instances a *glucose tolerance* test is necessary. That is, a fasting blood sugar is taken and the individual is given a measured amount of sugar to drink. Blood sugars are taken at hourly intervals thereafter. If there is an abnormal rise of blood sugar, and it remains increased for several hours, the individual is considered to have diabetes.

Symptoms. What are the symptoms of diabetes? The most frequent are increase in thirst, constant hunger, frequent urination, loss of weight, itching, especially around the groin, marked fatigue, changes in vision, and slow healing of cuts and scratches. The most likely persons to develop diabetes are those people who are overweight, over 40 years of age, and related to known diabetics. The best way to find out if you have diabetes is to report to your doctor or clinic and have him do the urine and blood test examinations.

MANAGEMENT OF THE DIABETIC PATIENT

Diet is still the keystone of treatment. The diets used today are those developed by the American Diabetes Association with the cooperation of the American Diabetic Association, and are available through all physicians or clinics. The diet is usually well balanced not only in carbohydrates, proteins, and fats, but also in vitamins. It is important that the diet be constant in food value for each day, rather than very high in carbohydrates one day and not so high the next day.

If an individual is overweight it is imperative that he lose weight and therefore eat fewer calories than an individual of normal weight. If an individual is underweight his diet must contain sufficient calories to increase his weight. These persons usually will need antidiabetic medication in conjunction with diet in order for them to maintain their weight. It is absolutely imperative that all people with diabetes maintain a normal weight at all times.

Regularity of food intake appears to promote ease of control of diabetes, particularly in those who are taking insulin to avoid insulin reactions. Whereas previously it was the trend to severely decrease carbohydrates in the diet of a diabetic, the recent tendency is to be more liberal in carbohydrate intake so that it is close to an average normal diet. However, it is necessary to reduce the dietary fat and cholesterol. This can be done easily by restricting the intake of meat fats, eggs, and cheese, and increasing the use of fish as a source of protein. It is felt that this modification of the diet may help to prevent the development of complications.

Exercise is also very important in controlling diabetes, because exercise burns sugar just like insulin. It is necessary to have a constant amount of exercise almost every day if possible. However, be careful to consult your doctor.

The discovery of *insulin* was the first breakthrough in saving the lives of many diabetic patients, and today it is still the most important form of treatment. As Dr. Charles H. Best, one of the discoverers of insulin, recently stated, "there have been at least 50,000 publications in the field of insulin, and yet we still do not know how this substance truly acts."

Insulin types. There are three main groups of insulin. The first group is the *rapid-acting type*. To this group belongs the Crystalline or Regular insulin. Its onset is one to two hours after injection and it reaches its peak in three to four hours, and lasts a total of six to eight hours. Also in this class is Semi-Lente insulin. It starts to work one or two hours after injection, reaching its peak six to eight hours after injection and lasts 12 to 14 hours.

The next main group is the *intermediate-acting insulins*. The onset of action of NPH is two hours after injection, which reaches its peak in nine hours and lasts 24 hours. Lente and Globin insulin have the same time action.

The third group of insulins is the *long-acting type*. In this group belong Protamine Zinc Insulin (PZI) and Ultra Lente. PZI onset of action is four to six hours after injection. It reaches its peak in 18 hours and lasts about 36 hours. The onset of action of Ultra Lente is in about four to six hours, reaching its peak in 18 hours and lasting 48 hours.

Insulin is vital in the treatment of (1) diabetic acidosis, (2) most juvenile and lean adult diabetics, and (3) diabetics with acute complications or associated conditions, such as infections, surgery, and pregnancy. Crystalline or regular insulin is primarily used for diabetic emergencies, such as acidosis, infections, and surgery, and occasionally to supplement the other insulins.

Many diabetics can be satisfactorily controlled by a single daily injection of one of the intermediate acting insulins. The most popular at the present time appear to be NPH and Lente Insulin. Patients with very unstable diabetes may require two or more injections of insulin daily for satisfactory control.

Individualization of doses. The type and dose of insulin for each patient must be determined by the physician according to the time and quantity of urine sugar excretion, the fasting and after-meal blood sugar levels, and other factors. These include the work schedule, the frequency in time of insulin reaction, allergic background, exercise, emotions, diet, etc.

With some of the diabetically unstable individuals the amount of insulin required may vary markedly with the amount of physical exercise that is taken. For example, if one engages in violent exercise or hard physical work, one's insulin requirements may be less on the days of marked exertion. The solution to this problem is either to take less insulin before undertaking strenuous activity or to eat more on such occasions. The answer to the individual's problems in this regard must be worked out with the aid of a doctor.

Any superimposed illness may alter insulin requirements. An increased demand for insulin by the body is a useful sign of the presence of some complication. When such increased demands are noted, unless the reason is obvious — for example a cold or mild respiratory infection—the patient must consult his doctor. Since so many factors are involved in individual insulin requirements, it is wise to leave the regulation of its amount in the hands of a skilled physician. Thus, when you are ill, do not attempt to regulate the insulin dose by checking only your personal feelings or urine tests— consult your physician.

Even when the diabetic is unable to eat any food, he will still require insulin. If the lack of appetite is due to an infection or intestinal upset he will ordinarily require his full daily dose of insulin, but in some instances it may be necessary to take only three-quarters of that dose. Your physician is the only guide to this problem. Regardless of the cause of not eating, unless it be a reaction, always take at least half a dose of insulin. Taking too much insulin for the body needs at a particular time may result in *insulin reactions*. These will be discussed later.

Oral Hypoglycemic Agents. Recently, several compounds (popularly called "diabetes pills") have been made available that can be taken by mouth.

None of these substances is insulin or even insulin-like, and there is no evidence that they will be of any value unless the patient's own pancreas is able to produce some insulin. Convenience and simplicity are the obvious advantages of the oral drugs. It is also quite rare that any patient taking these drugs will have an insulin-type reaction. Another advantage is that insulin should not be used in certain types of obese diabetic patients, and only the oral drugs should be used in this type of patient, as will be discussed later.

The first group of oral agents, known as the *sulfonylureas,* was discovered in Germany in 1942. At that time, while searching for a new "sulfa drug" to treat pneumonia, it was found that a certain group of drugs lowered the blood sugar. Since that time more than a thousand compounds belonging to this group have been synthesized, but at the present time only three of them are being used to treat diabetes.

The sulfonylurea group of drugs appears to act mainly by stimulating the cells of the pancreas to produce more insulin. In 1957 in the U. S. another new group of compounds, called the *biguanides,* were prepared in a laboratory. It was soon found that they also would lower blood sugar in certain types of patients with diabetes. These drugs have a different action from the sulfonylureas. They appear to help burn up the sugar rather than to increase the release of insulin from the pancreas.

The five oral hypoglycemic drugs now in current use are the sulfonylureas, called Orinase, Diabinese, and Tolinase; and the biguanides, called DBI and Meltrol. Studies in recent years called the "UGDP" study, which appeared to associate some of the oral agents with development of degenerative disease in the diabetic, have not been proved to be correct, in the judgment of many diabetes specialists; the oral drugs continue to be widely prescribed where their use is indicated.

Selection of oral agents. In order to select the most effective oral hypoglycemic agent for the individual diabetic patient, it is necessary to understand the physiological changes in the various forms of this disease, and to correlate these changes with the manner in which the oral hypoglycemic agent works in the body. Recently, several researchers in this country and in Europe were able to measure the amount of circulating insulin in the blood of diabetic patients. This has changed our concept regarding the regulation of the diabetes and selection of the proper oral agent.

In our clinics we have classified diabetic patients into three main groups: Group A is called the *keto-acidosis prone* or *insulin-dependent* class of diabetic patients, and includes those persons whose diabetes developed in childhood and a few adult patients who usually are quite thin or of normal weight. They tend to spill acetone in their urines quite frequently.

Recent work has shown that in this group of individuals there is truly a deficiency in the circulating insulin. Their pancreas does not make enough insulin to handle the needs of their bodies. This group is always dependent upon insulin by injection. Oral agents alone are not effective in this type of individual. Occasionally, insulin plus DBI or Meltrol may be helpful. This group has wide fluctuations of their blood sugars and in the morning may spill a lot of sugar in the urine and in the afternoon may be in an insulin reaction. When DBI or Meltrol is added to the insulin dosage, many of these individuals become more stabilized after a period of time.

The second group, Group B, is called the *keto-acidosis resistant* class, or *non-insulin dependent*. They comprise the stable adults in whom the condition develops after 40 years of age. These individuals often are overweight or tend toward overweight, and can have increased blood sugars and urinary sugars without developing acetone or going into acidosis.

Recent work has shown that these individuals have a normal amount of insulin produced by their pancreas, but that some of the insulin is inactivated by anti-insulin factors which prevent all the insulin they manufacture from burning up the sugars. That is why they have diabetes. It is this group of individuals that can be controlled adequately on DBI or Meltrol alone. DBI or Meltrol plus a weight reduction diet is very effective in a majority of this group of individuals. A few of them may need a combination of both DBI or Meltrol and a sulfonylurea.

The third group, or group AB, is the class that is *partially resistant to keto-acidosis*. They are individuals who may or may not be insulin dependent, and are adults usually under the age of 40, with a tendency to underweight, and in whom the disease has developed after maturity. These individuals are in good diabetic control with either very small doses of insulin, or an oral agent, but will develop acidosis under conditions of stress, such as during an infection, surgery, or emotional disturbances.

These individuals have a slight reduction in the amount of insulin produced by the pancreas and also a small amount of anti-insulin factors. Most of these diabetic individuals can be controlled on either a sulfonylurea or DBI or Meltrol.

All patients with diabetes must follow a proper diet. If they are overweight, they should reduce their weight to normal levels. If they are underweight, they should increase their weight to normal levels by an adequate diet.

What is good control in diabetes? Authorities list four points as evidence that a patient's diabetes is well controlled:

(1) The person feels well; (2) he maintains normal weight on a well-balanced diet; (3) his urine tests are usually negative; (4) his blood sugar tests are close to normal for his condition.

Urine tests. The patient with diabetes should learn how to test his own urine for *sugar* and *acetone*. Many doctors want a patient to do these tests before each meal and at bedtime for a period of time, so they can evaluate the type of diabetic control they have under various conditions on work days and holidays. A very popular method to test sugar in the urine has been the "Clinitest." This is a tablet which is dropped into the test tube which contains ten drops of water and five drops of the urine. The solution boils itself without a flame, and an orange color appears if there is a lot of sugar in the urine.

Another test for sugar in the urine is called "Tes-Tape." The directions for its use are printed on the package. It is only necessary to wet the very tip of the tape and to wait a full minute before comparing the color with the color chart on the package. If sugar is present a green color develops.

Another good test is called "Clinistix." This resembles a large cardboard match. It is dipped in the urine and color compared with the color chart on the package. All of these tests are very useful for recording the exact amount of sugar in the patient's urine.

There are two simple tests for *acetone* in the urine. "Acetest" consists of a white tablet. A drop of urine is placed on the tablet and within one minute a purple color appears if there is acetone in the urine. There is another good test for acetone. This is called "Ketostix." This is dipped in urine and the color compared with that on the color chart. All of these tests are very accurate. Another useful product is called "Keto-Diastix." This is referred to as a "dip test." It contains both tests for sugar and acetone on the same strip.

Complications. What are the complications of diabetes? One of the most serious is *diabetic coma.* Before the discovery of insulin, diabetic coma was the incurable and fatal outcome of diabetes. Thanks to the discovery of insulin, coma now rarely occurs.

Coma may follow *completely uncontrolled* diabetes frequently — that is, in persons who are not aware that they have the disease and therefore have not had treatment. It may also occur in individuals who have not kept themselves under good control. Any circumstance which causes a diabetic to suddenly lose body fluids, such as vomiting or diarrhea, may rapidly bring on coma. The prompt restoration of fluids, salt, and

insulin as a rule affords prompt relief. It may be said that today death from diabetic coma is a needless tragedy.

Every patient, his family as well as his physician, should be thoroughly informed on the simple steps to be followed in averting impending coma. In the case of either vomiting or diarrhea, all food and medicine by mouth should be stopped. There are no medicines of any kind to be taken orally which have the slightest value. Most of them do harm.

The most noticeable *signs of diabetic coma* are deep breathing or air hunger and a sweetish odor on the breath.

Diabetic coma never comes on suddenly. It is invariably preceded by one or several of the following symptoms: increased urination, vomiting, diarrhea, loss of weight, marked fatigue, thirst, continuous sugar in the urine.

As the coma develops, the patient becomes stuporous and his respirations become deep and labored and he develops a sweet odor to his breath. His skin becomes very dry and his face is flushed. It generally takes hours or even days for unconsciousness to occur, and treatment should be begun long before this happens.

If the urine has contained large amounts of sugar and acetone for 12 hours or more, it is imperative that the doctor be called immediately. Most cases of diabetic coma should be treated in the hospital. They are given intravenous fluids and large doses of insulin rapidly until consciousness is regained. They are given a soft diet and then a full diet, as soon as they are able to tolerate food.

Insulin reactions are just the opposite of diabetic coma. These reactions are the most frequent complications in patients taking insulin, and every diabetic taking insulin some time or other is likely to have one. Every organ in the body requires sugar for its proper function, which it gets through the blood stream. If the blood sugar is too low, the organs will rebel, producing definite symptoms.

Insulin reactions usually result when the patient either has eaten too little food, or has failed to digest what has been eaten, or has taken too large a dose of insulin. Unusual work or hard play or exercise may bring on a reaction, because increased muscular effort helps to burn up body sugar.

The first *symptoms* of an insulin reaction are extreme hunger, nervousness, heavy perspiration, palpitation of the heart, occasionally double vision, and there is usually no sugar in the urine. These reactions are most apt to come on late in the afternoon or early evening if the individual is taking one of the intermediate acting insulins like NPH, lente or globin insulins. Reactions from regular insulin usually occur three to four hours after injection of that type of insulin.

Unless reactions are well understood by both the patient and his family, they can be the cause of unnecessary alarm and expense. When these reactions occur the quickest relief can be obtained from eight ounces of orange juice to which has been added two teaspoonfuls of regular sugar. If this is not available, any sugar or carbohydrate-containing food, such as bread or crackers, may be taken. Even candy is very helpful in this condition.

Occasionally a reaction can be so severe that it may cause delirium, convulsions and unconsciousness. Never try to give solid food, milk, or fruit juices to unconscious diabetics or to those persons having difficulty swallowing. The food or juices may cause trouble if they get into the lungs.

The only way an unconscious patient can recover would be to be given an intravenous injection of glucose, or an injection of a substance called "Glucogon." Glucogon can be given by the patient's family in an ordinary insulin syringe. It may be obtained from any drug store and the full contents of the package injected into the individual, just like giving insulin. Within 15 to 20 minutes the patient will regain consciousness and then he may drink a glass of orange juice.

Glucogon works by taking the sugar that is stored in the liver and putting it in the blood stream where it is rapidly utilized by all the organs. This sugar is returned to the liver after the patient eats more carbohydrates in the form of orange juice or other food.

It is very wise for a diabetic patient to carry on his person a card stating that he is diabetic and giving directions for his care in an emergency. Sometimes with the onset of insulin reactions the person may stagger and appear as if under the influence of alcohol.

Blood vessel complications. Another complication that can occur in a patient with diabetes is *arteriosclerosis,* or hardening of the arteries. This usually occurs in older individuals who have not taken care of their diabetes. It may lead to trouble in various parts of the body — the legs, feet, heart, kidneys or brain.

Diabetics are also more susceptible to eye trouble. This is caused by tiny hemorrhages of the retina of the eye, the membrane that receives the image formed by the lens.

Among older diabetics, *gangrene,* particularly in the legs, must be carefully watched for. This condition is the result of poor circulation. Diabetics should give special attention to cuts and bruises, and particularly to any foot trouble, because they may be more subject to infection than the non-diabetic.

There are heartening aspects, however. First, most diabetics no longer die of their diabetes, but of some ailment or complication common to other people. Second, most authorities believe that the closer a diabetic follows the rules laid down by his doctor, the more likely he is to postpone or avoid complications.

Care of the feet. Because of the increased incidence of difficulty with the feet in the diabetic patient, there are important factors to consider to assure adequate foot care:

(1) Never wear tight or ill-fitting shoes. A small blister or corn may cause gangrene and loss of the extremity. Socks that are too small or too large may cause trouble. When "breaking in" new shoes, do not wear them more than 30 minutes the first day. Gradually increase the time worn and be certain they do not cause sores or blisters.

(2) If a blister or sore of any sort develops, it is important to institute treatment immediately. Such sores are usually painless. Nevertheless, the lack of pain should never give one any sense of security. Sores without pain are frequently more serious than if the pain were present.

(3) If a sore is present on your foot, clean it off with soap and water, and put on a dry sterile dressing. Stay off the foot and keep it elevated to the level of the body. Call a doctor immediately to be certain other procedures are not necessary. Even a small scratch or blister can cause serious trouble.

(4) Avoid chemical and heat injury. Never put strong medications such as iodine or carbolic acid on your feet without first consulting your doctor. Never use hot water bottles or heating pads on the feet. If your feet must be exposed to the cold, be sure they are wrapped warmly.

(5) Toenails should be trimmed once a week, cutting them straight across, being careful not to injure the flesh.

(6) If circulation is bad the skin may be shiny, dry, and very thin. Such skin develops calluses easily. If the feet are bathed in soap each night and rubbed with a turkish towel, calluses and the thick skin can be removed. After bathing, lanolin should be used to keep the skin soft.

(7) If circulation in the leg is bad, your doctor may advise you to do various exercises. To do these, lie flat on the bed, having a chair tipped upside down on the bed with a pillow lying on it so the legs may be elevated at a 45 degree angle. First place the legs on the back of the chair and keep them there until they become blanched or white. This usually takes from one to three minutes. Then let the feet hang over the side of the bed, working the toes and feet up and down like opening and closing the hand, for one minute longer than it takes for a good red color to develop. Then the feet should be placed flat in bed for from three to five minutes. The whole procedure is then repeated six or seven times once or twice a day.

Infections of any sort, whether a respiratory infection or infections of other parts of the body, almost always make the diabetes temporarily worse. This means you may have more sugar in the urine, and may require more insulin. Ordinarily, with mild infections, the maintenance of the usual dose of insulin or oral agents and eating lightly will be all that is necessary. If a high fever is present, if the infection persists over a period of two or three days, and large quantities of urine are passed, a physician should be notified.

Another complication that occurs occasionally is *neuritis*, or inflammation of the nerves. Neuritis consists of numbness and tingling or pains in the arms and legs. It is usually the result of poor control of the diabetes. If treated promptly by careful regulation and with the aid of certain medications, such as Vitamin B, the neuritis will usually respond to treatment.

Early diagnosis, prompt and proper treatment have prolonged the life of the diabetic considerably. Properly treated, diabetics can expect to live just about as long as anyone else and as usefully and happily. Proper treatment calls for a close working relationship between the diabetic patient and his physician.

Diet is still the basis of the treatment of diabetes. Insulin is needed in some individuals, but in a large proportion of patients, particularly older ones, the diabetes can be controlled by a diet and an oral drug. Successful treatment depends not only on diet, insulin and drugs, but also on the favorable outlook of the individual patient.

Diabetics do best when they put aside concern for their condition, trust in the doctor with whom they are cooperating, and lead normally active lives. Virtually every calling in life is open to them.

PREGNANCY AND CHILDBIRTH

by ROBERT LANDESMAN, M.D.

Diagnosis of Pregnancy • Changes the
Patient May Notice

PRE-NATAL CARE AND EXAMINATION
Care During Pregnancy

PREPARING FOR CHILDBIRTH

THE COURSE OF PREGNANCY
The First Trimester • The Second
Trimester • The Third Trimester

LABOR AND DELIVERY
As Labor Nears • Understanding Labor
• Pain Relief in Childbirth • Hospital
Procedures • Cesarean Section • The
Puerperium • Aftercare • After
Hospital Discharge

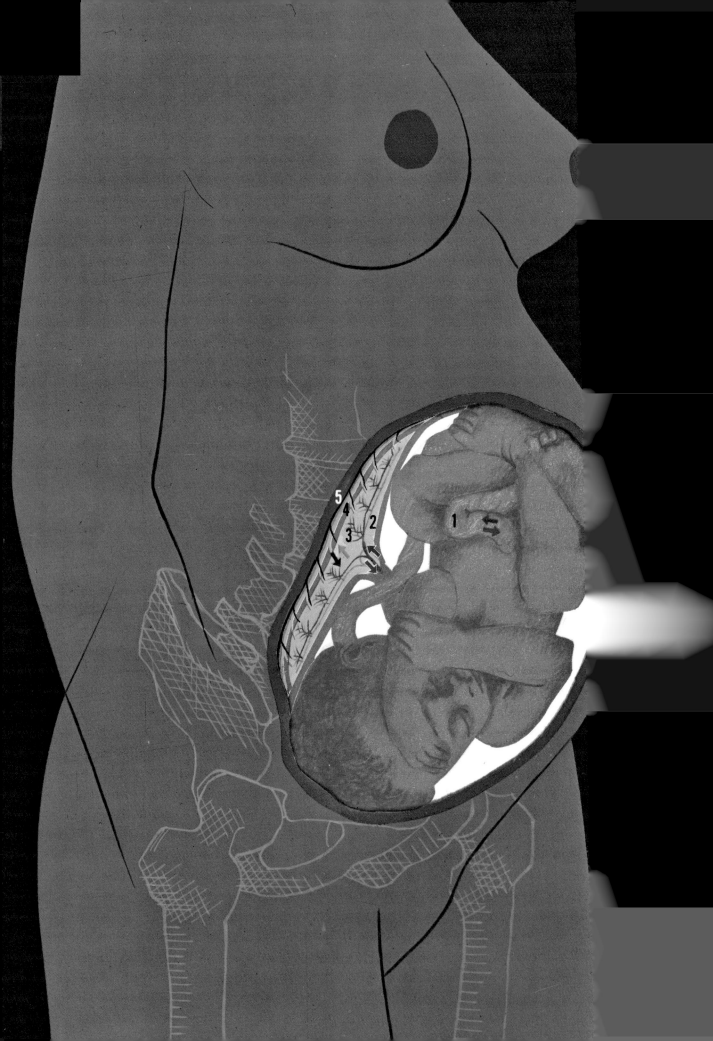

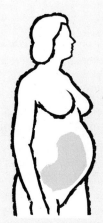

The intricate interlocking of maternal and fetal tissues in well-advanced pregnancy is shown diagrammatically in the color plate; the actual fine structures are bewildering microscopic mazes. The *placenta* (2) attached to the wall of the *uterus* (5) is the great temporary organ through which the fetus receives nourishment and disposes of the wastes. *Villi* (3) are profusely branched, minute fingerlike processes that merge into blood vessels of the *umbilical cord* (1). *Uterine vessels* (4) bring maternal blood to the placenta and drain it away.

Villi of the fetal side of the placenta float in maternal blood in excavated caverns fed by maternal arteries and emptied by maternal veins (blue arrows). These "caverns" are minute crevices between maternal and fetal tissues. Nutritional elements in maternal blood are diffused and absorbed across the villi into the fetal circulation. In the opposite direction, carbon dioxide and nitrogenous wastes of the fetus are diffused across the villi walls into the maternal circulation. Red arrows show the intake and output pathways of the fetal circulation. Usually there is no direct connection between the maternal and fetal circulations.

CHAPTER 10

PREGNANCY AND CHILDBIRTH

by ROBERT LANDESMAN, M. D.

Most women are anxious at times to know if they are pregnant. Difficulties of confirming pregnancy vary greatly from one patient to another.

Some women walk into a doctor's office and announce that they are pregnant. The evidence to them is perfectly obvious. They may complain of nausea, inability to eat a certain food or lack of morning appetite, or sudden distaste for cigarettes. Their menstrual period is several weeks late. They may have noticed an increase in breast size with a feeling of heaviness, darkening of the area surrounding the nipples, increased frequency of urination, and a feeling of heaviness in the pelvic area. Some have marked salivation — excess of saliva.

A "package" of all the above-mentioned symptoms would surely indicate to an anxious woman that she is probably pregnant. But to the physician these signs are not truly diagnostic of pregnancy.

Diagnosis of Pregnancy

At the present time there are four criteria for the presence of pregnancy. The *first criterion* is a *positive reaction to a biological test for pregnancy.*

Pregnancy tests. Hormonal products of conception, present in the urine of pregnant women, have a remarkably stimulating effect on the ovaries of young mice. This is the basis of the Ascheim-Zondek or AZ Test for pregnancy, first described over 30 years ago. The test is first definitely positive about four weeks after fertilization takes place, or six weeks after the last menstrual period.

The test requires a specimen of the patient's urine, taken first thing in the morning on awakening. Preferably the patient does not eat or drink after eight or nine p.m. the night before. The evening meal should be bland, without alcohol, drugs or seasoned foods which will leave products in the urine that can kill the test animals. Small amounts of urine are injected into mice over a three-day period. Pregnancy is indicated by obvious activity in ovaries of the mice. The test is most reliable, on the order of 95 to 98 per cent.

"Faster" tests have largely superseded the original AZ Test. The "rat test" and "rabbit test," almost as reliable as the original mouse test, take about 24 hours instead of three days. In the past decade the "frog test," performed in three to five hours, has become popular. These animal tests are usually performed with a urine specimen but they may be performed with blood.

Pregnancy tests are now regularly performed in the laboratory or in the doctor's office without animals. An agglutination test recognizes the presence of a hormone excreted by the placenta (chorionic gonadotrophin), which indicates pregnancy. The test is highly reliable and gives a dependable answer as early as ten to 14 days after the first missed menstrual period. The first, or early morning, urine provides a higher concentration of hormone and is more likely to be positive than more diluted specimens during the day. Drugs and alcohol are best omitted during the 12 hours prior to collection of the urine specimen. The test may be performed on a blood specimen, which may be desirable under rare circumstances when speed is essential.

A number of hormone preparations useful in diagnosing pregnancy are available. These are called *progestins* and are closely related to the natural hormone, *progesterone,* which is produced during every normal menstrual cycle. If one of these progestins is injected or given by mouth for four or five days, the patient, if *not* pregnant, will bleed two to seven days after the last dose. If she *is* pregnant there is no bleeding (called withdrawal bleeding), because her body and the early developing fetus are producing large amounts of progesterone, and the small amount given for the test does not significantly change the body level. In a non-pregnant woman, withdrawal of the progestin produces uterine bleeding just as occurs in a normal menstrual cycle. These compounds are not of the same degree of reliability as the biological tests for pregnancy.

Animal tests are very accurate, though an occasional doubtful result requires repetition. Usually, two or three animals are injected with the same urine specimen, and if all are "positive," pregnancy is virtually certain. It is important to use a laboratory that performs these tests every day, since accuracy is reduced if technicians do the tests infrequently.

The *second* positive test for pregnancy is the *presence of the fetal skeleton,* shown by direct x-ray film of the abdomen. It takes about four months of pregnancy for sufficient calcification to occur to make the fetal skeleton visible on an x-ray film.

The *third* reliable indicator of pregnancy is *fetal movements*. The patient may "feel life" between the sixteenth and twentieth weeks. She may misinterpret intestinal and muscular activity as movements of the fetus, but the trained physician may easily discern definitive movements of the infant by palpating the abdomen of the patient.

The *fourth* indicator of pregnancy is *the infant's heartbeat,* distinguishable at the eighteenth week (infrequently, the sixteenth week). With a stethoscope, the rapid fetal heart rate is easily distinguished from that of the mother.

Changes the Patient May Notice

There are a number of changes in the body and the way she feels that a woman may notice. These may or may not be associated with pregnancy.

Nausea and vomiting may occasionally begin even before the first missed menstrual period. The most frequent type is "morning sickness." Nausea may be worst at breakfast and may subside during the afternoon and recur in the evening. There are many reasons for nausea and vomiting; pregnancy is one of them. Nausea may continue with varying intensity for the first three months and then subside abruptly about the time the woman has missed her third menstrual period. Usually the patient with this nausea will not lose or gain weight, but a rare patient will refuse food and drink and lose much weight and require hospitalization. Serious complications from nausea and vomiting of pregnancy are rarely seen in this country.

Constipation is often but not always an associated complaint. Patients who have been troubled with constipation prior to pregnancy may have more difficulty as soon as pregnancy occurs. It is not a reliable symptom of pregnancy.

Congestion. Because of the increased amount of blood in the reproductive organs, associated with early pregnancy, many women often notice an increased feeling of weight in the pelvis. This feeling of weight, along with progressive slowing of intestinal activity, frequently leads to bloating of the lower abdomen. This bloating is not in any way related to enlarging of the uterus.

Pronounced exhaustion is very common during early pregnancy. Frequently, all the patient requires is reassurance that feelings of fatigue and exhaustion will pass away after several weeks. Such feelings are usually unrelated to anemia or any associated disease.

Frequent urination and an almost constant feeling of bladder fullness are related to the bloating and the increase of blood supply in the uterus and bladder.

Distaste for smoking is common in pregnancy. Frequently the patient will say she "can't look at another cigarette" although she may have been an inveterate smoker. This aversion usually subsides after the third month.

A "missed period" is frequently the first sign of pregnancy. In the great majority of women with a menstrual cycle of 25 to 30 days, being ten days late usually means the presence of pregnancy. However, a large number of women have great irregularity in their cycles (but still within the normal limits) and they may be 15, 20, or 30 days late before the next menstrual period appears. In general, if a woman is 14 days late it is pretty good evidence that she is pregnant. But it is not conclusive because, not uncommonly, some women will miss a menstrual period entirely (particularly during the summer months). This is true of very thin and very obese women.

Basal body temperature. Some patients, because of difficulty in becoming pregnant, are put on basal body temperature charts by their physician. The basal body temperature taken in the morning will, at or about the time of ovulation (fertile period), increase about one degree Fahrenheit. If this occurs and the temperature continues to stay up for 20 days consecutively, it is very good evidence of pregnancy, if the patient is not taking any of the progesterone drugs.

Breast changes may be a prominent sign of early pregnancy, but in a large number of women this is not the case. Characteristic breast changes are an increase in the size of the pigmented area around the nipple (areola), and the presence of enlarged glands in the area immediately surrounding the nipple. The breast may increase in size and weight so that a larger bra is usually required. This increase also happens prior to onset of a regular menstrual cycle, but the degree of breast change is much greater in pregnancy and is maintained longer than the usual two week interval of a normal menstrual cycle.

Medical criteria. The physician, in the great majority of instances, will be able to make the diagnosis on pelvic examination, about three weeks after the missed period. Not infrequently, he will notice the presence of a blue discoloration about the entrance to the vagina and on the neck of the uterus. This is called "Chadwick's sign," after the doctor who first described it. The doctor may find the uterus to be slightly enlarged and somewhat softened, suggesting the presence of pregnancy.

Certain situations make the diagnosis of pregnancy more difficult. About 25 per cent of women have some staining or slight bleeding early in pregnancy. This bleeding may indicate a threatened miscarriage. Profuse bleeding early in pregnancy often may indicate that the patient has miscarried and may require a cleaning of the uterus, or *curettage* (see Chapter 22). Or the uterus may not enlarge at all after the onset of pregnancy, suggesting the death of the ovum and the probability that the entire pregnancy will be discarded in a few days.

Early miscarriages which occur in ten per cent of pregnancies may complicate diagnosis, and require some reduction of the patient's activities. Rarely, an *ectopic* (outside the womb) *pregnancy* may take place in the Fallopian tube. The physician is alert to this if there is vaginal staining, a uterus not as large as it should be, and a small mass in the tubal area with lower abdominal pain.

A *mole* is another rare entity in which there is growth of the placenta without any fetus. This rare and important complication will terminate by itself, usually in the first part of pregnancy.

In all instances, diagnosis of pregnancy should be made by the time of the second missed period. If there are complicating factors, these should be explained to the patient; and if the pregnancy is perfectly normal, as it usually is, she should be given happy reassurance.

PRE-NATAL CARE AND EXAMINATION

A physical examination when the physician first meets the expectant mother is essential. This may pick up variations which are correctible, prevent later complications, and save the pregnant woman time in the hospital.

General examination. The blood pressure is taken to establish a baseline level. Elevated blood pressure may presage a complication known as toxemia which usually occurs in the last three months of pregnancy. The heart is examined for function, rate and rhythm. The breasts are examined to note the pattern of the nipples, their suitability for nursing at a later date, and to determine whether cysts or tumors are present.

Laboratory examinations on this visit include complete urinalysis, a hematocrit (amount of red cells in the blood), blood grouping (A, AB, or O), blood test to rule out syphilis and determination of the Rh factor. About 86 per cent of the population is Rh positive, 14 per cent Rh negative. If the blood is Rh negative, tests to determine the presence of antibodies will be done later.

A dentist should examine the teeth during the first three months of pregnancy (see Chapter 15). There is no real evidence of rapid destruction of teeth because of pregnancy, but frequently there is swelling and bleeding from the gum margins, which good dental treatment can minimize. There is some evidence to indicate that addition of small amounts of fluoride will be beneficial to the teeth of the developing fetus. Most of the new vitamin preparations for pregnancy have fluoride added.

Pelvic examination. The cervix or neck of the uterus is examined and Papanicolaou smears are taken (these are cells from the cervical area, which, stained and examined under a microscope, may reveal early and curable cancer of the cervix). The position of the ovaries and tubes is noted, as well as the size of the uterus at this initial visit. The physician can determine if the rate of growth of the uterus is normal during the early months of pregnancy.

Pelvic measurements may be done at the first visit, though it may be preferable to do this in the last two months of pregnancy, when the vagina is softer and larger and there is good rapport between physician and patient so the examination may be done without tension or muscular spasm. Measurements are made of the outlet between the two bones which rim the birth passage, as well as measurements made through the vagina to determine the distance across the pelvis through which the infant must pass to enter the world.

Predicting the birth date. As soon as pregnancy is confirmed, the patient's first question is usually "when will the baby be born?" The general formula is that birth occurs 280 days from the last menstrual period or 267 days from the time of last ovulation. But duration of pregnancy is highly variable, ranging from 250 to 310 days from the last menstrual period, and perhaps only one out of ten babies is born on the EDC (expected date of confinement). Frequently in a first pregnancy the baby is born a week or so beyond the expected date. Many mothers tend to repeat early or late delivery dates in subsequent pregnancies; but there is no general rule about it and there are many exceptions.

Miscarriage. Pregnancy that terminates prior to the twentieth week, with a fetus weighing less than one pound, invariably incapable of life, is, in medical language, an *abortion* — usually called a "miscarriage" by laymen. Spontaneous abortions occur in about ten per cent of pregnancies.

Pregnancies ending between the twentieth and twenty-eighth week produce a fetus or infant weighing between one and two and a half pounds. These are called *previable* infants, and all will require a long period of care in a premature nursery, with generally a ten to 25 per cent chance of survival.

Premature infants are born between the twenty-eighth and thirty-fifth week of pregnancy. Their weights run from two and a half to five pounds. Chances of survival for the largest prematures are 80 to 90 per cent.

The *term* or mature infant is born between the thirty-fifth and forty-fifth week. These infants have an excellent chance of survival and almost invariably may return to the home with the mother when she is discharged from the hospital.

Care During Pregnancy

Weight gain during the complete pregnancy should be on the order of 20 per cent or less of the pre-pregnancy weight. A woman who weighs 100 pounds should gain about 20 pounds during pregnancy. An underweight woman may be allowed to gain more. However, the weight gain is not "all baby."

The average baby weighs about seven pounds. The placenta or afterbirth weighs one pound. Amniotic fluid which surrounds the baby weighs about a pound and a half. Increased size of the uterus accounts for two pounds, increase of blood in the body is about two pounds, and increased breast size results in another pound. Increase in weight which is directly associated with the baby is some 14 to 15 pounds. About another ten pounds are accumulated over the entire body as fluid and fat. Any additional increase in weight is disadvantageous, impedes moving about in the last months of pregnancy, and may make delivery more difficult.

Diet. The average diet in the United States is quite adequate during pregnancy. The pregnant woman should avoid foods of high fat content, spicy foods such as pastrami and pickles, and foods such as cauliflower, cabbage, and baked beans that produce a lot of gas. In general her diet should include:

For breakfast: fresh fruit, orange juice, poached egg, one piece of toast, coffee with milk.

For lunch she might have a salad of tomatoes, lettuce, chopped chicken or fruit, or perhaps instead of salad, an open meat sandwich with one slice of bread and tea or coffee.

Dinner may include a clear soup, three or four ounces of broiled meat, two leafy vegetables, baked potato, gelatine dessert or fruit, with tea or coffee.

Ideally, the pregnant woman should have one portion of broiled meat a day, one egg, and two glasses of milk. Skim milk is entirely satisfactory, particularly for women who are overweight. Two glasses of milk will satisfy requirements for calcium and minerals necessary for building the infant's skeleton.

One of the vitamin products especially prepared for pregnancy should be taken, usually one dose daily. It is desirable that the product not contain iron, since this makes the capsule too large. There is a tendency for pregnant women to develop a relative anemia. After the third or fourth month, supplemental iron should be given and continued until delivery, and after if required, because of low blood count. A large reserve of iron in the liver, spleen, and bone marrow allows a much more rapid recovery from any iron deficiency.

If the patient is very obese, calorie-restricting techniques to lose weight, such as use of sugarless dietetic foods, may be used during pregnancy at times and circumstances when a physician prescribes them.

Two groups of women should be particularly cautioned about food intake and weight increase.

The obese woman may add weight very easily. This becomes a serious liability in labor. It is difficult for the obstetrician to determine the usual signs of progress of labor. The intense physical effort of labor is poorly tolerated and any procedure which includes anesthesia becomes more hazardous. Constant effort must be made to hold the weight gain to a minimum for maternal and infant safety, particularly in labor.

The second group consists of women who have high blood pressure, kidney disease, or previous toxemia of pregnancy. Rapid weight gain produced by a high salt diet with swelling or edema and elevation of blood pressure may precipitate a toxemia and constitute a grave threat to the unborn child. Rapid weight gain of more than two pounds in one week increases hazards to the fetus and may not be reversible by diuretics or restrictions in diet. Dietary regulation, if required by the obstetrician, may be for many months the most important medical therapy during pregnancy.

Bowel function. *Diarrhea* is undesirable because it is debilitating and may interfere with nutrition if prolonged. An occasional loose stool is not necessarily diarrhea. Pectin products or rice and potatoes may be used for mild diarrheas, but if the diarrhea is severe there should be no hesitation in using a prescribed drug such as paregoric to control it.

Constipation is almost universal during pregnancy. The simplest way of treating it is by liberal use of fruit juices, particularly prune, apricot, and orange juice. Laxative agents which increase the bulk of intestinal contents or very mild-acting chemicals such as senna products may be given.

Nausea and vomiting appear in most pregnancies during the first three months. The nausea subsides after the third missed period. Women should complain about this nausea to their physicians, who can assure them that it is related only to changes in the body associated with early pregnancy.

Eating dried fruits in small amounts and keeping the stomach slightly coated with food frequently helps to control nausea. Dried crackers, biscuits, or stale rye bread may be helpful early in the morning. Frequently, nausea is made worse by late rising and a rush to get to one's job. Relaxation and unhurried movements in the morning tend to minimize the nausea.

If nausea is severe, mild sedation may be helpful. At times, various anti-nausea drugs may provide relief when taken either orally or rectally, as directed by a physician. If the patient is not able to eat or drink for 24 hours, the doctor should be notified immediately.

Heartburn or burning pain in the area just below the ribs is frequent in the middle and later months of pregnancy. It is probably due to changes in the position of the stomach, related to the enlargement of the uterus, and to changes in acidity of the stomach. A quarter of a glass of skim milk will reduce the heartburn. Various standard antacid products may prove to be helpful, but bicarbonate of soda should be avoided because, although it will relieve heartburn, it can produce swelling of the entire body.

Spells of *shortness of breath* frequently occur in the later months of pregnancy, from pressure of the enlarging womb upon the diaphragm. This is not related to any disease of the lungs. Propping up the patient on two or three pillows frequently helps.

Flatulence or intestinal gas commonly occurs in pregnancy; the intestines are merely slowing down due to effects of hormones produced by the pregnancy. Discomfort may be reduced somewhat during pregnancy, by not consuming gas-forming foods such as cabbage, baked beans, cauliflower and broccoli.

Muscle cramps are frequent, particularly in the lower extremities, about the calves and thighs. These are associated with changes in the mineral content of the muscles during pregnancy. Limiting the consumption of milk to one glass a day for a week may reduce the cramps.

Back pain commonly occurs from changes induced by pregnancy. All the ligaments attached to bones become softened. The protruding abdomen and weakened abdominal muscles affect the posture or "stance" of the pregnant woman. Also, there are various neuromuscular relationships that may be affected by the advancing pregnancy.

Generally, the disturbing back pain can be lessened by good standing posture and sitting on hard well-shaped chairs rather than soft cushioned couches or chairs. Standard simple exercises of abdomen and back muscles ease the discomfort. The bed should have a hard mattress, perhaps even a board placed under the mattress. Frequent car riding may produce back pain. Hard backrests are available to support the back muscles and improve driving posture. Driving may have to be curtailed if back pain is very severe and none of these measures help. A light, well-fitted supporting garment may be used to improve posture in walking and sitting.

Sleeping habits of the pregnant woman may be upset. Emotional factors, such as worrying that something is wrong with the baby or that the baby is not moving, may keep her from falling asleep readily. Reassurance is important and worries should be talked out with doctor. Sleeping as well as breathing is easier in the last months of pregnancy if two or three pillows are used to prop the patient. In the last six weeks of pregnancy it is wise not to eat too late in the evening or to eat too large a meal. Mild sleep-inducing medications may be given safely if the sleeplessness is severe.

The beneficial effects of reasonable amounts of physical exercise in promoting conditions favorable to dropping to sleep at night should not be overlooked.

Faintness. The pregnant woman may get light-headed and possibly faint at least once during her pregnancy. If a fainting spell comes on, lie down or bend the head down between the legs and dizziness and faintness will subside quickly. Some women worry that they will "pass out" while driving a car. However, unless fainting spells occur with great frequency, driving is usually not forbidden. Premonitory sensations give a chance to pull over to the side of the road and lie down with the head at seat level. Carry a lump of sugar or piece of hard candy, chew on this, and dizziness and faintness will usually disappear. Fainting spells are at their maximum between the third and sixth months of pregnancy and rarely occur later.

Varicose veins often appear in pregnancy. The simplest way to prevent worsening of the varicosities is not to use constricting garters or rolled socks about the legs. When resting, elevate the legs on another chair or couch. If the veins are extensive, full-length elastic stockings may be worn, particularly when standing or walking for extended periods of time. Elastic stockings should fit tightly and are best put on by raising the leg far above the body and rolling them on from the foot. If a vein becomes tender, reddened and swollen it may be the early onset of phlebitis and the doctor should be consulted promptly for proper care. Surgery for removal of varicose veins is usually not recommended during pregnancy.

Hemorrhoids are quite common during pregnancy. Hemorrhoids are large veins about the opening of the rectum. Increased pressure of the enlarging abdomen and uterus tends to overdistend these veins. They may protrude outside the anus and be aggravated by hard or infrequent bowel movements. These are best treated by additional rest during the day and by cold compresses of diluted witch hazel. Discomfort may be relieved by anesthetic ointments prescribed by the doctor. Occasionally, a small hemorrhoid may become thrombosed (develop a blood clot in it) and be very painful. The doctor should be consulted and he will promptly relieve the discomfort. Surgery for hemorrhoids is not indicated during pregnancy.

Vaginal discharge is quite frequent during pregnancy. Moisture about the vaginal entrance tends to increase as pregnancy progresses toward the time of delivery. There are two common causes for abnormal vaginal discharge. A fungus called *monilia* causes a white flow. This is treated by specific drugs, either anti-fungal agents or gentian violet preparations. The other infection causes a foamy, bubbly discharge produced by *trichomonas* parasites. A new antitrichomonal drug which may be taken either by mouth or vaginally, is relatively specific for eradication of this condition.

Vaginal bleeding is quite frequently encountered during pregnancy. At the time of the first missed period, some staining and slight bleeding may be related to implantation of the fertilized egg in the wall of the uterus. This bleeding usually subsides in several days. If bleeding progresses it may be due to a threatened abortion and the doctor should be informed. Occasionally, bleeding is due to a benign growth at the neck of the uterus called a polyp, or by a softening of cervical tissue, called an erosion. This area bleeds easily on pressure. The doctor can control it. Occasionally, bleeding is produced by intercourse.

Exercise is important during pregnancy. Walking for a mile or so is fine for the average pregnant woman, but a long hike of four or five hours would be overdoing it. Dancing in its milder and less vigorous forms may be recommended. Sports such as tennis, golfing, or swimming, for short periods of time, are good relaxation for patients who are accustomed to them. This is too much activity for the final two months of pregnancy. More strenuous activities which are hazardous or fraught with tumbles, such as ice skating, skiing, horseback riding, diving, aqua-lunging and waterskiing are to be avoided during pregnancy. Even the exercises recommended are not advisable if the pregnancy is complicated by bleeding or cramps.

Every patient is an individual and the type of exercise good for her should be discussed with the physician.

Traveling is not hazardous for the normal pregnant woman. Airplane transport in pressurized cabins is the easiest form of travel. Rail travel is a little more difficult because of continuous pounding. Automobile travel for long distances is even more strenuous than train travel. Trips by car should be limited to two to three hundred miles a day, with frequent breaks to get out of the car, move around, and rest. Of course, some complication may make it unwise for a particular pregnant woman to travel; if so, the doctor will advise her.

It is not unusual for a woman in the first six months or so of pregnancy to make a long trip to a distant part of the country or even to go abroad. In such case she should have the name of an obstetrician who practices at her destination. She can also communicate with her own doctor by long distance telephone. In the final five or six weeks of pregnancy she should stay within 30 miles, or about an hour's easy traveling time, of the hospital.

Seat belts should be used at all times when driving or as a passenger in a car. The safety belt must *not* be placed high on the abdomen, but lower down, snug about the hipbones which can take the shock of a sudden stop.

Clothing should not fit tightly. Purchase lightweight undergarments that may be worn in both warm and cool weather. There is no reason why usual undergarments — a two-way stretch, for example — can't be worn in the early months of pregnancy, until they become too tight. When backache becomes troublesome, maternity girdles usually give considerable relief. High heels are an extra hazard when the abdomen enlarges and balance is precarious at best. However, a short woman married to a tall man may feel ill at ease in flats, and for morale reasons she may be permitted to wear moderately high heels if she is aware of the dangers involved.

Drugs should be used only for absolutely necessary reasons during pregnancy, particularly in the first three months when the vital structures and organs of the baby are being organized. The various antibiotics should not be used during pregnancy except for reasons the doctor considers compelling. Not only does the use of these drugs sometimes produce an annoying vaginal discharge, but strains of germs resistant to the drugs' actions may emerge. Such infections in a newborn infant are serious. Any drugs to which the patient is sensitive should be noted and used with caution if at all during pregnancy.

All drugs are forbidden during pregnancy except those specifically approved by the patient's doctor. The tragedy of thalidomide, a seemingly innocuous sedative which caused cruel birth deformities when taken by a mother during pregnancy, alerted the profession to unexpected hazards of drugs at critical stages of fetal development. Obstetricians generally have cut the use of medication during pregnancy to a bare minimum.

It is inadvisable to have extensive **x-ray diagnosis** performed during pregnancy, particularly during the first three months, because the embryo may be endangered by radiation. When x-rays are essential during pregnancy, the abdomen should be shielded with a lead apron and exposures kept to a minimum. Also, it is wise for a woman not to have postponable x-rays during the second part of her menstrual cycle because of the possibility that she has conceived.

If a pregnant woman eats raw meat or is in contact with cats, a test for *toxoplasmosis* (page 73) may be desirable.

Smoking during pregnancy has occasioned some furor. There is statistical evidence that infants tend to be smaller and the incidence of prematurity greater if the mother smokes excessively. It may be cruel, and frequently futile, to forbid cigarettes entirely to a woman who is accustomed to them, but nothing but good can come from cutting consumption from a pack or two a day to perhaps a half dozen cigarettes.

Infectious diseases may complicate pregnancy. It has been well publicized that an attack of German measles up to the ninth or tenth week of pregnancy may produce serious congenital malformations of the baby. If a pregnant woman has German measles or knows she has been exposed to the disease, she should consult her obstetrician immediately for advice on what to do.

Fortunately, there is now available a German measles (rubella) vaccine which is one of the important recent advances in obstetrics. Young girls who receive the vaccine through state programs or their doctors are immune to the viral infection and need never worry about the serious complications of German measles during a pregnancy in later years. It is recommended that all girls receive it before the age of ten.

A blood test to determine whether or not a woman is immune to German measles—many people have had the disease and become immune but do not know it or cannot remember—can be performed early in pregnancy. If the pregnant woman is not immune, she should avoid contact with anyone with a rash for the first three months. It is not considered safe at present to give the live-virus rubella vaccine during pregnancy because it might infect the fetus, but it may be given after the baby is born. The vaccine is an excellent immunizing agent that produces a high degree of immunity.

Poliomyelitis is a serious complication of pregnancy, but easily averted by vaccination as directed by the doctor. Influenza vaccination, though not recommended for everybody in the population, is an important protection for the pregnant woman.

All States in this country require a serologic test for syphilis in pregnant women. This is done routinely from a blood specimen obtained at the time of pre-natal examination. People can have syphilis without knowing it. The disease can be a serious complication for the baby, or result in late miscarriage, premature delivery, and even infant death. Syphilis discovered early in pregnancy can be cured readily with penicillin.

Most women have been vaccinated against smallpox, diphtheria and whooping cough, and many have acquired immunity to measles and chickenpox, by recovery from these diseases. However, it is prudent to avoid direct exposure to childhood diseases such as mumps, scarlet fever, and others. These diseases may not directly affect the fetus, but high fever may result in premature labor and termination of the pregnancy.

Pre-natal checkups. A physician cannot anticipate every question that may come up during the nine months of pregnancy. The intelligent patient will call her doctor at any time of the day or night when she considers it necessary. If a long trip is contemplated, the doctor should be informed. Old-wives' tales about pregnancy still persist, and the doctor can give reassurance about worrisome questions if they are asked.

The keystone of modern obstetrics is continued observation of the patient throughout pregnancy. Most of the complications of pregnancy, associated in the past with lack of medical attention, can be prevented when the patient is seen at frequent intervals.

During the first six months the patient should be seen every three to four weeks; during the seventh month, every three weeks; during the eighth month, every two weeks; and during the last month she should be seen every week.

The first visit to the physician includes a physical examination and blood-urine tests. Thereafter, visits include discussion of problems that may have come up, a review of the patient's progress, and a brief examination. This includes examination of the abdomen, listening for the fetal heart, palpating the size of the baby, and examination of a urine specimen. During the last month of pregnancy there is usually a weekly vaginal examination to determine the "ripening" of the neck of the uterus, the position of the baby, and the proximity of onset of labor.

PREPARING FOR CHILDBIRTH

Education for expectant parents has played an increasingly important role in recent years. In many obstetrical clinics throughout the country a series of six to eight sessions is given, usually at weekly intervals. These generally begin when the pregnancy is six to seven months along. Much of the mystery of the experience to come is cleared away by comforting understanding of the development of the fetus, body changes related to pregnancy, and the mechanism of labor. These courses are given by the American Red Cross, the Child Study Association of America, the Maternity Center Association of New York, and by most of the large teaching centers.

The expectant mother immediately gets heartening assurance that the risk of childbirth is scarcely greater than the risks of living without pregnancy. A half-hour trip by car on a congested highway is a distinctly greater hazard. The achievements of modern obstetrics are of course closely related to advances in all fields of medicine.

Exercises which develop muscles important in labor (principally of the abdomen, back, and pelvic floor) are practiced. *Breathing exercises* are particularly stressed as an aid during labor. The rhythmic activity of breathing has a calming effect, gives the woman in labor something to concentrate on, and helps to disassociate uterine contractions from overall tensions of the entire body. The *first stage* of labor is that during which contractions gradually increase in frequency and intensity. Slow, long, deep breathing is practiced for application in the early and middle parts of the first stage. Shallow, rapid breathing is substituted when first stage contractions become strong, on the verge of transition to the **second** stage of labor which terminates with expulsion of the baby. During the transition from first to second stage, a "pant, pant, blow" rhythm of breathing prevents pushing or bearing-down effort before the neck of the uterus is fully dilated. The "blow" part is exhalation through parted lips without contracting the abdomen.

Finally, in the second stage of labor, long "pushing" similar to that practiced with a bowel movement is substituted. As the baby's head is born, rapid panting breaths — begun at the obstetrician's command — help to prevent injury to the mother's tissues as the head emerges.

These well known special breathing rhythms are excellent for lessening the pain in labor by giving the mother a distracting and useful activity with assurance that everything is proceeding normally. Constant attention of an obstetrician or obstetrical nurse is necessary for best results with these techniques that the patient has practiced.

A great advantage of "training for childbirth" is that the need for sedatives at delivery is almost always reduced. High or even moderate doses of pain-relieving drugs may depress the onset of breathing in the newborn. Small amounts of sedation are necessary in most labors, but large or frequent doses are practically always unnecessary in the "educated" patient.

A woman may not desire or be able to attend formal preparation classes. The gap can be bridged very satisfactorily by conversations with the obstetrician and a "learn as you go" course guided by the obstetrical nurse during the actual progress of labor.

Hypnosis. True hypnosis goes far beyond suggestibility, distraction and reassurance instilled in preparation for childbirth classes. The obstetrician must

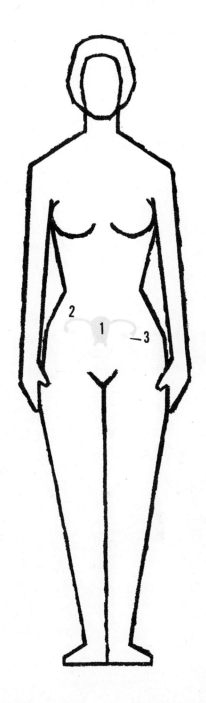

Orientation figure showing non-pregnant *uterus* (1), *Fallopian tubes* or *oviducts* (2), and *ovaries* (3). The ovary, analagous to the testis in the male, is attached by a rounded cord (ligament) to the upper side of the uterus behind the Fallopian tube. Actual position varies in individuals, with posture, and in women who have borne children.

spend a great deal of time in inducing and releasing the patient from the hypnotic state, and his almost constant attendance is necessary. Patients suit-

Fertilization and implantation of the ovum. The left side of the drawing shows an intact *uterus* (1); the cutaway right half shows some structures out of proportion, for clarification. The *ovary* (3) releases a mature *ovum* (5) from a burst follicle. The ovum encounters male germ cells in the tube (4) and *fertilization* (6) precipitates a series of *cell divisions* (7) which occur during the three or four day passage through the tube. It is thought that the microscopic cell-cluster remains free in the uterine cavity for several days and *implants* itself (8) in the *endometrium* or lining of the uterus (2) approximately 11 days after fertilization.

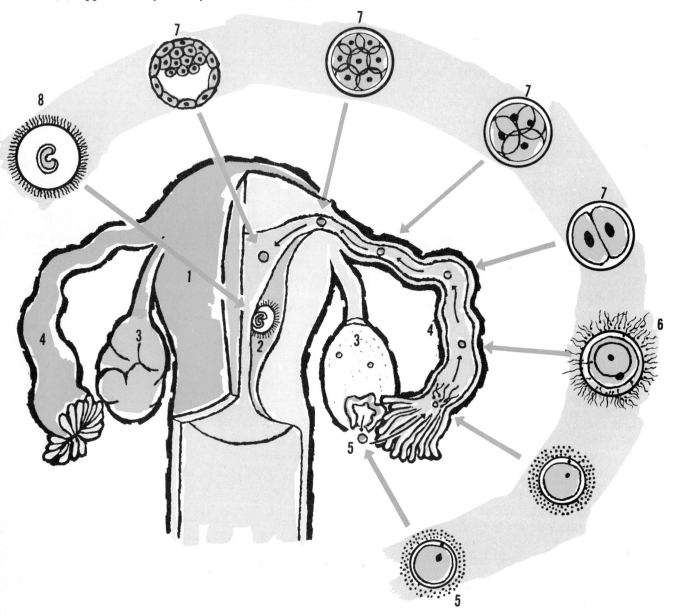

able for and desirous of hypnosis are usually rather carefully selected. Hypnosis, although dramatic in its relief of pain, is not a routine technique but one useful in particular circumstances.

There is a tendency for a patient prepared for a normal delivery to be taken by surprise by complications. She may wish and expect events to continue nor-mally although some complication may compel a departure from her expectations. Thus, childbirth preparation courses stress that there are particular considerations which may require anesthesia, forceps delivery, or even cesarean section, which are unpredictable but which the obstetrician will recognize and deal with effectively.

THE COURSE OF PREGNANCY

All pregnancies are divided into three parts (by the medical profession). Each part is a *trimester* — a period of three months, or more precisely, of 13 weeks. This division is useful because various events, signs, and developments tend to appear in different trimesters.

The First Trimester

During the first three months the uterus enlarges to about three times its non-pregnant size. This places it approximately at the pelvic brim so that it is usually not palpable (perceptible by touch) in the abdomen.

Bleeding of some severity is the most frequent unusual feature of the first trimester. About 20 per cent of women will stain or have a blood smudge on their underwear for one to three days. Usually this is "implantation bleeding" as the fertilized egg nests into the uterine wall after its descent down the Fallopian tube (oviduct) where fertilization occurs.

Implantation usually occurs about three weeks after the last menstrual period. At this stage the developing egg is barely visible to the naked eye, about the size of the point of a sharp pencil.

No further bleeding may occur. But if bleeding continues, with some slight cramps, there is **threatened abortion** with survival of the fetus in precarious balance. If cramps become severe and rhythmical, similar to labor contractions, bleeding becomes profuse, and on vaginal examination the doctor finds the neck of the uterus opening up, the condition is described as **inevitable abortion.**

If the fetus is expelled but the placenta remains, this is an **incomplete abortion.** This usually requires a curettage of the uterus to remove the remaining products of conception. Thereafter bleeding is usually moderate for a day or two and then staining ensues for several more days. Usually the uterus returns to its normal size in three to four weeks and a normal menstrual cycle intervenes at about the same time.

Early stage of implantation of the embryo, greatly enlarged (the structure shown in the squares would barely be visible to the naked eye). Once the *embryo* (1) with its *yolk sac* (2) is implanted, *villi* (3), originating from a membrane, the *chorion* (4), burrow into the lining of the uterus and form "roots" to anchor the embryo. At the same time, changes take place in the uterine lining and a *placenta* begins to develop.

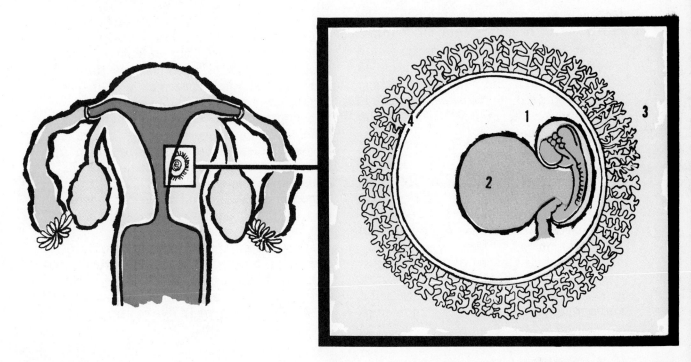

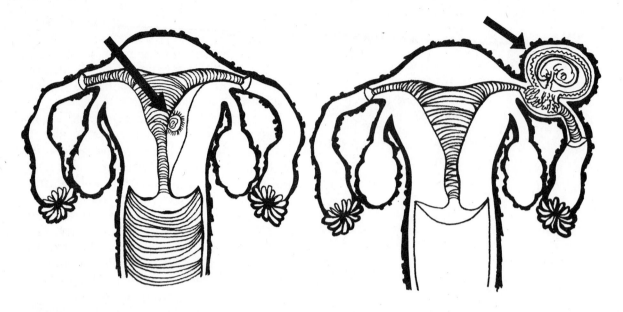

Normal pregnancy. Ovum rests in wall of womb, fetus grows in womb.

Ectopic pregnancy. Drawing shows embryo growing in Fallopian tube.

A *spontaneous abortion* — or "miscarriage" — is a natural process that occurs without artificial intervention. The vast majority of such abortions probably occur as a result of a developing egg with serious defects incompatible with life, or destined to give rise to a cruelly malformed fetus. The untimely occurrence of a spontaneous abortion is infinitely less of a burden than the presence of an infant that could not live long, and this is nature's way of ending a defective pregnancy and reestablishing the reproductive machinery for offspring.

Sometimes the fetus dies in the womb and the womb fails to grow. This is called *missed abortion,* and again, a curettage may be required. An *induced abortion* is one in which the uterus is emptied by human intervention. A *therapeutic abortion* is one justified in the eyes of the law, usually because continuation of pregnancy threatens the mother's life. Such indications are quite rare. If a woman has three or more consecutive spontaneous abortions, she is designated as an *habitual* aborter.

The embryo, a mere pinpoint in size at the beginning of the first trimester, grows to a length of some three inches and a weight of one ounce by the end of the third month. During this time, all of the vital organs — heart, lungs, intestines, brain, eyes, ears and skeleton—are formed. It is at this crucial period, when some women do not even know that they are pregnant, that outside insults such as drugs and illnesses of the mother can inflict disaster on the fetus. Once the basic structures are well developed, the fetus is somewhat better able to fend off insults of its environment.

Ectopic pregnancy usually occurs in the first trimester. The infinitesimal embryo is trapped in the blind alley of a Fallopian tube and will grow at this ectopic ("outside of the uterus") point. Space for growth in the narrow tube is very limited, and rupture usually ensues in the second or third month.

Symptoms of ectopic pregnancy begin when the tube is overdistended. There is severe one-sided pain, bleeding as in a miscarriage, and a small swelling in the tubal area may be felt by the doctor. Blood in the abdomen frequently reaches and irritates the diaphragm and this is felt as pain in the shoulder. Surgery to remove the portion of the tube containing the pregnancy is the only satisfactory treatment. Recovery is rapid and the patient will be walking about the hospital in one day and home in five or six.

Is normal pregnancy possible after an ectopic pregnancy? Yes, but it is not uncommon for a woman who has had one ectopic pregnancy to have another on the other side. The doctor will be alert for this possible complication if the patient has had an ectopic pregnancy.

The Second Trimester

The second trimester is the most peaceful time of pregnancy with the fewest complications.

Growth. From a length of three inches and a weight of one ounce, the fetus grows to some 14 inches and a weight of two and a quarter pounds at the end of the second trimester. The accommodating uterus enlarges steadily to an edge two and a half inches above the navel. Movements of the fetus ("quickening") become noticeable at about 20 weeks or midway in the second trimester. Usually the obstetrician will be able to hear the fetal heartbeat. The mother's weight gain is most rapid during these three months, averaging close to a pound a week.

Premature labor. The greatest hazard of this trimester is premature labor and delivery. The patient should report immediately any continued weak contractions, vaginal staining, or thin watery vaginal discharge. Any of these may suggest that the neck of the uterus is opening and a vaginal examination will confirm or deny it.

Premature labor results in a "preemie" (an infant below five pounds in weight) which usually requires special pediatric care, including use of an incubator and tube feeding. The obstetrician will do everything possible to maintain the infant in the uterus for the full period of normal gestation, to reduce risks to the infant. In general, bedrest, sedation, and abstinence from intercourse will be helpful in averting premature labor.

Premature birth in the second trimester ends unhappily with death of the infant nine times out of ten. The other ten per cent of larger "premies" survive after a long period of many months in an incubator. There is some hope that threatened premature birth when the

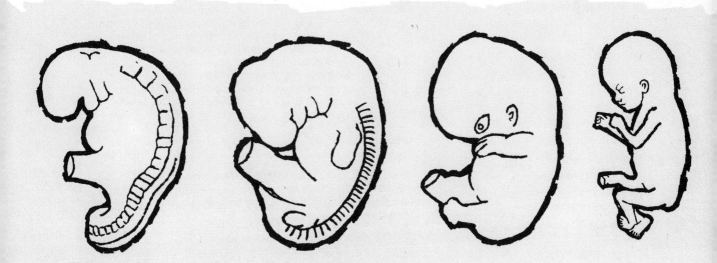

Rapid changes in development of the embryo and fetus are shown in four stages, from left to right: at two weeks, four weeks, eight weeks, and twelve weeks. Drawings do not show actual size. At four weeks the embryo is only about one-eighth of an inch "tall," at eight weeks, a little over half an inch. Organs such as the heart, ears, lungs, eyes and kidneys differentiate from primitive structures at critical stages of embryonic development. Injuries suffered by the embryo at such times may result in malformations of organs in process of development. By the third month, organ systems are quite well laid down and the fetus begins to look human.

TIMETABLE OF FETAL DEVELOPMENT

Only a few of the landmarks of growth of a new life in the womb can be given in the list below. Organs do not grow at uniform rates but surge forward, lag behind, come together, interact, change positions, and evince their earliest presence in the form of microscopic bulges and cell clusters that only an expert can recognize as the shape of things to come. Normally, conception occurs at the fimbriated end of the Fallopian tube (368) and it takes 3 or 4 days for the fertilized egg to reach the uterus.

AGE AFTER FERTILIZATION	STAGES OF GROWTH
5-9 DAYS	Remains free in uterine cavity.
10-11 DAYS	Attaches to and begins to become imbedded in the hormone-prepared lining of the uterus. Differentiation of embryonic germ layers (*ectoderm, mesoderm, endoderm*) from which specialized tissues will develop is well under way.
14 DAYS	Irregular, bloblike oval body with a faint longitudinal depression (*primitive streak*) from which cells are pushed continuously into enlarging body.
18-21 DAYS	Thickening of *neural plate*, forerunner of the central nervous system. The primitive heart is a simple tube. There are primitive lung buds. Two faint depressions are the sites of eyes. The embryo begins to curve head-to-tail to fit its environment.
4th WEEK	Beginning of gallbladder and liver tubules. Parts of brain begin differentiation. Local dilation indicates beginning of stomach. Heart tube becomes slightly bent with local bulges and constrictions. Nose parts suggested by pair of thickened bulges. There is a tiny liver prominence and belly stalk. Primitive head parts—mouth, brain, eyes, ears—are forming. Opening from mouth to gut breaks through; a little later, opening of anus. Primitive thyroid cells at floor of throat. Tiny rounded outgrowth suggests windpipe and larynx. The heart is under the chin. Its divisions are recognizable but it still operates as a simple tube. First heartbeats occur. Blood corpuscles form, circulation begins.
5th WEEK	Nasal pit, buds that will be arms and legs, cells that will develop into pancreas gland, tiny thickenings that will be tongue appear. The gut elongates. Primitive blood vessels function. Beginnings of eye lens, cranial nerves, retinal layer.
6th WEEK	Arm and leg buds lengthen, faint grooves suggest toes and fingers. Regional divisions of brain recognizable. Lung buds bifurcate. Primitive kidney parts established. Eyes far to either side of head. Epithelium and primitive ear parts begin to form. Nasal pits recognizable as nostrils. Stomach suggests adult form. Salivary glands identifiable. "Milk lines" from armpits to groin appear as slight thickening

from which breasts will later develop. Pre-cartilage cells laid down for parts of skeleton. Germ cells of gonads recognizable. First evidence of lymphatic system. Heart at critical stage of development; parts grow and fuse, its 4 chambers form.

7th WEEK

Distinct beginnings of fingers, toes, eyelids, delicate fibrils that will be muscles, autonomic nervous system. Nasal openings break through, optic nerve fibers extend, gallbladder elongates. Adrenal gland cells accumulate, thyroid cells start to move into position.

8th WEEK

Centers of bone growth established, formation of deeper lying bony structures begins, collar bone well ossified. Thumb and big toe begin to diverge. Local buds destined to be teeth appear. Rapid growth of nose and upper jaw. Bilateral parts of lips and palate meet and fuse. Human facial characteristics quite recognizable. Ears set very low on head. Externally, most of the changes from a minute oval body to a structure of recognizable human form (but not adult proportions) have been laid down.

3rd MONTH

Eyelids meet and fuse, eyes remain "closed" until seventh month. Bony parts of skull develop from base of skull upward. Ossification centers of jaws, nasal bones, ossicles of middle ear, occiput, are active. Inner ear structure almost completed. Eye lens formation proceeding rapidly. Primitive hair follicles and deeper-lying skin layers become distinct. External genitals evidenced by swellings; sex not obvious but distinguishable by an expert. Spots where nails will develop take shape. Buds of tear glands appear. Main lymphatic channels quite well marked. Vocal cords begin to take shape.

4th MONTH

Brain a recognizable miniature of adult brain; large bulge of forebrain distinguishable from cerebellum and brain stem. Paranasal sinuses have appeared. Buds of what will be sweat glands appear first on palms and soles. Bladder wall develops. Outer skin thickens into distinctive layers.

5th MONTH

Structures of testes and windpipe well established. Branching structures will become collecting tubules of kidney.

6th MONTH

Eyebrows, eyelashes begin to become visible. Fetus is coated with downy hair (*lanugo*). Skin ridges form on palms and soles, the lifelong basis of fingerprints and sole prints. The bronchial tree branches out actively, continues to do so after birth.

7th MONTH

Eyelids unfuse, that babies may be born with eyes open. Testes begin descent through inguinal ring to scrotum. Fat begins to be deposited under translucent skin layers and the fetus becomes plumper and plumper until birth.

A seven-month baby often is sufficiently well developed to survive. All of its vital systems have been established; what is lacking is the "finishing off" period of growth and maturation that normally occurs in the womb, but in the case of a premature infant has to take place in the outside world, requiring extra care. Every additional week in the womb, up to normal term, is of a plus value for the future life of the baby.

infant is too tiny to survive may be delayed by a Shirodkar operation, named for a doctor in India who had a patient who had three premature deliveries

Changes in size and contours of the uterus, abdomen, and breasts during the course of pregnancy. The uterus reaches progressively higher levels in the abdomen until about the middle of the last month. At that time, frequently during the first pregnancy, the head tends to settle deeper into the pelvis. This is called "*lightening*," from the sensation of decreased abdominal distention that is produced.

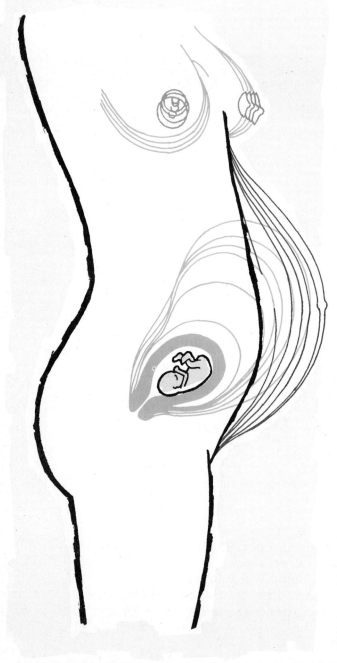

ending in stillbirths. In desperation, he placed a suture around the neck of the uterus and was able to maintain the pregnancy until the infant reached a weight of five pounds and survived. Occasionally the neck of the womb is closed carefully in selected patients and the technique has been considerably improved.

In recent years, intravenous alcohol has been effective in suppressing labor that has begun prematurely. Successful alcohol treatment may postpone labor for two to six weeks with delivery of a mature infant. Other drugs have been used for the same purpose in a small number of patients and some of them appear to be promising.

Toxemia may occur in the second trimester but is much more frequent in the last three months.

The Third Trimester

The last months of pregnancy are naturally subject to some increase in discomfort. The infant grows from a little over two pounds to seven pounds, on the average, and the uterus gradually continues to enlarge. There is almost constant activity of the womb's occupant, most noticeable to the hostess when she is inactive and most sensitive to internal gyrations, as when sitting, or just before going to bed, or waiting for a traffic light to change when driving.

Abnormal bleeding, again, is always something to report immediately to the doctor. There are two principal causes of such bleeding in the last trimester, and both arise from abnormalities that involve the placenta or afterbirth. Each occurs in about one out of 250 pregnancies.

Placenta previa is a mislocation of the placenta in an abnormally low position in the uterus. The placenta may be implanted directly over the outlet of the womb (central placenta previa), or it may be attached at the margin of the outlet or slightly higher on the uterine wall. As the neck of the uterus opens toward the end of pregnancy, a disruption of placental and uterine structures causes bleeding. The characteristic symptom is *painless vaginal bleeding*.

Bed rest in the hospital is usually compulsory. Transfusions may be necessary if bleeding is profuse, and cesarean section (delivery of the baby through the abdomen) may be required. Since every extra week of maturity counts heavily in the baby's favor, delivery is usually delayed until about the onset of the ninth month unless there are compelling reasons to the contrary. With careful obstetrical management, the outcome is usually happy for mother and baby. Placenta previa occurs somewhat more frequently in women who have had many children, especially in rapid succession, and in women who have had fibroid tumors.

Premature separation of the placenta is responsible for the second type of abnormal bleeding. In this instance a normally implanted placenta separates from its attachment to the wall of the uterus. Vaginal bleeding is usually accompanied by severe abdominal pain. The womb may become very hard. Frequently such separations are associated with high blood pressure.

Important abdominal pain and bleeding must be reported to the doctor immediately. Management of this condition calls for discriminating obstetrical judgment. Labor may be induced forthwith, or cesarean section may be required, depending upon individual circumstances.

There are other causes of bleeding in the third trimester, such as polyps and inflammation, but the important thing to remember is that every instance of vaginal bleeding should be reported to your doctor immediately.

Toxemia of pregnancy is another complication which is watched for in prenatal visits. The most frequent early sign is fluid retention, demonstrated by swelling of the fingers, tight wedding ring, swelling of the eyelids, tight shoes, and weight gain which may amount to five pounds in a week. (Some swelling of the feet at the end of the day, disappearing with rest, is common in normal pregnancies). There is abnormal protein in the urine. The more serious forms of toxemia are associated with *eclampsia* or convulsions.

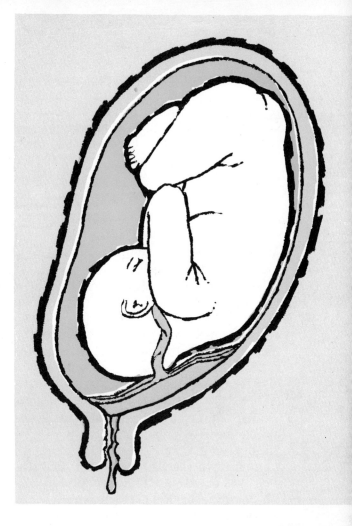

Implantation of the embryo may occur in abnormal sites, such as the Fallopian tube, resulting in an *ectopic* ("outside of the womb") pregnancy. Implantation may also occur in the uterus itself in such a position that the placenta covers the outlet of the womb completely or partially, as shown in the drawing. This is called *placenta previa*.

Toxemia is an increased danger to the baby and the mother. Hospitalization for one or two weeks, and sometimes early delivery, may be necessary. Milder signs of toxemia may be controlled less drastically. A low-salt diet is important (see page 32). Smoked meats, pickles, sea foods, pastries, cakes, sharp cheeses and cocktail snacks are forbidden. Long periods of rest, prolonged night sleep, and afternoon naps are helpful. Effective diuretic drugs are eminently successful in reducing fluid-swollen tissues.

Toxemia is more frequent in women with high blood pressure, previous toxemia or kidney trouble, or who have a twin pregnancy. It is much less severe in areas where good obstetrical care is the rule than in areas of poor nutrition and medi-ocre medical services. Acute onset of toxemia with severe headaches, convulsions, blurring of vision, and rapid rise in blood pressure and weight is rare in women who receive good pre-natal care at regular intervals.

Rh Factor. *Erythroblastosis* is a disease of newborn infants associated with the Rh blood factor. A blood factor is a physical substance which some people have in their blood and some do not. If a blood factor gets into the blood of a person who has not inherited it, it acts like a foreign protein, and the body creates antibodies that antagonize the factor, much the same as antibodies against measles viruses are built up to give immunity to measles. But some antibodies do not protect, but cause damage.

"Rh" gets its name from Rhesus monkeys, in which the factor was first discovered in 1940. About 85 per cent of women have the Rh factor and are Rh-positive or Rh+. The remainder are Rh-negative or RH-. If an Rh- mother and an Rh+ father conceive a baby, the fetus growing in the uterus produces Rh factor and some of it may pass into the mother's bloodstream. In that case the mother produces an antibody that is hostile to the Rh factor which to her body is a foreign substance. This antibody may cross back to the baby with destructive action on its red blood cells. The extent of this destruction determines the severity of "Rh disease" or erythroblastosis.

Most Rh- women with Rh+ husbands can produce one or two healthy babies or even more. Usually Rh disease does not manifest itself until the third or subsequent pregnancy. The maternal and fetal circulations do not intermingle, and it is thought that the back-and-forth transfer of Rh factor and antibodies may be effected by "leaks" in minute capillaries.

Blood studies of pregnant women determine their Rh status. If a patient is Rh+ there is nothing to worry about. If she is Rh- and has an Rh+ husband, the physician is watchful of a possible complication in an existing or future pregnancy. Even so, the odds are quite favorable. About five per cent of Rh-mothers, or one out of twenty, will have a baby with Rh disease, and this usually happens in a third or later pregnancy. Some evaluation can be made by frequent measurement of Rh levels in the mother's blood during the last two months of pregnancy. At the time of delivery a delicate test called the Coombs test may confirm the presence of erythroblastosis in the infant. If the disease is severe an exchange transfusion may be required at birth. This is done by replacing all the baby's blood with appropriate fresh blood of a donor. Occasionally, if the baby is alive in the womb and Rh disease appears to be worsening, early delivery at the thirty-fifth week may be indicated. A baby with Rh disease who is born in good condition will be watched carefully in the first few days after birth for signs of jaundice which may be due to a delay in onset of the disease.

Prevention of Rh disease has become possible in the past few years, through the use of Rhogam (immune human globulin containing anti-Rh antibodies). The globulin is not administered to Rh-positive mothers but may now be given routinely to Rh-negative mothers who have Rh-positive babies and who have not developed Rh antibodies from a previous pregnancy. The serum, given to the mother during the first 72 hours after delivery, destroys fetal cells in the maternal bloodstream and prevents erythroblastosis in subsequent pregnancies. As the number of mothers protected by the serum increases, the serious complication of Rh disease should become a rarity.

There are some other blood groups that may produce cross reactions somewhat similar to the Rh factor, but these are usually mild and disappear without requiring transfusions.

Contraception

Discussion of contraception, if desired, should begin in the hospital several days after childbirth, to allow time for consideration of methods most satisfactory

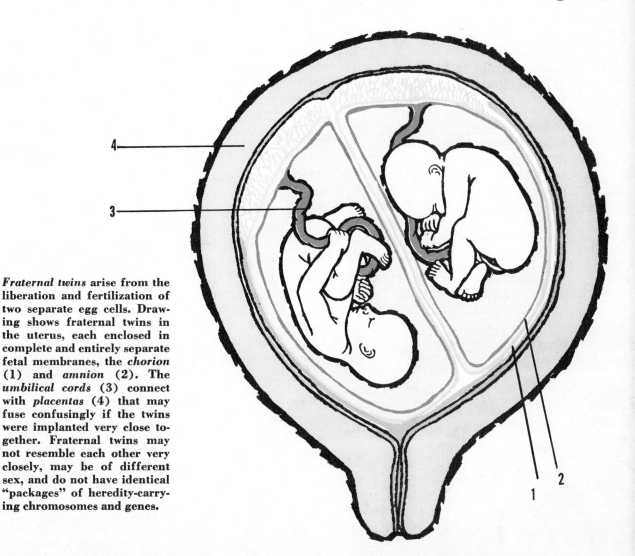

Fraternal twins arise from the liberation and fertilization of two separate egg cells. Drawing shows fraternal twins in the uterus, each enclosed in complete and entirely separate fetal membranes, the *chorion* (1) and *amnion* (2). The *umbilical cords* (3) connect with *placentas* (4) that may fuse confusingly if the twins were implanted very close together. Fraternal twins may not resemble each other very closely, may be of different sex, and do not have identical "packages" of heredity-carrying chromosomes and genes.

to the individual couple before marital relations are resumed. Intercourse may begin from four to seven weeks following a normal delivery.

The pill is not given to nursing mothers because it will dry up the milk. If the mother is not nursing, she may start on the pill four weeks after delivery and will be fully protected at six weeks. The pill is not recommended for women with a past history of phlebitis, facial pigmentation, or diabetes, and because of fluid retention factors is something of an additional handicap to women who want to lose weight.

Advances in shape and materials of intrauterine devices (IUD) have enhanced their usefulness and lessened side effects. A particularly good time for insertion of an intrauterine device is directly after childbirth, for it is easily placed in the enlarged uterus. The device

is not suitable if menstrual bleeding is excessive.

The diaphragm continues to satisfy many women but users have diminished somewhat in the past decade. Basal body temperature, including the use of rhythm, and condoms, have their adherents. (See page 343).

Spacing of infants in family planning often comes up for discussion. A two-year interval between babies is probably ideal; by then the first infant is usually toilet-trained. If the mother is over 35, closer spacing may be desirable.

TWINS

Twins present additional problems to the expectant mother, the obstetrician, and for that matter the father. The statistical chance of having twins is one to 92.

Identical twins (always of the same sex) develop from a single fertilized egg which divides in two early in its development. One identical twin is the mirror image of the other.

Fraternal twins originate from two separate eggs fertilized by two separate spermatozoa. The eggs arise from one or both ovaries, embed in the uterus separately, and grow independently. Fraternal twins may be of different sex and their relationship is no closer than that of brothers and sisters. They are more common (70 per cent) than identical twins.

Fraternal and identical twins cannot be positively identified from their appearance. The question can be settled at delivery by examination of the placenta and the membranes separating the twins. If two layers of membranes are present, the twins are identical; if four layers, they are fraternal. Also, study of their blood groups will usually distinguish the two types of twins. A tendency to produce fraternal twins (but not identical twins) seems to run in families.

Triplets occur about once in 9,000 births, quadruplets once in 500,000 births, and the odds against having quintuplets are about 40 million to one. Nevertheless, in 1963, thriving quintuplets were born to a family in South Dakota and another in Venezuela.

What makes a doctor suspect that a woman may have a twin or multiple pregnancy? For one thing, the uterus is usually much larger than expected for the stage of pregnancy. Rapid weight gain, sometimes ten pounds in three to four weeks, suggests possible twins. But these are only suspicions unless the

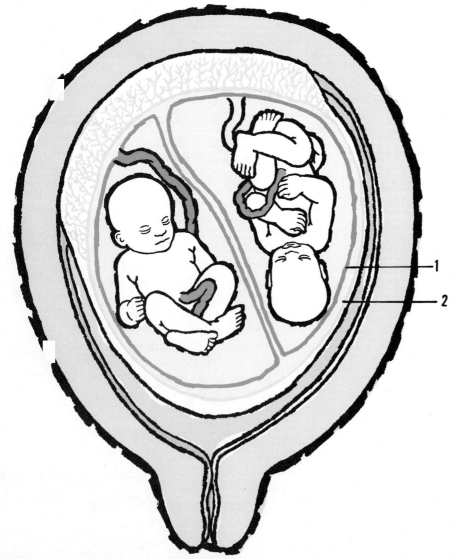

Identical twins arise from a single fertilized egg cell which divides into two independently growing cell masses, each of which develops into an individual. Since this division occurs after fertilization, identical twins have the same heredity elements, are always of the same sex, and resemble each other very closely. The drawing shows identical twins enclosed in the same *chorionic vesicle* (2), with separate *amnions* (1). Compare with membranes of fraternal twins, page 377. Fraternal or "two egg" twins are more common, and there seems to be some hereditary tendency for some women to produce more than one egg at a given ovulatory period. But the division of a single fertilized egg into identical twins appears to be a biological "accident" without known factors of causation.

obstetrician is able to feel two heads, two trunks, or to hear two independent fetal heartbeats. X-ray films which show two fetal skeletons clinch the diagnosis.

Multiple pregnancy is a weighty matter, notoriously uncomfortable. Labor usually begins about three weeks earlier than the expected date of delivery. Toxemia is a frequent but usually controllable complication of multiple pregnancy. Twins, individually, tend to be much smaller than a single-born infant. Twins at term may weigh five and a half to six pounds each, compared to seven to seven and a half pounds for a single infant.

The hazard to twins of very early labor and premature birth must always be kept in mind. Twins will be recognized relatively soon if the pregnant woman makes regular visits to her doctor, and not infrequently twins may be saved by simple measures to prevent prematurity.

Labor with twins tends to be long and slow. The large distended uterus does not contract with normal force. Usually the membranes of the lower twin will rupture, reducing the size of the uterus and improving uterine muscle contractions. Risks are slightly greater for the second twin. Occasionally the presence of twins is not known until the first baby is delivered and the uterus remains large and a second fetal heart is heard. In the very obese woman, or when the second baby is very small, or when the mother has had no pre-natal care, twins may easily be overlooked by the doctor.

LABOR AND DELIVERY

As Labor Nears

As pregnancy nears its end, there is natural concern about getting to the hospital in time and recognizing the signs of imminent events.

During the final weeks of pregnancy (thirty-eighth to fortieth weeks) there is frequently no increase in weight. Even the baby may seem to be preparing for his advent by some reduction of activity. The patient may notice an increased sense of well-being, less discomfort from heavy weight of the uterus, and more energy for her usual household activities.

Mild, fleeting, irregular uterine contractions coming every ten or 15 minutes or so and lasting ten or 15 seconds may be noted. Most women do not notice these mild contractions, but some feel slight pain, or occasional association with mild, transient low backache. If contractions come more frequently than every ten minutes, and last for 30 seconds, the obstetrician should be notified. It is advisable that neither fluids or solid food be taken once labor has begun.

A woman about to go into labor often notices the discharge of a mucus plug. This plug extrudes from the small remnant of the cervical canal which remains at the onset of labor, and when it is passed the surface of the fetal membranes is in direct contact with the vagina. Also, at the onset of labor there may be a discharge of clear watery material, which does not indicate rupture of the membranes but that rupture is imminent. A small amount of reddish or pink discharge known as "show" frequently indicates onset of labor.

Though **contractions at ten-minute intervals** are a warning to inform the doctor, the real beginning of labor is measured from the onset of contractions which occur at five-minute intervals and last at least 30 seconds. In general, a woman whose office examinations have been normal can wait at home until 30-second contractions occur every five or six minutes. However, if she has given birth before, it is advisable to have her in the hospital when contractions occur at ten-minute intervals.

In some patients (ten to 20 per cent) the membranes rupture spontaneously. This speeds up the entire mechanism of labor. If the membranes rupture and labor does not commence in a few hours, the doctor should examine the patient to determine whether labor is in progress. In a first pregnancy, the cervix may be long and thick and take two or three days to thin out. This is called *cervical effacement* which precedes the onset of labor.

Decisions as to whether the patient may stay at home, in bed or up and about, or in a hospital where frequent nursing observations can be made, are of course made by one's doctor. In a woman who has had more than one baby, labor usually commences from three to 25 hours after the membranes rupture.

Understanding Labor

It is important for a pregnant woman to have some understanding of the mechanism of labor, which means "work" — the bringing forth of a child.

Labor usually takes between six and 12 hours for a first baby, three to six hours in subsequent pregnancies. Labor under two hours, which is rare, is called very rapid labor and it is usually desirable to slow it down. A slow progressing type of labor is less likely to tear tissues than a fast labor.

The first stage of labor is the period from onset of dilation of the cervix, when complete thinning has taken place, to full dilation up to ten centimeters (one inch equals two and a half centimeters) to allow the baby's head to go through. Usually the head is down in the pelvis at about the level of the spine, a landmark about midway down the pelvis.

Intensity of contractions usually increases as the first stage progresses. When the cervix is slightly dilated, contractions will be mild to moderate but toward the end of the first stage will be more severe. Severe contractions last 40 to 50 seconds at the most, compared to ten to 20 seconds early in the first stage. If the membranes have not ruptured by the time the cervix is dilated about two inches, the doctor will rupture them. This improves the quality of contractions and lessens the duration of labor.

Transition in labor is the stage when the cervix is almost fully dilated. There is a tendency, even though dilation is not complete, for feelings of pressure and pushing to occur during contractions.

The second stage of labor is the time between full dilation of the cervix and the birth of the baby. This lasts from 30 minutes to two hours for a first baby, and from five or ten to 30 minutes in subsequent deliveries. The infant is born at the end of the second stage.

The third stage of labor is the period between the birth of the baby and delivery of the placenta. This usually takes five to ten minutes but may last as long as half an hour. If the placenta has not separated in half an hour, the obstetrician removes it manually. This manual removal usually requires ten or 15 minutes of general anesthesia.

Pain Relief in Childbirth

If the patient is well prepared and understands the mechanism of labor, effective results can usually be obtained with minimal amounts of pain-relieving agents. The physician assesses the progress of labor by frequent examinations and gives the medication most appropriate to the exact stage of labor the patient is in.

Barbiturates may be given orally or rectally early in labor to produce sleepiness and relaxation. After labor has progressed to cervical dilation of about two inches, various morphine derivatives can be used effectively. Meperidine is a popular agent which reduces the pain threshold and makes the patient more comfortable. She may even fall asleep between contractions and wake up only during the contractions.

If contractions become more violent, and the patient is somewhat apprehensive, scopolamine may be used. Scopolamine (called "twilight sleep" many years ago) is an *amnesic* or memory suppressing drug. Adequate amounts of it abolish the patient's memory of the pain of labor and delivery.

After the cervix has opened to seven or eight centimeters in the second stage of labor it is usually inadvisable to give sedation. Contractions then are less painful and there is a great desire to push or "bear down." The pushing sensation is similar to having a bowel movement. A large amount of sedation at this stage may make pushing less effective and slow the progress of labor.

At the time the baby is delivered a variety of anesthetic agents can be used. The simplest is a local anesthetic spread over the area in the lower vagina where the baby extrudes. This blocks the pain fibers and allows the mother to push and extrude the baby with a minimum of pain. Local anesthesia may be supplemented with nitrous oxide or "laughing gas" during the height of a contraction. At this same period, low spinal anesthesia or "saddle block" will give effective pain relief. Or *caudal anesthesia* (introduction of an anesthetic agent around membranes of the spinal canal) is also very effective. Each physician chooses the agents which, in his experience, are most satisfactory in serving the individual patient's needs.

Hospital Procedures

What is in store for the pregnant woman on the verge of childbirth when she arrives at the hospital?

Usually she is escorted to her room and is given a complete shave and an enema. The latter makes her more comfortable in labor and frequently stimulates contractions to greater effectiveness. After preparation the patient is taken to her own room on the delivery floor where a nurse trained in the care of labor patients is in constant attendance. From time to time the obstetrician will drop in to do a rectal or vaginal examination to determine the progress of labor and whether any medication is needed for comfort.

The waiting period in the labor room ends when a small part of the baby's head is visible at the entrance of the vagina, in a first pregnancy. The visible part of the head is usually about the size of a quarter or half dollar. However, a woman who has had children is taken to the delivery room with the onset of pushing sensations or when the cervix is dilated about four inches.

Delivery of the baby. The delivery room is virtually the same as an operating room. There are anesthesia machines with tanks of gases. Everybody wears a cap, gown, and mask. The large table on which the patient lies on her back has stirrups to support the legs fully. Metal handpieces or bars are available for the patient to push against during contractions. An overhead surgical light illuminates the birth area and an attached mirror allows the mother to watch the birth if she wishes.

As the patient's legs are being put into the stirrups, the lower part of the table is slid under the remaining part and the patient's vaginal area, lower abdomen and inner thighs are scrubbed with an antiseptic. The entire area is covered with a sheet with a window for the vaginal opening.

As the vagina becomes distended, the obstetrician usually does an **episiotomy.** This is an incision in the vaginal margin, done under local anesthesia. The purpose is to prevent the tearing of tissues as the baby's head is extruded.

The baby's head appears slowly during a contraction, with the face turned toward the floor. As the full head appears it rotates to the left or right. The shoulders are then born and the abdomen and lower extremities rapidly follow suit. Fluid remaining in the uterine cavity is expelled with a gush.

The baby, entering a world where it is "on its own" for the first time, begins to cry. Sometimes assistance is needed to initiate breathing. The umbilical cord is cut and the baby is placed in a heated crib. An identification tag identical to the one worn by the mother is placed on the baby's wrist.

A resident physician who is present at delivery examines the baby thoroughly. He examines the heart, lungs, abdomen, eyes, nose, palate, notes if the rectum is open and, in boy babies, that the testicles are descended into the scrotum. A rubber bulb with a glass catheter is used to suck out the baby's mouth, and frequently to draw fluid from the stomach to prevent it from being inadvertently inhaled into the baby's lungs.

After the delivery. Condition of newborn babies is often, though not universally, evaluated according to a score

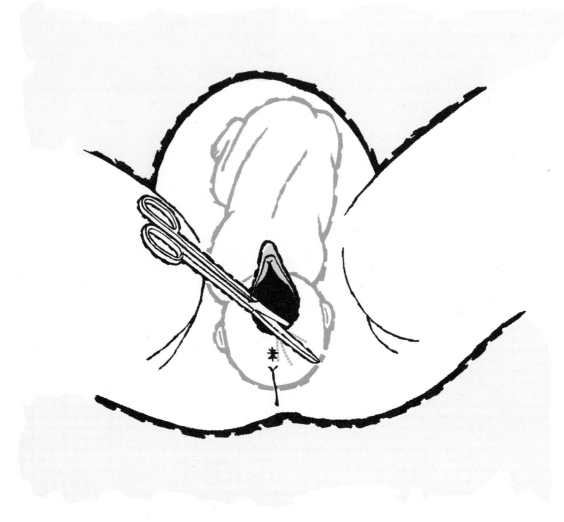

An *episiotomy* is an incision of the margin of the vulva, frequently done under local anesthesia as the baby's head distends the area. This in effect enlarges a constricted area through which the baby must pass. The purpose is to minimize or prevent lacerations or "childbirth injuries" that could be very troublesome and difficult to repair. The cleancut incision is directed in the midline toward the rectum or slightly to the right or left, as the obstetrician's judgment determines. After delivery the episiotomy is closed with sutures which need not be removed if absorbable materials are used.

named for Virginia Apgar, an anesthetist who devised it. Five factors are evaluated: heart rate, breathing, muscle tone, color, and coughing or sneezing in response to a catheter in the nose. The highest score is two points for each factor, or ten points for a very vigorous baby.

The baby is weighed and an antibacterial agent — silver nitrate solution or antibiotic ointment — is placed in each eye to prevent ocular infection by gonorrhea germs. This is routine procedure required by law. The baby is wrapped in blankets and placed in the warm crib for transportation to the nursery.

The episiotomy is sutured. The placenta usually separates spontaneously in five or ten minutes, and the nurse by gentle pushing on the uterus extrudes the placenta from the vagina. Before this is done it is advisable to take a specimen of umbilical cord blood to test for Rh sensitization of the baby. In many hospitals, whether the patient is Rh- or RH+, all bloods are tested for antibodies by a Coombs test.

After the episiotomy is sutured and things are going well, the uterus is continuously massaged, as it contracts in size. Immediately after delivery, oxytocic drugs may be given to contract the uterus. If everything after the delivery is satisfactory, the patient's legs are removed from the stirrups, the bottom part of the table is brought up into position, and the patient is observed for an hour in the delivery room before returning to her obstetrical floor.

Problems in delivery are fewer than they once were. Treatment has been most successful in overcoming poor labor con-

take a little longer to work, but in an hour or two mild contractions are replaced by strong contractions. Another labor stimulant is sparteine sulfate which may be given intramuscularly. Uniform doses every hour improve the contractions of the uterus.

Questions of *disproportion* of the baby's size in relation to the birth passage may be resolved by x-ray pelvimetry. These x-ray procedures may be done a week or two before labor, or more frequently during labor, when the exact dimensions of the head in proximity to pelvic parts through which it must pass can be determined more accurately.

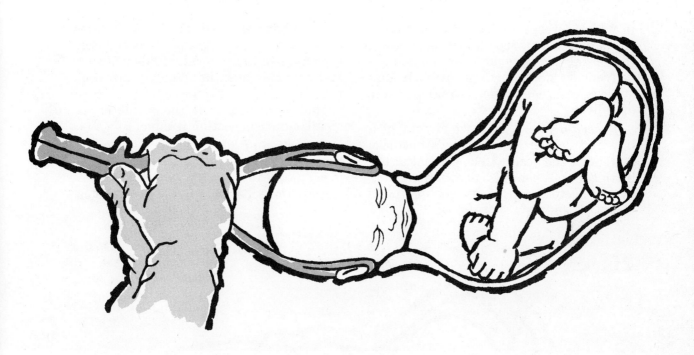

Obstetric forceps are instruments for extracting the baby's head without injury to the baby or the mother. The many types of forceps consist essentially of two curved flat blades (right and left) which are separately inserted around the baby's head with great care and joined by a lock. The drawing shows the application of forceps in principle. In practice, the blades of the forceps are usually parallel with the floor and the baby's face is toward the floor.

tractions. Oxytocin, a hormone of the pituitary gland which stimulates the uterus to contract, is now available in pure form. Small amounts of oxytocin, dripped slowly into a vein, almost invariably stimulate labor, insure adequate contractions, and a successful delivery. Oxytocin can also be given in tablets placed under the upper lip. The tablets

Forceps delivery. Not infrequently, because of the position of the baby or weak labor or other reasons, spontaneous delivery of the baby may not be possible or would be unnecessarily protracted. *Forceps* may be necessary. These are instruments with cuplike blades which are used with some form of anesthesia.

The use of forceps has greatly advanced

the art of obstetrics. These extracting instruments were introduced by the Chamberlen family in the seventeenth century and kept a family secret for over one hundred years. Not until 1726 were forceps generally introduced into obstetrical practice in England.

There are many types of forceps, depending on their uses. For instance, there are forceps for turning the baby's head if it is pointed in a wrong direction. The head may be rotated and delivered in the normal position. If the baby is in imminent danger, with poor heart action or extruding a great deal of stool (meconium), or if there is massive bleeding, labor can be promptly terminated by the use of forceps. There are circumstances in which forceps are not advisable — if the baby's head is too big for the mother, if the baby is very high, or immediate delivery is necessary. In such circumstances, cesarean section is a safer means of delivery.

Breech delivery. In three or four of a hundred deliveries, the baby's buttocks instead of the head will be present at the birth canal. When this condition is noted by the obstetrician, x-ray pelvimetry is done to determine if the mother's pelvis is of adequate size. If not, cesarean section is done before labor begins.

Labor in breech is usually longer than "headfirst" delivery. Usually the membranes are kept intact as long as possible to act as a wedge to dilate the cervix. There is a longer stage of pushing by the mother to bring the buttock down. Generally a large episiotomy is performed as soon as the buttock shows at the entrance to the vagina. As soon as the buttocks and extremities are delivered the patient is anesthetized and the trunk, upper extremities, and head are delivered.

The head may be born by pressure by the obstetrician on the inside of the baby's mouth, pressure by the nurse from above on the abdomen, pushing the head down and through the vagina, or special forceps applied to the head. If labor is slow and progress unsatisfactory in a breech presentation, or if the umbilical cord should protrude, or if the pelvis is too small, cesarean section is done.

Induction of labor (artificial stimulation of labor before it starts naturally) is sometimes necessary for medical reasons such as Rh sensitivity or diabetes.

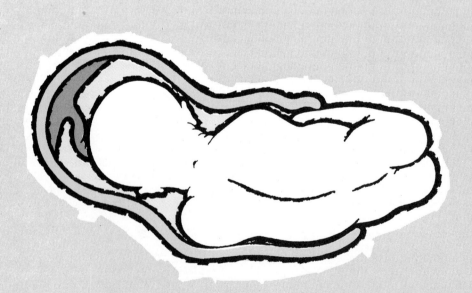

Breech presentation in which the baby's buttocks instead of the head present at the birth canal is not uncommon. Here the skills of the obstetrician are important in determining the best measures to deal with the situation, although many breech deliveries end without unusual manipulation. Usually the back of the baby is up with the face toward floor at the time of delivery.

However, induction may also be done for convenience when the time and the circumstances are right.

Labor is induced by rupturing the membranes, particularly in a woman who has had several children and whose cervix is dilated and completely effaced, or by the use of oxytocic (contraction-stimulating) drugs.

Induction will not work unless the cervix is "ripe" — thin and dilated. For medical indications, induction may require several days with use of oxytocin. An obstetrician knows when labor may be induced for the convenience of the patient. Induction for convenience can only be performed on a ripe cervix with an infant of sufficient size.

Cesarean Section

As recently as 50 years ago, *cesarean section* — surgical incision of the uterus and removal of the baby — was performed only in desperate emergencies with little hope of mother or infant survival. Today approximately 200,000 cesarean sections are performed in the United States every year, with a maternal death rate close to zero, and infant loss in uncomplicated cases about the same as in normal deliveries.

This record, achieved by improved surgical techniques, antibiotics and blood replacement, is all the more remarkable in light of the fact that cesarean section is a major abdominal operation often performed on an abnormal patient as an emergency procedure under less than ideal conditions.

Some of the indications for cesarean section have already been mentioned. In this country about half of these operations are done in patients who have had previous cesarean sections. Usually these are done as a safeguard to prevent the wall of the uterus from rupturing through the old scar during a labor contraction.

Before a first cesarean section is done, most hospitals require one or more obstetrical consultations. Except in emergencies, a "trial of labor" is usually allowed. Sometimes, good labor will overcome minor disproportions between the baby and the bony pelvis, and when labor starts spontaneously the doctor knows that it is the end of pregnancy and that the baby is mature.

How is the operation done? An incision is made through the abdominal wall below the navel. On entering the body cavity, the uterus is encountered. Its muscular wall is then incised and the baby and placenta are removed. The uterus is then closed and the abdominal wall sutured. The so-called "classical" cesarean section requires an incision high in the uterus. In the newer, generally performed operation the surgeon enters the uterus through a low incision. This low scar is much less subject to rupture in event of a future pregnancy.

A cesarean is not necessarily "the easy way to have a baby." The first few days after the operation are more uncomfortable for the patient than the first days after a normal delivery. Gas pains and transient bladder difficulties may persist for a while, but soon subside. The hospital stay for most cesarean patients is only a few days longer than for the vaginally delivered patient.

How many cesareans may a woman have? As many as ten have been reported, and instances of four or more cesareans are quite numerous. Some women who have had a cesarean are delivered in the normal way in a succeeding pregnancy, if the complication that required the original cesarean no longer exists. But it is much more likely that a repeat cesarean will be considered best for mother and infant. A cesarean operation does not usually interfere with future childbearing if the prospect of repeated sections is not in itself a deterrent.

The Puerperium
(The Six Weeks After Delivery)

The average maternity patient stays in the hospital three to five days after delivery, usually the longer period for the first baby. The day after delivery the patient may get out of bed to the bathroom but otherwise should remain in bed except for short periods of sitting in a chair. On the second and third day she may walk around the hospital floor and shower, and on the day of discharge may increase her activities. She may take a shower after the first day. It is not advisable to eat until three or four hours after delivery, but thereafter a regular hospital diet usually suffices.

Breast feeding. A decision as to whether the mother wishes to breast feed the baby must be made on the first day after delivery. Realistically, the decision is motivated by factors such as her background, whether she would really enjoy it, and the opinions of her husband and mother. The fact that it might be beneficial for her does not often predominate.

If the nipples are inverted or the baby is premature it is not advisable to breast feed. If the mother decides to nurse, the baby is brought to her about 12 hours after delivery and allowed to suck no more than five or ten minutes on each side. Usually the baby is not very desirous of sucking until the second or third day. Around the third day the breasts become engorged (very heavy and firm) and the milk comes in or is "let down."

Before each nursing session the breasts, and particularly the nipples, should be washed carefully with an antiseptic to prevent breast infection. The nurse will assist the mother. If there is scantiness of milk the baby should be brought out every four hours through the night. But if the milk is plentiful and the mother wishes to sleep, the two a. m. feeding may soon be eliminated, particularly if the baby is large.

The uterus and tissues of the nursing mother tend to recover their normal state more rapidly. Bleeding following delivery ceases sooner. However, lactation may prevent the menstrual period from returning for as long as six months (the average duration of breast feeding).

The only way to determine whether nursing is feasible is to try it. Capacity for milk production varies. Enthusiasm and encouragement by the husband help. If a woman is very active in social or other activities outside the house, nursing should be discouraged.

Pregnancy may occur during the nursing period even though menstruation does not. This is unusual but if pregnancy occurs, nursing should be stopped. The baby can be weaned by giving a bottle at alternate nursing periods and gradually diminishing breast feeding until feeding is completely by the bottle after a week or ten days.

Many mothers do not wish to nurse and for them there are various compounds that prevent the milk from coming in. These are principally the estrogens which prevent the pituitary gland from secreting lactogenic hormone that stimulates milk flow. If the estrogens are taken, usually by mouth, for ten days to two weeks, there is usually no engorgement of the breasts. Sometimes the breasts become engorged after the estrogens have been stopped. With breast engorgement, a tight brassiere should be worn and fluid intake should be restricted to a minimum. A little aspirin and codeine for 24 hours will alleviate the pain.

Aftercare

Care after delivery. Change in size of the uterus occurs rapidly after delivery. The day after delivery the uterus can be felt to be large and globular, about half way between the pubic bone (symphysis) and the navel. Over the next four or five weeks it returns to its pre-pregnancy size. Bleeding will cease after the first two weeks. Some ergot preparation is advisable for the first two days after delivery to keep the uterus firmly contracted and bleeding at a minimum. Gradually the bleeding will be replaced by *lochia,* a reddish and then white discharge which continues three or four weeks following delivery.

If a mother does not nurse, menstruation usually recurs six to ten weeks after delivery. But in the nursing mother, menstruation may not recur until a month or two after cessation of lactation. If menstruation does not occur after eight months, the patient should return to her doctor for an examination to determine the reason.

There may be severe contraction-like pains after delivery, quite variable from one patient to another. Some aspirin or codeine should relieve them and they should disappear after two or three days.

Episiotomy care. The patient usually wears a perineal pad to protect her clothing for the first week or two. A shower a day is all that is necessary as far as care of the episiotomy is concerned. No sutures need to be removed if absorbable material was used, and the area will heal satisfactorily. Sometimes a heat lamp or exposure to the air is beneficial. Occasionally, if there is uncomfortable swelling of the suture area, an ice pack or ice in a glove applied to the area of swelling will relieve discomfort.

Exercises. The abdominal wall may be very flaccid after delivery, but the muscles gradually regain their normal tone within six weeks. Simple exercises should be done in the first week or two. For instance, lie on back with knees bent; breathe in and out, pulling in the abdomen and holding it contracted for a few seconds. From the same position, reach for your knees without allowing the abdomen to bulge. While lying flat on the back with knees flat and tense abdomen, sit up and reach for toes. Perform straight leg-raising exercises. These or other simple exercises may be done as the doctor advises.

Elimination. Usually there is no difficulty in urinating after delivery. If there is, an attempt is best made while sitting on the toilet. If this is unsuccessful or the patient is very uncomfortable after six or eight hours, catheterization (drainage through a tube) may be necessary. This is rare in modern obstetrics.

If normal bowel movement has not occurred by the second night a mild cathartic such as milk of magnesia should be taken. If this is ineffective, and bowel movement does not occur by the third morning after delivery, an enema is given. There is a natural tendency to become markedly constipated after delivery. The patient should not be allowed to go without a bowel movement for more than three days at most.

After Hospital Discharge

The first days at home. It is best to stay in the house for a couple of weeks before venturing out into society or negotiating supermarkets. There are large blood vessels in the uterus that are blocked by clots. If these clots break away, considerable bleeding may occur. Usually there will be more blood than can be absorbed by one pad and as a consequence there will be staining of underwear or bedclothes.

Should this occur, do not eat or drink anything and notify the physician. If bleeding is not too excessive, several hours of bed rest with some hemorrhage-control preparation taken by mouth will stop the bleeding. But if bleeding is abnormally profuse, the patient is sent back to the hospital, possibly transfusions will be given, or the uterus may be cleaned out by curettage.

Rest. During the first week at home the mother should get at least eight or nine hours of sleep each night and take a morning and afternoon rest in bed. Streams of visitors, admiring though they be, are tiring. It is fine to socialize with a few close friends but a parade of company soon after delivery is a drain on the new mother.

Infections. Rarely, a patient may develop a fever following delivery. The vaginal pathway to the uterus is open and bacteria may invade it. An infection of the uterus can generally be brought under control by antibiotics in a day or two, and more often than not a return to the hospital will not be necessary.

Occasionally an infection will develop in the breast of a lactating mother. If there is a very hard, red area in one breast the doctor should be notified. Very likely he will suggest that nursing be stopped, and administer an antibiotic. This may be all that is necessary, but on occasion small abscesses form in the breast and require incision and drainage.

Complaints of burning and frequency of urination, related to a mild infection of the bladder or kidneys, are not infrequent. The doctor will usually prescribe an antibiotic which clears up the condition within 48 hours.

In all of these post-partum complications it is of the utmost importance to inform your doctor promptly. If he is called early the infection or bleeding will not get out of control.

Six-week checkup. Six weeks after delivery, the patient should return to the obstetrician's office for a checkup.

The teeth, neck, and abdomen are examined and the size of the uterus noted. The breasts are examined for possible infection if the patient is nursing. The vagina is examined and the presence of any discharge noted. Occasionally there may be erosion of a small area around the neck of the uterus which may need cauterization to prevent discharge. Papanicolaou smears to rule out very early cancer lesions of the cervix and uterus will be taken if this was not done at an earlier visit.

The mother's weight is usually five to ten pounds greater than it was before pregnancy. If she is very thin the gain is not disturbing, but if the extra poundage makes her obese, a weight reduction program restricted to a given number of calories should be put into effect.

Quite often the menses may not have started at the time of the six week checkup. She may be advised that if menstruation has not returned after another four or five weeks the physician should be informed. If she reports some pain with intercourse because of episiotomy sutures, it is encouraging to know that this gradually disappears. A hemoglobin checkup will reveal whether it is desirable to continue iron medication for another two or three months.

The post-partum checkup is an ideal time for doctor-and-patient discussion of future plans of the couple, such as their wish for more children or childspacing. Details of contraceptive methods will be explained if desired, including the rhythm method of timing the fertile period of ovulation, the diaphragm, and the oral progestin tablets (see Chapter 9). A new technique, still experimental, is the introduction of an inert plastic coil into the uterus. The coil does not interfere with menstruation but prevents nesting of the fertilized egg in the uterine wall. When pregnancy is desired the coil can be removed by the physician.

In conclusion, the patient is told that it is advisable to return once a year for a routine examination. Possible abnormalities may be recognized before the patient is aware of any symptoms, at an early stage when preventive and corrective treatment is most successful.

INFANT AND CHILD CARE

by MILTON I. LEVINE, M.D.

Growth Patterns • Infant and Adult Differences

DEVELOPMENT IN EARLY YEARS

Fever • Treatment of Fever • Disease Prevention • Vomiting • Treatment of Vomiting • Diarrhea • Treatment of Diarrhea • Constipation • Treatment of Constipation • Accident Prevention • Animal Bites • Bedwetting • Birthmarks • Breath-Holding • Colic • Convulsions • Cradle Cap • Croup • Cystic Fibrosis • Diaper Rash • Heart Murmurs • Hernias • Infantile Eczema • Intussuception • Mongolism • Pediculosis • Pylorospasm and Pyloric Stenosis • Teething • Thrush

CHART OF INFECTIOUS DISEASES

TONSILS AND ADENOIDS

Indication for Removal of Tonsils • Indications for Removal of Adenoids

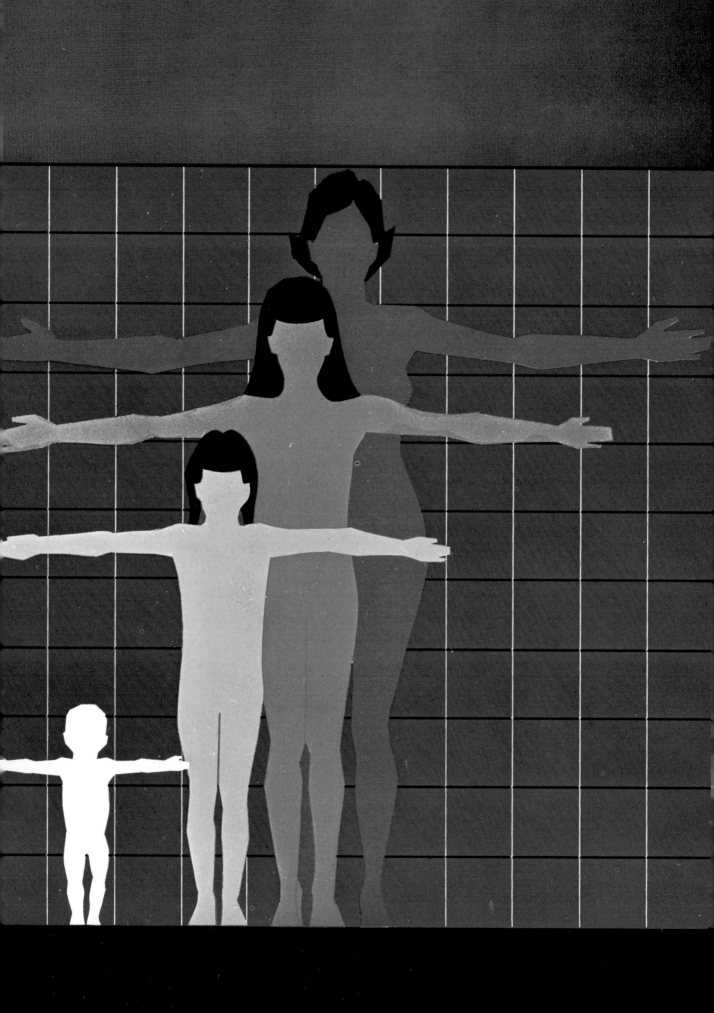

CHAPTER 11

INFANT AND CHILD CARE

by MILTON I. LEVINE, M.D.

It is good for new parents to know that a healthy baby is not so delicate, fragile, and "breakable" as he may seem. Healthy babies are remarkably "tough" little beings, but helpless in the sense that they can't say what they want or where it hurts, and that their needs must be satisfied by others who keep close watch, give loving care, and protect them against all sorts of hazards.

Newborn babies have a brief temporary immunity to a number of diseases, passively established by antibodies passed on to them by the mother before and immediately after birth. At the same time, infants are more susceptible than older children to skin and digestive disorders and some kinds of infections. Children are the special targets of so-called "childhood diseases" but are also subject to other afflictions, including rare ones, that also affect adults. We shall not attempt to mention every ailment that may affect an infant or child, since many are discussed elsewhere in this book (see *Index*).

Some disorders of children "behave" differently than in adults, or — like colic — do not occur in grownups, or require somewhat different treatment. It goes without saying that the skills of a physician and parental alertness to symptoms go hand in hand.

Growth Patterns

Never again in his life will a baby grow so rapidly as during his first year. Physical growth is easily measured in terms of weight and height. This gives a useful, though by no means exclusive, yardstick of general normal development. Disturbances or interruption of growth may accompany or give a clue to conditions that need correction. However, individual growth is an individual matter, sudden weight gain may be as ominous as weight loss, and what a worried mother takes to be the "skinniness" of a child who was previously chubby may be a normal phase of development.

Weight. In general, a baby weighs three times as much at the end of the first year as he did when he was born. His birth weight is doubled at approximately five months of age. Continuous weight gain during the first year is one index of good nutrition and, particularly during the

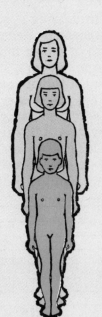

Growth patterns from birth to maturity not only produce familiar changes in height and weight, but marked changes in proportions of the body and maturation of organs.

Growth is most rapid in the first year of life, then gradually diminishes in rapidity until about age four. The color plate shows a child of about 18 months with head relatively smaller and limbs longer than a newborn baby.

From age four through prepuberty growth is steady but not so rapid as in infancy. Puberty brings a rapid spurt in growth. At maturity the growing ends of the bones close and skeletal growth ceases.

Only about one-fourth of a newborn's weight is muscle and its skeleton contains large amounts of cartilage rather than "hard bone." By age ten, proportion of muscle is the same as in adults, about one-half of body weight.

first few months, weight that remains stationary for a couple of months may be caused by illness or improper feeding.

Weight continues to increase during the second year, but at considerably less "velocity." Somewhat around two or three years of age, a child may look comparatively thin and undernourished to a worried mother, although his growth rate is normal. A great growth spurt comes with puberty, which begins at different ages in different children. Rapidly growing adolescents customarily consume, and need, more food than adults.

ing year until puberty brings a spurt in height as well as weight.

How tall will a child ultimately be? This is not only an interesting speculation, but sometimes a matter of concern to parents, one or both of whom may be unusually tall or unusually short. There are some rough formulas for predicting future height, such as the following: Measure the child's height at two years of age and multiply by two. Add slightly to this result if the child is a boy, subtract a little if the child is a girl. However, the answer cannot be taken too literally

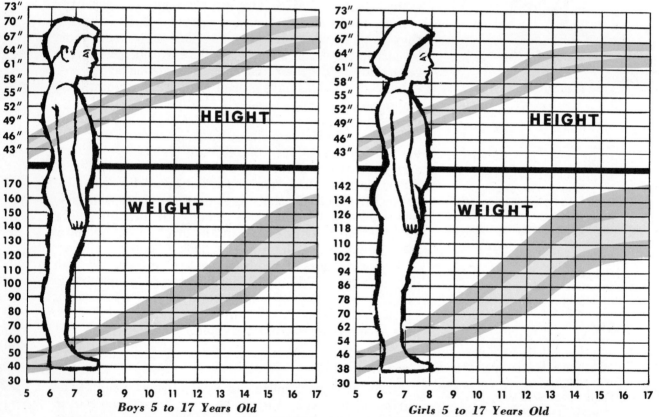

Boys 5 to 17 Years Old　　　*Girls 5 to 17 Years Old*

Chart shows average height in inches and weight in pounds of boys and girls at different ages. Wavy colored lines show normal range of variations between large and small children, with most common range shown in lighter-colored section in between. Whether a child falls within the "tall" or "short" zones shown above, or in a "heavy" or "light" zone, makes little difference to health, but unusual departures from averages should be investigated.

Height. In many homes, when a child is old enough to "stand tall" against something flat, there is a periodic ceremony of marking his height on a wall or door frame. If such records are kept year by year, it will generally be found that, although height continues to increase, the rate of increase after the age of three or four is slightly less with each succeed-

since growth is not a fixed process identical in everybody.

Sometimes, parents worry because a child "shoots up so fast" at a stage of growth that he seems headed for giantism, or, on the other hand, because he hardly seems to grow at all while playmates of the same age are growing out of their clothes. It must be remembered that puberty, with its great stimulus to growth, comes relatively early in some children and late in others. As a general thing, one may expect that effects of early or late maturation will level off, that the fast-grower will slow down and the slow-grower catch up, with ultimate height within a normal range.

Body proportions change remarkably from birth to maturity. At birth a baby's head is one-fourth the size of the body, the forehead is wider than the chin, the lower jaw small and receding. Growth lengthens the limbs and trunk so that at about two years of age the general body configuration is longer and thinner and the head is about one-fifth the size of the body. At six years, the body has stretched out further so that the head occupies about one-sixth of its length. The tendency to linear growth continues until puberty when the body tends to broaden relative to height. At about age 15 the head is one-seventh the size of the body and this proportion is maintained through life.

There are some sex differences in growth patterns. Boys are heavier and taller than girls at birth and up to about six years of age when girls weigh more than boys. Because boys usually mature a year or two later than girls, on the average, they are shorter and weigh less than girls until the early teens when they catch up and surpass girls (with respect to height and weight).

Infant and Adult Differences

There are considerable differences in proportions of water, bone, and muscle in infants and adults.

Water requirements of infants are higher than in adults, relative to size, not only because an infant's body is more "watery" but because a young baby breathes faster and loses more water from his lungs, especially in an over-heated dry environment. A baby can't ask for a drink, so his water supply — about 2½ oz. per pound of body weight — must be planned for. Most of this is furnished by his feedings.

Muscles constitute only about one-fourth of an infant's weight, compared to nearly half the weight of an adult. At about 18 months the skeletal muscles begin rather rapid development. The toddler age is a period of rapid muscle growth, with loss of "baby fat." This is an age when the arms and legs grow noticeably faster than the trunk, and the child's clothes become too short long before they become too narrow for his shoulders. At about 9 or 10 years of age, the proportion of muscle is about the same as in adults — approximately one-half of body weight.

Bones of a newborn infant contain much cartilage or gristle, and only the central sections of the long bones are mineralized. An x-ray film of a young baby's skeleton, showing only the mineralized part, looks like a collection of separate bones. One of the objective criteria of growth and development is "bone age" which measures the progressive mineralization of the child's skeleton.

Development in Early Years

It is always unwise to set hard-and-fast standards of infant and child development. Growth and development are largely determined by heredity plus the environment in which the child lives. Physical growth, time of sitting up, standing, walking, talking, and adolescent development, are usually inherited family traits, even though children in the same family may show differences. Development of qualities such as speech, sociability, and alertness to surroundings, is often largely dependent on the type of attention a child gets from his parents or parent substitutes.

An average normal child has ten to 15 words in his vocabulary at 18 months of age, but many children just as normal may not start talking until after two years of age. The average child is walking at 13 to 14 months of age, but many normal children may not walk unsupported until 15 or 16 months of age.

The chart of development in early years on page 392 is based on studies of average children and is not to be regarded as fixed or absolute.

DEVELOPMENT IN EARLY YEARS

Approximate Age	Activity	Vocal	Social
4 weeks	Stares indefinitely at rooms, lights, faces close by, etc. Looks at people but is just beginning to follow. Head sags forward on sitting. Hands grip on contact with objects. Will drop rattle immediately if placed in hand. Usually enjoys bath but cries when being dressed or undressed.	Little throaty noises	If infant cries, will usually stop crying if picked up. Reduces activity and usually calms down when talked to — especially by deep voice of man.
4 months	Lifts head up well when on stomach. Watches his hands and fingers. Plays with them. Grasps rattle or squeaky toy in hand and usually takes to mouth and bites. Interested in food. Follows lights.	Laughs and coos. Gurgles, growls, squeals, often even coughs to make sound.	Recognizes parents and others close to him. Smiles spontaneously, especially at those he knows. Enjoys people. Interest in other children. Likes rhythm. Enjoys being bounced on knee.
6 months	Sits up without support leaning forward. Bounces on feet when held by hands. Rolls over by self. Reaches for and grasps toy or rattle. Shakes rattle and bangs it. Transfers objects from one hand to the other.	Vocalizing a good deal.	Continues socializing. "Talks" to toys.
9 months	Sits up well. Creeps. Pulls self up on side of playpen. Holds bottle. Feeds self cracker. Often will walk with both hands held.	Often says "mama" and "dada." Enjoys sounds of his voice — often laughs at them.	Waves bye-bye and plays "How Big?" if these have been taught. Plays peekaboo. Likes to be with family in group. Enjoys carriage ride. May be shy with strangers.
12 months	Walks held by one hand. Stands alone for a moment. Plays well with objects. Short attention span. Throws things out of playpen. Enjoys putting things in and out of boxes, pails, etc. Likes to put things on head.	Usually has vocabulary of about 4 words, including "mama" and "dada."	Enjoys sociability greatly. Helps in dressing self. Usually coming out of shyness. Responds to "no! no!" but may continue, smiling. Still enjoys carriage. Much interested in dogs, autos, other children, etc.
15 months	Walks independently although unsteadily. Creeps upstairs. Throws objects. Looks at pictures in book.	Imitates sounds. Tries to say many things. Much gibberish.	Vocalizes wants and needs. Often will indicate when wanting to urinate or have a bowel movement.
18 months	Walks well. Rarely falls. Will climb into large chair or seat self in small chair. Throws or rolls ball. Builds 3 or 4 blocks. Pulls toys. Carries dolls and animals. Can carry out directions.	Has 10 to 15 words as a rule. Often names pictures in books.	Usually sociable and affable.
2 years	Runs well. Walks well up and down stairs. Builds 6 to 8 blocks. Carries out directions.	Sentences of 2 to 3 words. Starting to use pronouns.	Plays by other children rather than with them.

Fever

The first thing for a parent to remember is that the degree of fever is no indication of the severity of an illness. Some minor illnesses, such as roseola infantum, can be accompanied by a very high fever, whereas some very serious diseases, such as certain cases of diphtheria, may only have a low fever. The illness of a child should be judged more on the way he acts than the temperature registered on the thermometer.

A child's temperature should be taken by rectum with a rectal thermometer until he is between six and seven years of age. The rectal temperature is approximately one degree higher than the mouth temperature. Generally, the rectal temperature varies between 99° and 100°. It should be known, however, that a child's temperature fluctuates during the day, usually being higher in the late day and evening.

Occasionally, at the end of an infection the temperature may drop as low as 97°. This is no cause for concern as long as the child acts well. It will usually return to normal within 24 hours.

Not infrequently when children recover from an infection they may, for a period of a few weeks, run a low grade fever after activity. This has been called "action temperature." It is of no significance. It may readily be diagnosed by letting a child rest for 45 minutes and retaking the temperature. If it is only action temperature it will almost always return to normal after rest.

Treatment of Fever

If the fever is high or if it is making a child uncomfortable, efforts should be made to lower it. Aspirin can be given in tablets and by suppository. There is also a preparation like aspirin available in liquid form. The usual dosage would be one-half of a children's 1¼ grain tablet for infants under six months of age; one tablet (1¼ grains) for children six months to two years of age; two tablets (2½ grains) for two and three years of age; three tablets for children of four; and four tablets (five grains) for those five years and older. Aspirin suppositories should be given in the same dosages. Suppositories are of particular value when children are vomiting or when there is marked refusal to take medication by mouth. The preparations in liquid form will have an indication as to the amount that will equal the dosage of children's aspirin tablets (1¼ grains).

A warning must be given that an overdose of aspirin may be extremely dangerous to a child. Most of these preparations for children are flavored so as to make them attractive and acceptable. Too often, children, thinking them candy, will take large amounts with serious consequences. It follows that aspirin should be kept entirely out of reach of children.

Other means of reducing the temperature when the fever is very high (over 104° F.) are by alcohol sponge or by cool enemas.

An alcohol sponge is given by sponging a small part of the body at one time (about a six inch square). Pat the area gently with a sponge or soft cloth dipped in rubbing alcohol, then gently pat the area with a dry cloth. Then go to another area using the same procedure and continue on over most of the body. In this way the evaporation of the alcohol on the surface of the body takes down the fever and usually comforts the child at the same time. Most of the child's body can be kept lightly covered during this procedure.

The *cool enema* is usually very effective in reducing fever. Cold water is used with only the chill taken off. Bicarbonate of soda (one teaspoon to eight ounces of water) should be added to the water to make it more soothing internally. The amount given should be about four ounces to an infant, eight ounces for a child from one to three years of age, and one pint for children over the age of three. The contents of the enema should be inserted and the buttocks held together for at least three minutes to cool the body.

IMMUNIZATION RECORD

DISEASE:	Date of ORIGINAL IMMUNIZATION			Date of BOOSTERS			Physician
	1st Child	2nd Child	3rd Child	1st Child	2nd Child	3rd Child	
Diphtheria							
Tetanus							
Whooping Cough							
Poliomyelitis							
Measles							
Rubella (German measles)							
Mumps							
Smallpox				REVACCINATION			
Other immunizations such as influenza, typhoid, etc.							
Tuberculin Tests				RETESTS			

Disease Prevention

At the present time there are inoculations or oral preparations that in almost every instance will completely prevent most of the serious infectious diseases. The most important of these preventives are those against *diphtheria, tetanus, whooping cough, poliomyelitis* (infantile paralysis), *smallpox, and measles.*

In spite of this, there are still many children lacking these protective measures, either because their parents were indifferent, lazy, procrastinating, or because they believed that vitamins, diet, spinal manipulations or beliefs could prevent disease. Many children have died of these preventable diseases because of laxness on the part of their parents.

In areas where there has been laxity in giving vaccinations and inoculations, the diseases have appeared, disproving the idea that it is modern sanitation that is responsible for the present low rate of disease.

This is no time to live in the past. All children should have the benefits of modern protection from these deadly but preventable diseases. It is wise to keep a family record of immunizations in some permanent form, like the accompanying record-chart. It is easy to forget the dates of vaccinations and inoculations, but often it becomes important at some future time to know the date accurately. Families do move to different communities, members are treated by different doctors, a physician may cease practice, and altogether it is a wise idea to keep your immunization records where you can refer to them at any time. Remember, too, that immunizations "wear out" in time, and need boosting or renewal at intervals recommended by your doctor.

Formulas

There are various formulas in use today for the young infant who is not being breast fed. The aim of the physician in prescribing such formulas is to give the child a preparation of milk that will closely approximate breast milk in its nutritive values.

A simple formula can be made by a combination of whole milk or evaporated milk plus water and sugar. However, there are many commercial preparations available either in powder or liquid form, with which the simple addition of water provides an excellent formula simulating breast milk in almost every way. Some of the prepared formulas also include vitamins in their composition.

The physician usually determines the type of formula best suited to the individual infant, as well as the amount to be taken and the frequency of the feedings. Today most physicians allow considerable flexibility in the feeding schedule.

Feedings. Mothers should realize that the amount of formula prescribed by the physician is not to be held to too rigidly.

An infant who is on the breast may take four ounces at one feeding, six ounces at the next, and five ounces at another feeding. There is never a precise amount at each feeding. Likewise, simply because a doctor prescribes a five-ounce feeding, it does not mean that the baby must take the whole amount, or that the amount will necessarily satisfy the infant at every feeding. What physicians attempt to do is to prescribe a formula so that each bottle will contain the most that a baby is likely to desire.

Sterilization of the bottles is advisable for as long as the bottled formula is to be stored in a refrigerator. When the infant is placed on whole milk, the milk can be kept in a large container and poured into a clean but not sterilized infant's bottle just before it is to be used.

The size and type of nipple most successfully used again varies with the individual baby. The infant who sucks vigorously and finishes a bottle within five minutes will often get more satisfaction if given a slower-flowing nipple. On the other hand, the nipple hole should not be so small that the infant tires from the sucking effort or sucks in a great deal of air while attempting to suck milk from the nipple.

During feeding the nipple should be kept filled with milk. An infant sucks in air and may suffer from colic pains.

Vomiting

Vomiting in infants and children is very common since it may be associated with numerous conditions. Among the most frequent causes are allergy, car sickness, infections, cutting of teeth, gastrointestinal infections or upsets, pylorospasm, pyloric stenoses, poisons, intussusception and other intestinal obstructions, psychogenic causes, pressure on the brain, and lack of normal amount of sugar in the blood.

Vomiting is not to be confused with regurgitation, which is simply the spitting up of food after eating. This is usually caused by a bubble of air in the stomach. As a rule it is of no significance. It is very common in the newborn and young infant. Regurgitation of this type usually subsides and disappears before a child is six months of age. In a few instances it may continue as long as a year.

The time-honored method of preventing regurgitation due to air-swallowing is "burping the baby" — holding the infant upright over the shoulder and patting him gently on the back until he "brings up a bubble." A certain amount of air is bound to be swallowed with food, but things such as thumbsucking or a slow nipple may aggravate the condition.

There are a number of types of vomiting. Vomiting as such is due to the expulsive force of the stomach. If the force is very marked, as in pylorospasm or pyloric stenosis, the undigested or partly digested food is vomited out with such force that it is thrown one to two feet from the body. This is called *projectile vomiting*. Vomiting which is immediate would signify either an irritated or sensitive stomach, an allergy to a specific food, or a marked narrowing or closure of the esophagus (gullet).

Vomiting which is yellow signifies that in the course of stomach contractions bile has been sucked in from the intestines below.

Blood in the vomitus or "coffee-ground" vomitus may occur when capillaries bleed in the course of severe vomiting. It may also be a sign of a serious blood condition where capillaries are fragile. This is always an indication that a physician should be called.

Treatment of Vomiting

Simple vomiting from intestinal upsets can usually be arrested by the following steps:

1. Nothing by mouth for 1½ hours after last vomiting spell.
2. Then start with one-half tablespoon of medium strength tea, ginger ale or a cola drink. Increase by a half tablespoon every 20 minutes until four tablespoons are reached. Then cereal, crackers, toast or apple sauce may be offered. Gradually increase the diet but only if the child desires it. Do not give undiluted milk or orange juice until the stomach is settled.
3. There are a number of medications which can be given by mouth, rectum or by injection which are very effective in arresting a vomiting attack. These are prescribed by the physician.

Diarrhea

By diarrhea is meant a frequency of loose or watery stools. Breast fed babies in early infancy usually have loose bowel movements, often with each breast feeding. This is not diarrhea. An occasional loose movement in the average child, even if it is once or twice a day for a number of days, is not a diarrheal movement. But frequent loose or watery stools, especially when there is considerable water passed in the movements, is of significance and treatment should be under the direction of a physician.

Infants and small children are particularly susceptible to gastrointestinal upsets. In the small infant diarrhea can be of serious consequence. It is rarely dangerous after one year of age.

There are many causes of diarrhea, among which are infections, contaminated food, food allergies, laxatives or laxative foods, colitis, cystic fibrosis, celiac disease, and occasionally the cutting of teeth.

Treatment of Diarrhea

Most diarrheas can be cured with comparative ease if the cause is known. For instance, there are milk substitutes for infants who have a hypersensitivity to cow's milk; there are medications that will soothe an irritation of the gastro-intestinal tract; there are other medications that kill intestinal bacteria; the diet can be arranged to temporarily eliminate laxative foods such as spinach, prunes and apricots. Often a simple diarrhea may be eliminated quickly by bringing the child's milk to a boil and letting it simmer for 15 to 20 minutes (at times boiled skim milk produces faster results). Gradually solids may be added. In many cases of diarrhea, paregoric may be given to slow down the rapid action of the intestines. The dosage depends on the age and weight of the child and should be used at the direction of the child's doctor.

Diarrhea associated with ulcerative colitis, cystic fibrosis or celiac disease requires careful and specific medical care.

Constipation

By constipation is meant that the child's stools are hard and that there is difficulty in having a movement. Many normal children may have a stool of normal consistency every other day, and this should be of no concern if it causes the child no distress.

Unfortunately, there has been far too much emphasis placed on the supposed dangers of constipation. Not only have most people been brought up to believe that one has to have a daily bowel movement to remain in good health, but people are constantly being told by manufacturers and advertisers of laxatives that one must keep regular. But this is not true. There is no arbitrary necessity for a daily evacuation. Many perfectly healthy people normally have bowel movements every two or even three days.

Constipation in infants can usually be controlled with ease by regulating the child's diet as well as by the addition of substances that moisten the fecal matter, if necessary.

Constipation may be caused by a number of conditions, among which are improper diet, forced toilet training, chronic use of laxatives or suppositories, obstructive lesions, and anal tears (fissures) that cause severe pain on defecation.

It is a recognized fact that diet has a definite effect upon the consistency of the stool and regularity of the bowel movements. For instance, cow's milk is more constipating than breast milk. In early infancy, *breast fed* babies who develop constipation can usually be cured by giving the mother an increase of fruits and other laxative foods. In *bottle fed* babies, constipation may be treated by changing the sugar in the formula to one with more malt, by adding prune juice to the diet, or by adding malt extract to the formula.

All older infants and children of all ages require *bulk and roughage* for adequate functioning of the intestinal tract. This is attained through the addition of vegetables and fruits to the diet, which leave adequate residues.

The chronic use of laxatives and suppositories, although originally given to counteract constipation, eventually makes the digestive system so dependent on the abnormal stimulation that it will not function without it.

Toilet training. Forcing a child to sit on the toilet or potty against his will is one of the most common causes of constipation. The child tenses up and resists and often refuses to move his bowels, with resultant constipation. Parents should learn to relax while toilet-training a child. It should not be attempted too early — usually 15 to 18 months is early enough.

If a child resists, no force should be used, but each time the child soils he should be reminded of the toilet. Although he should not be scolded for soiling, he should be praised for using the toilet or potty. There is a time of toilet training readiness for each child which varies just as the time for sitting up, standing up, walking and talking varies from child to child. When a child is ready to be toilet-trained, he will usually train with ease if no force or scolding is employed.

Obstructive lesions are extremely rare in infants and children and are usually apparent at birth or shortly thereafter.

Anal tears (fissures) frequently bring about constipation. A large, hard stool distends the anal ring in defecation and tears the mucous membrane. These tears are excruciatingly painful whenever the anus opens. And so the child, fearing this pain, withholds his movement and develops constipation which often becomes chronic.

In such cases an anesthetic and healing ointment is applied to the anal tear several times a day and the stools are kept soft by large doses of mineral oil or a mineral oil product, using two to four tablespoons to insure lubrication and softening of the stool.

Treatment of Constipation

In minor cases of constipation it is advisable to regulate the child's bowels by the use of laxative fruits or by the addition of malt to the diet, either in the form of malt extract or as a sugar added to the formula. There are also several oral preparations available, which cause the stool to remain soft.

Suppositories and enemas should be resorted to only on rare occasions. At times, in severe constipation, a fecal mass in the rectum becomes large and impacted. This can be softened and passed without pain by the use of a new medicinal enema which comes already prepared in a plastic bottle with an enema tip. The tip is covered with any lubricant and inserted in the anus. Then the bottle is squeezed and the contents forced into the rectum. The buttocks are held together for about five minutes during which time the hard impaction is being softened.

Sometimes stronger cathartics are necessary for a time in addition to mineral oil or stool softeners. However, these cathartics should be given under the direction of a physician.

Accident Prevention

Accidents are the leading cause of death among children from one to 14 years of age. Ironically, it's still true that over 90 per cent of these accidents are preventable.

A physician can prevent a child from contracting diphtheria, tetanus, whooping cough, smallpox, typhoid, poliomyelitis and measles, but the prevention of accidents is almost entirely a responsibility of parents.

Nothing like a complete list of hazards can be given, but if parents will remember the following, as recommended by the American Academy of Pediatrics, they may save their children's lives or prevent serious accidents which could severely injure or disfigure for life.

Be Sure:

1. The handles of boiling pots can't be reached.
2. There are no open lamp sockets; cover them with safety plugs.
3. No poisonous medicines, including aspirin and sedatives, are available, even if on a high shelf. They should be locked away in a cabinet.
4. There are no dangerous substances on the kitchen or bathroom floor or shelves, or in unlocked closets; especially lye, ammonia, kerosene, furniture polish.
5. There are no mice seeds, ant buttons or insecticides around.
6. Safety gates are placed and kept closed on top of stairs and porches.
7. Bars or locked screens are placed outside windows.
8. Never to leave your child in the bathtub alone; he may turn on the hot water and be scalded, or may slip under the water.
9. To place non-skid mats or rubber guards under throw rugs.

10. To pick up toys, shoes and other objects which may cause accidents at night.

11. Never to give small children lollipops, unless they're sitting down, or sour balls at any time. The child with a lollipop may fall while walking and tear the roof of his mouth. The sour ball may be inhaled and completely close off the windpipe.

12. Any firearms are locked up and the key kept out of reach.

13. To watch out for Dad's razor and Mom's manicuring set and sewing basket with lethal scissors and needles.

14. To be careful of matches and cigarette lighters, a great potential danger.

15. Your child's furniture and toys are painted only with lead-free paint.

16. That doors open to potential danger are locked.

17. That pools, ponds and cisterns are fenced in or covered.

18. That toys have no sharp edges or exposed nails.

Animal Bites

Dog Bites. Children are not infrequently bitten by their own pet dogs who have been either annoyed, hurt or frightened. If the dog is healthy, has received his inoculations, and one knows that he has been momentarily upset by the child, the fear of rabies (see Chapter 2) can be almost entirely discounted. In such cases any wounds on the child's body should be well washed with soap and water and an antiseptic applied. The physician should be notified in all cases of dog bites.

If the child is bitten by a strange or unknown dog it is most important to find the animal, in order to be sure that he is not developing or suffering from rabies. Such dogs are kept under observation for one week. If rabies is developing it will become definitely apparent by the end of that time.

If a child is bitten on the face by an unknown dog or a dog that might be ill with rabies, inoculations should be started immediately since a bite on the face is close to the child's brain where the rabies virus takes hold. If, on the other hand, the child is bitten on the hand, arms or legs, one can wait through the first week before deciding if treatment is necessary. If the dog is known and is well at the end of the week, treatment started for face bites may be discontinued. If the dog is not found, children bitten on the hands, arms, or legs should receive the full course of anti-rabies inoculations. Most physicians also advise a tetanus toxoid booster shot for dog bites.

Squirrel and Hamster Bites. Children occasionally are bitten while feeding squirrels or feeding pet hamsters. Usually these bites need only be treated by washing well with soap and water and applying antiseptics locally. In some of the larger cities, park squirrels have occasionally been known to have died of rabies. It is wise in cases of squirrel bites to notify your physician, who will get necessary information from the local health department. Hamsters are usually bred at home or by special breeders and no possibility of rabies exists.

Snake Bites. The ability to differentiate the bite of a poisonous snake from the non-poisonous variety is extremely important. The bites may be differentiated by the marks they leave on the person's skin as well as by the local and general symptoms they produce.

The poisonous snakes — rattlesnakes, copperheads, moccasins and coral snakes — have two fangs in the forward portion of the upper jaw. These poisonous snakes have two rows of small sharp teeth in the upper jaw and two in the lower jaw. The two fang punctures are much larger than the punctures from the teeth and usually can be clearly seen after such bites. They appear at the end of the two lines of small bites due to the upper teeth.

Furthermore, the bites of rattlesnakes and other poisonous snakes cause a sudden, sharp, intense pain (the bite of a non-poisonous snake causes little pain). This is followed by local swelling within ten minutes and profuse bleeding, usually followed by nausea and faintness. Often there is shock.

The bite of a non-poisonous snake causes little pain and usually shows four rows of teeth marks from the upper jaw which contains four rows of teeth (in contrast to the two rows of upper teeth found in the poisonous snake) and two rows of teeth marks for the lower teeth.

For treatment of snake bites, see Chapter 25.

Insect Bites and Bee Stings. As a rule, insect bites and bee stings are only of temporary pain and discomfort. Usually prompt relief can be given by applying a paste made from a few drops of water in a tablespoon of bicarbonate of soda, or by applying a witch hazel dressing or a wet dressing of epsom salts. If this is inadequate in relieving the discomfort, an antihistamine cream or ointment may be applied.

For severe reactions from bee stings the child should receive antihistamines by mouth. If this is not followed rapidly by relief from the reaction, the child should receive injections of epinephrin or ACTH by the physician or let Isuprel tablets dissolve under the tongue.

Bedwetting (Enuresis)

Bladder control in normal children develops at different ages and depends upon the individual readiness of the child. Statistical studies on normal children have shown that 50 per cent of two-year-olds are dry at night; 75 per cent of three-year-olds, and 85 to 90 per cent of five-year-olds. In other words, bedwetting is not considered abnormal unless a child has passed the age of five, or when the child has been dry at night for a period of time and then reverts to wetting the bed.

Causes. Bedwetting which occurs past the age of five may be due to a number of organic causes.

1. The child may be perfectly normal but have late development of bladder control. This lateness of control is frequently familial, and is often in the history of one of the parents.
2. The size of the urinary bladder may be slow in development and may not hold as much urine as in the average child of five and over.
3. It is frequently associated with emotional insecurity or immaturity. Children who are unhappy in their home life and those that have anxieties are often bedwetters.

   It is commonly seen following hospitalization of children when the separation from their parents has proved traumatic. It was frequently observed during the last war when fathers left home for military service. It is often found among older children when new infants are born.
4. Mental retardation is an occasional cause of bedwetting since children suffering from this condition are usually delayed in the acquisition of mature habits.
5. Deep sleep has been considered as a cause of bedwetting, although this condition probably only occurs in certain children.
6. In situations where a child has been previously dry at night and then reverts to bedwetting, both organic as well as emotional factors should be considered. Although in the vast majority of such children the cause is psychological, organic disorders such as diabetes and kidney disease must not be overlooked.

Treatment. Organic causes of bedwetting such as diabetes, kidney disease, or some abnormality of the urinary tract, can be easily determined by a physician and necessary treatment advised.

But in the absence of organic causes the following measures may be taken to correct the condition:

1. ***The home and school environment*** should be investigated to determine if anything exists which produces great anxiety in the child. These should be

rectified as much as possible and the child should be reassured.

2. *Lifting a child* at 10 to 11 P.M. may be of considerable help if it does not upset the child too much. It may accustom the child to sleep dry for long periods of time and cause him to awaken when the bladder is full.

3. *Small bladder.* A recent study has demonstrated that a great many children over five years of age who are still bedwetters have urinary bladders that are considerably smaller than those of the average child of that age. These investigators were successful in curing enuresis in a considerable number of cases by having the children withhold as long as possible during the day, thereby gradually stretching the bladder. It may take three or four months to achieve success through this method.

4. *Apparatus.* A most successful method of treating the bedwetter who has reached the age of six is by means of an apparatus that rings an electric bell the moment a child starts wetting at night. It consists of a special pad placed under the child's sheet. This pad is connected by wires to an apparatus containing a bell or a buzzer. In some of these instruments a light turns on every time the bell or buzzer responds. As soon as the slightest amount of fluid reaches the

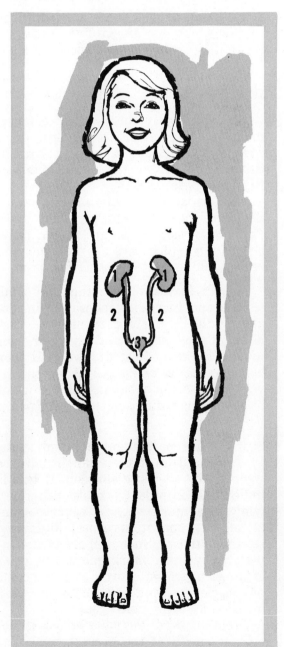

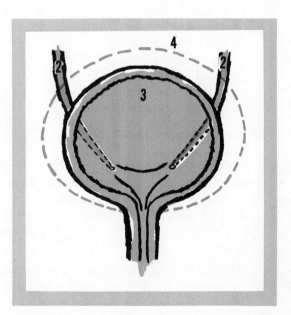

Some instances of enuresis (bedwetting) occur in children who have bladders of small capacity. In such cases the child is unable to control voiding normally because of small reservoir capacity. The figure shows *kidneys* (1), *ureters* (2), and a *bladder* (3) smaller than ordinary. Above, a small bladder (3), compared to a bladder of normal circumference, indicated by dotted lines (4).

pad the circuit is closed, the bell rings and the child wakens at once and goes to the bathroom.

This method has been found effective in 95 per cent of children over six who are still habitual bedwetters. In most cases the child sleeps through the night without wetting after the apparatus has been used only three to four weeks. A number of models are available, but an inexpensive one may be purchased from one of the large mail order houses.

This apparatus works by conditioning the child. At first, the urinating causes a bell to ring and the child wakens and immediately withholds. Later he learns to awaken when the bladder is full before the bell rings. Still later, he learns to sleep through the night without bedwetting and without awakening.

This method has also been found effective even in cases of enuresis due to emotional causes. Followups on many such children have shown that no emotional harm results from this method of treatment. As a matter of fact, most of the children are so delighted with their accomplishment that they are generally happier, reassured and much less anxious.

5. **Restricting of fluids** before bedtime. This is an old method of treatment, which unless practiced rationally may greatly upset the child. There is no question but that drinking a great deal of fluid before bed may overtax the small bladder of a child. A moderate limitation is often helpful.

6. **Extra salt** before bedtime. Some years ago it was found that an increase of salt in the blood prevented fluid from passing freely from the blood vessels into the kidneys. On this basis, the treatment of enuresis by a high salt diet was advised. It has proved of considerable help in many cases. Usually the children are given a large salty pretzel just before going to sleep. They will not get thirsty, for it takes about an hour before thirst sets in, and by that time they are usually asleep.

7. **Rewards and punishments.** These are not desirable, although some success has been noted when children are given gold stars for each dry night. In most instances a child is unable to control the bedwetting and although rewards may be greatly satisfying, punishments are very unfair.

8. **Drug treatment** has been used with a moderate degree of success in some instances. Previously, treatment was through the use of atropin. Its effect is questionable. The more recent treatment involves the use of tranquilizing drugs. These are helpful in cases where emotional upset or anxiety is the cause of the enuresis.

Birthmarks

Birthmarks are the result of enlargement of blood vessels in the skin, or of some extra pigment in the skin. Most of them occur during the development of the baby before birth.

Various types of birthmarks occur. Some are the dark red type, often raised *(hemangiomas)*, some are brown *(nevi or moles)*, and others are flat, varying from pink to purple *(portwine stains)*.

Hemangiomas often start as small lesions and increase moderately in size during the first eight or nine months. Many of these shrink and lose their color toward the end of the first year. If they do not subside adequately they can be very successfully treated with dry ice or by injections with a solution that shrinks blood vessels.

Moles are permanent pigment spots. If large and dark they can usually be removed by a plastic surgeon. If this is impossible or must be postponed for a while, the mark may be covered completely by preparations especially devised for this purpose. Such preparations completely cover the mark, match the color of the skin, are waterproof, will not come off on clothes, and remain on the skin until removed by cold cream.

Treatment of *portwine stains* is not too successful at the present time. The very pale portwine stains will often disappear within a few years after birth, but the darker stains remain. Although preparations to cover these birthmarks have been used very successfully, several new approaches have been reported, among which are tattooing the stains and sandpapering the area. A good dermatologist should be consulted.

Small children under the age of six are not as a rule bothered unduly by a birthmark and up to that age most playmates are not overly concerned about it. Occasionally a great deal is made of a birthmark by those around the child. Troubled parents speak of it in front of the youngster. Visits are made to doctors and discussions are carried on frequently about treatment or hospitalization.

Parents should avoid talk of the birthmark and warn friends also to do the same. Hospitalization and treatment should not be discussed until a day or so before it is to take place.

Breath-Holding

Some infants and small children have a tendency to suddenly hold their breath when frightened, hurt, or when crying vigorously. As a rule they respond by stopping breathing, turning blue, losing consciousness and occasionally getting convulsive seizures.

Practically all of these children cease these breath-holding attacks within a few minutes and are their normal selves again. And although these attacks are very frightening to adults around the child, they are not at all dangerous. The only danger is that many frightened parents tend to give in to a child in order to prevent such attacks. As a result, such children often become badly spoiled.

The brains and nervous systems of these children are perfectly normal, and most of these children cease having such attacks by the time they are four or five years old.

So far no drugs have been found effective in preventing breath-holding. Tranquilizers may help slightly by causing the child to relax.

Colic

Colic is a condition found most frequently in young infants, usually during the first three months. Colic is characterized by a tendency to frequent attacks of abdominal pain and as a rule, during these periods of pain, the abdomen is distended and the child's legs are drawn up on the body.

There are various causes of colic, among those which are most common are the following:

Allergy. Some colicky children are sensitive to cow's milk. If this is the case there is immediate relief once the baby is placed on a soy bean formula or a meat base formula or at times on goat's milk. Some children are sensitive to the sugar in the formula or cannot tolerate too much sugar. Both of these allergic factors can very easily be investigated and rectified if necessary.

Vitamin drops, usually of the multivitamin variety, are at times the cause of colic. To ascertain if these are the causative agents one has simply to omit vitamins for three or four days. It should be remembered, however, that many of the commercially prepared formulas, whether in powder or liquid form, already contain the vitamins within them. If one of these is being used, a preparation without vitamins should be substituted for a few days, or a simple formula of whole milk or evaporated milk with water and sugar may be given for the test period.

If it is determined that the infant is sensitive to the vitamin, a preparation containing only Vitamins A, C and D may be tried. If this still results in causing colic pains, then a preparation of A and D alone should be substituted and Vitamin C may be added later in one of the preparations containing it.

In the few cases in which an infant may be sensitive to the sugar in the formula or be unable to tolerate the amount of sugar or the amount of fat it contains, the physician can advise on the preparation of formulas to test this possibility.

Tension in the Baby. Many babies cry a great deal because they have an unsatisfied need for sucking satisfaction and are unable to relax until this need is met. This need for sucking varies in different infants and is separate from the sucking associated with feeding. A great many infants with so-called colic will cease crying and relax once they are given a pacifier.

Tensions are also carried over to the baby from the people who handle him. There are many instances where a tense crying infant, handled by a tense and nervous person, will quiet down and relax when placed in the care of a calm and relaxed individual.

Swallowing Excessive Air During Feedings. At times infants develop colic pains if the stomach is distended from air that is swallowed during feedings. This may result when the nipple does not fit the baby's mouth, or when the bottle is held too horizontally during feedings so that the nipple is only partially filled with milk when the baby sucks. In all of these situations, the air will be "burped up" when the baby is strongly patted on the back during and after feedings. If this bubbling is ineffective and the air is passed down from the stomach into the intestines, considerable pain as a result of colic usually results.

Pain from Rectal Fissure. Rectal fissures are cracks in the mucous membrane of the anus. These cracks produce intermittent or continuous pain. The pain is especially severe during the period when the baby is having a bowel movement and the anus is stretched. The possibility of an anal fissure should always be investigated in an infant who cries greatly at such a time. Treatment usually consists of keeping the movements soft and applying a healing anesthetic ointment to the fissure.

Hunger. The possibility of hunger must not be overlooked in investigation of causes of infant crying. Hunger is not infrequently the cause among infants who are breast fed. Many mothers rarely have accurate knowledge of the amount of milk taken by their infants. Most of these infants fall asleep at the breast, apparently satisfied, but awaken 30 minutes to an hour later crying from hunger. This crying is not relieved by a pacifier but often is temporarily relieved by giving warm water.

The possibility of lack of sufficient breast milk can be easily investigated by weighing a fully clothed baby immediately before nursing and again immediately after, without changing the diapers or any piece of clothing. This weighing should be repeated at four or five successive feedings before a decision is made as to the adequacy of the feeding.

Unknown Causes. The infants for whom no cause for crying can be found are comparatively rare. In such cases a physician will usually prescribe a medication which will relax the stomach and intestinal muscles. The amount can gradually be reduced after a baby is free of pain for several weeks.

Convulsions

One of the most frightening experiences for a parent is to see a child in convulsions. It occurs almost suddenly, the child becomes unconscious, the eyes are rolled up, the body first may twitch and then relax completely, so that many parents feel the child is dying. Breathing is heavy and coarse and there may be some frothing at the lips, and in rare instances soiling and urination.

But convulsions are almost always more frightening than dangerous. The attack usually lasts only a few minutes at the most, and as a rule has subsided completely by the time a doctor arrives.

Causes of Convulsions. The most common cause of convulsions in young children under the age of five is high fever which can accompany infections, such as contagious diseases, sore throats, inflamed ears, virus infections, etc. These are known as *febrile convulsions,* and only certain children respond to fevers in this manner. The reason for this is not entirely clear. Some physicians feel that in susceptible children the nervous

Babies may cry when they are tired, irritated, or hungry, but often they cry from good physical cause. An open safety pin in a diaper is an obvious physical cause, but other causes just as distressing may be overlooked. Cracks in the mucous membrane of the anus (rectal fissures) are painful, especially when the baby is having a bowel movement. Whoever manages the baby's toilet should be familiar with the normal appearance of the rectal area, shown at left below, to be able to recognize fissured areas, at right, which may be relatively inconspicuous but very painful.

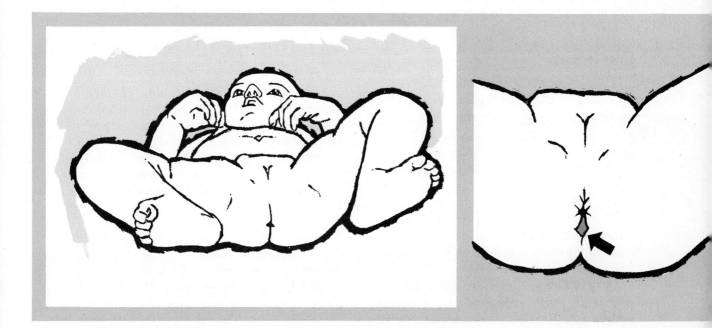

system is more irritable than in other children and adults. The tendency to have febrile convulsions is almost always outgrown by the time a child gets to four or five years of age.

This specific type of convulsion, which occurs only with fever, should not be confused with epilepsy, which can occur at almost any time, whether the child has a fever or not.

There is another type of convulsion that occurs in children who are breath-holders. These are children who when frightened or crying vigorously hold their breaths, turn blue, lose consciousness and at times have convulsive seizures. These are not dangerous at all and usually the tendency disappears by the time the child is four years of age.

Convulsions may also be caused by other less frequent conditions such as inflammation of the brain in certain infections, damage to the brain before or after birth, pressure on the brain, lead poisoning and kidney trouble.

Treatment. First telephone for a doctor. Don't get frantic. Remember that practically all convulsions subside without any danger to the child. But several suggestions may aid in limiting the duration of the seizures.

First, if the child is biting his tongue, force the mouth open and place a pencil or a clothes pin between the teeth.

If the child has a high fever, the temperature can be brought down quickly by giving an enema of cool water (room temperature), one teaspoon of bicarbonate of soda in an eight ounce glass of water. The enema is inserted and the buttocks held together for three minutes. This will usually lower the fever several degrees in 15 to 20 minutes. Sponging a child with half alcohol and half cool water is also effective in reducing the temperature. An application of an ice bag to the head or back of the neck may serve the same purpose.

The old procedure of placing a convulsive child in a cold bath is unnecessary and does no more than what can be accomplished by sponging or enemas. At times a child placed in a bathtub may be injured or inhale water during the convulsive seizure.

In children who have a tendency to convulsions with high fevers, the seizures may be prevented by combining sedatives with aspirin as soon as the temperature starts to elevate.

Cradle Cap

This is a condition commonly found in young infants. It appears as a thick scaling or greasy crusting over patchy areas or the whole scalp. It is due to a secretion from the oil glands in the skin, even in those babies whose scalps have been kept clean.

In most instances it may be successfully removed by oiling the scalp with baby oil, mineral oil, or petroleum jelly and then gently combing through with a fine-toothed comb.

If this is not successful, the infant's physician will prescribe an ointment which will dissolve the scales and crusts and will soothe any irritation which may be present on the baby's scalp.

Usually the scalp of a baby is shampooed twice a week. However, when a tendency to have cradle cap exists it can be washed every day or every other day.

Croup

There are two types of croup, one of which, although frightening, is not significantly dangerous. This is called *spasmodic croup*. The other type, extremely dangerous, is the croup due to a condition known as *laryngotracheobronchitis,* a serious inflammation of the larynx, trachea and bronchial tubes.

Spasmodic Croup. This condition usually arises without forewarning, although at times a child may have some nasal discharge and a slight hoarseness before going to bed. During the course of the night the child suddenly awakens from his sleep with severe difficulty in breathing and with the characteristic hard brassy cough (like the bark of a seal). Respirations are rapid and raspy and the child sits up, frightened and struggling to breathe. Usually there is very little, if any, fever.

With this condition the difficulty in breathing as well as the hard brassy cough can be rapidly relieved by the inhalation of warm steam. Some parents quickly bring the child to the bathroom and let him inhale the steam as hot water runs into the sink. With smaller children it is advisable to shut the bathroom door and turn on the hot water in the shower, keeping the child in the steamy room until the difficulty subsides. Older children, that is those between three and five, can usually inhale steam from a vaporizer. This hot steam usually relaxes the spasm of the muscles of the larynx.

If steaming is inadequate, the spasm can almost always be relieved by giving the child some syrup of ipecac. Usually a half teaspoonful is adequate for children under two and one teaspoon for older children. The ipecac causes vomiting and the muscle action of vomiting relaxes the spasm of the laryngeal muscles. *This type of croup is rarely seen after the age of five years.*

Usually the attack is confined to only one night, but occasionally it reappears on the succeeding night. During the day following an attack it is wise to give a simple expectorant cough medicine to produce mucus and prevent the dry cough so typical of croup. Occasional steaming should also be given during the day following an attack.

Laryngotracheobronchitis. This is one of the most serious conditions of infancy and early childhood. In its early stages it produces a croupy cough and difficulty in breathing similar to spasmodic croup. But it is most important to differentiate these two conditions, for laryngotracheobronchitis is progressive and may rapidly cause such difficulty in breathing that an extreme emergency results.

Both of these conditions produce croupy cough and raspy breathing, but usually there have been signs of a respiratory infection before the onset of laryngotracheobronchitis, the child as a rule has a fever which may range as high as 105°, he is much more toxic than in spasmodic croup, and is usually prostrated in contrast to the frightened and excited child with spasmodic croup.

The difficulty in breathing in this condition becomes more and more severe and is not relieved by steaming or vomiting. It is imperative that a doctor be called at once, for the child usually needs

The most serious form of croup (laryngotracheobronchitis) is an emergency requiring immediate medical attention to control obstructions to breathing that may be fatal if not relieved. Thick mucus may clog the *larynx* (1), the *trachea* (2), and the *bronchi* (3), obstructing passage of air to and from the lungs (4). Usually the infant has a high fever and respiratory infection preceding an acute attack.

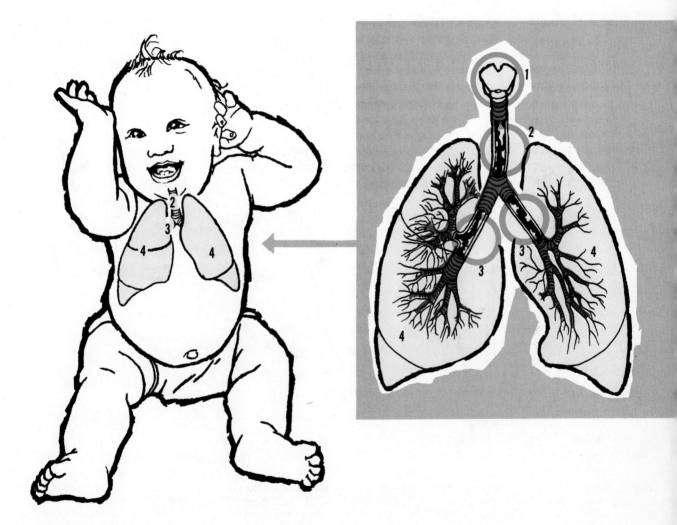

hospitalization where he can be watched very closely and receive treatment to loosen and dislodge the thick clogging mucus in the larynx, trachea and bronchial tubes and provide the much needed oxygen. At the same time, the child will receive antibiotic therapy to counteract the underlying infection.

This condition is one of the greatest emergencies in childhood and requires prompt medical attention.

Cystic Fibrosis

This is a comparatively rare familial disease characterized by serious and persistent lung infections, loose foul-smelling stools, and failure to gain weight.

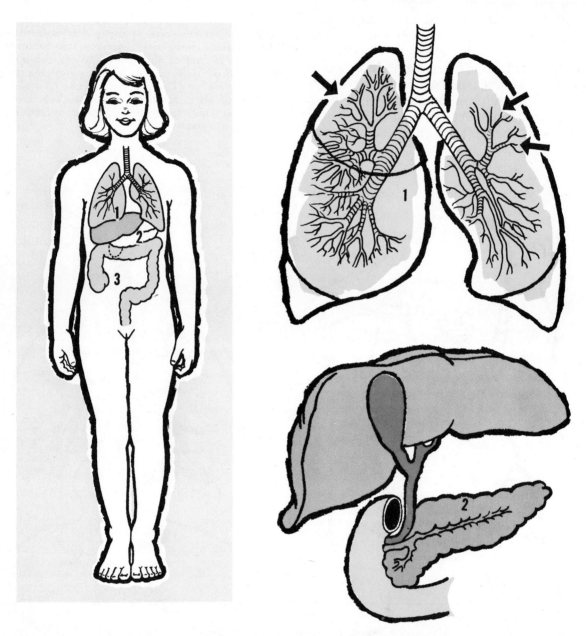

Cystic fibrosis is a generalized hereditary disease in which thick, viscid secretions affect many tissues and organs. Symptoms primarily involve the *lungs* (1), the *pancreas gland* (2), and the *gastrointestinal tract* (3). The "clogged" pancreas cannot produce sufficient amounts of digestive enzymes, and absorption of food is decreased. Thick mucus in the lungs impedes breathing and the patient is very susceptible to pulmonary infections.

The onset of symptoms occurs almost at birth, with difficult spasmodic coughing due to the thick mucus in the lungs, failure to gain weight, and usually, within a few weeks, foul-smelling stools.

In later stages of the disease the child becomes extremely thin with a large protuberant abdomen. There is a history of chronic lung infections with numerous attacks of pneumonia. And, as time goes on, most children with this condition develop shortness of breath and some difficulty in breathing due to the mucous plugging of the breathing tubes which makes the exchange of air in the lungs extremely difficult.

One other serious aspect of this condition is the tendency of these infants and children to lose a great deal of body salt through the skin in sweat. Because of this tendency these children lose large amounts of salt through sweating during the hot summer weather, and frequently develop heat prostration which is sometimes fatal.

The condition can be diagnosed with certainty by tests of salt in the body sweat, and by tests that show a lack of digestive juices from the pancreas.

Treatment must be under the close supervision of a physician for it entails proper diet to maintain nutrition, the prevention and control of pulmonary infections, the addition of salt to the diet, the addition of extra digestive medicines, and often the use of respiratory inhalation machines to bring air past the mucous plugs in the breathing tubes and to aid in the loosening and bringing up of these mucous plugs.

Diaper Rash

Almost every baby has a diaper rash at one time or another. It is not dangerous but can cause considerable discomfort. A diaper rash is really an ammonia burn. The urine, which does not contain ammonia when it is passed, is acted upon by bacteria on the outside of the body which break up the urine, causing the formation of ammonia.

A baby's skin is sensitive and needs protection to prevent diaper rash. A number of measures are helpful. Protecting the baby's skin by waterproof covering, preventing the urine from forming ammonia, killing the bacteria that break down the urine, using powders that absorb the moisture, and using ultra-absorbent diapers that aid in keeping the skin from getting too moist, are helpful measures.

The baby's skin can be protected from burning by several types of waterproofing. There are a number of good ointments available which are made specifically for this purpose, some of which also contain preparations that not only counteract ammonia but also kill bacteria on the skin. There are also ointments, lotions and powders containing silicone, a preparation that waterproofs the skin.

Occasionally, a diaper rash gets infected by certain of the bacteria present, resulting in the formation of pus heads. In this condition an antibiotic ointment is very effective, as well as the use of an antiseptic soap which not only kills bacteria but leaves an antiseptic coating on the skin. The best soap is a liquid one used by doctors in the operating room. It may be obtained from any drug store.

Many of the most severe diaper rashes are due to an infection by *fungi*, usually the type of fungus normally found in the feces. To treat this type of infection it is best to use an ointment that contains nystatin, a preparation that specifically kills these fungi. There are a number of these ointments available, some in combination with hydrocortisone which aids greatly in relieving the inflammation.

Diapers from a diaper service are almost always sterilized. If a mother washes her own diapers she should dry them in the sun, which kills all bacteria quickly, or she can boil them, or wash them and use a special diaper antiseptic in the last rinse.

There is also a special diaper marketed that absorbs the urine and passes it to the surface of the diaper, leaving the inner portion comparatively dry.

At times a diaper rash is due to loose stools which irritate the region around the anus. The treatment in this case should consist of trying to make the irritated area waterproof with one of the preparations previously described, and of changing the diaper quickly after it is soiled. Paper diaper linings are especially helpful in this situation.

Where very severe diaper rashes exist, it is often very helpful to remove the diaper completely for a few days while applying a healing ointment such as one containing cod liver oil.

Heart Murmurs

The fact that a child has a heart murmur is by itself no reason for a parent to be concerned or overanxious. Such murmurs may be heard in many normal children. As a matter of fact, between 50 and 75 per cent of all normal healthy children have heart murmurs at some time or another during their childhood. Often these murmurs are heard only when a child is anemic or when he has an infection and fever.

Doctors can usually diagnose three types of heart murmurs: *congenital, acquired,* and *functional.*

Congenital murmurs are heard at birth or shortly thereafter. Such murmurs are due to an imperfect formation or completion of the heart in its development. Frequently it is impossible for a physician to state from the sound of the murmur alone the cause of the murmur

or its eventual course. An electrocardiogram may be taken of the newborn or infant, but its results are usually suggestive rather than diagnostic. Most doctors prefer to wait until a child is approximately five years old before performing the specific diagnostic tests *(cardiac catheterization* and *angiocardiography).*

Parents of infants with congenital murmurs should realize that the important thing is not the murmur itself, but whether or not the defect produces signs or symptoms of cardiac difficulty. Such signs and symptoms would include blue spells, rapid breathing, extremely poor appetite and failure to thrive and grow normally.

In many instances the congenital cardiac defect may be entirely corrected by new cardiac operations, after which the

"Heart murmurs" are quite common in children, and many are no cause for concern. The most common infection that may damage the heart valves and result in acquired murmurs is rheumatic fever. The heart valves most often affected by this disease, shown below, are the *mitral* (1) and *aortic* (2) valves. The *tricuspid* valve (3) is rarely affected, the *pulmonary* (4) never. (See page 103.)

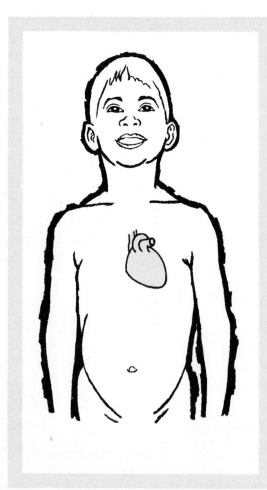

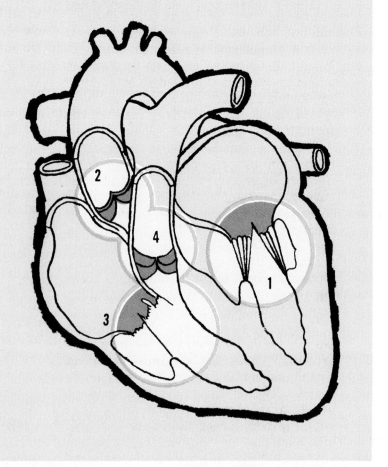

Umbilical hernias of various sizes (as shown below, a huge one) are protrusions of the intestines through a weakness in the abdominal wall in the region of the navel. If the protrusion can be pushed gently back into position it is said to be "reducible." If a non-reducible hernia is pinched by surrounding tissues so that its blood supply is cut off, it is said to be "strangulated" and immediate measures are necessary to prevent death of tissues.

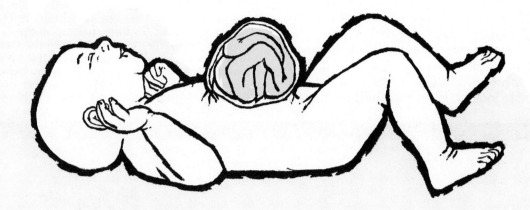

child will be as normal as any child born without cardiac defects.

Acquired cardiac murmurs are those that occur following an injury to the heart muscle or heart valve by an infection, most frequently rheumatic fever. In such case the physician would place a child on absolute bed rest and treat with drugs until all signs of the inflammation have subsided. The doctor can determine the activity of the infection and the damage to the heart muscle by such tests as the *electrocardiogram,* the *blood sedimentation* time, the *pulse rate,* and the *blood count.* The murmur may remain following an attack of rheumatic fever with resulting damage to the cardiac valves. Damage to the cardiac valves of such a degree that the heart function is disturbed can usually be corrected by cardiac operation.

Functional murmurs are those murmurs that occur off and on in children and are of no significance. They usually appear during fevers or when a child is anemic, and disappear when the condition has subsided or is corrected.

There is no reason to restrict the activities of a child with a cardiac murmur unless it is ordered by the physician. Most doctors will let a child with a murmur enter all activities as long as there is no sign of cardiac inflammation or weakness such as shortness of breath,

blueness, rapid cardiac rate, or an abnormality on cardiac tests indicating a weakness of the heart or an active inflammation of the heart muscle. Parents should do everything in their power to restrict a child as little as possible so that the child may not be damaged emotionally. The child should not develop a feeling of overanxiety nor one of weakness and hopelessness.

Hernias (Ruptures)

Hernias are due to a weakness of or an opening in the abdominal wall. The intestines beneath push through such areas and cause a bulging or ballooning. Such weaknesses or openings in the abdominal wall are almost always present from birth. But, although a weakness is there, the hernia may not push through until much later — in adolescence or even in adult life.

Two types of hernias are commonly found in infants and children. One is the *umbilical hernia* where the protrusion occurs at the region of the navel. The other is where the weakness is on either or both sides of the lower abdomen, causing a bulging where the abdomen is joined to the thigh. This type is called an *inguinal hernia.*

The danger of a hernia is greatest in situations where so much of the intestines may push through that it is difficult or impossible to push the protrusion back. This is called a *strangulated hernia* and is very dangerous, for when this occurs the blood supply to the strangulated portion is cut off and gangrene may occur.

It is vitally important that when an infant or child with a hernia *develops abdominal pain and later vomits,* the first place to look is in the region of the hernia

Hydrocele **(2) is an excessive accumulation of fluid in the sac that surrounds the** *testicle* **(1). Hydrocele present at birth usually disappears spontaneously before the infant is two years old. Sometimes the condition is complicated by an associated** *hernia* **(3), shown at right below. Congenital hydrocele may involve one or both sides of the scrotal sac.**

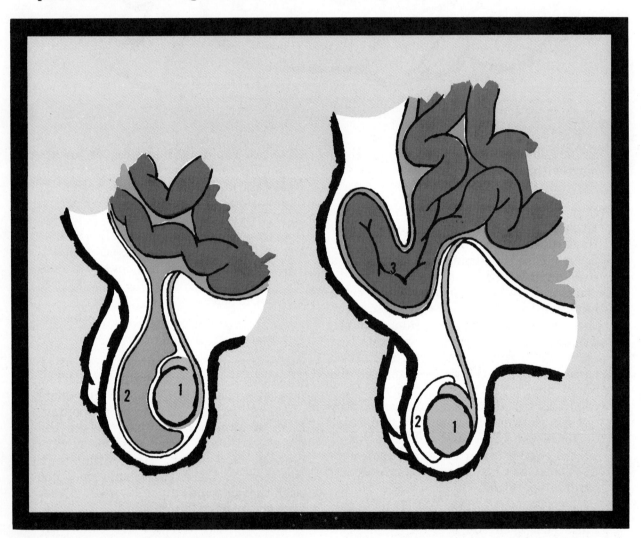

to see if it is protruding. If so, every effort should be made to quiet the child and push the protrusion back, for crying forces more of the intestines through the open or weakened area. If it is difficult to reduce the hernia with gentle pressure the child should be placed in a warm bath which usually relaxes the abdominal muscles. If this is unsuccessful a doctor should be called immediately.

The larger umbilical hernias are often strapped by physicians during the first year. Inguinal hernias may be temporarily treated by trusses. A very few inguinal hernias seem to heal spontaneously, but most physicians feel an operation is the first procedure, not only as a safety measure but also so as not to restrict the normal activities of a growing child. (See Chapter 22.)

Hydrocele

A good many male infants are born with a soft rounded swelling within one or both sides of the scrotal sac. This swelling is due to an extra amount of fluid in the sac around the testicle, where normally only a small amount is present. In almost every instance such hydroceles will subside and disappear spontaneously before the infant has reached two years of age.

At times a hydrocele in infancy may be associated with a hernia in the lower abdominal region. Such a possibility can be investigated by the child's physician.

In older boys, as in men, chronic hydroceles should be under the care of urologists since surgical treatment may be necessary. (See Chapter 8).

Infantile Eczema

Infantile allergic eczema is the most common skin disorder of infancy, with the one exception of diaper rashes. It is most usually due to a sensitivity to one or more foods that a child has eaten, or to direct contact of the skin with some substance to which it is sensitive.

In infancy it usually starts as a scattering of red pimples on the cheeks. The eruptions become more pronounced and spread to cover the whole face unless the cause is discovered and removed. If the condition gets more pronounced, the pimples form tiny blisters which break, causing a moist "weeping" eczema and finally a crusting. Usually there is considerable itching and the child becomes very irritable. The eczema, even if untreated, usually clears up almost entirely between one and two years of age, although some chronic eczematous lesions may continue to remain in the folds of the elbows and behind the knees.

Causes. In the first year of life the cause of eczema can usually be easily determined. If the eczema appears within the first month or six weeks of life it is usually due either to a sensitivity to cow's milk (if the infant is on a formula), to a sensitivity to the vitamin supplements the child is receiving or to a local irritant against the baby's tender skin, such as soap, baby oil or lotion, the cloth against which a baby's face lies, a woolen bonnet, sweater or blanket, or clothing that has been washed in bleaches that contain chlorine.

Treatment. A physician can usually prescribe an ointment that will relieve the condition, but the primary treatment lies in removing the offending substance whether it is in the infant's diet or directly in contact with the skin.

If the eczema is due to an allergy to cow's milk it is readily relieved by the substitution of goat's milk, or if that is inadequate, by a substitute preparation made of soy bean or meat-base formula, the last being an excellent substitute for milk although it is manufactured entirely from meat.

In older infants when foods are suspected as a cause of the eczema, an elimination diet should be attempted. (See Chapter 20). This may start with milk and gradual addition of a new food to the diet every four or five days to see if the eczema appears or becomes more intense with the addition of any particular food or foods. The most common foods responsible for eczema in the first years of life besides milk are eggs, wheat, and orange juice.

Where soap is suspected as an irritating agent, one could use hypo-allergenic soaps of which there are a number on the market. Various substitutes may be tried if baby oils, lotions, or powders are suspected of being the cause of the eczema. One should substitute an agent which does not include antiseptics or perfumes, either or both of which may be irritating.

Allergic skin tests which are so helpful in diagnosing the cause of most allergies are not particularly helpful or specific in infantile eczema due to food sensitivity, although occasionally patch tests against the skin are helpful in cases where a local irritant is suspected.

Intussusception

This is a very serious condition most commonly seen in children under the age

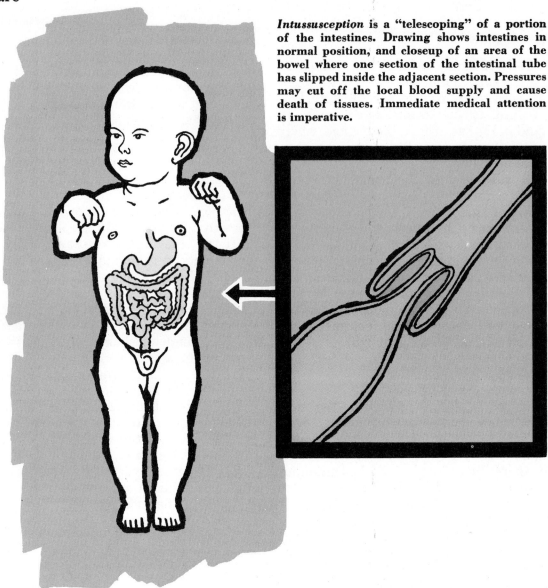

Intussusception is a "telescoping" of a portion of the intestines. Drawing shows intestines in normal position, and closeup of an area of the bowel where one section of the intestinal tube has slipped inside the adjacent section. Pressures may cut off the local blood supply and cause death of tissues. Immediate medical attention is imperative.

of two (the average age is seven months). It is caused by one portion of the intestine pushing inside the next segment. The pressure of the outside intestine compresses the blood vessels of the inner loop, cutting off the local blood supply. If not relieved quickly the inner portion of the loop may become gangrenous. This condition is two times more frequent in boys than in girls.

Symptoms. A child cries out suddenly with violent abdominal cramps and then starts vomiting. The cramps subside and then occur again at fairly regular intervals, generally leaving the child weak and almost flaccid.

But the telltale and most frequent sign of intussusception is blood in the stools. At times only a slight discharge of blood is passed by rectum, but more frequently there is a mixture of blood and mucus which because of its semblance to cranberry or currant jelly has been frequently called a "cranberry stool" or "currant jelly stool."

Treatment. This is an acute emergency and a doctor should be called immediately, for unless the intussusception is relieved it may prove fatal.

Often the physician can feel the mass in the abdomen caused by the condition. In rare instances it will subside under manipulation by the doctor. At other times it will subside when the child is given a diagnostic barium enema prior to x-ray or fluoroscopic examination. But if the intussusception is not relieved, an immediate operation is necessary. Time is very important, for if one waits too long and gangrene occurs, an amputation of a part of the intestine may be necessary. This is a very serious and critical operation for a small child already extremely ill and completely prostrated.

Mongolism

A Mongoloid child is a mentally retarded child whose features somewhat resemble those of the Mongolian race. The degree of mental retardation varies. Some of these children are severely retarded, while others can be educated to follow useful pursuits.

No one really knows why these children, who are of the white race or occasionally of the Negroid race, are born with Oriental-looking features, although considerable information has been gained in recent years as to the cause of the condition. In 1959 it was discovered that these children had an extra chromosome in the cells of their bodies. This would indicate that the condition is either familial or that something happens to the egg cell in the course of its development.

One fact about Mongolism is definitely established, and that is that older mothers are more likely to give birth to these children than younger mothers. Whereas statistically only about three in 1000 Mongoloid infants are born to mothers between the ages of 20 and 24 years, approximately 20 per thousand are born to older mothers—those between 40 and 50 years of age.

These children are usually not difficult to handle since they are almost always affectionate and of pleasant disposition. But being retarded, they are slower in development and need a good deal of extra care and help. They are generally more susceptible to respiratory infections such as colds, ear infections and pneumonia. These children may also have congenital heart lesions and often have hernias.

Pediculosis (Head Lice)

Infestation of the hair with head lice is a common condition, frequently found among school children, especially in large cities. The lice can jump from one child's head to another if the children are close together, or the condition can be contracted if one child wears the hat of a child already infested.

Once in the hair, the lice lay their eggs — tiny white pearly eggs — which become tightly glued to the hairs. These eggs look like dandruff to the naked eye, but cannot be brushed or combed out. Their pearly color can be seen under a magnifying glass.

The head lice are small insects which look something like tiny crabs. These bite the scalp, since they use blood for food, causing severe itching and at times even infections of the scalp.

There is no way of preventing a child from catching the condition. The aim should be to detect it quickly and clear it up as soon as possible. This can usually be done within 24 or 48 hours.

Treatment. There are two problems to be considered in treatment. The first is to kill the living lice, the second to kill and get rid of the eggs. At present there are a number of rapid and highly successful treatments. One of the best combines two insecticides, DDT and benzyl benzoate, with a wetting agent to loosen the eggs from their attachment to the hairs. Two applications are used, 12 hours apart — the first to kill the insects, the second to kill the eggs. The dead eggs can usually be removed by combing them out of the hair with a fine-toothed comb. If any eggs remain, a second treatment is advised a week later.

Another common method of treatment is by sprinkling DDT powder in a child's cap.

Pylorospasm and Pyloric Stenosis

At the end of the stomach where the food enters the intestines there is a circular muscle known as the *pylorus*. This remains contracted while the stomach is pumping and digesting food. When food is sufficiently mixed in the stomach, this muscle relaxes permitting the food to enter the intestines.

At times this muscle is in spasm and remains contracted. In such instances the stomach violently projects the stomach contents out of the mouth by projectile vomiting. The force may be sufficient to project material a foot or two.

This condition of *pylorospasm* is evident very shortly after birth and can usually be corrected easily by giving the child medication which relaxes the muscle. This permits the food to pass normally through the passage.

Atropine and its derivatives and small amounts of phenobarbital will usually relax the pylorus. As a rule, spasm-controlling medication can gradually be withdrawn after the muscle has been relaxed for two or three weeks.

Pyloric stenosis is a much more severe condition. In this condition the pyloric muscle is too thick and obstructs the opening at the end of the stomach so that food is unable to pass down into the intestines. The food is then vomited out projectilely. This condition is four times more common in boys than in girls. Vomiting usually does not commence until the infant is between eight and 14

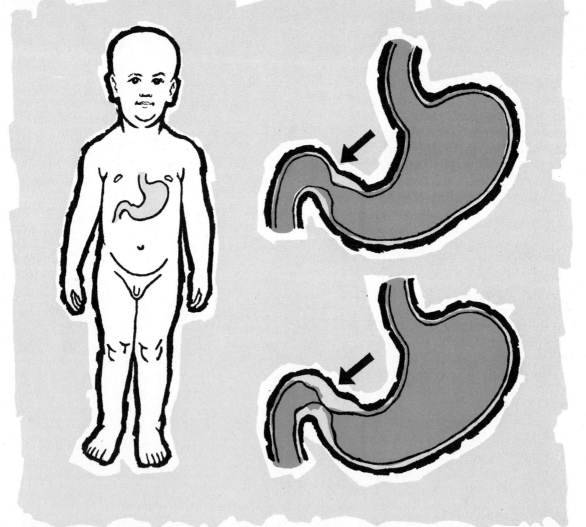

The *pylorus* is a ring of muscular tissue and mucous membrane which surrounds the opening between the stomach and the duodenum. The pylorus opens and closes periodically to control the passage of some of the stomach contents into the duodenum. In the top drawing above, the arrow points to a normal pylorus, and below it, to *pyloric stenosis* — an abnormal thickness of muscle at the outlet, preventing food from entering the intestines.

days of age, and from that time on the condition becomes more marked and projectile. Medication is rarely of help. The child becomes extremely hungry and the stools become very small and infrequent. There is progressive weight loss and dehydration becomes more and more pronounced.

On examination a physician can usually feel the pyloric mass.

The condition is completely relieved by an operation which cuts some of the muscle fibers of the pylorus.

The cause of pyloric stenosis is unknown. It may at times run in families.

Teething

Usually infants experience very little if any discomfort while cutting the first eight teeth — the middle four above and beneath. But the first four molars (the flat grinding teeth) that appear in the back of the mouth, usually between 12 and 18 months of age, are likely to cause some pain and upset.

The baby may be cranky and awaken during the night crying. He may lose his appetite, vomit easily, and may even have temporary diarrhea. Mothers used to call these back teeth "stomach teeth" because of their frequent effects on the child's digestive system during cutting. In many cases, rubbing the gums with paregoric or one of the analgesic teething creams or liquids will relieve the pain. The use of aspirin at this time is also helpful.

Occasionally infants develop fever during the course of teething. This is usually due to a throat infection rather than the teething itself. Some physicians feel that during the period of acute teething an infant's resistance to illness is lowered and the child is more prone to respiratory infections.

Thrush

Thrush is a fungus infection of the mucous membrane of the mouths of young infants. It often occurs while the infant is still in the nursery but may appear at home as well. The inner cheeks, lips, gums, soft palate, and tongue have scattered patches of grayish white color. The tongue is often heavily coated. These patches cannot be removed easily by rubbing, and when removed by greater pressure the denuded tissue beneath bleeds. The infected mouth is painful and infants so infected have difficulty in feeding.

Cause. Thrush is caused by an infection of the mucous membrane of the mouth by a fungus*(monilia)*. It is generally thought to be due to unclean nipples or other unclean objects that come into contact with an infant's mouth.

Treatment. The old and reliable treatment of swabbing the mouth two or three times a day with a one per cent aqueous solution of gentian violet is still to be recommended. The condition usually clears within a week.

A more recent, more specific, but more expensive treatment is the use of nystatin, the strength and dosage of which should be advised by a physician.

Chart of Infectious Diseases

Communicable diseases listed in the chart on the next page are for the most part preventable by timely vaccination. Some of the diseases are relatively uncommon and immunization is desirable only under conditions of susceptibility or exposure determined by a physician. Influenza vaccine is not used routinely but is generally restricted to high-risk patients and those with respiratory disease.

Several vaccines omitted from the chart (cholera, typhus fever, yellow fever) are mainly of concern to travelers in certain foreign countries (see page 52).

Routine smallpox vaccination of infants and children ceased in 1971.

Combinations of two or three specific vaccines reduce the number of "shots" required, lessening the anguish of patients and, not the least, of parents.

CHART OF INFECTIOUS DISEASES
For other infectious diseases and fuller descriptions, see Index.

Source	Mode of Transmission	Incubation Period	Period of Contagion	Type of Rash
CHICKENPOX Virus closely related to, if not the same as, the virus causing shingles (herpes zoster). In secretions of nose and throat of infected person.	By direct contact with person who has the disease.	12 to 19 days (usually 13th or 14th day)	From 1 day before appearance of rash to 6 days after appearance of rash.	Rash begins as small pink spots which develop into pinhead-size pimples. Then a tiny blister forms on top of pimple which turns to scab in about 4 days. Rash covers whole surface of body including scalp.
DIPHTHERIA Diphtheria bacillus. In secretions of nose and throat of infected person or carrier.	By direct contact with infected person or carrier, or by contact with articles infected by patient or carrier, or through contaminated milk.	Usually 2 to 6 days	Period of contagion varies—usually 2 weeks or less. Contagion considered over when 3 successive nose and throat cultures are negative at intervals of 24 hours.	None.
GERMAN MEASLES Virus in secretions of nose and throat of infected persons.	By direct contact with person who has the disease.	14 to 25 days (usually 17th or 18th day)	From start of symptoms to at least 4 days after. Contagion considered over 3 days after onset of rash.	Rash which may be mottled or made up of tiny pimples usually appears first on face and neck and works down, covering whole body in 12 to 24 hours.
HEPATITIS (Inf.) Hepatitis virus in feces and possibly in secretions of nose and throat of infected persons.	Mostly by feces of infected person. Possibly contracted by nose and throat secretions of infected person.	10 to 50 days (average 25 days)	Unknown. Virus may be in feces 2 to 3 weeks before onset of disease and at least during acute stage.	None.
INFLUENZA Influenza viruses. Usually Type A, Type B, or Asian type, in secretions of nose and throat of infected persons.	By direct contact with infected person, or by articles recently contaminated by infected person.	Usually 1 to 3 days	Shortly before and up to 1 week after onset of symptoms.	None.
MEASLES Virus in secretions of nose and throat of infected persons.	By direct contact with person who has the disease.	7 to 14 days (usually 10 days)	From 4 days before until 5 days after rash appears.	Mottled, slightly elevated pink rash appearing first on face and neck and extending down over whole body within 3 days. Then starts fading from head down.
MENINGITIS Meningococcus bacteria in secretions of nose and throat of infected persons.	By direct contact with infected person or carrier.	1 to 10 days (usually 3 to 7 days)	As long as the bacteria remain in the nose and throat of infected person.	Tiny dark red spots appearing mainly on trunk and buttocks in about 40 per cent of cases. May last only a few hours.
MUMPS Virus of mumps in saliva of infected persons.	By direct contact with person who has the disease.	14 to 21 days (average 17 days)	Until swelling of affected glands has completely subsided.	None.

Signs and Symptoms	Treatment	Care of Exposed People	Immunization (Prophylactic)
CHICKENPOX Usually fever and headache, followed by appearance of rash within 24 hours. Rash fully out in 2 to 3 days, followed by drop in temperature. Itching of lesions usually subsides by 4th day.	No specific treatment. Cut fingernails, apply drying and anti-itching lotion such as calamine lotion with 10 per cent phenol, anti-itching baths. Antihistamines by mouth may also be very helpful.	None.	None.
DIPHTHERIA Headache, fever and severe sore throat with confluent white exudate forming over tonsils, throat and soft palate. Fever 101° to 103°. There may be difficult swallowing, a croupy cough, and bloody discharge from nose.	1. Diphtheria antitoxin. 2. Penicillin. 3. Erythromycin.	Penicillin by injection and also by mouth for 5 to 7 days.	Diphtheria toxoid with booster inoculations given at periodic intervals.
GERMAN MEASLES Symptoms usually mild, with low grade fever and occasionally headache. There are usually swollen glands behind neck and on back of head. These appear either before or during appearance of rash. Eyes may be slightly inflamed.	No specific treatment.	Usually none given or desired except for exposed women in first 3 months of pregnancy who have not, to their knowledge, had German measles. A blood test should be made to see whether or not they have immunity.	Live German measles virus vaccine will immunize for long periods of time but the degree and duration of immunity is not fully determined. It should be given to all children and especially to girls approaching puberty.
HEPATITIS (Infectious) Early signs are malaise, weakness, headache and loss of appetite. Then right upper abdominal discomfort and pain, nausea and vomiting, usually occur. Urine is dark, feces light colored. Soon afterward, jaundice appears.	None specific. In severe cases with liver damage, corticosteroids may be used.	Injections of gamma globulin usually protect for 5 weeks or longer.	Temporary immunization for 5 weeks or longer may be obtained with injections of gamma globulin.
INFLUENZA Usually sudden onset with headache, malaise, chills, and aches and pains in arms, legs and back. Nose congested. Hard, dry cough common. Duration approximately 3 days.	No specific treatment.	None.	Polyvalent vaccine against known viruses causing influenza. Yearly booster injection to maintain immunity.
MEASLES Fever usually 3 or 4 days, followed by hard, dry cough, red eyes and running nose. Tiny white spots (Koplik spots) then appear on inner cheeks, gums and palate. Then fever rises high as rash appears and continues for several days until rash has covered body. Then fever drops, cough subsides, and eyes clear as rash subsides.	No specific treatment. Antibiotics often used to prevent complications.	Measles may be prevented or modified by injections of gamma globulin during incubation period. Treatment must be early to prevent the disease. Gamma globulin of no help once symptoms have appeared.	Live measles virus vaccine will immunize for long period, possibly for life. May develop a fever in 6 to 8 days. Killed measles virus vaccine protects for 2 to 3 years. No reactions.
MENINGITIS Fever, headache, vomiting. Later, delirium and loss of consciousness. Stiffness of neck is a fairly constant sign, the child being unable to put chin on chest.	Penicillin or a sulfa preparation are quickly effective if given in early stages.	Penicillin or sulfonamides by mouth as prescribed by physician.	None.
MUMPS Occasionally fever and vomiting, but often no signs or symptoms before tender swelling appears in front of and below ear. Usually on one side first, swelling on other side of face appearing in 2 or 3 days, or at times not appearing.	No specific treatment recommended in infants and children.	Immediate immunization of susceptible persons is provided by hyperimmune mumps globulin. This immunity is temporary, lasting only a few weeks.	Live mumps virus vaccine gives long immunity, probably for life. It should be given to all children, especially boys, before puberty.

CHART OF INFECTIOUS DISEASES

Source	Mode of Transmission	Incubation Period	Period of Contagion	Type of Rash
PARATYPHOID Salmonella bacteria in feces and urine of infected person or carrier.	From feces and urine of infected persons and carriers, either directly or indirectly from contaminated milk, food, shellfish, etc.	1 to 10 days	As long as patient or carrier harbors the organisms.	Usually a pimply and mottled pink rash (rose spots) on trunk and extremities.
POLIOMYELITIS Poliomyelitis virus in feces and material from nose and throat of patients and carriers.	By direct contact with patient or carrier, or by contact with feces of patient.	Usually 7 to 14 days but may be less	Not known. At least 5 days from nose and throat secretions. Virus may be present in feces for several weeks.	None.
ROCKY MOUNTAIN SPOTTED FEVER Infected ticks.	By bite of infected tick.	2 to 12 days (usually 4 to 8 days)	Not contagious.	Rash which usually appears about the 5th or 6th day is a mottled bright red color, scattered first over wrists and ankles. Later, rash becomes darker and covers abdomen and back until rash disappears. Brown pigment remains for a time.
ROSEOLA INFANTUM Virus probably in nose and throat secretions of infected persons or carriers.	Not known, but probably by direct contact with infected person or carrier.	Not known	Not known.	A mottled measles-like rash which may be faint or bright pink, usually covering the body within 24 hours after appearance.
SCARLET FEVER—see page 425.				
SMALLPOX Virus of smallpox.	Contact with patient, either direct or indirect. Infection may come from lesions of patient, clothing of patient, air surrounding patient, etc.	8 to 16 days (usually 12 days)	From first symptoms until all scabs have been shed.	First, small dark red spots appear over body which form pimples. On the 5th or 6th day fluid appears in these lesions and blisters form, each about the size of a pea and surrounded by red area. Blisters are dimpled. By the 9th day, fluid turns to pus. Then pus dries and foul-smelling scabs form.
TYPHOID FEVER Typhoid bacteria.	Feces and urine of patient or carrier.	7 to 21 days (average 14 days)	As long as patient or carrier harbors the typhoid organisms.	Usually pimply and pink-patched rash on trunks and extremities (rose spots) a few days after onset of symptoms.
TETANUS Tetanus bacillus.	Usually occurs through infected wounds.	3 to 21 days (average 10 days)	None.	None.

Signs and Symptoms	Treatment	Care of Exposed People	Immunization (Prophylactic)
PARATYPHOID FEVER			
Fever, headache, malaise, loss of appetite, vomiting, and usually diarrhea containing blood and mucus. Abdominal pain is usually also present.	Antibiotics not generally used. In long-drawn-out cases, ampicillin is the drug of choice.	Removal from contact.	3 doses of paratyphoid A and B vaccine given by injection at weekly intervals. Booster every 2 years.
POLIOMYELITIS			
Usually starts with fever, vomiting and irritability. These may subside after several days. Then usually a flareup occurs after 2 or 3 days, with severe headache, fever of 102° to 103°, and a stiffness of neck and back. Pain in affected muscles follows. Paralysis occurs in 10 to 15 per cent of cases.	None specific.	None of proved value. Gamma globulin has been used but effectiveness is questionable.	Sabin oral live polio vaccine may protect for life. Salk killed polio vaccine (booster every 2 years).
ROCKY MOUNTAIN SPOTTED FEVER			
Acute onset with chills, fever, severe headache and pains in joints and bones. Rash appearing about the 5th or 6th day. Fever may remain high for 3 weeks. In severe types there may be convulsions, spasm, and coma.	Chloramphenicol and tetracycline are effective in treatment, especially if given early.	None.	3 doses of vaccine given by injection at 5 to 7 day intervals, repeated yearly.
ROSEOLA INFANTUM			
Sudden onset of high fever, often 104° to 106°. Usually child does not appear very ill. No physical signs as a rule, except slight red throat. After 3 or 4 days of high fever, temperature drops to normal, rash appears and child is well.	No specific treatment.	None.	None.
SMALLPOX			
Onset with high fever, headache, backache, vomiting and delirium. Child appears very ill. Rash appears after 3 days. Pustules form scabs in 8 to 10 days. Scabs drop off within 3 weeks.	Marboran has been found to be effective almost 100 per cent in preventing smallpox in those exposed to the disease, when given during the incubation period.	Revaccination. Prompt vaccination if not vaccinated.	Vaccination with live cowpox virus vaccine. In 1971 the routine vaccination of all children was discontinued in the United States on recommendation of the United States Public Health Service.
TYPHOID FEVER			
Onset usually with fever, headache, malaise, loss of appetite, vomiting, and occasionally chills. Diarrhea is usually present but not always. Mild abdominal tenderness and distention also are common symptoms. Condition usually lasts 1 to 3 weeks.	Chloramphenicol is the drug of choice in treatment.	None. Family contacts excluded as food handlers until 3 successive negative tests.	3 doses of typhoid vaccine given by injection at weekly intervals. Booster every 2 years.
TETANUS			
Increasing stiffness of jaw until difficult to open mouth. Later, stiffness of back and abdominal muscles with neck thrown back and back curved in. Spasms of muscles are excruciatingly painful.	Tetanus antitoxin.	Not necessary.	Tetanus toxoid, 2 injections at intervals of 1 month. Booster every few years. For immediate immunization of those not protected by tetanus toxoid, tetanus antitoxin is given.

CHART OF INFECTIOUS DISEASES

Source	Mode of Transmission	Incubation Period	Period of Contagion	Type of Rash
TUBERCULOSIS Tubercle bacillus from sputum of infected persons.	Cough droplets from sputum of infected person. Can also be spread through articles contaminated by such sputum or bacteria therefrom.	Approximately 3 to 8 weeks from time of infection to signs of tuberculin allergy as shown by skin tests.	Children with first infection type of tuberculosis are generally not contagious. Children who develop tuberculous lung cavities (very rare) or with draining tuberculous sinuses are contagious as long as tubercle bacilli are present in sputum or drainage.	None.
WHOOPING COUGH Whooping cough (pertussis) bacillus.	Discharges from mouth and cough of infected persons. Almost always by direct contact or by objects freshly moistened.	5 to 21 days (usually under 10 days)	Contagiousness greatest in early stages before severe cough becomes paroxysmal (repetitive). Contagion is believed to last 6 weeks from onset.	None.

Revised Schedule for Active Immunization and Tuberculin Testing of Normal Infants and Children

AGE	IMMUNIZATION OR TEST
2 months	**DTP:** diphtheria and tetanus toxoids combined with pertussis (whooping cough) vaccine. **TOPV:** trivalent oral polio virus vaccine. Suitable for breast-fed as well as bottle-fed infants.
4 months	**DTP** **TOPV**
6 months	**DTP** **TOPV**
1 year	**Measles.** May be given as Measles-Rubella (German measles) or Measles-Mumps-Rubella combined vaccines. **Tuberculin Test.** Frequency of repeated tuberculin tests depends on risk of exposure of the child and the prevalence of tuberculosis in the population group.
1 to 12 years	**Rubella** **Mumps** Physician will determine age of administration.
1½ years	**DTP** **TOPV**
4 to 6 years	**DTP** **TOPV**
14 to 16 years	Combined tetanus and diphtheria toxoids of the adult type. Repeat thereafter every 10 years.

It is important that infants and children be immunized at the proper time. Schedules are well observed if children are under the care of a pediatrician, but considerable numbers of preschool and school children do not have all the recommended vaccinations or booster "shots." Measles vaccine is highly effective but a rising incidence of the disease indicates that many children have not been vaccinated. Parents should make sure that the immunization procedures listed above are given at the proper time.

Signs and Symptoms	Treatment	Care of Exposed People	Immunization (Prophylactic)
TUBERCULOSIS			
Usually little or no specific signs or symptoms of the first infection type of tuberculosis, the type usually seen in children. The signs and symptoms may be only those of a mild viral infection with low grade fever and a dry cough. Complications such as an infection through the blood stream will produce more severe symptoms.	INH (isoniazid) is the treatment of choice and should be given for at least a year. A newer drug, rifampin, has shown great effectiveness in tuberculosis. In severe cases, one of the drugs may be combined with streptomycin and para-amino-salicyclic acid	Repeated tuberculin tests and x-rays if tests are found positive.	BCG vaccine is advised for children with negative tuberculin tests who have a great probability of exposure to a person with active contagious tuberculosis.
WHOOPING COUGH			
Onset insidious with simple dry cough. As disease progresses, cough gets more severe at night. At about the third week cough becomes very severe, spasmodic and paroxysmal (repetitive), during which child may lose breath and become blue. At end of paroxysmal cough there is a long crowing inspiration (the whoop of whooping cough). Improvement usually occurs from 5th week on.	Tetracycline or chloramphenicol may be helpful in preventing complications. Severe cases should receive pertussis immune anti-serum or hyperimmune pertussis gamma globulin.	Children who have received pertussis vaccine should have a booster dose. If child has not been protected by the vaccine he should receive either an inoculation of pertussis immune anti-serum or hyperimmune pertussis gamma globulin.	3 doses of pertussis vaccine injected at intervals of 1 month. If quicker immunity is necessary the inoculations may be given at 1 week intervals. For immediate protection either pertussis immune anti-serum or hyperimmune pertussis gamma globulin may be given with 4 to 5 week protection.

Tonsils and Adenoids

The removal of tonsils and adenoids is probably the most frequent operation performed on children. Today it is generally accepted that healthy tonsils and adenoids serve as protective agents in the human body, as a defense against the invasion of bacteria into the bronchial tubes and the lungs. They serve as fortresses holding the infection in the nose and throat.

The decision as to removal of tonsils and adenoids then rests on whether these bodies have become a menace rather than a means of protection. If an operation is felt necessary, most pediatricians prefer to hold off the tonsillectomy until a child is approximately three years of age, for if they are removed too early there is often a regrowth of the tissue. Adenoidectomy when indicated may be performed at any age.

Since there may be separate indications for the removal of tonsils and the removal of adenoids, it is wise to consider each category separately.

Indication for Removal of Tonsils

1. *Size of Tonsils.* The size of tonsils is rarely an indication for their removal. Only two conditions may be considered. When tonsils are so large as to obstruct the swallowing of food a tonsillectomy is definitely indicated. At other times tonsils are very large and swell up during infections to such a degree that they almost close the throat passage and make breathing very difficult. In such cases a physician must make the choice between immediate removal or treating every infection quickly with antibiotics in an attempt at control before the tonsils enlarge so greatly. Many physicians prefer to try to hold off removal of the tonsils if it is at all possible, because many tonsils shrink in size between the age of three and ten years.

2. *Repeated attacks of tonsillitis or chronic infection of the tonsils.* Repeated attacks of tonsillitis or chronic infection of the tonsils may be con-

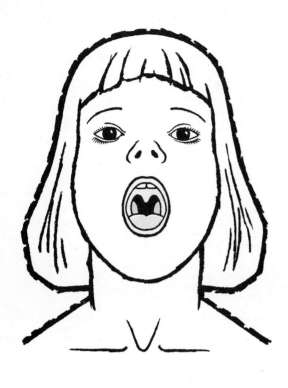
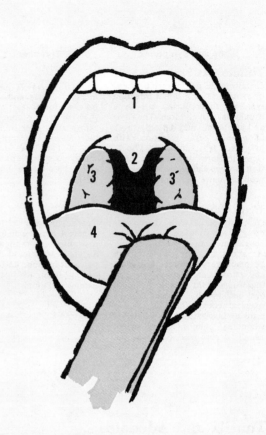

Tonsils (3) are easily seen, especially if enlarged. The small structure that hangs down from the back of the *palate* (1) is the *uvula* (2), above and behind the base of the *tongue* (4). Adenoids (also called pharyngeal tonsils) lie at the back of the nasal passages and upper throat near the Eustachian tube opening.

sidered as legitimate reasons for their removal. In such conditions it seems obvious that the tonsils, instead of serving as protective agents have become the seat of infection. The child is not only constantly being run down by the infections but, if he is of school age, misses a great many days of education and contact with his companions. In these children there is usually a quick and remarkable improvement in the child's general health following the removal of the tonsils.

Occasionally one hears that children who have had rheumatic fever and nephritis should have tonsillectomies. This is not at all an indication for the operation. There is no evidence that, if tonsils are healthy, their removal gives such children any added protection against subsequent attacks of these diseases. The indications for tonsillectomy in such children should be the same as for all children. Prophylaxis of recurrent rheumatic fever attacks is discussed elsewhere in this book.

Indications for Removal of Adenoids

There are only two indications for removal of adenoids.

1. *Frequent infections.* Frequent infections, which in turn cause frequent attacks of ear inflammation, is one indication. The earaches of childhood

are almost always due to infection and swelling of adenoid tissue at the opening of the Eustachian tubes (the tubes that connect the inner ear with the naso-pharynx). Repeated infections of the ear may permanently damage the mechanisms necessary for adequate hearing, and a lasting partial deafness may result.

2. *Tissue is so large that it obstructs breathing or* obstructs the Eustachian tubes. Obstruction of the naso-pharynx, which is evidenced by constant mouth breathing and snoring at night, has a number of detrimental results. In the first place, the nose is important in breathing, for it not only filters the air inhaled, but moistens it and warms it before it reaches the throat, trachea and bronchial tubes. Breathing through the mouth tends to dry the mucous membrane of the throat and respiratory tubes, especially during the winter months when the air in the average home is extremely dry. The dryness of these tubes, plus the cold air inhaled, at times makes the respiratory tree very susceptible to all manner of infections.

One other aspect of obstructive adenoids, often overlooked, is that they tend to spoil a child's appetite by preventing full taste of food to a great extent. If one has experienced the loss of taste when a cold occludes breathing through the nose, he will understand just how much of the pleasure of eating is lost by lack of smell. Following adenoidectomy, most children who have had obstructive adenoids eat with eagerness and gain weight from the increase in the amount of food eaten.

Many pediatricians advise only removal of adenoids if indicated, leaving the tonsils intact if they are healthy and cause no difficulties.

Congenital Disorders

Any abnormality that is present at birth is congenital, but not necessarily hereditary. Many birth defects are accidents that are most unlikely to recur in subsequent children. Some defects and disorders, however, are genetic, transmitted by interaction of the genes of the parents. This does not necessarily mean that every child of the same parents will have the same overt defect.

Should some abnormality be present in a child at birth, or be recognized in infancy or early childhood, parents worry and wonder about the risks of having other children. The obstetrician, pediatrician, or family doctor can frequently set fears at rest. Some conditions, however, do carry variable risks of repetition which may make special genetic counseling advisable. The mechanisms of heredity are complicated indeed; for fuller discussion see Chapter 25.

SCARLET FEVER (scarlatina)

Scarlet fever is an infection caused by strains of streptococcus germs which produce a toxin to which some children are susceptible and some are not. The distinctive feature is a red rash followed by peeling of the skin. Otherwise, the manifestations of scarlet fever are the same as those of other streptococcal infections such as "strep" sore throat. In fact, strep throat can be thought of as scarlet fever without a rash.

Symptoms of scarlet fever—irritability, fever, sore throat, vomiting—usually are rather sudden in onset. These are followed in a day or so by the appearance of bright red spots and rash, usually beginning in the neck, chest, and back areas, which may spread to the entire body except the head. Skin around the mouth is pale, the tongue bright red. After the rash fades, in about a week, the skin begins to peel off in fine flakes or in larger pieces. Thick parts of the skin may continue to peel for several weeks.

In addition to bed rest, treatment generally includes use of an antibiotic to which strep germs are susceptible. The antibiotic has no effect on the toxin that causes the rash, but it does limit to some degree the infection.

Most cases of scarlet fever today are quite mild. Sometimes the rash is such a slight blush that it is barely perceptible. For reasons unknown, scarlet fever has become a much "tamer" disease than it used to be in past generations when it was greatly feared. Nowadays, serious complications are uncommon, although proper care to watch for and prevent them is, of course, important.

Earache or inflamed glands of the neck are possible complications that parents should watch for. Rarely, scarlet fever or strep throat may be followed by rheumatic fever or may reactivate the disease. Patients should be under a physician's care. There is no preventive of scarlet fever or strep throat, but antibiotics may limit advance of the disease following exposure and restrict its spread within the household.

SPECIAL CONCERNS OF WOMEN

**by DANIEL G. MORTON, M.D.,
ROBERT H. FAGAN, M.D., and
HOWARD C. BARON, M.D.**

Childhood Problems · The Adolescent
Girl · Dysmenorrhea · Maturity ·
Feminine Hygiene · Pelvic Infections
· Vaginal Discharge · Cervicitis ·
Fibroid Tumors · Ovarian Cysts ·
Endometriosis · Uterine Displacements
· Vaginal Relaxations

PELVIC MALIGNANCY

Cancer of the Cervix · Cancer of the
Ovary · Post-Menopausal Complaints
· About "Female Operations" · About
Symptoms

CANCER OF THE BREAST

Dangerous Fallacies

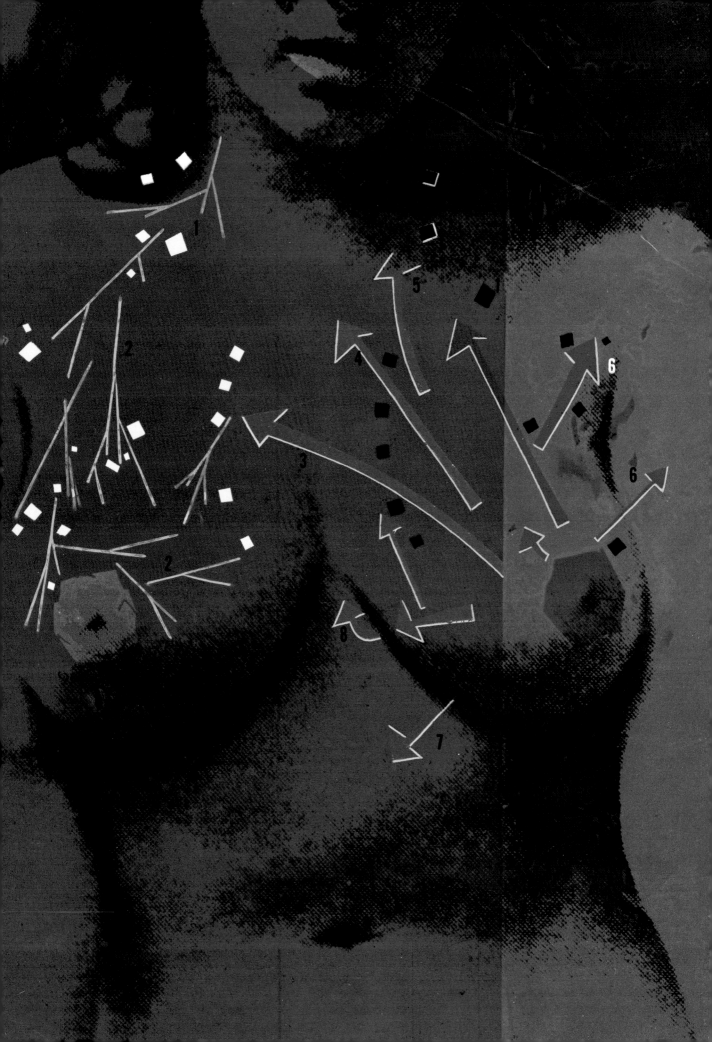

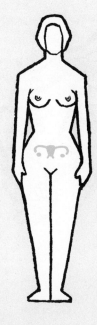

This chapter is concerned with *gynecology*, the branch of medicine which treats diseases of women, especially of the sexual organs.

The color plate shows diagrammatically the pathways by which cancer of the breast may invade other parts of the body if cancer is not detected and treated early while it is still localized.

Lymph nodes (1) are shown as white and black squares. The lymph glands are connected by *communicating channels* (2), shown on the left side of the drawing. The principal lymphatic drainage route from the breast is toward the neck where vessels empty into major veins which go to the heart and then throughout the body. Malignant cells from the breast may be carried in these channels.

Numbered arrows on the right side of the drawing show different directions of spread and drainage: (3) to the opposite *breast and axilla*; (4) to the *internal chest nodes*; (5) to the *neck* and general circulation; (6) to the *axilla and chest wall*; (7) to the *liver and nodes of the stomach area*; (8) to the *chest and lungs*.

CHAPTER 12

SPECIAL CONCERNS OF WOMEN

by DANIEL G. MORTON, M.D., and ROBERT H. FAGAN, M.D.

Gynecology is the branch of medical science which especially concerns the reproductive organs of the female sex. It encompasses the health, diseases, and treatment of female patients from babyhood through advanced old age.

Childhood Problems

Anatomical defects. Occasionally it happens that the sexual organs of a newborn baby show some deviation from normal. Happily, such congenital malformations are most unusual. If there is some defect of the external genital structures, this will be apparent to the doctor when he inspects the baby.

For example, the clitoris, which is analogous in the female to the penis in the male, may be enlarged and actually resemble a small penis. However, it rarely happens that the true sex of the infant cannot be established immediately at birth. In uncertain cases it is important that the true sex be determined early enough so that a female will not be "brought up" as a male or vice versa.

The hymen, the thin membrane at the opening of the vagina, may be very thick or have no opening in it *(imperforate hymen)*. This may cause no difficulty until the girl begins to menstruate. The flow of blood cannot escape and gradually accumulates behind the imperforate hymen. The correction is simple surgical incision.

There may be a band of fibrous tissue in the center of the vagina, forming two compartments instead of one *(septate vagina)*. More rarely, there is complete absence of the vagina. In many instances, plastic operations can create an artificial vagina with satisfactory function.

At other times there are duplications or partial duplications of internal genital structures. For example, the

427

Concerns of Women

The female figure shows internal sex organs. At right, top drawing shows normal structures: *uterine cavity* (1); *Fallopian tubes* (2); *ovaries* (3); *cervix* (4); *vagina* (5). Lower drawing shows uterus with two chambers and one cervix, resulting from failure of parts to fuse properly during fetal development.

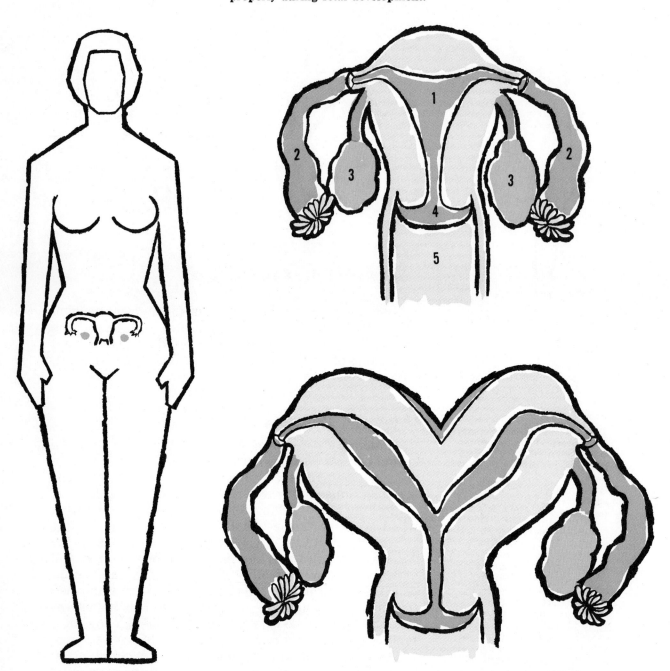

uterus may have two chambers instead of one, with only one cervix, or there may be a complete halving of the uterus, cervix, and vagina, producing a doubling or pairing of these organs, one on each side. These conditions due to faulty development are sometimes incompatible with pregnancy, but not always.

Tumors of the reproductive organs are uncommon in infancy and childhood.

Tumors may be benign or malignant, and are treated the same as tumors in adults — that is, by surgical removal when this is feasible, or by irradiation. Early diagnosis is urgently required.

Certain kinds of tumors may stimulate early growth of the sexual organs. Rarely, a girl eight years of age or younger may undergo the characteristic changes of puberty and onset of menstruation. The breasts enlarge, pubic hair appears, and in many respects a miniature woman exists in a child's body with a child's mind. Such precocious puberty creates psychological problems for the child and the parents which must be handled intelligently. Determination of the particular cause of premature sexual development is obviously important since the underlying condition may be correctible.

Hygiene of the girl infant and child is of great importance, and not at all complicated. The external genitals may become irritated, inflamed, and swollen if they are not regularly and properly cleansed with an ordinary mild soap and water solution. There is a secretion from the folds of tissue surrounding the clitoris and vagina called *smegma*. This is sticky and irritating if not removed. In infants this may be done with a tuft of cotton or a cotton-tipped applicator dipped in a neutral oil. Smegma may accumulate at any age.

The lips on either side of the vagina may become adherent due to inflammatory processes. Correction by a doctor is quite simple. As children grow older, small foreign bodies such as pebbles, bobby pins, pieces of wood or metal, may be inserted into the vagina and become lodged there, causing local irritation. The only outward sign may be a troublesome vaginal discharge, if the foreign object has "disappeared" and is not apparent on external examination. When search for the cause of unexplained vaginal discharge leads to discovery of an unsuspected foreign body, its removal corrects the condition.

As little girls grow older and begin to take over their own personal hygiene responsibilities, they should be instructed in proper habits of cleanliness.

The Adolescent Girl

Normal growth of the sexual organs during childhood gradually brings about the changes we recognize as puberty and adolescence, culminating in menstruation, ovulation (egg-cell release), and capacity for motherhood.

Before these culminating changes are established and stabilized, other changes in the young girl's body are apparent. Her hitherto boylike body begins to assume feminine contours, the breasts begin to enlarge, the vulval folds become more pronounced and pubic and axillary hair appear. At the same time the girl's personality frequently changes. She may become moody, more serious, display emotional instability, burst into tears suddenly, feel misunderstood, and she may become, temporarily at least, a somewhat "difficult" member of the family.

Such changes are quite natural consequences of hormonal rhythms and surges and organic changes that have not had time to "settle down" into well-established patterns of full maturity. It is highly important that an understanding adult ease a young girl's transition into womanhood by explaining these changes and their significance before they occur, so the girl will not be taken by surprise but will be prepared for them as natural and anticipated aspects of becoming an adult. The ideal person to explain matters is the mother — provided that there is a good mother-daughter relationship and that the mother herself has proper understanding and attitudes about womanly functions.

A girl's reactions to menstruation tend to follow the patterns she observes in her immediate environment. If menstruation is referred to as "the curse," a painful monthly "sickness" that must be endured, an unfair burden on her sex, it is quite natural for a girl to regard it with dread and to resent stirring changes in her body that she is powerless to control or prohibit. On the other hand, if menstruation is depicted as a process of health and normality, an index of vital, charming womanhood with normal capacity for love and parenthood, the girl's adjustment to transition into womanhood will be much better.

Onset of menstruation. The age at which menstruation first occurs in perfectly normal girls may vary from ten to 16 years or even more.

During the first few years the periods may be irregular, perhaps skipping several months at a time. There may also be differences in the amount and duration of the flow. "Heavy" or profuse periods may occur when menstruation is becoming established because ovulation, or release of an ovum from the ovary, does not occur each month. The ovarian hormone, progesterone, which forms only after ovulation, is important in controlling the menstrual flow. If progesterone is not present, the periods may be abnormal, profuse, and prolonged, but the underlying cause — failure to ovulate — is not itself abnormal or uncommon when the menstrual cycle is becoming stabilized in young girls.

The principal danger here is that a succession of heavy periods may cause sufficient blood loss to produce anemia. Therefore, excessive periods should be reported to one's physician and efforts should be made to control them. Erratic periods during adolescence are not at all unusual. It is interesting to note

Development of the breast: Left, rudimentary ducts in infancy and childhood; Center, elongation of ducts and tissue growth; Right, adult breast with milk-secreting lobules. Lower drawing shows external female genitals of a child, left, and adult, right: (1) *labium major*; (2) *labium minor*; (3) *clitoris*; (4) *urethral orifice*; (5) *vagina*. The hymen is a membranous partition which partially blocks the orifice of the vagina.

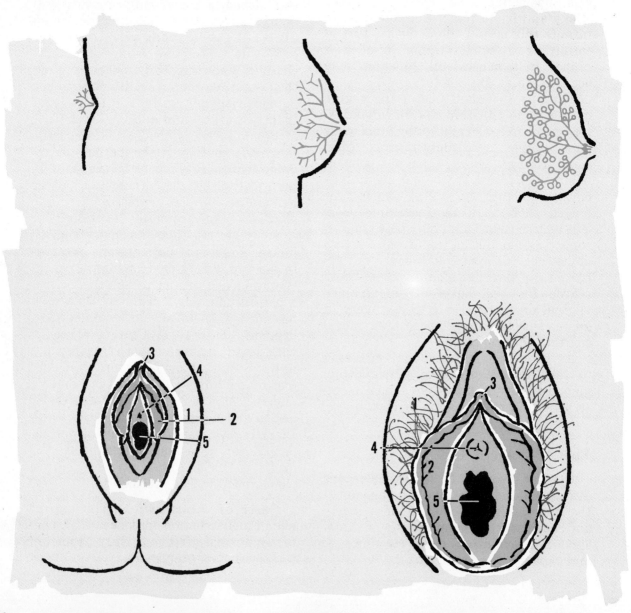

that irregular periods and emotional problems are also common at the other end of the childbearing years, just prior to the menopause.

Dysmenorrhea (Painful Menstruation)

A fairly common problem during adolescence is the occurrence of painful periods *(dysmenorrhea)*. Not uncommonly the complaint continues into adulthood.

The less common type of dysmenorrhea is *secondary* to such conditions as pelvic inflammation, endometriosis, polypoid growths within the uterus, and a variety of other disorders in which the painful periods are symptoms of some underlying disease process. Successful treatment of the basic disease corrects a physical cause of dysmenorrhea.

Much more often, however, dysmenorrhea occurs without any abnormality of the organs or any detectable disease. This most common type of periodic pain is called *primary* dysmenorrhea.

Symptoms. The characteristic complaint is cramps — as if the uterus were attempting to expel the menstrual blood through a tightly closed, unwilling cervix; cramps continue until the seeming obstruction has been overcome. The cramps (some patients liken them to labor pains) occur at the onset of the period and for the first several days of the period.

Curiously enough, this type of dysmenorrhea occurs only in cycles in which ovulation has taken place. Dysmenorrhea of this type is a disturbance of function, not a pathological condition, and it is influenced by a great variety of physiological and psychological events. It is more common and more severe in high-strung, nervous girls and women, especially those of excessive sensitivity who tend to over-react, and to whom as a consequence of early training the psychologic import of menstruation is that of being "sick" or "unwell."

Dysmenorrhea accounts for a good deal of incapacitating bed rest for a day or two during the month.

Treatment. Dysmenorrhea has been combated by so many different measures, with greater or less success, that it is obvious that no single treatment is specific. Mild pain relievers are commonly used in self-medication. Bending and swaying exercises, theoretically intended to "loosen up" constricted areas, are dubious as far as any deep physiological effects are concerned but they have the value of positive action and encourage activity instead of bed rest. Hot tub baths may be comforting.

Although obstruction of the cervical canal is practically never present in primary dysmenorrhea, repeated dilations of the cervix have sometimes been done in an attempt to relieve symptoms — a treatment that may well be worse than the disease! Since dysmenorrhea occurs only in ovulatory cycles, hormones to suppress ovulation have been used, but this is unwise on a long-term basis. Even surgical removal of a segment of the sympathetic nerves serving the uterus and cervix has been done in extreme cases.

The most effective "treatment" of primary dysmenorrhea is sympathetic factual explanation of the menstrual process, the undoing of superstitious or resentful attitudes, such as that menstruation is a "curse" or a "sickness" (rather than an index of normal womanhood), and encouragement to be up and active rather than taking to one's bed for a day or two at "that time of month."

Instruction. As children grow into the teen age, girls as well as boys become more interested in sex. It is during these years that parents usually warn their children about undesirable sexual activities. It is highly desirable that information come from a respected parental source, but it is possible that evil aspects of sexual activities may be dwelt upon so exclusively as to handicap the child's later sexual adjustments in marriage. It is indeed true that sexual promiscuity may lead to venereal disease, unwed motherhood, and difficulties that leave scars for a lifetime. It is also true that sexual happiness is essential to marital happiness, and that the positive side should not be overlooked, or minor misbehaviors magnified out of true proportion, in helping teenagers through a difficult time of growing up.

Maturity

Marriage is the natural expectation of most young women. The present divorce rate, plus unknown numbers of unhappy marriages that do not culminate in divorce, indicates that many marriages are entered into with little real understanding of the problems, adjustments, and responsibilities involved. The medical professions, and the gynecologist especially, may play an important role in attaining happy marriage by giving premarital advice and examination.

It is wise for one contemplating marriage to give thought to fundamental questions:

1. Is there mutual physical attraction?
2. Is there deep devotion between the two?
3. Is each willing to accept the other as a co-parent if and when children arrive?
4. Is there mutual respect?
5. Is each willing to assume the responsibilities of marriage?
6. Are there common interests, kindred activities?

Affirmative answers to these questions suggest that the marriage will rest on a firm foundation.

A *physical examination* before marriage is always advisable.

What is meant by a gynecological examination? This consists of the usual physical examination with emphasis on examination of the breasts, abdominal and pelvic organs, and a smear test of the vaginal secretions (Papanicolaou test). The pelvic examination may disclose conditions that should be corrected. Sometimes the vaginal orifice may be found to be so constricted that intercourse would not be possible without prior dilation. At other times, conditions such as ovarian cysts or fibroids of the uterus, which may influence pregnancies,

are found. The physician may feel that laboratory tests such as a blood count, urinalysis, or x-rays of the chest are indicated for proper diagnosis.

The prospective bride should be helped to understand her sexual responsibilities in marriage. The gynecologist is particularly qualified to answer certain of her questions, or to discuss matters that she may not think of inquiring about, such as any differences in the sexuality of men and women.

The prospective bride usually is interested in information about family planning and child-spacing. The gynecologist is expertly qualified to give important information about all aspects of fertility and infertility if he is invited to do so. (See Chapters 9 and 10.)

Feminine Hygiene

Douches have a place in a woman's personal hygiene, although some women never use vaginal douches. Many do so only at the end of a period, or after sexual relations, or if there is an increased vaginal discharge.

Harm may result from douches only if irritating substances are used in the water. If one chooses to douche for personal hygiene, it is desirable to use a harmless aromatic powder or liquid, of the sorts marketed by many pharmaceutical companies. The addition of white vinegar to the water is a time-honored habit, but the odor of vinegar is not particularly pleasant and the package is bulky for traveling on a holiday.

The acidity or alkalinity of a douche is of virtually no importance because the solution is in contact with the vagina for too short a time to modify the existing environment.

Many women have long hairs which tend to become matted in a moist environment and to impede sexual relations. It is unwise to attempt to shave the pubic area but it is desirable to keep long hairs trimmed and feminine care here is as important as care of the axilla and legs.

Orgasm, the successful culmination of the sexual act, is always desirable but not always attained by some women. Many factors enter into this failure — fatigue, hurt feelings, abruptness, worries, lack of careful hygiene on the part of the sexual partner, and many other psychic and physical factors.

Often there is little understanding of the complex mechanisms involved. As a woman becomes sexually aroused there is an increased blood supply to the sexual organs, the clitoris and vaginal folds become more distended, the pelvic organs become congested with blood, and the cervical and Bartholin's glands secrete more lubricating mucus. The peak of excitation causes the muscles surrounding the outer portion of the vagina to contract and the inner portion to balloon. These involuntary contractions continue for several seconds, forcing the blood supply to diminish to the normal state, with feelings of relief and comfort.

Repeated failures to achieve this state leave the woman with an uncomfortably congested pelvis and emotional frustration. Long-continued failure may become a source of marital unhappiness and indeed one of the major factors leading to divorce. The "fault," if such it be, is not always, or often, solely that of the wife; the husband's role is vital to mutual satisfaction; and it is in such areas that unhappy couples who seek competent professional counsel may be greatly helped.

Dyspareunia, or painful intercourse, is another cause of marital unhappiness and frustration. There are many possible causes. Fear of injury, not necessarily a rational or conscious fear, may cause a painful prohibitory constriction or spasm of pelvic muscles, called *vaginismus*. Or intercourse may be painful because of physical reasons, such as infection of the vagina or cervix or tumors of the pelvic organs. In such circumstances it is obvious that medical help is urgently needed, and that the dyspareunia is merely a symptom of a physical disorder that needs correction.

Pelvic Infections

Infections in the pelvis are quite common, and may affect any or all of the pelvic organs as well as the skin surrounding the vagina.

Sometimes the skin becomes inflamed, burning, and itching due to a local allergy. Some women, especially those who perspire rather profusely, find nylon panties to be irritating, since nylon does not absorb moisture. In such an instance, shifting to undergarments made of different materials relieves the condition. At other times, harsh soaps, deodorants, and bath powders prove irritating.

If the skin is broken due to scratching, bacteria may enter, causing *vulvitis*. The Bartholin's glands, on either side of the vaginal opening, may become infected, causing considerable swelling and pain. Skene's glands, located under the urethra, may also become infected, causing painful urination. Numerous kinds of infecting organisms may enter the vagina and cervix, causing them to become painful, itchy, and swollen. Organisms of gonorrhea and syphilis may gain entry through the vagina (see Chapter 2).

Virus infections may cause painful warty growths *(condyloma acuminata)* on the skin surrounding the vulva and anus. They are not venereal. They are usually removed by electrocoagulation under local anesthesia, using an instrument with a wire loop heated by an electric current.

Many other non-venereal types of infection may gain entry to the body through the vagina. Some of these may spread upward and infect the uterus, Fallopian tubes, ovaries, and even the lining of the pelvic cavity. Appropriate treatment should be instituted early, which means that the infected patient must be alert to symptoms and signs of anything out of the ordinary and report these to her physician.

Vaginal Discharge

Normally the vagina is moist, occasionally to the extent that a vaginal discharge that stains the underclothing may be noticeable. This normal moisture consists of a mucoid substance produced by the glands in the cervix and an exudation from the vaginal walls. The color is white and there is no odor.

If discharge is more than minimal it is probably due to abnormal conditions such as an infection or ulceration of the cervix or one of several different forms of vaginal infections. In the latter case the discharge is rather profuse and usually causes itching, burning and inflammation, and irritation of the vulval skin.

Three of the most common types of vaginal infections which are not considered to be venereal diseases, but are most annoying, are the *yeast* infections (candida albicans), *trichomonad* infestations, and *hemophilus vaginalis* infections. All of these cause leukorrhea (increased vaginal discharge) with itching and burning. Occasionally, all three types of organisms are present at the same time. The diagnosis is made by microscopic examination of discharge material smeared on a glass slide.

Yeast infections are rather common in pregnancy, in the elderly, in association with diabetes, and following the use of some antibiotics. The discharge is white and cheesy and often occurs in plaques in the vagina and sometimes on the vulva. The diagnosis is simple and several forms of treatment are effective.

Trichomoniasis. This quite common form of vaginitis is caused by a one-celled microscopic organism, a protozoon or member of the animal kingdom (rather than of the plant kingdom, as bacteria are) called *trichomonas vaginalis*. The minute creature is pear-shaped, highly infectious, and capable of vigorous movement, using its whip-like flagellae as propellers. Infestation of the vagina produces a thin, white, foamy vaginal discharge of offensive odor. The discharge causes diffuse redness of the vagina which is usually associated with burning, irritation and chafing of skin in the vulval region, and, especially at onset, itching.

The affected patient often complains of painful intercourse (dyspareunia), painful urination, and soreness. Some believe that there are emotional causes for trichomoniasis (the organism may be recovered from the vaginal secretions of women who have no overt symptoms) and it appears to be more common in women who are emotionally upset, especially over sexual frustrations. Established infection at least tends to intensify such frustrations because of the soreness involved and the disagreeable profuse discharge.

The condition often responds quite satisfactorily to any one of numerous preparations (powders, jellies, suppositories, tablets) but has a pronounced tendency to recur. The organism is often harbored in the male, who is unaware of any symptoms, so that wives are frequently reinfected by their husbands. A relatively new drug called *metronidazole*, which has recently become available to physicians, is highly effective in eradicating this infection from both partners.

Hemophilus vaginalis vaginitis causes much the same symptoms as the conditions described above, but is slightly less common. The causative organism is a small bacillus. Antibiotic creme is usually effective.

It is important to distinguish between the various types of vaginal infections in order to institute effective treatment, and this obviously requires the diagnostic skills of a physician. In the event of excessive vaginal discharge, pelvic examination and examination of the discharge material are demanded. Any bloody or blood-stained discharge, apart from menstruation, calls for prompt examination by a physician.

Cervicitis

Infection of the cervix, the neck of the uterus, is quite common. **Cervicitis** may be due to gonorrhea, syphilis, or some specific infection. The more usual form of chronic cervicitis is a protracted inflammatory process associated in a nonspecific way with many and varied strains of organisms that may inhabit the vagina. A cervix lacerated at childbirth is more susceptible to bacterial invasion. The cervical canal may be involved, with cervical discharge and impairment of fertility. These infections are usually cured quite readily in the doctor's office or a hospital by cauterization.

Polyps (small fleshy growths) may occasionally develop in the cervix or uterus. These small growths are almost always benign, but should be removed and examined under a microscope because in rare instances they may show malignant changes.

Fibroids may be as small as a garden pea or as large as a full-term pregnancy, although huge sizes are rarely seen today because the growths are usually recognized and removed before attaining tremendous dimensions.

Frequently the tumors are multiple and knobby, and cause the womb to be not unlike a lumpy potato, with nodules buried in its wall.

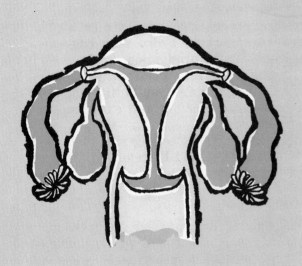

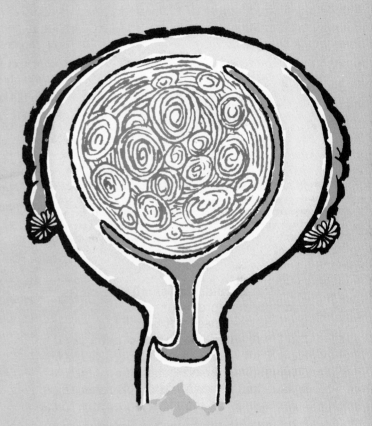

Fibroid tumors of the uterus (*myomas*) are probably the commonest tumors found in women. Fibroids are benign growths (noncancerous) consisting of smooth muscle and connective tissue. The tumors may distort the wall of the uterus or project into the uterine cavity. Below, normal uterus, and at right, uterus distended by a large fibroid tumor.

Fibroid Tumors (Myomas)

Fibroid tumors of the uterus are tumors of muscle and connective tissues. They constitute the most common type of pelvic tumor, occurring in about 20 per cent of women of 35 years of age or older. They are characteristic of sexual maturity. The vast majority of them occur in middle life, commonly in the third, fourth and fifth decades.

Symptoms. Often a fibroid tumor is discovered in a routine physical examination of a woman who has experienced no symptoms. The growths are painless, in absence of complications, and may be present for many years without causing distress. If enlargement is sufficient to exert pressures on nearby structures, various symptoms depending on size and location may occur — difficult urination, constipation, vague feelings of "heaviness," disturbances of menstruation.

435

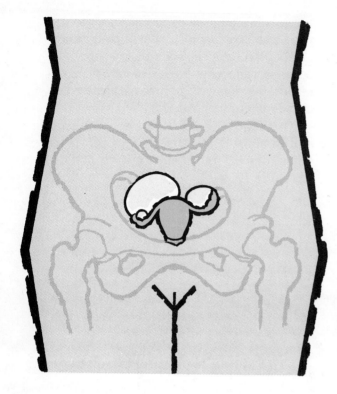

Ovarian cysts protruding into the pelvic portion of the peritoneal cavity. Cysts are fluid-containing sacs which may rupture and release irritating material into the abdominal cavity. Some cysts have *pedicles* (stemlike attachments) which may become twisted and cause severe pain.

If the fibroids are small and cause no pressure symptoms or menstrual abnormalities, they need not be treated actively, but there should be an examination every six months or so to keep watch on the situation. Otherwise, the usual treatment is surgical removal. Many factors affect the decision in the case of an individual patient, as evaluated by the doctor. In a procedure called *myomectomy*, the tumors are removed from their beds and the cavities closed. This operation may be preferred in young women who desire to become pregnant.

In women who are near or past the menopause, the entire uterus may be removed (hysterectomy) instead of excising individual tumors. Tumors of moderate size that cause no symptoms in women near the menopause may just be left alone and watched, since there is some tendency for fibroids to regress after the change of life. When surgery is considered too hazardous for a particular patient, treatment by radiation (x-ray) tends to shrink the tumors.

Ovarian Cysts

The ovary may be the site of various types of tumors, many of which are benign. Some are malignant (See *Pelvic Malignancy*, this Chapter).

A *cyst* is a sac containing fluid or mucoid material. Several varieties may arise in the ovary. Small cysts sometimes disappear without treatment, but if they enlarge or become twisted they must be removed. A cyst that has a slender stem *(pedicle)* may twist tightly around the stem, causing intense abdominal pain that may arouse suspicion of appendicitis.

The ovary, as well as being a producer of eggs, produces sex hormones. The ovary secretes estrogen, necessary for feminine development, and progesterone, which is necessary for preparing the uterus for pregnancy (see Chapter 9). Some tumors of the ovary may cause excessive hormone production.

It is not possible to determine the exact nature of an ovarian cyst until it has been removed surgically and examined under a microscope.

Generally, cysts exceeding size of an average orange should be removed.

Endometriosis

This is a condition in which fragments of *endometrium,* the tissue which lines the uterus, migrate to other parts of the body and become implanted there. In effect, the displaced tissue acts very much like a miniature uterus in a place where it has no business to be.

Under the influence of ovarian hormones, the displaced tissue bleeds (or "menstruates") like normal endometrium lining the cavity of the uterus. This causes chemical irritation. Nature's attempt to wall off these pockets of menstruating tissue results in formation of cysts filled with blood. The cysts may rupture and release tissue which forms additional implants.

These cysts are commonly in the ovaries, tubes, uterus, or the peritoneum lining the pelvic cavity. Endometrial implants in the ovary commonly cause so-called "chocolate cysts," filled with chocolate-colored material.

The cysts continue to grow under continued stimulation by the ovaries. Endometriosis may cause painful periods, profuse and prolonged periods, or pelvic adhesions that result in various symptoms, depending on the location of tissues that become adherent. Endometriosis is frequently a factor in complaints of inability to become pregnant.

Endometriosis is fairly common in young women. Diagnosis may be difficult since there are rarely any external signs, although sometimes a vaginal examination may disclose local lesions. A number of other pelvic conditions which may produce somewhat similar symptoms must be distinguished. Positive diagnosis may require surgical exploration.

Treatment of endometriosis is not necessarily surgical. There is a great range in severity of symptoms. Small areas of endometriosis may cause few if any symptoms. Frequently explanation of the situation will encourage some patients to endure some pre-menstrual and pelvic discomfort if it is not severe.

Uterine Displacements

These conditions are often referred to as a "tipped uterus."

Such conditions are very common in women and rarely cause any serious symptoms. The great majority of women who have a uterus somewhat out of theoretically "ideal" position do not report any symptoms.

A normal uterus is directed forward. Occasionally a large boggy uterus that is tipped backward (retroverted) may cause some feeling of heaviness in the

Prolapse of the uterus is an extreme form of displacement in which the womb "drops" or "falls" into the lower part of the vagina and protrudes through the opening. At left below, structures in normal position: (1) *bladder*; (2) *uterus*; (3) *rectum*; (4) *vagina*. Compare with *prolapsed uterus* (2) at right. Repair by surgery is usually preferable, but sometimes supporting devices may be used.

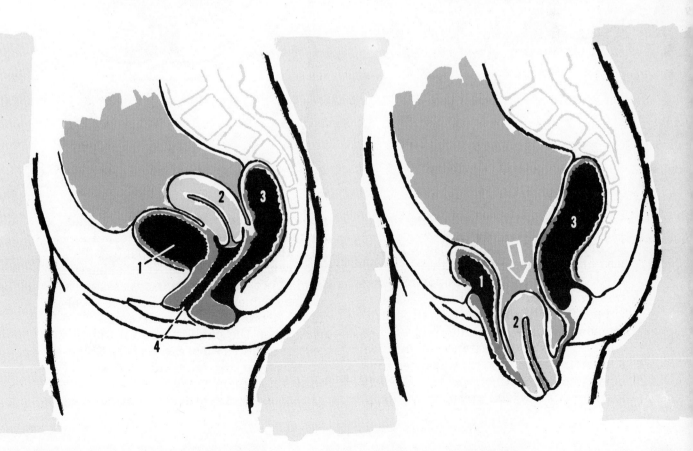

Concerns of Women

pelvis, sometimes backache, and make pregnancy less likely but by no means impossible. A physician can usually replace a uterus and insert a supporting device (pessary) which holds it in satisfactory position, to see if symptoms complained of will be relieved.

into the lower part of the vaginal canal. This is usually associated with some variety of uterine displacement previously mentioned. Occasionally the uterus may actually protrude through the vaginal opening. This condition is known as *prolapse* of the uterus.

At left below, a *cystocele* — bulging of the base of the bladder into the vaginal canal. Arrow shows direction of protrusion of *bladder* (1); *uterus*, (2); *rectum* (3). At right, a *rectocele*, a similar bulging of the rectum through the rear wall of the vagina. The *rectum* (3) bulges into vagina as shown by arrow; *bladder* (1); *uterus* (2). Cystoceles and rectoceles can be corrected surgically.

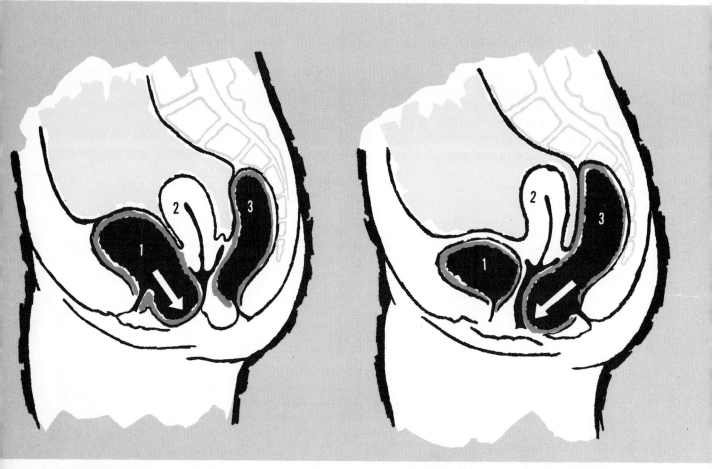

Vaginal Relaxations

These occur commonly as women become older and their tissues become less firm and muscular. Although childbirth injuries may be important contributing factors, relaxation of adequate support of pelvic structures may occur in women who have not borne children, presumably due to inheritance of deficient supporting tissues. With weakened muscular tone and with stresses such as lifting and gravity, the uterus may "drop"

If supporting structures of the bladder become weakened, the base of the bladder may sag into the vaginal canal and bulge through the vaginal opening. This is known as a *cystocele*. It is a partial hernia. As the condition progresses there may be frequency of urination and involuntary passage of a small amount of urine when the patient is in an upright position. There is increased risk of bladder infection *(cystitis)* which may spread to the upper urinary tract.

In similar fashion, if supporting

438

tissues of the lower bowel and rectum become weakened, this organ bulges (herniates) through the rear wall of the vagina. This is called a *rectocele*. It may cause pain and difficulties in defecation, although a mild herniation may not be particularly troublesome.

Cystoceles and rectoceles can be corrected surgically. Some women refuse surgical repair. Occasionally, the general physical condition of the patient may preclude the stresses of surgery, but this is quite rare today, for with modern surgery and local types of anesthesia, elderly women tolerate reconstructive vaginal surgery very well.

There are non-surgical methods of support which may be used successfully, although permanent repair by surgery is usually preferable. Devices used to support the uterus and/or the vaginal walls are called *pessaries*. These are usually made of rubber or plastic material in a variety of shapes suited to individual need. Pessaries require careful fitting and removal at frequent intervals. Some women find it helpful, in giving some support to sagging uterus or vaginal structures, to insert into the vagina every morning a large cotton tampon with string attachment, which is removed and discarded at night.

PELVIC MALIGNANCY

Cancer is a malignant growth — that is, it spreads through tissues of the body in uncontrolled fashion and eventually involves near or distant structures, in contrast to benign growths which may get larger locally but do not invade neighboring organs and therefore usually do not kill.

The invasion route of cancer is via the lymph and blood vessels to lymph glands and distant organs. Once the disease is widespread it is difficult if not impossible to control it successfully. That is why early discovery of cancer, when it is still localized and can be removed surgically or destroyed by irradiation before it can spread hopelessly, is of such vital importance. The cause of cancer is unknown.

There is some evidence of genetic predisposition to some forms of cancer, but people do not inherit cancer as such.

Cancer may affect any of the genital organs of women. Malignancy of the genitalia is not common before age 20, and does not reach its greatest frequency until the mid-forties and on. The order of frequency of cancer of the female reproductive organs is:

Cervix (or neck of the uterus)
Endometrium (or lining of the uterus)
Ovary
Vulva
Vagina
Oviduct (or Fallopian tube)

Cancer of the first two organs is by all odds the most common and accounts for

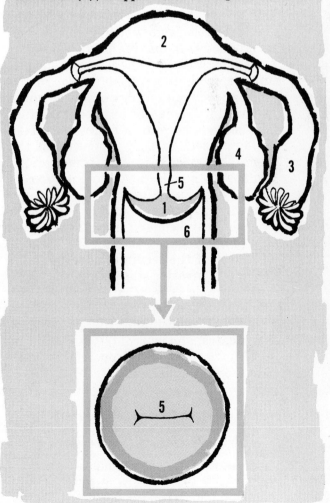

The *cervix* (1) is the lower and narrow end ("neck") of the *uterus* (2), shown in relation to other structures: *Fallopian tubes* (3); *ovaries* (4); *cervical os*, orifice of the cervix (5); *vagina* (6). In square, underside of the cervical os (5), at upper end of the vagina.

approximately one-fourth of the deaths from cancer of all types in women. (Cancer of the breast is discussed elsewhere in this chapter).

Cancer of the Cervix

This is malignant growth in the neck or mouth of the uterus, the part that occupies the upper end of the vaginal canal. Cancer of the cervix is more common in women who have borne children.

Cancer of the cervix often exists in an incipient, symptomless form (cancer *in situ*) for many years before the fullblown disease develops. In its incipient stage when no indication of disease is evident to the naked eye, the diagnosis can often be suggested by the Papanicolaou or "Pap" smear test, which is immensely important as a screening test for cancer of the cervix and endometrium.

The "Pap" test is a painless procedure. The cervix is exposed by a vaginal *speculum,* an instrument which dilates this cavity to make the interior more easily visible, and which gynecologists use regularly in making pelvic examinations. The surface of the cervix is scraped and material dipped from the top of the vagina is spread onto glass slides which are fixed immediately for later staining. The secretions contain many materials, including cells cast off by tissues of the tract. Cancer cells in such preparations can usually be recognized by their excessively dark staining and irregularly shaped nuclei. A presumptive diagnosis of cancer can be made from the recognition of such cells in the smears.

Cancer of the cervix discovered in its early, non-invasive stage is almost invariably curable. The "Pap" test has been responsible for diagnosis of cancer of the cervix in its incipient stage in many, many cases, and has contributed immeasurably to a marked drop in the death rate from this disease.

Early discovery of cancer of the cervix (as from a "Pap" smear test) with prompt treatment almost invariably results in cure. Normal structures shown in top drawing; Center, cervical cancer invading *bladder* (1), *uterus* (2), *rectum* (4); the *cervix* is (3), spread to *lymphatics* (5). In circle, advanced cervical cancer as seen in vagina.

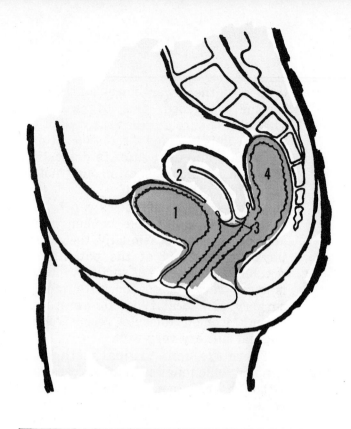

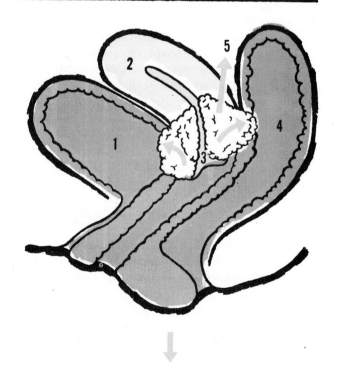

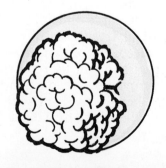

Other tests also may help in making an early diagnosis. A positive or suspicious "Pap" smear calls for a confirmatory repeat test, and then a biopsy of the cervix. A biopsy is done by removing a sample of tissue from the cervix, preparing it for staining, and studying it under the microscope.

All women should have a pelvic examination and "Pap" smear test at least every year, and preferably every six months. This measure can be a part of one's general checkup examination.

When cervical cancer becomes invasive or "fullblown," an ulcer or papillary (nipplelike) outcropping develops first. This is associated with a watery, and later bloody, discharge, especially noticeable after intercourse. There is no pain until very late in the disease.

Appearance of symptoms demands immediate gynecologic examination, including the procedures described above. A biopsy is the final important step in positive diagnosis, although many of the fullblown growths are recognized by the physician in ordinary office examination.

The earlier the diagnosis, the better the outlook for cure. Treatment may be surgical removal of the uterus and surrounding tissues in the early stages, or radiation (combinations of radium and supervoltage x-rays, or cobalt 60, or cesium, or the linear accelerator). There are *no* other forms of treatment worthy of considering at the present time.

Cancer of the lining of the uterus (endometrium) is a disease of older women. The average age at diagnosis is 57 years.

The most typical early symptom is *bleeding*. If the patient has passed the menopause, conclusive diagnosis usually requires that tissue be obtained from the interior of the uterus. In every instance of vaginal bleeding after the menopause, a diagnostic curettage or scraping of the interior of the uterus and a biopsy of the cervix are indicated.

The best approved treatment of this form of cancer is radiation with radium in the uterus, followed by removal of the entire uterus and cervix (total hysterectomy) some weeks later. If the uterus is very small, the operation may be performed without preliminary radium. The outlook is relatively good if symptoms have existed for a short time only.

Cancer of the Ovary

These small female organs are essential to perpetuation of the race through their production of fertilizable egg cells. They also produce the female sex hormones that are vital to feminine attributes and functions, and are analogues of the testes in the male.

The ovaries — normally two to every woman — are elongated, solid, almond-shaped organs about one and a half inches long. They lie deep in the pelvis against its side walls where they are well protected from harm.

In the older years especially, the ovaries become subject to cyst formation (previously described) and occasionally to malignant changes. Sometimes these changes are heralded by pain, by menstrual disturbances, or by progressive enlargement of the abdomen. But often such changes are insidious and "silent."

Diagnosis of cancer of the ovary depends almost entirely upon discoveries made at pelvic examination—convincing proof of the importance of periodic pelvic examination. Conclusive diagnosis may only be possible after opening the abdomen.

Treatment is surgical removal and suppressive radiation therapy. In some cases, chemotherapy is also helpful.

Cancer of the vulva is almost entirely a disease of old age. It occurs as an ulcer or warty excrescence of the skin of these parts. It is painless in the early stages. The diagnosis is usually suggested by the physical findings and confirmed by biopsy.

One should never neglect a sore place on the vulval skin which does not soon heal. Vulval cancer very often occurs in an irritated area of whitened vulval skin *(leukoplakic vulvitis)*, a condition which is often accompanied by severe itching. This is not to say that all thickened, whitened, itching skin areas lead to cancer, but it is urged that medical assistance should be sought.

As with other forms of cancer, the prospect of success in treating cancer of the vulva depends upon making a diagnosis in an early stage of the disease. The treatment is surgical removal.

Cancer of the vagina is very much like cancer of the cervix, except that it is comparatively infrequent. The symptoms are the same and the findings are those of an ulcer or an indurated or cauliflower-like mass in the vaginal wall. Cancer of the vagina usually occurs only in old age. The treatment is radiological or surgical, depending upon location in the vaginal wall and the extent of the growth.

Cancer of the oviduct (Fallopian tube) is very rare, and simulates cancer of the ovary or inflammatory disease of the pelvic organs. The diagnosis is rarely made until the time of surgical opening of the abdomen. The treatment is surgical removal. The outlook is not good, because of the usually late diagnosis.

Precautionary measures. With respect to the female genital organs in general, the best prophylactic measure is to have regular periodic examinations, including the vaginal smear or "Pap" test not less often than once a year.

In addition, one should consult a gynecologist at once should there be bleeding or bloody discharge between periods, or after the menopause, or a persistent watery discharge, or an enlarging lump or mass in the abdomen or on the external parts, or if a persistent ulceration or irritated area should appear. Prompt attention to these matters may make the difference between life and death.

Post-Menopausal Complaints

Changes in a woman's body during the menopause and after are described elsewhere (see Chapter 9).

Some menopausal women are depressed from brooding about getting older, that youth is irretrievably gone, the children more independent and mother not so managerially necessary to them, and perhaps that the husband's romantic interest in his wife is somewhat tempered. Actually, none of these morbid circumstances may be valid.

A menopausal woman need not lose her attractiveness, her sexual appeal, or her sexual ability. In a good marriage she should become more attractive to her husband (who isn't so young as he once was, either) as the embodiment of the happiness they have known together. Her children need her—not so much as a parent as an experienced well-loved friend.

Women should face the "change of life" with the determination to pursue hobbies and activities that were out of the question in the past because of the ceaseless duties of child care and managing a busy if not hectic household. There is, too, a diminishing possibility of pregnancy at this time, and not infrequently this gives a new sense of freedom and resurgence in husband-wife relationships. It is most unusual for a woman to become pregnant after 47 years of age. The time when pregnancy is no longer possible for a menopausal woman may be reasonably estimated at the time when no periods have occurred for six months.

At this time of life some women develop symptoms due to prolapse of the vaginal walls and bladder with urinary incontinence. Others develop menstrual irregularities and unusual periods, sometimes of flooding proportions, sometimes spotting.

Various complaints may occur long after cessation of the menses. Problems of prolapse often become more marked, especially in women who lift their heavy grandchildren. Due to estrogen deprivation, the vagina becomes less elastic, more easily irritated, and bleeding may occur from an inflammation of the vagina, or there may be tenderness, burning, and itching. When such conditions are due to lack of estrogen, as is common, proper hormone therapy can correct them. However, post-menopausal bleeding may be due to some threatening growth such as cancer of the cervix or uterus, and it is imperative that the patient be examined and the cause of the bleeding determined.

About "Female Operations"

Patients are sometimes confused about operative procedures. When is surgery really necessary and when may medical treatment suffice? These decisions are not made about patients in general, but about a particular patient, in light of all the circumstances relevant to that patient. Decisions should be based on recommendations of the physician who has observed the patient and who will explain to her and her family the reasons for his recommendations.

One of the most common minor gynecologic operations is the "D. & C.," which means dilating the cervix and curetting or scraping the lining of the uterus (see Chapter 22). This is essentially a diagnostic procedure. The patient need remain in the hospital only a day or two.

Hysterectomy is another common operation in gynecology that often is not well understood by patients. A number of conditions in which removal of the uterus is advisable or imperative have been discussed elsewhere in this chapter, and there are other conditions not mentioned.

"Hysterectomy" refers to removal of the uterus only. It does not imply that the ovaries will be removed too. To be sure, the ovaries may be removed if they are found to be diseased. Usually, the body of the uterus and the cervix are both removed. This is known as a *total hysterectomy*. Removal of the uterus per se does not cause one to gain weight nor does it cause imbalance of hormones or destroy the capacity for sexual relations.

The conscientious physician recommends surgical procedure only when he would advise it if the patient were a member of his own family. This is a pretty safe rule that all conscientious doctors follow.

Sterilization operations are performed in cases in which a medical condition makes future pregnancy dangerous; for instance, in a patient with incurable mental disease. In the female, this involves cutting out a section of the Fallopian tubes to shut out the egg cell from the uterus. Since the tubes are within the pelvic portion of the peritoneal cavity, *Fallopian tube resection* is considered a major abdominal operation.

About Symptoms

Symptoms which bring a woman to a gynecologist are usually pain, unusual bleeding, or a swelling in the pelvic area. These symptoms may occur separately or together. For example, inflammations of the vulva, Bartholin's or Skene's glands, the vagina, cervix, uterus, tubes, and ovaries, all cause pain, and there is usually some associated swelling.

In large tumors of the uterus or ovaries, pain may be due to pressure on surrounding organs. If an ovarian tumor becomes twisted, the pain is intense even though the tumor may not be large.

Irregular bleeding, spotting between periods, or after intercourse, is always cause for a careful examination. Such bleeding may be due to infections, to early malignant changes, to an abnormal pregnancy or an imbalance of hormones. Great emotional stress may cause bleeding resembling a period.

Swelling of the lower abdomen, when not due to a pregnancy, may be due to large tumors of the uterus or ovaries. The most common non-pregnant swelling of the lower abdomen which gradually extends quite high is — you're right! — obesity. Watch your weight!

CANCER OF THE BREAST

by HOWARD C. BARON, M.D.

Not long ago an attractive woman in her forties, obviously embarrassed and a bit timid, hesitantly approached a saleswoman in a large urban department store. She gestured toward a small sign reading: "Women with Breast Surgery — Ask for Miss Smith."

"I've had one of my . . . ah . . ." the shopper began.

The saleswoman smiled understandingly and interrupted her. "It's no problem. Will you step this way? It takes about 15 minutes."

The shopper, who was my patient, was elated when she told me this story. "That saleswoman's attitude cured me of all my complexes," she said. "I realized only then that there is nothing strange or different about me since the mastectomy. My problem is an adjustment in my bra."

Mastectomy is the medical term for surgical removal of a breast, usually because of cancer. My patient was right. Her loss is neither "odd" nor "different." More than 50,000 American women had a breast removed for cancer last year, and another 50,000 will undergo the same surgical procedure before the present year is over.

A million or more women in the United States alone wear some sort of surgical breast form. Some of them are glamorous personalities of the theatrical world and famous women in many walks of life whose friends and acquaintances never suspect that they have had a breast removed, or in some instances both breasts, or even dream that these active and vigorous women suffer any handicap, as indeed they do not.

Cancer of the breast most frequently strikes women in the prime of life, between 40 and 60 years of age. One out of every 18 American women is destined to develop breast cancer at some time during the average life span of 72 years. At this moment, radical mastectomy is the best chance that medical science can offer

Structures of adult female breast. Below: *Milk ducts* **(2); radiate spoke-like from** *nipple* **(1). Milk-storing** *sinuses* **(3); branch into** *tubules* **(4); connected with milk-secreting glands or** *lobules* **(5). At right, vertical cross section shows** *nipple* **(1);** *fatty tissue* **(2);** *milk glands* **(3).**

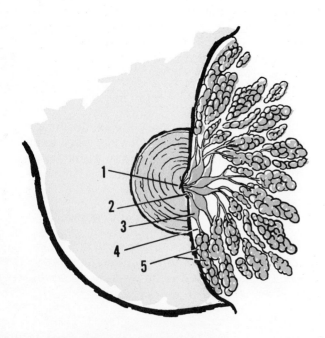

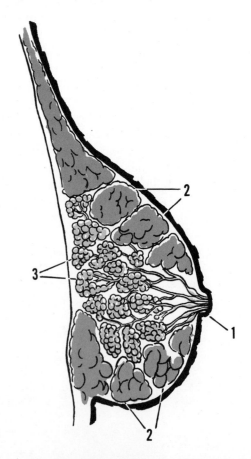

of saving their lives. "Radical" means complete removal of the breast and of some associated tissues, particularly in the armpit area, to lessen the possibility that cancer cells might migrate to other parts of the body and establish themselves there.

Despite significant advances against breast cancer fatalities achieved by weapons of surgery, x-ray, and certain drugs, there has been no decrease in breast cancer *incidence*. Early detection offers the woman with breast cancer her best hope of survival. No form of cancer springs into full bloom overnight. Yet after decades of campaigns aimed at getting women to seek medical attention at the first sign of a suspicious "lump" in the breast, an average of 15 months elapses between the time a woman discovers a lump and the time when she goes to her doctor for an examination.

During that wasted 15 months a malignant growth can make a great deal of disastrous progress. Insidious cancer has two fatally evil characteristics: it grows, sometimes rapidly, at the site where it starts; and its treacherous cells can also spin off through the rest of the body, setting up satellite areas of cancerous growth called *metastasis*.

Self-detection. Some 98 per cent of women with cancer of the breast discover evidence of the tumor themselves, usually while bathing. The most common self-discovered sign is a painless "lump," frequently in the upper outward area of the breast. Yet most women who make this discovery wait a year or more before they consult a doctor, and in the meantime the lump, should it be malignant, is spreading its tentacles toward other parts of the body.

Ignorance and *delay* account largely for many deaths from cancer of the breast that would not have happened if a small suspicious lump had been called immediately to a physician's attention, at a time when the malignant tumor is localized and chances of cure by surgical removal are excellent.

It must be emphasized that not every suspicious lump in the breast means cancer. Just as there are many types of cancer cells, so are there many kinds of lumps that may appear in the breasts. Fortunately, most of these lumps prove to be harmless tumors or cysts. Yet fear that "a lump in the breast" invariably means cancer may provoke paralyzing panic and sad and possibly fatal delay in consulting a physician to find out what the lump actually does mean.

Discovery of a lump in the breast does not always mean that cancer is present. But it does always mean that you should see your doctor without delay.

Many doctors encourage their intelligent women patients to examine their breasts every month in a routinized way, suggested by the accompanying drawing, and give instructions in how to do so. A woman's familiarity with the normal feel and texture of her breasts assists in recognizing changes that may occur. In some instances, self-examination procedures may perpetuate harmful "cancer phobias" that are quite unreasonable, but there is little risk of this in intelligent women who are properly informed by their competent doctors.

Other symptoms than a lump to be aware of are:

Any alteration in the usual shape of the breast.

Elevation or sinking of the nipple.

Slight dimpling of the skin of the breast.

Discharge, bleeding, or a rash around the nipple.

Early breast cancer is practically always painless — too often a patient says, "why, yes, I've noticed a lump there for months but it hasn't bothered me at all." *Pain* is not a reliable "early warning" signal of breast cancer. Pain in the breast is usually a symptom of some other trouble altogether, or of a malignant tumor in a late stage of growth.

The doctor's examination. Diagnosis of breast cancer of course requires the skills of a physician. Far advanced breast cancer is sadly obvious, but early stages are not. Examination of the breasts with a view to early detection of anything

445

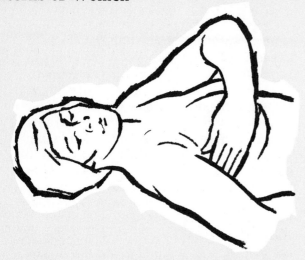

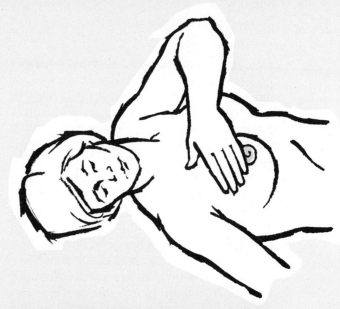

Many doctors instruct their women patients in monthly self-examination of the breasts. This is best done after the menstrual period. The woman lies on her back in bed with a pillow under the shoulders. The armpit and entire area of each breast should be felt with the flat of the fingers.

About one-half of breast cancers occur in the upper outside quarter of the breast, the general area shown being examined above. Familiarity with the normal "feel" of the breasts, gained by regular monthly self-examination, makes it easier to recognize any unusual change.

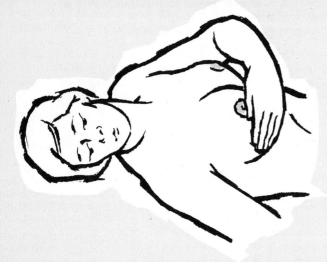

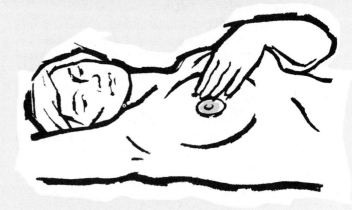

A step-by-step routine of self-examination to cover the lower, outer, inner and upper aspects of the breast, and the armpit areas, as suggested in these drawings, is desirable. Sequences are not arbitrary as long as the examination covers the entire breast and associated areas.

Skill in self-examination is soon acquired by practice. Discovery of a "lump" in the breast does not necessarily, or usually, mean cancer, but it does mean that a doctor should determine the nature of the lump.

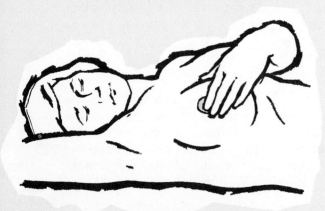

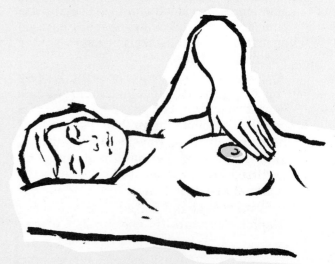

abnormal is a part of regular physical checkups. More often than not the doctor is happily able to assure the patient, to her great peace of mind, that all is well. The nature of a small lump or other symptom, reported by the patient or discovered by a doctor, must be determined.

The doctor examines and palpates the breasts in a number of positions: standing, with arms overhead, lying on the examining table. He also examines the armpits which contain some of the lymph channels and lymph glands leading from the breast, a pathway which cancer cells frequently take in spreading.

A comparatively new technique the doctor may elect to use for detecting breast tumors, employing x-rays, is called *mammography*. Recent refinements of this technique have given mammography an accuracy score of about 90 per cent. Some of the tumors discovered by this x-ray process have been so minute that they eluded the experienced fingertip examination by the physician. Mammography is far from being a substitute for physical diagnosis, but most doctors regard it as a valuable aid in the detection and diagnosis of breast cancer.

Final diagnosis of whether a suspicious breast tumor is benign or malignant rests upon surgical biopsy—removal of a sample of tissue from the suspicious lump for microscopic examination by a pathologist. This is done under anesthesia in the operating room. The tissue sample goes immediately to the laboratory, and while the surgeons wait, the specimen is frozen with liquid carbon dioxide so that a tissue-thin slice may be obtained for microscopic scrutiny.

Should this microscopic examination prove the tumor to be benign, the tumor alone is removed by a fairly simple operation and the breast itself is left intact with little or no disfigurement.

Breast cancer surgery. A biopsy specimen that proves to be malignant means radical surgery — that is, complete removal of the breast, and of adjacent lymph nodes near the armpit and collarbone, and sections of the arm and chest muscles beneath the breast. The surgeon cannot take chances. He must get *all* of the malignancy to save and prolong his patient's life.

In the two to five-hour operation, the surgeon usually makes an elliptically-shaped incision and removes the breast and surrounding tissue in a single bloc. This technique is considered less likely to disturb and spread loose cancer cells and it also entails less disfigurement than some of the older procedures.

With sutures and skin grafts, the surgeon is able to close the "window" or incision with a minimum of scarring. As in other surgery, the pink lines of incisions become smoother and paler with the passage of time.

It would be fatuous to minimize the seriousness or complexity of this operation. Patience, delicacy, and great skill are essential. But let the apprehensive woman realize that it constitutes the removal of an *external* organ only, one which she can forfeit without major organic change or injury to her health or general well-being. The operation is literally superficial (by definition, "on the surface"). No major cavity of the body is invaded or affected.

After surgery. Following the operation, most surgeons advise treatment of the chest area with x-rays, or one of the new anti-cancer drugs, or both. The purpose of this is to kill any stray cancer cells that might be too deep-seated to be discoverable by any sort of inspection. The whole area where the tumor existed is suspect and no chances are taken.

The so-called "magic bullet" which could destroy cancer cells wherever they hide without harming the normal cells of the body is still a hope of the future. But we do possess drugs which show heartening results against some cancers, notably of the prostate, uterus, and breast. Female breast cancer is classified as a "hormone dependent" type — that is, the rate of growth of existing breast cancer is affected by female hormones, although this is not to say that hormones incited the cancer in the first place. Similarly, cancer of the prostate is affected by male sex hormones. Use of antagonistic hormones (male hormones in breast cancer, female hormones in prostate cancer) or hormone doses and removal of hormone producing organs by castration, has proved to be of considerable palliative benefit in appropriate cases, but is not to

comfortable and useful life. Among such drugs are nitrogen mustard, thio-tepa, 5-fluorouracil, and a number of others well known to doctors, and promising new ones emerge from time to time from a vast cancer chemotherapy research program which to date has screened more

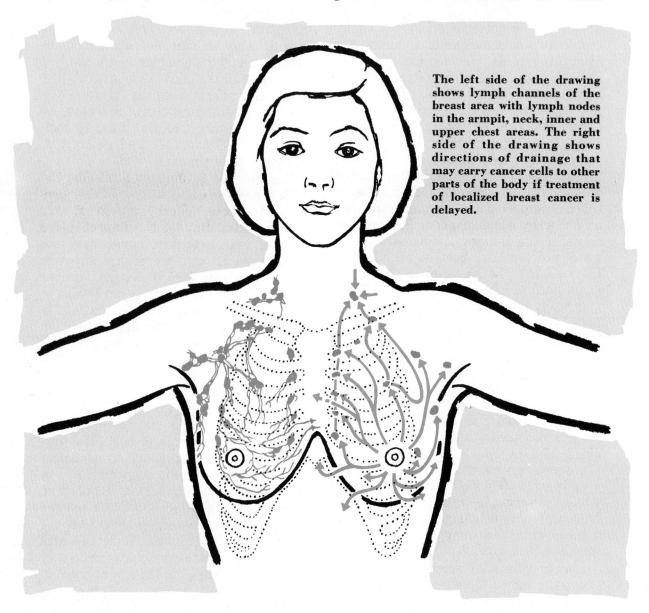

The left side of the drawing shows lymph channels of the breast area with lymph nodes in the armpit, neck, inner and upper chest areas. The right side of the drawing shows directions of drainage that may carry cancer cells to other parts of the body if treatment of localized breast cancer is delayed.

be looked upon as a cure, and never as an alternative to recommended surgery.

Unhappily, there are cases of "inoperable" breast cancer — disease so far advanced or so widespread that surgery cannot be curative. But even in these cases, drugs now available can usually relieve pain, delay cancer spread, prolong

than 75,000 anti-cancer compounds in animal cancer experimentation.

In some cases, one or another of available drugs has made possible the more effective use of surgery and radiotherapy. Medical journals are filled with case history reports of marked improvement when certain drugs are used with certain breast cancer patients. Each patient's needs are of course different and meticulous medical teamwork is necessary in order that the individual patient may have the best therapies in the light of present knowledge.

Dangerous Fallacies

Why do so many women with breast cancer — 25,000 of them every year in this country — delay so long in seeking medical help that the doctor or surgeon can do little to save their lives?

Fear, groundless fear, half-truths, phobias, and old wives' tales undoubtedly play a sad part in delaying treatment until malignancy is far advanced.

One of the most frustrating of all fallacies is the mistaken belief that a diagnosis of breast malignancy is a death sentence. The truth is that more than 65 per cent of women who have had a diseased breast removed are living active, useful lives. Everyone seems to hear of the occasional patient who does not do well after mastectomy, but there are no headlines for the thousands every year whose lives are unchanged or improved by mastectomy, because that is not news any longer.

Another common fallacy is the belief that mastectomy demands a visit to a famous medical center located in a big city and employment of the country's highest paid, most difficult to obtain surgeon. There may have been some truth in this 30 years ago, but today's excellent surgical training programs are producing skillful surgeons eminently capable of providing this same service in the majority of the community hospitals throughout the country.

Fear of mastectomy is fed, too, by a warmly human trait that we would all be the worse for if it were wiped out: vanity, the admirable desire always to look one's best. One of my patients once told me:

"Doctor, you'll be shocked to hear about my first thought after you operated and while I was still in the recovery room. It wasn't 'did you get all the cancer?' but 'what do I look like?'"

Fear of disfigurement is very real and never to be treated lightly. But apprehension is outmoded by modern refinements in surgical techniques. With an eye to physical appearance as well as complete excision of malignancy, surgical procedures these days are wielded so cleanly and skillfully that even when skin grafting is necessary there is a minimum of scarring.

Deep-seated psychological fears are most difficult to rout, and often enough are unexpressed and known only to the woman herself. A woman faced with mastectomy understandably shrinks from being "different." Will her husband still love her? Will her family and friends view her as a "freak"?

Actually, not a whit of her femininity is lost. Mastectomy per se effects no change in personality or character traits. There is no interference with hormone production and womanly functions. The patient is the same wife, the same mother, the same career girl that she was before the operation. Her physical attractiveness is not diminished; as a matter of fact, most women who have undergone mastectomy compensate by attention to makeup and grooming, making them more attractive than ever.

The young or middle-aged woman worries particularly about the attitude of the man in her life. Is she still desirable? The honest male animal will assure her that a man's attitude is based largely on a woman's image of herself, and her desirability is in direct proportion to her interest in *him!* There is more truth than fancy in this, that the woman who becomes more absorbed in the man in her life and his needs becomes more physically attractive to him irrespective of her surgical experience.

Prosthetic devices. This is not to minimize adjustments, physical and emotional, that must be made by the patient.

Her first shock, and it is a shock, comes when she tries to walk for the first time after her operation, a short and timorous trip down the hospital corridor. She will feel "off balance," strangely lopsided, but while she is still in the hospital she will receive aid and training to restore graceful coordination in walking.

Another aspect of her adjustment will be in learning about "prosthetic devices," breast forms and cosmetics that visually replace the missing breast contours quite perfectly. These forms, made of foam rubber, dacron and other components, can be bought for as little as three dollars. Bathing suit designers now create garments with provision for insertion of these forms. And women who have been accustomed to sleeping on their stomachs need not change their habits. Manufacturers of bedding now offer a specially designed but low-priced pillow for complete comfort. These devices are now sold in most specialty shops and in every large department store in the nation.

The specific cause of breast cancer (and other cancer) is unknown. We know that there is a higher incidence of breast cancer among childless women, among those who have fewer than two children, and among those who have never breastfed a baby. But these are admittedly negative findings, and a truly enormous amount of cancer research continues unceasingly to augment our knowledge of disordered processes of cells that are involved in malignant changes.

If and when some marvelous "cancer drug" is discovered, physicians all over the world will know about it. There are no "secret cures" for cancer. Unfortunately, there is cancer quackery, with promises of benefit from some mysterious medicine or treatment not employed by responsible physicians. The greatest tragedy is not the loss of money spent on worthless treatments, but that delay in seeking competent treatment may be so prolonged that chances of cure are hopeless.

Early surgery is still the major means of saving the patient with breast cancer at this writing, and it is safe to predict that radical mastectomy will continue to play a dominant role in the foreseeable future. But mammography, x-ray, and the new drugs have supporting roles that continue to increase in importance.

A woman can direct her own defenses against cancer in a number of simple ways. Her annual physical examination in the doctor's office is of paramount importance. The doctor may advise that she examine her own breasts each month, particularly after the menstrual period, for any abnormality. Discovery of a lump or any suspicious change should cause her to consult immediately with her doctor.

THE DIGESTIVE SYSTEM

by J. ALFRED RIDER, M.D.

Mouth and Esophagus • The Stomach •
The Small Intestine • The Large
Intestine • Liver and Gallbladder

DIAGNOSTIC TESTS AND INSTRUMENTS

THE MOUTH

THE ESOPHAGUS

Congenital Defects • Diverticulum •
Esophagitis • Stricture • Ulcer of the
Esophagus • Hiatus Hernia •
Achalasia • Varices • Tumors •
Perforation or Rupture

STOMACH

Heartburn • Indigestion • Gastritis
• Stomach Ulcer • Tumors of the
Stomach • Stomach Cancer • Pyloric
Stenosis • Postgastrectomy Syndrome

DUODENUM

Duodenal Ulcer • Duodenitis • Tumors
• Diverticulum

THE LIVER

THE GALLBLADDER

Cholecystitis • Gallstones •
Postcholecystectomy Syndrome •
Cholangitis • Tumors

THE PANCREAS

THE SMALL BOWEL

THE COLON AND RECTUM

Functional Disturbances • Megacolon
• Constipation • Diarrhea •
Diverticulosis •Appendicitis • Ulcerative
Colitis • Tumors

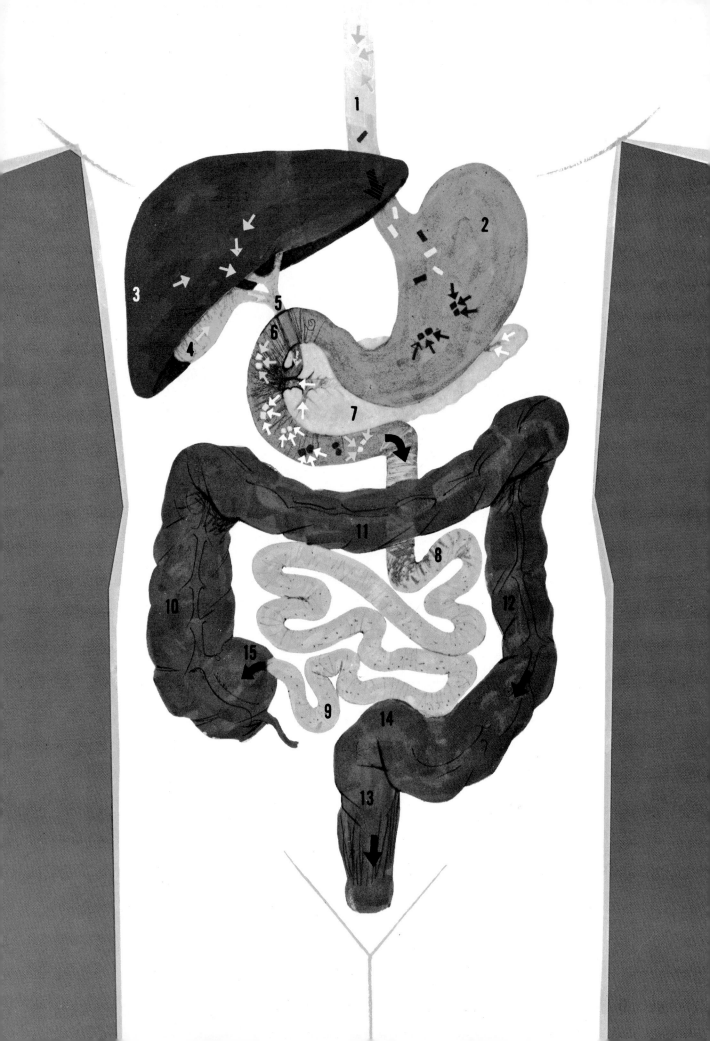

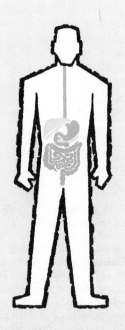

The colorplate shows organs in "exploded" view for clarity. *Esophagus* (1); *stomach* (2); *liver* (3); *gallbladder* (4); *common duct* (5); *duodenum* (6); *pancreas* (7); *jejunum* (8); *ileum* (9); *ascending colon* (10); *transverse colon* (11); *descending colon* (12); *rectum* (13); *sigmoid* (14); *cecum* (15).

Beginning in the esophagus, colored squares represent *carbohydrates* (blue), *proteins* (red), *fats* (yellow). In the stomach, proteins are partially digested by gastric juices (red arrows). *Bile* which emulsifies fats (green arrows) is produced in the liver, stored in the gallbladder, and released into the duodenum. Digestive enzymes of the pancreas (white arrows) enter the duodenum and further digest carbohydrates, proteins and fats. Virtually all absorption of nutrients occurs in the small intestine (8, 9), from the duodenum to the junction with the colon, where a valve controls the flow of contents into the colon.

Direction of flow of contents of the alimentary canal is shown by heavy black arrows.

CHAPTER 13

THE DIGESTIVE SYSTEM

by J. ALFRED RIDER, M.D.

The digestive tract is an open-end muscular tube which passes through the body. Wastes excreted through it have never been "in" the body but have merely been surrounded by it. Digestion occurs outside you. The inside of your mouth, or stomach, or intestines, is really outside you. Only what passes through the walls of the tract gets inside the body.

The digestive tube is more than 30 feet long from one open end to the other. It is continuous but its various bulges, turns, and regions have special names, such as "stomach." It has muscular mechanisms which propel materials along its course, and valves which regulate delivery of partially processed materials at different points on the "conveyor belt." Here and there, chemicals produced by specialized tissues are introduced through connecting tubes or surfaces. Digestion is a process of continuous chemical simplification of materials that enter via the mouth. Materials are split into smaller and simpler chemical fragments which can then be absorbed through the walls of the tract and thus, finally, enter into the body.

In this way, a building block of what entered the mouth as beefsteak may help to build insulin, or a fingernail, or an enzyme, and what entered as a piece of bread may furnish some of the energy for hitting a golf ball for long yardage on the fairways.

Mouth and Esophagus

Digestion begins in the mouth, with grinding of food by the teeth and admixture of saliva. Here we encounter the first of many enzymes that catalyze chemical processes in the digestive tract. *Ptyalin* is an enzyme in saliva which begins to split starches into simple sugars. There are three saliva-producing glands on each side of

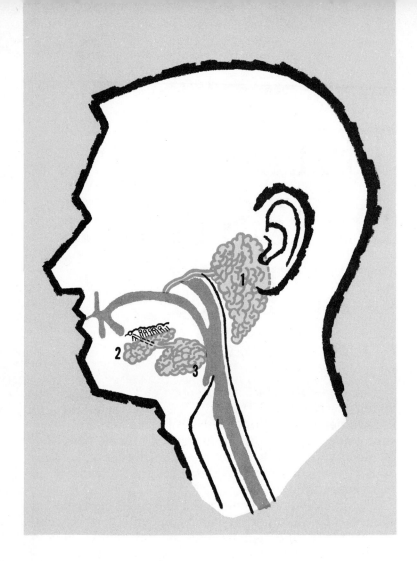

The saliva-producing glands are the *parotid gland* (1) in front and below the ear, the *sublingual gland* (2), and the *submaxillary gland* (3), also called *submandibular*. The glands are paired on each side of the face. Saliva contains an enzyme, *ptyalin*, which begins to split starches into simple sugars.

the face. The *parotid gland* in front of and below the ear is the one that swells painfully if one has mumps. The *sublingual gland* lies under the tongue and the *submandibular gland* a little below and behind it.

A portion *(bolus)* of masticated food is forced to the back of the oral cavity and into the *esophagus* or gullet, a muscular tube. Here a characteristic activity of the digestive tract known as *peristalsis* comes into play. This is a kneading, "milking" constriction and relaxation of muscles that propels material through the tube. Encircling muscles constrict behind a mass of material, squeeze it forward, while the muscles in front of the material relax in rhythmic waves. The mechanical principle is about the same as that of a milking machine.

To prevent backflow of materials, and to time their release to the conveyor belt when a processing step is sufficiently well advanced, the digestive tract is equipped with valves at important junctions. These are pursestring muscles or sphincters which tighten to hold back material and relax to eject materials at appropriate times. The first of these ringlike muscle-valves is the *cardia*, at the point where the esophagus opens into the stomach. It takes 3 or 4 seconds for a bolus of food to be "milked" down the esophagus, or up it, if one swallows upside down.

The Stomach

The biggest bulge in the digestive tract is the stomach. It is located rather higher than some people think, lying mainly behind the lower ribs, not under the navel, and does not occupy the belly, a region for which "stomach" is sometimes a misused euphemism.

There is no fixed shape of the stomach. It is a flexible bag enclosed by restless muscles, constantly changing form. It is a flabby wrinkled tube when empty and an impressive pear-shaped organ when distended by a couple of quarts of food and drink. However, it is customary to describe the stomach as shaped like a J, lying more obliquely than vertically, and this facilitates description of parts.

The "body" of the stomach, roughly, is the shaft of the J, and the upper part, around the area of the esophagus opening, is the *fundus*. This is a region where gas bubbles collect and necessitate burping, in a baby, or belching in an adult, or eructation if one prefers a discreet medical term. The lower part of the stomach tapers without sharp differentiation to the pyloric end, or outlet. The *pylorus* is a sort of bottleneck with a strong sphincter which contracts and relaxes at appropriate times to eject a quota of stomach content into the adjacent duodenum. A familiar portrait of Napoleon shows him with his left hand lying across his lower chest in the area of the pylorus (he had trouble there).

Thick, resilient stomach walls are multi-layered. Three muscle layers run in circular, longitudinal, and oblique directions, so the stomach can writhe and squeeze quite powerfully. Swallowed food arrives in the fundus area and is kneaded, squeezed, mixed with juices and made more liquid. Virtually nothing is absorbed through the stomach walls except alcohol. Watery materials such as soup leave the stomach quite rapidly. Fats remain in the stomach considerably longer. The "staying power" of a meal depends largely on quantities and proportions of carbohydrates, proteins, and fats that compose it. An ordinary mixed

Orientation of the stomach, and cross section showing structures. The stomach wall has three layers of muscle running in different directions: *circular* (1); *longitudinal* (2); and *oblique* (3). Foods enter the *fundus* (6) from the esophagus, at the *cardia* (5), and contents are discharged at intervals through the *pylorus* (4) into the duodenum. The "lesser curvature" is the shorter portion of the stomach wall, at left; the "greater curvature," the opposite and longer length of the stomach wall.

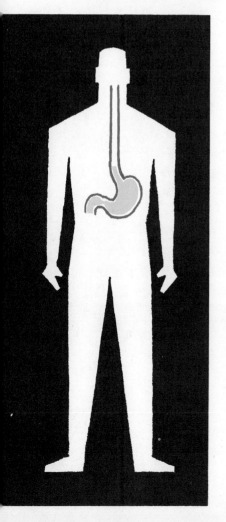

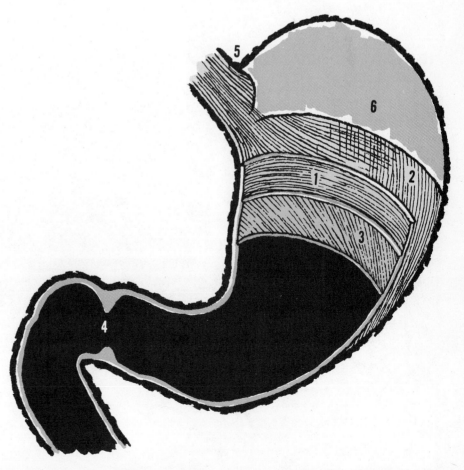

diet meal is emptied from an ordinary stomach in three to five hours.

The stomach is lined with a slick mucous membrane, creased and folded, and with some resemblance to a honeycomb. Under a microscope the surface is seen to have myriads of tiny pits. These are depressions where glands — about 35,000,000 of them — exude their secretions. Stomach glands and specialized cells produce mucus, enzymes, hydrochloric acid, and a factor that enables Vitamin B_{12} to be dissolved through intestinal walls into the circulation.

Gastric juice is a complex mixture of many substances. The predominant enzyme of the stomach, *pepsin,* is a potent digester of meats and proteins. Another enzyme, *rennin,* has the sole task of curdling milk. Pepsin is active only in an acid medium. A normal stomach is definitely on the acid side. Hydrochloric acid produced by stomach cells is a highly corrosive mineral acid. A drop of it on the skin would inflict a bad burn. Gastric juice containing hydrochloric acid and flesh-digesting pepsin is corrosive. A frequent question is, "Why doesn't the stomach digest itself?" An important protective mechanism is the film of mucus that coats the stomach wall. And hydrochloric acid is considerably diluted

Magnified structures of the stomach lining from areas of the *cardia* (1); *fundus* (2); and *pylorus* (3). Special secretory cells of the cardia produce mucus; pepsin and hydrochloric acid are produced by cells of the fundus; cells of the pylorus are mucus-secreting. The stomach also produces intrinsic factor, essential for absorption of Vitamin B_{12}.

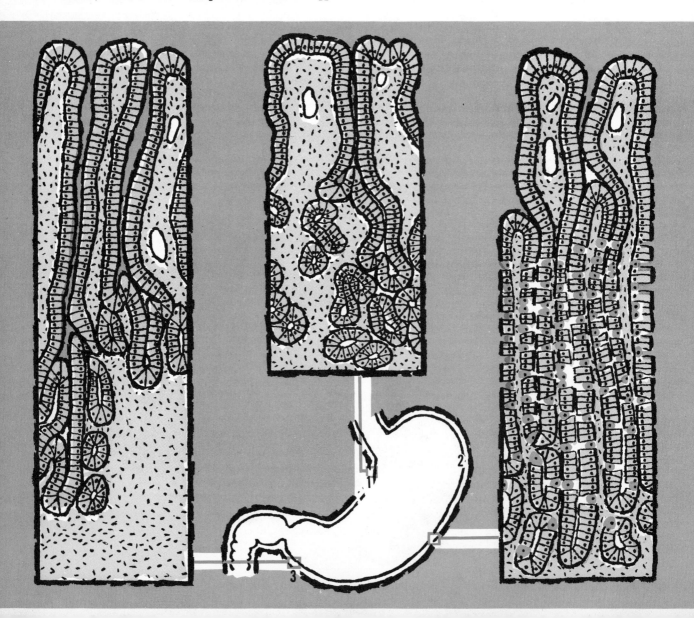

when its quantity is in proper proportion to stomach contents that it works upon.

The stomach is nearly always free of bacteria. Few germs can survive its acid bath. Some parasites, however, successfully resist destruction.

A convenient food-reservoir is lost if the stomach or a large part of it has to be removed. Frequent small feedings then become necessary. But the stomach is not absolutely indispensable to digestion. Most of the process occurs beyond it.

tapers to about one inch diameter at its lower end. The tube is continuous but its areas are somewhat arbitrarily named and we shall consider them in sequence.

The duodenum begins at the stomach outlet where the pyloric sphincter periodically disgorges jets of material. The name means "12 fingerbreadths long" — 8 to 10 inches. The duodenum makes such a sharp horseshoe curve that its starting point and termination are very close to-

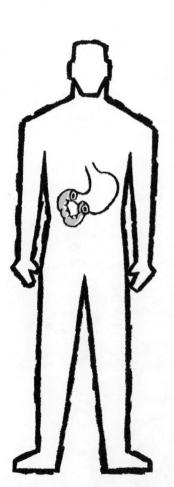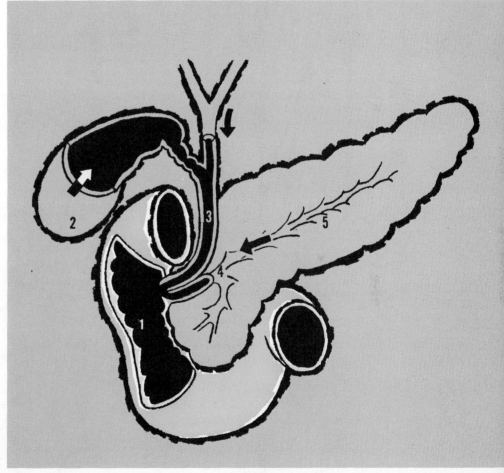

The *duodenum* (1), the beginning of the small intestine, is an area of great chemical activity, where bile from the *gallbladder* (2) and hepatic ducts enters via the *common duct* (3). Protein, fat, and carbohydrate-splitting enzymes of the *pancreas gland* (5) enter the duodenum through the *pancreatic duct* (4). In the duodenum, the environment is alkaline, in contrast to the acid stomach.

The Small Intestine

Digestion is completed in the small intestine and virtually all absorption of nutrients occurs there. The 22-foot or greater length of the small intestine is compactly wound into the abdomen. It

gether. A significant change in environment of materials to be digested begins to take place in the duodenum. The acid environment of the stomach gives way to an alkaline environment in the small intestine. This is largely brought about by highly alkaline bile, pancreatic juice,

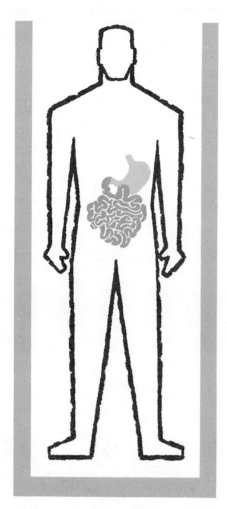

poses, we may consider the function of the small intestine as a whole.

The mucosal lining is raised in circular folds which increase its surface. Thousands of microscopic, round-ended, fingerlike projections called *villi* stud the intestinal wall. These are like the pile of an exceedingly fine carpet and give the feel of velvet. Glands which open at the bases of the villi discharge enzymes, mucus, and other constituents of alkaline intestinal juice.

Below, the small intestine looks externally like a simple tube, but its muscular walls knead food mechanically in segmental contractions, shift food backward and forward in pendulum movements, and propel the food column by peristaltic action.

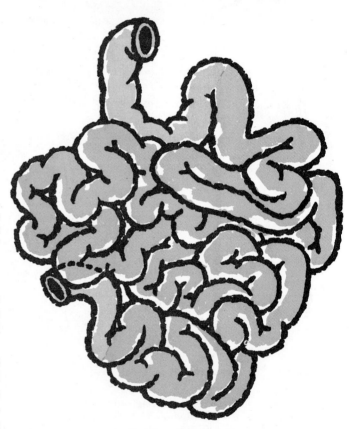

Above, the *jejunum* continues from the duodenum. Considerable portions of the small intestine can be removed surgically, if diseased, but some functioning portion of the small bowel is essential since major processes of digestion and assimilation occur here.

and local secretions of intestinal walls. It is in an alkaline environment that the most important work of digestion and absorption is done.

The general area of the duodenum is a busy focus of chemical deliveries and structural junctions. Ducts bringing bile from the liver and juices from the pancreas open into the duodenum at about the midpoint of its horseshoe bend. The gallbladder, areas of the liver, the head of the pancreas gland, and the writhing pylorus are in close proximity.

The duodenum joins with the *jejunum,* which is about ten feet long, and the jejunum with the *ileum* which is ten to 12 feet long and constitutes the rest of the small intestine. For practical pur-

Opposite page: The small intestine, particularly the ileal portion, is richly lined with microscopic *villi* which give a velvety "feel." Villi are fingerlike projections which vastly increase the surface area in contact with foodstuffs. Glands at the base of the villi secrete intestinal juices. Each villus has a capillary network and a central *lacteal* (lymph channel). Cross-section of three villi in foreground of drawing shows, from left to right, blood supply *to* villus, blood supply *from* villus, and a *lacteal* structure which absorbs fat into the lymph. Small arrows indicate absorption into villi; vertical arrows, direction of absorption.

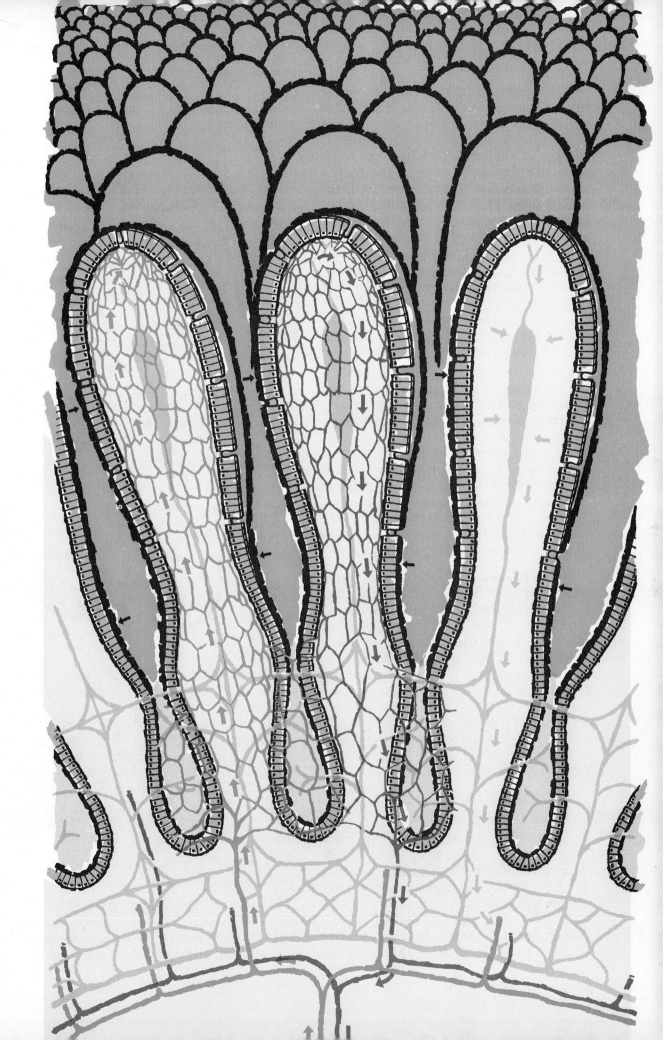

Digestive Tract

It has been estimated that the small intestine contains 5,000,000 villi. These multitudes of projections increase the surface area enormously. The internal surface of the small intestine has more than five times the area of the body's skin surface. But the villi are not inert little knobs. They lash and sway ceaselessly, lengthen and shorten, swell and shrink, agitate fluids in their vicinity.

Semi-liquid contents of the small intestine are kneaded, churned, and moved along by bursts of peristaltic action and rhythmic constrictions of segments of the intestine. Sometimes the results are audible as rumblings, for which there is a fascinating medical word: *borborygmi.*

Beginning at the end of the duodenum, the small intestine is supported by the *mesentery.* This is a flat structure, attached at the back of the abdomen, which radiates outward like an open fan. The curved edge of the fan is attached to the intestines which are supported like guy wires strung from a tentpole. The mesentery carries nerves and blood vessels to the small intestine and gives loose, flexible support that permits freedom of movement by the slippery tube.

Digestion and absorption. The intestinal wall is impermeable to large fat, carbohydrate, and protein molecules of foodstuffs, or for that matter to other large molecules. Digestion is a chemical process of converting nutrient materials, by enzymatic action, into smaller and simpler units which can penetrate barriers and enter the body. Enzymes perform quite specific tasks. One enzyme cannot do a different enzyme's work. The most important digestive enzymes are furnished by the pancreas gland and small intestine. In broad classification, *lipases* split fats, *proteases* split proteins, and *amylases* split starches.

Collectively, digestive enzymes perform quite staggering feats that we take for granted. Theoretically, chemists could "digest" an ordinary meal by applying high temperatures, pressures, and cracking procedures quite intolerable to the human body. But it would take weeks or months to imitate what the digestive

Digested elements of carbohydrates and proteins that pass into the villi are absorbed into networks of blood vessels—*stomach* (1); *duodenum* (2); *jejunum* (3)—and are collected into the *portal vein* (4) which carries them to the *liver* (5). Assimilated fats pass for the most part into lymph channels.

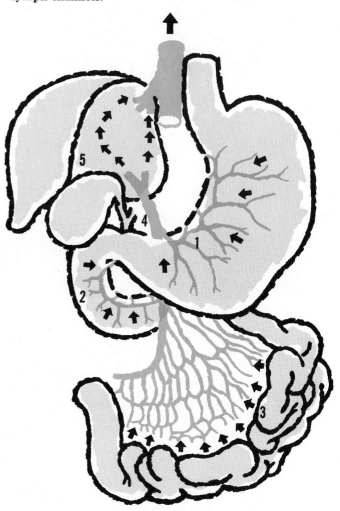

tract accomplishes in a few hours with comfort and with no little satisfaction to the owner.

Digested elements of carbohydrates and proteins are absorbed into networks of blood vessels and collected into the portal vein which carries them to the liver. Villi contain a central lacteal or lymphatic vessel, and fat elements for the most part enter the body through lymphatic channels.

The Large Intestine

If you put the flat of your right hand over the lower right abdomen, inside the hipbone area, you cover the general area where the small and large intestines join.

Here the inch-wide ileum opens into a much broader tube, the *cecum,* which below the junction has a blind pouch from which dangles a wormlike structure, the vermiform *appendix.* The large intestine above the cecum is the *colon.* The large intestine crosses over the underlying small intestine in a sort of square arc; its bends are called flexures.

The general course of the large intestine is approximated if you move your right hand upward from the appendix region, along the *ascending* colon, make a left turn at the rib corner and sweep across the abdomen to the left side along the *transverse* colon, then make a left turn downward along the *descending* colon. Below this the colon takes an S-shaped turn *(sigmoid flexure),* becomes the *rectum,* and terminates in the *anus.*

Material entering the cecum from the ileum is quite watery. At this junction a muscular valve prevents backflow. There are no villi in the large intestine and very little is absorbed from it except water. Primarily, the colon is a storage and dehydrating organ. Material which enters in a liquid state becomes semi-solid as water is absorbed. It takes 12 to 14 hours for contents to make the circuit

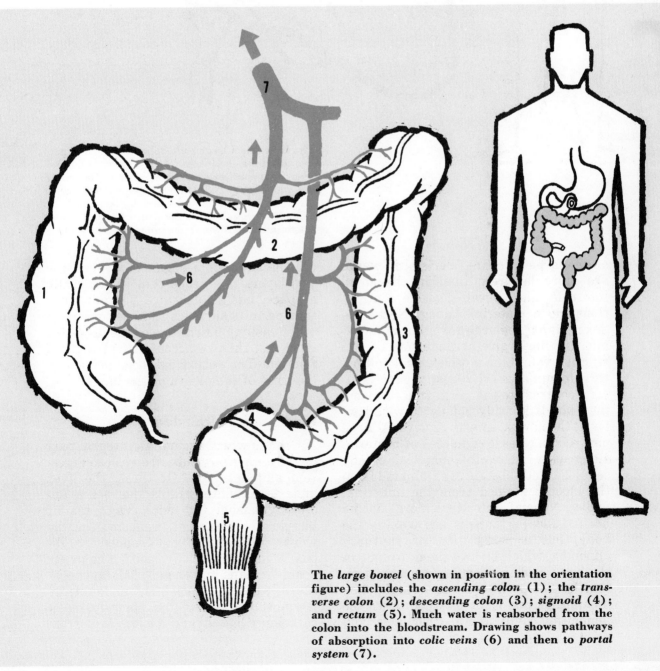

The *large bowel* (shown in position in the orientation figure) includes the *ascending colon* (1); the *transverse colon* (2); *descending colon* (3); *sigmoid* (4); and *rectum* (5). Much water is reabsorbed from the colon into the bloodstream. Drawing shows pathways of absorption into *colic veins* (6) and then to *portal system* (7).

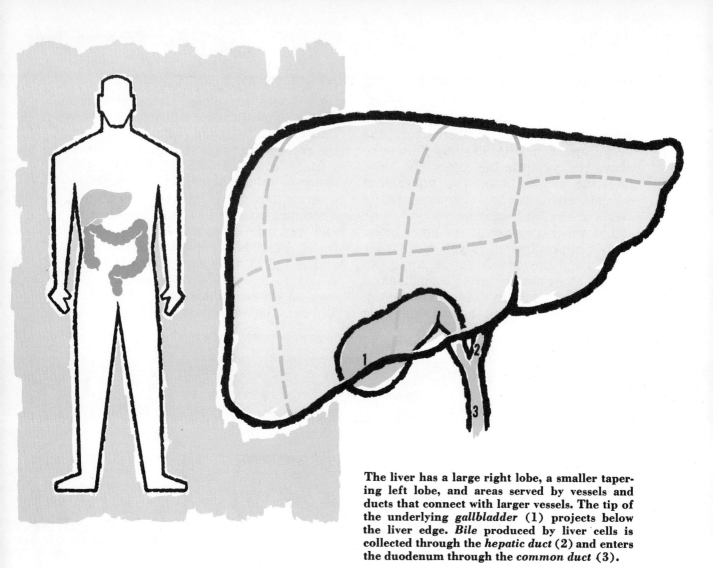

The liver has a large right lobe, a smaller tapering left lobe, and areas served by vessels and ducts that connect with larger vessels. The tip of the underlying *gallbladder* (1) projects below the liver edge. *Bile* produced by liver cells is collected through the *hepatic duct* (2) and enters the duodenum through the *common duct* (3).

of the large intestine. Peristaltic waves are more leisurely than in the small intestine, and overall massive contractions move materials along. Nerve reflexes signal the urge for a bowel movement. A final valve arrangement of two ringlike voluntary muscles, anal sphincters, terminates the digestive tract.

In contrast to the germ-free stomach, the colon is lavishly populated with bacteria, the normal intestinal flora. A large part of the feces is composed of bacteria, along with indigestible material, chiefly cellulose, and substances eliminated from the blood and shed from the intestinal walls. Normal intestinal flora do no harm, since organisms are outside the body, but a perforation or ruptured appendix which strews them around in the body causes infections such as peritonitis. The *peritoneum* is a tough, slick membrane, one layer of which lines the abdominal cavity and another layer cov-

ers the abdominal organs. Between the two layers is a space that is not really a space, but a lubricated contact point that permits surfaces to slide over each other easily. Squirmings of the digestive tract can thus be accomplished without friction. The peritoneal arrangement is like that of the pleura of the lungs.

Liver and Gallbladder

Organs which are not an integral part of the alimentary tube are vital to digestion and nutrition. Of these, the liver and its satellite gallbladder were anciently associated with vagaries of human temperament, reflected in the words "choleric," "melancholy," "bilious," "jaundiced," "liverish." The prefix "chol-" means bile or gall. "Melancholy" literally means "black bile," undoubtedly the most depressing kind. Happily, medical science has advanced a long way from the time when human dispositions were thought to result from combinations of the four humors — blood, phlegm, black and yellow bile.

The liver, the largest solid organ of the body, weighs about four pounds and occupies the upper part of the abdomen beneath the diaphragm. Most of it lies on the right side. It is divided by a fissure into a large right lobe and a smaller, tapered left lobe, the tip of which overlies the stomach near the esophageal junction. As anyone who has bought liver from a meat market knows, the maroon-colored organ appears to be rubbery and homogeneous. Only under a microscope do vast numbers of minute, polygonal structures called *lobules* become evident. Each lobule contains hundreds of liver cells, arranged like fine spokes radiating out from a central vein. The lobule is interlaced with minute bile and blood capillaries.

The liver is an incomparable chemical plant. It can modify almost any chemical structure. It is a powerful detoxifying organ, breaking down many kinds of

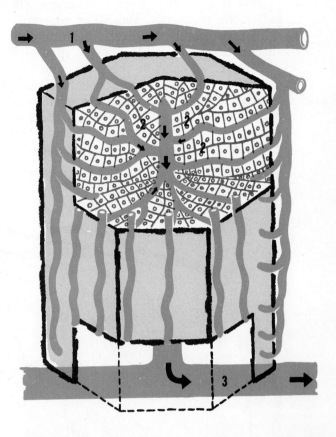

Closeup of a *liver lobule*: Fine branches of *portal vein* (1) bring blood with nutrients picked up in digestive tract. Blood runs through "stacks" of liver cells (2) which synthesize substances and perform intricate chemical processes. Blood with "processed" materials enters fine branches of *vena cava* (3) for transport to general circulation.

toxic molecules and making them harmless. It is a blood reservoir and a storage organ for some vitamins and for digested carbohydrate (glycogen) which is released to sustain blood sugar levels. It is a manufacturing site for enzymes, cholesterol, proteins, Vitamin A (from carotene), blood coagulation factors, and other elements. In some circumstances it can resume its embryonic function of red blood cell production.

And the liver produces bile which assists digestion. *Bile* is an orange-yellow fluid, bitter as gall (which is another name for it), secreted by liver cells and collected through networks of fine channels into the *hepatic duct*. This joins with the *cystic duct* from the gallbladder to form the *common bile duct* which opens into the duodenum.

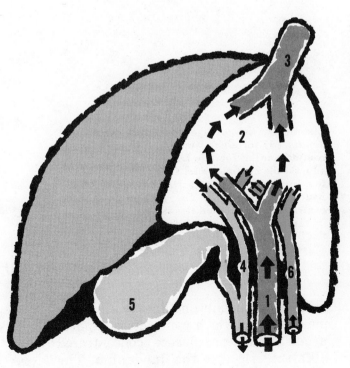

"Flow chart" of substances to and from the liver: The *portal vein* (1) brings food elements to the liver (2), for assimilation, and the *inferior vena cava* (3) carries elements in the blood to the general circulation. Bile drains from the liver via the *hepatic duct* (4) and is stored in *gallbladder* (5). The *hepatic artery* (6) supplies blood to liver tissue.

461

Bile is a complex fluid containing bile salts, bile pigments, and other constituents. The pigments, derived from disintegration of red blood cells, give the yellow-brown color of the feces, and are excreted. Bile salts are reabsorbed and reused. These salts promote efficient digestion of fats by detergent action which gives very fine emulsification of fatty materials. This not only assists

the pancreatic duct there is another of the many sphincters or muscular valves that nature uses to control the flow of materials. When this valve is closed, accumulating fluid pressure forces bile up the cystic duct into the gallbladder on the underside of the liver. The gallbladder is a saclike storage organ about three inches long. It holds bile, modifies it chemically, and concentrates it about

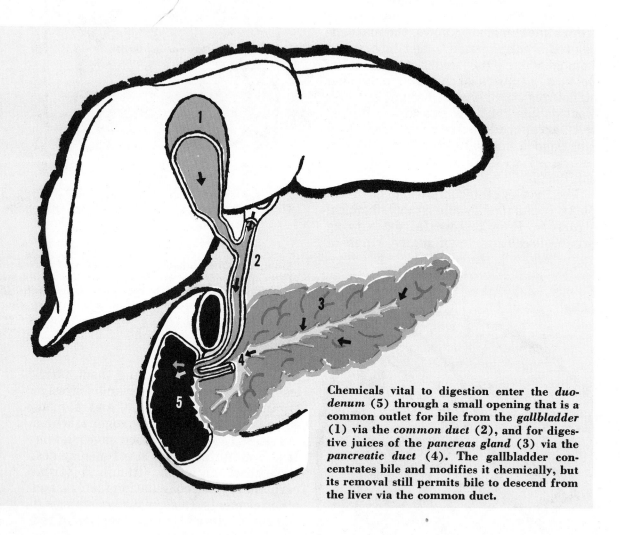

Chemicals vital to digestion enter the *duodenum* (5) through a small opening that is a common outlet for bile from the *gallbladder* (1) via the *common duct* (2), and for digestive juices of the *pancreas gland* (3) via the *pancreatic duct* (4). The gallbladder concentrates bile and modifies it chemically, but its removal still permits bile to descend from the liver via the common duct.

digestion, but gives, perhaps more importantly, efficient absorption of fat elements by villi of the intestines. Bile aids in alkalinization of the intestines.

The gallbladder. Bile is made continuously by the liver but does not drip steadily into the intestines. At the duodenal outlet of the common bile duct and

tenfold. Its membrane-lined wall has a muscle layer which contracts at appropriate times to squeeze concentrated alkaline bile into the duodenum. The sight or taste of food may be sufficient to empty the gallbladder. It is particularly stimulated to powerful contraction by a high-fat meal, and a cupful of cream is often given to a patient in tests of gall-bladder function. Constituents of gall-bladder fluids sometimes crystallize and form gallstones.

The pancreas gland is a racemose structure ("like grapes on a stalk") which lies mostly behind the stomach. It is about six inches long and has a broad right end, or head, which nestles into the curve of the duodenum. The rest of the pancreas trails off to a tail at the left of the body.

The pancreas is a double purpose gland. Its clusters of islet cells secrete insulin into the blood, not into the digestive tract. Insulin is concerned not with digestion of sugars but with their utilization. Entirely different pancreas cells produce clear, watery pancreatic juice which contains enzymes that split fats, proteins, and carbohydrates. The juice is collected into a central pancreatic duct which joins with the common bile duct in a chamber that opens into the duodenum.

DIAGNOSTIC TESTS AND INSTRUMENTS

Certain special tests and instruments are used to obtain information necessary for accurate diagnosis of gastrointestinal diseases. Of course the particular tests used in an individual patient will be determined by the nature of his difficulty. Some special gastroenterological tests and procedures are described below. Descriptions of other examinations and tests that may be given will be found in chapters of this book discussing *x-rays* and *laboratory tests*.

Esophagoscopy is a direct visual examination of the esophagus performed with a special instrument called the *esophago-scope*. This instrument is a hollow tube equipped with a light and a lens so that the entire area of the esophagus may be examined. The instrument is inserted gently into the esophagus and observations made as it progresses toward the stomach. The slender tube is about a foot and a half long and its inner diameter is approximately a quarter of an inch.

Gastroscopy. Gastroscopy is a visual examination of the stomach performed with the aid of a special instrument called a "gastroscope." Two types of instruments are frequently used. The *flexible gastroscope* is a long, slender, round device which contains numerous lenses placed so that a moderate amount of bending of the instrument will not produce distortion of the image. The other is a newer instrument called the *gastroduodenal fiberscope*. Instead of lenses, the image is carried by means of thousands of individual glass fibers. This instrument is approximately a yard long and its inner diameter is a little less than a half inch.

Before either instrument is inserted, the patient's throat is anesthetized. The instrument is then inserted into the mouth and moved into the stomach, in a manner similar to that used by a sword swallower. It is an easy procedure and relatively painless. The instrument affords an excellent view of 80 to 90 per cent of the stomach.

Gastroscopy is especially valuable in detecting lesions, such as ulcers or tumors, not seen at an x-ray examination. It is also valuable for confirming the presence of lesions seen at x-ray examination and for permitting a better evaluation of lesions merely suspected on the basis of x-ray examination.

The gastroduodenal fiberscope permits an examination of almost the entire inside of the stomach. The optics are better than those of the gastroscope and it is much more flexible. Because of its flexibility it causes less discomfort to the patient than the gastroscope and is probably somewhat safer.

Proctosigmoidoscopy is the direct visual examination of the rectum and the sigmoid colon, performed with the aid of a hollow metal tube called a *procto-scope*. This instrument is approximately one foot long and a half inch in internal diameter. It is equipped with a light source at one or the other end, depending upon the type of instrument used. The proctoscope permits the inner lining of the bowel wall to be seen directly.

Digestive Tract

Proctosigmoidoscopy enables the inner lining of the lower bowel to be seen directly with a viewing instrument, the *proctosigmoidoscope*. The top drawing at the right shows the bowel area *rectum* (1), and *sigmoid colon* (2), accessible to the instrument, and below, the instrument in place, with a view of bowel *polyps* as seen by the examiner. A large percentage of pre-cancerous, cancerous, and other lesions of the bowel lie within a few inches of the "outside" (the rectal outlet), and proctosigmoidoscopic inspection as a part of regular physical examinations is an important measure for early detection and treatment.

This examination is an *indispensable part of routine physical examination*. It is especially indicated in the examination of any person who has gastrointestinal symptoms. Cancer, polyps, ulcers, and inflammation of parts of the bowel are readily diagnosed, as they can be directly seen with the aid of the proctoscope.

It is also possible, if there is a question of any abnormality, to introduce a pair of long forceps through the proctoscope in order to snip off a small segment of the bowel wall. This small piece is examined under a microscope in order to detect any disease that may be present.

Peritoneoscopy is a procedure that is little used in the United States, but is popular in some other countries. The instrument used in performing this examination is like a small gastroscope.

An incision is made through the abdominal skin and abdominal wall, and the instrument is forced through the abdominal wall into the peritoneal cavity (the space between the intestine and the abdominal muscles). It is possible thus to see the liver, part of the stomach, intestine, colon, and the ovaries.

The results of this procedure are valuable in determining whether disease is present in any of these organs. It is, however, somewhat difficult and borders on being a surgical procedure. The usual precautions required before surgical operation must be taken.

Liver Biopsy. This is a special technique for obtaining and examining a specimen of liver tissue. After the skin is anesthetized a needle is inserted into the liver

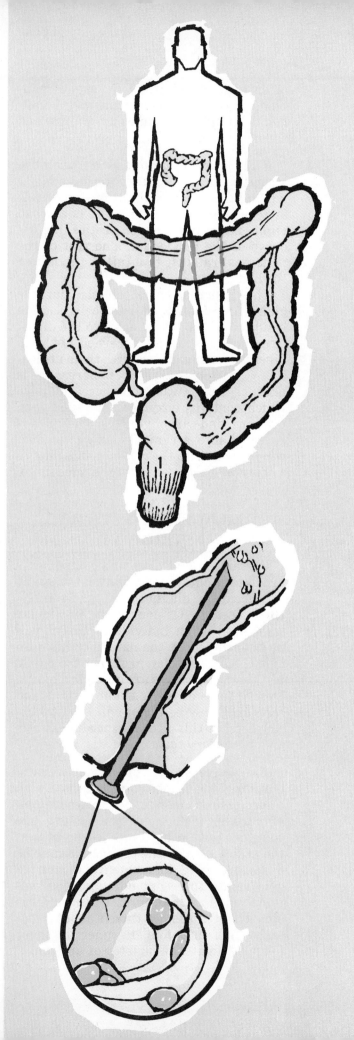

464

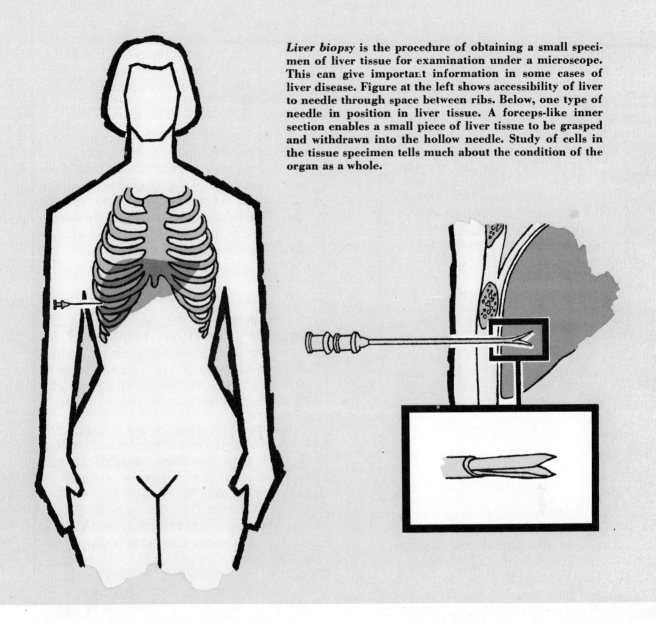

Liver biopsy is the procedure of obtaining a small specimen of liver tissue for examination under a microscope. This can give important information in some cases of liver disease. Figure at the left shows accessibility of liver to needle through space between ribs. Below, one type of needle in position in liver tissue. A forceps-like inner section enables a small piece of liver tissue to be grasped and withdrawn into the hollow needle. Study of cells in the tissue specimen tells much about the condition of the organ as a whole.

substance entering from the right side in one of the spaces between the lower ribs on the right side, or in the region of the upper abdomen.

Two types of needles are available. One type permits a small forceps-like inner core to be forced into the liver substance, and a segment of liver tissue is grasped and withdrawn. Another type of needle works on the principle of suction. After it is inserted into the substance of the liver, suction is applied through a small glass syringe and a segment of liver is drawn up into the bore of the needle.

Liver biopsy is almost painless and involves little hazard or risk of complication. It provides extremely rewarding information concerning liver structures that could not be obtained otherwise except by resorting to surgery. Malignancies, cirrhosis, and hepatitis are readily diagnosed on the basis of the results of this examination.

Small Bowel Biopsy. In this procedure a long, hollow plastic tube, on the end of which is a small metal capsule with an opening on the side across which a small knife can be drawn from the inside of the tube, is used. The tube is swallowed and is allowed to progress, by means of peristaltic movements, into the small bowel. The position of the tube is checked by means of fluoroscopic examination. When the proper level is reached, suction is applied to draw a small piece of bowel into the end of the capsule. The knife is then drawn across the segment and a small piece of tissue is cut off. The specimen of bowel tissue thus obtained is examined under the microscope.

This microscopic examination is especially valuable in the diagnosis of tropical and nontropical sprue as well as of other diseases of the small bowel. The procedure is painless and generally creates little risk, if any, of complications.

Gastric Analysis. In this procedure, a small plastic or rubber tube is passed through the nose or mouth into the patient's stomach. Gastric juice is then aspirated by means of a syringe or other suction device. This juice is analyzed to determine the degree of gastric acidity, and by means of a special cell-staining technique, the presence of malignant cells may be determined. The amount of gastric acidity is invariably high in patients with duodenal ulcer and absent in patients with pernicious anemia.

Duodenal Drainage. In performing duodenal drainage, a long rubber tube is passed through the nose or mouth into the duodenum. The duodenal juices are then aspirated and analyzed to determine the presence and the amount of the duodenal enzymes present.

The sediment can be given a special stain and analyzed under the microscope to determine the presence of malignant cells in the duodenum. This part of the procedure may be of the utmost value in the detection of cancer of the pancreas, gallbladder, or duodenum.

Examination of stools or feces. It is important to determine whether parasites or bacteria are present in the feces if they are suspected as a cause of disease. To perform this examination, a fresh stool is collected in a clean container. It is immediately examined under a microscope in order to see whether

worms, or parts of worms, or eggs (ova), are present. Ameba and other parasites are readily discovered by this means also. A portion of the stool may be cultured to determine whether bacteria are present.

All patients with gastrointestinal disturbances should have their stools analyzed to determine whether evidence of blood is present. The most common test for presence of blood in the stool is called the *guaiac test*. A person on a meat-free diet should not have chemical evidence of blood in his stools. The demonstration of chemical or occult blood in the stools may be the first indication of a malignancy or a bleeding ulcer.

THE MOUTH

The mouth is the beginning of the digestive tract. Here, preparation for digestion of food begins with shredding and grinding of food into small pieces so that digestive steps can proceed efficiently when particles reach the intestine.

Salivary Secretion. Saliva moistens the food and prepares for efficient digestion. It tends also to soften and lubricate the food bolus so that it passes easily down the esophagus.

Saliva comes from the *parotid* glands (in front of the ear) and from the *submaxillary* (below the angle of the lower jaw) and *sublingual* (under the tongue) glands. Saliva contains an enzyme, *ptyalin*, which initiates the hydrolysis or digestion of starch. This action can take place only in an alkaline medium.

As soon as the food reaches the stomach, where there is acid, this process of hydrolysis originating in the mouth is stopped and non-salivary enzymes take over. Normal persons may secrete a quart to a quart and a half of saliva per day.

An *increase* in salivation may be secondary to an ulcer of the stomach or duodenum, or it may be a symptom of poisoning (as by mercury or lead), or it may be caused by nervous tension. A *decrease* in saliva production may result from causes associated with old age or it may be a symptom of extreme nervousness and tension, that is, an anxiety state.

THE ESOPHAGUS

Congenital Defects

Atresia. In esophageal atresia the esophagus ends in a blind pouch just below the throat junction. This condition is evident as soon after birth as an infant attempts to take liquids. There is sudden regurgitation along with a cough caused by aspiration of the liquids. In an x-ray film of the esophagus plain air will be seen in the upper portion. Further x-rays may be taken after administration of a radio-opaque substance to outline the extent of the pouch. This condition can be corrected by surgery.

Congenital Stenosis. A fibrous narrowing of the esophagus which can occur at any level. Symptoms, diagnosis, and treatment are similar to those of atresia.

Webs or Bands. A membrane which blocks off the esophagus. Symptoms and diagnosis are the same as those of other congenital lesions. Diagnosis is made after x-ray examination and examination of the lesion with a special instrument which can be used for examination of the esophagus (esophagoscope).

Diverticulum

A *diverticulum* is an outpocketing of all the layers of the esophagus so that a pouch or sac leading off from the main tube is produced. This may be caused by increasing pressure or by infectious diseases. The symptoms are a sensation of pressure upon swallowing, regurgitation of previously ingested food, and sometimes a feeling of a lump in the esophagus. X-ray examination shows a typical outpocketing filled with barium. Treatment is surgical excision of the sac.

Esophagitis

Esophagitis is an inflammatory process involving the lining of the esophagus.

Acute esophagitis may be caused by the swallowing of chicken or fish bones, severe vomiting, regurgitation of acid gastric juice, infectious diseases, or the use of a gastric tube after surgery. Symptoms are severe pain below the breastbone or a burning sensation upon swallowing.

Definitive diagnosis is made after esophagoscopy which reveals an intense inflammatory reaction. Removal or treatment of the primary cause is indicated. In the case of burns, ordinary antidotes such as sodium bicarbonate for acid and vinegar for lye are used. In general, antacids are helpful. Antibiotics may be necessary if there is subsequent infection.

Chronic esophagitis is most commonly caused by regurgitation of acid gastric juice from a herniation of the stomach into the esophagus. Other causes are chronic ingestion of irritating foods or spices, the use of tobacco or alcohol, vitamin deficiency, chronic infectious diseases, and diseases which interfere with normal esophageal peristalsis.

Chronic esophagitis may interfere with the normal passage of foods just as an ulcer or a tumor does. The symptom is chronic pain below the breastbone that is always worsened by swallowing.

An x-ray examination may show some disturbance in the mucosal pattern of the esophagus. Viewing the tissues through an esophagoscope, necessary to make a definite diagnosis, one sees that the lining of the esophagus is bleeding, reddened, and contains ulcerations or erosions with adherent mucus. The first aim in treatment is to remove or treat the primary cause. A bland diet and the use of antacids are frequently of benefit.

Stricture

Stricture is narrowing of the esophagus resulting from acute or chronic esophagitis or secondary to a tumor. Difficult, painful swallowing, especially when coarse foods are swallowed, is the chief symptom. X-ray examination shows a characteristic narrowing of the esophagus that is confirmed by esophagoscopy.

Treatment is dilation of the esophagus by inserting a series of slender olive-shaped metal instruments (bougies), gradually increased in size, through the area of stricture. However difficult this may appear, surgery is rarely necessary unless a tumor is present.

Ulcer of the Esophagus

An *esophageal ulcer* usually occurs in the lower esophagus and is caused by the regurgitation of acid gastric juice. The symptom is severe pain below the breastbone immediately after eating or swallowing. Vomiting is common and hemorrhage may occur. Rupture of the ulcer is a rare but serious complication. X-ray examination will show a sharply punched-out outpocketing. An esophagoscopic examination will usually reveal a typical small ulceration.

Treatment is similar to the treatment of any ulcer and includes a bland diet, antacids, and milk every hour. At times the use of a local oral anesthetic is helpful to relieve pain. Results of treatment are good if the primary cause can be removed.

Hiatus Hernia

The protrusion of part of the stomach into or next to the esophagus is called a *hiatus hernia.* In most cases the hernia itself does not cause severe symptoms, but the herniation may cause pain under the breastbone, burning, or the regurgitation of foods or liquids. The condition is often associated with chronic esophagitis. The symptoms seem to be worse after meals or during straining or stooping. X-ray examination will reveal a

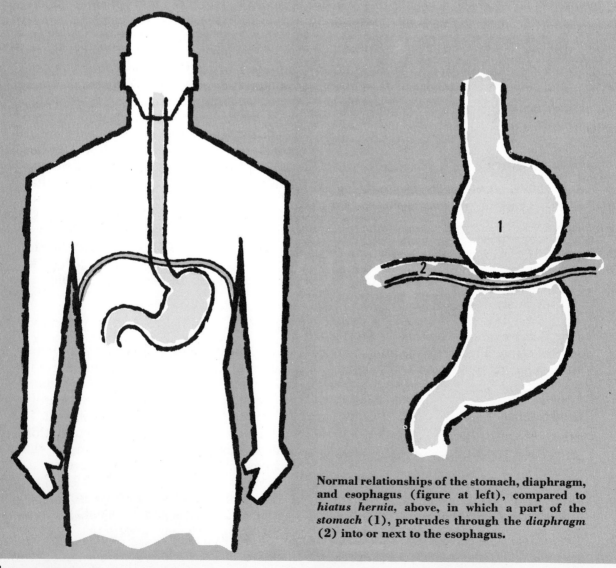

Normal relationships of the stomach, diaphragm, and esophagus (figure at left), compared to *hiatus hernia,* above, in which a part of the *stomach* (1), protrudes through the *diaphragm* (2) into or next to the esophagus.

hernia pouch, which may also be seen with an esophagoscope.

Treatment is diet to reduce weight in obese patients, antacids, and elevation of the head of the bed four to six inches at night. If necessary, the hiatal ring may be tightened up by surgery performed through the thorax or abdomen.

Achalasia (Cardiospasm)

In *achalasia,* a disturbance of normal peristalsis of the esophagus causes foods to stick at the junction of the esophagus and the stomach. This area lacks the

Treatment is dilation of the junction by means of a pneumatic rubber balloon which reaches a circumference of approximately four and a half inches. For patients who do not respond to this treatment a type of surgery is necessary in which the muscle layer of the esophagus at this junction is cut.

Globus Hystericus ("lump in the throat"). This is a psychiatric disorder characterized by a feeling of a lump in the throat which does not disappear upon swallowing. The x-ray appearance is normal. This condition is best treated by

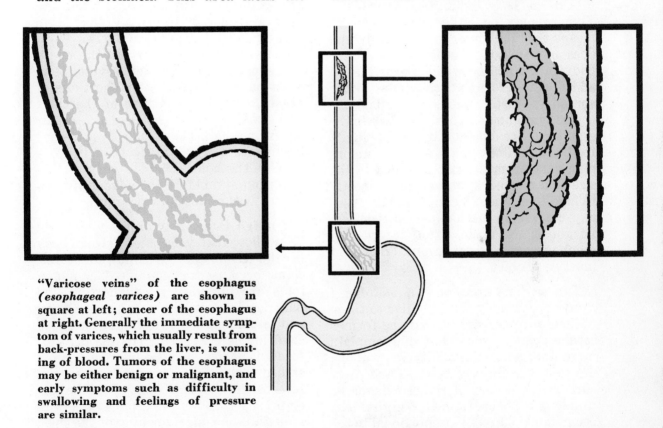

"Varicose veins" of the esophagus (esophageal varices) are shown in square at left; cancer of the esophagus at right. Generally the immediate symptom of varices, which usually result from back-pressures from the liver, is vomiting of blood. Tumors of the esophagus may be either benign or malignant, and early symptoms such as difficulty in swallowing and feelings of pressure are similar.

normal ability to "open up" when a bolus of food arrives. The chief symptom is difficulty in swallowing food into the stomach. There is a feeling that food sticks at the junction of the esophagus and the stomach, and frequently undigested food is regurgitated. In making a diagnosis, an x-ray will show a smooth narrowing of the junction of the esophagus and stomach (the *cardia*). An esophagoscopy may only reveal chronic esophagitis in that area.

a qualified psychiatrist if the symptoms are not relieved promptly by medications and reassurance of the patient.

Varices

Varices of the esophagus are in reality varicose veins and are caused by back flow pressures from the liver. Varices are usually secondary to cirrhosis or some obstruction of the blood flow into the liver.

The first symptom is usually vomiting of blood. The diagnosis is made after x-ray examination reveals the varices, or by esophagoscopy which will also show the varicose veins.

The first step in treatment is to stop the bleeding. This may be accomplished by the insertion of a tamponading ("plugging") balloon into the esophagus. In most cases, however, surgery is necessary to prevent future hemorrhages.

Tumors

A *tumor* is, by definition, any growth. Tumors may be either *benign*, which means that the tumor grows locally and does not spread to other parts of the body, or *malignant*, which means that in addition to growing locally, the tumor spreads to distant parts of the body.

The symptoms of a *benign tumor* in the esophagus are difficulty in swallowing, a feeling of fullness, or pressure. Tumors may vary from the size of a pea to the size of a marble. Symptoms are directly related to size and location and are usually caused by mechanical obstruction. Diagnosis is made after x-ray and esophagoscopic examinations. Treatment must be surgery.

Cancer. The symptoms of *malignant tumor* or carcinoma are similar to those of benign tumor except that the former become steadily worse. Patients complain more and more of inability to swallow. There are feelings of fullness and pressure in the region of the esophagus or under the breastbone. Weight loss occurs and is directly proportional to the degree and duration of swallowing difficulty and mechanical obstruction. Other symptoms may be hemorrhage or perforation into the lung, in which case pneumonia results.

Diagnosis is made after x-ray examination, which will show an irregular filling defect. Esophagoscopy confirms this finding and biopsy makes the diagnosis positive. Quite frequently the esophagus is rinsed with a special solution, in which, when examined under a microscope, cancer cells are seen.

The only definitive treatment is surgical, although x-ray therapy may give temporary palliative relief. Certain chronic diseases of the esophagus, such as chronic esophagitis, or chemical injuries such as those caused by lye, may predispose the tissues to cancer.

Perforation or Rupture

A hole in the wall of the esophagus may result from many causes. Instrumentation, and swallowing of a foreign body, such as a chicken bone or fish bone, are examples. Rupture or perforation may also occur following increased pressure such as may result from vomiting or a crushing injury to the chest. The symptoms are sudden, severe, deep, chest pain associated with shortness of breath, and shock. X-rays of the chest will usually reveal the presence of air or air and fluid. The treatment is always immediate surgical intervention in order to close the hole. This is a very serious condition and before the advent of antibiotics was almost always fatal.

Foreign Body. Any object which can be swallowed may become a foreign body in the esophagus — bones, dentures, coins, or pins, for example. The symptoms are difficulty in swallowing and pain localized in the esophagus. X-ray and esophagoscopic examinations will confirm the diagnosis. The majority of foreign bodies can be removed by a skilled esophagoscopist utilizing special forceps. However, if removal of the foreign body through the esophagoscope is impossible, surgical opening of the chest and esophagus is necessary.

STOMACH

Heartburn (Pyrosis)

One of the most common symptoms of gastric distress is **heartburn,** a burning sensation which usually begins in the "pit of the stomach" and extends up into the esophagus, and frequently into the throat, and is accompanied by a sour eructation (the non-Latin word is "belch"). It is usually caused by pressure in or distention of the lower esophagus, such as that caused by belching or regurgitation of gastric juices, or by irritation from the gastric juice.

Heartburn may be associated with organic diseases, such as ulcer or gastritis, or it may be secondary to functional spasms in a nervous or tense person. The symptoms are only important if they are associated with an organic disease. The treatment consists of measures designed to remove the primary cause.

Indigestion

Many people who have heartburn, or who experience pain or discomfort in the upper abdomen, or who belch, or have a feeling of being "gassy" and bloated, will say that they have "indigestion." As in the case of heartburn, "indigestion" is a nonspecific symptom and may be associated with organic diseases or may result from functional spasm or aerophagia (swallowing of air) in a nervous or tense individual with poor eating habits.

There is no specific diagnostic test, although the tests commonly used for diagnosing organic disease of the stomach should be employed (for example, x-ray and gastroscopy in order to rule out the presence of gastric disease). If there is an organic cause, treatment is directed toward it. If the disturbance is functional, the patient may be assisted or helped by mild sedatives, reassurance, tranquilizers, bland diet, simple antacids, and at times by use of a special silicone preparation that enables him to belch more easily and thus to relieve pressure caused by gas.

Gastritis (inflammation of the stomach)

There are several different kinds of gastritis. *Acute gastritis* may be caused by some specific irritant, for example, alcohol, a caustic, or certain medications. The symptoms are burning pain over the stomach, nausea, and vomiting. Diagnosis usually is made on the basis of the patient's history or by looking into the stomach with a gastroscope.

It is usually sufficient to remove causes such as tobacco, coffee, alcohol, or drugs. In cases of acute caustic irritants, appropriate antidotes such as bicarbonate of soda for acids, lemon or vinegar for alkalis, and starch for iodine must be used. The stomach should be evacuated immediately by stomach pump or vomiting. If treatment is prompt, the outlook is usually good. If there has been overwhelming damage to the stomach, perforation, with catastrophic consequences, can occur.

Chronic gastritis is inflammation of the stomach which has persisted for many weeks, months, or even years. Most causes of chronic gastritis are unknown. In some instances, however, chronic gastritis may follow acute gastritis or long-term ingestion of gastric irritants such as alcohol, drugs, tobacco, or coffee.

Symptoms may be absent, mild stomach distress may be experienced, or the symptoms may be of such severity as to cause constant nausea with frequent episodes of vomiting and burning epigastric pain similar to that caused by peptic ulcer. Chronic gastritis may be *superficial, atrophic,* or *hypertrophic*. Diagnosis is most conclusively made after gastroscopic examination of the stomach.

In *chronic superficial gastritis* the lining of the stomach is edematous (fluid-swollen), bleeds easily, and is seen to have reddened patches and mucus adhering to it.

The gastroscopic appearance of the stomach in *chronic atrophic gastritis* is that of graying and thinning of the mucosa and conspicuous bluish blood vessels. Atrophic gastritis invariably occurs in persons suffering from pernicious anemia, but a person who has atrophic gastritis does not necessarily have pernicious anemia.

Early in the course of *chronic hypertrophic gastritis*, the stomach, as seen through the gastroscope, exhibits a velvety appearance. As hypertrophy or morbid overgrowth increases, granular nodules can usually be seen. Creases and

471

crevices form the boundaries of irregular polygons of different sizes, creating a cobblestone appearance. Frequently areas of hemorrhaging mucosa are seen.

Treatment of patients with gastritis is to remove the cause of the symptoms. The patient must then be treated similarly to a patient with an ulcer. (See discussions of *gastric ulcer* and *duodenal ulcer*.) A patient with atrophic gastritis may respond symptomatically at times to injections of Vitamin B_{12}.

Stomach Ulcer

An ulcer is literally a sore—a localized erosion of mucous membrane with gradual disintegration of tissues and loss of substance. "Peptic ulcer" is a general term for ulcers that occur in the stomach or, as is more common, in the duodenum (*duodenal ulcer*).

A *gastric ulcer* (also called stomach ulcer) is one which is seated in the wall of the stomach. A prominent symptom is burning pain in the stomach area which is relieved by taking food, milk or antacids. Pain usually occurs when the stomach is empty or when hunger causes awakening at night. Vomiting may occur. Occasionally a massive hemorrhage occurs; emergency medical treatment including blood transfusion or surgery may be required.

Diagnosis of gastric ulcer is made on the basis of the appearance of the stomach at the time of an x-ray examination. The patient swallows a suspension of barium before the examination and a pocket of barium remains in the ulcer and is seen by means of the x-ray. The typical x-ray appearance of a benign ulcer is a sharply punched-out pocket of barium projecting away from the cavity of the stomach.

Most ulcers of the stomach are benign — that is, not cancerous. Gastroscopic study is important to confirm the presence and character of the ulcer. Stomach fluids are examined under the microscope to determine whether malignant cells are present (gastric cytology).

Peptic ulcers include ulcers of the stomach and of the duodenum. There has been some decrease in the incidence of stomach cancer in recent years. The drawing shows a *gastric ulcer* (1) in the wall of the stomach; cancer of the *pylorus* (2) causing obstruction, and *duodenal ulcer* (3) in a common location in the bulb of the duodenum. Ulcers may erode the stomach or duodenal wall to various depths; a complete perforation permits contents to seep into the abdominal cavity.

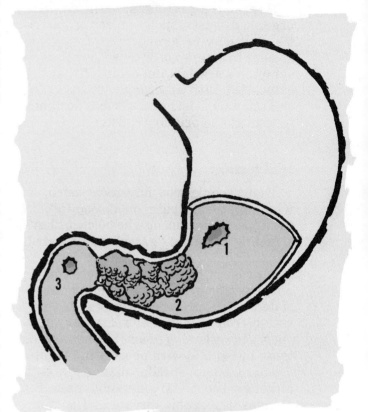

Treatment of a patient with a gastric ulcer depends first of all on absolute neutralization of gastric acid. Free hydrochloric acid is present in the stomachs of all patients with benign ulcers. In general, a bland diet that prescribes *lean meat*, *two cooked fruits* and *two cooked vegetables*, and abstinence from fried foods, spices, and roughage such as turnips and cabbage and onions, is helpful. It is not necessary to follow a strict milk and cream diet, although it may be necessary for the first few days to eat only soft foods. Rest, both physical and mental, is important. Abstinence, or at least a great decrease in consumption of things which increase gastric acid, such as alcohol, coffee, and cigarettes, is of great importance. Sedatives or tranquilizers are helpful. In some patients psychotherapy is necessary, as persons with ulcers are frequently nervous, tense, hard-driving individuals.

Drugs such as atropine or agents which act like atropine decrease production of gastric acid. Many new antisecretory or anticholinergic agents are of great value in decreasing acid formation.

The sheet anchor of ulcer therapy is still the use of agents which chemically *neutralize* gastric acidity. Milk or milk and cream is the most common antacid. The most common medications are aluminum hydroxide combined with magnesium compounds, and calcium carbonate.

In the administration of *antacids* two difficulties are often encountered: the antacids frequently are not given in large enough amounts or not given often enough; and they may cause constipation (in case of calcium carbonate) or diarrhea (in the case of the magnesium compound). It is essential, at least at the start of treatment for an ulcer, to give these agents in amounts of one to two grams every one half to one to two hours, or to prescribe a half glass of milk or milk and cream every one to two hours. Since recurrence of ulcer attacks is frequent, it is recommended that patients continue to follow a modified diet and take antacids from one to several years before treatment is discontinued.

Gastric freezing is a relatively new technique that has been developed for treatment of patients with ulcer. A balloon is placed in the stomach and then joined to a freezing apparatus. The balloon is filled to approximately quart size with 95 per cent alcohol. The lining of the stomach is then superficially frozen for about one hour. A decrease in gastric acidity results. This technique is so new it cannot yet be predicted how effective it will be on a long-term basis.

For the five to ten per cent of patients who do not respond to the medical treatment of ulcer, for those in whom there is a question of malignancy, and for those in whom there is malignant ulcer, surgery is necessary. This consists of surgical removal of half to two-thirds, or in rare cases, the whole stomach. Most patients are at least temporarily cured by medical management. Those patients who undergo surgery for a gastric ulcer

are usually cured. However, this is not true in cases of duodenal ulcer where new ulcerations tend to occur.

Complications that may occur as the result of an ulcer are *perforation, massive hemorrhage,* or *obstruction.* Treatment of massive hemorrhage is replacement of blood, strict ulcer program, and careful observation. If hemorrhage continues, surgical operation is necessary.

In cases of perforation, surgical operation consists of sewing up the rent in the stomach; in cases of obstruction, a part of the stomach is removed or a new opening into the stomach is made.

Tumors of the Stomach

Benign tumors of the stomach are relatively rare and usually do not cause symptoms except as a result of their location — for example, at the inlet or outlet of the stomach. Symptoms of obstruction are nausea, vomiting, and at times vague abdominal disturbance. Diagnosis is made by means of x-ray examination which shows a defect in the inner wall of the stomach. Gastroscopic examination is necessary to confirm the type and location of the tumor.

The treatment is surgical removal, after which the outlook is excellent. There are no recurrences. Except for possible surgical complications, the treatment should involve little if any risk. Benign tumors include leiomyoma, fibromyoma, aberrant pancreas, and others.

Stomach Cancer

The most common **malignant tumor** of the stomach is carcinoma, although several other malignant tumors such as sarcoma, lymphosarcoma, and Hodgkin's disease, must be considered in making a diagnosis.

Symptoms are very indefinite. Any indigestion or abdominal discomfort must be viewed with suspicion, especially if it persists. Loss of appetite, loss of weight, and mild intermittent stomach distress, which may become continuous, are frequent symptoms. A feeling of fullness and discomfort induced by eating may also be experienced. Symptoms may be like those of ulcer: burning distress that is relieved by food. Vomiting is not uncommon and the vomited material may contain blood that looks like coffee grounds (because blood that has been acted upon by gastric acid changes in color and appearance). Anemia is very frequent and chemical evidence of blood is often found in the stools.

Diagnosis may be made in some ten per cent of cases by physical examination which reveals a hard mass in the upper abdomen, enlargement of the liver, or lymph glands in the neck. A tumor mass in the rectum (or on the ovaries in women) indicates spread of the cancer.

In most instances, however, the x-ray examination will reveal either a mass, which may or may not be irregular, projecting into the cavity of the stomach, or an ulcer. A cancerous ulcer typically is surrounded by a tumor border and this can be seen by means of x-ray. In early cases the border may be sharp and indistinguishable from that of a benign gastric ulcer.

A gastroscopic examination is very important as a means of better evaluation of the lesion. It is possible to obtain a specimen of a suspicious lesion by biopsy through the gastroscope in order to examine it microscopically. A cytologic examination of fluids obtained from the stomach should always be done.

Treatment in cases of cancer is surgery with removal of the lesion and as much of the surrounding margin as possible. For patients in whom the tumor has been found to be sarcoma, lymphosarcoma, or Hodgkin's disease, treatment is surgical and x-ray therapy should follow. The immediate prognosis for a patient with a cancerous lesion of the stomach is usually good but the five-year survival ranges from five to 25 per cent. In selected cases of the other malignant tumors the prognosis is usually better and the survival may be five to ten years. There is a somewhat higher incidence of cancer of the stomach in patients with pernicious anemia.

Pyloric Stenosis

In this condition the outlet of the stomach is narrowed. The abnormality is usually congenital and is most common in a first-born male child. It is characterized by projectile vomiting (forceful ejection) and pain in the stomach region. (See Chapter 11, pyloric stenosis in infants).

In the adult patient, pyloric stenosis can develop after long-standing ulcer of the duodenum. Symptoms are frequent vomiting of undigested food after eating. Diagnosis is made upon the x-ray appearance of a thick pylorus. Treatment is surgical. Relief from symptoms should be complete.

Postgastrectomy Syndrome

Symptoms referred to collectively as the *postgastrectomy syndrome* follow partial removal of the stomach. Some of the symptoms result from the surgery itself and occur simply as a result of disturbing the normal physiology of the stomach. Mechanical difficulty may occur as a result of scar formation or the twisting of a loop of bowel. These conditions usually cause pain and vomiting soon after surgery. Treatment is surgical correction.

The most common type of postgastrectomy syndrome is the *dumping syndrome*. This is a symptom complex that occurs soon after eating. The patient may feel bloated or full, may have diarrhea, and may vomit food. Frequently, feelings of warmth, weakness, rapid heartbeat, and chilly perspiration occur immediately after meals. Symptoms disappear in 30 to 60 minutes and are lessened if the patient lies down immediately after eating. The symptoms may be ameliorated if the patient eats bland foods and avoids rich foods or sweets. Frequent small meals, high in protein, moderate in fat, and low in starch are helpful. Fluids should be limited. Anticholinergic drugs may give additional benefit.

Marginal ulcer. A marginal ulcer forms either just inside or just outside the outlet of the stomach in five to ten per cent of patients who have had part of the stomach removed. The symptoms are quite similar to those of ulcer distress. Treatment consists of following a strict medical program (described under gastric and duodenal ulcer), or surgical removal of the ulcer and more of the stomach, or x-ray therapy of the stomach to decrease gastric acidity, or undergoing gastric freezing, a new technique, which is described under ulcer treatment.

DUODENUM

Duodenal Ulcer

The most common disease of the duodenum is *duodenal ulcer.* The ulcer is a sharply punched-out defect in the duodenum wall, commonly about the size of a dime, that is caused by the digestive action of the gastric juice.

An ulcer may occur at any age, but it is most common between the ages of 20 and 50 and is more common in males than females. It has been estimated that ten per cent of the people in the United States have a duodenal ulcer at one time or another. Ulcers are more common in nervous, tense, hard-driving persons with great ambition and numerous frustrations than in more relaxed "easy-going" persons. For practical purposes, a duodenal ulcer is always benign and *does not become cancerous.*

Symptoms. Epigastric pain or distress is the most characteristic symptom. The type of pain is quite variable, and may be aching, gnawing, hurting, burning, cramping, or hunger-like. It is usually restricted to an area an inch or two in diameter about the navel. The pain usually occurs an hour or two after meals or when the stomach is empty, is generally chronic, and recurs frequently. The pain is usually promptly relieved after taking milk, or antacids. Ulcer attacks seem to occur more frequently in spring and fall than in summer and winter. Diagnosis of duodenal ulcer is usually made on the basis of history, physical examination, which might reveal point tenderness in the upper middle portion of the abdomen, and x-ray examination.

When the ulcer is chronic, in addition to the punched-out crater there is a deformity of the duodenum so that its bulb looks like a clover leaf instead of a chocolate drop on an x-ray film.

Treatment of duodenal ulcer consists of attempts to remove factors which contribute to its production. Coffee, tea, cigarettes, alcohol, and irritating spicy foods should be eliminated. Relief from nervous tension should be sought. Regular hours for meals, sleep, and rest are very important. In addition, measures to neutralize acid gastric juice should be taken (see *gastric ulcer*).

It is usually not difficult to relieve symptoms promptly and to heal an acute duodenal ulcer. Recurrence and exacerbation are, however, the rule.

Complications that may occur as a result of duodenal ulcer are perforation, massive hemorrhage, and obstruction. The canal of the normal duodenal bulb is slightly greater or less than an inch in diameter. If this diameter is constricted to, perhaps, a quarter of an inch, there is usually some enlargement or expansion of the stomach and overvigorous peristalsis with vomiting.

Surgery. Approximately 80 to 90 per cent of patients with duodenal ulcer should respond well to medical management. For those who do not, or who have complications such as obstruction or massive, uncontrollable hemorrhage, surgery may be necessary. Surgery is usually one of two types: One type effects a "mass action" by removing one-half to two-thirds of the stomach, thus decreasing the amount of tissue in which acid producing cells are located. The second type is a *bilateral vagotomy* which means cutting the vagus nerves, thereby abolishing nervous stimuli to gastric secretion. Following surgery 75 to 80 per cent of the patients are well, another 20 to 25 per cent will have various symptoms, and perhaps five to ten per cent may develop another ulcer.

Gastric hypothermia is a new technique which has been developed to freeze the stomach lining briefly to decrease acid production (see *gastric ulcer*).

In selected cases, x-ray therapy to the stomach has been used to eliminate gastric acid and enable the duodenal ulcer to heal.

In general, treatment by medication and strict diet is preferred since in itself it does not produce any complications or increased risk of mortality.

Duodenitis

Duodenitis is closely related to duodenal ulcer. The diagnosis is usually made on the basis of symptoms and results of x-ray examination. On instrumental visualization an irregularity of the lining of the duodenum, not sufficient for diagnosis of duodenal ulcer, is seen. The symptoms are quite similar to those of duodenal ulcer, and treatment is, in general outline, the same.

Tumors

Tumors of the duodenum are extremely rare. The symptoms of tumor, whether benign or malignant, are those of obstruction: a feeling of pressure, cramplike pain, and vomiting. X-rays show the duodenal passageway to be narrowed and it may be smooth or highly irregular. Treatment is always removal of the tumor by surgical operation.

Diverticulum

Diverticulum of the duodenum, relatively uncommon, is an outpocketing from the central canal. It usually causes no symptoms and is only diagnosed after x-ray examination. A suspension of barium, swallowed by the patient before the examination, will outline the pocket. Occasionally a diverticulum bleeds or perforates or becomes acutely inflamed in the same way as the appendix. With the exception of complications or the rare case in which the diverticulum produces symptoms of obstruction, no treatment is indicated or necessary.

Superior mesenteric artery syndrome. This is a condition in which a part of the duodenum is compressed at the point that it passes the spine by the artery that serves the small intestine and upper half of the colon. The condition usually occurs in thin people with a forward curve in the backbone that projects it toward the abdominal contents, and with a lack of tonus so that the abdominal organs tend to fall. The symptoms are those of chronic obstruction and are characterized by a feeling of distention, cramps, and vomiting. X-ray examination will show that the duodenum is greatly dilated immediately before the point of obstruction. Exercises or the wearing of a special belt may be of benefit. For those who do not respond well to these measures, surgery may be necessary.

THE LIVER

The liver is the largest organ in the body and performs more functions than any other organ. It is essential for the metabolism of carbohydrates, proteins, fats, and minerals; it plays a major part in detoxifying poisons and drugs; it manufactures cholesterol; it is concerned with iron storage and the manufacture of the elements essentially necessary for blood clotting; it converts glucose to glycogen and stores the latter as a source of energy. One of its primary functions is the destruction of old red blood cells and conversion of the hemoglobin molecule into *bilirubin*.

Jaundice is the most common finding in any derangement of the liver. Jaundice refers to a yellowing of the skin caused by an excess of bile pigments in the circulatory system and in all the tissues of the body. Jaundice may occur when the outflow of bile has been blocked and when liver substance itself is inflamed. When such inflammation occurs, the small bile ducts within the liver become obstructed; as a result a large portion of the bile that is produced by the liver is absorbed directly into the blood stream because it cannot flow normally out of the bile ducts into the duodenum.

"Jaundice" comes from a word meaning "yellow," and the common expression, "yellow jaundice," is a redundancy.

Cirrhosis of the Liver

Cirrhosis is characterized by inflammation of the liver substance itself. Fibrosis and scarring are frequent subsequent occurrences. *Portal cirrhosis,* the most common type, is also referred to as *Laennec's cirrhosis,* "gin drinkers' cirrhosis," or "alcoholic cirrhosis." It is present in about 2 or 3 per cent of adults in the United States.

The exact cause of the condition is unknown, although it appears to be related to the ingestion of alcohol and poor nutrition. It also may be caused by exposure to chronic poisons such as carbon

condition progresses, weight loss, nausea, vomiting, complaints of indigestion, and inability to tolerate fats usually occur. If the condition continues to become worse, jaundice develops, and other signs of liver disease, such as the presence of prominent vascular networks or "spiders" over the head and upper body, may develop. Dilated veins over the abdomen may also be seen.

As the cirrhosis becomes progressively worse, fluid in the abdomen (ascites), evidenced by a large, protuberant abdomen, develops. X-ray examination reveals that the protuberance is caused by fluid. Noticeable swelling of the legs

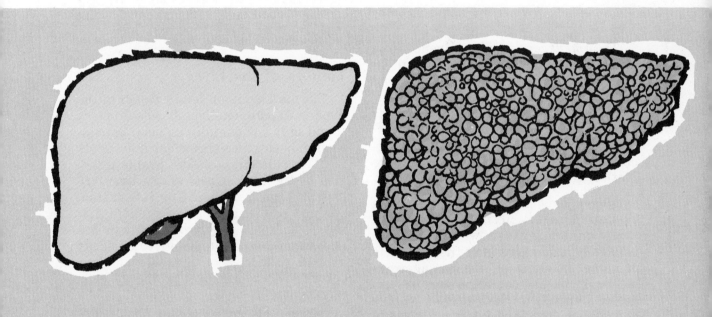

The surface of a normal liver is smooth. The most common type of *cirrhosis of the liver,* at right above, produces nodules of pinhead to bean-size, giving a hobnailed appearance (hence the term, "hobnail liver"). Such livers may be enlarged or smaller than normal. Increase in fibrous tissue distorts liver lobules and causes various degrees of obstruction of the portal circulation.

tetrachloride and phosphorus. It may be associated with chronic diseases of the bowel, such as chronic ulcerative colitis or regional enteritis.

Symptoms. At first the symptoms of cirrhosis may be very slight and its presence may only be apparent when the physician discovers, upon physical examination, that the liver is enlarged. As the

(edema), which usually results from a decreased ability to handle salt, an increase in pressure in the portal vein, and a decrease in circulating proteins in the blood, may also occur. Other complications such as enlarged veins in the esophagus (see *esophageal varices*) may occur. These varices may bleed and cause hemorrhages. Hemorrhoids may become another manifestation of liver disease.

Diagnosis is usually made on finding a large liver on physical examination; results of special chemical tests reveal the presence of liver damage. Other chemical tests confirm the presence of increased bile pigment (bilirubin) in the blood stream that has produced the jaundice. Diagnosis is made most definitive, however, by liver biopsy. In this procedure a needle is inserted into the liver and a small piece of liver is drawn up into the bore of the needle by means of a syringe and then examined under the microscope. Inflammation and degeneration of liver cells caused by an increase in fibrous tissue, characteristic of cirrhosis, are readily apparent when a specimen of liver tissue is examined under a microscope.

Treatment consists of abstinence from alcohol, consumption of foods high in protein and carbohydrates, bed rest and restriction of salt intake. Further treatment using diuretics or cortisone is prescribed for severe cases and complications are treated as necessary. The prognosis varies from complete recovery to death from liver failure or complications.

Biliary cirrhosis. Biliary cirrhosis is similar to portal cirrhosis in terms of symptoms and signs; however, the cause is usually inflammation of the bile ducts or stones blocking off the passageways of bile ducts. The condition may be suggested by basis of the patient's history and the results of special liver tests. But the results of a liver biopsy or even, at times, surgical exploration of the liver and the bile tubes, must be evaluated in order to make the proper diagnosis. Treatment is to remove the cause if possible, otherwise it is similar to that of the common type, portal cirrhosis.

Infectious Hepatitis. This is one of the most common liver diseases and also a cause of jaundice. It is described in detail in another chapter.

Postnecrotic cirrhosis. This condition refers to cirrhosis that occurs after infectious hepatitis. The symptoms and signs of this condition are quite similar to those of portal cirrhosis but the cause is inflammation of the liver caused by the presence of a virus rather than the presence of toxins. The treatment is similar to the treatment for portal cirrhosis. In general, the condition is more severe than portal cirrhosis, since the offending cause cannot be removed.

Cardiac cirrhosis may occur in patients with chronic heart failure. In this condition congestion of the liver has been present for a period of several months or years and has produced fibrous and inflammatory changes. In general, the changes are not as severe as those produced in portal cirrhosis; the distinction can be made by microscopic examination of tissue removed at liver biopsy. Appropriate treatment is treatment for the basic disease, chronic heart failure.

Tumors of the Liver

The most common *benign tumor* of the liver is **hepatoma.** Usually hepatoma is found only incidentally at necropsy, although hepatomas may occur in patients with chronic cirrhosis or chronic infection of the liver. *Cysts* of the liver are usually caused by parasitic infestation, such as echinococciasis (hydatid disease). The cysts may grow slowly in size and may become completely calcified. If growth continues or pressure changes occur, surgical removal of the cysts is imperative.

Almost *any disease* caused by infestation, such as tuberculosis, leprosy, brucellosis, and infectious mononucleosis, as well as amebiasis, may affect the liver and cause swelling and enlargement or damage to the liver cells. When these diseases occur, appropriate bacteriologic and cultural methods must be used in order to make a correct diagnosis. Appropriate treatment consists in treatment for the disease itself.

Malignant tumor or cancer that originates in the liver is relatively rare. It is usually not diagnosed until the patient has noticed a great increase in the size of his liver, or the presence of a large mass in the right part of his upper abdomen, or that he has become jaundiced. No treatment for this condition is effective. Most cancers of the liver, however, are not primary, but have spread to the liver from some other source in the body. Unfortunately, treatment in this case is also hopeless, since the liver is a vital organ and no one can survive its removal.

THE GALLBLADDER

The gallbladder is a sac-like structure which stores and concentrates the bile constantly being secreted by the liver. The gallbladder is not essential to health. It is a common misconception that flatulence, or "gassiness," and abdominal distention are related to gallbladder disease.

A medical word for the gallbladder is *cholecyst*, from *cholo-*, a combining form meaning gall or bile, and *cyst* for bladder. Thus, "cholecystitis" is inflammation of the gallbladder.

The outstanding symptom of gallbladder disease is colicky pain in the right upper quadrant of the abdomen. This pain is usually brought on or aggravated by a fatty meal. The pain is usually sudden and severe, and extends through the back and up into the right shoulder.

Cholecystitis

Acute cholecystitis is an acute inflammation of the gallbladder. There is a bacterial invasion of the gallbladder, as in appendicitis. The patient has a high fever, increased numbers of white blood cells, severe pain in the right upper quadrant of the abdomen, nausea, and vomiting. Jaundice may also be observed. Sometimes there is a palpable gallbladder mass. X-ray examination will frequently show areas of calcification indicative of stones in the region of the gallbladder. Treatment of acute cholecystitis generally is immediate surgical removal of the gallbladder.

Chronic cholecystitis is a chronic, inflammatory condition of the gallbladder that is almost invariably associated with *gallstones*. Symptoms are repeated attacks of pain in the right upper quadrant of the abdomen, nausea, and vomiting frequently brought on by ingestion of a fatty meal.

Diagnosis may be made on the basis of an x-ray examination of the gallbladder after the patient swallows a special iodine dye. This dye is concentrated in the gallbladder and gives a radio-opaque shadow. It often happens, however, in people with chronic cholecystitis, that the gallbladder has lost its capacity for concentrating the dye, or it may be so filled with stones that there is no space for the dye. Treatment of chronic cholecystitis is also surgical removal.

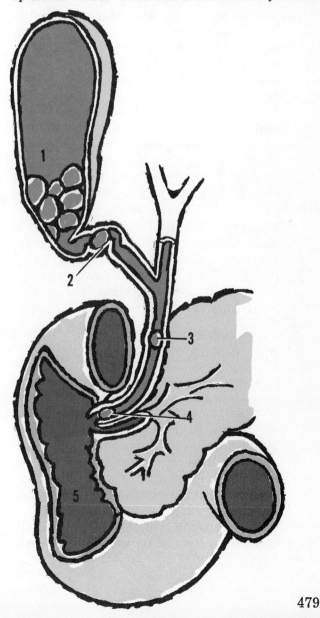

Gallstones in the *gallbladder* (1) may remain there, or may pass into the *duodenum* (5), causing colicky pain, or a stone may become lodged in the *cystic duct* (2), the *common duct* (3), or lower in the duct (4). *Bile* may back up behind a stone in common duct and cause jaundice.

Gallstones

It has been estimated that about ten per cent of the adult population has **gallstones.** Gallstones are rare in people under the age of 20, but their incidence increases with age. Credible estimates are that after the age of 40, gallstones are present in 50 per cent of women and 20 per cent of men.

The exact cause of gallstones is unknown, but many theories have been proposed. Conditions which lead to increased concentration of the bile and possible precipitation of the bile salts, cholesterol or calcium; infection; excessive ingestion of fat, and liver disease may play roles.

Persons with gallstones may or may not have symptoms. Frequently the diagnosis can be made only after an x-ray examination, but about half the patients have some symptoms indicating gallstones. These symptoms are quite similar to those of chronic cholecystitis. Jaundice may be present if a gallstone blocks off the common bile duct.

When gallstones occur in young or middle-aged patients, and especially if symptoms are present, the gallstones should be surgically removed. If the gallstones are an incidental finding in an elderly patient, it may be best for the patient not to undergo surgery. For the elderly patient or the patient who is a poor surgical risk, or refuses surgery, certain medical measures may be of benefit. These include the avoidance of fatty foods, loss of weight, and use of anticholinergic or antispasmodic drugs.

Postcholecystectomy Syndrome

There is considerable controversy as to whether this condition really exists, but, as the name implies, it refers to symptoms which occur after the gallbladder has been removed.

A small number of patients are, to some degree, apparently unable to tolerate fatty foods after the gallbladder has been removed. This has been thought to result from the fact that after the gallbladder — the storage sac for bile — has been removed, there is no mechanism for suddenly increasing the amount of bile released into the duodenum after a fatty meal has been eaten. A few patients with this syndrome will respond favorably to the ingestion of bile salts with meals, but most patients who are thought to have postcholecystectomy syndrome are really suffering from other conditions.

Cholangitis

Cholangitis refers to an acute inflammation of the bile tube which leads from the gallbladder to the duodenum (common bile duct). This inflammation is probably caused by invasion of bacteria from the intestinal tract or from the blood stream. It can be quite a serious condition, manifested by chills and fever, and pain in the right upper quadrant of the abdomen. If infection progresses it will involve the liver or block off the bile tubes, in which case the patient will become jaundiced.

Treatment is usually administration of antibiotics and removal of stones in the gallbladder or in the common bile duct if they are present.

Chronic cholangitis. Chronic inflammation of the common bile duct is usually brought on by stones which have passed out of the gallbladder and have become embedded in the common bile duct, causing a decrease in bile flow with associated growth of bacteria. Symptoms, not as severe as those of acute cholangitis, are recurring chills and fever and attacks of pain in the right upper quadrant of the abdomen. In many cases jaundice is associated with these symptoms.

Stricture of the common bile duct is a narrowing · or actual blocking of the common bile tube which leads to the duodenum. This occurs as a result of the presence of a stone, or severe inflammation, or occurs after surgery for removal of the gallbladder, during which the common bile duct may have been damaged. This damage then causes scar formation and contraction of an area of the common bile duct. The treatment for this condition is surgical repair.

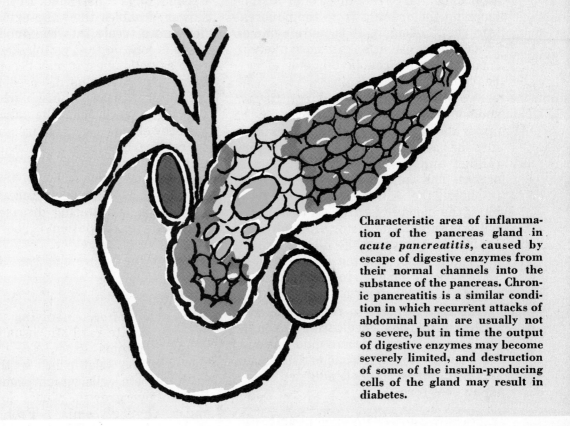

Characteristic area of inflammation of the pancreas gland in *acute pancreatitis*, caused by escape of digestive enzymes from their normal channels into the substance of the pancreas. Chronic pancreatitis is a similar condition in which recurrent attacks of abdominal pain are usually not so severe, but in time the output of digestive enzymes may become severely limited, and destruction of some of the insulin-producing cells of the gland may result in diabetes.

Tumors

Benign tumors, for practical purposes, are polyps or small growths which are present in the wall of the gallbladder and project into its cavity. They usually do not cause symptoms, although at times they may be associated with chronic inflammation. X-ray examination shows a projection from the wall of the gallbladder into the cavity. The treatment is surgical removal of the gallbladder.

Cancer of the gallbladder rarely occurs except in patients who have had gallstones or chronic inflammation for many years. The patient has pain in the right upper quadrant of the abdomen that is usually associated with jaundice, since the cancer, by the time it causes symptoms, has almost always spread to involve the bile ducts. The treatment is surgical, but the expectation of cure is almost nil.

THE PANCREAS

The pancreas is composed of two kinds of tissue. One is concerned with internal secretions, or hormones. This tissue is present in the Islands or Islets of Langerhans where there are three types of cells (alpha, beta, and gamma). The most important are the *beta* cells which secrete insulin. Disturbance in insulin production causes metabolic disease, such as *diabetes* if insulin production is low, and *hypoglycemia* (low blood-sugar) if production is high (see Chapter 9).

The other tissue component of the pancreas produces digestive enzymes. The *alveoli* are small tubules which are lined with groups of cells that secrete these enzymes which find their way from the pancreatic ducts into the duodenum.

Pancreatitis

Acute pancreatitis is a sudden, severe, acute, inflammatory process in the pancreas. It is caused by the escape of pancreatic enzymes from the alveoli into the pancreatic substance itself. This usually results from some obstruction to the outflow of the pancreatic juice, such as adjacent biliary tract disease or a stone blocking the opening from the pancreas into the duodenum. It is more common in alcoholics. An attack is more likely to occur after an alcoholic binge or after a heavy meal.

Symptoms of acute pancreatitis are sudden, acute, excruciating pain in the upper abdomen which frequently extends into the back. The upper abdomen is very tender and severe vomiting usually occurs. The patient often appears to be in shock: the skin is cold, clammy, and blue; the blood pressure is low; and the pulse is rapid. The history and physical examination suggest the diagnosis, and laboratory tests showing serum amylase (a pancreatic enzyme) to be significantly elevated usually confirm it.

The treatment is to relieve the pain with appropriate medication, prohibit oral ingestion of foods and fluids, administer intravenous fluids, and advise strict bed rest. Surgery is not indicated unless an abscess forms.

Chronic pancreatitis is similar to the acute form but recurrent attacks of abdominal pain are not ordinarily as severe as in acute pancreatitis. As the disease progresses, digestion may become significantly disturbed since the output of digestive juice may become very limited. Furthermore, as the disease advances, the Islet cells are destroyed and diabetes may develop.

The condition is suggested by a history of recurring attacks and evidences of disturbance of digestion, such as the presence of fat in the stool, and especially, diarrhea. The concentration of serum amylase is persistently elevated. X-rays of the abdomen frequently show areas of calcification in the region of the pancreas.

Treatment of chronic pancreatitis is bland diet, abstinence from alcohol, use of anticholinergic drugs or agents which suppress the output of pancreatic juice, and supplemental enzymes to correct the digestive disturbance.

Surgery may be of benefit in selected cases in which a stone is present or if the pancreatic duct, which enters the duodenum, is constricted. In these cases, surgery enables the pancreatic juice to flow more freely into the duodenum. If there is concomitant gallbladder disease, such as gallstones, it may become necessary to remove this diseased organ. A special surgical procedure in which a new opening is made from the pancreas into the bowel (called a marsupialization operation) has recently been developed. This should be resorted to only in severe cases.

In general, chronic pancreatitis is a severe and debilitating disease and the prognosis for the patient is poor from the standpoint of longevity.

Tumors

Benign tumors involving the pancreas are quite rare and usually do not cause symptoms, except for those that occur in the Islet cells. If the tumor involves beta cells which produce insulin, an overgrowth causes low blood-sugar (hypoglycemia). Probably less than 10 per cent of these tumors are malignant.

Usually patients with this type of tumor experience attacks associated with low blood-sugar occurring when they are hungry or several hours after meals. The attacks consist of weakness, rapid heart beat, cold, clammy perspiration, trembling, dizziness, apprehension, irritability, restlessness, and at times actual convulsion. Treatment is surgical removal of the tumor.

Recently a non beta-cell Islet tumor has been shown to be responsible for the production of resistant gastric or duodenal ulcers. Patients with this type of tumor secrete large quantities of acid. Since it is difficult to remove the entire involved area of the pancreas, the general treatment is surgical removal of the entire stomach to prevent recurrent stomach or duodenal ulcers.

Cancer of the pancreas is an almost hopeless disease. It is more common in older males. The symptoms are usually steadily increasing, vague, upper abdominal distress, indigestion, and weight loss. Diarrhea with excessive fat in the stools may also occur. Upon x-ray examination of the duodenal loop after a patient has swallowed a suspension of barium, an irregularity in the region of the pancreas or a widening of the duodenal loop indicating that something is growing in the region, may be seen.

About 20 per cent of people with a malignant tumor of the pancreas present themselves to a physician because of jaundice. This jaundice is caused when the tumor is located in such a way that it presses upon the common bile duct where it enters the duodenum. Diagnosis of malignant tumor may be made after aspirated juice from the duodenum, studied under the microscope, is found to contain malignant cells. In approximately 10 per cent of patients with pancreatic tumor, a tumor mass in the abdomen may be felt upon physical examination. Treatment is surgical removal of the pancreas if possible, but the cure rate is just about zero.

THE SMALL BOWEL

Congenital Defects

In *faulty rotation* of the small bowel a person is born with most of the small bowel on the right side of the abdomen rather than on the left side. Although it is usually of no clinical significance, it may cause confusion at the time of an x-ray examination. This anomaly occasionally favors the development of an internal hernia in later life.

A *congenital occlusion* is a condition discovered in the first few days of life in which the bowel is blocked off. Symptoms are persistent vomiting and distention of the bowel. Treatment is surgical repair.

Meckel's diverticulum is an outpouching from the ileum and is a remnant of the tube which connected the primitive intestine with the umbilical vesicle. It is estimated to be present in two per cent of all people. The pouch of the diverticulum is usually two to five inches long. In some cases, gastric mucosa which may secrete

acid and produce ulceration, hemorrhage, perforation and obstruction is present. Acute inflammation may occur and is indistinguishable from acute appendicitis. Surgical exploration is usually required to make the diagnosis and surgical correction is usually the only treatment for this congenital anomaly.

Intestinal Obstruction

Obstruction of the intestine is any condition which interferes with the passing of intestinal contents through the bowel passageway. The most common cause is adhesions resulting from previous surgery. Symptoms are cramping, colicky, severe, sharp, abdominal pain, abdominal distention, and vomiting. At times peristaltic movements across the abdomen are visible and at times a palpable mass is present. An x-ray examination of the abdomen will usually reveal distended loops of bowel.

If the obstruction is not complete, it may respond to aspiration of the bowel contents with a long intestinal tube. If this does not relieve the obstruction promptly, surgery is necessary.

Another less common type of obstruction is *paralytic ileus.* In this condition peristaltic activity of the bowel is significantly decreased. As a result, the bowel distends because food products are not propelled through the bowel. This condition is fairly common after surgical procedures or severe injury to the bowel. The passage of a long intestinal tube to decompress the bowel is successful treatment in most cases.

Intussusception is a condition in which one loop of bowel "telescopes" into the canal of another loop of bowel. In the condition known as *volvulus* the bowel twists on itself as a rubber balloon is twisted to keep air in it. In both of these conditions the symptoms are quite similar: sudden, severe, cramping, sharp, localized, abdominal pain associated with nausea and vomiting. Surgical treatment for both is required unless the condition promptly relieves itself, as occurs after the passage of a long tube.

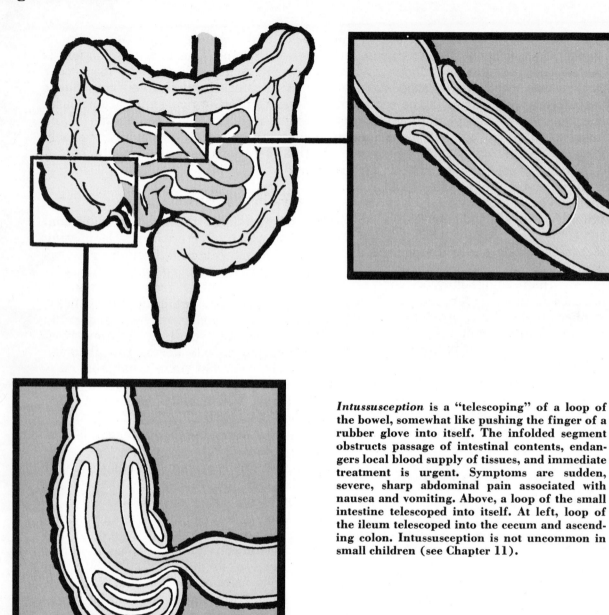

Intussusception is a "telescoping" of a loop of the bowel, somewhat like pushing the finger of a rubber glove into itself. The infolded segment obstructs passage of intestinal contents, endangers local blood supply of tissues, and immediate treatment is urgent. Symptoms are sudden, severe, sharp abdominal pain associated with nausea and vomiting. Above, a loop of the small intestine telescoped into itself. At left, loop of the ileum telescoped into the cecum and ascending colon. Intussusception is not uncommon in small children (see Chapter 11).

Regional Enteritis

Regional enteritis is an inflammatory disease which involves the small bowel and is manifested by diarrhea, abdominal cramping, pain, fever, anemia, and weight loss. It is of unknown cause, although in some cases allergy or hypersensitivity factors appear to be involved.

Usually the inflammation begins in the terminal ileum and spreads towards the jejunum. There may be numerous "skip areas," which means that the bowel may not be wholly involved. The inflammation frequently leads to narrowing of the bowel, or stricture formation.

The diagnosis of regional enteritis is suggested by a history of diarrhea, which may be bloody, abdominal pain and fever, and at times a palpable mass in the right lower abdomen in the region of the appendix. X-ray examination will show a thickened, inflamed small bowel with an area of stricture. Some areas of stricture are so pronounced that they give the appearance of a "string."

Treatment is medical: a strict, bland diet, avoidance of allergens if allergy is a contributing factor. Sulfa drugs or antibiotics may be of benefit. ACTH or cortisone and its derivatives are of use in severe cases. In general, physical and emotional rest are important to the patient. Surgical operation is resorted to for complications of the disease.

Specific infections may produce signs and symptoms similar to the signs and symptoms of regional enteritis, namely, diarrhea, cramping, abdominal pain, fever, and anemia. However, in general, these are not chronic, although they may be very severe at onset. The diagnosis is usually made on the basis of culture of the stool and specific treatment depends upon the nature of the organism found.

Malabsorption Syndrome

This syndrome describes the inability of a patient to absorb normal amounts of various constituents in the diet. The symptoms are diarrhea characterized by the passage of soft or watery, greasy, frothy, foul-smelling stools in which excessive amounts of fat are present; weight loss; malnutrition; and secondary manifestations of impaired digestion or absorption such as severe vitamin deficiencies, decreased calcium in the bones, and skin diseases. Accurate diagnosis is essential in order to treat this condition properly.

These conditions fall into two main categories: (1) those in which *digestion* is impaired but absorption is normal; (2) those in which *absorption* is impaired but digestion is normal.

The first type may result from diseases of the pancreas, severe liver disease, surgical removal of a large portion of the stomach, or some disturbance in normal physiology as a result of surgery. As a consequence, foods are not broken down sufficiently to allow the small bowel to absorb them normally. Treatment is directed entirely to the primary disease and the prognosis depends upon the severity and cause of the condition.

Of all the diseases of the small intestine that cause malabsorption, the most common is the **sprue syndrome.** In this condition the intestinal villi, the small finger-like projections of the internal bowel wall, are decreased in number, blunted, and shortened so that the absorptive area available to the digested food products is significantly decreased. When this condition occurs in children, it is known as *celiac disease.* When it occurs in the temperate zone, the disease is referred to as *nontropical sprue.* Tropical and nontropical sprue are quite similar; however, in tropical sprue infection appears to be present.

The diagnosis is made by special chemical tests to determine how effective absorption of various food products is. Upon x-ray examination of the small bowel, an abnormal pattern is usually seen; the most definitive diagnostic method is to cut out a small piece of the bowel by means of a special suction biopsy tube which is passed through the mouth into the small bowel. This specimen is then examined under the microscope for diagnosis.

Treatment. It has been found that these patients respond well to a diet free of *gluten,* a substance that is present in wheat and rye. The patients with tropical sprue may be given antibiotics in addition to the diet. Other nonspecific measures may be a low-fat diet and supplemental vitamins. In certain instances the use of cortisone or its derivatives may be necessary to improve absorption. Other causes of malabsorption are various diseases of the small bowel, such as regional enteritis or tuberculosis, or malignant diseases such as lymphosarcoma. The syndrome may also occur after removal of 50 per cent of the small intestine, or after massive exposure of the small bowel to x-rays.

Tumors

Tumors of the small bowel are rather rare. Benign tumors may produce symptoms of obstruction if they become large enough. Diagnosis is made on the basis of x-ray examination, and treatment is surgery. *Malignant tumors* are more rare than benign tumors, and the symptoms are also primarily those of obstruction. In addition, hemorrhage and malnutrition with increasing weight loss is common. The diagnosis again is made on the basis of x-ray examination and treatment is surgical removal of the malignant tumor with as wide a margin of surrounding tissue as possible.

Peritonitis

Peritonitis is an acute inflammation of the abdomen. The peritoneum includes the outer lining of the bowel and the inner lining of the abdominal cavity. Inflammation occurs when infection is introduced into the peritoneum by direct injury, perforation of the bowel such as may occur with intestinal obstruction or a perforating ulcer, malignancy, or infection. Peritonitis may also occur if infection of the uterus or Fallopian tubes follows childbirth.

The most common cause, however, is *rupture of the appendix* following appendicitis. This produces an acute inflammatory reaction in the peritoneum. The symptoms are nausea, vomiting, and severe abdominal pain. The abdominal muscles become very rigid and are tender to pressure. Body temperature invariably rises. The number of white cells in the blood also increases. Diagnosis is made on the basis of x-ray and physical examinations of the patient's abdomen, body temperature, and white blood cell count. The treatment is generally surgical operation to remove the cause if possible, followed by drainage of the peritoneum and intensive antibiotic therapy.

THE COLON AND RECTUM

Functional Disturbances

Irritable colon, spastic colon, and *spastic colitis* are terms referring to the same condition, which is functional and not organic.

One of the most common causes of lower abdominal pain is the irritable colon syndrome. In this condition the colon overreacts to various stimuli, such as emotions or certain foods. Symptoms may include cramping pain in the lower abdomen, bloating, passing of gas, distention, or a generalized abdominal ache. Results of x-ray and proctoscopic examinations are negative, except for some evidence of increased spasm in the colon.

Treatment consists of reassuring the patient that the condition is not serious, administering sedatives, tranquilizers, prescribing a bland diet, and, at times, giving small doses of atropine or belladonna. Anticholinergic or antispasmodic agents may in some cases be of benefit. When intestinal gas or bloating is particularly distressing, further relief may be obtained by the use of a special "gas-relieving" silicone derivative.

Mucous colitis is a variant of the irritable colon syndrome. Symptoms are the same as described above except that a large amount of mucus (harmless) is passed with the bowel movement.

Megacolon

This congenital condition is caused by the absence of certain nerve cells (ganglion cells) in the region of the sigmoid colon. As a result, peristalsis through this region is not normal and fecal matter backs up, and causes the colon to dilate greatly. It is extremely difficult for a person with a megacolon to have a normal bowel movement. In fact, it is not uncommon for children with this condition to go a month without a bowel movement. Treatment is surgical removal of the segment of the colon in which the ganglion cells are absent. The results are excellent and the patient is usually cured.

Constipation

Constipation is the difficult or infrequent passage of stools. It must be remembered that the range of variability of bowel habits in normal people is wide and that it is not essential to have a bowel movement every day. Constipation may, however, be a sign of obstruction of the

Megacolon ("giant colon") is a congenital condition that may result from malformation of anal and rectal structures, causing mechanical obstruction. The more common form of megacolon (also called *Hirschsprung's disease*) results from congenital absence in a part of the colon of nerve cells necessary for propulsion of intestinal contents. Normal stimulation to have a bowel movement is lacking, and backed-up fecal matter causes great dilation of the colon and distention of the abdomen, as shown in the two figures below.

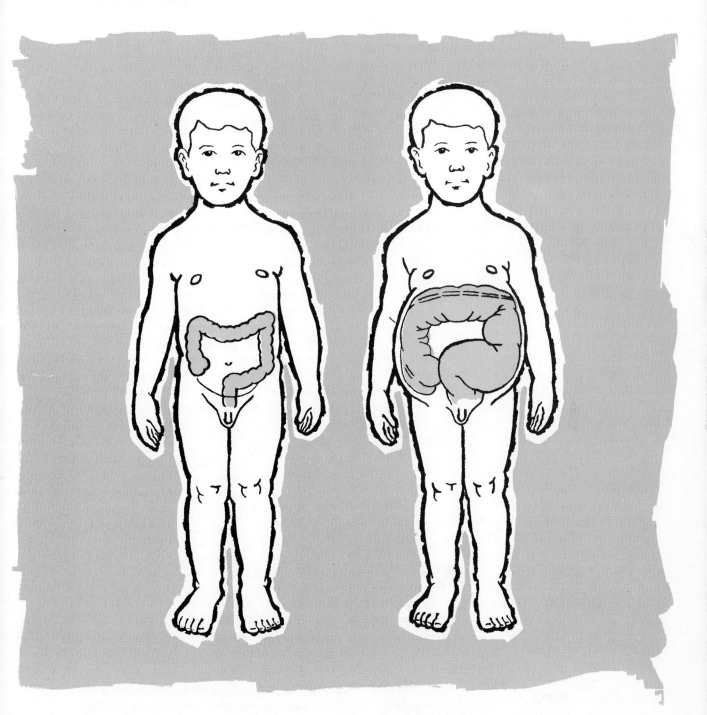

colon caused by a tumor or a cancer. A person suffering from constipation should have a complete physical examination and an x-ray examination of the colon. In most instances, constipation is caused by one or more of the following factors: psychoneurosis, presence of hard fecal material, a relaxed (atonic) colon, and spastic colon. Treatment is based upon the cause. If the cause is neurosis or anxiety, it must be treated with appropriate sedatives, tranquilizers, or psychotherapy.

Diet is of great importance in that certain foods such as prunes, dates, and raisins, exert a laxative effect by means of direct chemical irritation. Other foods, such as cereals and leafy vegetables, provide bulk and thus soften the stool.

In the case of atonic colon, certain stimulating foods or medications, such as cascara or senna, are of benefit. In the case of spastic colon, sedatives and tranquilizers may be more helpful. For those cases in which hard fecal material is the cause, bulk-producing foods or artificial bulk-producers such as methylcellulose and psyllium are effective. Agents such as milk of magnesia or magnesium carbonate are of benefit in relieving most forms of constipation, but since they may cause excessive loss of fluids, they are not recommended for habitual use.

Diarrhea

Diarrhea is abnormal frequency and liquidity of stools. The passage of frequent soft or watery stools may be associated with low, cramping, abdominal pain and a feeling of urgency, or relatively few symptoms may be present.

There are several main causes of diarrhea. Diarrhea may occur as a nonspecific response to numerous agents that irritate the small and large bowel. Diarrhea occurs as a result of many *infections* of the intestinal tract, such as dysentery, or eating of spoiled food, in which case bacteria or toxins from the bacteria may be present. Diarrhea occurs as a result of a partial obstruction of the colon or small bowel, inflammatory disease of the bowel, toxins, certain medicines, or an overdose of laxatives. High on the list of causes of diarrhea are those conditions primarily based upon nervousness and anxiety.

Acute diarrhea may be treated symptomatically with agents such as bismuth and paregoric. If diarrhea persists more than a day or two, specific diagnostic investigation should be undertaken.

The treatment of diarrhea caused by a disease depends entirely upon the nature of the disease. For those patients in whom the condition appears to be a functional disturbance brought on by nervous tension or anxiety the liberal use of sedatives, tranquilizers, and anticholinergic agents gives benefit by reducing the motility of the bowel. Constipating powders such as calcium carbonate or bismuth carbonate are also of benefit. Needless to say, the main treatment must be directed toward the primary cause.

Diverticulosis

This is a condition in which small outpockets form on part of the colonic wall. They are like blebs or sacs. There may be numerous small pockets which give the appearance of grapes. They occur in a weakened area of the bowel wall similar to a weakened area in a rubber balloon or the inner tube of a tire. They are usually multiple and are diagnosed only after an x-ray examination. They are more common in people who have chronic constipation and strain at stool. They cause no symptoms unless there is a complication such as an inflammation or perforation. No treatment is necessary unless a complication occurs.

Diverticulitis is an inflammation or infection in one or more of the diverticula. Symptoms are low, cramping, abdominal pain, and tenderness in the area of involvement. If the condition is severe, chills and fever and development of an inflammatory mass which produces an obstruction of the bowel may occur. Diagnosis is made on the basis of x-ray appearance of an irregular saw-toothed bowel wall and by the clinical history of the patient.

Treatment of acute cases is usually medical and consists of administration of antibiotics and a liquid diet. For people with chronic diverticulitis it is important to develop good bowel habits and to abstain from roughage or irritating foods. In those people in whom symptoms persist or obstruction occurs, surgical resection of the area of involvement is warranted.

Appendicitis

Appendicitis is an acute inflammation of the appendix. The appendix is a vestigial organ of no use to human beings. It is only important when it becomes inflamed and infected. Immediate surgery is then necessary in order to remove this appendage.

The symptoms of appendicitis are pain in the right lower portion of the abdomen, and usually fever and nausea. Vomiting, constipation, and diarrhea may occur. The number of white cells in the blood is elevated. If the correct diagnosis is made and surgical operation is performed within 24 to 48 hours after the onset of symptoms of appendicitis, there are usually no complications and the risk is no greater than in removing tonsils. There is probably no such thing as chronic appendicitis.

The *vermiform appendix* ("worm-shaped") is a small, narrow, blind tube projecting from the cecum. A distended, inflamed appendix, shown on left, may rupture, release toxic materials, and cause peritonitis. The appendix is served by a single artery, and inflammation may impair local blood supply and cause death of tissues (gangrene). Symptoms of appendicitis, especially in infants and children, are not always typical, or discrimination may be difficult. *Laxatives should never be given to a person who has abdominal pain.*

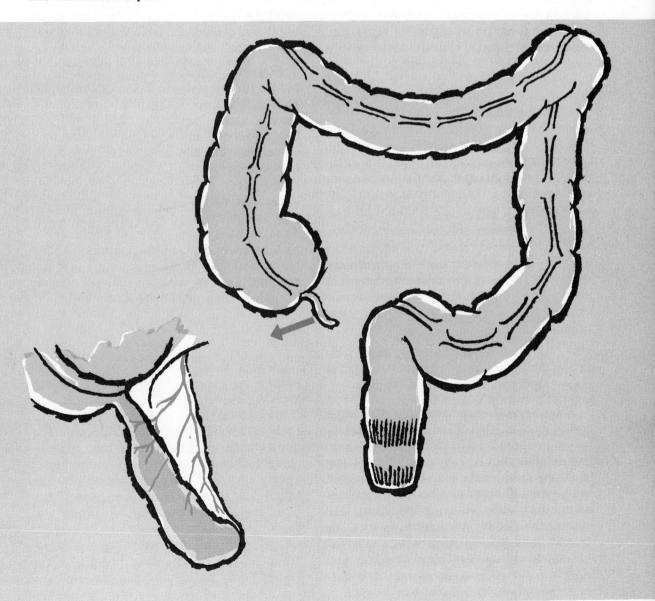

Ulcerative Colitis

Ulcerative colitis is an acute or chronic inflammatory disease involving the colon and the rectum, characterized by bloody diarrhea. It is attended by ulcerations of various size in the area of involvement. The disease may be mild or severe. Complications such as anemia, perforation, generalized infection, arthritis, and skin lesions are fairly common. The cause is unknown but evidence is accumulating to indicate that this may be an allergic or hypersensitivity disease.

A definitive diagnosis is made on the basis of x-ray or proctoscopic examination. X-ray examination of the colon will reveal fine ulcerations, thickening of the colon, a loss of the normal pliability and peristalsis. The term "lead-pipe colon" has been used to describe this appearance. Proctoscopic examination reveals bleeding, inflamed rectal mucosa.

Treatment must be individualized from patient to patient. A bland diet and in some instances the removal of milk, wheat, and eggs from the diet, especially if allergy or hypersensitivity is suspected, may be of great benefit. Various sulfa drugs have been used, but in severe cases cortisone and its derivatives, or ACTH, are necessary and often produce dramatic improvement. The disease is characterized by exacerbations and remissions and may last for many years. It may be of a gradually worsening nature or a complete cure may be obtained.

Proctitis. Proctitis is a nonspecific inflammatory disease confined to the rectum. It is usually caused by some irritation or infection. Treatment depends upon the cause, which is not serious.

Hemorrhoids are probably the most common condition affecting the gastrointestinal tract. Basically, a hemorrhoid is a dilated vein accompanied by clotting of blood or thrombus. It also consists of subcutaneous tissue and skin and is associated with chronic infection and scarring. Most hemorrhoids can be treated medically by improving the bowel habits, avoiding straining at stool, and keeping the anal area clean. Hot Sitz baths and suppositories may be prescribed for acute hemorrhoids. At times surgical excision of blood clots is necessary to relieve exquisite pain. Chronic hemorrhoids that cause symptoms are best excised surgically. (See Chapter 22).

Fistulas. A fistula in the gastrointestinal tract is an abnormal connection between one loop of bowel and another loop of bowel, or the bowel and the skin. This penetration is caused by infection or inflammation and allows discharge of fecal material. A visible opening to the skin may be present. An x-ray examination will reveal the presence of a bowel-to-bowel fistula and its extent. Treatment must first be directed toward the primary cause of the disease. This by itself may produce a cure; however, in other cases extensive surgical excision of the fistula may be necessary.

Fissure. A fissure is a small ulcer or break in the skin in the region of the anal-rectal line. Symptoms are usually severe, sharp, burning, aching pain in the region of the anus, accentuated by bowel movements and persisting after bowel movements. A diagnosis can be made after direct visualization of the area. The cause is usually constipation and the passage of a large, hard stool. Treatment is improved bowel habits; hot Sitz baths and antibiotic ointments may be helpful. For those cases which do not respond to the measures listed above, surgical excision is necessary.

Tumors

Benign tumors of the colon are also known as *polyps*. A polyp is a growth which projects into the canal of the bowel. It varies in size from one-quarter inch to several inches in diameter. The projections may be flat, or they may be marble-shaped and project into the bowel cavity on a thin stalk, or they may be like small raspberries in appearance. Approximately five per cent of adults will be found to have a polyp of the rectum or colon. Small polyps cause no symptoms. Large polyps may bleed and the patient may notice blood in his stool and

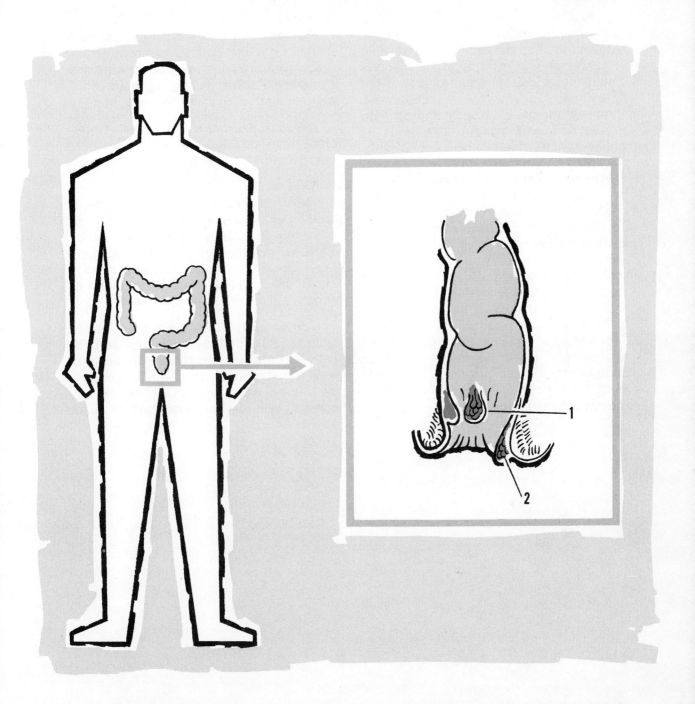

Hemorrhoids (piles) are dilated veins in the region of the anus. *Internal hemorrhoids* (1) originate fairly high in the rectum. *External hemorrhoids* (2), are situated outside of the sphincter muscles that control the outlet.

may have cramping pain in his abdomen. When a polyp is discovered it should be surgically removed because it may grow and obstruct the bowel or it may develop into cancer of the colon.

Malignant tumors. Symptoms of *cancer of the colon* depend somewhat on the loca-tion of the tumor and the rate of growth. If the mass grows slowly, symptoms may not be apparent until evidence of obstruc-tion, characterized by constipation or ina-bility to have a bowel movement, occurs.

A cancerous growth on the right side of the colon or cecum is usually charac-terized by diarrhea, because it interferes with the absorption of water from the fecal material in the colon. The symptom of cancer on the left side of the colon is usually constipation, because part of the passage is blocked off by the growth. Other symptoms may be cramping pain in the abdomen, weight loss, and the presence of visible or chemical blood in the stool.

Many *cancers of the rectum* can be felt by the physician upon performing a digital examination. Cancers higher up are diagnosed on the basis of x-ray examination revealing an irregular mass projecting into the bowel passage, or a constricted segment of the rectum or colon. If the mass is within the reach of a proctoscope, a small segment of the growth may be removed by a special forceps. This segment is examined microscopically to determine whether malignant cells are present. The treatment for cancer of the colon is surgery, the sooner the better.

Parasitic infestations. Numerous parasites may infect the gastrointestinal tract. Symptoms of all such manifestations are similar: cramping pain in the abdomen and diarrhea. (See Chapter 2.)

Bacterial infections with gastrointestinal manifestations such as nausea and vomiting are discussed in Chapter 2.

Nonspecific viral enteritis is a general term for several types of viral disease usually characterized by sudden, severe, acute diarrhea and fever. These conditions are usually self-limiting and there is no specific treatment. Supportive measures as outlined under treatment of functional diarrhea are indicated.

Gastrointestinal allergy is discussed in Chapter 20, but it is important to indicate that allergies to foods may produce severe gastrointestinal disturbances such as nausea, vomiting, diarrhea, or any combination of these symptoms.

NUTRITION

by WILLIAM J. DARBY, M.D.

Recommended Daily Dietary Allowances
• Understanding Foods • Vitamins •
Minimum Daily Requirements Compared
with Recommended Dietary Allowances

DEFICIENCY DISEASES

OVERWEIGHT

Standards of Average Weights in Pounds
for American Adults • Calorie and Food
Composition Table • Reducing Diets •
1200 Calorie Diet • Underweight •
Harmful Excesses

NUTRITION DURING GROWTH

Nutrition in Childhood

NUTRITIONAL NEEDS OF THE MOTHER

Pregnancy

FOOD FADS AND FALLACIES

THERAPEUTIC DIETS

Food Storage

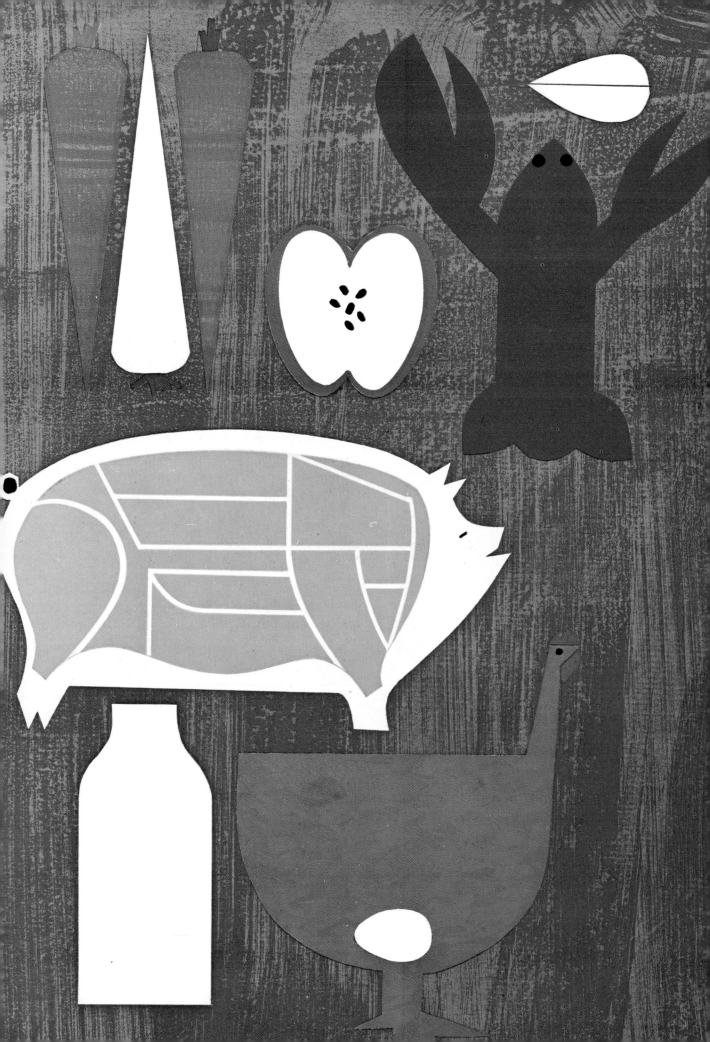

CHAPTER 14

NUTRITION

by WILLIAM J. DARBY, M.D.

Proper food is essential for the maintenance or restoration of health. Disease may result from lack of nutrients, from consumption of a diet unsuitable for a particular disease or person, or, rarely, from ingestion of harmful quantities of unusual substances which may be associated with certain foods.

Nutrients in foods are chemical substances of known composition and structure. They are classified as *carbohydrates* (such as sugar, starch, glycogen) ; *lipids*, loosely called *"fats"*; *proteins* (large molecules which contain nitrogen and are built of amino acid units) ; *inorganic elements or salts* (such as compounds containing iron, calcium and phosphorus) ; and *vitamins*. The latter are a chemically unrelated group of organic compounds needed in trace to small quantities by the body.

Calories. Carbohydrates contain carbon, hydrogen, and oxygen, and their "burning" is the body's usual source of energy for muscular work, body heat, breathing, and other functions. The *calorie* is not a nutrient or a substance, but a unit for expressing an amount of energy. In nutrition, one calorie is the amount of heat energy that will increase the temperature of 2.2 pounds of water one degree Centigrade.

Carbohydrates and fats are the chief sources of calories; proteins may also furnish calories. One gram (one-thirtieth of an ounce) of these nutrients, when burned in the body, supplies the following number of calories:

Carbohydrate	4 calories
Fat	9 calories
Protein	4 calories

It is evident that fat is a concentrated source of calories. Since a gram of fat provides more than twice as much energy as an equal amount of either carbohydrate or protein, it is easy to understand why reduced intake of fats (as rich gravies, cream dressings, greasy foods and fat spreads) is advised for those who are overweight and wish to reduce. *Alcohol* likewise is a concentrated source of calories, supplying 7 calories per gram. Since all of these categories of nutrients can furnish calories, it is evident why the total food intake must be decreased in reducing diets.

Proteins. Amino acids which are linked together to form proteins contain nitrogen and sometimes sulfur in addition to carbon, hydrogen, and oxygen. There are more than 20 amino acids which differ from each other in their structures. These building blocks are linked together in various patterns and combinations in the protein molecule, which sometimes contains substances in addition to amino acids. This makes possible an almost unlimited number of different proteins, much as combinations and sequences of letters of the alphabet make possible an almost limitless number of words. Each protein does not necessarily contain every amino acid, just as different words do not contain all the letters of the alphabet.

The body can manufacture more than half of the individual amino acids, but certain ones cannot be synthesized by the body, at least in amounts necessary for growth and health. These amino acids which the body cannot manufacture are known as *essential amino acids* — essential because they must be supplied by the foods we eat every day.

Drawing shows scheme of carbohydrate, protein, and fat digestion, in numbered squares: (1) some starches and sugars begin to be broken into simple sugars in the mouth by an enzyme in saliva; (2) proteins are partially digested in the stomach, some carbohydrate digestion continues, fats are little affected; (3) in the duodenum, bile from the gallbladder emulsifies fats, and digestive enzymes from the pancreas gland attack carbohydrates, proteins and fats; (4) in the small intestine, elements are further broken down and absorbed.

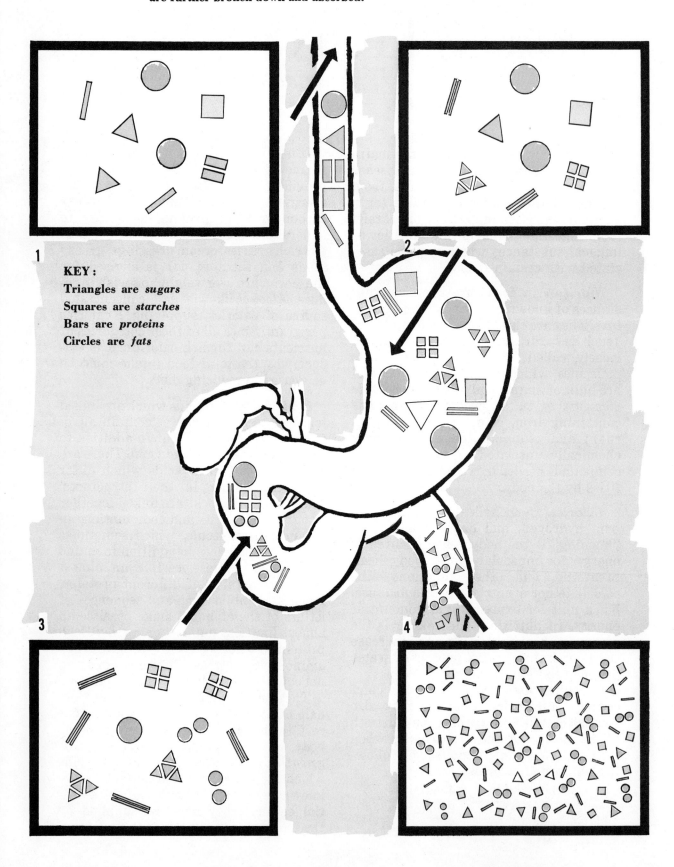

KEY:
Triangles are *sugars*
Squares are *starches*
Bars are *proteins*
Circles are *fats*

The nutritional value of a protein depends on the number and kind of individual amino acids it contains, but especially of the essential amino acids. Dietary protein is broken down by the body into its constituent amino acids and these are "reassembled" to make body proteins. Clearly, the right kinds and amounts of amino acids must be present as raw materials if the body's protein factories are to put together a specific molecule.

Our hosts of body proteins serve many functions. They are parts of the structure of skin, hair, nails, connective tissue, and innumerable other organs. Many hormones are proteins or derivatives of amino acids. The vast array of enzymes in the body are proteins. The word "protein" signifies "of first importance," and one can readily understand why.

Fats are less complex than proteins, but likewise are constituted of fundamental units — fatty acids and glycerol (glycerine). Again, certain fatty acids cannot be synthesized by the body and hence must be supplied by the diet. These are known as *essential fatty acids*. Since their chemical structure is characterized in part by various numbers of chemical bonds which contain fewer hydrogen links than they would if "completely saturated," they are often referred to as *polyunsaturated fatty acids*. Not all polyunsaturated fatty acids are required by the body. The organism breaks down ingested fat and resynthesizes it into fats characteristic of its tissues.

Carbohydrates similarly are broken down and rebuilt in the body. Common simple carbohydrate building blocks are glucose, galactose, and fructose. Numerous carbohydrates and derivatives exist in foods and in the body. We can synthesize from other available materials all the carbohydrate we need. But the body must have sufficient precursors of the many so-called non-essential nutrients to enable it to synthesize the carbohydrates, fats, and proteins necessary for proper functioning. That is one reason why a *variety* of foodstuffs must be consumed to feed the metabolic mill which produces new compounds.

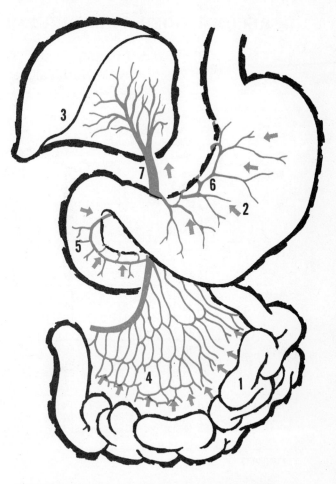

Pathways of assimilation. (1) *Small intestine*, (2) *stomach*, (3) *liver*. The *mesenteric veins* (4), *duodenal veins* (5) and *gastric veins* (6) merge into the *portal vein* (7) which carries many absorbed nutrients to the liver. Most assimilated fats pass into lymph channels.

The body makes many chemical substances by converting constituents of foods. For example, it can transform carbohydrates into fat, or into a portion of the protein building blocks. It synthesizes milk sugar and converts certain amino acids to hormones. However, there are other substances than those already noted which the body must have and which it cannot synthesize. *Vitamins* and required *minerals* must come from diet.

The accompanying table of Recommended Daily Dietary Allowances summarizes the major essential nutrients in foods and indicates the amount of each which is judged to be desirable for health by the Food and Nutrition Board of the National Academy of Sciences—National Research Council.

RECOMMENDED DAILY DIETARY ALLOWANCES (Revised 1968)

Food and Nutrition Board, National Academy of Sciences—
National Research Council

	Age years	Weight pounds	Height inches	Calories	Protein grams	FAT SOLUBLE VITAMINS		
						Vitamin A I.U.	Vitamin D I.U.	Vitamin E I.U.
Children	1 to 2	26	32	1100	25	2000	400	10
	2 to 3	31	36	1250	25	2000	400	10
	3 to 4	35	39	1400	30	2500	400	10
	4 to 6	42	43	1600	30	2500	400	10
	6 to 8	51	48	2000	35	3500	400	15
	8 to 10	62	52	2200	40	3500	400	15
Boys	10 to 12	77	55	2500	45	4500	400	20
	12 to 14	95	59	2700	50	5000	400	20
	14 to 18	130	67	3000	60	5000	400	25
Girls	10 to 12	77	56	2250	50	4500	400	20
	12 to 14	97	61	2300	50	5000	400	20
	14 to 16	114	62	2400	55	5000	400	25
	16 to 18	119	63	2300	55	5000	400	25
Men	18 to 22	147	69	2800	60	5000	400	30
	22 to 35	154	69	2800	65	5000	—	30
	35 to 55	154	68	2600	65	5000	—	30
	55 to 75+	154	67	2400	65	5000	—	30
Women	18 to 22	128	64	2000	55	5000	400	25
	22 to 35	128	64	2000	55	5000	—	25
	35 to 55	128	63	1850	55	5000	—	25
	55 to 75+	128	62	1700	55	5000	—	25
Pregnancy				+200	65	6000	400	30
Lactation				+1000	75	8000	400	30

Vitamins. These nutrients, which cannot be synthesized by the body, are needed in such exceedingly small amounts that it is evident that they are not sources of energy. They serve instead as catalysts for bringing about many transformations and reactions in the tissues. To use a mechanical analogy, a catalyst is somewhat like the lubricant in a car engine — it permits the engine to run smoothly and at a greater rate. The source of energy in the engine is gasoline, not the lubricant. Very little lubricant is consumed in proportion to gasoline, but without a lubricant the engine soon begins to knock and show signs of malfunction. So it is with vitamins. Without a particular vitamin there occurs a given set of symptoms or a recognized deficiency disease.

There is nothing "magic" about vitamins. They do not possess wondrous stimulating properties often claimed for them. A normal, healthy individual needs no more vitamins than he gets from a good usual diet, and the same applies to minerals, including "trace" minerals. Additional intakes of vitamins above his dietary allowances will not benefit him. Supplementary vitamins promoted for self-administration by healthy people are usually of no benefit. Critical studies of such products have shown that in general beneficial effects ascribed to them by persons taking them can be duplicated by giving those same people inactive pills or placebos.

Most vitamins act as co-enzymes— small but essential parts of an enzyme that catalyzes some body process.

The American Medical Association, through its Council on Foods and Nutrition, has considered the usefulness of multivitamins, and in a report in the

The allowance levels are intended to cover
individual variations among most normal persons
as they live in the U. S. under usual
environmental stresses.

WATER SOLUBLE VITAMINS

Vitamin C mg.	Folacin mg.	Niacin mg.	Riboflavin mg.	Thiamine mg.	Vitamin B_6 mg.	Vitamin B_{12} microgram
40	0.1	8	0.6	0.6	0.5	2.0
40	0.2	8	0.7	0.6	0.6	2.5
40	0.2	9	0.8	0.7	0.7	3
40	0.2	11	0.9	0.8	0.9	4
40	0.2	13	1.1	1.0	1.0	4
40	0.3	15	1.2	1.1	1.2	5
40	0.4	17	1.3	1.3	1.4	5
45	0.4	18	1.4	1.4	1.6	5
55	0.4	20	1.5	1.5	1.8	5
40	0.4	15	1.3	1.1	1.4	5
45	0.4	15	1.4	1.2	1.6	5
50	0.4	16	1.4	1.2	1.8	5
50	0.4	15	1.5	1.2	2.0	5
60	0.4	18	1.6	1.4	2.0	5
60	0.4	18	1.7	1.4	2.0	5
60	0.4	17	1.7	1.3	2.0	5
60	0.4	14	1.7	1.2	2.0	6
55	0.4	13	1.5	1.0	2.0	5
55	0.4	13	1.5	1.0	2.0	5
55	0.4	13	1.5	1.0	2.0	5
55	0.4	13	1.5	1.0	2.0	6
60	0.8	15	1.8	+0.1	2.5	8
60	0.5	20	2.0	+0.5	2.5	6

MINERALS

	Age years	Calcium gm.	Phosphorus gm.	Iodine microgram	Iron mg.	Magnesium mg.
Children	1 to 2	0.7	0.7	55	15	100
	2 to 3	0.8	0.8	60	15	150
	3 to 4	0.8	0.8	70	10	200
	4 to 6	0.8	0.8	80	10	200
	6 to 8	0.9	0.9	100	10	250
	8 to 10	1.0	1.0	110	10	250
Boys	10 to 12	1.2	1.2	125	10	300
	12 to 14	1.4	1.4	135	18	350
	14 to 18	1.4	1.4	150	18	400
Girls	10 to 12	1.2	1.2	110	18	300
	12 to 14	1.3	1.3	115	18	350
	14 to 16	1.3	1.3	120	18	350
	16 to 18	1.3	1.3	115	18	350
Men	18 to 22	0.8	0.8	140	10	400
	22 to 35	0.8	0.8	140	10	350
	35 to 55	0.8	0.8	125	10	350
	55 to 75+	0.8	0.8	110	10	350
Women	18 to 22	0.8	0.8	100	18	350
	22 to 35	0.8	0.8	100	18	300
	35 to 55	0.8	0.8	90	18	300
	55 to 75+	0.8	0.8	80	10	300
Pregnancy		+0.4	+0.4	125	18	450
Lactation		+0.5	+0.5	150	18	450

MAJOR VITAMINS: THEIR NAMES, ACTIONS and SOURCES

Vitamin	Other Names	Some Things it Does	Important Sources
VITAMIN A Large amounts can be stored in the liver. Dietary deficiency uncommon. Infants may need supplements before they begin to eat vegetables and egg yolk.	Axerophthol	Needed for growth of bones and teeth; for healthy epithelial cells (skin, mucous membranes); for normal vision (it is part of visual pigments of the retina). Part of an enzyme concerned with production of adrenal hormones.	Preformed Vitamin A occurs only in foods of animal origin; best sources are liver, kidney, eggs, whole milk, cream, cheddar cheese, butter, fortified margarine, fish liver oils. Plant pigments known as carotenes are converted by the body into Vitamin A. Best vegetable sources are dark green leafy and yellow vegetables.
VITAMIN B1	Thiamine; aneurin	Part of enzyme systems that release energy from carbohydrate foods. Necessary for proper function of the heart and nervous system and many tissues.	Pork, including ham, most meats, poultry, milk, eggs, green peas, whole grain or enriched breads and cereals, peanuts, peanut butter, wheat germ, brewer's yeast.
VITAMIN B2 Easily destroyed by light.	Riboflavin; lactoflavin	Essential for normal growth and respiration ("breathing") of cells. Participates in protein metabolism.	Milk (rich source), organ meats, lean meats, fish, poultry, cheese, eggs, green leafy vegetables, yellow vegetables, enriched breads, cereals.
NIACIN Tryptophane, an amino acid of protein foods, can be converted into niacin by the body.	Nicotinic acid; nicotinamide; pellagra preventive factor	Participates in enzyme systems that convert food into energy. Prevents pellagra.	Liver, lean meats, enriched or whole grain breads and cereals, poultry, fish, peanuts, potatoes, milk.
PANTOTHENIC ACID	Filtrate factor	Needed for synthesis of adrenal hormones, production of antibodies, healthy nervous system and integrity of many tissues.	Widely distributed in virtually all plant and animal tissues; ordinary diet provides enough. Good sources are liver, meat, eggs, green leafy vegetables, nuts, whole grain cereals.
VITAMIN B6 Human requirements not established; average diets furnish enough.	Pyridoxine, Pyridoxamine, Pyridoxal	Participates in metabolism of amino acids, fatty acids, and protein synthesis. Necessary for synthesis of adrenal hormones, blood cells.	Meat, liver, vegetables, whole grain cereals, bran.
VITAMIN B12 The molecule is biologically unique, in that it contains cobalt.	Cobalamin; cyanocobalamin.	Needed for normal development of red blood cells, prevention of pernicious anemia, health of nervous system, proper growth.	Food of animal origin; lean meat, fish, oysters, milk.
FOLIC ACID Dietary deficiencies rare	Pteroylglutamic Acid	Needed for formation of red blood cells and proper intestinal functioning	Most common foods contain the vitamin. Good sources are green leafy vegetables and meats.
VITAMIN C Daily needs relatively large.	Ascorbic Acid	Participates in adrenal gland functions, use of some protein elements, absorption of iron, formation of collagen framework of bones and teeth, integrity of blood vessels.	Found in most fresh plant foods; most abundant in tart "acid" fruits. Good sources are fruits, juices, berries, dark green leafy vegetables, broccoli, peppers, cabbage, new potatoes.
VITAMIN D Produced by action of ultraviolet rays on substances in the skin.	Calciferol, Viosterol, Ergocalciferol	Needed for normal bone growth, proper use of calcium and phosphorus. Prevents rickets.	Small amounts in eggs, tuna, salmon, sardines, herring. Substantial amounts in fish livers, irradiated milk and other fortified foods.
VITAMIN E	Tocopherol	Protects Vitamin A from destruction by oxidation, necessary for normal red blood cells, appears to prevent abnormal changes in fatty tissues.	Provided in ordinary diets. Good sources are whole grain cereals, lettuce, vegetable oils, wheat germ.
VITAMIN K	Menadione; coagulation vitamin	Enables the liver to form substances that help blood to clot.	Normally furnished by intestinal bacteria that synthesize it. Leafy vegetables are good food sources.

Journal of the American Medical Association it recognizes that the usual source of vitamins is food and that all of the nutrients essential to health in the normal individual are supplied by adequate diets which meet the recommended dietary allowances of the table on page 496. There are, of course, certain well recognized medical needs for vitamin supplementation that will be discussed later.

Understanding Foods

Some understanding of the nutritive value of foods is essential in planning proper meals and developing good dietary habits. But it is not necessary to remember in minute detail the amount of nutrients in individual foods or groups. It is sufficient to know that foods of certain groups are similar in their content of major nutrients, and to recognize the group to which various foods belong.

One might classify foods into many groups. But as a practical matter of diet planning and education, a *convenient guide to the composition of an adequate diet* is that prepared by the U. S. Department of Agriculture, in which common foods are divided into four basic groups,

each of which has similar nutritive values. Selection of foods as indicated in the accompanying table provides adequate amounts of important nutrients more or less automatically.

This plan will supply an adult with one-half to two-thirds of his calorie allowance, four-fifths of his iron and thiamine, nine-tenths of his niacin, and all of his riboflavin allowances. Other foods normally included in the daily intake but not specifically mentioned in the plan raise the supply of these nutrients to the recommended allowances and provide other nutrients as well. These foods include such items as butter, margarine, other fats and oils, sugars, desserts, jellies, and unenriched grain products.

The *milk group* provides abundant quantities of excellent quality protein, calcium, and riboflavin, as well as good portions of several other nutrients. Indeed, milk contains significant amounts of most of the nutrients required by man except iron and variable amounts of Vitamins A, C, and D. For practical purposes one may use whole milk, buttermilk, skim milk, or cottage cheese interchangeably in a mixed diet. Hard cheeses

"FOOD GROUP PLAN" FOR INSURING ADEQUATE DIETS

MILK GROUP
(some milk daily)

Children	3 to 4 cups
Teenagers	4 or more cups
Adults	2 or more cups
Pregnant women	4 or more cups
Nursing mothers	6 or more cups

(Cheese and ice cream can replace part of the milk)

VEGETABLE-FRUIT GROUP
(four or more servings)

Including:

A dark green or deep yellow vegetable, important for Vitamin A, at least every other day.

A citrus fruit or other fruit important for Vitamin C, daily.

Other fruits and vegetables including potatoes.

MEAT GROUP
(two or more servings)

Including beef, veal, pork, lamb, poultry, fish, eggs, with dry beans and peas and nuts as alternates.

BREAD-CEREALS GROUP
(four or more servings)

Whole grain, enriched, restored.

and ice cream may be considered equivalent for some of the milk group portions.

The *meat group* includes all lean red meats, specialty meats, fish, eggs, poultry, and dried legumes (beans, peas) or nuts. All of these foods are rich in good quality protein, contain some fat, and provide good supplies of thiamine, niacin, riboflavin and iron, among other nutrients. Meats, especially organ meats, are good sources of Vitamin B_{12}.

Vegetables and fruits are important sources of Vitamin A and carotene, of Vitamin C, and provide significant quantities of riboflavin, thiamine, calcium, iron, and folic acid.

Breads and cereals provide a highly acceptable source of calories, with B vitamins and protein as well as iron.

For those who wish to determine calories and amounts of nutrients of various foods in greater detail, a table of food composition is given on page 507. Figures in this table are for foods as consumed, and have taken into account the expected loss of nutrients in food preparation.

Effects of cooking on food values have been widely studied. In most cases there is relatively little loss of nutritional value when proper methods of food preparation are used. The proportion of the original nutrient retained in a prepared food varies with the nutrient as well as the food and the method of preparation.

The calorie, fat, carbohydrate, protein, and mineral contents of foods are little reduced by cooking unless there is excessive leaching of some of the water-soluble minerals and vitamins, or unusual dry heat which may reduce the protein nutritional value somewhat. In general, riboflavin, niacin, and Vitamin D are quite stable. Vitamins A and C and thiamine may be reduced during cooking if heating is prolonged and there is free exposure to air. The loss of these nutrients is usually not greater than 25 to 30 per cent.

As a rule, cooking losses can be minimized by reducing the period of heating, using covered cooking vessels, and minimizing the amount of water that is added and discarded.

Canned and frozen foods. Present day commercial canning and freezing processes consistently retain very high percentages of nutrients originally present in the raw product. Indeed, the ability to process fresh fruits and vegetables immediately, directly from the field, allows harvesting of the crop at the peak of nutritional value. This may give greater nutritive value than one would obtain from a fresh fruit or vegetable harvested with primary consideration of shipping endurance, followed by a period of display at a produce counter.

Processed foods. Procedures such as milling remove certain of the nutrients which were present in the whole grain — so does the peeling of potatoes, discarding of organs in dressing meat animals, paring of fruits, and many other acts of food preparation. The milling of wheat, for example, removes the rough outer coat and considerable quantities of fiber as well as the oily endosperm. This enables flour to be stored longer without developing rancidity, and is necessary to supply high grade flour to our urbanized society. Properly milled flour as is commonly available is a valuable foodstuff and its nutritional value is enhanced by enrichment.

Scientific knowledge of nutrition is not only applicable in preserving the nutritive value of foods but allows the nutritional improvement of many. Examples are the fortification of milk with Vitamin D, of margarine and other fats with Vitamin A, the addition of iron to infant cereals, of Vitamin C to apple and other juices, the iodinization of salt, the enrichment of flour and cereal products with thiamine, riboflavin, iron and calcium. A very considerable part of the vitamin and mineral intake of the public comes from enriched and fortified foods.

Other examples of enhanced nutritional quality are the use of protein concentrates in infant foods, breadstuffs and cereals; modification of the chemical composition of some fats to more desirable patterns; and the addition of certain amino acids to enhance the nutritive value of grain products used in foods and feeds. These measures improve our diets and nutritional health.

Modern food technology. Significant advances in the technology of food processing have made possible a wide variety of prepared or partially prepared foods, ranging from "mixes" to ready-to-eat frozen or packaged food. Common foods such as fats and bread now have much improved keeping qualities. Many of these improvements are due to new and better packaging materials and the use of safe chemical additives which prevent fat from becoming rancid (anti-oxidants), retard the development of molds in breads (mold inhibitors), and otherwise improve quality. Vitamin C, for instance, is added to peaches and other fruits during the freezing process to preserve the color of the fresh product.

Such beneficial use of chemical additives to improve foods is very different from practices of half a century or more ago when various agents were misused in an unsafe, deceitful, or debasing manner. Unfortunately, there is failure to distinguish between these two eras among many who lack scientific understanding of such matters. The present day use of chemicals in food (foods themselves are chemical substances) is an essential part of our application of science to human betterment. It is well regulated by responsible food and chemical industries. Legal controls at both Federal and State levels assure constant monitoring in the public interest. This is very much in contrast to the era before passage of pure food and drug laws and the development of scientific knowledge of foods and nutrition.

Vitamins

Sometimes confused with the Recommended Dietary Allowances (page 496) is another set of standards known as the *Minimum Daily Requirements*. These are established by the U. S. Food and Drug Administration for purposes of product labeling. It is these standards which are usually referred to on labels that state that items provide a stated per cent of the minimum daily requirements. The accompanying table compares the two standards.

Supplementary vitamins at certain periods of life, such as during pregnancy and lactation, may be beneficial for healthy persons whose diets are ordinarily adequate. Certain supplementation of the diet of infants likewise may be desirable. Supplements may be of value to persons with prolonged illnesses associated with poor appetite and poor eating habits. In such instances, however, it is important that a physician determine the need and consider the type of vitamin preparation appropriate to the patient's needs.

Vitamin supplements differ in the variety and amounts of vitamins they contain. In some instances the formulas are designed to serve well-recognized uses widely advised by physicians. In other instances formulas may be designed to (a) supplement restricted dietary intakes; (b) to treat individuals who have clearcut deficiencies; or (c) in a few instances to be used for some non-nutritional therapeutic purpose. The latter two categories of vitamins should certainly not be taken except on a physician's recommendation, since toxic amounts of some vitamins, particularly A and D, can be injurious.

The Council on Foods and Nutrition of the American Medical Association notes that an artificially fed infant should receive supplements of Vitamins C and D if the diet does not supply 30 mg. of ascorbic acid and 400 U.S.P. units of Vitamin D. Many prepared infant formulas provide these nutrients, and all of the evaporated milk used in infant feeding in this country is fortified with Vitamin D. Since an intake of this vitamin approximately four times greater than the recommended allowance can cause decrease in appetite and reduction in growth of the infant, the amount of Vitamin D given to an infant should not exceed the supplementation recommended by the pediatrician.

Minimum Daily Requirements Compared with Recommended Dietary Allowances

Vitamin	M. D. R. Adults	R. D. A. Man, Aged 25	M. D. R. Children, 6-11 Yr.	R. D. A. Children 9-12 Yr.
Vitamin A, U. S. P. units	4,000	5,000	3,000	4,500
Thiamine, mg.	1.0	1.4	0.75	1.1-1.3
Riboflavin, mg.	1.2	1.7	0.9	1.3-1.4
Vitamin C, mg.	30	60	20	40
Vitamin D, U. S. P. units	400	——	400	400

Healthy children who are fed adequate wholesome foods need no supplemental vitamins except Vitamin D. This is provided in adequate amounts throughout the growth period if the child consumes one and a half to two pints daily of Vitamin D-fortified milk. Relative to other vitamins, the Council on Foods and Nutrition of the American Medical Association "believes that preparations containing the B-complex are not needed for routine use but would be of value for children with special problems. *It is important that the growing child be introduced to a wide variety of wholesome foods*, since food is the normal source of nutrients."

Many supplements are mixtures of minerals with vitamins. The same Council report comments concerning these that "although certain supplemental vitamin mixtures with calcium, iron, or with both minerals have proved useful, there is no good evidence to support the inclusion of the 12 or more mineral elements essential for man. Few of these minerals are likely to be lacking even in restricted diets. When iron is needed as a dietary supplement, it should be given as such in most instances . . . "

Overdosage. Ingestion of excessive amounts of fat-soluble Vitamins A and D and of carotene (an orange pigment which can be converted into Vitamin A in the body) is potentially hazardous since these vitamins are not readily excreted and tend to accumulate in the body. Thus, children who receive an overdose of Vitamin A in excess of 50,000 U.S.P. units daily may develop loss of appetite, loss of weight, become fretful and irritable, complain of itching of the skin, and develop cracks at the corners of the mouth and of the lips. Loss of hair and changes in bones may occur.

Similarly, a daily intake of 1,800 U.S.P. units of Vitamin D continued over long periods of time may produce loss of appetite, nausea, headache, diarrhea, and lassitude in children, and later, weakness, tiredness, and in severe cases, anemia. Excessive ingestion of carotene, either as a carotene-containing supplement or by overenthusiastic feeding to infants and young children of carotene-rich yellow and green fruits and vegetables (especially carrots, peaches and greens) may result in a yellowish discoloration of the skin, most readily visible over the palms of the hands and the soles of the feet. This discoloration may easily be mistaken for jaundice, but it does not appear in the whites of the eyes.

These considerations emphasize the desirability of properly selected diets as the primary basis of good nutrition and that dependence not be placed upon one or another supplement that may be incomplete, unnecessary, or useless in a given situation, or even, at times, harmful.

DEFICIENCY DISEASES

Lack of any essential nutrient over an extended period can so deplete body stores that injury results. The body normally stores enough vitamins to see it through brief periods of dietary deprivation. For all vitamins, normal stores may be depended upon to maintain an adult for several weeks and a child for a few weeks. In the case of Vitamins A, D, and B_{12}, the normal stores of a well fed person are so large that months or years may pass before deficiency signs are manifest.

Severe classic deficiency diseases, especially those due to lack of a vitamin, have largely disappeared from the United States. Important deficiency diseases which may occur in this country or are of wide international concern at present include the following:

Calorie deficiency is semi-starvation and is recognizable as excessive leanness, and in children, growth retardation. It may be accompanied by other symptoms such as lack of appetite, lassitude, easy fatigability, other evidences of chronic disease. It may be secondary to chronic illness (rheumatic fever, tuberculosis, psychologic illness and hyperactive thyroid), in which case its correction depends largely upon recognition and treatment of the primary disease.

Protein deficiency as it most often occurs is really a lack of both protein and calories. The most severe form, known as *kwashiorkor,* occurs in infants and children between the ages of six months and four or five years. It is rare in the United States and Europe.

Kwashiorkor develops in infants and children who are fed exclusively on diets high in carbohydrates and low in protein or with protein of poor quality. Such diets consist principally of sugar, corn, manioc flour, plantain, or other single cereal or starchy tuber. Since the nutritional value of proteins depends on their amino acid composition, which varies from one protein to another, the nutritive value of a *combination* of proteins eaten at one meal is superior.

Scurvy. A lack of Vitamin C or ascorbic acid results in scurvy, a disease in which small blood vessels are easily ruptured, giving rise to small to large red spots under the skin at sites of trauma and to swollen red gums which bleed easily. Scurvy is rare in the United States due to the widespread use of fruits, juices, and vegetables, and the early introduction of fruits and vegetables into the diet of the infant. However, it is still seen in the rare "tea and toast granny," the low income bachelor who lives alone, or the occasional person with unduly restricted diet.

It is usually seen in bottle-fed infants of 6 to 18 months whose mothers have failed to supplement their diet with fruits, juices, or vegetables. Some cases have resulted from the mistaken belief that an orange-flavored drink is identical with orange juice.

Rickets is a disease due to lack of Vitamin D, which results in poor absorption of calcium from food and consequent improper mineralization of bone. In severe cases the soft bones are deformed and may even suffer fractures. Tetany (spasms of the muscles) may occasionally occur.

The rarity of rickets in the United States may be attributed largely to the wide availability of canned evaporated milk or fresh homogenized milk fortified with Vitamin D. Such milk provides 400 units of the vitamin per quart of fresh milk or of reconstructed canned or dried milk. For many years, pediatricians have also recommended supplementary oil preparations containing Vitamin D during the first few months of life. The latter practice is still common although many infants get adequate Vitamin D in their milk-based formula. This duplication of sources may lead to unnecessarily high intake of the vitamin. If unusually large amounts of the vitamin are taken, calcium is laid down in abnormal amounts in parts of the body, including the kidneys.

Foods are not the sole source of Vitamin D. This nutrient is formed from precursors in the skin under the influence of certain ultraviolet wavelengths of light. These wavelengths are present in unfiltered sunlight. Hence, direct exposure to the sun increases the body's supply of this vitamin and helps to prevent rickets.

Vitamin A deficiency. This vitamin is necessary for proper functioning of the light-sensitive retina of the eye, and is involved in the visual mechanism which makes it possible to distinguish various shades of gray. A deficiency of this vitamin is manifested as "night blindness" and reduced ability to adapt to the dark after exposure to bright light. In severe cases, the cornea of the eye (the clear "window" at the front of the eyeball) may undergo dissolution or softening (keratomalacia), and excessive dryness of the eye (xerophthalmia) may be evident. In severe deficiency of this vitamin there may be tissue changes in the respiratory tract, but Vitamin A does not have any anti-infective or cold-preventing properties as is sometimes claimed.

Pellagra and beriberi are usually associated with monotonous diets consisting primarily of corn (maize) in the case of pellagra, or white rice in the case of beriberi. Pellagra occurred widely in the United States, especially in the South, until about 1940, but is now a rare disease in this country, seen only in persons with bizarre food habits, alcoholics, or in rare medical situations. Pellagra results from a lack of nicotinic acid or its precursor amino acid (tryptophane) in the diet; beriberi, from a lack of thiamine, (Vitamin B_1). Often associated with these deficiencies is that of another B vitamin, riboflavin.

Pellagra is manifest by rough, thickened, or blisterlike lesions of the skin of the hands, feet, and face, soreness of the mouth and tongue, and other symptoms. Riboflavin deficiency also produces lesions of the lips and tongue. Beriberi produces changes in nerves of the extremities, especially the legs, often with some loss of motor function; edema; and increase in size of the heart and cardiac failure. Some psychological changes may occur in either beriberi or pellagra, but

neither niacin nor thiamine should be thought of as specific remedies for neurotic complaints, "nervousness," or other nerve disorders.

All three of these nutrients are contained in the flour enrichment mixture, and hence enriched cereal products make important contributions to total intake.

Nutritional anemias. There are many causes of anemia, only some of which are nutritional in origin. For full discussion of iron-deficiency and other anemias, see Chapter 4.

Extreme deficiencies of essential nutrients can damage many body systems. *Beriberi*, a deficiency disease, may chiefly affect the peripheral nervous system (below), with early symptoms of tingling of the hands and feet and weakness of the legs, or heart damage may be sudden and predominant.

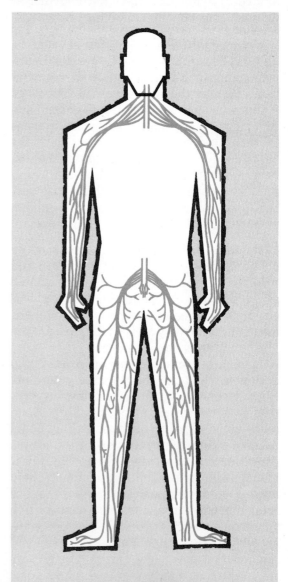

Iodine deficiency leads to an enlargement of the thyroid gland in the neck known as simple goiter. For discussion, see Chapter 9.

Dental caries, or tooth decay, is associated with the quality of the diet. For full discussion, see Chapter 15.

Water and salt deficiencies. When loss of water from the body is excessive relative to intake, one may become dehydrated. This is particularly likely to occur in infants and young children during acute bouts of diarrhea and vomiting, especially in hot weather or in tropical climates. It is to be guarded against by offering frequent dilute clear liquids (tea, carbonated beverages, juices, clear broth, bouillon) and water.

Patients with diarrhea and vomiting, especially infants, may become deficient in potassium. Replacement of this salt requires careful medical supervision.

Under conditions of strenuous physical effort with profuse sweating in hot environments, sufficient salt (sodium chloride) may be lost to create a salt deficiency. This condition is characterized by weakness, abdominal cramps, and faintness, and will be relieved by taking salt tablets or other forms of ordinary salt. On the other hand, excessive intake of salt can be harmful. It is especially important to guard against accidental administration of large amounts of salt to young infants, as may happen by accidentally giving salt instead of sugar because of similar containers. It is safest in the home to keep salt in its original package or in an obvious container such as a salt shaker.

OVERWEIGHT

Obesity is an excessive proportion of fat in the body. A practical index of obesity is body weight in relation to height and age. In a few diseases there is a tendency for the body to retain excessive amounts of water, with an increase in weight which does not indicate excessive body fat, but edema. Such changes are readily recognized, usually by the subject but certainly by his physi-

Standards of Average Weights in Pounds for American Adults

Applicable from 25 years of age
(Adapted from Build and Blood Pressure Study, Society of Actuaries, 1959)

Height ft. in.	Women (pounds)	Men (pounds)
4' 10"	104	
11"	107	
5' 0"	110	125
1"	114	128
2"	117	131
3"	120	135
4"	123	138
5"	127	142
6"	131	145
7"	134	148
8"	138	152
9"	142	156
10"	146	160
11"	151	164
6' 0"	156	169
1"		173
2"		178
3"		182
4"		186

cian, as being different from obesity. In women of reproductive age there may be relatively small cyclic increases in body weight for a few days before the onset of the menses, due to water retention. This premenstrual edema does not reflect an increase in body fat.

What constitutes "normal" or standard weight? When does one begin to consider weight excessive? For reasons to be discussed later, the average weight of men and women in their mid-twenties — approximately 25 years of age — is a better "yardstick" than the changing averages in later years of life. The accompanying table based on a recent study does not attempt to make allowances for different body builds. Most people don't know accurately whether they have a "heavy," "medium," or "light" skeleton and musculature. Weight that is ten per cent greater or less than the figures given in the table may be quite in keeping with the physical characteristics of a given individual.

Overweight children. A study of draft records during the last war showed that a greater percentage of boys who as children were ten percent or more overweight were physically acceptable for the draft than those who were underweight or average in weight as youngsters. This would imply that for children the maintenance of average weight or slightly overweight may not be harmful and may even be beneficial as they become adults. Nevertheless, even for children, gross overweight of 20 per cent or more is undesirable, if for no other reason than a tendency for them to feel set apart from their social group. Gross obesity in children is frequently a sign of maladjustment which of itself requires attention.

Overweight adults. A great body of evidence points to the undesirability of following the average trend to accumulate weight gradually from the age of 25 years onward. Over the years this may "pile on" six to 10 per cent more weight than the average weight at age 25. The weight gain reflects increased fat content of the body, and is due to failure to restrict calorie intake to the level of calorie expenditure.

Body fat cannot accumulate if the intake of calories just equals the expenditure of energy. *To gain weight one must consume more calories than are expended.*

For most people, their basic expenditure of energy — maintaining body temperature, circulation, digestion and breathing — is the largest component of total energy (or calorie) expenditure. The amount of calories needed to maintain these basal functions decreases with age, but often there is not a similar decrease in appetite and the individual consumes calories in excess of his energy requirements. This accounts in large part for the average increase in weight from the late twenties onward.

Exercise. There are wide differences in the number of calories expended in exercise. A sedentary office worker may expend 400 or so calories a day in his activities, while a man doing hard labor may expend three times that many calories or more. The average adult in today's society seldom exercises in a manner comparable to an athletic teenage boy or laborer of yesterday. Unfortunately, the appetite-regulating mechanism does not usually reduce food intake to the level of lessened energy expenditure, and excessive calories are converted into fat and stored in the body.

Vital statistics reveal that the mortality rate is lowest for adults who are five to ten per cent below average weight. This relationship is quite striking with respect to a number of specific diseases. All such evidence points to the desirability of maintaining body weight at approximately that which is standard or average for the population at age 25.

Prevention of obesity is easier and probably more beneficial to long-term health than reduction of excess weight. Prevention is accomplished by modest adjustments in diet and exercise. It is relatively easy to remove or "keep off" two to five pounds of body fat by some reduction of calorie intake and comparatively mild exercise such as walking, swimming, or participation in sports. Riding around a golf course instead of walking, or lying on a beach instead of swimming, should not be mistaken for active participation.

Conscious efforts to increase activity should be made. For instance, make it a rule to walk upstairs instead of taking an elevator, to walk an additional two miles a day, to mow the lawn yourself instead of hiring it done. At times a program of exercise in a supervised gymnasium may be desirable to insure regular activity. Exercise not only increases caloric expenditure but improves fitness and muscle tone and, when part of an enjoyed hobby, provides mental relaxation.

CALORIE AND FOOD COMPOSITION TABLE

Short method of dietary analysis. Values for servings take account of cooking losses. Where listings mention, for instance, "add 1 serving of fat," add calorie and other values for that item to the food listed. Compute values of mixed dishes (e.g., macaroni and cheese) on basis of foods in the combination. Adapted from Vanderbilt Food Composition Tables.

FOOD	Calories	MINERALS				VITAMINS			
		Calcium (gm.)	Phosphorus (gm.)	Iron (mg.)	Vit. A (I. U.)	Vit. C (mg.)	Thiamine (mg.)	Riboflavin (mg.)	Niacin (mg.)
CEREAL PRODUCTS									
(Refined)									
1 slice bread (1 oz.)	80	.01	.02	.2	—	—	.02	.02	.3
½ cup cooked cereal and cereal products									
½ - 1 cup prepared cereal									
3 soda crackers									
1½ cups popcorn									
1 griddle cake									
whole grain and enriched:									
1 slice bread	80	.02	.03	.6	—	—	.07	.04	.6
½ cup cooked cereal									
½ - 1 cup prepared cereal									
2 graham crackers									
DAIRY PRODUCTS									
1 tsp. butter	35	—	—	—	165	—	—	—	—
1 cu. in. Cheddar type cheese	125	.22	.15	.3	420	—	.01	.13	—
½ cup cottage cheese, skim	95	.10	.19	.3	20	—	.02	.31	.1
⅛ cup light cream (for heavy cream, add ½ serving butter)	60	.03	.02	—	250	—	.01	.04	—
½ cup custard	150	.15	.16	.6	440	—	.06	.26	.1
1 medium egg	80	.03	.10	1.4	570	—	.05	.14	.1
½ cup ice cream	165	.10	.08	.1	420	1	.03	.15	.1
1 cup skim or buttermilk	85	.30	.23	.2	—	2	.10	.43	.2
1 cup whole milk	165	.28	.22	.2	385	2	.10	.41	.2
DESSERTS									
1 piece plain, chocolate cake, 2½ x 2½ x 2½, (2½ oz.); for iced, add 1 serving sweets	250	.09	.10	.4	140	—	.02	.06	.2
1 waffle, 6 in. diameter (2 oz.)									
2½ doughnuts, cake type (add 1 serving fat)									
2 medium plain cookies	175	.01	.03	.4	100	—	.02	.02	.2
⅙ single shell pie crust	110	—	.01	.4	—	—	.05	.04	.5
½ cup puddings, cream fillings	150	.14	.13	.1	225	—	.04	.22	.1
FATS									
2 slices bacon (⅔ oz. raw)	105	—	.01	.02	15	—	.03	.02	.4
1 tablespoon fat (½ oz.)									
1 tablespoon mayonnaise (½ oz.)									
1 cu. in. salt pork (½ oz.)									
2 tablespoons French dressing (1 oz.)									

CALORIE AND FOOD COMPOSITION TABLE

FOOD		MINERALS				VITAMINS			
	Calories	Calcium (gm.)	Phosphorus (gm.)	Iron (mg.)	Vit. A (I. U.)	Vit. C (mg.)	Thiamine (mg.)	Riboflavin (mg.)	Niacin (mg.)
FISH									
1 medium serving cooked cod, haddock	55	.01	.15	.4	—	1	.04	.06	1.6
1 medium serving tuna (2 oz.)	115	.01	.19	.8	60	—	.04	.06	6.0
1 medium serving cooked halibut, herring, whitefish (2½ oz.)									
1 medium serving canned salmon	125	.11	.23	.8	135	—	.02	.12	5.6
FRUITS									
1 small banana	90	.01	.03	.6	430	10	.04	.05	.7
½ cantaloupe, 4½ in. diameter	30	.02	.02	.6	5130	50	.07	.06	.8
Citrus Fruits:									
1 medium orange	45	.03	.02	.4	115	45	.06	.02	.2
½ medium grapefruit									
½ cup juice									
1 medium large lemon									
1 fresh medium peach (3 oz.)	70	.01	.03	.6	910	6	.01	.03	1.0
2 - 3 fresh apricots									
3 fresh plums (dried 1 oz.) (for sweetened, canned, dried, or fresh, add ½ serving sweets)									
3 - 4 dried dates	80	.03	.03	.9	15	—	.04	.03	.3
1½ - 2 small dried figs									
1½ - 2 dried apple									
¼ cup raisins									
½ cup other fresh and canned fruits	55	.01	.01	.4	95	4	.04	.03	.2
GRAVY, WHITE SAUCE									
¼ cup	105	.07	.06	.2	225	—	.04	.11	.2
LEGUMES									
½ cup cooked beans, peas; (dried 1 oz.)	100	.05	.13	2.0	10	1	.19	.07	.7
½ cup cooked soybeans; (dried 1 oz.)	105	.07	.18	2.4	35	—	.32	.09	.7
MEAT									
1 medium serving cooked beef, lamb, veal	185	.01	.15	2.3	—	—	.07	.17	3.7
1 medium serving cooked fowl	150	.01	.16	1.7	—	—	.04	.08	5.2
1 small serving cooked liver	125	.01	.29	4.7	32,100	19	.16	2.38	8.9
2 slices cooked sausage, minced ham, dried beef, luncheon roll (1 oz.)	85	.01	.05	.9	—	—	.08	.08	.8
½ cooked frankfurter									
1 medium serving cooked pork, ham	180	.01	.16	2.2	—	—	.47	.17	3.5

CALORIE AND FOOD COMPOSITION TABLE

FOOD	Calories	MINERALS				VITAMINS			
		Calcium (gm.)	Phosphorus (gm.)	Iron (mg.)	Vit. A (I. U.)	Vit. C (mg.)	Thiamine (mg.)	Riboflavin (mg.)	Niacin (mg.)
NUTS									
1 tablespoon peanut butter	90	.01	.06	.3	—	—	.04	.02	2.3
8 - 15 walnut halves									
16 peanuts									
12 - 15 almonds									
12 pecan halves									
SWEETS									
1 tablespoon sugar, jelly, jam, syrup, honey	55	—	—	—	—	—	—	—	—
1 serving plain Jello									
1 serving plain fondant or mint (½ oz.)									
6 oz. bottle soft drink									
1 2 - oz. chocolate coated candy bar	290	.06	.09	1.1	65	—	.04	.17	1.1
1 tablespoon molasses or sorghum	50	.04	.01	1.8	—	—	.02	.03	.6
VEGETABLES									
⅔ cup cooked cabbage	25	.05	.03	.5	90	30	.05	.05	.3
⅖ cup cooked sauerkraut									
1 cup raw cabbage	15	.02	.03	.5	50	22	.04	.04	.2
⅔ cup cooked cauliflower									
½ cup cooked corn	85	.03	.07	.6	195	10	.07	.09	.6
1 large cooked parsnip									
⅔ cup cooked asparagus	20	.02	.05	1.0	1,040	18	.13	.17	1.2
⅔ cup cooked broccoli	30	.13	.08	1.3	3,400	74	.07	.15	.8
⅔ cup cooked carrots	30	.03	.03	.6	12,500	4	.05	.05	.4
½ cup cooked green beans	25	.04	.02	.7	660	14	.07	.10	.5
⅔ cup cooked spinach, turnip, kale, leafy greens	30	.20	.05	2.7	10,400	33	.08	.21	.6
½ cup cooked or canned peas	70	.02	.09	1.8	630	15	.25	.14	2.3
½ large cooked sweet potato	140	.03	.05	.8	8,605	22	.10	.06	.7
1 small cooked potato (4 oz.) (for fried, add 1 - 2 servings fat; for half quantity French fried, add 1 - 2 servings fat)	85	.01	.06	.7	20	14	.09	.03	1.0
½ cup canned tomato or tomato juice	20	.01	.02	.5	1,305	18	.05	.03	.8
1 small fresh tomato (4 oz.) (for 2½ tablespoons catsup, add ½ serving sweets)									
½ cup cooked beets, eggplant, onions, etc.	40	.03	.05	.6	80	8	.03	.04	.3
2 pieces celery	10	.02	.02	.2	105	4	.02	.03	.2
8 slices cucumber									
⅓ head lettuce									

A physician's appraisal will settle the matter as to whether deviation from weight standards is significant. At the same time a physical examination may reveal some disorder that needs treatment. Any moderately sudden unexplained weight gain or loss is an indication to have a checkup to determine the cause.

Reducing Diets

Reducing the number of calories taken in per day is relatively simple, though it usually requires some will power, or perhaps "won't power." It also requires some knowledge of the caloric potencies of different foods so that those low in calories may be consciously chosen. This does not require a precise calorie count of every serving. General knowledge that fats and oils are the most concentrated source of calories, alcohol is next, and that relatively pure carbohydrates such as syrups and sugars provide few nutrients other than calories, indicates that it is important to limit the quantities of these foods in a reducing diet.

At the same time, it is usually necessary to reduce the total quantity of most other foods by taking smaller and fewer servings. Calorie values given in the food composition table on page 507 are helpful in meal planning.

Fruits and vegetables, for the most part, are relatively low in calories, with some exceptions (fruits canned in heavy syrup, vegetables served with oils, and fats). Hence, their intake need not be greatly reduced, and may even be increased by substituting them for a calorie-rich dessert.

Bread and cereals should be limited to not more than four servings per day, and these should be whole grain or enriched forms to improve the nutrient quality of the diet.

Meat, fish or poultry should be included daily, choosing leaner cuts such as leg of lamb, ground beef, lean ground round, lean rump, lean loin of pork, lean well trimmed ham. Cottage cheese, preferably uncreamed, may be used as a meat substitute.

Skim milk, buttermilk, or cottage cheese from the milk group are relatively low in calories due to removal of fat. Since some cheeses and ice creams are quite high in fat, they must be selected with care. "Ice milk" instead of ice cream slightly reduces the calories per serving.

To be avoided are foods such as whipped cream, gravies, cream soups, fried foods, casseroles and mixed dishes, creamed foods, puddings and cakes, and "gooey" desserts. Butter or margarine should be limited to one serving two times per day.

Any drastic reduction of caloric intake should not be undertaken without the counsel of a physician. Weight control requires personal discipline to adhere to a pattern of regular exercise and dietary limitation, restriction of alcoholic beverages, and foregoing of between-meal and before bedtime snacks.

For most overweight persons, a 1200-calorie diet gives gratifying non-drastic weight reduction. It is of course important that the diet provide all nutritional essentials except calories. This is best achieved by a variety of well-chosen foods from the four basic food groups. The American Heart Association suggests that a balanced 1200-calorie diet include the following:

1 pint of skim milk

3 or more servings of vegetables

3 servings of fruit

4 servings of breads and cereals

5 ounces (cooked) of meat, fish or poultry

2 level tablespoons of fat

4 eggs each *week,* not daily

Sugars and sweets to be used only as a substitute for one serving of bread or cereal

A great variety of appetizing, common, and seasonable foods can be included in this framework. Each day's menu can be varied. A sample menu for a 1200-calorie diet, cited from the diet manual of the Vanderbilt University Hospital, is an example. This should not be followed unvaryingly, but is used as an illustration of the principles set forth.

1200 CALORIE DIET

Sample Menu Pattern

Breakfast

Grapefruit half
Poached egg
1 slice bacon
½ cup oatmeal
1 slice enriched white toast
Coffee with saccharin
¼ cup half-and-half

Dinner

2 ozs. roast beef with natural gravy
½ cup quartered potatoes
Stewed tomatoes, as desired
Tossed salad with fat-free dressing,
    as desired
1 tsp. fortified margarine
1 medium fresh peach
1 cup skim milk

Supper

3 oz. broiled chicken
½ cup carrot dollars
Turnip greens with vinegar, as
    desired
Cole slaw with fat-free dressing
1 slice enriched white bread
1 tsp. fortified margarine
½ cup dietetic canned applesauce
1 cup buttermilk

Beverages are sometimes overlooked as a source of calories. Carbonated soft drinks of the ordinary type contain 70 to 100 calories per serving. Coffee with a tablespoonful of cream and a teaspoon of sugar approximates 45 calories. Beer provides 120 calories per eight ounces; wines, 80 to 120 calories per four ounces; distilled spirits (whiskey, rum, gin, brandy) approximately 80 calories per ounce; cocktails, 180 to 220 calories; eggnog, 300 to 400 calories per serving. Unwise intake of beverages may make the difference between success and failure in weight control.

Underweight

Excessive leanness is associated with increased morbidity and may itself be a manifestation of illness which needs guidance from one's physician. A planned program for weight gain should be approved by him. To gain weight is sometimes as difficult as for an overweight person to lose it, and success requires as much discipline as weight reduction.

What has been said about reducing diets is an excellent guide to what *not* to do in dietary adjustment to gain weight. A dietary program to *increase* weight aims to increase the daily intake of calories appreciably above caloric expenditure. This is done by eating more of all food groups, but particularly of foods high in calories.

The fundamental plan for a balanced weight-gain diet should adhere to the basic food groups outlined on page 499. From the *milk* group one should take four or more cups per day of whole milk, augmented by servings of cheese and ice cream. From the *meat* group one should eat two or more servings of meat, poultry, or fish, including the fatter cuts. One or more eggs per day and servings of the meat alternatives can add an appetizing variety.

Little can be done to enhance caloric intake from the *vegetable-fruit* group other than to serve vegetables with creams, butter, salad oils, and to prepare battered and fried forms of appropriate foods, to augment the fat calories. Fruits can be used with sugar or heavy syrup, with the addition of cream whips.

A common difficulty in efforts to gain weight is rapid appetite satiation, or a feeling of "getting filled up too fast." Appetizing, appealing, flavorsome foods may coax the light eater, and developing an interest in foods and their preparation sometimes provides additional motivation. Snacks or extra meals — mid-morning, mid-afternoon, bedtime — effectively increase caloric intake, particularly if it is difficult for the lean subject to increase his intake at regular meals. The snacks can be sandwiches with beverage, milk and egg drinks, milk shakes, and for the accustomed a cocktail at lunch or dinner may be a further stimulus to eating.

Harmful Excesses

Sufficient *overdosage* of at least nine nutrients—Vitamins A and D, carotene, calories, iodine, salt, potassium, fluoride, iron — is harmful. To this list one may add a number of trace elements, such as cobalt, zinc, and selenium, which are required in animals but whose role in human nutrition is not completely defined. Even such familiar nutrients as sugar, water, and certain amino acids are toxic when taken in excess. There is an optimal range of intake of many essential nutrients, and the concept of a harmful or toxic substance *must be related to amount rather than to a particular substance as such*. It is important to consider the toxic potentialities of even essential nutrients before taking supplements or preparations which could increase the intake of various substances far above the level of safety.

Metabolic disturbances may impair the body's ability to use commonplace and harmless nutrients, with the result that harmful breakdown products accumulate in the body and do damage. Several congenital diseases of this sort are known as "inborn errors of metabolism."

In *galactosemia,* the infant has a defective enzyme system and cannot handle common sugars — lactose (milk sugar) and galactose (one of the sugars resulting from digestion of lactose) — with the result that these sugars do serious harm. The infant fails to gain weight, is irritable, the liver becomes enlarged, jaundice may occur, and cataracts develop if the condition is untreated. Other serious consequences include mental retardation. When recognized early this condition may be treated successfully by using special diets or formulas free of the offending sugars.

Phenylketonuria is another "inborn error" which can be modified by diet. Here the inherited defect is absence of a liver enzyme, which makes it impossible for the infant to handle phenylalanine, a common amino acid of protein foods. Certain breakdown products accumulate in the blood, damage the developing central nervous system, and lead to mental retardation unless the condition is detected and treated early. Treatment consists of restricting the intake of phenylalanine through use of a special digest of protein from which the amino acid has been removed, along with appropriate intake of low protein foods (vegetables, fruits) and supplements judged necessary by the physician.

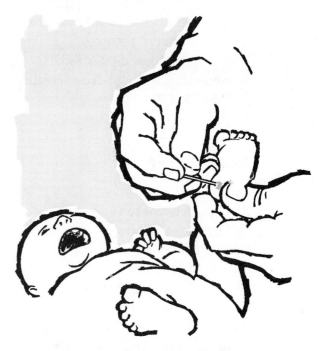

In the *Guthrie test*, a drop of blood taken from a newborn baby's heel and studied in a laboratory tells whether or not the infant has *phenylketonuria* — an inborn inability to metabolize an amino acid of common protein foods. Prompt use of a special diet promises to prevent brain damage in affected infants.

There are many other congenital inborn errors of metabolism, in most of which dietary therapy is of little avail. A rare disorder known as *Wilson's disease* involves a defect in which copper is absorbed in excessive and harmful quantities. Promising attempts at treatment by reducing the copper content of the diet and use of agents which reduce absorption and increase excretion of the trace element are being made.

NUTRITION DURING GROWTH

Growth increases requirements for dietary protein, carbohydrate, fat, vitamins, and minerals in excess of quantities needed merely to maintain the body at a fixed size. Also, during periods of rapid growth the requirements for basal metabolism are higher per unit of body weight than in the adult, and activity—expenditure of calories — is higher, particularly during preadolescence and adolescence.

To meet these large nutritional requirements, the child — especially the older child and adolescent — consumes what might appear to be inordinate quantities of food. But this also applies to infants when one considers relative body size. During early life an infant may consume 50 calories per pound of body weight. If a 170-pound man ate at the same rate per pound he would consume 8,500 calories a day — three to four times the calories that an average man of that weight actually consumes!

Growth is most rapid during fetal development. Simultaneously with rapid growth of the fetus there are growth changes in the mother's body — growth of the uterus and related structures, increase in breast size, and other increases in body tissue. After the child is born the nursing mother provides practically all the nutrients the infant requires during the first few months of life, and this accounts for her increased nutritional needs during lactation.

Infant nutrition. An infant will almost triple his weight during the first year. He consumes somewhat more calories per pound of body weight during the first half of the first year than during the second half. He tends to adjust food intake himself, refusing food when he is satisfied or being satisfied with fewer feedings. The new mother may interpret this as an indication that the baby isn't eating properly and that something is wrong with him, but as long as the infant appears satisfied, healthy, and gains at a steady rate, there is no cause for concern.

Rapid infant growth demands relatively high intake of calories, protein, vitamins and minerals. For the breastfed infant, all of these needs will be met by an adequate supply of breast milk, except for Vitamin D. Neither mother's milk nor ordinary cow's milk is a necessarily dependable source of this vitamin. However, supplementation with Vitamin D concentrates is simple and routine for breastfed infants, and may or may not be necessary in bottle-fed infants, depending on whether the milk or formula has been fortified with this factor.

Foods rich in Vitamin C (orange juice or other juices), or supplements, are usually introduced early, especially if the infant is artificially fed. All types of cow's milk are undependable sources of this factor, and amounts originally present in the raw products are reduced by heat-sterilization procedures.

Thus the usual pattern of infant feeding is early introduction of sources of Vitamins C and D, and usually at a slightly later period, iron-rich foods such as infant cereals, meats, egg yolk, and greens. Failure to provide these additions to a milk-based diet may lead to development of scurvy, rickets, or iron-deficiency anemia. The latter is not uncommon and results from failure to add appropriate foods to an infant's diet of milk. The milk-fed, anemic, iron-deficient infant has been called a "milkaholic," implying addiction to milk to the exclusion of other foods.

Breast milk is considered the most desirable infant food, and the "early" milk (colostrum) transmits some immunologic substances from mother to infant. An adequate amount of breast milk will satisfy the requirements of the infant for approximately the first six months, except for Vitamin D and iron. However, it is desirable to introduce additional foods or supplementary feedings before the sixth month, to assure caloric and nutritional adequacy, to develop acceptance for other foods, and to relieve the mother of regular confining nursing schedules.

Successful breast-feeding is a source of psychological satisfaction to mother and infant, and provides a safe food with less risk of infection to the infant than artificial feeding when carelessness or

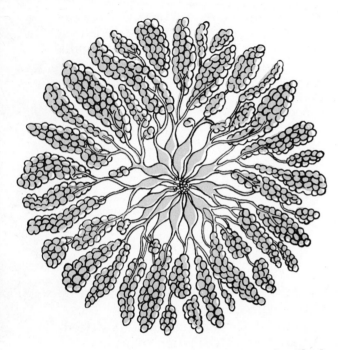

Internal structures of the breast, the ideal source of infant nutrition. The bunched clusters of tiny lobules at the periphery are the milk-secreting glands, draining into ducts which swell into a small reservoir, narrow again, and collect at the nipple. Changes occur during pregnancy which make milk production possible.

circumstances make proper sterilization of formulas difficult.

Artificial or bottle-feeding of infants has been greatly improved in recent years. The pediatrician has a wide choice of formulas suited to needs of individual infants. Milk-based formulas usually use canned evaporated milk, appropriately diluted, with addition of ordinary sugar, corn syrup, starch, dextri-maltose, or rice or barley flour, to adjust the carbohydrate and calorie content. The bottled formula is commonly heated by *terminal sterilization* — that is, the container and its contents are heated all at once — assuring freedom from harmful bacteria and at the same time improving the digestibility of the milk.

Many varieties of prepared formulas are available and may be prescribed by the pediatrician. These are convenient and dependable, but generally more expensive than home-prepared formulas. Various specialized proprietary formulas contain added Vitamin C, Vitamin D, may be enriched with iron, or contain unusual amounts of iron for use in special situations. There are a number of milk-free formulas for infants who are sensitive to milk. Special formulas should be used only on the advice of a physician.

The *feeding schedule* recommended by the physician should be followed. Commonly, these are scheduled at four-hour intervals, but there is considerable acceptance of "demand feeding"—giving the baby his bottle when he is hungry. The time for introducing vitamin supplements and iron-rich foods varies considerably. The trend in recent years has been toward earlier introduction of a large variety of foods such as cereals, egg yolk, pureed meats, vegetables and fruits. As the child's experience with foods is widened, the mother should continue to encourage the use of protein-rich meats, eggs, vegetables and fruits, rather than desserts, puddings, noodles, macaroni and pasta mixtures.

Water needs of infants must not be overlooked. Remember that a baby's requirement for water is relatively high and is greater when more concentrated formulas are used. In warm weather the requirement for water is increased. Finally, the infant is particularly sensitive to losses of water and salts resulting from diarrhea and vomiting.

Nutrition in Childhood

The major nutritional problem during this period is one of developing and maintaining sound food habits despite the pressures and emotional changes which occur in the growing child and young adolescent. Major difficulties include:

Deviations in eating habits induced by conflicts and jealousies, which may lead to rejection of foods and underweight, or overconsumption and obesity.

Establishment of unhealthful food habits. A child may reject meat, milk, or some other important food that he "does not like." This may be an expression of negativism or revolt against parental admonition or some emotional situation, or a reflection of group pressures, such as rejection of milk by a teenage girl because her friends think milk is fattening.

Failure to eat an adequate breakfast. This may result from a too-rushed morning program or poor breakfast patterns in families.

Inadequate lunches and unwise expenditure of lunch money for excessive amounts of sweets, soft drinks, and other items that tend to dilute the nutritional quality of the day's food intake.

Children frequently go on "food binges" and for a period of several meals, eat enthusiastically of some temporarily favored food but reject others. These temporary patterns usually correct themselves unless they are overemphasized by parents to a point of conflict with the child. It is a wise parent who distinguishes between a temporary food binge that will pass and a more deep-rooted alteration in food habits that may become nutritionally harmful.

Informed adult guidance and example are very important in establishing good eating habits in the young.

NUTRITIONAL NEEDS OF THE MOTHER

Pregnancy

Rapid growth during pregnancy enhances the need for diet of high quality to avoid depletion of the mother, prepare her for lactation, and assure the best possible nutritional status for both mother and infant. Increased needs, in general, are met by some increase in milk consumption, use of Vitamin D fortified milk, regular inclusion in the diet of seafoods, fish, poultry, and lean meats, use of iodized salt, enriched bread and cereals, and liberal use of fresh fruits and vegetables. Some pre-natal finding by the obstetrician may indicate the desirability of some specific supplement or alteration in the diet, such as iron supplementation.

Excessive weight gain in pregnancy is not uncommon, during the later months. Weight control in pregnancy by caloric restriction is the same in principle as weight control under other circumstances, discussed under "Obesity"

earlier in this chapter. It is vital that the weight control diet be of high quality, reduced only in calories. As a practical matter, this means curtailment of sources of calories that are not accompanied by particularly good protein and vitamin values — reduced intake of fats and oils, cream gravies, fat meats, soft drinks, sweet desserts and the like. Skim milk may desirably be substituted for whole milk.

Sometimes the physician warns the patient to reduce her intake of salt, usually because of increased retention of water with edema and rapid weight gain, changes in blood pressure, or other evidence from laboratory findings. Frequently the salt intake can be reduced sufficiently by merely refraining from adding salt to food and by avoiding obviously salt-treated foods such as ham, bacon, olives, salted fish and bouillon cubes. (For list of low-sodium foods, see diets on page 32).

Extreme reduction of the salt content of the diet should be undertaken only under the guidance and counsel of a physician, who will institute appropriate checks and perhaps prescribe a rigid special diet and a salt substitute.

"Morning sickness" of early pregnancy (see Chapter 10) may frequently be alleviated by taking a relatively dry, small breakfast and sometimes by eating a small piece of dry toast before rising in the morning. It is not unusual for a certain amount of "indigestion" to be experienced even in late pregnancy. This may be helped by reducing the amount of food normally eaten at regular meals and dividing the usual day's food intake into five or six smaller meals.

Congenital defects. There is a great deal of interest in the possibility of preventing congenital defects in infants by proper nutrition of the pregnant woman. It is well established by animal experiments that interference with nutrition of the developing embryo, from deficiency of certain nutrients (Vitamin A, riboflavin, Vitamin B_6, folic acid), can result in a variety of congenital defects.

These malformations range from defective development of the eye, nervous system, or bones, to death of the fetus.

To produce these defects experimentally, the nutrient deficiency must be adjusted very critically, both as to intake level and stage of gestation. The nutritional level of the female at which malformation can be induced is so low that her general health is not good. If an even greater deficiency is created, the female may not be able to become pregnant or the fetus may die.

A few studies have been interpreted to indicate that a small percentage of human congenital defects may be of similar origin. However, more extensive studies made at such centers as Vanderbilt University fail to show such a relationship at the nutritional level of mothers in the United States.

It seems unlikely that dietary deficiency in mothers in this country plays any significant part in formation of congenital abnormalities in their offspring. Certainly there is no evidence of such relationship if the mother's diet approaches the levels of Recommended Dietary Allowances, and there is no reason to believe that vitamin or other nutritional supplements during pregnancy can reduce the likelihood of a congenitally abnormal infant, in a woman taking a reasonably good diet.

It has sometimes been proposed that malnutrition, especially protein deficiency, is responsible for toxemia of pregnancy — a condition characterized by elevated blood pressure, edema, laboratory evidence of impaired kidney function, and in extreme cases, convulsions. Critically designed studies have failed to sustain this hypothesis. A good diet relatively high in protein is useful in treating this condition, but there is not good evidence that a poor diet is responsible for its development.

Birth size. Is it possible to influence the size of the baby by controlling the caloric intake of the mother? There is some relationship between size of the newborn and the mother's intake of calories. For example, in Holland during the Nazi occupation there was a decrease in the birth weight of infants born to mothers subjected to semi-starvation during pregnancy. It has been found in studies at Vanderbilt University that infants born to obese women have a greater birth weight than those born to women of average weight or less. These influences on birth weight, however, are smaller and less pronounced than other influences, such as body build of the parents, except under extreme conditions.

Lactation imposes similar nutritional requirements as pregnancy except that the need for total calories and for calcium is greater. These enhanced needs can be met readily by increased consumption of the four basic food groups, with special emphasis on milk, meats, vegetables and fruits, in keeping with appetite (unless appetite is excessive). Probably the best guide to calorie intake is weight adjustment. Within four weeks or so after delivery the mother should have returned to her pre-pregnancy weight or slightly above, and should not gain additionally during lactation.

It is usually advised that the lactating woman take an additional pint of milk daily and some increase in fluid intake is probably desirable since during lactation there is an appreciable secretion of water in the milk.

FOOD FADS AND FALLACIES

There are many unsound beliefs about foods. Some of these may be associated with social groups and reflect cultural attitudes or traditional patterns. Various traditional misconceptions, though lacking in scientific validity, do no particular harm since there are many ways of compensating and adapting when a liberal choice of high quality foods in a mixed diet is available.

Quite different misconceptions are promoted by the food faddist, who may be sincere but uninformed, but more often has a financial rather than an altruistic motivation. The food faddist is not new, but he takes advantage of modern methods of communication and exhortation. Frequently he is represented to be an "outstanding authority" or "expert" and does not deny it, although a check of his credentials often reveals an absence of the scientific training he professes to possess. Often he identifies himself with famous or glamorous persons by "name-dropping" at some point in his writings or presentations.

His persuasive pitch may be aimed to convince customers of the remarkable effectiveness of his product, or on the other hand, to view with alarm the disastrous consequences to health of allegedly toxic or "devitalized" everyday foods other than those he promotes. The latter device leads his converts to distrust foods which by scientific evidence are beneficial and healthful.

Some fads and fallacies of the past occasionally reappear in the same or another guise, and new ones arise. Examples of fads and fallacious beliefs include the alleged harmfulness of alum in baking powder; the alleged production of cancer from eating foods cooked in aluminum utensils; the cure of many diseases by eating common or unusual food products; the false idea that calories taken in some particular form cannot produce body fat and hence do not count toward the total energy content of the diet; that one may remove calories from such things as potato chips; that some foods "make fat melt away."

Other examples of fads and fallacies include the notion that chemical fertilizers produce foods with less nutritional value than does "natural manure"; the attribution to certain foods of mystic powers of promoting longevity; the belief that a so-called "natural" food or vitamin is more healthful or beneficial than a processed or synthetic one; the promotion of capsules and preparations containing dozens of trace substances and exotic-sounding components.

Faddish misinformation interferes with building sound food patterns, and may even lead to malnourishment by excesses or deficiencies if the convert slavishly follows a rigid program of limited special products. Harm can be done by harmless and even beneficial foods and products if faith that they will cure some condition leads to delay in seeking medical attention that may be needed grievously. Finally, faddist foods and products are almost always much more expensive than excellent foods and products available everywhere in the open market.

THERAPEUTIC DIETS

Therapeutic diets are modifications of adequate, normal diets, designed to provide for some unusual need of a particular patient. This need may be temporary, such as a period of convalescence from an operation, or it may be a permanent need that continues for years or even a lifetime.

Not all dietary instruction received from a physician should be interpreted as "placing the patient on a diet." In many instances the advised diet may be an aspect of educating the patient as to what constitutes an adequate diet and how to attain it. This is the case when a patient obviously has been following an inadequate diet or when a mother receives advice about feeding of her child.

When, however, some abnormal condition such as peptic ulcer, diabetes, some types of heart disease or other illness exists, the objective is to modify a normal adequate diet to provide for an unusual need of the patient. The patient should regard such diets as redirection of his dietary habits rather than as some special therapy that sets him apart from others. The physician or dietician is attempting to assure the patient of adequate dietary intake with a minimum of inconvenience.

In most situations, a modified diet useful in management of a given condition is not to be regarded as a single measure of cure. Usually a therapeutic diet is but one of the therapeutic measures the physician or dietician employs. On the other hand, diets for weight control, or for elimination of something that is harmful to an individual (as in galactosemia or some allergic conditions) are rather specific therapeutic tools.

The physician may give detailed dietary instructions himself, or he may determine the characteristics of a diet needed by the patient and indicate these to a competent dietician who is especially trained in the field of foods and diet therapy and can effectively guide the patient in establishing his new dietary habits.

Basic considerations which underlie various types of therapeutic diets may be illustrated by examples. The principle of *caloric adjustment* has been discussed in the sections on obesity and leanness. The principle of *elimination or reduction* of a single substance harmful to the patient has been discussed under metabolic disturbances. The same principle is applied in diets used in management of food allergies, the difference being that it is sometimes difficult for the allergist to identify the offending foods. This is usually done by temporary *elimination diets* (see Chapter 20). *Diets for diabetics* are discussed in Chapter 9.

Gastrointestinal disorders. Slightly different considerations are involved in therapeutic diets for treatment of gastrointestinal disorders. Here one is concerned with the amount of food consumed

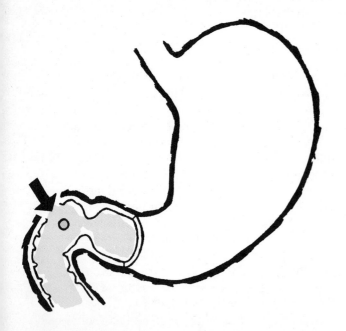

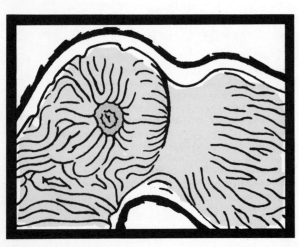

Duodenal ulcer is one of many conditions in which prescribed diets may play a role in treatment. At left, arrow points to typical location and relative size of an ulcer in the duodenum, just beyond the stomach outlet. Below at left, the ulcer surrounded by the normal, many-folded mucosal lining of the duodenum. At right below, an ulcer has eroded through the mucosa and muscle layers almost to the point of perforation. Dietary treatment aims to minimize acid secretion by the stomach and to encourage healing by frequent feedings of bland non-irritating foods.

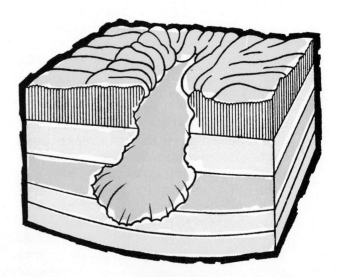

at a time, the texture and physical properties of the diet, and with properties which may influence the reaction of the gastrointestinal tract to food.

For example, the patient with *duodenal ulcer* may be put on a schedule of frequent small feedings of bland foods with little fiber or roughness (see page 32). Such a diet is designed to minimize acid secretion by the stomach and to assure as much neutralization as may be obtained. In acute *gastrointestinal infections* with diarrhea, the object of dietary change is to reduce the overstimulation of the gastrointestinal tract. To this end, relatively small quantities of bland foods are advised, with a liberal supply of fluids through frequent taking of moderate quantities of tea, clear broth, carbonated beverages and the like.

In **gallbladder disease** with attacks of gallbladder colic and in a number of conditions in which there is *poor absorption of fat* from the gastrointestinal tract, the physician may prescribe a diet with reduced fat content. Similar diets may be indicated in some cases where there is excessive cholesterol or fats (triglycerides) in the blood. The principal foods which contribute fat to the diet are *meats, whole milk, butter, ice cream, margarine, lard* and other *shortenings, cooking oils* and *salad dressings.* Any appreciable alteration of fat intake will require reduction in consumption of these fat-rich foods, in such a manner that the diet continues to be nutritionally adequate. In other words, foods such as meat and milk should not be eliminated from the diet, but lean meats, skim milk, and cottage cheese should be used to minimize fat intake from food groups.

Polyunsaturated fats. When the physician judges it desirable to increase the ratio of polyunsaturated to saturated fats, the diet must be designed not only to adjust the total *amount* of dietary fat but also to adjust the *sources.*

Vegetable oils such as corn, cottonseed, soya, and safflower are rich sources of polyunsaturated fats, especially linoleic acid. Accordingly, these vegetable fats may be advised for use in cooking meats, fish and eggs, in salad oils, in vegetables or baked products. If it is judged desirable to reduce the saturated fat in the diet, this will mean a decrease in fat derived from dairy products and meat. Only non-fat milk may be allowed, no cream, and the amount of eggs limited. To make such adjustments while maintaining the nutritional quality of the diet requires professional guidance, since uninformed dietary manipulation may deprive one of some essential nutrient or nutrients.

When a physician advises an increase in polyunsaturated fat intake, it must be remembered that the polyunsaturates are a *replacement* of some of the other fats, not an addition to total fat intake.

Salt- or sodium-restricted diets are frequently prescribed in the treatment of some types of high blood pressure, cardiovascular or kidney disease. Sodium (contained in ordinary salt, sodium chloride) is an essential nutrient and too-drastic restriction can produce deficiency symptoms. It is important that a person on a rigid low-sodium diet be under the surveillance of a physician.

There are three common levels of dietary sodium restriction. The first permits some 1,500 to 3,000 mg. of sodium per day, approximately half of the usual intake. This may be attained by simply refraining from adding salt to foods as served and by eliminating salted foods and condiments. The lower level of 1,500 mg. may be obtained by not adding any salt to foods during cooking or to foods as served. To reduce sodium intake to the commonly employed lower levels of 500 and 200 mg., it is necessary to impose strict limits on both the quantity of many common foods and the kind of foods that may be included. These low levels require careful guidance.

Unrecognized sources may increase the sodium content of a rigidly restricted diet. In some communities, the local water supply may contain significant amounts of sodium, and a number of common medicines contain some sodium.

A rigid low-sodium diet tends to be tasteless and flat. Agents which impart a salt-like flavor but add little or no sodium to the diet have been developed. These salt substitutes are primarily potassium chloride plus ammonium chloride or amino acid derivatives. The formulas vary. It is wise to check with one's physician to be sure that a particular salt substitute is suitable, since those which contain potassium may be harmful or improper in the treatment of some types of kidney disease.

Food Storage

How long can perishable foods stored in a refrigerator maintain "high quality life"? Some approximate yardsticks have been issued by the U. S. Department of Agriculture:

1 or 2 days

Meats: ground meats, variety meats (liver, kidney, brains), poultry, cut-up and whole, fish, leftover cooked meats and meat dishes.

Fruit: berries, ripe tomatoes.

Vegetables: sweet corn, asparagus, broccoli, lima beans (shelled), Brussels sprouts, spinach and other green leafy vegetables, lettuce, green onions, green peas.

3 to 5 days

Dairy products: milk and cream, cottage cheese.

Fruit: cherries, grapes, peaches, apricots.

Meats: fresh meat cuts, cold cuts, corned beef, ham slice, half ham.

Vegetables: cabbage, cauliflower, lima beans (unshelled), snap beans, celery, carrots, tops removed.

1 week

Meat: bacon, sliced.

Poultry products: shell eggs.

Fruit: apples, eating ripe, oranges, grapefruit, lemons.

2 weeks

Dairy products: butter, soft cheeses other than cottage cheese.

Meats: cured ham, whole; dried beef, sliced.

Well-wrapped hard cheeses keep indefinitely at refrigerator temperature. Butter should be stored tightly wrapped. Fresh berries lose food value and spoil more rapidly if washed before refrigeration. Bananas, melons, avocados and pineapples are best stored at cool room temperature. Carrots, beets, and radishes keep best in the refrigerator when the tops and root tips are removed.

THE TEETH AND THEIR CARE

by ROBERT G. KESEL, D.D.S.

What Teeth Are For • Tooth Structure • How Teeth Develop • Timetable of Tooth Eruption • Teething • Shedding the Baby Teeth

DENTAL CARIES

Prevention of Tooth Decay

PERIODONTAL DISEASE

Dental Erosion • Dental X-rays • Abscessed and Pulpless Teeth

DENTURES

Tooth Extraction

ORTHODONTICS

TUMORS OF THE MOUTH

Temporo-Mandibular Joint Disturbances • Pregnancy and Teeth • Dentifrices • Thumbsucking and Other Habits • Halitosis • Fallacies About Teeth

MODERN DENTAL PRACTICE

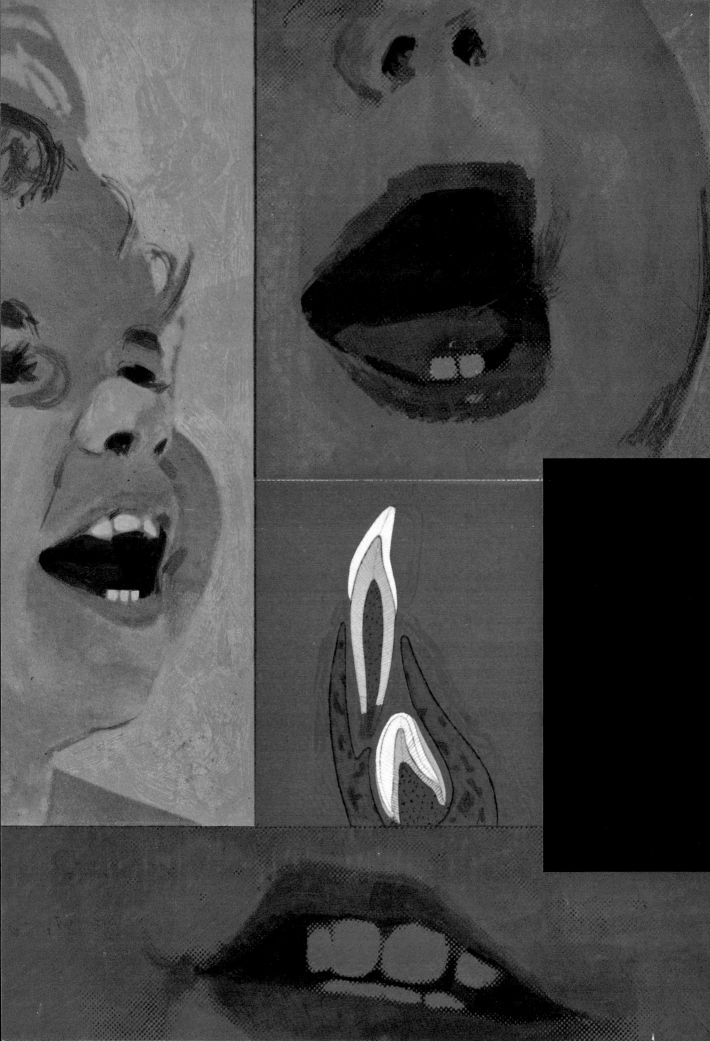

CHAPTER 15

THE TEETH AND THEIR CARE

by ROBERT G. KESEL, D. D. S.

Hardly anyone goes through life without a dental problem of some type. Well over 20,000,000 people in the United States have lost all of their natural teeth. Dental caries (tooth decay) strikes over 90 per cent of our population. Periodontal disease (gum disease, pyorrhea) affects over half of the adult population and is the major cause of tooth loss after age 35. About one-third of the child population could benefit from treatment that corrects the misalignment of the teeth (orthodontics).

Dental diseases and disorders, untreated, lead to toothache, tooth loss, possible health impairment and costly replacement services. New dental tissue cannot be grown to heal the wounds that have occurred. Even when properly treated, the diseases leave a permanent "scar" in the form of a filling, a bridge, a missing tooth, a loss of gum tissue, or an artificial denture.

Knowledge that is now available can do much to reduce the extent of dental troubles — *if it is understood and conscientiously applied.* Such information is given in this chapter for the consideration of everyone who is sensibly concerned about an often neglected aspect of physical and psychological health.

What Teeth Are For

The main function of teeth, of course, is the preparation of food for good digestion. A full complement of healthy teeth permits a wide selection of food and encourages a better balanced diet. Poor teeth may limit food selection to soft, mushy, or semi-liquid kinds that need little or no chewing, and lead to a monotonous diet or malnutrition.

Personal appearance. The "winning smile" depends on good healthy teeth. Many individuals become socially withdrawn because of poorly arranged or unsightly, diseased teeth.

The appearance of the lower half of the face is determined to a large extent by the teeth. The receding (Andy Gump) chin, the protruding (lantern) jaw, the sagging cheeks and sunken lips are the result of misplaced or missing teeth.

Speech. Teeth are important for proper speech. Many of the speech sounds are "shaped" by the position of the tongue and lips against the teeth. People without upper front teeth may be quite unable to speak distinctly. Thus, the mouth with its teeth, tongue and lips is an important organ of expression. Any serious impairment of these organs not only disrupts the first stage of good digestion but can inflict hurtful wounds of the personality.

Tooth Structure

The tooth has a crown and a root. The *crown* is the part that is visible when the mouth is open. The *root* is usually two or three times longer than the crown and it fits into a bony socket in the jaw.

Teeth

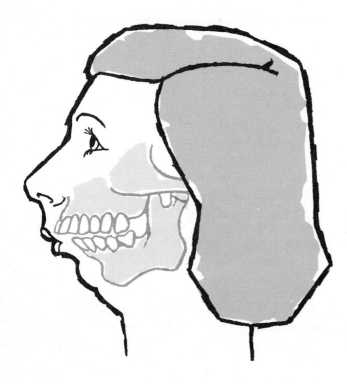

the center of the tooth. This construction provides some elasticity which the harder and more brittle enamel does not have. The small channel that runs through the center of the tooth from the crown to the root tip contains the *dental pulp*. In the crown this channel widens to form the *pulp chamber* and in the root it is called the *root canal*.

The pulp is composed of soft tissue containing small blood vessels and nerve fibers. It contains the remains of the dentin-forming organ and provides moisture to the dentin through the dentinal tubules. If the pulp is destroyed by disease or accident, the dentin dries out and becomes more brittle.

The soft tissue comprising the pulp serves as a cushion which allows slight changes in the circulation of the blood into the pulp without noticeable pres-

Appearance of the lower half of the face is determined to a large extent by the teeth. Improper "meshing" or contact of upper and lower teeth may intensify a receding chin (above) or a protruding jaw; missing, drifted, or malpositioned teeth may distort the shape of the lips, mouth and cheeks.

The root is attached to the bony crypt by a tough membrane or ligament. There is a constriction in the contour of the tooth where the crown and root join. This area is called the *neck* of the tooth. The root tapers or rounds off at its terminal end and this is known as the *apex* (plural, *apices*) of the root.

The tooth is composed of four tissues: *enamel, cementum, dentin* and *pulp*. The hardest tissue in the human body — the dental *enamel* — covers the crown. The root is covered with a bone-like substance called *cementum*. The ends of the fibers in the ligament that attaches the tooth to the jaw are embedded in this substance. The tough fibrous attachment is called the *periodontal* (around the tooth) *membrane* or ligament.

The bulk of the tooth beneath both the covering enamel and cementum is made of an ivory-like material known as *dentin*. The dentin contains many minute tubules arranged in a near parallel fashion that extend to the enamel and cementum from the pulp, which lies in

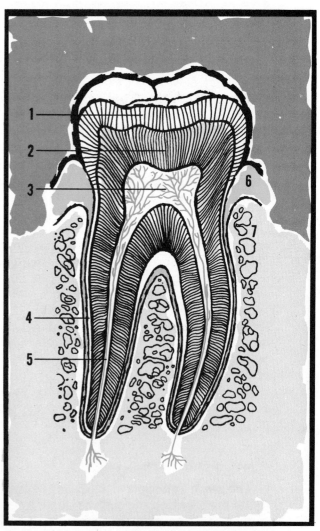

Structure of a tooth in cross section: (1) *enamel*; (2) *dentin*; (3) *pulp* containing blood vessels and nerve fibers; (4) *cementum*; (5) *root canal*; (6) *gum*; (7) surrounding *bone* of jaw. The crown is the visible portion of the tooth above the gum line.

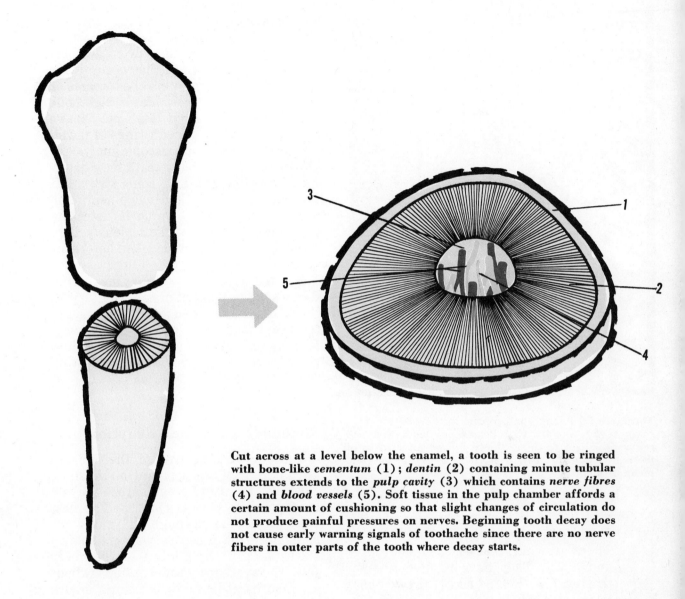

Cut across at a level below the enamel, a tooth is seen to be ringed with bone-like *cementum* (1); *dentin* (2) containing minute tubular structures extends to the *pulp cavity* (3) which contains *nerve fibres* (4) and *blood vessels* (5). Soft tissue in the pulp chamber affords a certain amount of cushioning so that slight changes of circulation do not produce painful pressures on nerves. Beginning tooth decay does not cause early warning signals of toothache since there are no nerve fibers in outer parts of the tooth where decay starts.

sure on the nerve fibers. The blood flow can be altered by the irritation of very hot or very cold food or by the infection that accompanies tooth decay. If the irritation is very severe or prolonged, the pressure that develops, because of the unyielding dentinal wall surrounding the pulp, causes pressure on the nerve fibers. This pressure is interpreted as pulsating or throbbing pain — in short, there is a toothache.

How Teeth Develop

"Baby teeth." We develop two sets of teeth during our lifetime. The first set is called *primary (deciduous, "baby", "milk")* teeth.

There are 20 of them. The four in the front of both the upper and lower jaw are called *incisors*. They have a cutting edge to shear or bite off particles of food. Next in line as we proceed away from the

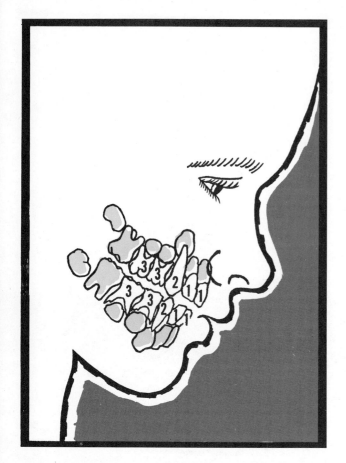

There are 20 "baby" or primary teeth: *incisors* (1); *canines* (2); *molars* (3). Permanent teeth that will replace the baby teeth are shown in color. Early loss of the baby teeth can prevent proper growth and development of the jaws.

Growth rings. The mineral salts that harden the teeth are laid down in microscopic layers or rings, like the annual growth rings of trees. The rings that are forming at the time of birth (known as *neonatal rings)* are more prominent because of body changes that occur when an infant first encounters the stresses of independent existence. Major metabolic stresses encountered later may leave their mark on the growth rings of developing teeth. Thus, microscopic analysis of shed or extracted baby teeth may determine the time at which some stress left its imprint on tooth development, and yield information of value in detecting the causes of some of the seriously crippling disorders that develop before or shortly after birth.

The teeth also are excellent measuring devices of the amount of radioactivity an individual was exposed to during the tooth-hardening or calcifying process. Radioactive mineral elements locked into the growing teeth provide a long-lasting record of the exposure level.

Timetable of Tooth Eruption

Although the crowns of the incisors are fairly well developed at birth, these teeth do not usually erupt through the gum pad for several months. The first teeth to appear through the gums are usually the lower central incisors, one on either side of the midline of the lower jaw. The average age of eruption is about six months after birth. Within a month the lateral incisors usually appear alongside of the centrals. The upper central incisors usually come into the mouth at about seven and a half months, followed by the lateral incisors at nine months.

The first molar teeth ordinarily erupt before the canines, leaving a space between the incisors and the molars. The lower first molars come in at about the age of one year and the upper first molars about two months later. The canines come into the space reserved for them between the sixteenth and eighteenth month and the second molars make their appearance at about the twenty-fourth month.

midline of the jaws are the *canines* *(cuspids, "eye teeth", "dog teeth").* There are four, one on each side upper and lower. They have pointed tips for tearing food. Behind them are two molar teeth on each side of both jaws. The molars have the largest crowns and are so arranged that when the jaws close their broad chewing surfaces mesh together to produce a grinding action.

When a baby is born usually no teeth are visible, but within the jaws there are 20 developing primary or "baby" teeth (eight incisors, four canines, and eight molars). These teeth grow from buds which begin to form about six weeks after conception. Mineral salts, mainly calcium phosphate and carbonate, begin to be deposited in these buds at about the sixteenth week of prenatal life.

The eruption time and sequence vary with the individual child. In rare instances the baby may be born with the lower incisors already visible in the mouth. This may create a nursing problem which must be solved by the pediatrician and the dentist. In some children, tooth eruption may be slow. A delay of three or four months may have no significance; however, if tooth eruption is markedly delayed a dentist or a physician should be consulted.

The primary teeth are important. Some parents assume that these teeth can be neglected because they will be replaced by a second set. This attitude has doomed too many children to becoming dental cripples in adult life. Neglect not only can cause infection and pain from diseased primary teeth, but the early loss of primary teeth can prevent proper growth and development of the jaws. The resulting collapse in the size of the jaws can produce crowding and irregularities in the position of the permanent teeth. This malpositioning may make the permanent teeth more susceptible to the diseases and disorders that cause trouble during adolescent and adult life. Parents should realize that the primary teeth are intended to function until the permanent teeth are ready to take over.

The permanent teeth. There are normally 32 permanent teeth. The increase is produced by the addition of eight bicuspid teeth and four third molars ("wisdom teeth"). The eight bicuspids replace the eight primary molars usually during the ten- to 12-year period.

The bicuspids, as the name implies, have two cusps or pointed edges, one on the cheek side of the chewing surfaces and the other toward the tongue. These teeth, two on each side of the upper and lower jaws, intermesh when the jaws are closed and increase the shearing and grinding action. The twelve permanent molars do not replace any primary teeth. There are three on each side in each jaw. They provide the surface area for most of the grinding and maceration of food.

The *first permanent molar* is already forming at the time of birth. It makes its

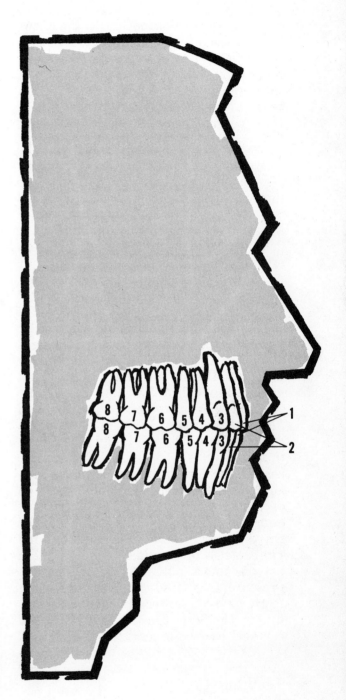

There are **32 permanent teeth**: *central incisors* (1); *lateral incisors* (2); *canines* (3); *first bicuspids* (4); *second bicuspids* (5); *first molars* (6); *second molars* (7); *third molars* or wisdom teeth (8). The first permanent molar erupts at about 6 years of age.

appearance behind the last "baby" molar at about six years of age, and is often called "six-year molar." Although it is considerably larger than the primary molars, many parents do not realize that *it is a permanent tooth intended to last for a lifetime.* These first molars are usually the most susceptible to decay of all the permanent teeth. Dental caries (tooth decay) frequently begins in the pits and fissures (grooves) in the chewing surfaces of these molars. Over 25 percent of children, six to seven years old, have beginning cavities in one or more of these molar teeth. If this decay is not found and corrected with a proper filling, the decay will cause the loss of the tooth.

The first permanent molar is the "keystone" of the dental arch. Its early loss can cause other teeth to shift into improper positions. Changes so produced can impair jaw development, facial appearance, and set up a chain reaction detrimental to the future dental and general health of the individual. The first permanent molar is an important permanent tooth and *it should receive careful attention beginning at age six.*

The second permanent molars usually make their appearance between the ages of 11 and 13 years, and the third molar between 17 and 21 years. The third molars are called "wisdom teeth", by equating wisdom, sometimes rashly, with physical maturity. Wisdom teeth often cause trouble. The jaws may be so small that one or all of these third molars remain completely embedded in the jawbone. In other instances, only a portion of the crown may erupt and a flap of gum tissue may overlap much of the third molar enamel. These embedded (impacted) or partially erupted teeth may become a source of trouble from the pressure they produce on the adjacent teeth or from infection that develops under the gum flap. Their surgical removal may be necessary.

Teething

A baby usually fusses during the times that he is erupting (cutting) his primary teeth. The cutting and pushing of the sharp edges of newly formed teeth through the gum tissue is an uncomfortable experience. Some infants react more vigorously than others. It is very important at these times to make sure that the irritability of the child is not the sign of a real illness mistakenly thought to be the symptoms of teething.

During teething a baby may drool, bite, chew, and gnaw on anything he can place in his mouth. He may work his lower jaw forward and from side to side trying to rub the gum pads together over the erupting tooth. Teething rings and other objects of suitable size and firmness will help satisfy the baby in his urge to push the teeth through the overlying gum tissue. At first he may need help in learning to handle these objects. He may be given hard foods to chew on such as celery, carrot sticks, and toasted bread so that he can use his gums.

The primary teeth cause more trouble in their erupting than do the permanent teeth. Most of the permanent teeth replace primary teeth that have been shed recently so they have a path to follow. The 12 permanent molars do not have any primary teeth to succeed. But when they erupt around the ages of 6, 12 and 17 the discomfort they cause is not as annoying, because at those ages youngsters are occupied with a wider range of mental and physical activity and a slightly sore gum is not very disturbing.

Shedding the Baby Teeth

The pressure that develops gradually on the roots of the primary teeth from the permanent teeth growing beneath causes the baby-tooth roots to be absorbed gradually. The attachments remain sturdy enough for these teeth to function properly until just before the permanent teeth replace them. If, for some reason, a permanent tooth does not form, the primary tooth root does not resorb and the baby tooth may continue to serve throughout life unless it is lost because of accident or disease.

The tooth-shedding process usually begins with the lower front teeth at the age of about six to seven years. The upper front teeth loosen and come out about the same time. This is that period in family life when the child lisps, can't eat corn on the cob, and is often nerved to the sacrifice by expectation that the departed baby tooth, placed under the pillow, will during sleep be changed by the "tooth fairy" into a dime, or, if the fairy is very thrifty, a nickel or a penny.

The *lower* canines are normally the next primary teeth to be shed, at about nine and a half years, preceding the shedding of the *upper* canines by as much as two years. The first primary molars are usually shed at about 10 to 11 years of age and the second molars around 11, which makes the upper canine the last baby tooth to be lost.

There are times when a primary tooth does not resorb properly or fails to resorb. This delays the eruption of its successor tooth which may come into the mouth in an abnormal position. If any baby teeth remain in the mouth for several months beyond the time that they are normally shed, a dentist should be consulted. He will probably want to make an x-ray examination to determine if a permanent tooth is developing and what its position is in the jaw.

Absent and extra teeth. In very rare instances neither primary or permanent teeth may form. This condition is known as *anodontia* (without teeth). It is usually accompanied by other abnormalities in the skin structures, such as faulty hair and sweat gland development. The jaws never reach a normal contour because of the failure of the teeth to produce the necessary expansion in growth. At an early age, full dentures may be constructed for affected children to improve chewing function, speech and appearance. It might be thought that dentures would act as splints and prevent any jaw development. The jaws do continue to grow, however, but not to the extent that they would if natural teeth were present. The dentures for these individuals have to be replaced periodically to accommodate the amount of growth that does occur.

Occasionally one or several teeth fail to develop. Such a condition is known as *partial anodontia*. This may happen with either primary or permanent teeth. If a primary tooth does not form, it means that there will be no corresponding permanent tooth. The formative bud for the permanent tooth comes from the same stem that produces the primary tooth. Although the primary teeth may all form, something may happen to prevent or arrest the development of the formative bud for one or more of the permanent teeth. The permanent tooth most frequently missing through failure to develop is the third molar (wisdom tooth). Usually its absence does no harm.

It has been speculated that evolution is reducing the number of human teeth, even as "soft" modern diets which require little chewing reduce the need for them. It may be that lack of exercise for the teeth and jaws deprives these structures of stimuli for growth and good alignment of the teeth. In many instances, the wisdom teeth are already dispensable and should be removed when they develop in useless and trouble-making ways. Perhaps wisdom teeth are the first victims of a genetic trend toward fewer teeth, but as yet there is no proof to support this line of reasoning.

On the other hand, some persons may develop more than the normal number of 32 teeth. These extras are called *supernumerary teeth* and they can develop anywhere in the jaws. They are most frequently found in the upper front area of the mouth. They may remain embedded in the bone or they may erupt and seek a place in the alignment of the teeth. Usually they produce crowding or pressure on the regular teeth and should be removed by the dentist.

"Third sets" of teeth. Sometimes we hear of a person who appears to be getting a third set of teeth. Usually this is an older individual who has lost his teeth and is wearing full dentures. Suddenly he becomes aware of a new tooth coming through the gums. This phenomenon is invariably a supernumerary tooth or perhaps one of the regular teeth that remained trapped in the bone because of a crowded dental arch. After the teeth are extracted these buried teeth may follow their natural inclination to erupt. The pressure from a denture placed over them may be a further stimulus to eruption. The appearance of these teeth gives the false impression that they are part of a third set.

Modern dentistry requires that an x-ray examination be made of the jaws before dentures are constructed to detect unerupted teeth, broken-off roots, residual infection or any abnormality in the jaw bones. We will hear less about the third set of teeth as the routine of x-raying the jaws before constructing dentures is more widely practiced.

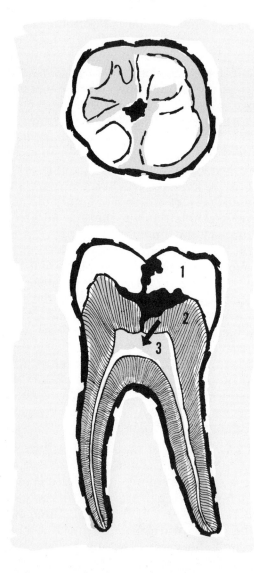

Tooth decay begins with acid action that dissolves *enamel* (1) of a tooth. At this stage a dentist can remove the decayed part, fill the cavity, and stop the progress of decay. Otherwise, decay progresses into the *dentin* (2) and finally infects the *pulp cavity* (3), at which stage it may be too late to save the tooth.

DENTAL CARIES
(Tooth Decay)

The major cause of toothache is *dental caries* (tooth decay). This disease at some time attacks almost everyone. It is more prevalent during childhood and adolescence. About 50 per cent of all two-year-old children have at least one decaying tooth. When the age of 16 years is reached, the average youth will have seven decayed, missing or filled teeth. It is estimated that less than four per cent of pupils attending high school have no decayed teeth.

Cavities begin to form at the tooth surface in areas where bacteria and food debris accumulate and remain undisturbed for prolonged periods of time. These areas are usually the pits and grooves in the chewing surfaces of the molar teeth, between the teeth on the surfaces that touch each other, and in the area along the gum line next to the lips and cheeks. These areas are not easily cleansed by the washing effect of the saliva, by the rubbing action of food passing over the surfaces of the teeth while chewing, or by brushing the teeth.

There is abundant evidence that a tooth cavity is produced largely by the action of bacteria on carbohydrate (starch and sugar) food residues, with the production of acids that can dissolve the enamel.

Many factors may exert an indirect influence on dental caries. These include inherited resistance or susceptibility to decay, the contour and composition of the teeth, their position in the mouth, the character and the amount of saliva. Some observers believe that emotional factors such as a tendency to fret and worry contribute to tooth decay. But there is general agreement that the direct cause of cavity formation is the dissolution of the hard enamel and dentin by acids that are formed from the action of bacteria on readily fermentable carbohydrates.

Prevention of Tooth Decay

There are several ways by which the destructive processes of tooth decay can be significantly lessened. Preventive measures are directed toward (1) reducing the exposure of the teeth to fermentable carbohydrates (dietary control), (2) controlling the bacteria associated with the disease (oral hygiene, immunization), (3) increasing the resistance of the teeth (fluoridation). Many investigations have demonstrated the ability of these methods to obtain desirable results but in order to be effective they must be conscientiously and consistently applied.

Dietary Control. One of the most effective means of reducing the activity of dental decay is a dietary program that sharply reduces the amount and frequency of sugar consumption. The average person in the United States eats about 100 pounds of sugar per year. Twenty-five to 40 pounds would be sufficient to supply all the calories needed from a carbohydrate source for good nutrition. Excessive sugar is detrimental for several reasons. It appeases appetite, "fills one up," lessens the desire (and room) for foods of more nutritional value, and in this way can contribute to malnutrition — especially in children, who are high sugar consumers, and also are in the age when the tooth decay process is most active.

Much excess sugar is consumed in "hidden" form, in candy, pastries and jams. Such items are often eaten between meals and perhaps several times a day. Thus the teeth are exposed frequently to the material that can be the basis for harmful acid formation. The starches are not as readily converted into acid in the mouth as are the sugars and therefore they do not contribute so greatly to the dental decay process.

Snacks and "timing." Control of tooth decay through cutting down on excessive consumption of sugar is difficult for many people. But it is well worth the effort to *substitute* nutritious and less fermentable foods such as fresh fruit, nuts and cheese, for highly concentrated sugars. This is particularly true for between-meal snacks.

If you are going to consume ten teaspoons of sugar in a day, it is better for your teeth if you take all the sugar at one time. The sheltered areas on the teeth where fermentation occurs can hold only so much sugar at one time. When these areas become saturated with fermentable material any extra is swallowed and eliminated from the mouth. Thus the bulk of the ten teaspoons of sugar taken at one meal would pass through the mouth without affecting the teeth. However, if the same amount of sugar is taken in two-teaspoonful "doses" at five different times, the sheltered surfaces of the teeth will have five exposures to acid attack instead of one. Efforts to lessen decay activity by dietary measures should not only lower the amount of sugar consumed but also should reduce the number of exposures of the teeth to sweetened edibles during the course of a day.

Toothbrushing. Does toothbrushing prevent tooth decay? There is some skepticism because tooth decay is widespread despite the increased sale of toothbrushes and dentifrices.

However, there are reasons for this paradox. One is that the toothbrush is usually not used at the time when it could be most effective. Acid formation on the tooth surface begins within moments after sugar has entered the secluded areas and reaches a maximum in 15 to 30 minutes. This is why the toothbrush should be used *immediately after eating* if it is going to exert its greatest effect in disrupting acid formation. Brushing the teeth just after getting up or before going to bed has a beneficial cosmetic effect and a stimulating action on the gum tissue, but is not of much help in controlling tooth decay.

If the teeth cannot be brushed promptly after meals or snacks that have a high sugar content, *rinse the mouth thoroughly with water*. The flushing action of the water can remove the soluble, fermentable sugar from the sheltered areas before the teeth can be attacked by acid.

Another reason why the toothbrush has not been more helpful in caries control is that generally it is not used correctly. Too often, particularly in children, the brush comes into contact with only the prominent surfaces of the teeth that are naturally cleaned by the food gliding over them. The harder-to-reach areas where bacteria and food debris can accumulate — the areas vulnerable to decay—are not well-cleaned by the usual kind of brushing.

Personal toothbrushing techniques can be improved by a simple "seeing is believing" demonstration. To "get at" decay-vulnerable areas with a toothbrush, one must know where these areas exist in the mouth. A so-called "disclosing solution," a harmless dye, will reveal colorless films and deposits on the teeth. Once an individual sees where these vulnerable areas are in his own mouth, he can do a more effective job with the toothbrush in reducing or eliminating deposits, thereby lessening the acid-manufacturing process involved in tooth decay.

If the toothbrush is used more effectively to keep teeth clean, and if it is employed at the strategic time for disrupting acid formation, it can do more to prevent cavity formation than it has actually done for most people.

Bacteria control. Certain types of bacteria are found in the mouth when teeth are decaying but are absent when there is no dental caries. Whether these microbes are the cause of decay, or are merely present because the decay process supports their growth, is not positively known.

Several dentifrices designed to rid the mouth of these bacteria have been developed, but evidence as to whether they actually lessen cavity formation is conflicting. Definitive studies are difficult because large numbers of subjects must be observed for a year or two, unflagging cooperation in prescribed use of a dentifrice is hard to obtain, and any effectiveness of the dentifrice may be overcome by the high caries-producing diets consumed by most of the subjects.

Recent research has shown that animals without tooth decay develop cavities when inoculated with certain bacteria obtained from an animal with carious teeth. Some of the inoculated animals, however, remain resistant to tooth decay, presumably because of immunological mechanisms that prevent the bacteria from growing in their mouths. Continuing research seeks to identify specific bacteria that may produce human tooth decay and to find practical methods of immunizing against dental caries.

Tooth resistance. The methods for controlling caries require conscientious cooperation of the individual. From a realistic point of view, any procedure that denies something enjoyable (such as sugar) or requires performance of a strict ritual day after day (careful brushing after meals) will not be followed with sustained enthusiasm by large numbers of people. But an agent that can give partial protection without the slightest personal effort is *fluoridation* of the public water supply.

In the early 1930's it was discovered that excessive amounts of fluorine naturally present in the drinking water in some communities caused a condition known as "mottled enamel," a spotty discoloration of the teeth. The element interfered with proper enamel development, but produced the mottled defect only in persons who used the water during the age period of enamel development. Despite the mottling, residents of communities where this disturbance occurred had less tooth decay.

Subsequent research showed that a level higher than one part of fluoride to a million parts of water was necessary to develop mottled enamel. A number of surveys were made correlating the fluoride content of the water supply with the dental condition of the residents who had been born and raised in the respective communities. In those areas where the water contained from 0.8 to 1.2 parts per million of fluorides, the native residents were found to have much less tooth decay and no obvious mottled enamel. This finding encouraged dental investigators to begin studies to determine what the results would be when the fluoride level in a deficient water supply was raised to the recognized optimal amount of one part per million.

Several of these carefully conducted studies have been under way for more than ten years. They have shown a reduction of up to 60 percent in the amount of dental caries when compared with other communities that have less than 0.5 parts per million of fluoride in their water. The greatest benefit is obtained by children who are conceived, born, and raised after the water fluoride content has been raised to the optimal amount.

Intensive study of the natives in those areas where the fluorides occur naturally in the water and where they have been adjusted to the protective level have revealed no adverse or harmful result. At the level of one part of fluoride per million parts of water the only demonstrable result has been a significant improvement in dental health.

How fluorides work. The element fluorine has a strong affinity for calcium which is a major component of the tooth substance. The fluorine combines with the calcium to produce a substance that is less soluble in acids such as those associated with tooth decay. This resistance is the major factor in the protective action of fluorides. If the protective fluorides are present in the body fluids during the period of tooth formation, they are built into the tooth substance. This is the most effective means of providing fluorine element and the reason why most children who have received the optimal water fluorides from before birth show the greatest benefit.

Topical fluorides. Fluorides also may provide a significant amount of protection when applied periodically to the surfaces of the teeth. Here again advantage is taken of the affinity of fluorine and calcium. The surface layer of the enamel can take up fluorine ions placed in direct contact with it and thus make the surface layer more resistant to acid dissolution. Individuals residing where the water supply is not fluoridated can have fluoride solutions applied to their teeth by their dentist. Various technics and solutions of fluorides are used. The so-called topical application of fluorides requires some time, effort, expense, and the results usually are not as beneficial as those obtained through water fluoridation.

However, it is recommended for children who live where they cannot benefit from water fluoridation.

Fluorides are also being applied topically in the form of dentifrices. Studies indicate that a definite reduction in the amount of tooth decay can be obtained through the daily application of a fluoride-containing dentifrice during the routine toothbrushing procedures.

Fluoride limitations. It must be remembered that increasing the resistance of the tooth against decay through the use of fluorides is not completely effective. At best the average reduction in the number of cavities is little more than 50 percent. Other agents are being sought that will be harmless and yet more effective than fluorides but to date no better agent has been discovered.

The public must not develop any false sense of security and assume that once they have the protection of fluoridation, their dental problems are over. They cannot relax their vigilance in regard to caries control. They cannot go on sugar binges or neglect their oral hygiene. They must continue to visit the dentist periodically so that he may care for the cavities that still may occur.

Periodic Dental Inspection. The surest way of preventing the loss of teeth from dental decay is regular examination by the dentist for the detection of small cavities and their correction with proper fillings. The inspections should begin about the child's *third birthday*. This is about one year after all of the primary teeth have erupted, and almost half of the children at this age will already have at least one cavity started. It is desirable to have the child visit the dentist and become acquainted with him before there is need for any extensive treatment.

Visits to the dentist should be placed on a routine basis. Every six months is sufficient for most people. Some may need treatment at more frequent intervals and others may require only an annual checkup to keep in good dental health. The frequency of the inspections can only be determined by experience and the judgment of the family dentist. The main purpose, of course, is to detect early any deviations from normal and to treat them before extensive and expensive damage occurs. Periodic inspection and treatment is the most certain preventive procedure that can be followed. Pursuing this periodic dental inspection from early childhood is the surest way to avoid tooth loss and becoming an adult dental cripple from accumulated neglect.

PERIODONTAL DISEASE
("Pyorrhea")

More teeth are lost by people over 35 because of *periodontal disease* (so-called *pyorrhea)* than from any other cause. Over half of our population beyond age 35 has developed some form of this disease. Many of these people are unaware of this condition because usually it is painless and slowly progressive.

There are several types of periodontal disease which, as the name implies, develop in the tissues immediately surrounding the teeth — *gingivae* (gums), *periodontal membranes*, (bone).

Gingivitis. The simplest and most common form is an inflammation of the gums known as *gingivitis*. It begins with a slight swelling along the gum margin of one or more teeth. The gum tissue in the area may have a slightly different color. As the condition grows worse the puffiness and color change become more pronounced, the "collar" of gum tissue loses its tight adaptation to the tooth surface, and the tissue bleeds on slight pressure. Usually there is no pain and, unfortunately, the person is not conscious of the trouble that is brewing. He only knows that his gums sometimes bleed when he brushes his teeth. At this point treatment is usually simple and effective in checking the disease.

"Pyorrhea." If the disturbance is not treated, the gum tissue may gradually separate from the tooth and a pocket may form between the soft gum tissue and the hard tooth surface. The gingivitis, which is more superficial, has now developed into a more deep-seated condition called *periodontitis*.

Bacteria, saliva and food debris collect in the pockets and intensify the destructive process. Pus usually forms and that is why this condition has been known as *pyorrhea*, which means "pus flowing". The bone adjacent to this area disappears, more attaching tissue is lost and the pocket deepens and widens. Eventually the tooth loosens and its movement in chewing sets up additional irritation.

The effect is comparable to rocking a fence post back and forth in the ground — it becomes more and more movable in its socket. When teeth become noticeably loose or begin to shift with spaces develing between them, considerable damage has been done. Too many people do not become aware of their periodontal problem until this stage is reached.

Treatment. In these later stages treatment becomes more difficult because the destroyed tissue cannot be regrown. The dentist, with the patient's cooperation, attempts to arrest the destruction and preserve the remaining supporting tissue. His efforts may include a variety of preventive procedures.

Tartar removal. One of the most important is his meticulous cleaning and polishing of the tooth surfaces, particularly those surfaces adjacent to or beneath the gum tissue. In most mouths there is a tendency for this debris to harden into a substance called dental *calculus* (tartar). Calcium and other mineral salts contained in saliva deposit in a matrix formed by bacteria, food particles and salivary sediment.

This matrix is attached to the tooth surface in secluded areas along the gum line and between the teeth. Here, by a mechanism not yet understood, the mineral deposits solidify when poor oral hygiene permits stagnation to occur. Good brushing and other means of tooth cleaning can remove much of the deposits while they are in the soft state, but after they have been allowed to stagnate for 24 or more hours ordinary hygienic methods may not remove them.

These solidified mineral deposits are particularly irritating to the gums and underlying bone. They tend to intensify the destructive process in the adjacent gum and bone tissues and they act as a center for the further collection of debris. If some effective, easily applied method could be found for harmlessly preventing these hard accumulations from forming on the teeth, it would be the greatest possible single discovery for the preservation of the teeth of the adult population. The chemical composition of these calcified deposits is so similar to that of the teeth that finding a solvent which would remove or prevent their formation, yet not cause any detrimental action on the teeth, is extremely difficult.

The hard and soft accumulations must be removed by a dentist or a dental dentist can best decide and he or the hygienist can best instruct in the method that should be followed by the individual who has gingival or periodontal disease. *Conscientious and sustained home care by the patient is extremely important to combat this condition.*

Gum surgery. Tooth cleaning may not suffice to prevent or cure periodontal disease in some instances. The dentist may have to remove surgically the gum tissue that has been separated from the teeth during pocket formation. This procedure eliminates areas of stagnation and irritation, and while it produces greater surface areas on the teeth to be kept clean by

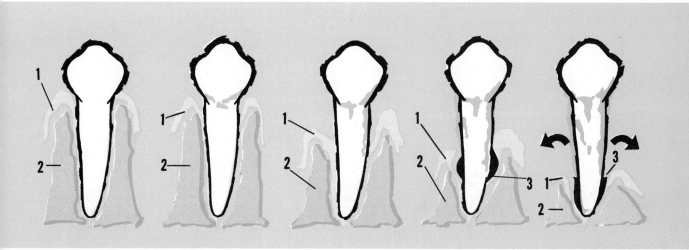

Stages in which a tooth, perhaps one without a cavity, is lost because of "pyorrhea" (periodontal disease). Hard deposits of tartar, shown in color, are irritating to gums and underlying bone. Pockets form between *gum tissue* (1) and tooth surface, become wider and deeper, gums and adjacent *bone* (2) recede, pus forms in *pockets* (3). The tooth becomes wobbly in its socket and in the final stage is lost from lack of support. Tartar cannot be removed by ordinary toothbrushing but must be removed by a dentist or dental hygienist with the aid of special equipment.

hygienist—both are trained to do the job and have the equipment to accomplish this important end.

Once the deposits have been removed, the patient can prevent or slow their recurrence by following faithfully the cleaning procedures that are prescribed by his dentist or dental hygienist. There is no one routine that can be prescribed for use by all individuals because of the differences in mouths, in the accumulation of debris, and other variables. The the patient and dentist, it makes these surfaces more accessible to good cleaning and prevention of disease.

Occlusion. The dentist will check the *occlusion*, that is, the way in which the upper and lower teeth meet and intermesh when the jaws close. It may be that a few teeth strike each other early and thus are subjected to excessive pressure. Or, some teeth may be in such position that the force delivered when the teeth contact is not directed toward the end of the root, but instead tends to wedge the teeth sideways. Such movement tends to put abnormal stress on the bony attachment.

The dentist may adjust the occlusion by carefully grinding certain tooth surfaces in order to obtain a more equal distribution of the "biting" pressures. He may even make some changes in the alignment of the teeth to secure relief from improper chewing stress. He sometimes constructs *splints* of various types that hold two or more adjacent teeth together, providing them with mutual support against the biting strains. Splints are usually employed only when teeth have become quite loose. They are essentially helpful in preserving some teeth for a further period of service.

Tooth-clenching. Some people have a habit of clenching or grinding their teeth particularly during sleep. This habit is known as *bruxism* and the undue stress it places on the supporting tissues of the teeth can be very damaging. It is sometimes necessary to make an appliance to be worn, particularly at night, to relieve this strain and eliminate the habit.

Adjacent teeth tend to drift toward the space left by loss of a tooth. The drawing shows teeth shifting to fill a gap left by loss of a first molar. "Drifted," out-of-position teeth are less able to tolerate chewing stresses; spaces in which food particles accumulate may open between them, causing irritation of gum and bone. Thus when a tooth is lost it is usually important to place a bridge or appliance as soon as possible to keep other teeth in normal position.

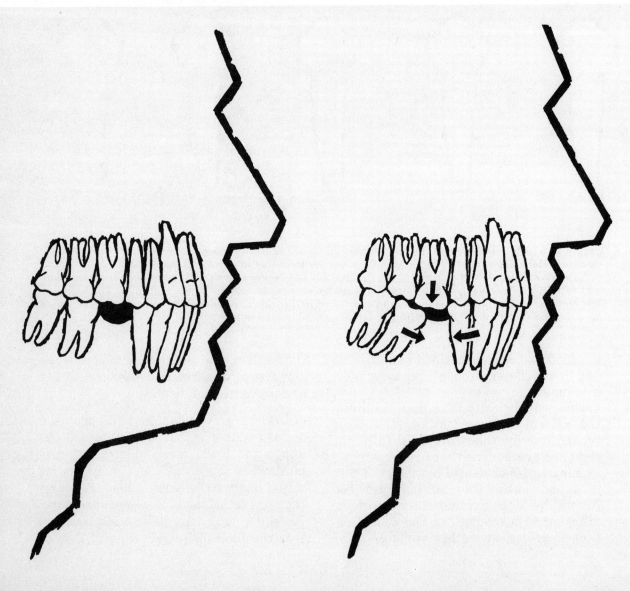

Tooth-drift. If a tooth or several teeth are lost, there is a tendency for the neighboring teeth to shift toward the space created by the loss of the tooth. This movement may place teeth in such a position that they are less able to tolerate the stress of chewing. Also, such tooth migration may open spaces between the remaining teeth. Thus food fibers and particles may pass between the teeth and pack against gum tissue, setting up an irritation that can cause destruction of gum tissue and even bone. This is the reason why it is usually important to place a bridge to substitute for the missing tooth or teeth as soon as possible.

The rough margins of dental cavities along the gum line cause irritation that can progress to the destruction of deeper tissues. The edges of poorly fitting crowns or fillings can have the same effect and these defects must be corrected if good dental health is to be maintained.

Trench mouth. Sometimes the gingivae become acutely infected with a condition known as *necrotizing gingivitis (trench mouth, Vincent's infection)*. The gums are painful, swollen, inflamed. A greyish yellow membrane usually covers the inflamed areas. The breath has a foul odor. This disease requires treatment by the dentist as soon as possible and proper care usually brings relief within 24 to 48 hours. Further treatment will be necessary to clear the condition and to prevent recurrence.

There is another condition frequently confused with necrotizing gingivitis, especially in children. This is *aphthous stomatitis*. It is extremely painful and has a somewhat similar appearance. However, the lesions may appear in other areas of the mouth besides the gums. It is believed to be a viral infection; it is more stubborn to treat and usually follows a predetermined course of one week to ten days. The *aphthous ulcer* or troublesome "canker sore" is a form of this condition. This lesion usually occurs on the inside of the cheek or lips or in the area where the cheek and gum joins.

The dentist will also consider the general health of the individual who has gingivitis or periodontal disease. Consultation with a physician may be necessary. Any condition such as diabetes or blood disorders that lessen the resistance of the tissues to infection or to the irritations that may exist around the teeth will need treatment. Improper diet or any disorder that interferes with good nutrition can predispose or contribute to gingivitis and periodontal disease.

Pregnancy can also affect the gum tissue, as demonstrated by inflamed swellings that bleed profusely which may occur about the teeth. This form of gingivitis usually disappears after the baby is delivered. The gingivitis associated with a systemic condition can be lessened or prevented by good oral hygiene and by eliminating any gum irritants that may be present. Dentists can learn much about the general health of an individual through the diseases and disorders that may affect the gum tissue.

Dental Erosion

Dental erosion is a peculiar disease that effects the teeth of some people. It begins on the outer surface of the tooth in localized areas and causes the tooth substance to disappear. The eroding surface remains smooth, hard, and highly polished throughout the course of the disease. This feature differentiates it from dental caries in which the surface is soft, sticky or roughened.

Erosion can affect any tooth and can be confined to one or two teeth or to a series of teeth. If it is found on one side of the mouth, it usually will be found on the opposite side also, although not necessarily to the same extent. The surfaces most frequently involved are the cheek and lip sides in the area near the gum line. It does not usually spread beyond the surface on which it begins, that is, it does not travel around corners onto other surfaces and it rarely occurs in the areas between the teeth.

The disease usually goes unnoticed until the enamel is penetrated and the eroding process begins to invade the underlying dentin. Then the involved tooth or teeth may become very sensitive to hot or cold food and drink and the eroded surface may be painful to the touch of even a toothbrush. The affected person often is unaware of erosion's presence until this sensitivity develops. The destructive process progresses slowly and intermittently. However, it sometimes may cut through the dentin so rapidly that within a few months the pulp within the tooth becomes exposed. It can cut so deeply that within a few years the undermined crown will break off from its root during the chewing of food.

The cause of dental erosion is not understood. It is likely that some unknown chemical process weakens the tooth surface. This chemical action, combined with a mechanical or frictional process, rubs away the tooth substance and produces the smooth polished surface.

Contact with concentrated acid substances, such as undiluted lemon juice, may play some part in the erosive process.

Treatment is based on this concept. Vigorous toothbrushing in areas of erosion must be avoided. Gentle brushing with a soft brush or wiping the involved areas with cotton or gauze may be employed for oral hygiene. Acid foods or drinks that might contribute to the softening of the tooth substance should be limited or removed from the diet. Frequently the erosion process stops spontaneously and may remain inactive. If the erosion continues or discomfort persists, a filling may have to be placed to check the deepening process. The erosion can continue around the surface margins of the filling, however, and if this happens a full crown will probably be needed to save the tooth.

It is variously estimated that dental erosion affects from one to ten percent of our population. It occurs most frequently in the fourth to fifth decade of life. It should not be confused with so-called *dental attrition* — which is the wearing down of the biting surfaces of the crowns by vigorous chewing. Nor should it be confused with the abrasion that results solely from mechanical action, such as that produced by too vigorous tooth brushing or the wear that is caused by the pipe stem of an habitual pipe smoker, or the rubbing of a movable dental appliance against the tooth surface.

Typical erosion is a human disease; it is not found in animals. There is evidence that erosion is on the increase and that it is found most frequently in individuals who hold positions of responsibility and are subject to mental tension.

Dental X-rays

Good *x-ray pictures* often reveal the early development of disturbances in the teeth and jaws that the dentist is unable to detect by looking in the mouth. Beginning decay in hidden surfaces between the teeth, or beneath a filling, or at the bottom of a narrow pit or groove in the chewing surface, may be revealed by x-rays long before it is otherwise detectable. The height of the bone surrounding and supporting the teeth, the amount of bone that has been destroyed by periodontal disease, the development of root abscesses and cysts, the presence of unerupted teeth or broken root fragments embedded in the bone, can be determined by taking x-ray pictures, since such abnormalities are hidden from view.

It is usually desirable to have an x-ray examination at periodic intervals so that the dentist can have a continuing record of any change that may occur in the teeth and the bone around them. Comparison of the series of pictures may lead to the earlier detection of disease and permits the dentist to check on the effectiveness of previous treatments.

With modern shielded apparatus and high speed x-ray film, only a very small amount of x-ray radiation is required to take a complete set of dental pictures. The very small fraction that could possibly reach the more sensitive cells of the body is less than everyone receives routinely from cosmic rays from outer space, radioactive sand and stones, and the illuminated numerals and hands on clock and watch faces. Literally millions of dental x-ray examinations are made annually without the observation of injury to any patient.

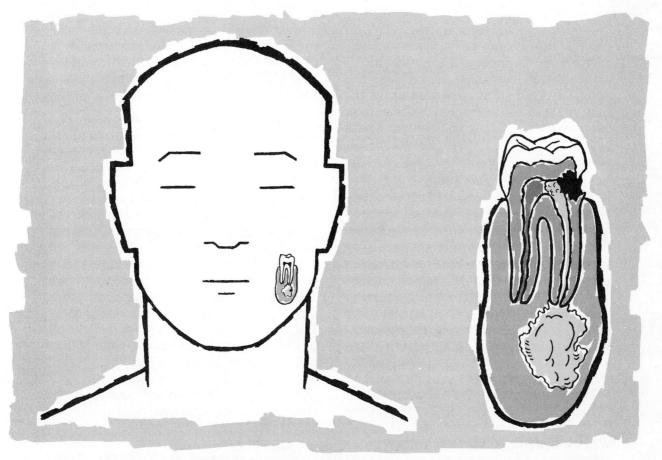

An abscess at the root of a tooth may result from infection from deep decay, as shown in the drawing, or from other causes. If the pulp is "dead," the patient may feel no pain and the abscess may be discovered in the course of routine x-ray examination. Infected pulp tissue may cause bone around the root of the tooth to be resorbed, and treatment or extraction of an abscessed tooth is important.

Abscessed and Pulpless ("Dead") Teeth

An x-ray examination often reveals an abscessed tooth, frequently to the amazement of the patient. The pulp or "nerve" within the tooth may have died because of some irritation, or infection from deep decay, or from a hard bump on the tooth that the individual may have forgotten. The death of the pulp can occur painlessly or it can cause excruciating pain. As a result of the dead and usually infected pulp tissue within the root canal, the bone around the end of the root may be resorbed. This area from which the bone has disappeared shows as a dark shadow in the x-ray picture. These teeth require treatment or extraction and the sooner they are detected and cared for the better for the patient.

Toothache. Generally when the pulp within a tooth becomes irritated it will ache and this means some form of treatment is required. Years ago it usually meant extraction of the tooth but more and more of these teeth are now being saved by that new branch of dentistry known as *endodontics* (*endo* meaning "within" and *odontus*, "the tooth"). The treatment is the removal of the pulp under local anesthesia followed by the preparation and filling of the root canal. The cause for the irritated pulp and the symptom of toothache most often is a deep cavity.

Sometimes, particularly in children, before the root has fully developed, it is possible to clean out the decayed material and cover over the pulpal area with a medicated cement. The procedure is known as *pulp capping*. In other circumstances, the portion of the pulp near the cavity may be removed and the medicated cement carefully placed over the amputated pulp stump remaining in the root canal. This treatment is known as *pulpotomy* or *pulp amputation*. These technics may keep the pulp alive until the root is fully formed, thus making the conventional type of root filling at a later time possible. In some instances pulps protected by these capping procedures may stay vital and require no further treatment by the dentist.

Saving a "dying" tooth. Pulp irritation may be so severe that the pulp tissue dies or will die if left in the tooth. The treatment then required, if the tooth is to be saved, is removal of the pulp tissue, medication and mechanical preparation of the canal, followed by the obliteration of the canal with a *root filling*.

When the pulp has been dead for some time and has not been removed, changes in the bone around the root take place. When there has been a considerable amount of bone destroyed, and perhaps the end of the root also shows signs of resorption or roughening, an operation known as *periapical surgery (root resection, root amputation, or apicoectomy)* may be performed to save the tooth.

This operation requires the exposure of the root end by making an opening through the overlying gum and bone. The small mass of inflamed tissue is scraped out of the bony cavity at the root end, the root end itself may be smoothed, and then the window in the gum is closed with sutures. Periapical surgery is usually done on the readily accessible and single-rooted front teeth. This operation has been highly successful in the saving of many of these diseased teeth that otherwise would have to be extracted.

Broken teeth. When a tooth is fractured its dental pulp chamber often will be exposed. If it is, and enough of the tooth remains in the jaw to permit the crown portion to be restored with an artificial substitute, the pulp must be removed and the root canal filled. If the pulp is not exposed, a protective cement may be placed in contact with the fractured dentin surface and the repair is "watched" to see if the pulp will survive the injury. This observation period may vary from days to months.

Replacing a "knocked-out" tooth. If a tooth is accidentally knocked out of its socket, the tooth and the victim should be taken to the dentist just as soon as possible. Such teeth may be successfully replaced, but success depends to a large extent upon the speed with which the tooth is properly treated and anchored back in its socket.

The pulp in these teeth dies and so they usually are removed and the roots are filled before the replacement is done. After the root-filled tooth has been carefully cleaned it is placed in its socket and tightly splinted to the adjacent teeth. The splint is left in place until the treated tooth has become firm in the jaw.

Sometimes the re-attachment of tooth and jaw is completely successful and the tooth remains in the mouth. More frequently, however, the root slowly resorbs and when most of the root has disappeared from the jaw, the tooth will eventually loosen and come out. This process usually takes several years and the accident victim has the use of his own tooth for a worthwhile interval.

Discolorations. Sometimes the crowns of teeth darken after the root has been filled. This discoloration often is caused by blood that seeped into the dentin before the root canal was filled, or from oral secretions invading the dentin beneath a crown filling that does not tightly seal the cavity. Such discolorations can be corrected by the dentist through a process known as bleaching. The technique is a fairly simple one. Bleaching agents are applied within the tooth to remove stains that are in the dentin. Bleaching is not for the removal of superficial stains that may be polished off on the enamel surface of the tooth.

The bleaching process is usually successful but sometimes the discoloration may reappear after a few years and then another bleaching will be required. The process is quite harmless.

DENTURES

Over 20 million Americans wear complete upper and lower dentures ("plates" or "false teeth"). Some individuals have to have them before they are 20 years old. It has been estimated that by age 60, one out of every four persons wears complete dentures.

Dentures made today are much superior to those of 30 or more years ago. The materials have been greatly improved, making dentures much more lifelike, more durable, less bulky and less porous — therefore, less likely to absorb fluids and emit an offensive odor. Refinements in technique have helped with the fitting of dentures and with establishing the right "bite," which is the proper relation between the upper and lower jaws as the teeth are closed.

For convenience and efficiency, generally, there are no teeth like one's own. But when the natural ones become diseased, or weakened through repeated and extensive filling, or when they have been badly worn, broken, discolored, or are misaligned, modern artificial dentures can be a definite improvement. Many people look better with their false teeth than they did with decrepit ones of their own.

Adjusting to dentures. Most people become accustomed to their complete dentures within a short time. New dentures may cause some soreness and require adjustment. If the soreness becomes severe, the dentures should be removed and the mouth rested. When reporting to the dentist for an adjustment, however, the teeth should be worn for the preceding 24 hours. This will permit the tender spots to redevelop so the dentist can see where the adjustments need to be made.

Chewing. In chewing with new dentures, it will be easier to start with soft foods, taking small bites and eating slowly. Chewing should be done on both sides of the mouth. Sometimes the wearing of dentures will cause an increase in the saliva flow and a feeling of fullness or nausea. Relief may be obtained by putting a candy mint in the mouth or by rinsing the mouth with cold water. The unpleasant symptoms should diminish and gradually disappear.

Speech. It frequently is necessary to make some speech adjustment in learning to speak with dentures in the mouth. The tongue and lips have to become adjusted to their contact with the new teeth in making certain sounds. Learning to make these adjustments will be facilitated by reading aloud, speaking slowly and deliberately. The amount of time required to master the artificial teeth depends to a large degree on the attitude and cooperation of the individual.

Wear and care. The dentures must be handled with care and must be kept clean. It is well to wash them after every meal. They should be scrubbed with a soft brush, soap, or a denture cleanser and water. The water should not be hot, since heat can alter the shape of the denture. The cleaning should be done over a bowl well filled with water so if the denture is dropped accidentally it will not crack or break by striking a hard surface.

For the first few weeks, it may be well to wear the new dentures day and night. This procedure helps in adjusting to the new teeth. Later the dentures may be removed at night so that the saliva can contact all of the gum and palate surfaces. When dentures are removed for the night they should be kept in water.

Some people, unfortunately, have very little bony ridge left after all of their teeth have been removed. Sometimes what little ridge is left on the upper or lower jaw is soft and flabby. Such individuals invariably have difficulty in wearing dentures because of the lack of rigid support. An extended period of practice in using the dentures is required before these unfortunates are able to manage them. There are a variety of adhesive powders and devices available for assisting in "anchorage," but the dentist should advise and direct their use. Psychology and experience probably are the most effective aids.

Implant dentures. A method called "implant dentures" has been developed to help denture wearers with so little or flabby ridges that it is impossible for them to wear the conventional type.

The gums are opened surgically and a perforated saddle made of an inert metal is adapted to the surface of the jaw bone. Attached to the saddle is a projection of metal that has a small button of the metal at its end. The gum tissue is placed back over the metal saddle, leaving the button protruding into the mouth.

This procedure may be performed on both sides of the mouth. After the gums have healed sufficiently a denture is made, containing little receptacles on the gum side that will fasten over the metal buttons protruding through the gum. The denture is inserted into the mouth and receptacles snapped over the buttons, in much the same way as with snap-fasteners of a garment. This gives the denture stability. The denture can be unsnapped for removal.

Implant technics are still under study and are not widely used. Considerable precision is required in aligning the receptacles with the buttons, and the permanence of such attachments is difficult to predict accurately. Most people who have lost all of their teeth have sufficient bony ridge remaining in the jaw so that resorting to such implant procedures is usually unnecessary.

A *partial denture* is a removable appliance that substitutes for one or several missing natural teeth. It is held in the mouth by attachments that grip the natural teeth adjacent to the space left by the missing teeth. These attachments are called clasps.

A partial denture should not be worn at night unless the dentist advises doing so for a special reason. Partial dentures also should be cleaned after each meal and special attention should be given to cleaning the inside of the clasps. Food residues trapped under these clasps can be harmful to the natural teeth. The natural teeth also should be carefully cleaned after eating in order to remove any food debris that could stagnate under the cover afforded by the partial denture in the mouth.

A partial denture should not be left out of the mouth for any extended period. Teeth remaining in the jaw can shift their position within a few days, ruining the fit of a partial denture and making it necessary to remake the denture.

Denture adjustment. Because the structures in the mouth are living they are subject to change. These changes may affect the wearing of either a partial or a complete denture. It is important to have a dentist conduct a periodic examination of the mouth and the dentures to make sure that trouble is not developing. Certain adjustment may have to be made.

Many times the bone under a complete denture resorbs. When this happens the denture may loosen, but its fit may be improved by "relining" or "rebasing". This process consists of adding denture material on the surface that contacts the gums, thereby filling in for the lost bone and readapting the denture's fit.

The denture itself is used as the tray for taking an impression of the jaw ridge. The areas of change in the ridge contour are recorded in the plastic impression material that adheres to the jaw side of the denture when it is removed from the mouth. The amount and location of the additional denture material needed to refit the denture is determined in this way. Relining is done only to improve the fit. It does not help if changes have occurred in the biting or chewing relationship of the dentures.

"Immediate dentures." So-called "immediate dentures" frequently are constructed to avoid embarrassment caused by having to go without teeth for days or weeks while the gums heal following teeth extraction.

In this procedure, the teeth back of the canines or cuspids are removed and a period of time allotted for the gums to heal and the bony ridges to smooth out and become firm. Sometimes it is necessary to contour the bone and remove sharp prominences by surgical procedures. This is simple and painless under local anesthesia. It is known as *alveolectomy* or "bone trimming," and leaves a desirably shaped surface.

When the gums are healed, impressions of the jaws are taken with the front teeth still in place. Models are made from these impressions and then the teeth are cut off from these models and the models shaped to the approximate contour that the gums will have after the natural teeth are extracted. Dentures are made to fit the models that have been so prepared. The patient's front teeth are carefully removed and any necessary bone trimming and gum suturing performed. After the bleeding has been controlled, the dentures are inserted and the individual is given instructions for wearing them.

Healing beneath the immediate dentures is usually uneventful. One might expect pain to result from wearing a denture over an area from which teeth recently had been extracted, but just the opposite occurs. The immediate denture acts as a protective covering for the jaw as it is healing. After a few weeks or months there may be enough bone shrinkage to loosen the denture. Then it may be necessary to reline or remake the denture to compensate for bone loss and reestablish the fit. The artificial teeth can be set in the denture to so resemble the shape, color, and position of the natural teeth that even close friends are not likely to detect the transition.

Denture fabrication. Much of the *fabrication* of the modern denture is done in a dental laboratory by a person who is called a dental technician.

The dentist diagnoses the oral conditions, making sure that there are no abnormalities or conditions that would interfere with wearing a denture. He takes the impression of the jaw. He studies and records the manner in which the teeth should close for efficient chewing and for the proper distribution of the biting force over the jaw ridges for comfort and for the preservation of the underlying bone. He selects the type and color for the artificial teeth and then prescribes how the dental technician should construct the dentures.

After they are fabricated, the dentist places the dentures in the mouth, checks their fit, function and appearance, and gives instructions in their use and care. He has the responsibility for making any adjustments that may be necessary and for periodically examining the denture wearer to make sure that the dentures are functioning properly and the underlying supporting tissues are healthy.

The *technician* becomes expert in the fabrication of dentures because he continually repeats this mechanical process. He is able to save the dentist a considerable amount of time and permit the dentist to spend more time providing professional care at his operating chair.

Some technicians may take improper advantage of their mechanical training and offer to perform denture service to people without the direction of a dentist. He can offer the service at a lower fee than a dentist would charge because he does not have the investment in education and equipment that a dentist is required to have. Because he lacks education and training in diagnosis, denture designing, and prevention of the dangers arising from wearing improperly constructed dentures, the direct dealing of the technician with the public is hazardous and is illegal in the United States.

A practice, formerly used, of having an edentulous (toothless) person take impressions of his own jaws by biting into softened wax and sending the impressions to a laboratory for the construction of dentures also is illegal. This so-called "mail order denture" business has been outlawed by an Act of Congress. While the cost of dentures obtained from irresponsible sources may be less initially, the price paid later for the replacement that will be necessary and the irreparable damage that may be done to the underlying bone and soft tissue makes the ultimate cost exceedingly high. Cancer of the mouth frequently results from the irritation and damage caused by poorly fitting dentures.

Tooth Extraction

Following the extraction of a tooth, the wound in the jaw usually heals within a few days without complications. Cooperation in following the instructions given by the dentist will help avoid trouble. It is desirable to slow down in one's activity for several hours following an extraction. The purpose of remaining quiet is to slow blood circulation, thereby reducing bleeding and helping a firm blood clot to form in the socket.

Aftercare. Often some swelling develops in the face following an extraction. This reaction usually is nothing to worry about and it can be minimized or prevented by the application of cold. As soon as possible after extraction an ice bag or a moist cloth wrung out with cold water should be applied to the face in the affected region. It should be kept in place for 15 minutes out of each hour and repeated for several hours.

The mouth should not be rinsed after the extraction until the following day. This is in order to let the blood clot remain undisturbed while it is solidifying. After the first day the mouth can be gently rinsed with warm salt water. The salt solution is made by dissolving one-half teaspoonful of salt in a glass of warm water. Routine but careful brushing of the remaining teeth should be continued the day following the extraction in order to keep the mouth clean and lessen the possibility of infection.

If bleeding persists. Actual bleeding should stop shortly after tooth removal. Some oozing or actual bleeding may continue for several hours or even persist into the next day. If much bleeding does continue it may be controlled in the following way:

Use a clean piece of gauze to wipe away gently the blood that may have collected in the area of the wound. Then, a clean piece of gauze can be folded into a pad of sufficient size so that when placed over the wound the teeth can be tightly closed and firm pressure made by pressing the gauze with the teeth against the bleeding area. The pressure should be maintained for half an hour and can be repeated, if necessary. When bleeding persists or occurs in considerable amount the dentist should be consulted.

Eating should continue without interruption (except of course between meals) after tooth extraction. An effort should be made not to miss a meal. It will be necessary to eat soft foods so as not to disturb the blood clot. Such nutritious foods as soft boiled eggs, soups, custards and ground meat are on the recommended list. Solid foods should be added to the diet as soon as they can be chewed comfortably and without dislodging the clot.

Most extraction wounds heal without complications. If considerable swelling, continued bleeding, severe or prolonged pain should develop, instructions for their relief should be obtained by the patient from the dentist.

Dry socket is a complication that sometimes develops following the extraction of a tooth. As the name implies, the blood clot that normally forms in the socket shortly after tooth removal fails to develop or is lost. This leaves the bony wall of the *alveolus* (socket) bare and unprotected. The bone is exposed to the oral environment including bacteria, saliva and food debris. The lining of the alveolus contains many sensory nerve endings and when these are bared to this irritating environment a great amount of pain can develop.

About all that can be done is to prescribe sedative medication to reduce the pain, keep the area as clean as possible, and place an anesthetic dressing of some type into the open socket until nature develops a protective covering for the exposed bone. Healing usually is delayed and several days pass before all of the pain disappears.

The reasons why a dry socket forms are not fully known. Some believe it results from a rapid bacterial action, others because of a fault in the blood clotting mechanism. Too vigorous rinsing of the mouth following extractions or sucking on the area or manipulations by the tongue all tend to dislodge the clot. That is why it is recommended that the area about the extraction should not be disturbed during the 24 hours after tooth removal and, if the mouth must be rinsed, it should be done very gently with cold water.

ORTHODONTICS
("Tooth Straightening")

Orthodontics is that branch of dental science that treats the malalignment of the teeth and jaws — so-called "crooked teeth." A dentist who specializes in such treatment is known as an *orthodontist*.

primary teeth, dietary and growth disorders, and undesirable habits such as prolonged thumb sucking.

Teeth out of position can interfere with the proper chewing of food, impair appearance and may lead to psychological problems. Improper relationship of the teeth toward each other may make

"Before and after" drawings of a child who has had orthodontic (tooth-straightening) treatment. At left, protruding front teeth, and at right, restoration of normal "bite" by use of orthodontic appliances such as braces which gently reposition the teeth, and retaining devices which permit the muscles and jaws to become adjusted to the new position of teeth. Orthodontic treatment can be given successfully to adults as well as children although procedures usually take longer to complete.

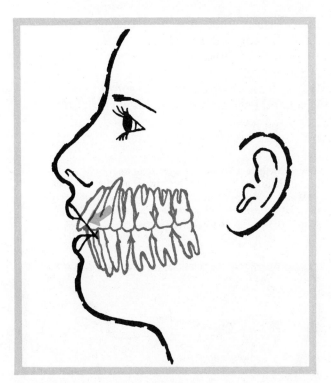 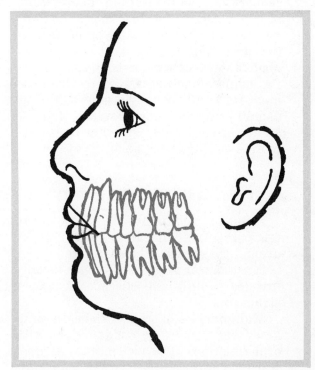

He is primarily concerned with the detection, prevention and correction of irregularities in the position of the teeth, the improper relationship of the jaws, and the associated facial deformities and speech imperfections.

Heredity is one of the most important factors producing the crowding or spacing of the teeth and the improper way in which the upper teeth mesh with the lowers when the jaws are closed. Other factors that influence the development of these irregularities (known as *malocclusion)* may be the early loss of the

them more vulnerable to attack by decay or periodontal disease. Usually the irregularities are not outgrown but can only be corrected by orthodontic treatment.

A number of devices have been developed for applying gentle pressure to move the teeth. They are called *bands* and are used along with other means to reposition the teeth and to influence the growth and contour of the jaws. The proper time for starting treatment and the length of time required to complete treatment vary with the type and extent of the malocclusion.

Some conditions require treatment soon after the primary teeth have erupted. Others should wait until the permanent teeth are in place. When tooth repositioning has been completed, *retaining* appliances are usually worn for a period of time sufficient to permit the muscles and jaws to become adjusted to the new position of the teeth.

Not for children only. There is no adult age limit for receiving orthodontic treatment. Persons in the 40 to 60 age bracket have benefited by the judicious movement of teeth that are in a position which jeopardizes their retention. The severity of the malocclusion, the amount of damage already inflicted, and other factors influence the orthodontist's judgment about the success of orthodontic service for adults. The process of tooth movement for adults usually is slow. Children usually respond more rapidly than do adults because their growing bones are more susceptible to molding.

TUMORS OF THE MOUTH

It has been estimated that from five to ten percent of all cancers occur in or around the mouth. The cure rate is poor because cancer around the mouth usually invades rapidly and spreads to deeper structures.

Malignancies in the mouth begin painlessly and usually do not interfere with oral functions. The victim may be unaware of cancer's presence for some time and this delay in recognition and treatment permits the complicating penetration. The earlier that malignancies in the lip, tongue, cheek, palate and gums are detected and removed, the more favorable the chances of long survival.

One of the great challenges to modern dentistry is the early recognition of tumor growths or non-healing sores in the mouth area. This can be accomplished only if people have regular semi-annual dental examinations. The examination for this condition should include not only an inspection of the teeth but a careful appraisal of all the tissues lining and adjacent to the oral cavity.

Irritation appears to be associated with cancer development. That is why rough edges on teeth or fillings should be corrected as soon as possible. The same holds for bridges or dentures that are loose or do not fit properly. The prolonged consumption of extremely hot drinks or highly spiced foods can be hazardous. Excessive smoking undoubtedly is irritating to the oral membranes. Overexposure to sunlight or weather is a causative factor in cancer of the lower lip.

Precancerous lesions should be watched for. One of these is called *leukoplakia*. It appears as a white patch or patches anywhere on the mucous membrane lining the mouth or covering the tongue. The surface of the area may be smooth and thin or it may be raised and thick. The surface may become roughened and fissured or it may ulcerate. Leukoplakia results from irritation and if not treated it tends to become malignant.

The mouth is a frequent site of cancer and early recognition of tumors (below, a papilloma) as well as precancerous lesions is an important benefit of regular dental examinations. Rough edges of teeth, fillings, or dentures that cause irritation should be corrected as soon as possible.

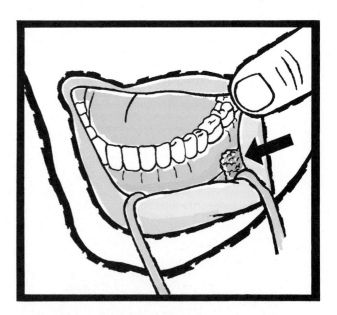

Pre-malignant growths such as *polyps* and *papillomas* also occur in the oral cavity. These outgrowths of soft tissue are often subjected to irritation during chewing or toothbrushing. While these tumors are not malignant, they sometimes become so and should be kept under strict observation. If they are in a position where they are frequently irritated, they should be removed for patient comfort and to avoid possible danger.

Ulcers occasionally occur about the mouth from some irritation such as the sharp edge of a cavity, the too vigorous use of a new toothbrush, or biting the cheek or lip in chewing food. These all heal within a few days if the irritant is removed. Any ulcer that does not heal within two weeks after the irritant has been eliminated should be regarded with suspicion and should be examined by a dentist or a physician.

The presence of a cancer is confirmed by a biopsy. Cytologic (cell structure) studies of cells obtained by gently scraping the surface of suspicious oral areas are also being applied. This simplified technique may detect cancer much earlier than other procedures, and may also help to allay the fears of persons with cancer phobia who fear that any slight deviation from normal that they detect is an early cancer. The techniques involving the study of cells under a microscope are described elsewhere.

Temporo-Mandibular Joint Disturbances

Disturbances related to the joints connecting the lower to the upper jaw create problems that sometimes are difficult to diagnose and that may have a dental origin. These joints, which are two in number, one on the right side and one on the left, are called *temporo-mandibular joints*. They are located just in front of the external opening of the ears. They consist of an extension upward of the lower jaw (mandible) which has a rounded end that fits into a socket in the base of the skull. These bony parts are held together by ligaments and muscles. The arrangement of the temporo-mandibular joints is responsible for the wide variety of movements that the lower jaw can make and they permit freedom to chew, swallow and talk.

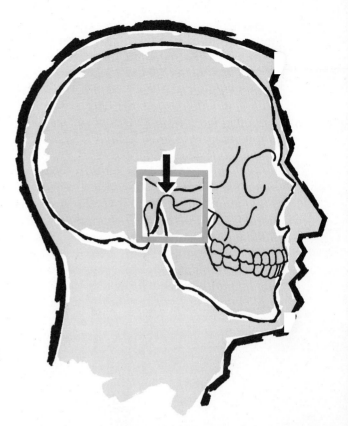

The temporo-mandibular joint is a hinge in which the lower jaw or mandible moves in a socket formed by bones at the base of the skull. Disturbances in this joint, closely related to the teeth, may cause pain, deviation of the lower jaw, clicking noises when chewing, and other disturbing symptoms.

Like other joints in the body, they are susceptible to systemic diseases such as arthritis and tumor formation. Their close relationship to the teeth, however, often brings about changes in them that are not common in other body joints.

Symptoms. These changes may involve such things as: a clicking noise upon opening the mouth or while chewing, an inability to open the mouth fully, a deviation of the lower jaw to one side or the other upon opening the mouth, pain when opening the mouth, soreness in the side of the face, pain in the region of one or both joints when chewing, and in some instances recurrent headaches. Pains in the neck and back may have their origin in the area of the temporo-mandibular joints. The lower jaw may be susceptible to recurrent dislocation of the joints when the mouth is opened widely because of a weakness in the joint structure.

Dental conditions which may contribute to or cause these disturbances and complaints are malocclusion of the teeth, or uneven bite. (Bite is the relation between the upper and lower teeth when the mouth is closed and the teeth are brought into contact.) Other causes are: overclosure of the bite, overopening of the bite, poorly fitting dental restorations, and habits such as grinding, clinching, or gritting the teeth.

In examining a person with the above complaints the dentist usually takes special x-rays of the joint and carefully studies the patient's bite, any prosthetic appliances he may be wearing, his dental habits, and his general health.

Treatment for these conditions may involve grinding of the patient's teeth to adjust an uneven bite, replacement of the improper restorations, special appliances to correct habits, corrections of malocclusion, use of physical therapy such as massage and special exercises, and in some severe cases a complete reconstruction of the patient's occlusion.

Pregnancy and Teeth

A misconception still persists that the developing fetus can withdraw calcium from the mother's teeth and thus cause cavities. The old wives' tale, "For every child, a tooth", is not true. While the fetus does require calcium and will rob the mother of her calcium if the supply from the diet is not sufficient, the mineral does not come from the dental enamel. Instead there is a much more available supply in the mother's skeletal bones. The mineral contained in the enamel cannot be withdrawn into the bloodstream and circulated to another tissue, organ or to the growing fetus. Calcium is fixed in the enamel and can only be removed by external action such as acid forming on the tooth surface as in dental caries or by cutting with dental instruments.

There is no evidence that women who have borne large families have experienced more dental decay than have comparable women of similar ages who have never been pregnant. If caries becomes more active during pregnancy, it is more likely to be because of a letdown in oral hygiene, particularly where there has been an increase in between-meal snacks and milk drinking. If there has been frequent acid regurgitation with bouts of so-called morning sickness, the natural acid-neutralizing agents in the mouth may be used up or less able to combat the acids formed by fermenting food. That is why the pregnant woman should practice meticulous oral hygiene and rinse the mouth thoroughly with water if it is inconvenient for her to brush after eating.

The pregnant woman may experience some inflammation of the gums as mentioned in the gingivitis section of this chapter. Here again the degree of cleanliness and the removal of calculus (tartar) deposits, rough cavity margins, and other sources of irritation will reduce the amount of swelling and inflammation. When the teeth are in good condition the gum tissue usually returns to normal within a short time after the baby is delivered and the hormonal balance returns to normal.

Dentifrices

Dentifrices are used to help the tooth brush clean the teeth. They also provide flavor to make brushing more pleasant. Of the two types of dentifrices in general use — powders and pastes — the paste form is more popular. Powders and pastes have essentially the same composition except that pastes have glycerine or some similar fluid added to provide a paste consistency.

The principal ingredients in a dentifrice are a mildly abrasive substance such as powdered chalk and a detergent (foaming agent) both of which assist the cleansing action of the brush. A non-sugar sweetening agent, such as saccharin, and flavoring oils are added to encourage toothbrushing by making the act more pleasant. No superiority in cleansing efficiency between the two types has been established.

Whatever the properties of a particular dentifrice, it must be used according to directions, the restriction of dietary carbohydrates must not be relaxed, and the periodic examinations by the dentist must be continued to detect and correct the cavities that will still develop. In other words, we should not put all our faith and confidence in a dentifrice as the sole means for preserving oral health. For one thing, toothbrushing alone is unlikely to completely prevent deposits of tartar on the teeth, and it cannot remove hardened deposits.

Thumbsucking and Other Habits

Infants are born with a natural instinct for sucking. Thumbs and fingers are ready objects for satisfying this need. Generally this action produces no lasting effect on the arrangement of the permanent teeth and the development of the jaws unless the habit continues *after the age of four*. Then the extent of the deformity depends on the frequency, intensity, and duration of the sucking procedure. Persistent thumbsucking results most frequently in unsightly spacing and protrusion of the upper front teeth.

Parents who are overly concerned with the early breaking of this habit actually may contribute to its continuance. The constant admonition and irritating demands to keep the thumbs or fingers out of the mouth may cause the habit to continue well beyond four years. Children aware of the parental concern may suck defiantly or as an attention-getter.

Tongue-thrusting. Sometimes children develop a habit of biting the lips or of thrusting the tongue between the teeth during times of tension. While these habits usually do not noticeably irritate the tongue or lips, the lips or the heavily muscled tongue can exert sufficient pressure over a period of time to alter the position of the teeth and cause a malformation of the jaws. Such habits usually develop in older children after a number of their permanent teeth have erupted. As soon as the habit is recognized a dentist should be consulted. He may need to construct an appliance to protect the teeth or to help break the habit.

Mint sucking. Sometimes adults develop a habit of carrying a candy mint in the mouth between the cheek and the teeth. They may do this to stimulate saliva, to help break a smoking habit, or because they believe it will sweeten their breath or for some other reason. These candies usually have a high sugar content. When allowed to dissolve slowly, and if used frequently, they can keep a high concentration of acid-producing material in close contact with the teeth. These adults usually have some gum recession which allows the exposed root surface, or thin enamel near the gum line, in the area close to where the candy is held, to suffer a rapid attack of dental decay.

Acid drinks. The excessive use of acid drinks such as lemon juice also can damage adult teeth. The acid in itself may be sufficiently strong if the drinks are used frequently to dissolve the tooth substance, or the acid may neutralize or reduce the natural effectiveness of the saliva in protecting the teeth.

Objects. Adults can also injure their gums by the injudicious use of tooth picks or dental floss. These agents are helpful in cleaning the areas between the teeth but they must be used carefully.

The mouth should not be used for holding or carrying objects such as nails by carpenters or tacks by upholsterers. Such habits if prolonged can cause harmful and unsightly wear on the teeth. Nor should teeth be used for such heavy duty as removing bottle caps or cracking nuts. Teeth can withstand considerable force, but when the wrong leverage is applied, the enamel may be chipped or the teeth themselves may be broken.

Halitosis

People with halitosis or bad breath usually are searching for a mouth wash that will cure their problem. Mouth washes, however, are designed primarily to mask the odor and do not correct the cause of the trouble. The origin of the odor is more deep-seated and as a rule cannot be eliminated or even reached by rinsing the mouth or gargling.

Odors emanating from the teeth come from deep cavities containing decaying matter, from areas between the teeth where food becomes impacted and putrefies, and from deep pockets containing pus and debris under the gums along the roots of the teeth. These conditions require treatment by the dentist to eliminate the source of odor as well as to preserve the teeth.

Sometimes the bad breath results from congestion or infection in the nasal cavity or the sinuses or it may have its origin in the respiratory or alimentary tract. Unless persistent halitosis results from the habitual consumption of foods that produce an offensive odor it indicates an abnormal condition that should be searched out and treated by a doctor.

Fallacies About Teeth

Erroneous beliefs about the teeth may do harm indirectly by discouraging the proper personal or professional care.

It is not a "fact of life" that several or all of the permanent teeth have to be lost as we grow older. Except for accidents or malformations, teeth are lost as a consequence of decay or periodontal (gum and bone) disease, conditions which can be prevented or arrested by timely and proper care. The primary cause of loss of teeth is neglect.

A toothache that "goes away by itself" does not mean that the tooth has recovered from whatever affects it. Pain is a warning signal that something is wrong and that no time should be lost in consulting a dentist.

Large fillings do not weaken the teeth. The truth is that unfilled cavities weaken the teeth, and if neglected lead to loss of a tooth which timely filling could have completely prevented.

Drinking lots of milk does not prevent tooth decay. Milk is the richest dietary source of calcium, needed for teeth and bone-building, and an excellent food, but milk cannot arrest the process of tooth decay or prevent its inception. Diet has relatively little effect on fully formed teeth except in a detrimental way if there is an excess of concentrated sugars that play a part in the decay process.

MODERN DENTAL PRACTICE

High speed "drills." Tremendous improvements have been made in the efficiency of dental service. An example is the equipment used to prepare the teeth for fillings and crowns. For years dentists have used rotary tools (drills) for this purpose. These cutting instruments rotated at a top speed of 5,000 revolutions per minute. Discomfort was often felt from the vibration, pressure, and heat that developed in the use of these instruments.

Today, improvements in the motors that turn the instruments and the use of the turbine principle permit speeds of up to 300,000 revolutions per minute. Only a very light touch is required to cut enamel and dentin at these high speeds. The rotations are so rapid that the sense of vibration is eliminated. Of course heat is generated by such rapid cutting, but the instruments are devised so that a spray of water and air is directed at the area being cut, keeping the temperature at a comfortable level. With the advent of this high speed, new types of cutting tools had to be developed to prevent their rapid wear and loss of cutting efficiency. These improvements add up to more speed and comfort in dental operations.

Medications. Research has improved the medications used in dental treatments. Antibiotics are now available for preventing or speedily eliminating dental infections that were exceedingly painful and dangerous to manage a few years ago. Dentists long have been interested in lessening the pain associated with dental operations. It was a dentist, H. G. Wells, who first demonstrated the possibility of overcoming pain during a surgical operation by the use of nitrous oxide (laughing gas) as a general anesthetic. The local anesthetics widely used in dental practice are continually being improved. Tranquilizers and sedatives provided to patients before and after treatments have done much to remove apprehension, discomfort and pain from improved dental service.

Dental Materials. The materials used to fill and replace teeth also have been improved. These materials must meet a number of exacting requirements. They must be strong enough to withstand the strains and stress placed on them in the process of chewing. Some people can exert as much as 200 pounds of pressure when their teeth are clenched. The restorative material must not be dissolved, discolored, or permeated by the fluids in the mouth. Filling material must not expand or shrink appreciably after it is placed in a cavity. These materials must be non-poisonous. If possible, they should resemble the color and appearance of natural teeth or gums.

The ideal filling material has not yet been developed. Current research is seeking a material that can be placed in a cavity in a soft or plastic state, that will fuse or bond with the tooth substance so that it cannot be washed out or dislodged from the cavity, and that will have the appearance and the resistance to wear of natural enamel. The goal is an ambitious one but modern science may eventually produce the material.

There are several materials that are widely used by the dental profession for restorative purpose. They include gold, silver, porcelain, synthetic porcelain, and acrylic resins. Gold has had extensive use. Originally small increments of very thin strips of pure gold called foil were malleted into a cavity. The purity and malleability of the gold under pressure allowed the increments to fuse together into one solid mass of gold filling the cavity. These so-called gold foil restorations make excellent and durable fillings. However, many patients object to the malleting procedure and to the appearance of a gold cavity filling.

The *gold inlay* was introduced as a cavity filling in the early 1900's. It was based on the development of a precision casting process. The prepared cavity is filled with softened wax which is then carved to the proper shape for the tooth.

A mold is made of the wax pattern, the wax is eliminated, and molten gold cast into the empty mold. The materials and technic for making this type of restoration have been greatly refined and today the cast inlay made of a hard gold alloy is in wide use. While the inlay is made to fit the cavity accurately, it must be sealed into the tooth with dental cement.

The *silver filling* is really an alloy (amalgam) of silver, tin and mercury. It is produced by mixing a combination of powdered tin and silver with mercury to form a soft mass. Small bits of this are carried into a cavity and packed against each other until the cavity is filled and the excess mercury squeezed out. This amalgam hardens in a short time and while it is hardening it can be carved to the desired contour. These silver or amalgam fillings are more brittle than gold restorations and if not mixed properly they may tend to shrink or expand.

Porcelain is used as a cavity filling material or in the construction of a porcelain jacket crown. The porcelain is a mixture of clay-like materials blended together in powder form to resemble the appearance of natural tooth substance. The blended powders are made into a plastic state by moistening them and the mass is contoured into the desired form. It is then solidified by baking at a high temperature. While the porcelain restoration is natural in appearance, it has the disadvantage of being more fragile than one made from a metallic mixture. A "jacket crown," as the name implies, requires the removal of the natural enamel and replacement with a jacket of baked porcelain that builds the surface of the crown back to its original contour.

Synthetic porcelain or *silicate cement* fillings are usually placed in the front part of the mouth because of their natural appearance. They are made from porcelain-like powders that are mixed with a liquid, usually phosphoric acid. The mixture is packed into a cavity and sets into a solid cystalline mass within a few minutes. While it makes a pleasing restoration because it is hard to detect from the natural enamel, it has a tendency to wash away and therefore is not as durable as most other filling materials.

The *acrylic resins* were developed for dental restorative purposes about the time of World War II. The recently improved forms are widely used in denture construction. They have about completely replaced the rubber or vulcanite denture material. Their big advantage is their lifelike appearance for gum replacement and their density which reduces the absorption of fluids from the mouth and the odors that often resulted.

The modern dentist has improved equipment and material with which to perform his service. He is usually guided in making his diagnosis and conducting his treatment by x-ray pictures of the mouth and teeth. He uses other diagnostic equipment and tests that permit him to observe much more than the crowns of the teeth in the mouth. He is educated and equipped to prevent serious trouble from occurring in the oral cavity. He can provide the competent treatment and the advice that will usually permit most individuals who seek his care to secure a lifetime of efficient, healthy service from their natural teeth.

THE EYES

by DERRICK VAIL, M.D.

A Small Ball With Muscles • Teamwork of Muscles • Structures for Seeing • Focusing Machinery • Making Light Visible • Our Two Seeing-Systems • Nerve Paths of Vision • Tears Without End

EYE EXAMINATIONS

Eyeglasses

CARE OF THE EYES

Home Measures • Allergies

CHILDREN'S EYES

Ocular Muscle Imbalance

INFECTIONS OF THE EYES

THE RED EYE

The Mechanism of Glaucoma • Congenital Glaucoma • Cataract • Detached Retina • Cancer of the Eye • Systemic Diseases that Affect the Eyes • Headaches • Eye Exercises • Floating Spots

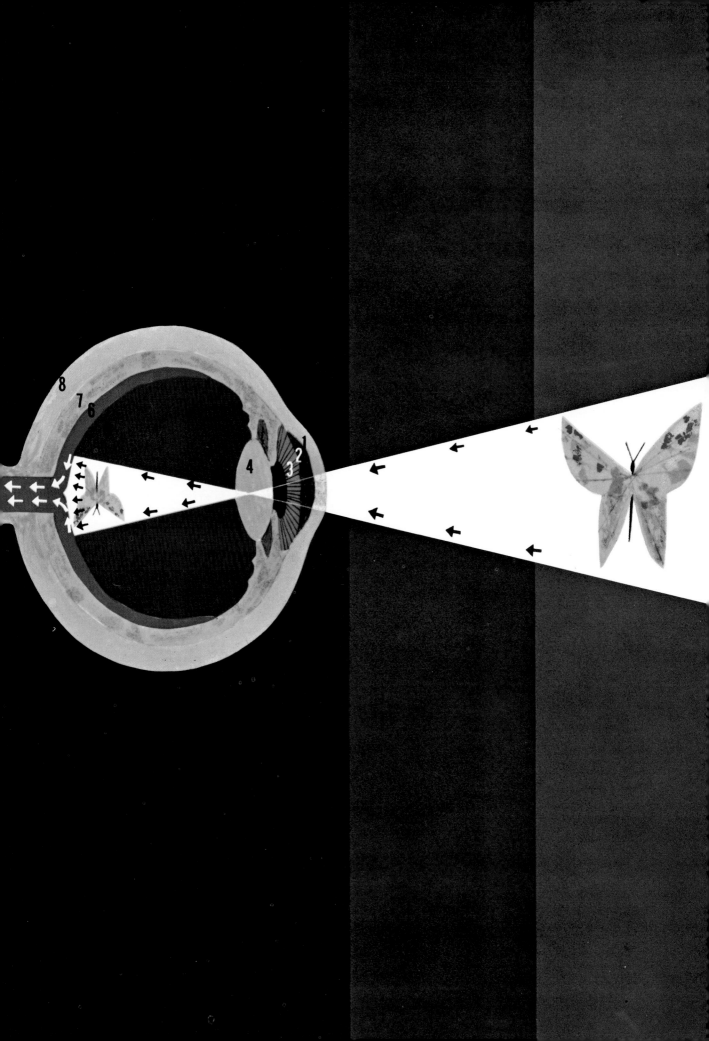

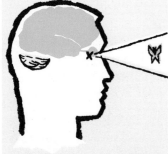

The color plate shows major structures and mechanisms of the human eye, diagrammatically.

Light waves from a butterfly are transmitted to the retina (6) at the back of the eye as shown by black arrows. As in a camera, the image is upside down. Light waves are bent as they pass through the transparent window of the eye, the *cornea* (1), and the *crystalline lens* (4), which changes shape for the focusing. The *iris* (3), the colored part of the eye, has a hole in its center (the pupil) which adjusts to admit more or less light. The *anterior chamber* (2) contains watery fluid and the *posterior chamber* (5) contains semifluid vitreous humor.

The *sclera* (8) is the strong outer coat of the eye, underlaid by the *choroid* (7), a thin layer with many blood vessels.

In the retina, light stimulates nerve endings, and nerve impulses (white arrows) travel over the *optic nerve* (9) to the brain which interprets or "sees" these impulses as a butterfly in upright position.

CHAPTER 16

THE EYES

by DERRICK VAIL, M.D.

When we say "I see," we usually mean that we understand something. To speak of men and women of vision, whose views are farsighted and perceptive, is more often to compliment their characters than their keen eyesight. Thus does our sense of sight intertwine with all our waking activities, and leave sensory imprints that in sleep we jumble into dreams. Through our eyes, awareness of near and far away events streams instantly and constantly into the decision-making mind, and alone of the senses, sight can turn from the page you are reading to a star a million light years away.

Whether or not eye defects are more common today than in the past, there is no doubt that the need for efficient, comfortable sight — in driving cars, reading and learning and doing the close eyework of civilization, dodging traffic — is more critical than when primitive men hunted by day and, having no lights to turn on, bedded down at twilight. Neanderthal man didn't wear glasses, nor fill out income tax forms.

Our eyes are quite well protected, cushioned in hard sockets, self-cleansing, self-lubricating, shuttered and self-adjusting. But the eyes may reflect ill health elsewhere in the body, and they are subject to defects, accidents, and disorders of their own. Some disorders creep up insidiously and cause blindness, and many others may cause great discomfort or minor or major handicaps of defective vision that often are correctible or preventable if treated properly and promptly. The prince of senses deserves nothing less than skilled professional attention and sensible care by the owner.

A Small Ball With Muscles

The eyeball *(globe)* is a resilient sphere about one inch in diameter, mildly inflated by internal fluids, turned by its own muscles.

The eyeball rests in a bony socket *(orbit)* that tapers from front to back like a cone. Beneath the eyebrows a ridge of bone gives considerable protection against frontal blows. The bony socket wall above, below, and to noseward of the eye is very close to the sinuses of the facial bones. The socket shell is pitted to receive structure attachments, and is pierced to admit nerves and

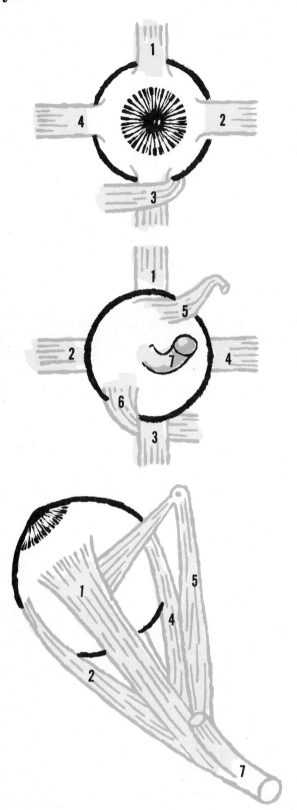

Movements of the eyeball are produced by six muscles, shown in drawings (top to bottom) in front and rear view of left eye and looking down upon it. There are four *rectus* ("straight") muscles attached to the upper, outer, under, and inner sides of the eyeball (1, 2, 3, 4 respectively) and an upper and lower *oblique* muscle (5, 6). Also shown is the *optic nerve* (7).

blood vessels. The tip of the cone has an opening through which the optic nerve passes from the back of the eye to make complicated connections with the brain. A semi-fluid mass of fat gives cushioning support to the eye and allows it to move with easy freedom.

Man is among the few mammals that can fix the gaze upon an object by turning the eyes without turning the entire head. This convenient shifting is done by six muscles attached externally to each eyeball. Four straplike muscles are attached to the top, bottom, and sides of the eyeball, not far behind the visible white of the eye. Farther back, attached to the side farthest from the nose, are two other muscles. When one muscle group contracts, an opposing group relaxes.

Teamwork of Muscles

Collectively, the half-dozen muscles rotate the eye and turn it up, down, or sideways. They also hold the eyes straight. This is complicated by the fact that we have two eyes that must work together, like binoculars. An eye that does not follow its partner is at risk of becoming an unseeing eye. The problem has been likened to that of driving a team of horses with an intricate set of reins. The reins represent muscles; the "driver" is the flow of nerve impulses which directs various combinations of reins to pull this way or that way, so the "horses" turn in unison and do not go off in different directions. Conditions of eye-muscle imbalance are rather common, and in milder forms than obviously "unteamed" eyes the patient may not even be aware of the condition.

We are either right-eyed or left-eyed. There is always a dominant eye. One can easily determine which it is by making a circle with thumb and forefinger and looking through it with *both* eyes open at an object across the room. Without moving thumb and forefinger, first close one eye, and then the other. The eye which still sees the object through the circle is dominant. Dominance is unconsciously expressed in many ways, as in choosing the eye to sight a rifle.

Structures for Seeing

A vertical cross-section of the eye shows the arrangement of major parts but scarcely conveys the marvel of vision.

The outer coat of the eye, the *sclera,* is strong, elastic connective tissue, visible in front as the "white of the eye." At the very front of the eye, the transparent window, which bulges out a little, is the *cornea,* a modified continuation of the sclera. The middle coat of the eye, the *choroid,* is a thin pigmented layer composed largely of interlaced blood vessels, vital to the eye's nutrition. A specialized continuation of the choroid is the *iris,* which gives our eyes their color. The pupil is a hole in the iris, and it is black because the inside of the eye is dark. The innermost coat is the *retina,* a gossamer light-sensitive tissue which covers the back of the eye and curves forward like a deep rounded cup. Retinal nerves converge into the large optic nerve.

The *crystalline lens* is suspended just behind the iris and is attached to the *ciliary body,* which is principally muscle. The lens and associated structures divide the eye into two compartments. The larger chamber behind the lens is filled with semi-liquid transparent *vitreous* ("glassy") *humor* which "inflates" the eye. The much smaller space between the cornea and lens is filled with watery liquid, the *aqueous humor.*

Much of the mechanical part of seeing is accomplished by structures of the frontal part of the eye, called the *anterior segment.* An enlarged view shows structures in greater detail. The lens is delicately slung, somewhat like a hammock, by fine ligaments *(zonules)* connected to the ciliary body. The only internal muscles of the eye are the *ciliary* (hair-like) *muscles* which change the shape of the lens and muscles of the iris. The iris hangs from a ciliary attachment and rests lightly on the lens. The angle at the junction of the cornea and iris is an important area. Nearby, minute passages called the

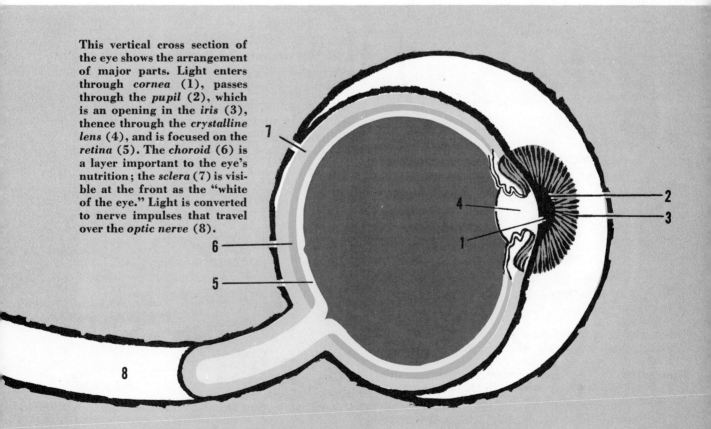

This vertical cross section of the eye shows the arrangement of major parts. Light enters through *cornea* (1), passes through the *pupil* (2), which is an opening in the *iris* (3), thence through the *crystalline lens* (4), and is focused on the *retina* (5). The *choroid* (6) is a layer important to the eye's nutrition; the *sclera* (7) is visible at the front as the "white of the eye." Light is converted to nerve impulses that travel over the *optic nerve* (8).

canals of Schlemm permit drainage of internal eye-fluids and act as safety valves to prevent pressures from building up disastrously and destroying vision, as in glaucoma.

Focusing Machinery

The collaborative functions of eye structures are to bring an image into focus on the retina, convert the stimuli of light into nerve impulses, and transmit torrents of electric currents over the optic nerves to the back of the brain where what we see is actually seen. By far the most common eye defects are errors of refraction — nearsightedness, farsightedness, astigmatism — in which an image does not rest squarely on the retina.

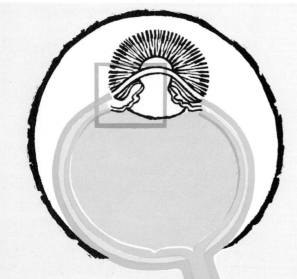

The curved cornea does a major part of the light-focusing. It is like a fixed lens that does not change its focus. Fine hair-line focusing is accomplished by the crystalline lens, which is made of modified skin cells that are glass-clear. When we look at close objects, up to about 20 feet away, focusing help is necessary to see them sharply. The lens does this by changing its thickness and curvature. This is called *accommodation*.

The lens is enclosed in a capsule slung by ligaments to ciliary muscles. Contraction of these muscles relaxes the ligaments, the lens becomes thicker and more curved, and near objects come into focus. Ordinarily, these muscles are active only when we are looking at objects closer than 20 feet. Thus, when doing close work, it is restful to pause occasionally and look out a window into the distance.

Many complaints of eye fatigue are actually complaints about tired ciliary muscles. Farsighted persons often can see fine print distinctly, but at cost of a great deal of ciliary-muscle energy that is tiring and could be eased by glasses. With increasing age, the lens gradually loses some of its accommodative powers and no amount of ciliary effort will avert the telltale need of holding a book at arm's length to read it. Nearsighted persons usually are able to read effortlessly for hours on end, since their natural focal length is for close work, but distant objects are fuzzy.

Above, location of structures shown in enlarged view of anterior segment of the eye at right. The *iris* (1) rests on the *lens* (2), which, with the *cornea* (3), enclose the *anterior chamber* (4) which is filled with aqueous fluid. The lens is delicately suspended by fine *ligaments* or *zonules* (5) attached to the *ciliary body* (6). The *ciliary muscles* (7) change the shape of the lens for focusing.

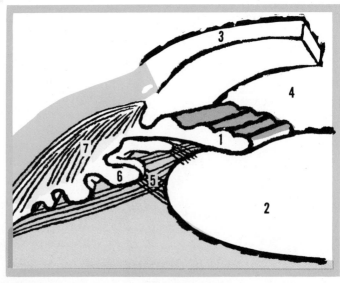

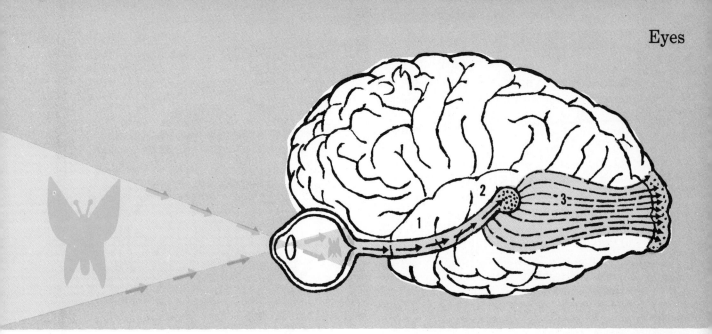

Nerve pathways of vision in the brain. Rays of light falling as an inverted image of a butterfly on the retina excite nerve impulses in rods and cones of the retina. Nerve impulses follow pathways of arrows in *optic nerve* (1) to midbrain area (2) and in fibers (3) called *visual radiations* that make intricate connections in the occipital lobes at the back of the head.

The iris controls the amount of light entering the eye by adjusting the diameter of the pupil, as the diaphragm of a camera enlarges or reduces the light opening. The iris is a circular pigmented sheet of muscle tissue with opposing circular and radial muscles which automatically constrict or expand the pupil in accordance with the brightness of light that strikes the eye. A fully expanded pupil exposes about 17 times more area than a constricted one.

Making Light Visible

The tissue-thin layer of the retina converts light-energy that falls upon it into nerve energy that we see in the back of our heads. Physically, light waves are neither visible nor colored, any more than radio waves of the electromagnetic spectrum. The marvel of vision is that a very narrow range of this spectrum can be seen as a brilliant sunset or the face of a child or an onrushing car giving distant warning to get out of the way.

The retina develops from part of the brain wall converted into a cup, and in this sense our brains are continuously exposed to the outside world. Layered retinal tissue, no larger than a teaspoon, is a mosaic of hundreds of thousands of nerve endings with intricate connections in depth. The nerve endings are either *cones,* named for their shape, or *cylindrical rods.* Oddly, the nerve endings are

pointed away from the source of light, toward the back of the eyeball. The cones are connected individually, the rods more collectively, to cells which terminate in fibers which collect into the huge bundle of fibers that is the *optic nerve.*

There are no sense receptors at the point where the optic nerve enters the back of the eye. Consequently this small spot is blind. This is shown by looking at a black dot on a printed page with one eye only, and moving the eye slowly noseward until the dot disappears. Light falls directly upon the optic nerve but the "message" of visibility does not get through because conversion machinery has been bypassed. This photo-chemical machinery is very complicated, but the result is that light energy which stimulates the rods and cones is transformed into nerve impulses. There is no difference between nerve impulses we hear as sound, or feel as pain, or taste as flavors, but receptor tissues are different. Stimuli which excite the retina are not wiped out instantaneously; there is brief persistence of the image. This phenomenon sustains the motion picture and television industries.

Everything we look at directly, to see it most sharply, comes to focus on the

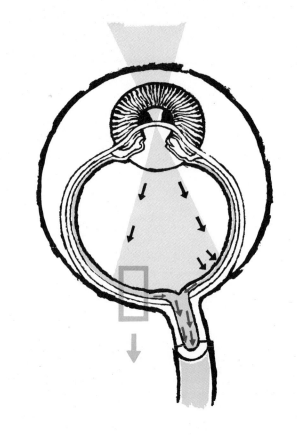

fovea, an area near the center of the retina that is smaller than a pinhead. Surrounding it is a slightly larger area called the *macula lutea,* from its yellowish color when seen through an ophthalmoscope. All our finely detailed seeing is done here. Man and primates alone possess this ultra-discriminating area.

The fovea is composed only of cones, so tightly compacted — on the order of 150,000 to a square millimeter — that they are squeezed almost to the thinness of rods. Beyond the macula, cones dwindle and rods take over. Each retina has something over 100,000,000 rods and between 6,000,000 and 7,000,000 cones. The different capacities of these two kinds of nerve endings control aspects of seeing that we experience all the time without thinking much about it.

Our Two Seeing-Systems

At dusk all landscapes are gray, and so are cats, and we cannot always even be sure it is a cat. We may not even see the cat in dim light, unless it moves and we catch a glimpse of motion from the corner of our eyes. This is "twilight seeing" or night vision, effected almost entirely by the rods of the retina, which are much more sensitive to light than the cones but cannot distinguish colors or fine details.

We see best in dim light not by looking directly at an object but to one side of it. On a clear night look into the heavens at any star you fancy. Somewhere off to one side there will be a very faint star that is barely discernible. Look directly at the faint star and it disappears. Move your eyes a little away and you see it again. When you look at it the light falls on the fovea, which has only cones, which are too insensitive to respond to light so dim.

A substance called *visual purple* which breaks down when exposed to light plays a part in night vision. It comes into play when your eyes slowly adjust to the dark of a movie theater as you grope for a seat. After a few minutes you can see many empty seats — if there are any. Visual purple is produced only by the rods. A product of its breakdown is Vitamin A, which is also needed for its regeneration.

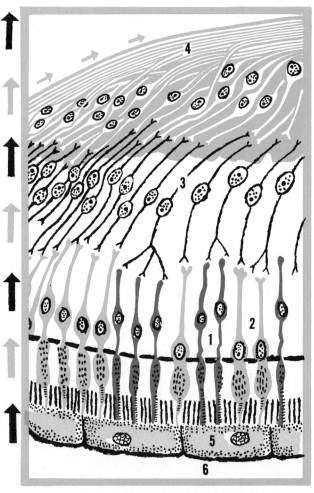

Drawing shows light rays impinging on retina, and enlarged section of the tissue-thin retina. *Rods* (1) and *cones* (2) connect with *bipolar cells* (3) and *fibers* (4) that collectively form the optic nerve. Also shown are the *pigment* (5) and *choroid* (6) layers.

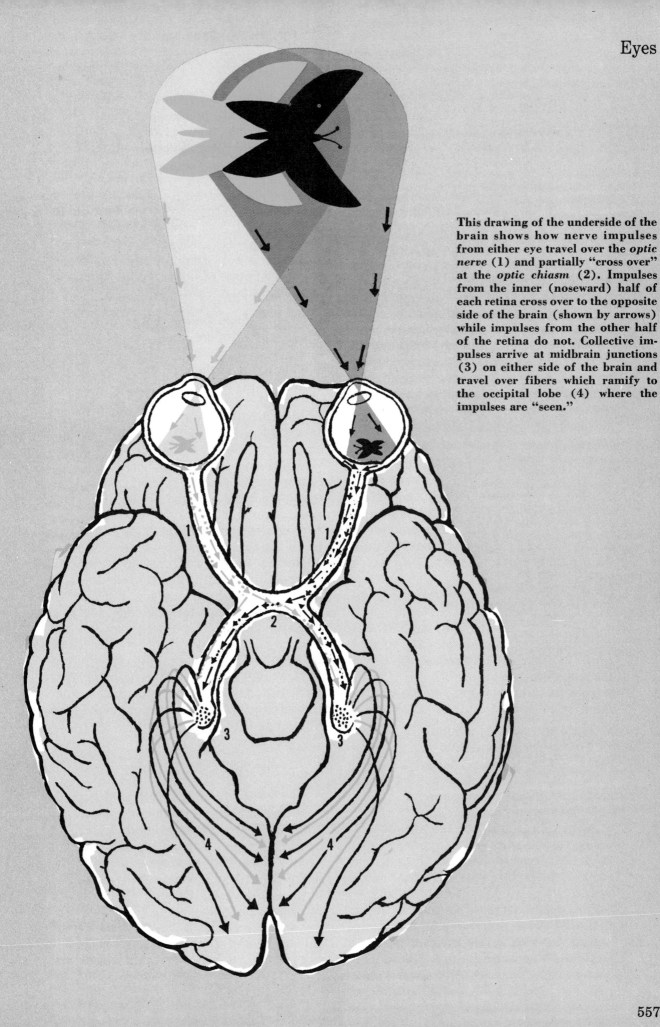

This drawing of the underside of the brain shows how nerve impulses from either eye travel over the *optic nerve* (1) and partially "cross over" at the *optic chiasm* (2). Impulses from the inner (noseward) half of each retina cross over to the opposite side of the brain (shown by arrows) while impulses from the other half of the retina do not. Collective impulses arrive at midbrain junctions (3) on either side of the brain and travel over fibers which ramify to the occipital lobe (4) where the impulses are "seen."

"Night blindness" is failure to see as well as one should in dim light, and involves the rod department of the visual system.

Cones are for bright-light seeing, and only cones can distinguish colors. The eye can distinguish about 7,500,000 barely perceptible differences of hue (no wonder painters have trouble matching colors to please a housewife). Color blindness is most likely a reduction or absence of cones sensitive to certain wavelengths of light.

Human beings alone can distinguish the full color range of the spectrum. Bees can see ultra-violet light, but to them red is blackness, and red flowers are not pollinated by bees. Chickens have mostly cones, can't see well in dim light, and roost at sunset. On the other hand, some owls are well equipped with rods, and naturally are night owls.

The visual field is the breadth of area encompassed by vision when the gaze is fixed straight ahead. The field area varies somewhat for colors, being largest for blue and smallest for green. Symptoms of "tunnel vision" and other distortions of the visual field are of value in diagnosing certain eye disorders.

Nerve Paths of Vision

Everything we see is created from a mere series of signals streaming over nerve pathways. The eye may be physically perfect and yet be blind if there is interruption of the optic nerve and its ramifications.

The optic nerve is a bundle of about a million fibers individually connected to parts of the retina. It is not a typical nerve, but an extension of the brain, embedded in that great organ for much of its length, and fraying out in its rearward ramifications to make uncountable connections in the *visual cortex,* which is in the occipital lobe at the extreme rear of the brain. It is here that nerve impulses are transformed into vision.

The optic nerves from each retina partially criss-cross a short distance behind the eyes in a curious way, in an area called the *optic chiasm.* Fibers from the half of each retina that is closest to the nose cross to the opposite side, but fibers from the temple side of each retina do not. The collected bundles continue to junctions at either side of an imaginary midline through the head, from which the fibers *(visual radiations)* fray out and spread toward the rear of the head where they make thousands of connections in the region of a fissure in the occipital lobes. It is here that the brain provides mental images of what we see, pictures conjured up by electrical impulses.

Upside-down image. The eye projects an inverted image upon the retina, and the question of why we don't see things upside down is seemingly baffling. However, the problem is not a real one. We do not see the retinal image per se, but billions of nerve impulses that coalesce in visual centers of the brain. We associate sights of the outside world, and relate them to "realities," with patterns of nerve activities stimulated through the eyes. We have to learn to see. A person blind from birth, suddenly given sight, does not immediately "see" that an object is an orange or that a box is square.

Nerves in the retina send orders to contract or expand the pupil. Automatic nerve-orders direct ciliary muscles to change the shape of the lens for fine focusing. We can turn both eyes inward toward the nose by voluntary effort, but to keep both eyes straight, turning in unison, like a team of horses in perfect harness, is an unconscious neuro-muscular function in which we have invested a good deal of learning.

Tears Without End

Our eyes are quite well equipped to take care of themselves in normal circumstances. Tears are continually produced by the *lacrimal apparatus,* and only in excess does the product roll pitifully down the cheeks. To be literally dry-eyed is to be threatened with blindness. Tears lubricate the eyes, cleanse them by flushing small particles toward the corner of the eyes, and contain an antibacterial substance *(lysozyme)* that inhibits germs.

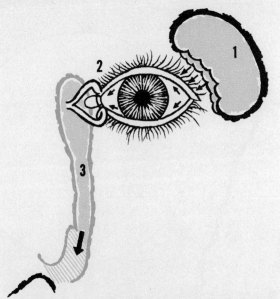

Tears produced constantly by the *lacrimal gland* (1) in the upper part of the eye socket flow over the front of the eye, collect in the *conjunctival sac* (2) at the inner corner of the eye, and drain through a channel (3) which opens into the nose. Thus weeping is followed by sniffling.

The tear glands, about the size and shape of almonds, are located — one to an eye — just within the upper outside part of the socket. The gland secretes tears which flow through half a dozen short ducts, along which there are accessory glands, and follow a channel which delivers them into the conjunctival sac — the tiny wedge of pink tissue at the nose-corner of each eye. The tears are spread by blinking the eyelids, which are lined inside by delicate tissue, the *conjunctiva*, which continues around to enwrap the front part of the eyeball.

From the inner corner of the eyes, the tears drain through a channel which opens into the nose, which is why profuse weeping is accompanied by sniffling. As far as is known, man is the only creature that weeps from emotion, if we except crocodile tears.

The whole operation of the tear glands is like that of windshield wipers using antibacterial tear-water.

EYE EXAMINATIONS

If you want to have your eyes examined you should seek out either an *ophthalmologist* (oculist) or an *optometrist*.

There is much confusion regarding these labels. An *ophthalmologist* (oculist) is a Doctor of Medicine, who, while licensed to practice all branches of medicine and surgery, has specialized in the examination of the eye and its related structures and in the prevention, diagnosis and medical and surgical treatment of their defects and diseases, prescribing whatever is required, including eyeglasses and contact lenses. His education and training qualify him to relate findings observed in an examination of the eye to those diseases in other parts and systems of the body which may have an effect on the eye.

An *optometrist* is one whose education, training and licensure qualify him to examine eyes, without the use of drugs, for abnormal visual problems not due to disease, since he is not a physician. He may prescribe, fit and supply eyeglasses and contact lenses. While he is not qualified to diagnose disease or treat disease, if his examination leads him to suspect a defect or disease requiring medical or surgical treatment, as it well may do, he should refer the patient to a professional source of medical care.

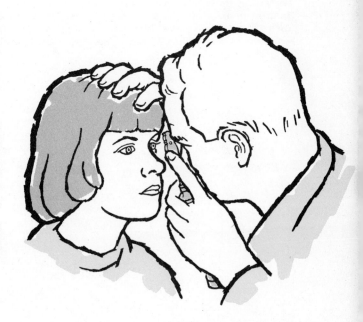

The ophthalmoscope consists essentially of a perforated mirror with which light is reflected into the patient's eye, enabling the interior of the eye to be visually inspected by the examiner.

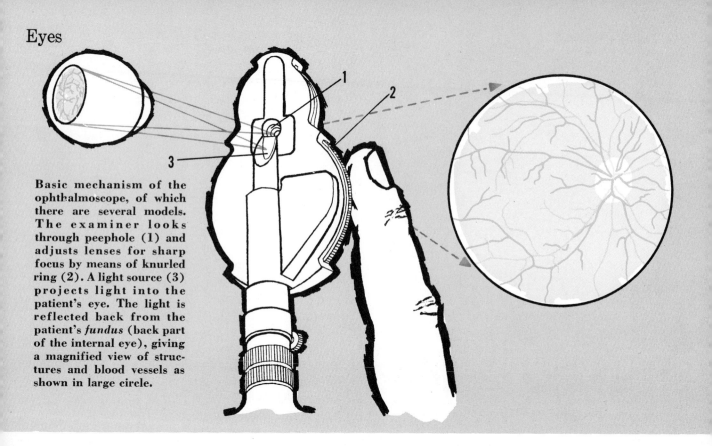

Basic mechanism of the ophthalmoscope, of which there are several models. The examiner looks through peephole (1) and adjusts lenses for sharp focus by means of knurled ring (2). A light source (3) projects light into the patient's eye. The light is reflected back from the patient's *fundus* (back part of the internal eye), giving a magnified view of structures and blood vessels as shown in large circle.

An *optician* is a skilled technician who is qualified to fill the lens prescription.

Examining instruments. A competent examination of the eyes requires the use of a number of special bits of apparatus.

Important examining instruments are:

An *ophthalmoscope,* permitting the observer to study the interior structures of the eye. A *slit lamp microscope,* to study with high magnification the structures in the anterior part of the eye.

The visual field is the area of central and peripheral vision perceived by either eye gazing upon a fixation point. Below is a standard chart with normal visual fields of left and right eyes shown in unshaded areas. The slightly off-center dots are "blind spots" where the optic nerve enters. Constrictions or distortions of the visual fields are significant in the diagnosis of certain diseases.

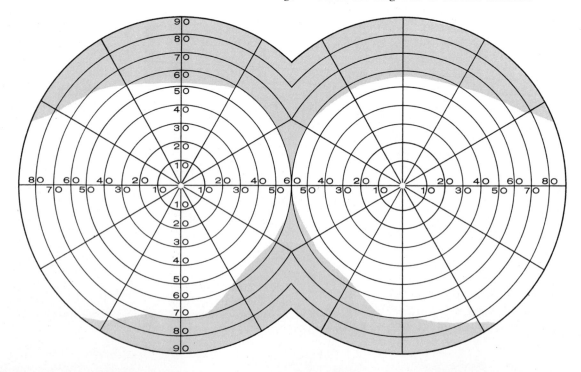

A *tonometer,* to measure pressures within the eye (somewhat like a tire gauge).

A *perimeter,* to map the limits of the fields of vision.

A *gonioscope,* to study the angle of the chamber of the eye where the outflow drainage apparatus of the eye is to be found.

A *retinoscope* or other instrument, to disclose any refractive aberration of the eye (e.g. myopia and astigmatism), or various modifications of the above; and a set of test lenses to find which one or ones fit the eyes.

Last but of most importance, is the chart for measuring visual acuity and the set of lenses used in testing the acuity and improving it if possible. The entire procedure is known as a *refraction* of the eye, and it is upon the findings of an oculist or optometrist yielded by this testing of visual acuity that the prescription for eyeglasses is based.

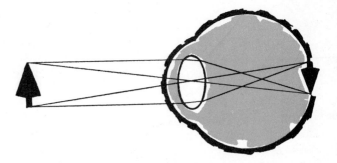

Parallel light rays from a distant object (arrow head) are refracted into sharp focus on the retina of a normal eye. Light rays from objects closer than 20 feet are not parallel and must be brought into focus on the retina by a change in the shape of the lens (accommodation).

neither diverge nor converge. If the object is closer than 20 feet the light rays diverge and must be made parallel by action of the lens within the eye or by the addition of a supplementary lens held in front of the eye, otherwise they will not come to a sharp focus on the area of central visual acuity of the retina.

The bending of the parallel rays to converge to a focus on the retina is done by the cornea and the lens of the eye (just as a "burning" glass bends the rays of the sun onto a piece of paper). Looking at an object at 20 feet or more, the normal lens is relaxed into its normal biconvex shape. The parallel rays of light "bent" (refracted) by the cornea and lens cross at the nodal point of the eye (about seven millimeters back of the cornea) and continuing their straight course fall upon the retina, forming an inverted image of the object.

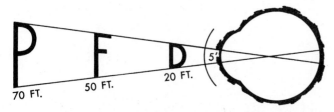

Letters of the familiar "eye test chart" are so designed that their different sizes at various distances are equivalent to a chord of identical size across an arc (5-degree visual angle). Thus a letter 20 feet away will appear to be the same size as larger letters if the latter were viewed, as indicated, from a distance of 50 or 70 feet.

The *test chart* consists, essentially, of block letters in diminishing sizes so that at various distances the appropriate letter will subtend a visual angle of five minutes at the nodal point of the eye. Thus the top large letter on the chart will appear to be of the same size when it is 200 feet away as will the standard (five minute letter) at 20 feet. A glance at the diagram explains this better than words can do.

For all practical purposes, the distance of 20 feet is considered to be infinity (consider your camera). This means that the rays of light coming from an illuminated object are parallel. That is, they

Nearsightedness and farsightedness. However, if the eye is too long from front to back, as it is in *nearsightedness* or *myopia,* the image of an object 20 feet or more away falls somewhere in front of the retina, and can only be sharply focused by holding in front of the eye a concave lens which diverges the rays coming from the object. A myopic person, however, by squeezing his lids together to produce a slit or pinhole effect, can get a fairly sharp focus (similar to a pinhole camera). Such a nearsighted person, by bringing the object near enough to his eyes, can get a good focus on his retina.

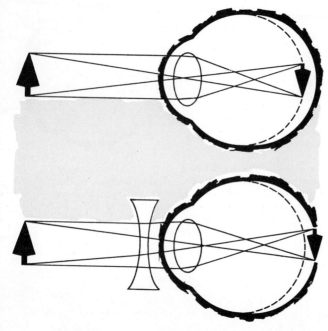

In *myopia* or nearsightedness, the image of an object (unless it is held close to the eyes) falls in front of the retina instead of upon it, and the object is seen indistinctly. The condition is corrected by placing a concave lens of proper curvature to bring the image into focus on the retina.

If the eyeball is too short from front to back, as it is in *farsightedness or hyperopia,* the image of an object 20 feet or less away is focused behind the retina. Such a person by *accommodation*—that is, thickening the lens by action of the inner muscle of the eye—can shorten the focus so that the image is sharply seen. But even for objects 20 feet or more

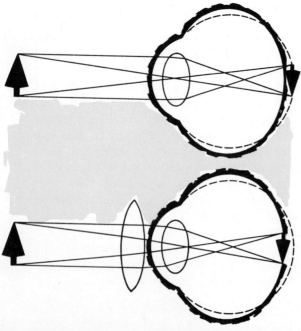

away, the relaxed normal state of the lens is not sufficient to focus the image properly. Accommodation is necessary to accomplish this. The nearer the object is brought, the more accommodation is required. The constant contraction of the inner muscle of the eye necessary to focus, in such an eye, will lead to fatigue and eyestrain. Hyperopia then should be corrected by placing the appropriate convex lens in front of the eye to assist the relaxation of the human lens.

The closer an object is brought to the eye, the more convex the human lens must become in order to focus it. As we age the human lens loses its elasticity and its power of thickening, so that by the time we are in our forties "our arms are too short" to read a telephone book. This condition is called *presbyopia,* and is overcome by the wearing of convex lenses (often in a bifocal), which need to be made a little stronger from time to time as we grow older.

Astigmatism. If the curvature of the cornea is irregular so that some rays of light are bent more in one diameter than in another, the resultant image is blurred because, if one part of the ray is focused, the other part is not. This is something like the distortion produced by a wavy pane of glass. This is called *astigmatism.* It is corrected by using a lens that bends the rays of light in only one diameter (axis). This is called a *cylinder.* A cylindrical lens can be turned in the trial frame to its proper axis to even up the focusing of the rays of light in all parts.

A **prescription for glasses** may look something like this:

+ (or plus) 2.0 D ◯ + (or plus) 0.50 cyl ax 90

What does this mean? "Plus" or the sign "+" indicates a *convex* lens suitable for a farsighted person. "Minus" or the

In *hyperopia* or farsightedness, the image of an object is focused behind the retina of an eyeball that is too short. A convex lens brings the light rays into focus on the retina. Although hyperopic persons may be able to see things sharply by thickening the lens of the eye (accommodation), this involves effort of inner muscles of the eye and may cause eye fatigue.

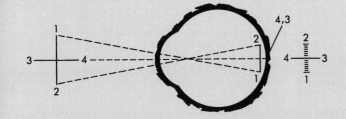

sign "—" indicates a *concave* lens for a myopic person. The "D" is an abbreviation for *diopter* which indicates the "strength" or power of the lens. A diopter is a unit of measurement of the refractive or light-bending power of a lens. (The normal human lens in its relaxed biconvex shape has a power of about ten diopters.) The symbol ⌒ means "combined with."

Thus, the prescription given as an example means that the optician grinds a convex spherical lens of two (2.0) diopters combined with a convex cylindrical lens of half a diopter (0.50) situated vertically (axis 90°). Lens prescriptions may look strange, but opticians anywhere know just what they mean.

Incidentally, it's a good idea to carry your lens prescription with you when traveling away from home, in case your glasses are lost or smashed. A spare set of glasses is good insurance, too, particularly for persons who would be seriously handicapped in getting along without them in case of loss.

Eyeglasses

What do glasses do? They help in focusing the rays of light onto the retina. The eye is a receiving organ only and the image on the retina is carried back into the brain and interpreted there.

Glasses cannot change the eye in any way or produce any disease even if they are very badly fitted. Wrong glasses can make you uncomfortable, blur your vision, make your eyes feel irritated and "sandy", and by blurring your sight can cause headaches and even nausea, but in spite of this they do not produce any damage. So if you hear that wrong glasses can ruin your eyes, this is not so.

Nor is it true that once you have begun to wear glasses you will always need them. You need them perhaps to see properly, but the wearing of glasses does not make things worse.

Tinted glasses and *sunglasses* are worn to cut down the glare of light, and it is true that some eyes are more sensitive to glare than are others. But the normal human eye is designed by nature to appreciate light, especially in the temperate zones. Besides, the eye requires more light as we get older. Thus the wearing of tinted glasses is not advisable except on the beach, in the high mountains, in snow, and in driving cars over concrete highways in bright light. They should never be worn after dark or in the house. Myopic women and some men, neurotic people, and some movie stars wear dark glasses all the time. It seems to be a psychological necessity and even a status symbol.

Contact lenses have been remarkably developed in the past few years. When properly fitted to a person who has a strong desire and motivation to wear them, or has poor vision from ocular disease that could be benefited (such as a distorted cornea, for example, shaped like a cone), or after cataract surgery on one eye when the other eye has good vision, they can usually be worn for many hours without difficulty. However, the lenses must be most accurately fitted. If not, they can rub against the cornea, abrade it, and lead to discomfort and even serious trouble.

Contact lenses are expensive because of the meticulous care and skill and the time required to make and fit them. They are easily lost, and sometimes get caught

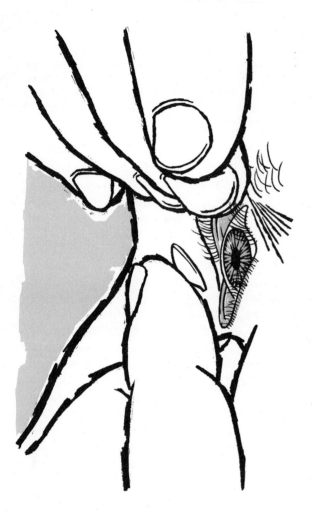

A contact lens, shown at left being applied, is a tiny lens worn over the cornea of the eye in lieu of glasses, frequently for conditions that glasses cannot correct so satisfactorily. Contact lenses are relatively expensive, since meticulous care is necessary to shape and fit the lenses to individual eyes for safety and comfort.

into use. Soft-contact lenses which absorb moisture from the eye may be more comfortable to wear.

Telescopic lenses and strong "magnifying" glasses are most useful in some cases of low vision due to ocular disease. There are a number of these "visual aids", as they are called, some of them more complex and therefore more expensive than others. As so often is the case, the simplest one is often the best.

CARE OF THE EYES

Although it is remarkable how well the sturdy eyeball is protected against hostile forces, it is still vulnerable. The fact that most eye injuries are preventable requires constant attention and awareness by each individual. National and local societies for the prevention of blindness are doing their job day in and out, but each of us is also an "island" in this respect.

If you must rub your eyes, use clean disposable tissue for this purpose, never your fingers. Wear your glasses as directed by your physician. Read in a good light that comes from over your shoulder, preferably the left one. Remove your dark glasses after sundown and never drive your car with them on at night.

under the upper lid and are hard to remove by the patient, especially in cases after a cataract operation.

In spite of these and other disturbing events, contact lenses are wonderful visual aids, and as they become better and better, more people are using them with delight and benefit. Newer forms of contact lenses are beginning to come

Special "visual aids" may be useful for persons with extreme or unusual disorders of vision, and for the working comfort of people with normal vision in some circumstances. The drawing shows a type of magnifying binocular spectacles which permit conveniently longer working distances in dentistry, surgery, and other situations.

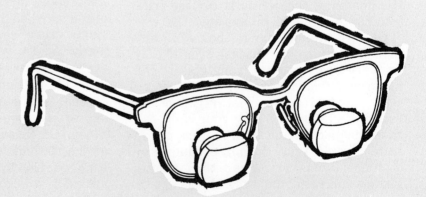

If your work or your hobbies expose your eyes to the danger of flying particles, wear protective goggles.

If you think you have something in your eye, you probably do, so see your physician right away. Irritable and "sandy" eyes may be caused by lack of sleep, too much drinking or smoking, or a faulty diet as well as by the need for proper glasses or by the wearing of improper ones.

Home Measures

A simple and effective *eye wash* can be easily made by adding a level teaspoonful of salt to a pint of boiled water. A cotton pad soaked in the salt solution at room temperature and placed upon the closed eyelids for four or five minutes is remarkably soothing to tired eyes, particularly so if you fall asleep while this is going on, for you may need the rest.

After reading steadily for a half hour or so, look away at a distant object for a few moments and change the focus.

You should have your eyes checked about every two to three years to see if you need glasses or a change in the ones you are wearing, but particularly to see if any disease is present or developing. This is especially important after 40 years of age.

If a chemical is rubbed or splashed into your eye, immediately hold your head, with the eyes open, directly under a gently running stream of water from the nearest tap. Do this at once and for at least five minutes. Then run to your nearest physician or ophthalmologist as an emergency. Chemical burns of the eyes are terribly serious affairs and once the chemical gets into the ocular tissues, washing the eyes won't do much good, for the action continues deeper and deeper into the structures. This is truly an emergency, as much or more so than is a ruptured appendix.

Allergies

The irritated, running eyes of the hay fever victim are well known to everyone. What is not quite so well known is that allergic irritation to the eyes and lids can be caused by drugs or medicines, environmental dust, cosmetics, newsprint, carbon paper, foods and many other things.

Itching and redness of the eyes or the lids are the chief symptoms of allergy, and shortly after this the involved tissues become swollen and watery. Don't try to treat yourself, for the job of discovering the villain can be a most difficult task even for the expert in this field, and the treatment can be as varied as the cause. (See Chapter 20).

CHILDREN'S EYES

The eyes of the newborn infant do not focus or work together until five or six months after birth and then they may wander a bit for another six months. If they do not appear straight or parallel by then, consult your ophthalmologist for advice and treatment.

If there is a discharge from the baby's eyes it may be due to the silver nitrate that is instilled at birth, or to an infection (conjunctivitis or pink eye). It may also be due to the blockage of the passage of tears into the nose. The blockage is due to a thin strand of tissue. This strand usually disappears shortly after birth, but may persist. If so, the ophthalmologist will probe the passage and open it up. Generally that is all that is needed.

The baby's pupils should be black. If not, or if there is a white pupil, it should be seen by your physician. This may mean that there is a cataract present, or something else wrong inside the eye of more serious nature. One should not delay in finding out what is wrong and doing something about it.

The pre-school child should have the eyes examined to see what is going on. Glasses may or may not be indicated. The ocular muscles may or may not be working normally together. Certain defects, congenital, familial, or acquired may be present. The parents should know about these things and do something about it without delay, instead of waiting for the child to complain.

Ocular Muscle Imbalance
(Cross-eye, wall-eye)

The eyes may be crossed or divergent from birth or not become obviously so until later. These conditions require early study, diagnosis and proper care.

An eye that turns in or out in early childhood may lose its vision unless

Squint. Because there are six muscles in each eye that have to do with motility of the eyes, and the two eyes must work together as a pair, the problem of *strabismus* (squint, heterotropia) can become very complex. It is not unusual to find that in addition to the horizontal eye muscles not working together, there is a vertical imbalance as well. Also we

Below, two eyes that see as one. At left, both eyes turn slightly inward toward each other (converge) as they focus on an object held close to the eyes. At right, the eyes become more parallel as they focus together upon a more distant object. The separate images from each eye are seen as one; this is called *fusion*. This complex process of fusion gives stereoscopic or three-dimensional vision for judgments of depth and distance. Movements of each eye are controlled by muscles attached to the eyeball.

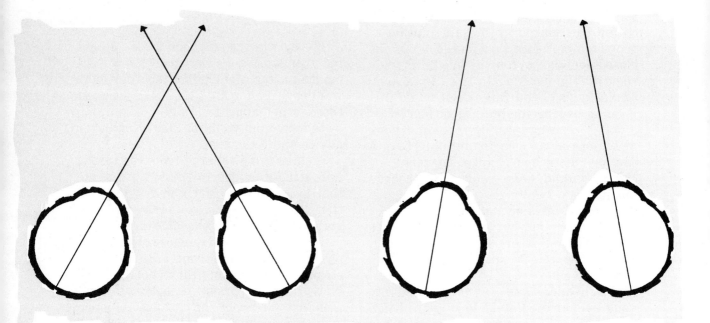

treated. This is known as *amblyopia from non-use.* If discovered early a lot can be done to restore vision in many instances — for example, by glasses or covering the good eye, or by muscle exercises and other measures. It is obvious why an early examination and exact diagnosis is of the greatest importance. No child will "outgrow" a cross or wall eye and parents should be aware of this.

It is well too for the parent to be prepared for the physician to say that surgery is necessary, for it is so in most instances, and often the earlier the better. Modern surgery is a far cry from what was done even twenty years ago and the results are uniformly good.

find in some cases that an eye will become askew only in a certain position of gaze.

By *fusion* we mean that the image seen with one eye fuses with the image seen with the other. Fusion is essential for stereoscopic, or three-dimensional vision. Normally it is present early in childhood. But if one eye is defective, or if there is a muscle askew, fusion does not take place.

It happens in some instances that a child has an alternating strabismus even if the vision is perfect in each eye. For example, when he looks at an object with his right eye, the left turns in, and vice versa. Such patients do not have fusion, nor do many of them develop it even after

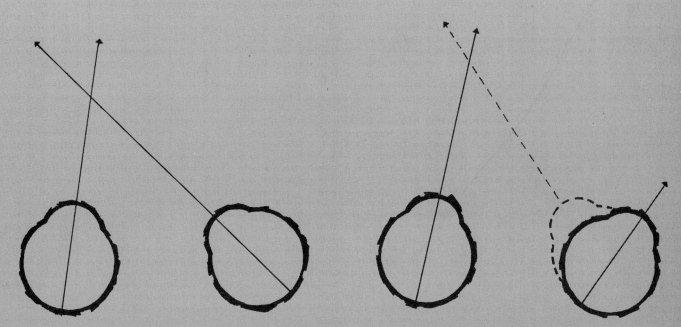

Cross-eye or convergent squint is shown at left above. The right eye is turned inward upon the left eye that is properly focused on an object. At right, *wall-eye* or divergent squint, in which the right eye is turned outward from the normally focused left eye. The most common form of squint is "concomitant convergent strabismus," shown in the drawing of the child below. There is an inward turn of the left eye and the faulty relationship of the axes is maintained in every direction of turn (hence, "concomitant"). The condition is often associated with hyperopia or farsightedness.

surgery. In this instance surgery is frequently successful in making the eyes appear to be straight and cosmetically satisfactory, but the vision is still alternated between the two eyes.

It is nice to have fusion, but it is not absolutely necessary in order to get along in normal life. It is most helpful in judging distances between objects, but a child without fusion does very well through practical experience.

Ocular muscle exercises (orthoptics) are designed to stimulate fusion and to increase its amplitude. If one succeeds in this endeavor the eyes will maintain their correct position and relationship, one with another. This is why, following surgery as a rule, orthoptic exercises are frequently prescribed by an oculist. They may or may not work.

Amblyopia, or the suppression of the vision of an eye from non-use, becomes

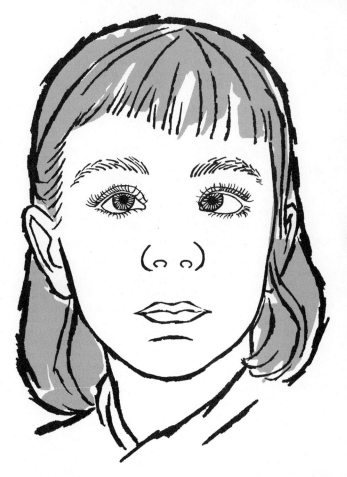

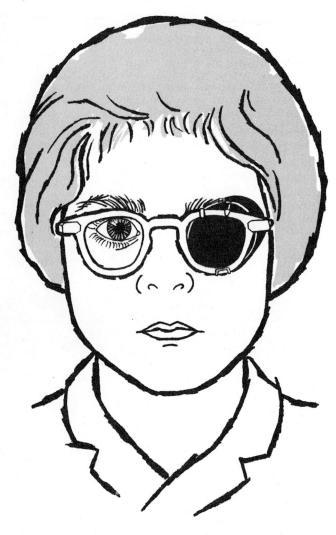

The image from a crossed eye tends to be suppressed and the eye to become incapable of seeing although there are no organic changes (amblyopia). As part of the early treatment of such a condition, a patch or a blacked-out spectacle lens may be worn over the good eye for several weeks or months, to compel the weaker eye to do the work of seeing and hopefully to improve its vision.

more difficult to overcome as the child gets older. There is a saying that after the age of six, amblyopia cannot be corrected. However, it is comforting to know that this is not strictly true of all cases, and there are instances where treatment of the amblyopia even later in life has been successful. So keep plugging away and follow directions, no matter how much the patient may object, or in what way he shows his dislike of the business. Occlusion or covering of a child's eye may often be harder for the parent to take than it is for the child.

INFECTIONS OF THE EYES

Bacteria (e.g., streptococcus), *molds* (e.g., penicillin) or *viruses* (e.g., the virus of fever blisters) get into our eyes all the time. If the organism is stronger than the immunity or resistance of the ocular tissue, or if there is a break or cut into the structures, infection takes place. If it attacks the white of the eye (the conjunctiva) the eye becomes red, feels sandy, and there is a discharge that varies from being watery, mucous, or full of pus. In any event, the discharge sticks the eyelashes together. This is especially noticed on arising in the morning. The vision is not disturbed except by the discharge getting into the cornea.

"Pink eye." The condition is known as pink eye or *acute conjunctivitis*. The causative agent can be transferred from one eye to the other or to the eyes of another person by fingers or cloth, because the discharge contains the contagious and infectious organisms.

Acute conjunctivitis should be treated early and by an expert. Fortunately, many antibiotics and some of the sulfa preparations are most effective. Once in awhile, however, the organism is resistant to the drug, or may not be susceptible to it (for example, viruses), and other measures of treatment are then used for relief of this condition.

Stye. If organisms, especially bacteria, get into the roots of the eyelashes a local infection takes place known as a *hordeolum* or *stye*. If, on the other hand, the infectious agent gets into one of the grease or sweat glands of the eyelids a swelling forms due to a breakdown of the greasy material and some pus. This forms a cyst or *chalazion* of the lid. Styes and chalazions need to be opened up and drained of their contents.

An embedded *foreign body* in the cornea can cause serious infection and an ulcer that can perforate and cause loss of the eye. Or the infection can get into the deeper structure of the eye and cause the inside to be full of pus and result in blindness.

The *conjunctiva* is a thin mucous membrane that covers the insides of the eyelids and is reflected over the "white of the eye" and is continuous with the epithelial lining of the cornea. The cross-section drawing of the eyeball shows its location (size exaggerated). The top drawing shows a normal eye, and below it, *conjunctivitis*—inflammation of the conjunctiva, with characteristic congestion and enlargement of blood vessels giving a red or "bloodshot" eye. Conjunctivitis may result from local infection, allergies, irritation, or from inflammation within the eye itself.

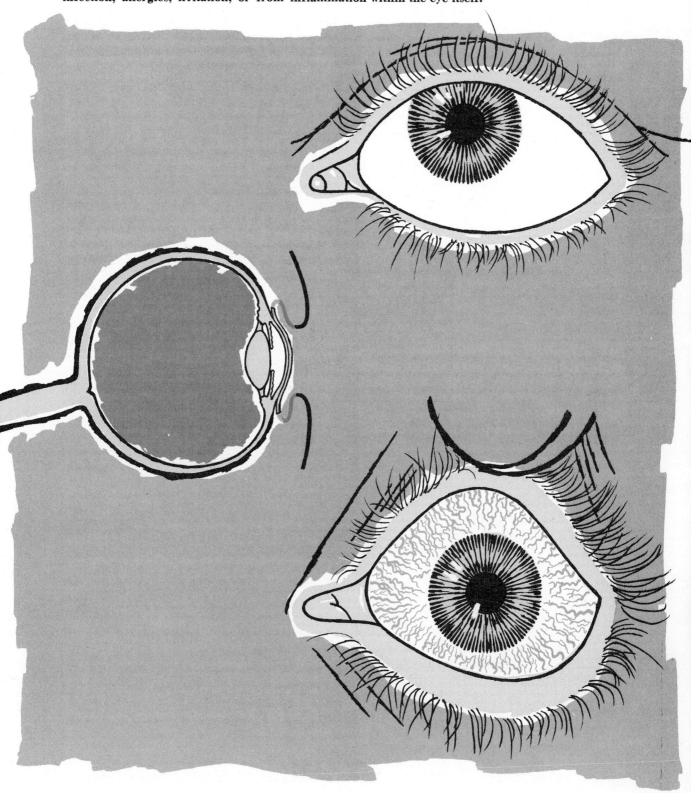

A *stye* is an infection, usually by staphylococcus organisms, of one of the glands of the eyelid margin. Application of hot compresses usually brings the stye to a head and pus escapes. If styes occur in repeated crops, a general health checkup is advisable.

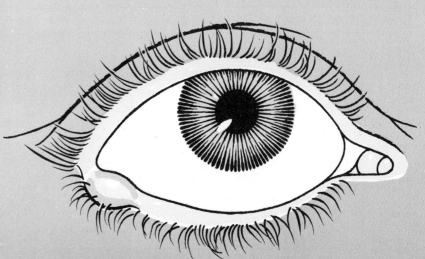

Thus a *perforating injury* of the eye (for example a knife wound, a BB shot, and a host of other ocular lethal things) can cause blindness not only as the result of the direct injury, but also because bacteria are carried into the eye.

Trachoma. Certain viruses, notably the *trachoma* virus, attack the conjunctiva, especially that of the upper and lower lids, causing a form of granulation. This is a chronic, steadily progressive disease which leads to blindness eventually, due to ulceration and scarring of the cornea.

We don't encounter much trachoma any more in our country, but it is a common cause of blindness in the Middle East, Africa and some parts of Asia today. Filth, lack of hygiene, malnutrition, close personal contact, all of these factors and others make a fertile host for the trachoma virus to grow in and develop, setting the stage for blindness.

Trachoma vaccines have been developed and are being tried out with indications of success. But the disease can be eradicated, as it has been in our country, through obeying the laws of cleanliness and hygiene. Running water and the free use of soap in each home has done more to get rid of trachoma than has any other measure so far.

THE RED EYE

Without pain or blurred vision.

This may mean that a hemorrhage from a ruptured small blood vessel under the conjunctiva has taken place. It is a very common affair that more often occurs in older people. It may follow a sneeze, or a sudden compression of the abdomen as happens on lifting or straining. It looks awful, but the patient may not be aware of it unless he sees himself in a mirror or is startled by an exclamation of a friend.

It is deep red at first, and then changes to purple, green, yellow, and finally in about six days or so fades away. There is no treatment and the condition is usually unimportant.

If a person has many subconjunctival hemorrhages it is wise to have a medical checkup in order to rule out some general medical condition that may be underlying.

Acute conjunctivitis (or pink eye) has already been described. The eye is red and there is no pain as a rule, but there always is a gritty or sandy sensation, a discharge, and the lids are always stuck together on awakening.

Unless reddened eyes result from something as obvious as exposure to smoke, the cause should be investigated.

With pain and blurred vision.

There are two major conditions that produce these signs and symptoms. These are *acute iritis* and *acute glaucoma.*

Iritis is an inflammation of the iris, the colored part of the eye. The cause is frequently obscure, although it is certain that the tissues of the iris and the ciliary body as well as the choroid (these three structures are known as the *uvea)*

later, as an outpouring of fighting cells takes place inside the eye, especially in the anterior chamber).

A red painful eye needs immediate expert attention.

Acute iritis and acute glaucoma can cause the patient to have somewhat the same signs and symptoms. The treatment of the two conditions is quite different.

Acute glaucoma often begins as a congested eye with mildly blurred vision,

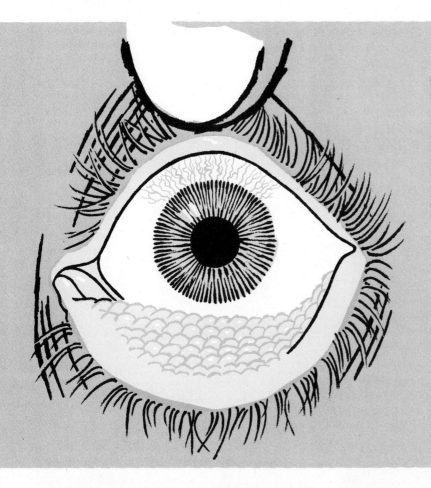

Trachoma is an infectious disease of the eyes associated with lack of cleanliness. It is caused by a virus. As the disease progresses, the insides of the eyelids take on a raspberry-like appearance (granulation) and the upper portion of the cornea becomes involved, as shown in drawing. Ulceration and scarring of the cornea eventually cause blindness or gross impairment of vision.

become sensitized to a protein from some source, usually bacterial, in the body. Attacks occur therefore when the toxic agent comes in contact with the sensitized iris tissue.

In an acute attack of iritis the eye is red and this redness is mostly concentrated around the periphery of the cornea. The eyeball is tender to touch and movement. Pain in and around the eye is sometimes exquisite and the vision may or may not be blurred (this usually comes

associated with headache in and especially around and behind the eyeball. A regular but not constant symptom is the seeing of rainbow rings (halos) around street lamps at night. The attack may subside spontaneously on rest and sleep. Or it may increase in severity. The congestion gets worse, the vision fades and may even disappear, the pain becomes quite terrible, and the patient may go into a form of shock consisting of pallor, sweating, fainting and vomiting.

Every time an acute attack occurs more and more damage takes place. So even the mild attacks, which are always recurrent, necessitate immediate emergency medical care.

The treatment is surgical (*iridectomy*) and this is almost 100 percent effective, so that no further attacks occur and the patient is rescued from certain blindness.

Because sooner or later acute glaucoma affects both eyes, prophylactic surgery is advised for the other so far unaffected eye. This is difficult for the average person to understand, but is always

There are several types of *corneal ulcer*; top drawing below shows a dendritic ulcer resulting from infection by the herpes simplex virus, the cause of the common cold sore. Lower drawing shows different stages of ulcer erosion, left to right: invasion of superficial layer of the cornea, then of deeper layers of the cornea, and finally, perforation.

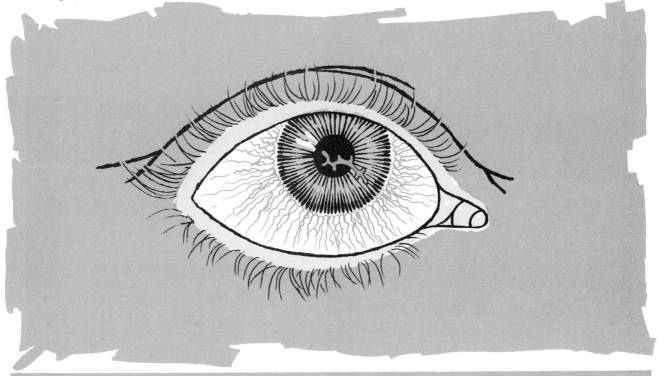

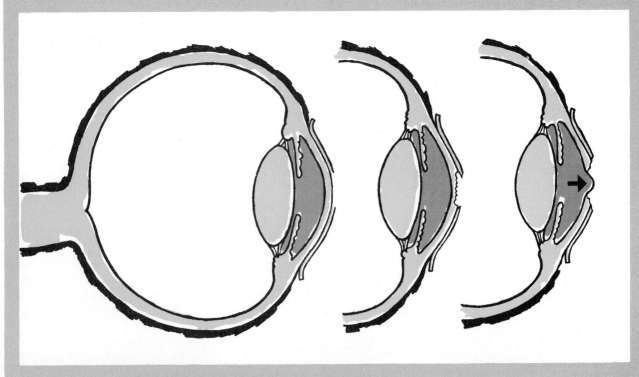

considered necessary by the modern ophthalmic surgeon.

The mechanism of this form of glaucoma and the other form known as *wide angle* or *simple* glaucoma will be considered separately.

An **ulcer of the cornea,** either from bacteria or a virus, causes pain, congestion and blurred vision.

Diseases of the cornea itself, such as interstitial keratitis (inflammation of the cornea) due to syphilis, tuberculosis, or other things, produces pain, redness, tenderness and blurred vision.

Sensitivity to light *(photophobia)* which can be quite intense, usually associated with watering eyes, occurs in acute iritis and glaucoma but is much more evident in corneal diseases.

The painless white eye with disturbed vision.

A number of things, all taking place within the eyeball, cause these symptoms. The loss of vision may be gradual, as in the development and progression of a cataract or simple glaucoma. Or it may be due to an inflammation of the *choroid* (choroiditis, uveitis), in which event an inflammation, usually pimple-like, hits the choroid and produces a reaction calling out the fighting cells which may fill the vitreous, or by eroding a choroidal or retinal blood vessel produce bleeding within the eye, or both. It is obvious that these responses will reduce one's vision, sometimes gradually, at other times quite violently.

Another cause of partial painless loss of vision, gradually getting worse, is the development of a tumor within the eye.

The loss of vision may be sudden. This happens when a blood vessel within the eye, almost always a retinal one, becomes ruptured, blocked off (thrombosis) or plugged (embolus). It is also a symptom of detached or separated retina, although in this event the patient is apt first to notice a shower of black particles floating in his sight, flashes of light, followed by a developing veil or curtain which, unless taken care of surgically, will lead to eventual blindness.

Another cause of painless, non-congestive, sudden blurring of vision or blindness, is disease of the optic nerve (optic neuritis, retrobulbar optic neuritis).

These and several other conditions, some in the eye, others in the brain, all require careful study and expert diagnosis and must be considered as urgent medical affairs, not to be fooled with.

The Mechanism of Glaucoma

The signs and symptoms of the two main forms of glaucoma have been described.

Glaucoma means essentially an increased pressure within the eye. Normally, the rate of formation of the intraocular fluid and its outflow are in balance. The fluid, formed by the ciliary cells, bathes the interior of the eye and nourishes it and then flows forward around the lens into the anterior chamber. It is evacuated through the minute drainage canals situated in the angle of the anterior chamber. From here it goes into the veins of the sclera and conjunctiva and then into the general circulation.

If more fluid is formed than can be carried away, or if, as is most often the case, the outflow channels become narrowed with age, or blocked up by a swollen iris and dilated pupil, the pressure within the eye becomes elevated.

If the blockage is sudden, as it is in acute glaucoma, it is because the angle is narrow, often genetically so. The root of the iris in these cases becomes thickened when the pupil dilates as it does in the dark, after certain drugs, and exciting or emotional events (marital quarrel, death in the family, anger, or even after an exciting game of cards). The thickened root of the iris fills up the narrowed angle, blocks off the outflow channels and dams back the inflow. The natural mechanical result therefore is an increase in intraocular pressure (glaucoma).

In older people (about two per cent of all of us over 40 years of age) the blockage of the outflow is more gradual, as the outflow channels become more and more narrowed with age. The mechanics

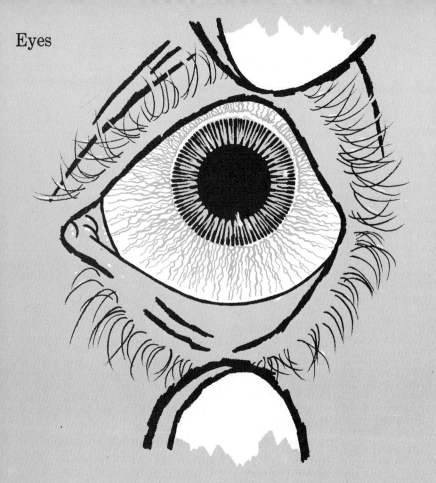

Acute or insidious forms of *glau-coma* damage vision through the buildup of fluid pressures within the eyeball, like an overinflated tire. At left, drawing shows dilated pupil and reddened eye in acute glaucoma. Some common forms of glaucoma do not cause early symptoms and the condition is detected in routine examinations which give the best chance of pre-venting possible blindness. Draw-ings below show the anterior segment of the eye and mechan-isms of glaucoma. In top rectan-gle, fluid produced by *ciliary cells* (1) flows around *iris* (2) to angle where it enters *canal* (3) and is absorbed in *veins* (4). Unob-structed flow maintains normal fluid pressures. Bottom rectangle shows closed angle, blocking out-flow of fluid, with back-up result-ing in destructive pressures.

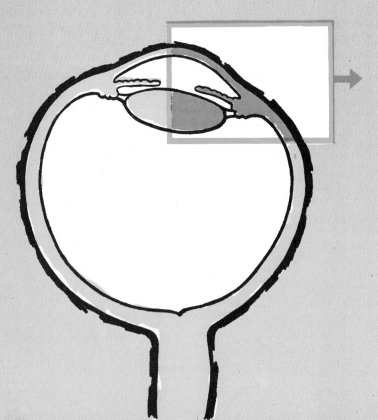

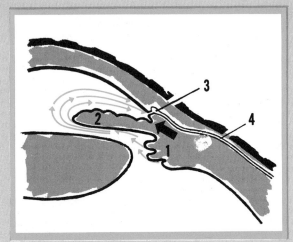

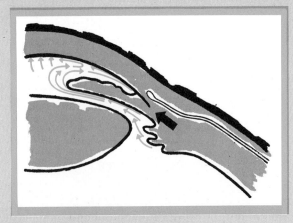

and the immediate results are quite different because of the gradual versus the sudden occlusion of the outflow apparatus. This form of glaucoma is known as the *wide angle* (in contrast to the narrow or acutely blocked angle) form, or as *chronic simple glaucoma* or *non-congestive glaucoma.*

This is a very insidious and therefore dangerous form of glaucoma. It can steal away some of the vision, by pressure on the optic nerve, retinal cells and blood vessels, before the patient becomes aware of it. Remember, it is painless and the eye remains white.

The increased pressure within the eye pushes back the soft pulp of the optic nerve and depresses it into a cup. The compressed nerve fibers can't live long, any more than flowers under a stone can. The decreased blood flow injures the precious retinal cells.

So it is that often the first thing a person with this form of glaucoma notices, is a blurring of vision on the side towards the nose, which spreads to involve other parts of the field of vision until, unless recognized and properly treated, total and hopeless blindness ensues (absolute glaucoma).

Because of the insidious serious nature of this disease in the patient who is unaware of it, it has become routine practice by every ophthalmologist, and it is hoped by every general practitioner, to measure the intraocular pressure or ocular tension of the eyes of everyone over 40 who comes into the office. Indeed, nowadays increasing efforts are made to set up tension (tonometry) stations everywhere by local, state and federal actions under medical direction, so that more and more individuals over 40 can at least have the tensions of their eyes measured. If tension is found to be higher than normal the individual is referred to an ophthalmologist or an eye clinic.

Ocular tension is measured by an instrument called a *tonometer*. It can be compared crudely to an ordinary tire gauge, and everyone knows that an abnormal amount of air in a tire can raise the dickens with a tire.

After the eye is anesthetized with a drop of a local anesthetic, the base of the instrument is placed on the cornea, and the amount of indentation of the instrument gives a fairly good reading of the ocular tension. (Compare kicking of a tire to see if it is soft or hard.)

But tonometry is only one phase, perhaps the most important one however, in the study of an eye to see if chronic simple glaucoma is present. Determinations of visual acuity, the mapping out of the boundaries of the field of vision *(perimetry)*, the study of the appearance of the optic nerve *(ophthalmoscopy)* and an observation of the anatomy and appearance of the angle of the anterior chamber, *gonioscopy,* are necessary tests.

The **treatment** of chronic simple glaucoma is either medical (drops) or surgical. In this event a new outflow channel is made (e.g. trephine opening). Surgery is usually not performed until a trial of drugs is made. If these medications don't work, and there are a large variety of them to try, then surgery must be done (see Chapter 22).

Surgery is effective in about 85 per cent of the cases of glaucoma. It will not restore the vision that is lost. This is gone forever. But if it is successful it will check the progress, otherwise relentless, of the disease. It will put out the fire but not rebuild the house.

Congenital Glaucoma

This is a form of glaucoma that occurs in babies and children under two. The symptoms are sensitivity to light, spasm of the lids and watering eyes. Sometimes there may be pain which the child shows by fretting, refusing feedings and being obviously miserable. An unusually large cornea, often cloudy or hazy, which increases in size, and a deep anterior chamber are signs demanding attention.

The cause is a faulty development of the anterior chamber angle associated with aberrant tissue that covers and blocks the outflow channels.

The treatment is always surgical.

Diagram of the principle of tonometry. The *plunger* (1) of the instrument is supported by the *footplate* (2) that rests on the anesthetized eyeball. Pressures of fluid in the *anterior chamber* of the eye (3) raise the plunger to varying degrees. Excessive pressures within the eye can inflict irreparable damage on the *optic nerve*(4).

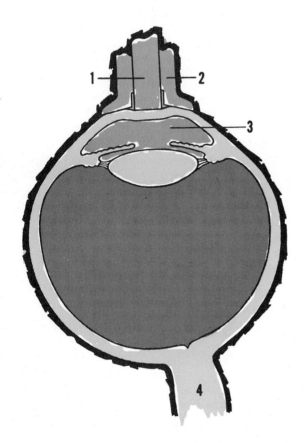

Cataract

The lens of the eye, situated just behind the pupil, is a remarkable structure. In health it is clear and focuses the rays of light as has already been described.

With age and in such diseases as diabetes and uveitis, it loses this transparency and becomes more and more opaque, gradually shutting out the vision as does an increasingly dirty window.

This is known as *cataract*. It is not a growth but a biochemical change in the lens. Small opacities are the rule in age and occur in all animals. They may increase in number, coalesce and make the lens completely opaque, producing a "white pupil". This is known as a "ripe" cataract. It may take many years to arrive at this stage and during this time the vision gets worse and worse until the patient is able only to recognize light, dark and colored lights.

Nowadays it is not necessary to wait until the cataractous lens becomes completely ripe in order to remove it surgically. Incidentally, there is no medicine that will absorb, retard or prevent the relentless progress of cataract, and the unethical advice to use such preparations is a form of quackery.

Cataract is an opacity of the crystalline lens of the eye or its capsule which acts like a curtain to prevent light rays from reaching the retina. Some forms are congenital; the more common forms occur after middle age. Opacities may be small or they may coalesce and opacify the entire lens, producing a "white pupil," as shown at the right below, in contrast with a normal eye. Removal of the opaque lens restores clear vision, but requires spectacles or contact lenses to substitute for the human lens.

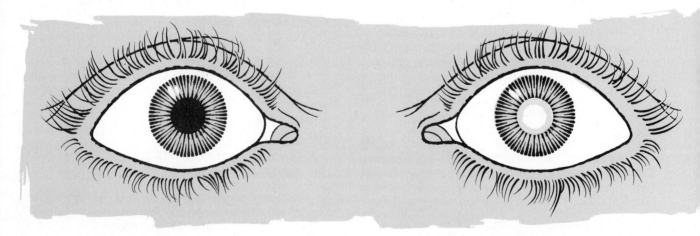

Modern cataract surgery has reached a high state of perfection. It is almost always successful. New technics, anesthetics, drugs, nursing care, equipment, instruments and the training of eye surgeons for this purpose are superb. It is not a painful operation to fear unduly and the patient's recovery from it is generally without trouble (see Chapter 22).

The operation itself consists of incising the anesthetized eye, making a small hole in the iris, removing the cataractous lens with forceps or suction apparatus through the dilated pupil, and sewing up the wound.

As in any operation, there may be complications, but fortunately these are usually minor in nature and yield to modern care and treatment. About one eye in a thousand is completely lost as the result of the operation. But since a cataractous eye is doomed to blindness anyway, the odds are all in favor of the patient. There is no operation that has

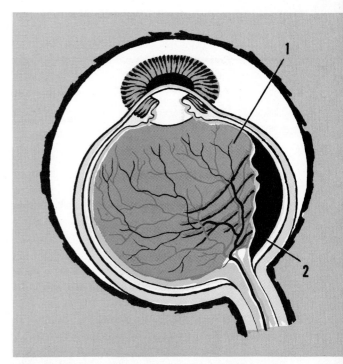

Diagram of *detached retina*. The *retina* (1) separates from the underlying *choroid* (2), usually because a tear in the retina permits fluid to seep under it and lift it up. Various surgical methods of "spot welding" the tissue-thin retina to reattach it are often successful.

given so much happiness to so many people as has the removal of a cataract.

Glasses after cataract surgery. After cataract surgery the lens is gone and an eye without a lens can't focus. It is necessary to supply this lack by "cataract glasses". These are necessarily thick and sometimes heavy. The wearing of them at first can be disturbing, because the vision is not quite the same in width, and objects seem to be bigger than they were before.

The vast majority of patients, however, soon become adjusted to these disturbances and return to daily visual activities.

Modern contact lenses are increasingly being used by the aphakic patient (i.e. one who has had a cataract removed) with comfort and safety, if these are properly fitted. Some aphakics cannot wear the contact lenses for some reason or other, but those who can have a more efficient and wider vision than do those who wear the usual correcting spectacles.

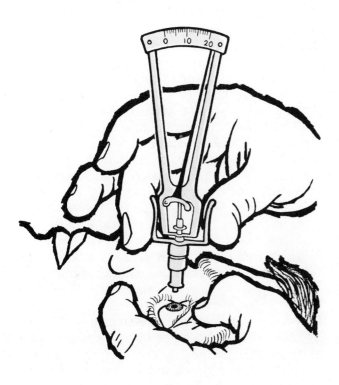

Measuring internal pressures of the eye with a *tonometer*. A small plunger at the bottom of the instrument, pressed upon the anesthetized cornea, is connected to a scale-lever which registers the amount of indentation.

Detached Retina

The subject of **detached** or **separated retina** has already been touched upon. The condition is diagnosed by careful study of the interior of the eye by means of the ophthalmoscope. There is almost always a hole or tear in the retina. This is responsible for its separation from its bed, because the intraocular fluid gets through the hole and lifts it up just as water beneath wallpaper could do.

The cause of the hole or holes is not entirely known, but it is believed to be due to traction on a diseased or degenerated part of the retina by bands of tissue in the contracting diseased vitreous. Sometimes holes are the result of severe ocular concussion or perforation.

The treatment is always surgical. Each hole or tear in the retina is sealed off, something like spot welding, in various ways (diathermy, coagulation, buckling of the eyeball, light coagulation).

The operation is successful in about 80 percent of cases, and the earlier the operation is performed, as a rule, the better is the chance of success.

Cancer of the Eye

Malignant tumors can develop in the eye as elsewhere in the body, either directly in the tissues or as the result of metastases from a tumor elsewhere.

The usual forms seen by ophthalmologists are those arising from the retina in young children (*retinoblastoma*) or those of pigmented nature arising in the uvea (iris, ciliary body and choroid), generally in adults.

These are fatal, unless the eye is removed early, although in some rare instances the tumor can be destroyed by radiant energy or some form of cauterization or destructive chemicals or drugs.

Systemic Diseases that Affect the Eyes

Some diseases of the general system affect the eyes. These constitute a large and growing number of cases often leading to total blindness.

The chief of these is *diabetes*. Diabetics are kept alive longer than ever before because of the advances of medical treatment in this area. This is good.

What isn't so good is the fact that with this lengthened span of life of the diabetic, changes occur in the blood vessels of the retina. As a result, repeated hemorrhages into the retina and the vitreous occur and each time they do, more and more damage to sight takes place. These vascular changes lead to the outpouring of exudates of various sorts and the development of proliferating scar tissue in the retina and vitreous. The formation of cataract is but a part of the entire process.

This is a most complex problem and is the subject of continuous research throughout the world to discover the underlying causes and mechanisms involved, to find some preventive measure and to discover a satisfactory method of treatment.

So far efforts along these lines have not been entirely successful, but progress is being made. Some day these problems will be solved. At the present time, the only measure of which we are certain, to prevent and to retard the more or less relentless advance of the retinal vessel disease, is to insist that the affected patient follow his physician's directions meticulously. Any diabetic will agree that this is a very hard thing to do and is contrary to human nature. But there must be no let up at any time.

As one gets older the relentless course of *arteriosclerosis* or "hardening of the arteries" takes place. This process occurs in the retinal vessels as well. They break, resulting in hemorrhages, usually small. They dry up or become occluded. When this happens nutrition to the retinal cells is lost and the area of the retina supplied by these vessels becomes blind, atrophic and scarred. If the central or major vessel no longer functions, the inner eye, deprived of its blood supply, becomes entirely blind, often in a matter of seconds.

On the other hand, if only a branch of the central vessels is involved, only that sector of the retina supplied by the affected vessel becomes blind.

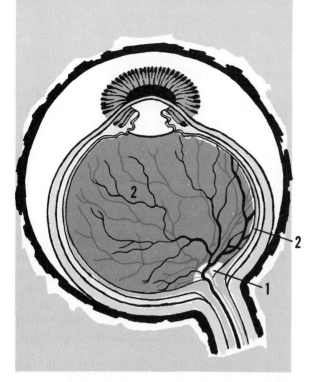

Blood vessel patterns in the fundus (back) of a normal eye. The *optic disk* (1) is the area from which the optic nerve emerges; the *retina* (2) is shown in cross section and with its vessels. Direct view of these vessels through an ophthalmoscope gives important diagnostic information.

central part of the retina *(macular degeneration)*. The vessels in the underlying choroid are the ones that are involved.

This results in a blind area in the central vision, the part of the vision that is used in looking directly at an object. One can no longer read, recognize faces, or the colors of objects.

The side vision remains good, so that these unfortunate people always see to get about and to avoid obstructions. They do not become blind in the usual sense.

Nothing can be done to restore the function of the macula. Ordinary glasses do not help. Sometimes optical aids, known as "visual aids", that are essentially magnifiers, may be of some help. A number of clinics having to do with the fitting of these "visual aids" are springing up here and there. They are most valuable.

If the arteriosclerosis is combined with high blood pressure the outlook is more serious.

A peculiar form of this vascular disease (sclerosis) that is very common, and always in the elderly, is the deprivation of the blood supply exclusively to the

Arteriosclerosis, often accompanied by high blood pressure, afflicts retinal vessels as well as other vessels of the body. At left below, view of a normal retina as seen through the ophthalmoscope. *Arteries* (1) are smooth branching vessels; *veins* (2) are shown in gray; (3) is the *optic disk*. At right, arteriosclerotic changes: arteries become congested and straighten out like a garden hose under high pressure. Underlying veins are compressed and breaks may occur, with tiny hemorrhages and obstruction of local circulation. Visual symptoms vary with the part of the retina that is affected.

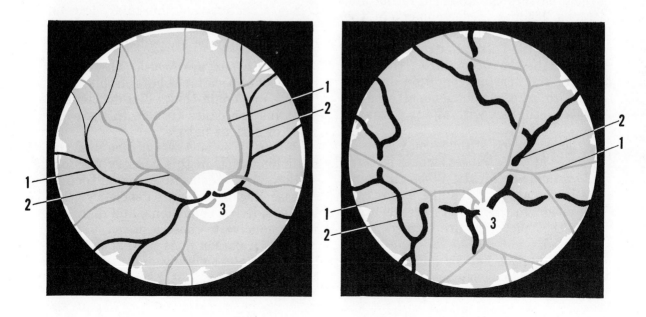

Diseases of the blood, such as leukemia, pernicious anemia, and a host of things falling into the growing discipline of hematology, sometimes lead to retinal hemorrhages. The vision can be affected to a degree compatible with the duration, extent and location of these hemorrhages.

Congenital and familial diseases affecting the retina through its blood supply are found now and then. A typical example of this is *retinitis pigmentosa.*

Here the blood vessels of the peripheral part (sides) of the retina and choroid become narrowed in the course of time. The ophthalmologist sees pigment deposits in the involved zone of the retina, which come closer and closer to the macula. The latter is usually not involved, so that central vision may remain good for a long time. But the peripheral vision closes down and the sight is as if one were looking through a tube of a gun barrel.

Retrolental fibroplasia. Quite rare today is the condition known as *retrolental fibroplasia.* In 1942 it was discovered that some premature infants who had been kept alive in oxygen incubators developed a white membrane behind the lens and were blind. In the ensuing 12 years many hundreds of these babies were afflicted before it was shown that excess oxygen was to blame. The oxygen was toxic and led to new blood vessels developing into the anterior retina and vitreous, leading to detachment of the retina and fibrous tissue. After this discovery and the better control of oxygen delivered to the prematures, the incidence of this terrible condition dropped almost to zero. An occasional case is, however, still met with and is puzzling.

Arteriosclerosis of the blood vessels of the brain at times causes strokes or cerebral vascular accidents. When this happens in the areas of the fibers that conduct vision to the centers of the brain where the "pictures" are formed, sight is affected.

Usually only a half or quarter of the field of vision in each eye is affected and this is indeed most disturbing to the patient, who may feel that he is wearing horse blinkers.

Tumors of the brain, by pressing on these areas either directly or on the blood vessels, may give the same effect.

Headaches

Headache is perhaps the most common human complaint. It is a subjective symptom, disturbing to patient and his physician. There are many causes for it and its severity is no indication of the seriousness of the cause.

Eyestrain is only one of the causes, although it is a common one. It is, however, the simplest to determine by a careful eye examination and if found, usually can be easily alleviated.

In all cases of headache, therefore, it is necessary to rule out ocular conditions as a contributing cause.

Eyestrain due to refractive errors and ocular muscle defects shows itself by burning, tearing, or a sandy sensation in the eyes. The eyes may ache, and pain in and behind the eyes may be present. Patients often complain of a "pulling sensation". They may fatigue easily, may be cross and irritable, and show distaste for reading or studying. Drowsiness and the symptoms of eyestrain are usually absent during the morning hours.

I suppose that in the last analysis eyestrain is the result of the effort to overcome refractive and muscular defects. Motivation plays a large role, and neurotic signs may be present too.

Vitamins and eye health. There have been a lot of peculiar beliefs on this topic. There is no doubt that a diet deficient in vitamins can cause trouble in the eyes, some of serious nature.

But it is indeed very rare for the opthalmologist, in this country particularly, to find definite cases of ocular disease due to vitamin deficiency. Our hygiene, living conditions, and diets are not conducive to these lesions.

When a person does not eat properly (for example, smoking and drinking at the expense of his diet) or has a debilitating disease, or one that prevents proper assimilation of foods, deficiency develops and if severe enough can lead to ocular trouble such as *night blindness* (retina), *dryness* of the eyes, *optic nerve* disorders (e.g. tobacco-alcohol blindness) or *ulcers* of the cornea.

A well balanced assimilated diet is essential, and if not present must be supplemented with manufactured vitamins in therapeutic doses.

Eye Exercises

These words have come to have several meanings. The scientific term for exercising the eye muscles, but particularly for strengthening ocular fusion, is *orthoptics*. This is a perfectly legitimate field and is often successful.

The non-scientific term "eye exercises" usually means an endeavor to relieve myopia and avoid the need of wearing glasses, notoriously by "palming". There is no way short of surgery that can alter the shape or length of the eyeball. However, it has been shown that a person can be taught to pay more attention to the shape of things and recognize them more readily. This is a sharpening of vision to be sure, but it is psychological.

During the war it was claimed by some non-medical technicians that color blindness could be cured by "exercise". That is, a color blind person could be taught to recognize the difference between red and green, for example. This turned out to be fallacious and was discarded even by the enthusiasts who had to yield to the truth that color blindness is an anatomical anomaly of the retinal cells that cannot be altered by exercise.

Color blindness is a congenital, inherited, sex-linked (i.e., passed down by female carriers to their sons) defect. It is not a disease and cannot be cured.

The most common form is *red-green* color blindness, which affects about four per cent of males. Red and green are seen as shades of yellow, yellowish-brown, and gray. The condition does not impair sharpness of vision and the affected person is usually unaware of being color blind until the defect is revealed by tests involving discrimination of colors.

Red-green color blindness is a handicap in certain occupations where discrimination of color signals is important, as in piloting an airplane or driving a locomotive, and it rules out some vocations such as mixing pigments or matching printing inks or advising about interior decoration. But as a rule a color blind person is not particularly handicapped in his daily affairs, except that, if left to his own choices, he may select neckties, shirts and socks of gaudily clashing colors which to him look quite neutral and harmonious.

Since color discrimination is a normal function of the cones of the retina, color blindness involves some inherited and irreversible defect of these structures, probably an absence of retinal cones sensitive to particular wavelengths of light.

Floating Spots

The vitreous in health is a solid transparent jelly, "like mother used to make". This is so in health and up to middle age. Then aging makes the vitreous more fluid. When this happens, cells and normal strands of tissue can float around with eye movements. As they do so, they cast shadows on the retina and these are observed as floating spots, especially in the nearsighted.

They are annoying and worrisome. There isn't anything we can do about it, except to study them against the sky or a blank wall and "enjoy" the phenomenon. Sometimes a more careful change in glasses will make them less obvious.

Sometimes they conglomerate and fall to the floor of the inner eye where they remain unless shaken up, as one does with old fashioned snowflakes in a paper weight.

But sometimes these floating spots mean trouble going on inside the eye, especially as a forerunner of retinal detachment. Then, too, hemorrhages and exudates in the vitreous show themselves as floating spots, threads or strands.

So if you notice these floating objects, see your ophthalmologist to find out for sure whether they are due to old man time or to a disease process at work.

Bags under the eyes. Since the skin of lids is very soft and loose (pinch it up for yourself and see) fluid accumulated in the body for a number of reasons will settle under the skin of the lids. Hence bags.

Loss of weight, menstruation, kidney and heart disease, overactive thyroid, disorders of other glands, hard drinking, loss of sleep, and other things can cause this excess of fluid beneath the skin.

If the color or texture of the skin is conducive, the bags are discolored and give the "dark circles" under the eyes that are cherished by the beatniks as a badge of something or other.

Bulging eyes. These may be a familial trait where the eyes are larger than usual. But if the condition comes on rather suddenly and progresses it could mean some thyroid trouble. (See Chapter 9). If one or both eyes bulge unduly, the patient should be seen as soon as possible by his physician for diagnosis and treatment.

All facts pertaining to the eyes and vision cannot possibly be discussed. It is attempted here to give information that may help to understand the anatomy and function of the visual apparatus and to answer questions pertaining to ocular disorders that are most commonly experienced.

The eye is a glorious part of the body and intimately shows all of its experiences in health and disease.

So important is vision to us that there cannot possibly be any "do it yourself" kit in taking care of it.

EARS, NOSE AND THROAT

by ALBERT P. SELTZER, M.D.

Mid-Ear Amplifiers · From Sound
Waves to Sound · Centers of
Equilibrium · Bone and Air
Conduction

IMPAIRED HEARING

Varieties of Impairment · Tests of
Hearing · Do You Hear Well? · Deaf
Infants and Children · Surgery for
Otosclerosis · Hearing Aids

INFECTIONS OF THE EAR

Earache · External Ear Infection ·
Middle Ear Infection · Mastoiditis ·
Perforated Eardrum · Tinnitus ·
Wax in the Ears · Dizziness, Deafness
· Protruding Ears

THE NOSE AND SINUSES

The External Nose · The Nasal Cavity
· Organs of Smell and Taste ·
Pathways of Sensation · The Nasal
Sinuses · Mouth and Throat ·
Postnasal Drip · Nose Drops · Nasal
Polyps · How to Blow the Nose ·
Deviated Septum · Plastic Surgery of
the Nose · "Sinus Trouble" ·
Hoarseness · Laryngitis · "Bad
Breath" · Cleft Lip and Cleft Palate

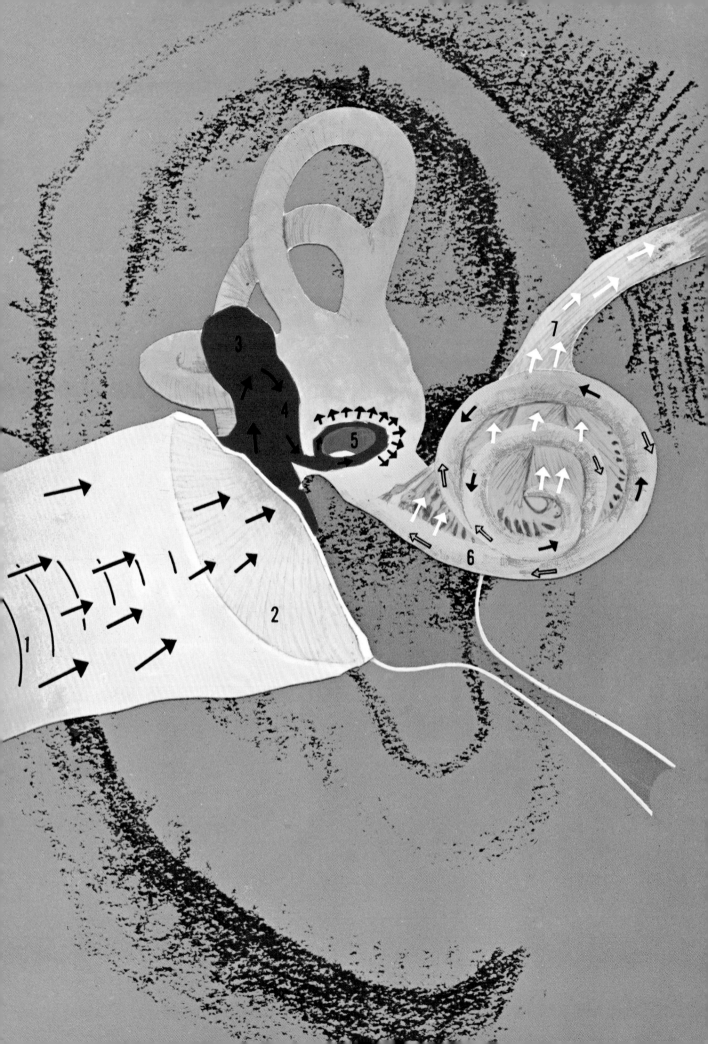

CHAPTER 17

EARS, NOSE AND THROAT

by ALBERT P. SELTZER, M.D.

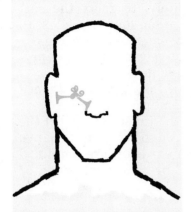

The color plate shows how sound waves are converted into nerve impulses, interpreted as hearing.

Sound waves entering the *external ear canal* (1) cause the *eardrum* (2) to vibrate. In the middle ear, vibrations are amplified and transmitted by a chain of *ossicles* (tiny bones): *malleus* or hammer (3), *incus* or anvil (4), and *stapes* or stirrup (5). The malleus is attached to the eardrum.

The footplate of the stapes, in contact with the oval window of the *cochlea* (6), transmits vibrations to fluid in the labyrinth. The cochlea ("snail-shaped") is lined with a membrane containing feathery hair cells tuned to vibrate to different frequencies. Nerve endings transmit impulses via the *acoustic nerve* (7) to receiving areas in the brain.

Black arrows show direction of physical vibrations; white arrows, of nerve impulses. Air pressure on either side of the eardrum is equalized by the Eustachian tube which opens into the throat.

A familiar trick question asks, "If a tree crashes to the ground in a forest where there is nobody to hear it, does it make a noise?" The answer is no. Sound is something perceived by a human or animal brain. Sound waves, in absence of organs to perceive them, are soundless, although they may be powerful enough to set objects to trembling.

Sound waves are vibrations of air or other media. What we hear begins as "shook-up" air which is amplified, and converted to fluid waves which excite nerve endings that carry impulses to the brain where sound is heard. Many sounds we hear arrive via our bones as well as by air. Our auditory system is one of the most sensitive and discriminating of senses, able to distinguish puffs of air coming from a familiar voice or from a particular instrument in a symphony orchestra. It is well protected by the location of its most delicate structures within hard bony areas of the head.

The external ear is largely ornamental (in many instances), but it helps a little to direct sound waves into the ear canal. This little canal penetrates about an inch into the head, with the *eardrum (tympanic membrane)* at its end. The *middle ear* is an air-filled cavity sealed by the eardrum and surrounded by thin bony walls. There is an opening which leads to the *mastoid bone,* and a tubular passage about an inch and a half long which opens into the throat, called the *Eustachian tube.* Air on either side of the pale-pink concave eardrum must be at equal pressures for the drum to vibrate freely. A partial vacuum in the middle ear, for instance, would pull upon the eardrum like a suction cup and restrict its movement. Pressures are normally equalized by air which can move both ways through the Eustachian tube.

"Popping" of the ears when we go up in a high-speed elevator is a familiar sensation. Atmospheric pressure is less at the top of a skyscraper; consequently, air trapped inside the middle ear expands and pushes

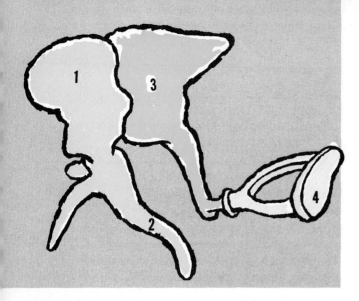

Conducting system of the middle ear: the *malleus* (1) has a *handle* (2) attached to the eardrum. Vibrations pass from malleus to *incus* (3) to footplate of *stapes* (4), thence to fluids of inner ear.

its way out through the Eustachian tube. Obstruction of the tube can cause difficulties, and germs traveling up it may cause infections and even spread to the mastoid bone behind the external ear.

Mid-Ear Amplifiers

Sound waves strike the eardrum and cause it to vibrate, but the vibrations are incredibly small. At some frequencies, vibrations as small as one-billionth of a centimeter — much less than the diameter of a single hydrogen atom — can be detected. A remarkable amplifying system is built into the middle ear. It consists of a chain of three tiny bones, the *ossicles,* the smallest bones in the body. Altogether they occupy about as much space as a small carpet tack.

From a fancied resemblance to familiar objects, the ossicles are called the *hammer (malleus), anvil (incus),* and *stirrup (stapes).* The hammer-handle is in contact with the eardrum. Its "hammering" parts vibrate against the anvil-bone. In turn, anvil blows move the stirrup bone. In this way, sound wave energies are greatly amplified and we can sometimes hear whispers we are not supposed to.

There are tiny muscles and ligaments in the middle ear which assist and help to protect hearing. One set of muscles

pulls the hammer-bone inward and increases the tension of the eardrum, like tightening the head of a snare drum. Another muscle attached to the stirrup-bone acts oppositely, to relax the eardrum, especially when loud noises assail it. Thus the movements of middle-ear parts are protectively adjusted in proportion to the volume of sound.

The footplate of the stirrup is attached to a flexible membrane which covers an opening into the inner ear, called the *oval window.* Through the ossicle chains, pressures on the eardrum are amplified to much greater pressures on fluids of the inner ear.

From Sound Waves to Sound

The inner ear is a complex bony structure filled with fluid and delicate parts. When we hear, the footplate of the stirrup-bone strikes against the oval window like a piston, or an extraordinarily fast pile-driver, and the vibrations continue as fluid waves in the inner ear. Near the oval window, another membrane-covered opening, the round window, cushions and dampens the fluid.

Waves in the inner ear excite an apparatus of surpassing complexity

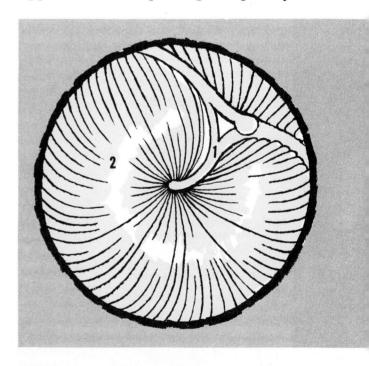

Drawing shows *handle of malleus* (1) attached to inner aspect of *eardrum* (2). Tiny sets of muscles increase or relax the tension of eardrum.

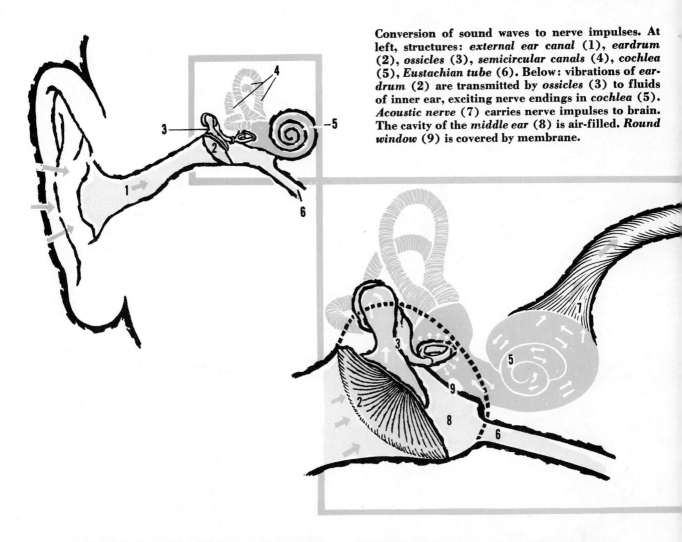

Conversion of sound waves to nerve impulses. At left, structures: *external ear canal* (1), *eardrum* (2), *ossicles* (3), *semicircular canals* (4), *cochlea* (5), *Eustachian tube* (6). Below: vibrations of *eardrum* (2) are transmitted by *ossicles* (3) to fluids of inner ear, exciting nerve endings in *cochlea* (5). *Acoustic nerve* (7) carries nerve impulses to brain. The cavity of the *middle ear* (8) is air-filled. *Round window* (9) is covered by membrane.

which might be compared in a very rough way to a piano keyboard with keys arranged in graduated steps from treble to bass. However, the inner ear console has more than 20,000 "keys," and is not laid out flat like a piano keyboard but is coiled in a spiral like a snail shell. Indeed, the *cochlea*, as the organ is called, gets its name from the Latin word for snail. It is a tubular bony structure lined with a membrane containing thousands of feathery hair cells tuned to vibrate to different sounds. Nerve endings are contained in a complex, slightly elevated structure over the floor of the tube forming the cochlea. This area *(organ of Corti)* is the center of the sense of hearing.

Sensitive hair cells are "shaken" by oscillations of fluid around them, which has been made to oscillate by pulsations of the stirrup-bone which was set to vibrating by sound waves that struck the eardrum. The hair cells stimulate indi-

vidual nerve endings whose fibers merge into the nerve of hearing *(acoustic nerve)* which carries impulses to auditory centers of the brain, where sound is heard. What begins as physical vibrations becomes the music of a symphony orchestra, the squawkings of a bluejay, or the gurglings of a baby.

If straightened out, the spiral canal of the cochlea would be about an inch and a half long, but rolled up like a snail shell, it occupies a space about the size of a pea. In this tiny area with its nerve-lines to the brain we make thousands and millions and billions of exquisite discriminations between infinitely complex and endlessly different patterns of sound waves that touch our eardrums. Nerve receptors for the deepest of deep bass notes—about 16 cycles per second—are located at the very end of the innermost turn of the cochlear spiral. From here, if we imagine the spiral unwinding, the keyboard

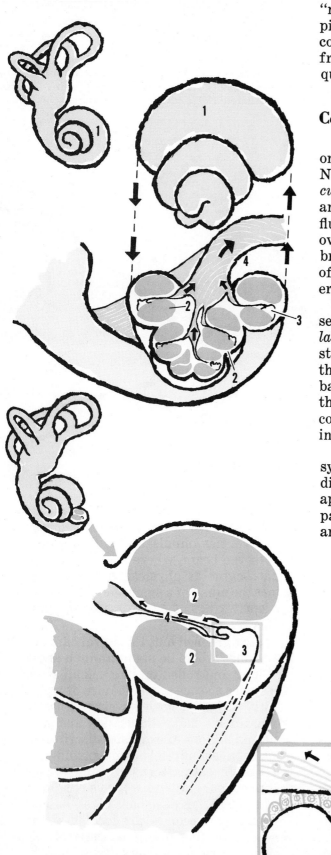

"notes" are increasingly tuned to higher-pitched sounds, until at the big end of the cochlea we may hear very high notes with frequencies of 20,000 cycles per second or quite possibly even more.

Centers of Equilibrium

Our sense of balance is not dependent on hearing, but organs of equilibrium. Near the cochlea are the three *semicircular canals,* which lie in planes at right angles to each other. The canals contain fluid which responds to movements and, over intricate nerve pathways to the brain, gives information about positions of the body — a sort of automatic governor of body balance.

The cochlea, semi-circular canals, and several small structures comprise the *labyrinth,* a very appropriate name. The structures weave a labyrinthine course through bony ducts and spaces and are bathed in fluids of membranous parts that surround them, a veritable maze of complicated, delicate, inter-communicating units of great sensitivity.

Inflammations of the labyrinth cause symptoms of dizziness, vomiting, and disturbances of balance, which may disappear in a few days, or advance to severe pain, fever, deafness in the affected ear, and other serious complications.

Centers of the sense of hearing. Top drawing at left, closeup view of *cochlea* (1), with *chambers* (2), which carry fluids in contact with the *organ of Corti* (3), from which nerve impulses are carried to the cochlear branch of the *acoustic nerve* (4). Lower drawing at left, closeup of *organ of Corti* (3) in relation to *chambers* (2) and *cochlear duct* (3); *nerve fibers* (4). Below, microscopic view of organ of Corti showing *hair cells* (5) that communicate with *nerve fibers* (6) going to brain.

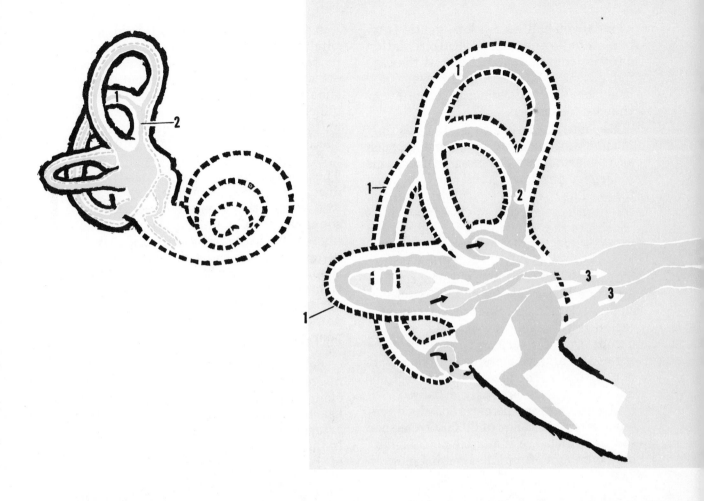

Organs concerned with equilibrium of the body. The *semicircular canals* (1) at right angles to each other contain fluid in the *semicircular duct* (2). Our sense of balance is maintained by fluid movement in the semicircular canals that affects nerve endings of the *vestibular nerve* (3) going to the brain.

Bone and Air Conduction

Any vibration that stimulates the acoustic nerves becomes audible. Vibrations can reach the nerves over bony structures of the head, as well as by sound waves that strike the eardrum. We use both bone and air conduction all the time, although air conduction predominates in general listening. Bone conduction is especially related to speaking.

Practically everyone is astonished, and sometimes shocked, the first time he hears his voice on a tape recording. It sounds like a stranger's voice, not at all like the voice the speaker thinks is his. The reason why our voices don't sound to us as they do to others is that a good deal of the sound we hear is bone-conducted. Auditors — and tape recorders — hear only what is air-conducted. Lower frequencies tend to be accentuated by bone conduction and the voice may sound more powerful than it really is. In voice training, recordings that reproduce the voice as others hear it are very helpful.

Air and bone conduction differences are important in making tests of hearing. If a patient hears air-conducted sounds poorly, but bone-conducted ones quite well, the site of trouble is probably in the middle ear. If he cannot hear bone-conducted vibrations, he suffers from nerve-deafness with impairment of structures of the inner ear.

If our ears were only a little more sensitive to low frequencies, we would constantly hear the noise of the body, which is pretty noisy. If you close both ears with your fingertips, to shut out air-borne sounds, you can hear a low, gentle rumbling tone — the noise of local circulation and tiny muscle contractions. If the ears did not have a cut-off point, we would hear some sort of thudding sound every time we took a step.

Repeated exposure to loud noises may in time cause hearing impairments, such as "boilermaker's deafness." Often, this is largely a reduced ability to hear high tones. The "treble" end of the cochlea, the high-note section of its keyboard, is nearest to the oval window through which sound waves are hammered by the stirrup-bone. Some loss of perception of high tones is inevitable, too, with increasing age, partly because of loss of youthful elasticity of tissues. But ordinary conversation is relatively low-pitched, and the dampening of a screamingly shrill voice is not an unmixed blessing. Physically, if not critically, the ideal listener to high-fidelity music is probably a baby. Good hi-fi sets and records can reproduce frequencies in the range of 20,000 cycles per second which are inaudible to considerable numbers of middle-aged listeners.

IMPAIRED HEARING

Totally deaf people are relatively few. But large numbers — an estimated 6,000,000 in this country — have some degree of hearing loss. There is indeed a steady loss of hearing acuity as we grow older. The normal young ear can hear tones within a range of 16 cycles per second — the lowest bass note of a pipe organ — up to high-pitched sounds of 20,000 cycles per second and even more. A person in his sixties is lucky if he can hear sounds of 12,000 cycles per second.

This loss is limited to high-frequency sounds and must be considered normal since it happens to practically everybody as the years roll on. It is probably related to gradual loss of tissue elasticity in the hearing apparatus, not unlike that shown by the familiar "pinch test" of the skin of the back of the hand. Young skin, pinched together, snaps back with alacrity but in older people returns slowly to position.

A slight loss of perception of high-pitched sounds is not a complete catastrophe. It muffles some of the shrillness of the world. But impairment severe enough to make ordinary conversation difficult or impossible to understand is quite another matter. The pitch of human speech ranges between 300 and 4,000 cycles (wave frequencies) per second. These are the cycles most vital to the conduct of human affairs. Inability to hear well within this range is a serious personal and social handicap. Hard of hearing persons are often blamed unfairly for being crotchety, cantankerous, rude and suspicious, if they do not answer questions, or seem to think people are whispering behind their backs, because they do not hear what is going on, and have poor discrimination.

Severe hearing loss in the elderly cannot be attributed merely to aging. Many older people have perfectly adequate hearing. Except for degenerative and arteriosclerotic changes which increase in incidence with age, most of the causes of hearing impairment are similar in younger persons. What can be done for the person who is hard of hearing — and in most cases a great deal can be done — depends upon the nature of the impairment and its timely recognition.

Varieties of Impairment

In the most general way, there are two types of hearing loss: *conduction deafness* and *nerve* or *perceptive deafness*. Sometimes there is mixed impairment involving both the conductive and nervous apparatus. There is also a functional sort of deafness ("hysterical deafness") in which the hearing apparatus is physically intact, and the cause must be sought in psychic areas.

Different impairments affect different structures of the ear. Conduction deafness is failure of airborne sound waves to be conducted efficiently through and over external and middle ear structures, so that adequate messages do not reach the nerves of the inner ear. Perceptive deafness is failure of the auditory nerves to accept, perceive and transmit messages to hearing centers in the brain.

Conductive loss may be caused by so simple and correctible a thing as a lump of ear wax which obstructs air vibrations. But the most important conductive defects lie in and around the middle ear, where chains of tiny bones augment and transmit vibrations from the eardrum to the inner ear. Pus-forming middle ear infections may damage delicate structures, or these may be malformed at birth. A rather common cause of hearing

pitched sounds tend to be affected first so that considerable good hearing remains in the lower-pitched regions. However, nerve damage may be complete, sudden or insidious, and is never repairable.

Causes. The ears, like other organs, are subject to wear and tear, congenital malformation, infection, injury and insult. Infection of the mother during pregnancy with German measles and perhaps other virus infections, Rh blood incompatibility, and some complications of labor and birth, are associated with high incidence

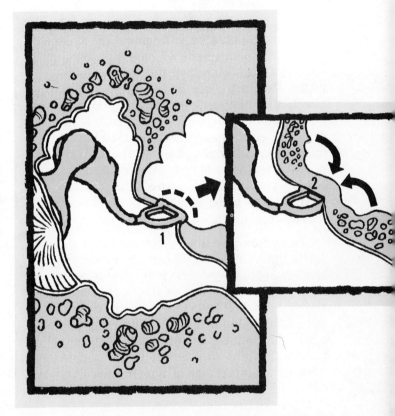

The larger drawing shows a normal *stapes* (1) transmitting vibrations freely to fluids beyond (arrow). Smaller drawing shows the mechanism of *otosclerosis*, a form of hearing impairment caused by overgrowth of bone which prevents the foot of the *stapes* (2) from vibrating freely. Abnormal bone growth which dampens vibrations and dulls hearing may occur in the footplate of the stapes as well as the surrounding area.

loss is *otosclerosis*, a painless overgrowth of bone in the region where the footplate of the delicate stirrup-shaped ossicle delivers its pistonlike vibrations to the inner ear. Bone surrounds and "freezes" the footplate so that it cannot vibrate, and the auditory nerves receive no message or a badly muffled one.

Nerve deafness varies according to the location and extent of damage. Often there is partial, indeed quite good hearing; fibers concerned with the highest-

of ear defects and often total deafness in newborn babies. High fevers, meningitis, mumps and measles and other infections in infants and children may be followed by severe hearing loss.

Certain drugs such as quinine and streptomycin can inflict permanent injury upon the auditory nerves. Blows and skull fractures can damage ear structures. Advanced infections of the middle ear are less common since the advent of antibiotics, but are still a significant cause of hearing impairment. Tendencies to some ear defects seem to run in families. This is true of otosclerosis, which has a hereditary component.

Noise is a more pervasive, insidious cause of ear-nerve injury than most of us realize, for it causes no particular pain unless it is as loud as a cannon blast. The ears have considerable comeback power from temporary brief exposure to noise and ordinarily recover overnight. However, prolonged exposure to intense noise gradually damages the inner ear.

Tests of Hearing

Early recognition of deafness in infants is extremely important (see below). Measurement of hearing acuity requires some standard unit of the loudness of sound. This is the *decibel*. For practical purposes, we may say that a whisper is "20 decibels loud"; conversation, 60 decibels; subway noise, 100 decibels; a jet airplane, 140 decibels. How much of the noise is heard depends on the ears. Standardized techniques enable hearing loss to be measured in terms of loss of decibels.

An audiometer is an instrument which emits pure tones which can be turned up louder, decibel by decibel. With it a physician can make an *audiogram* which shows how well the patient hears different sound frequencies. If a sound must be made 20 decibels louder than standard for the patient to hear it, he is said to have a 20-decibel loss of hearing for that sound frequency.

If an audiogram shows, for instance, that a patient has a 20-decibel hearing loss, it means that he probably does not hear distinctly in a theater or meeting hall, and no doubt knows it or thinks that the acoustics are bad or that everybody has taken up mumbling. A loss of more than 30 decibels usually means that a hearing aid is necessary to hear conversation distinctly, and of 50 or so that it is hard to hear over the telephone.

There are a number of other testing devices, some of them highly specialized. The latter are most likely to be used by *otologists* (ear physicians) and audio clinics maintained in many large hospitals and medical centers in large communities. Devices as simple as a watch or tuning fork give valuable information to those who are trained to use them and interpret the results.

Often the family physician is the first to be consulted about and to determine the general nature of a hearing impairment. A good deal can be learned about the nature of a hearing impairment by taking a careful history, examining, and making fairly simple tests. For instance, a vibrating tuning fork can distinguish between conduction and nerve deafness, if it is placed on bone behind the patient's ear and the results interpreted. If he hears bone-conducted sound, the difficulty lies somewhere in the sound-wave conducting system; if he does not, the hearing nerves are affected.

Do You Hear Well?

One cannot self-diagnose ear troubles, but simple self-tests of hearing like those below may indicate that you do not hear as well as you should and encourage you to consult your doctor who may refer you to an ear specialist.

Do you hear speech more distinctly over the telephone than speech in a room?

Can you hear a soft sound such as a faucet dripping in a room?

Do you frequently miss words or phrases that others listening to the same radio or TV program seem to catch?

Can you — literally — hear someone who is talking behind your back?

Do you often ask someone to "say that again"?

Do you have to strain or "cock one ear" to hear what is being said?

Deaf Infants and Children

Some infants are born totally deaf or with serious hearing loss. Surprising numbers of pre-school children are handicapped by defective hearing. A study conducted by the Kansas Medical Society Committee on Conservation of Hearing and Speech showed that about one out of 20 children of pre-school age had deafness or seriously defective hearing. All were cases that had come to the attention of a physician, and many neglected cases were undoubtedly missed.

Unless deafness is detected and treated early, an infant's entire life is cast in unnecessary tragedy. Normal development of speech and understanding of language requires adequate hearing. Sounds not heard cannot be imitated and no meaning can be associated with special sounds we call the spoken word. If no help is given at the proper time, the child may be thought to be — and in fact behaves as if he were — stupid, inattentive, listless, disobedient, or mentally retarded.

Signs in infants. How does one suspect loss of hearing in an infant? One of the most obvious things is absence of the startle reflex. That is, a sudden loud noise, like a bang on a pan, does not startle him or make him cry. This sign can be detected quite early, certainly by the age of 6 months. By the time he is nine or ten months old, a normal baby localizes sound quite well, and turns his head or otherwise indicates that he knows where the sound is coming from. A deafened infant does not. A "good baby" who sleeps undisturbed through all sorts of household din and clatter may simply not hear the noise. Loud voices do not awaken or disturb him.

Another important sign is that the child does not develop speech at the normal time. A deaf infant may go through the babbling stage like any other baby but he soon gives it up if he cannot hear the sounds he makes. He is shut out from the meaningful world of sound, and as he grows older can only communicate in grunts and gestures.

A baby may be born with normal hearing but acquire deafness after birth as a sequel to scarlet fever, mumps, measles, other infections or injuries. The family doctor who attends the child is alert to such possibilities of deafness.

Observations by the family that a baby or child apparently does not hear well should be reported at once to the family doctor. He will examine the child, give tests, and if the hearing defect can be treated medically he will do so. If not, he will refer you to a hearing specialist and help you to get in touch with reliable sources of help and information.

Treatment. As in adults, impaired hearing in infants—excluding irreparable congenital malformations — is of the conductive or of the perceptive variety. The conductive type of loss usually can be improved to a very satisfactory degree with hearing aids and occasionally by surgery.

The problem is more serious if the infant has nerve deafness with total or almost total inability to hear any sounds at all. One must give up any hope that the child's hearing can be improved. It is important that the situation be recognized early, because the child can never learn to talk in the normal way because he hears no sounds to imitate. He can see a dog, but cannot learn that a certain pattern of sound waves always means "dog" when spoken.

But the situation isn't hopeless. The child can be taught "unnaturally" to speak, by special and difficult training techniques. Training is a long, slow process which requires patience, love, and co-operation on the part of the parents. Costly types of equipment, training aids, and teaching skills are necessary, and facilities generally are available only in large urban centers.

The earlier the handicap is discovered, the earlier the youngster can be referred to a specialist teacher of the deaf, a school for the deaf, or a speech and hearing clinic conducted at a university or medical center. The ideal time to start training is in the second year of life when children are most teachable.

Surgery for Otosclerosis

As mentioned above, *otosclerosis* is a condition of bony overgrowth which interferes with free movement at the end of the tiny chain of ossicles which deliver vibrations to the membrane-covered oval window that opens into the inner ear. It is not a simple enlargement of bone. Normal compact bone in the area is replaced with spongy bone filled with networks of blood vessels. Consequences vary with the encroachment of bone which may obliterate the oval window, immobilize the *stapes* (the terminal stirrup-shaped ossicle), and interrupt the entire chain of sound conduction. It is much like what happens if a vibrating tuning fork is pinched between the fingers. The vibrations are dampened and stopped.

Of itself, otosclerosis is a form of conduction deafness, the most common form in adults, although it is sometimes found in children. Otosclerosis is a chronic and progressive condition, causing increasing loss of hearing.

Symptoms commonly appear between 15 and 40 years of age; early onset is most usual. The first symptom may be some difficulty in understanding whispers, or voices at a distance. The patient usually hears his own voice well by bone conduction, and in fact it seems quite loud to him so he tends to speak softly. The same bone conduction mechanism exaggerates the sounds of chewing, so the patient may hear poorly at the dinner table, feel shut out from family chatter, and tires of asking members to repeat what they have said. As the condition worsens the patient tends to become more withdrawn and secluded.

Otosclerosis usually is correctible with hearing aids. It is also the one common form of impaired hearing that is most amenable to correction by surgery. Candidates for surgery must be carefully evaluated and selected. Little benefit could be expected, for instance, if there is associated nerve deafness which would make restoration of conductive pathways of no avail.

Several operative procedures have the same general objective: to restore free vibrating movement to sound-conducting pathways. The operation is not a simple one; all the techniques require great skill. The surgeon, in effect, has to operate in-

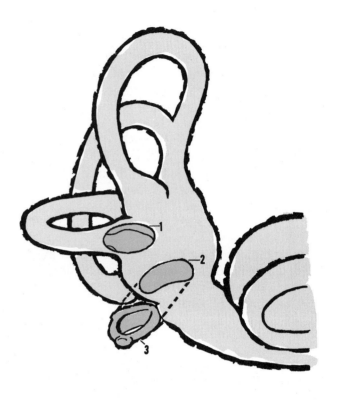

The fenestration operation for otosclerosis creates a new *oval window* (1) by surgery in place of normal *oval window* (2) where the *stapes* (3) has become firmly fixed, frozen in position, and is unable to transmit vibrations freely.

side a hard-to-reach pea which contains very delicate structures. This specialized surgery has been greatly improved by advances in magnifying accessories, headlights, and special instruments. Chances of restoring good or excellent hearing in selected patients are good, although success of course cannot be guaranteed by the surgeon.

The fenestration operation creates a new bony window opening with fine drilling instruments not unlike those of a dentist. Another approach is *stapes mobilization* — the tiny stirrup bone is "unfrozen" from surroundings that congeal its movements, so free vibratory motion is restored. There are several techniques of doing this. In another relatively new procedure, the stapes is removed along with some of the otosclerotic bone that surrounds it. A strip of tissue taken from one of the patient's veins is grafted over the oval window, and a plastic substitute no bigger than the tip of a ballpoint pen replaces the removed stirrup bone. Refinements of technique have made this the procedure preferred by many ear surgeons; the fenestration operation is less often performed today.

Continuing improvements in operative techniques and methods have greatly brightened the outlook for permanent improvement of hearing in properly selected patients in skilled hands. There are still a few failures, but on the average about three-fourths of suitable patients attain very satisfactory long-term improvement of hearing and the ratio is increasing steadily.

Hearing Aids

Well-fitted modern hearing aids could benefit more hard-of-hearing people than they actually do. Reasons why a hearing aid is never tried or is kept unused in a bureau drawer are all too human. Often the affected person does not want to admit that he does not hear well, and is reluctant to "advertise" it by wearing an instrument he fears is conspicuous. He may buy a hearing aid of sorts because someone in the family insists on it, but wear the instrument only under duress.

A poorly fitted aid may not actually improve his hearing deficit, so he can't be blamed for not using it. But even an excellent aid may seem bad to him because he has forgotten what sounds are like and he has difficulty in interpreting many overlapping noises.

Modern hearing aids are remarkable electronic devices, compact almost to the vanishing point. Essentially, they are amplifying devices that make sounds louder. However, if the wrong sound frequencies are intensified and the right ones are not, the results will be anything but ideal. Hence there is no such thing as a good-for-everybody hearing aid. Selection, and assurance that the aid is working properly after it has been tried for a while, requires the counsel of an ear doctor who knows all about a particular patient's trouble. In buying a hearing aid, it is important to deal with a responsible company servicing the product of a responsible manufacturer.

Hearing aids usually are of great benefit in simple conduction deafness. Air-conduction types are worn in the ear, bone-conduction types in contact with bone. The ear doctor will advise which is better in a given instance. There are ingenious ways of making the devices inconspicuous, such as incorporating the

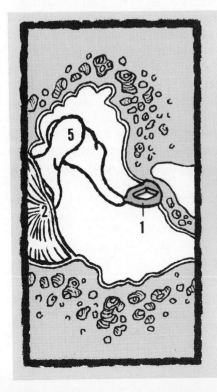

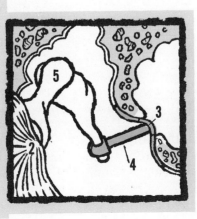

Various surgical techniques for correction of impaired hearing resulting from otosclerosis have been developed. Larger drawing shows *otosclerotic stapes* (1) held immovable by surrounding bone. Smaller drawing shows oval window replaced by *vein graft* or other substitute (3) with replacement of stapes by a *polyethylene tube* (4). In another technique, a hole is made through the stapes and a piston-type element inserted to transmit vibrations. Other structures shown include *ear drum* (2) and *ossicles* (5).

mechanism into the side frames of eyeglasses. Girls are said to prefer devices which are worn in the ear, which permits them to remove their glasses for the sake of appearances when out in society.

Often, one ear is better than the other and an aid need only be worn in one ear, the poorer one. But sometimes the opposite is the case, and hearing is better and sounds are more natural if devices are worn in both ears.

Some degree of nerve deafness, with or without conduction deafness, makes the selection of the proper hearing aid a bit more critical. Frequently, the patient hears certain sound frequencies quite well and others poorly. It is as if groups of keys of a piano keyboard were muffled so there would be gaps in a composition played on it. A suitable hearing aid should fill in the gaps and not magnify sounds that are already loud enough.

Sometimes, even with an excellent and well-fitted aid, sudden return of long-forgotten sounds may disturb the wearer temporarily. Patience and a period of relearning may be necessary (as when a person first puts on bifocal glasses) until it becomes comfortable to wear the aid. In extreme cases, hearing may have been impaired so long that some training in recognizing the sounds of speech is necessary. The combination of an appropriate hearing aid and explanation, counsel and assistance of an ear doctor can often re-open a wonderful world of sound.

INFECTIONS OF THE EAR

Earache

Earache is a pain in the ear and there may be many causes for it. It is a warning sign that something is wrong. Most types of earache are not especially dangerous, but some are. It is not a symptom to be treated for long by homely measures such as dropping warm (not hot) olive oil into the ear canal. This may possibly ease pain a bit but cannot correct the cause. If pain in the ear does not subside in 24 hours or so, disturbs the patient's sleep

at night, and makes him conscious at all times that he has an ear, a physician should be consulted for relief.

External Ear Infection
(Otitis Externa)

Few things are more painful than boils in the ear canal. These are of the same nature as boils elsewhere in the body, and are usually caused by staphylococcus organisms which inhabit the skin. Swelling within the narrow, confined ear canal may be excruciating and seem to radiate to nearby parts of the face. A physician may have to drain the boils to relieve pressures, and at the same time give treatment to control infection and prevent recurrences.

The habit of poking and picking at the ear opening with a pencil, match, hairpin or anything else is a nefarious practice which can scratch and irritate delicate skin, invite infections of various sorts, and even puncture the eardrum. The old rule is "never put anything in your ear smaller than your elbow." Infections and inflammations may also come about from foreign bodies lodged in the ear.

Fungus infections of the ear are not uncommon. The condition is sometimes called "swimmer's ear" since contaminated water and incompletely drained water tend to set up moist and soggy conditions favorable to fungal growth. The normal condition of the ear canal is to be filled with air, not fluid, and it is well to keep it dry at all times. A fungus infection of the external ear is very much like misplaced "athlete's foot." It affects the skin, usually is itchy, crusted, and weepy, and can be painful if there is swelling of the ear canal.

Various ointments and solutions are effective in controlling external ear infections but there are different kinds of causative organisms and selection of the proper medicine should be left to one's physician.

It is important to drain the ears properly whenever water gets into them.

Middle Ear Infection

(Otitis Media)

The middle ear is a small bony box containing the chains of ossicles which conduct sound vibrations. Products of infection trapped in the middle ear press against the eardrum and distend it, and may force their way into the spongy mastoid process (the bony area which can be felt behind the external ear), and even reach the coverings of the brain. The real danger in middle ear infections is the complications. There is a threat to hearing as well as to health. Pus that fills the middle ear can damage the sound-conducting chains of tiny bones. A good deal of conductive deafness results from neglected middle ear infection.

Children are especially liable to middle ear infections because their Eustachian tubes are shorter and straighter than in adults. Respiratory infections often precede middle ear infections. The Eustachian tube affords upward passage to germs from the nose and throat. It is also possible for middle ear infection to enter through the auditory canal if there is an opening in the eardrum.

Acute middle ear infection signifies its presence by intense stabbing pain. A doctor using a viewing instrument *(otoscope)* can see the eardrum bulging from pressure of fluids behind it. Middle ear infections are not so common as they once were because timely treatment with antimicrobial drugs prevents many infections from progressing to the ear. Antibiotics and similar drugs may cause an acute middle ear infection to subside uneventfully if therapy is begun in time.

Not infrequently, pus breaks through the eardrum and drains from the ear canal. This naturally relieves feelings of pain and pressure, but a doctor's care is necessary to be sure that the infection is actually cleared up and that there are no after-effects which need attention. The broken eardrum may heal satisfactorily or it may not, depending on the extent and location of the break and other factors. If the doctor sees the patient when perforation of the drum seems

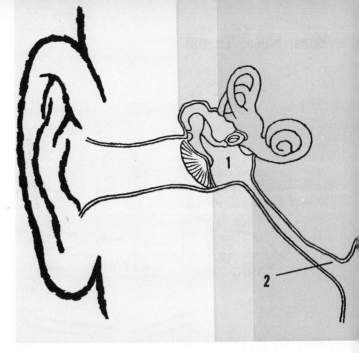

The *middle ear* (1) is an air-filled bony cavity communicating with the throat via the *Eustachian tube* (2). Germ-laden material may ascend to the middle ear from the throat area and cause infection, with formation of pus that may be trapped there.

imminent but has not yet occurred, and symptoms indicate that infection is advancing toward the mastoid cells, he may make a small incision in the eardrum *(myringotomy)* for drainage. Healing and hearing after this carefully placed surgical incision for drainage are usually good, but a spontaneous perforation does not always turn out so well.

Chronic middle ear infection may follow acute infection, or be associated with obstructed or infected tonsils and adenoids, or with allergies, or recurrent discharge through a perforated drum that failed to heal. There is a tendency for membranes to become thickened and for Eustachian tubes to constrict. Ear physicians distinguish several forms of chronic otitis media of varying seriousness. Early diagnosis and treatment are important to avert the threat of impaired hearing. In one form of inflammation the middle ear is filled with sterile fluid which tends to cause scar tissue and adhesions.

Chronic drainage — a "running ear" — is a warning to consult an ear physician promptly. The symptom is easy to ignore because it is usually painless. But a *draining ear* is like a time bomb. It may "explode" at any time into the mastoid areas. Low-grade infection produces just

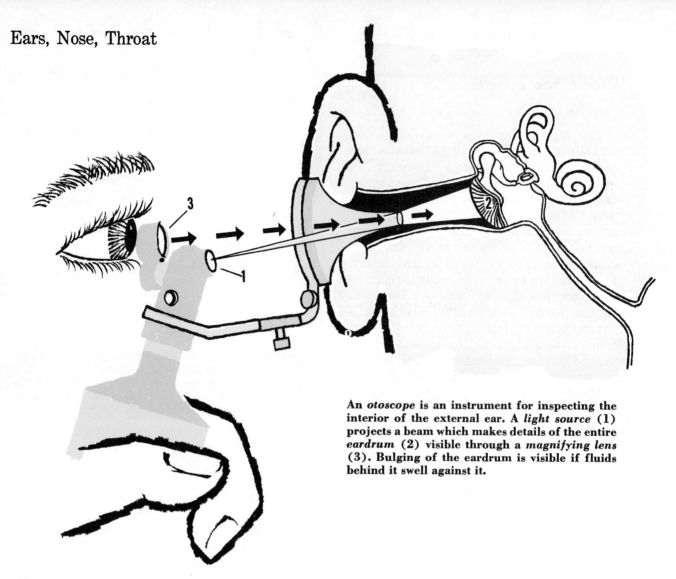

An *otoscope* is an instrument for inspecting the interior of the external ear. A *light source* (1) projects a beam which makes details of the entire *eardrum* (2) visible through a *magnifying lens* (3). Bulging of the eardrum is visible if fluids behind it swell against it.

enough secretion to prevent the eardrum from healing completely but usually not enough to stimulate the patient to get much needed medical help. Constant drainage irritates tissues, may cause polyps to grow, and skin of the ear canal may grow through the perforated eardrum into the middle ear, with formation of a fatty mass containing nests of epithelium (*cholesteatoma*) which requires fairly radical surgery. In addition, the middle ear is directly accessible to bacteria through the perforated drum.

The doctor may take a culture to determine the proper antibiotic to eliminate the infecting organisms. A draining ear must be kept clean and dry at all times, and it is especially dangerous for the patient to go swimming, even in heated indoor pools in the winter.

A hearing test of children who have middle ear infections, or after they have had scarlet fever, measles, or other childhood diseases often associated with such infections, is important in order to discover abnormal conditions of the middle ear which may be corrected in time to avoid permanent loss of hearing.

Mastoiditis

"Mastoid trouble" once was a quite common and feared complication of middle ear infections. And trouble it was: extension of infection to mastoid air cells in bony parts surrounding the ear canal and middle ear, softening and destruction of bone by pus, danger of infection of brain membranes causing fatal meningitis.

Antibiotic drugs have almost made mastoiditis a thing of the past, but not quite. Timely treatment of middle ear infections, or of infections which could extend to the middle ear, prevents pus from being forced into the mastoid area, so the patient is never aware of trouble that could have happened. Neglect or unusual circumstances still lead to occasional cases of mastoiditis. Treatment for mastoiditis is surgical, usually through an incision behind the ear that exposes infected bone which is carefully cleaned out by the surgeon.

Perforated Eardrum

As we have seen, the eardrum may be perforated by infections. The punctures may be tiny pinholes through which

that are delayed for a considerable time. Sometimes, in suitable patients, a persistent perforation can be closed by an operation known as *tympanoplasty,* in which a piece of skin from the ear canal is grafted over the eardrum.

It is very important that a person with a perforated eardrum or draining ear abstain from diving, swimming, and water sports in general. Ear plugs cannot be depended on to protect the ear completely. At best, nature did not design the human ear for submersion, and a perforated drum is an added handicap.

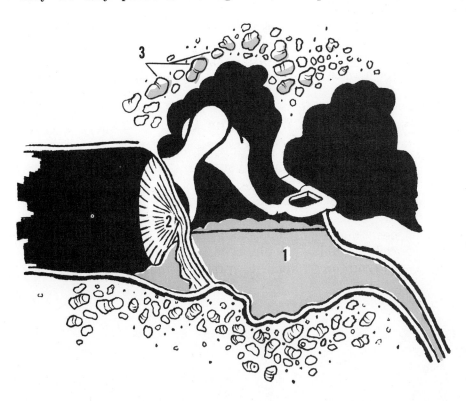

Possible consequences of neglected middle ear infection *(otitis media)*: Pus from *middle ear* (1) breaks through *eardrum* (2); infection may spread to *mastoid cells* (3) in surrounding bony parts. Acute middle ear infection causes intense pain ("earache") unless drainage is accomplished; a chronic "running ear," even though painless, should have prompt medical care to avert complications.

drainage occurs. Some chronic infections may enlarge the perforations and make them permanent. The eardrum may also be torn by shattering blasts or punctured by sharp objects unwisely inserted into the ear. The eardrum is closer to the external opening of the ear than most people realize.

A perforated eardrum may heal and repair itself and never cause any future trouble, but this is not necessarily the case and there may be complications involving other structures than the drum, so that supervision by a physician is important. There may be after-effects

Tinnitus *(Head Noises)*

Some sounds which do not originate from ordinary sound waves but are nevertheless heard may be imaginary, but most likely they are real enough and quite distressing to the person who hears them. Such sounds, heard by the patient but not by others, are symptoms of *tinnitus*—ringing, roaring, clicking or hissing sounds in the ears.

Tinnitus is not a disease of the ear, but is frequently a feature of various ear diseases — or of no detectable disease at all. For instance, a person with a perforated eardrum often has tinnitus which probably disappears when the drum heals. Tinnitus is a common symptom of otosclerosis and many other middle ear conditions or infections, and persons with impaired hearing often complain of it. But tinnitus can arise anywhere along the nervous pathways of hearing and the tissues serving them, and it is exceedingly difficult, and often impossible, to pinpoint the site of trouble with precision.

Sometimes head noises (a more serviceable word than tinnitus) can be cured by so simple a measure as removing hard masses of wax from the ears. Other local causes may be found. Clicking and ticking noises may be produced by contraction of small muscles, or in the Eustachian tube by sticky mucoid material which can snap like a rubber band when the tube opens and closes. Drugs such as quinine and aspirin, and abuses of alcohol and tobacco, may cause tinnitus. Various treatments to remove local causes of head noises — medicines to reduce mucoid secretions, unblock the tubes, control allergies, remove fluids from the middle ear — may be successful.

Often, specific causes of head noises cannot be found, but a search should always be made. Frequently the symptom accompanies ear disorders which themselves require primary treatment. Head noises sometimes disappear spontaneously or after various forms of treatment, none of which is successful in all instances. Tinnitus associated with hardening of small blood vessels in the auditory system is likely to be permanent.

Head noises are hissing, ringing, whistling, whizzing, roaring, booming sounds but the kind most frequently described by patients is "like steam coming out of a kettle," or "fog horn," or "bells." The patient with tinnitus usually works at peace in noisy surroundings which drown out his head noises, and the condition may be most annoying at night when the room is quiet.

Wax in the Ears

The amount of wax *(cerumen)* you have in your ears depends on the activity of wax-secreting glands in the external canal. The wax serves a lubricating, protecting and cleansing function and entraps small particles like flypaper. Some people, especially those with oily skins, tend to produce more ear wax than

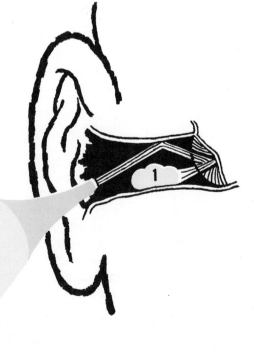

"Ear wax" *(cerumen)* may collect in the ear canal and form a *hard mass* (1) that hinders sound waves from reaching the eardrum, so that hearing is dulled. Removal by a doctor who injects warm fluid, as shown, in such a way that fluid presses against the eardrum and forces out the wax, is relatively simple. Matches, toothpicks, or other small objects should never be inserted into the ear, because of danger of injuring the eardrum and the skin of the ear canal.

others. When first formed, the wax is soft and oily. Older wax is brown and may become quite hard. The wax may emerge quite unnoticed from the ear opening or tiny fragments may collect near the ear opening and be removed by ordinary face-washing.

Occasionally, a hard mass — literally a ball of wax — collects close to or in contact with the eardrum at the inner end of the ear canal and does not budge. The mass obstructs sound waves and the patient may think he is losing his hearing. There may also be discomfort from pressures.

Wax is rather easily removed by a doctor—but not by a patient using bobby pins, matches, even door keys, to dig at the ear. The doctor takes a warm solution of water into an irrigating syringe, places a curved basin snugly beneath the bottom of the ear, and (in an adult) pulls the ear upward to straighten out the ear canal. He then presses the syringe plunger and squirts water into the ear in such a way that it rebounds from the eardrum and forces out the wax. Usually this does the job, although in stubborn cases it may be necessary to make an opening in the edge of the wax so that water can get behind it. Although it sounds simple, the washing should be done by a doctor since it is quite possible to rupture the eardrum if a stream of water is misdirected against it.

Dizziness, Deafness
(Meniere's Syndrome)

There are many causes of dizziness and one must not jump to the conclusion that an attack is caused by disease of the inner ear. Dizziness is but one of the symptoms of a disorder, not uncommon in persons of middle age and older, that is loosely called Meniere's syndrome, after the physician who described it.

There are three classic symptoms: tinnitus or head noises, usually the first to be noticed; attacks of dizziness; increasing deafness.

Some hearing loss is usually present before attacks of dizziness or vertigo set in, but the patient may not be particularly aware of it. Attacks of dizziness are generally abrupt, "out of the blue." Attacks may be momentary, recur frequently or be spaced a long time apart, or they may be continuous for weeks, months or years. Dizziness may or may not be accompanied by severe nausea and vomiting.

The cause of the disorder is not known. There is considerable controversy as to what constitutes a case of Meniere's syndrome, and expert evaluation is important. There appears to be disturbance of function, perhaps because of excess fluids, of the labyrinth, the semi-circular canals and intercommunicating cavities of the inner ear concerned with our sense of balance.

Various medical treatments are based on different theories as to causes of the disorder. Among these measures are diuretic drugs and low-salt diets, aimed to reduce swollen fluid pressures in the inner ear; anti-motion sickness and antihistamine drugs; sedatives and blood vessel dilators. One or another measure may be quite helpful in an individual patient but this usually has to be discovered by trial since no single measure is universally successful in all cases. If medical measures fail, and disability is very severe and deafness well advanced, destruction of the labyrinth by surgery or ultrasound may be employed as a last resort to prevent severe attacks.

Protruding Ears

The visible ear helps to collect sound vibrations to some extent, but is mostly a cosmetic embellishment. Various malformations of the ear, present at birth, range from its total absence to quite insignificant abnormalities. Plastic surgery can reshape and correct most malformations quite satisfactorily, although perfect results cannot be guaranteed. Perhaps the most frequent candidates for such correction are persons with protruding ears that stand out too far from the head. Corrective surgery to draw the ears close to the head is relatively simple, as operations go, although it must be remembered that no operation is a minor one as far as the patient is concerned.

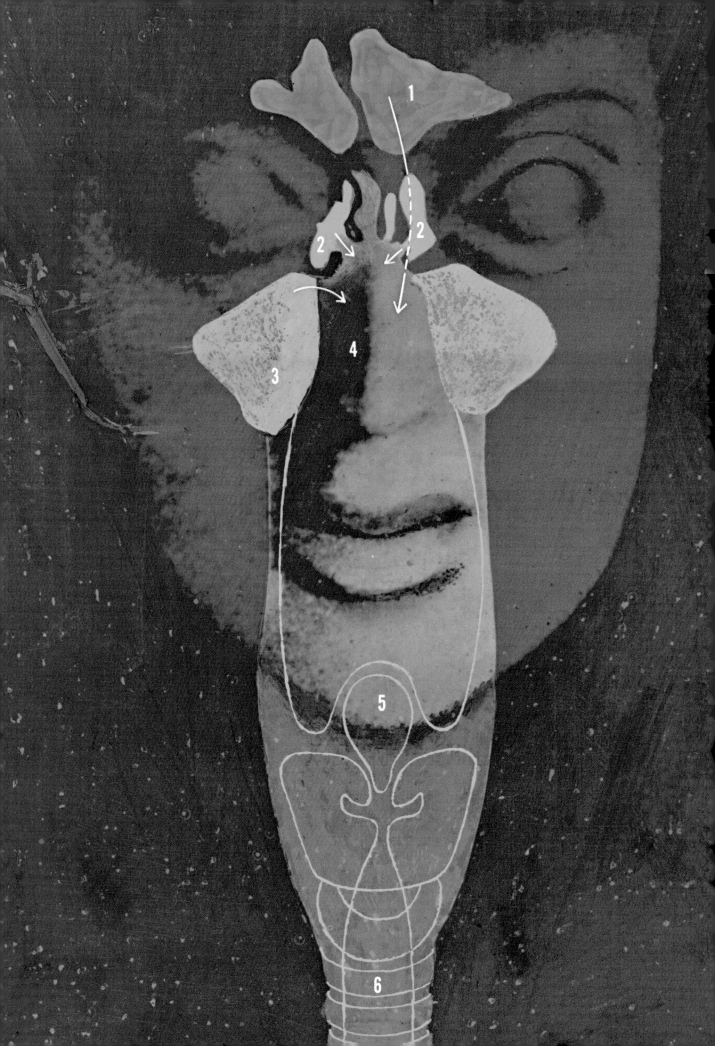

THE NOSE
AND SINUSES

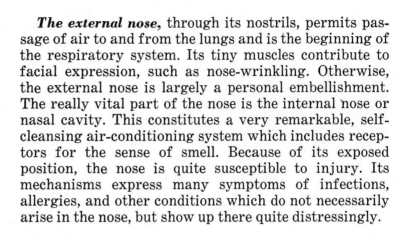

The external nose, through its nostrils, permits passage of air to and from the lungs and is the beginning of the respiratory system. Its tiny muscles contribute to facial expression, such as nose-wrinkling. Otherwise, the external nose is largely a personal embellishment. The really vital part of the nose is the internal nose or nasal cavity. This constitutes a very remarkable, self-cleansing air-conditioning system which includes receptors for the sense of smell. Because of its exposed position, the nose is quite susceptible to injury. Its mechanisms express many symptoms of infections, allergies, and other conditions which do not necessarily arise in the nose, but show up there quite distressingly.

The External Nose

Only the upper part of the nose is underlaid with bones, two of them, one on each side of the midline. The bones help to form the bridge of the nose, which supports the nose-pieces of glasses. The skin in this area is quite thin and the outline of underlying bone can be felt easily by a fingertip. The framework of parts in front of the bone, including the tip of the nose and flares around the nostrils, is mostly built of tough cartilage, with some small muscles and fatty cushioning, covered with skin.

Between the two nostrils is a fleshy part, called the *columella,* which feels soft if pressed between the fingers. Immediately behind it is a flexible but harder structure, the *septum,* which runs between the two nostrils to the floor of the skull at the back of the nasal cavity. The septum is largely cartilage but has a bony segment farther back. The septum is a wall which divides the nose into two chambers from front to back, a right and a left cavity, each served by its own nostril. Most of the structures of the nose are paired, but for purposes of discussion, a description of one is a description of its partner.

Injuries of the external nose are quite common, since it is outstanding in a literal as well as a figurative sense. The nose is part of the bony structures that surround and protect the eyes, and there may be some consolation in reflecting that some injuries are better absorbed by the nose than by the delicate eyeball. Damage to the nose should have the prompt attention of a doctor, for even injuries that seem slight and heal without much trouble may result in distortions of parts, leading to discomforts in breathing and sometimes to mouthbreathing.

There is a great range in the size and shape of the nose, but in general the length of the nose corresponds

The *paranasal sinuses* ("lying beside the nose") are air spaces of variable size and shape in bony structures which nearly surround the nasal cavity. The sinuses are lined with mucous membrane continuous with that of the nasal cavity, into which the sinuses drain. The sinuses normally are paired on either side of the midline of the face.

The color plate shows the *frontal sinuses* (1) above and behind the root of the nose; at a slightly lower level, honeycomb-like *ethmoid sinuses* (2) of the ethmoid ("sieve-like") bone; and the *maxillary sinuses* (3) in the cheekbones. The *sphenoid* sinuses are not shown here.

Secretions of the sinuses normally drain through tiny passages into the *nasal cavity* (4). Also shown in front view is the *epiglottis* (5) and the *trachea* (6).

Various symptoms and degrees of "sinus trouble" may arise if drainage is obstructed, infection enters, and germ-laden material accumulates. Sinusitis may be acute or chronic.

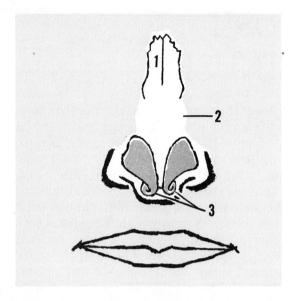

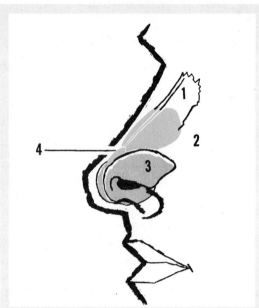

directly with the height of the whole face. Also in general, the long, narrow type of nose is represented by the white races, and the flat, broad type by the colored races. The long nose usually has a straight or convex profile, with a straight, comparatively pointed tip. The flat-nosed profile is concave, with the tip broad and turned upward.

Geography seems to have something to do with the width-length ratio of the nose (the *nasal index*). Noses of the flat, broad type are common in ethnic groups in hot equatorial regions, and in general noses tend to be narrower in proportion to distance from the equator. This probably reflects efficient adaptation to environment, and the evolution of the nose to properly air-condition a generally hot or cold environment.

Individually, of course, there is great variation in the nasal profile, within perfectly normal range. There is no reason to accept the nose as an index of character, particularly since the shape of the nose has diametrically opposite meanings to various fanciful interpreters. Tahitians, for instance, consider it an insult to be called long-nosed. But Napoleon always chose men with large noses for important missions, and Pascal wrote: "If the nose of Cleopatra had been shorter, the whole face of the earth would have been changed."

Structures of the nose. Above: *nasal bone* (1); *upper lateral cartilage* (2); *lower lateral cartilage* (3); *septum* (4). **At right, the lower lateral cartilages and medial cartilages form the** *columella* **or "little column," the fleshy lower part between the nostrils. Only the upper part of the external nose is underlaid with bone; the rest is largely cartilage or gristle, with a few small muscles, covered with skin.**

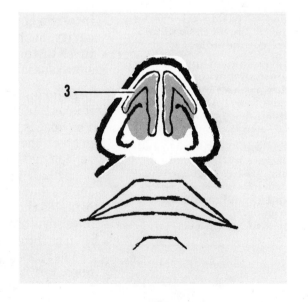

The Nasal Cavity

The main cavity of the nose lies between the floor of the brain cavity and the roof of the mouth. On the outer sidewall are three scroll-shaped bones called *turbinates,* which are covered and surrounded by soft spongy tissue with a rich blood supply. These shelf-like projections enlarge the surface with which air is in contact on its way to the lungs. Their air conditioning efficiency is remarkable.

Incoming air picks up any needed moisture from surrounding moist membranes. At the same time, the air is almost instantly warmed to the temperature of circulating blood. Even on a bitterly cold day, inhaled air does not freeze the lungs, because it is as warm as the lungs when it reaches them. These air-conditioning benefits are largely lost by mouth-breathing.

Membranes that line the passage secrete mucus and fluids continuously. Overly dry membranes are not only uncomfortable, but dryness impairs important protective functions of the nose — hence the desirability of adding moisture to room air which tends to become excessively dry when homes are heated in the winter. Nasal secretions have two main functions: to humidify inspired air, and to help keep the nose clean.

A normal nose is self-cleaning. A runny nose drains from the front a little too exuberantly, but normally there is a more modest output which on occasion leads to useful blowing of the nose. Coarse hairs inside the nostrils, called *vibrissae* (the same name is given to cats' whiskers) filter relatively coarse particles from inhaled air, and finer hairs trap many finer particles, as is obvious from secretions produced after one has been working in dusty or smoky surroundings.

Sticky mucus of the internal nose traps fine particles and many bacteria and moves them to the junction of the nasal cavity and throat *(nasopharynx)* by "riding" on the feathery tips of tiny whip-like cells called cilia. The cilia with beating, sweeping movements keep a film of mucus and entrapped particles flowing toward the throat. Normally, the secre-

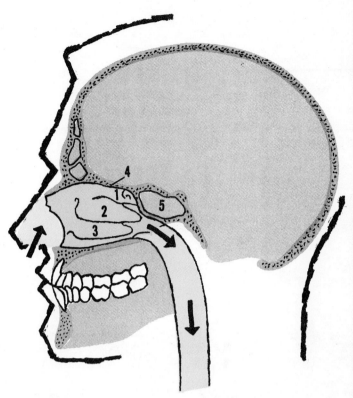

The *superior* (1), *middle* (2), and *inferior* (3) *turbinates* are scroll-shaped bones of the outer sidewalls of the nasal cavity, covered by spongy tissue which moistens and "air conditions" inhaled air. Also shown: *ethmoid bone* (4) which forms floor of brain and roof of nasal cavity, and *sphenoid sinus* (5).

tions are unconsciously swallowed and disposed of harmlessly via the stomach. Many bacteria are destroyed by stomach juices. Nasal secretions contain an antibacterial substance, lysozyme, which is also present in tears. Lysozyme acts against the more common forms of bacteria inhaled with air.

The system is not perfect, of course. Some persons who are not necessarily ill carry colonies of "resistant staph" germs in their noses. These may spread via the air or more directly and cause infections that do not respond to commonly used antibiotics. Tissue of the turbinates is erectile — that is, it swells and becomes engorged under some circumstances. "Sniffles" that follow the inhalation of cold air are a common experience. Congestion and excessive secretion usually subside promptly in a normal nose. But under some circumstances, such as a bad head cold, tissues do not "rebound" and stuffed-up congestion may ensue.

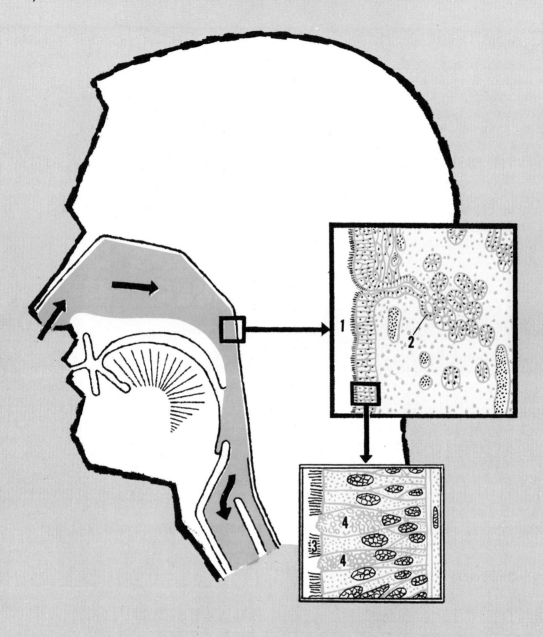

Arrows in profile drawing show path of inhaled air. An enlarged section of the mucosal lining of the throat shows layer of *ciliated epithelium* (1) and *mucus-secreting gland* (2), and, in greater enlargement, *cilia* (3) and *goblet cells* (4) that secrete mucus. Cilia are fine hairlike processes that move incessantly in sweeping motions that propel a moving film of mucus with entrapped particles toward the outside.

Organs of Smell and Taste

The first mammals were tiny creatures with noses close to the ground. The sense of smell, in pursuing food and detecting dangers, was vital to the survival of many primitive organisms, and it is still very important to most creatures, with the notable exception of man. Our smell apparatus is greatly inferior to that of dogs, but good enough to warn us of a gas leak or spoiled food, and to sustain a considerable traffic in perfumes and deodorants or other odorous materials.

Our smell-receptors are located in a small patch of tissue, about one-half inch square, located at the very top of the nasal cavity near the inner end of the upper throat. The patch has a yellowish tinge, in contrast to surrounding pink tissue, and it consists of several million tiny endings of the *olfactory nerve* whose bundles pass through the *cribriform plate* (meaning "perforated like a sieve") and enter the farthest forward extensions of the brain.

Anything that is smellable must be volatile enough to be airborne and probably soluble enough to be dissolved in mucous materials of the nose. However, the smell-patch is quite well shielded from air currents which pass below it in the ordinary course of breathing. The process of sniffing, to smell a faint odor better, sets up currents and air swirls which bring odorous materials into more effective contact with nerves which carry impulses to the brain where they are recognized as scents.

The sense of smell fatigues quite rapidly. Upon entering a room in which some strong odor is present, we are at first very much aware of it, but in a little while we almost cease to perceive it. There are subtle differences in people's abilities to detect different odors. Substances which have definite odor to some people may be odorless to others. These are normal variations; the rare inability to smell anything at all *(anosmia)* is abnormal but of itself carries no threat to health or life. Except, of course, when the odor of a gas leak or smoke is a warning to take emergency action.

Much of what we think we taste, we smell. Anybody who has a heavy cold notices that flavorsome foods of many kinds seem bland and tasteless, but the taste organs are not affected. What happens is that congestion prevents odorous air-swirls, created by chewing and swallowing, from reaching the smell-patch high in the nasal cavity, because of congestion. Taste buds, which are cells that are chemical receptors of taste sensations, are located in the tongue but are not spread about evenly.

Taste buds are not the minute "pimples" or *papillae* we see when we look at the tongue, but flask-shaped structures in the walls of the papillae. There are about 250 taste buds per papilla, diminishing to 90 in old age.

Unlike the sense of smell, which is so complex that no system of classifying stimuli has been successful, taste is compounded of but four sensations: bitter, salt, sweet, and sour. A particular taste-bud is sensitive to only one of these. As shown in the drawing, the four kinds of taste receptors are concentrated in different regions of the tongue. There is some decrease of taste-bud sensitivities with increasing age, which may explain why a wife's pie doesn't taste like the pie that mother used to bake.

Receptors for the sense of smell are located in a small patch of tissue (1) at the top of the nasal cavity; nerves pass through apertures in the *ethmoid bone* (2) to the brain. Details in drawing on following page.

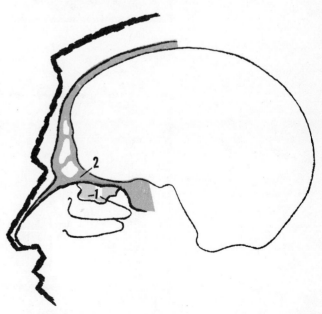

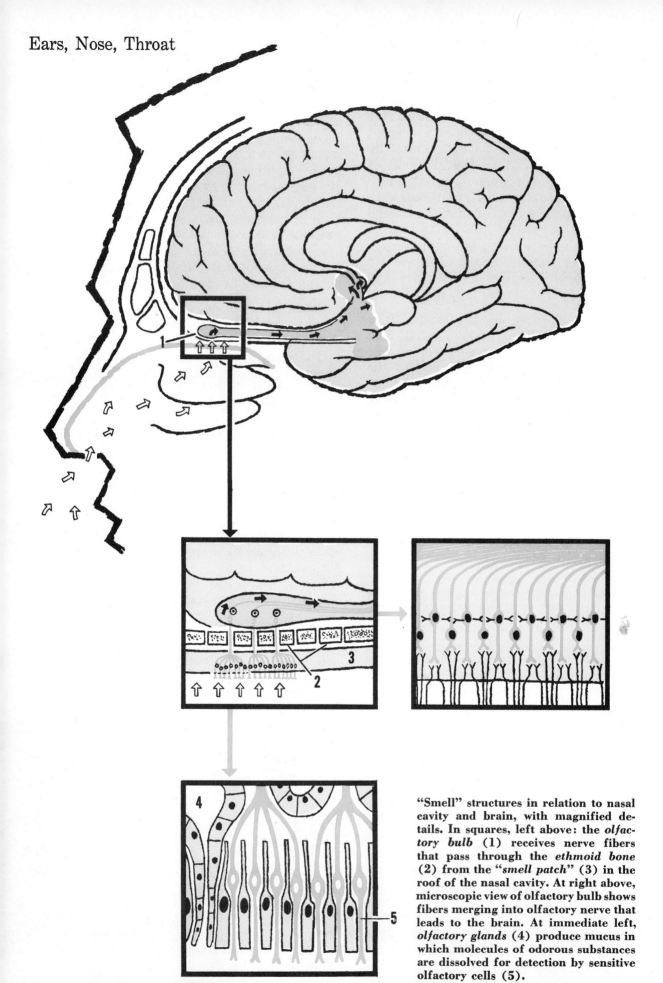

"Smell" structures in relation to nasal cavity and brain, with magnified details. In squares, left above: the *olfactory bulb* (1) receives nerve fibers that pass through the *ethmoid bone* (2) from the *"smell patch"* (3) in the roof of the nasal cavity. At right above, microscopic view of olfactory bulb shows fibers merging into olfactory nerve that leads to the brain. At immediate left, *olfactory glands* (4) produce mucus in which molecules of odorous substances are dissolved for detection by sensitive olfactory cells (5).

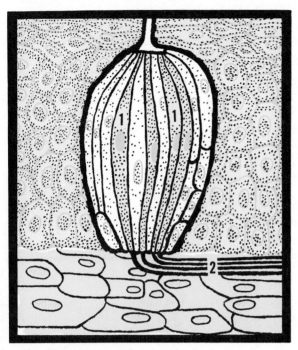

Section through a taste bud. Dissolved substances on the surface make contact with spindle-shaped *gustatory cells* (1) and impulses travel over *nerve fibers* (2) to the brain.

Pathways of Sensation

The senses of smell and taste are "chemical senses." What is perceived in the brain as an odor or flavor is the presence of certain molecules in fluids that are in contact with receptor organs of smell and taste. Thus there is some direct contact with whatever we smell or taste. A bone-dry nose or tongue would be unable to smell or taste anything. Chemicals have to be dissolved in local mucus or fluids to become tastable or smellable, but in the case of some substances, such as mercaptan (exuded by skunks) a very few molecules are quite enough to produce a disagreeable impression.

The "smell brain" is a very ancient part of the brain called the *rhinencephalon,* from Greek words meaning "nose brain." This primitive part of the brain in human beings is very small and is quite overwhelmed by the massive cerebrum, but is relatively large in many animals and reptiles that depend a great deal on the sense of smell to tell them what is going on in their environment. Dogs, for instance, obviously can see and hear, but they depend a great deal on their noses for reliable information and undoubtedly can smell things we cannot.

Just above the bone which separates the top of the nasal cavity from the brain, the undersurface of the *olfactory bulb* receives nerve fibers which pass upward from the small "smell patch" in the roof of the nose through tiny holes in the thin bone. The drawing on the opposite page shows details of how chemical stimuli from the outside world are interpreted as odors.

Taste buds, shown on this page, look alike under the microscope, but each is capable of registering only a single sensation — either sour, salt, sweet, or bitter. How an individual taste bud can be so exclusively discriminating is not known, but it is probably a matter of different enzymes produced in the different buds. We taste (or gourmets think they do) countless subtle flavors, but all are compounded of the four basic sensations, greatly enhanced and subtly refined by the sense of smell.

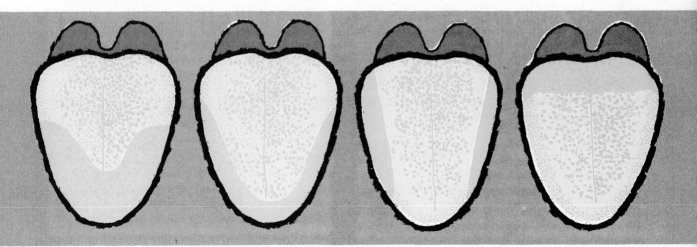

A single taste bud is sensitive to only one of the four primary sensations of taste. The taste buds of the tongue are not uniformly distributed. Colored areas in drawing, from left to right, show concentrations of taste buds sensitive to *salt, sweet, sour,* and *bitter,* respectively. Taste buds are most numerous in young children and their numbers are greatly diminished in old age.

Location of the major paranasal sinuses, front and side views: *frontal sinus* (1); *ethmoid cells* (2); *maxillary sinus* (3); *sphenoid sinus* (4); *turbinates* (5). Direction of drainage of the various sinuses is shown by arrows. All the sinuses normally drain into the nasal cavity.

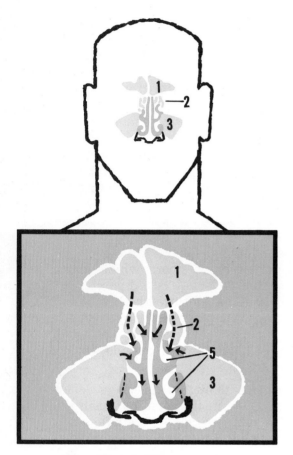

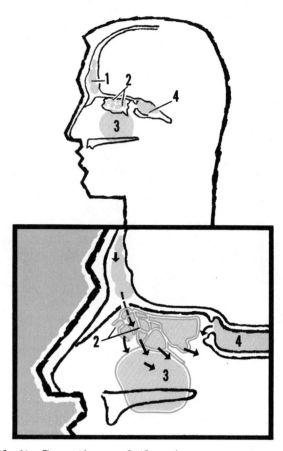

The Nasal Sinuses

The nasal sinuses are a series of air spaces which nearly surround the nasal cavity within the skull. They are literally holes in the head, and why nature gave them to us is not known. The sinuses make us a little lighter-headed than if bone were solid; possibly they serve as honeycomb insulators of the nearby brain cage, and perhaps limit the excursion of local fractures. But the paranasal ("lying beside the nose") sinuses are not essential to life. A few people, who may never know it, lack certain sinuses, but this does no harm and may even do good: they can't get sinusitis in those areas.

The sinuses normally come in pairs so that one-half of each pair lies on either side of the midline of the face. These empty, irregular air spaces are surrounded by thin bony walls, and are lined with mucous membrane which is like that of the internal nose and is continuous with it. Secretions of the sinuses normally drain through tiny passages into the nasal cavity. Under ordinary circumstances, the interior of the sinuses is free of germs, but it is possible for germs to enter from the nasal cavity and cause infections, or for obstructed outlets to dam up fluids, or for other variants of what is loosely called "sinus trouble" to arise.

There are four major pairs of sinuses. The *frontal sinus* lies in bone just above and behind the root of the nose, about on a level with the eyebrows. The sinuses lie on either side of a thin bony partition, and each cavity is usually divided into several small compartments. However, the frontal sinus is quite variable in size and shape, and the space on one side is commonly larger than on the other. Sometimes there are one or as many as six independent cavities, each with its own separate connection with the nasal chamber, and occasionally a sinus may be present only on one side, or both may be entirely lacking. The average capacity of both frontal sinuses is about 3½ teaspoonfuls.

Immediately behind the frontal sinuses, but on a lower level, is the *ethmoid* ("sieve-like") *bone*. It contains many small honeycomb-like cavities and is pierced with small holes for the passage of the "smell nerves" from the nasal cavity to the brain. These honeycomb spaces, or ethmoid cells, vary from three to eighteen in number, and sometimes the compartments may extend into the bony framework of the turbinates and even into the bony palate.

Behind the ethmoid and at a still lower level is the *sphenoid* ("wedge-shaped") *bone*. It is shaped somewhat like a large butterfly, with a middle part, called the body, from which wing-shaped processes diverge. The sphenoid bone touches parts of most of the other bones of the skull, and it is intricately pierced by openings for the passage of blood vessels and nerves. The "body" of the bone rests against the ethmoid, and within this part are the *sphenoid sinuses*, which may extend into the wings of the bone and exhibit great diversity of size and shape.

In the cheekbone is the *maxillary sinus*, largest of all. Commonly, the cavity has the rough shape of a pyramid, but there is considerable variation of form and size. The floor of the maxillary sinus is close to roots of the teeth.

Mouth and Throat

The mouth, opened wide as for a dentist, is rather easily inspected with aid of a mirror. The hard palate, or roof of the mouth, merges with the soft palate at a point which can be felt with the tip of the tongue. A small peninsula of tissue, the *uvula*, hangs down from the soft palate into the throat. These soft structures can be set in vibration by air passing over them during sleep, producing the phenomenon of snoring, which frequently causes a good deal of distress to other persons but never to the owner.

Tonsils, unless they have been removed, can be seen as somewhat oval, flattened bodies over either side of the passageway into the throat. Their exposed surfaces are covered with mucous membrane in which there are a number of small pits that open into saclike cavities called crypts or follicles. The deep unexposed surface of the tonsil is covered by a fibrous capsule which attaches the tonsil to the wall. This arrangement makes its surgical removal relatively easy. By cutting through the mucous membrane, the gland can be "shelled out."

Throat. For descriptive purposes, the *pharynx*, or throat, is divided into upper, middle, and lower regions. Actually, it is a membrane-lined muscular tube which is continuous with the back of the nasal cavity, where it forms a blind pouch and turns downward to merge with the windpipe and *esophagus*. The upper part *(nasopharynx)* is concerned with passage of air through the nose, the middle and lower parts with passage of air and food, and thus the throat is part of both the respiratory and digestive systems.

Openings of the Eustachian tubes which permit air to enter and leave the middle ear to equalize pressures are in the upper pharynx. In this region, too, are collections of lymphoid tissue, especially prominent in children, which are called *pharyngeal tonsils* but are more familiarly known as *adenoids* when the tissues become infected and enlarged.

The lowest part of the throat leads in front to the *larynx*, or voice-box, and the windpipe or *trachea*. A special structure in the upper part of the larynx contains delicate folds of elastic tissue separated by a narrow fore-and-aft slit. These folds are the *vocal cords*, which stand out from the walls somewhat like shelves. Muscles control the tension and rate of vibration of the cords as air passes through them, modifying the sounds of the voice. This part of the larynx is called the *glottis*.

Just behind the opening into the larynx, and continuous with the back wall of the throat, is the upper end of the esophagus which connects the throat with the stomach. Both air and food travel the passages above, but it is vital that food particles be kept out of the windpipe and lungs. Nature takes care of this automatically—

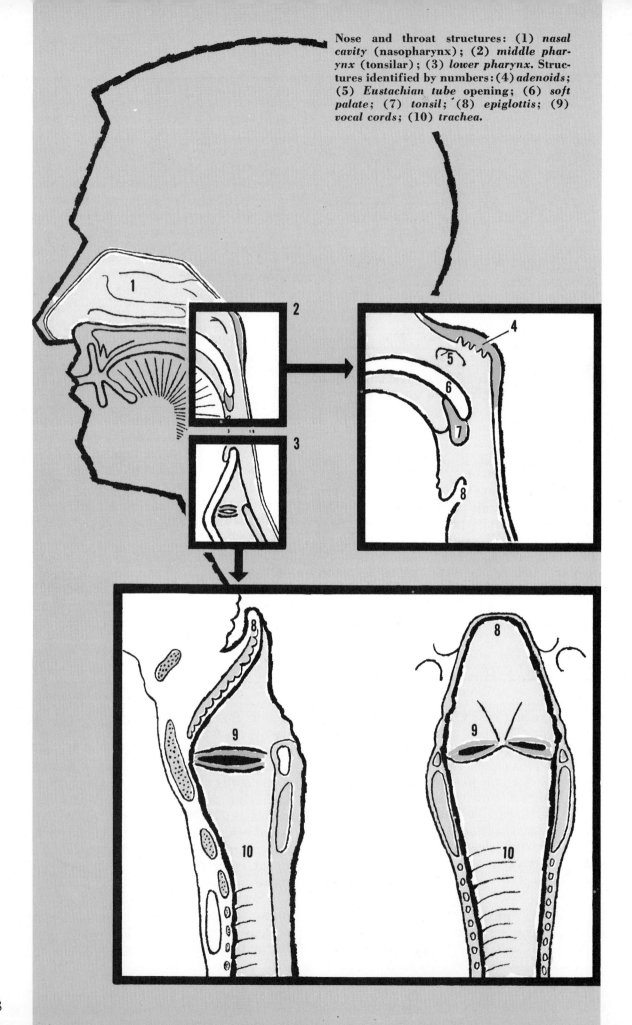

Nose and throat structures: (1) *nasal cavity* (nasopharynx); (2) *middle pharynx* (tonsilar); (3) *lower pharynx*. Structures identified by numbers: (4) *adenoids*; (5) *Eustachian tube* opening; (6) *soft palate*; (7) *tonsil*; (8) *epiglottis*; (9) *vocal cords*; (10) *trachea*.

except when we "swallow something the wrong way," and choke and sputter until we get rid of it — by an ingenious lid or trapdoor, the *epiglottis*. This tonguelike bit of tissue in the upper rim of the larynx opens when we breathe, and permits air to enter the windpipe, but snaps shut when we swallow so that food passes over it into the nearby esophagus without falling into the larynx. Swallowing, incidentally, is accomplished not by gravity but by muscles. We can swallow just as efficiently if we hang by our feet.

Postnasal Drip

Secretions of the nasal passages that are not expelled by nose-blowing drip down the back of the throat and are swallowed harmlessly. This is a natural way of getting rid of what doesn't drain from the front of the nose. When secretions are excessive, constant, or persistent, a person is likely to be uncomfortably aware of them. There is much hacking, coughing, hawking, and clearing of the throat, and some people ease their embarrassment by attributing matters to a popular affliction known as "postnasal drip." We all have some back-of-the-nose drainage of which we are normally unaware. A patient may be excessively aware of a drainage system that is not abnormal, or secretions may actually be excessive (as whenever we have a cold).

Causes of exaggerated postnasal drip include sinus infections, colds, allergies, long soft palate that tickles the throat, obstructions, irritation of membranes by smoke, dust, or fumes, infections, emotional disturbances, and excessive and prolonged self-medication with various "nose medicines."

Excessive postnasal drip is a symptom which, if not caused by something so obvious as a cold, should be investigated to determine and remove the causes if possible. Very often the patient is constantly aware of and worried about a condition that is not serious, and needs reassurance that postnasal drip, though unpleasant, is harmless. Some persons are so aware of an irritation that causes

them to cough or clear their throats frequently that they fear they have cancer. Assuring them that they have a simple postnasal drip takes the weight of the world off their shoulders.

Prevention. One can do several things to minimize postnasal drip:

Overheating and poor ventilation in winter result in low humidity and drying of the nasal membranes. Secretions tend to become thicker, are not carried off normally, and droplets fall into the back of the throat. Vaporizers or devices which add moisture to overheated dry air help to keep nasal membranes normal.

Sleeping on a high pillow instead of a low flat one often helps to reduce postnasal drip.

Some people have a habit of drawing secretions into the back of the throat. Sometimes a postnasal drip can be cleared by so simple a measure as telling the patient to blow his nose more often.

Nose Drops

Medicines that are inhaled, sprayed, or dropped into the nose can be very effective in shrinking swollen membranes. But the drugs are quite potent and it is important to follow a doctor's directions for their use very carefully. For instance, doses should not be taken too close together. This is apt in time to cause "rebound" congestion which makes matters worse and invites more frequent and more closely spaced doses. Overuse or unnecessary use of medicinal sprays can also cause postnasal drip, by forcing secretions backward into the throat.

Nose drops with oily bases are best avoided. Fine droplets may be inhaled into the lungs, especially by infants, and oils which cannot be absorbed by tissues can cause a stubborn form of respiratory tract disease known as lipoid pneumonia.

Nasal Polyps

Persons with allergies are especially likely to have *nasal polyps* — soft, moist, pendulous outgrowths from mucous membranes which line the nose. Whether the underlying cause is an allergic reaction, some inflammatory process in the membranes, or both, is not positively known. Common nasal polyps may be small and numerous or large and single. The usual symptom of their presence is obstruction of nasal airways on one or both sides. Severe obstruction encourages mouth-breathing, with undesirable consequences. Obstructive polyps should be removed. Common nasal polyps are almost always benign — that is, not cancerous—and a pathologist's confirmation of this from examination of removed tissue is very reassuring.

How to Blow the Nose

One might think that the art of nose-blowing is instinctive and needs no teaching. However, the self-taught noseblower commonly pinches both nostrils between the folds of a handkerchief, takes a deep breath, and lets go with a bang. Too often this forces germ-laden secretions into the Eustachian tubes, whence they may work their way into the middle ear and set up infections. A better nose-blowing technique is the following: with handkerchief or tissue beneath the nose, grasp the bridge of the nose between thumb and and fingers, at a point where underlying bone prevents either nostril from being pinched shut. Blow.

Deviated Septum

The *septum*, or wall, that divides the nose into two equal parts normally extends in a straight line from the front between the two nostrils to the floor of the skull at the back. But it is not at all uncommon for the septum to deviate from a straight line. A deviated septum may be congenital, but is more often caused by blows, injuries in contact sports such as football, and crushing fractures suffered in automobile and other accidents.

A crooked, deviated septum may not be apparent on the outside. Its effects vary with the nature of the deformity. Air passages may be partly or wholly stopped up, making breathing difficult.

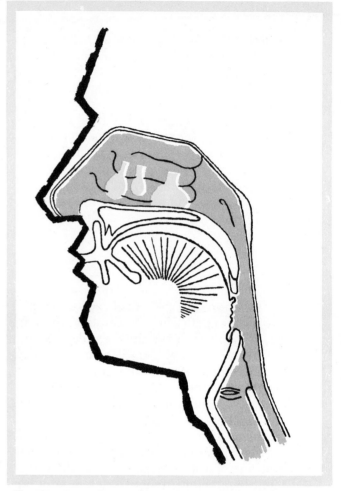

Nasal polyps, shown above, are soft, pendulous outgrowths from lining membranes of the nose. Polyps, often associated with allergies, may be of sufficient size to cause obstructive symptoms.

If mouth-breathing results, inhaled air is not cleaned, warmed, and moistened as it would be by normal passage through the nose. Air currents in the nose may be slowed or deflected so that sinus outlets do not have the "stroking" benefits of air passing over them, an action which normally helps to keep pressures within the sinuses at proper levels. A crooked septum may deflect secretions from the front of the nose toward the back and cause excessive postnasal drip.

To correct deformities of the septum it is often necessary to cut out the bent portion so the rest may fall into a straight line. The operation is done inside the nose and does not leave any external scars or deformities. Most often a local anesthetic is used. Dressings within the nose are generally removed the next day, the patient is told not to blow his nose for a few days, and within a short time the newly-aligned septum settles down to do its work quietly for a lifetime.

Plastic Surgery of the Nose (Rhinoplasty)

Many deformities of the nose do not interfere seriously if at all with the health of the owner. Some deformities are conspicuous, but many are departures from some ideal or desired shape of the nose rather than true deformities. Probably few human beings are completely satisfied with the shapes of their noses. A competent plastic surgeon can correct gross deformities of the nose well enough to revolutionize the lives of persons who have been seriously handicapped in society and business. He can also re-sculpture noses so slightly misshapen that hardly anyone notices them except the owner, who may be unhappy and depressed about an organ that dominates the features.

Surgery for cosmetic purposes needs no justification, of course. At the same time, there are a few persons who feel that the entire course of their lives will be miraculously changed for the better if their noses are straightened, shortened, or otherwise modified. Since even a perfect result cannot guarantee romantic, social and vocational conquests, a surgeon sometimes rejects a neurotic patient who clearly expects unreasonable miracles from correction of a cosmetic "defect" so trifling as to be virtually unnoticeable.

With models, sketches, photographs, physical examination, measurements, the surgeon explains what an operation may reasonably be expected to accomplish.

A quite common objective is to remove a bony hump, shorten the nose, narrow the bridge, lift or narrow the nasal tip, in varying combinations. A bony hump (a small hump is more difficult for the surgeon than a large one) is cut down from within the nose and excess tissue removed. At the same time the bridge of the nose must be narrowed to accommodate the new shape. Pieces of bone or cartilage may be used like sculpturing materials. The nose tip may droop or overhang too much. The tip is mostly cartilage and can be shortened, narrowed, or given a pert tilt.

What is the patient in for? About a week in a hospital, and probably another week before he or she feels like returning to routines of work and living. For one thing, the operation inevitably leaves some swelling and discoloration around the eyes, and the patient temporarily looks as if he had got the worst of it in combat. Immediately after surgery the patient is kept on his back without a pillow with his head between sandbags (to prevent jarring motions) for a couple of days. Chewing might disturb healing so he is given a liquid diet. In about six days the patient goes home from the hospital, but returns to the surgeon's office for after-care until dressings are removed around the twelfth day. Altogether, it is well to plan a two-week "vacation" from ordinary affairs.

Other plastic procedures, such as correction of saddle-block deformity (conspicuous depression of the bridge of the nose) require addition rather than subtraction of tissue and involve extensive grafting, sometimes even as extensive as providing a new nose in cases where the organ has been largely destroyed by disease or injury. A condition known as *rhinophyma* — huge, reddish, bulbous, knobby overgrowth of the end of the nose — is corrected by surgically shaving down the excess tissue.

"Sinus Trouble"

Every nasal infection involves the nasal sinuses to some degree. All the air-filled cavities of the sinuses open into the nasal passages and membrane linings are continuous with those of the nose and throat. Thus, *sinusitis* (inflammation of the sinuses) is virtually a universal ailment that everybody experiences when, for instance, one has a head cold. Usually the condition is mild and short-lasting even if untreated, and disappears along with the respiratory infection that accompanies it—provided that secretions can drain freely from the sinuses. If there are obstructions to free drainage,

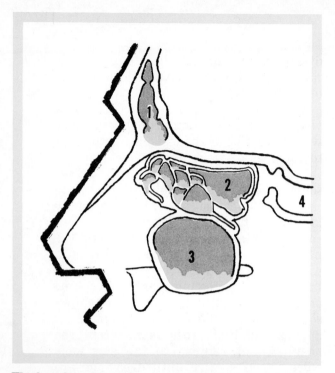

Thick, infected secretions may collect in any of the sinus cavities if drainage is obstructed. Drawing shows purulent material in *frontal sinus* (1); *ethmoid sinuses* (2); *maxillary sinus* (3); *sphenoid sinus* (4). The immediate concern is to provide free drainage.

acute and chronic conditions popularly known as "sinus trouble" can become established if not treated.

Sinus headaches. Not all headaches can be blamed on the sinuses by any means, but mild or severe headache is a common symptom of sinus trouble, although it may be entirely absent. Sinus headaches are almost always at their worst in the early morning or on arising. Headache may be very painful if the frontal sinuses are involved. Ethmoid disorder may be accompanied by dull headache and sense of fullness between or above the eyes. Infection of the sphenoid sinuses may cause dull headache and a vague sensation of pressure.

Sinusitis may be acute or chronic. If sinus infection is not thoroughly eradicated it is apt to become chronic, with permanent changes in membranes and successive remissions and recurrences of trouble. Thick, sticky, pus-containing discharges from sinus openings indicate infection. There may be local pain and tenderness, especially if the maxillary sinus is involved. Material that cannot escape freely from the sinuses builds up

pressures and may cause inflammation of nearby structures.

What causes attacks of sinusitis? A sinus outlet may be obstructed by a deviated septum or polyps that have arisen within the sinus after recurrent attacks. The most common condition that favors sinus disorder is swelling and congestion of membranes, such as occurs with a head cold. Nasal allergies may cause similar congestion which cuts off the means of escape of sinus secretions.

Treatment. The immediate concern is to provide free drainage for sinus secretions. In general, simplest measures are tried first, such as nose drops which constrict tissues and help to open up obstructed openings. Antihistamine drugs may help if there is a history of allergy. If there is fever or evidence of extension of infection, antibiotics may be used. If response is not satisfactory and the patient is very uncomfortable, secretions may be sucked out of the affected sinus through a tube connected to a vacuum device. Occasionally, irrigation of the sinus with saline solution is helpful in the chronic stage, but is rarely necessary. Correction of conditions which lead to chronic sinusitis is usually undertaken after the acute stage is over.

Sinusitis in children. There are about as many runny noses in children as there are noses. Generally the runniness subsides uneventfully, but sinusitis may occasionally result from neglect. Simple measures are worth applying to any child whose nasal discharge persists beyond three days.

Warm packs and steam humidification help to ventilate the sinuses so that drainage can take place. Warm packs can be prepared by soaking thick cloths in hot water and wringing them out, taking care that the pack is not too hot to be applied to the skin. A vaporizer which delivers large amounts of warm water vapor is a good investment. Home-made measures of delivering steam are valuable too, but care must be taken to make sure that there is no danger of direct contact with a hot vessel or with scalding vapor that can cause serious burns.

Hoarseness

Hoarseness is a *symptom* which may mean no more than that one has yelled too much at a football game. Most often the cause of temporary hoarseness is simple and obvious, such as a cold with congestion of throat structures. But persistent unexplained hoarseness may at times be a symptom of some serious systemic condition. Hoarseness that persists longer than three weeks is a warning that a doctor should be consulted without fail to determine the cause.

Laryngitis

Inflammation of the larynx or voice box is known as *laryngitis*. The predominating symptom is unmistakable. You can't speak above a whisper, if at all. *Simple acute laryngitis* is usually caused either by infection or by overuse or strain of the voice.

Laryngitis from abuse of the voice is an occupational hazard of auctioneers, orators, singers and others who use the voice loud and long. It also occurs in screaming children and mothers who have to shout to be heard above the din or after a short period of vocal abuse such as running a noisy convention meeting or leading a cheering section or making one's self heard at a party where everybody talks at once.

The other form of simple acute laryngitis is associated with the common cold and has the same sort of reaction in the larynx as occurs in the nose, throat, and bronchi in a cold: inflammation, swelling, redness and increased flow of secretions.

Complete recovery can be expected in a few days if you follow the admonition: "Whisper, please." Don't speak a word aloud. Rest the voice as you would rest a broken arm in a splint. Heat, drugs, or other measures may be prescribed by a doctor as circumstances warrant. Smoking and dusty atmospheres are irritating to the injured larynx and should be avoided if possible.

Chronic forms of laryngitis which recur frequently without respiratory infection or voice strain have the same symptom — hoarseness — but a variety of possible causes. Loss of the voice may occur without physical disease of any nature of the larynx, as from hysterical states, remote affection of nerves serving the voice, or some systemic diseases not localized to the larynx. Tuberculosis and syphilis are occasionally in the background of chronic laryngitis. Hoarseness may also result from any sort of mass pressing from the outside against the larynx. Allergic reactions may cause swelling of laryngeal tissues with hoarseness.

Benign tumors of the larynx are not uncommon. These may be polyps, cysts, or fibrous growths. Nodules may form where abused vocal cords strike too vigorously together. These are not unlike corns or calluses produced by pressure and friction, and at times they become ulcerated. Surgical removal of benign tumors may sometimes be necessary and results are usually excellent.

Cancer of the larynx is not rare; it accounts for about two per cent of malignancies. Early cancer of the throat causes little more than a slight huskiness of the voice: no pain, no bleeding, no loss of feelings of well-being. Hoarseness may be the only symptom indicating cancer of the larynx at an early stage when it is most curable.

All diseases of the larynx produce the characteristic symptom of hoarseness. If you are hoarse, there are two important things to remember:

Whisper, please. And see your doctor.

"Bad Breath"

Most often the cause of foul breath will be found in the mouth or upper respiratory tract. Decaying teeth and unhealthy gums are common causes. Longstanding mouthbreathing due to nasal blockage may cause offensive breath by drying out normal secretions and facilitating the entrance of microorganisms. Infection in the nasal cavity can cause bad breath. Chronic low-grade inflammations of the nose and upper throat can lead to loss of normal ciliary action (flow of secretions) with unpleasant breath odor.

In such cases odor can be stopped only by locating and correcting the pathologic condition. Rinsing the mouth with a solution of a teaspoonful of salt mixed in a glass of water is a simple hygienic measure. There are some people who have a quite unwarranted obsession about bad breath and some who are not aware that their breath is unpleasant.

Cleft Lip and Cleft Palate

In general practice some 35 years ago there was nothing that gave me such a sad feeling as the delivery of a baby with a cleft palate. Parents ask "why did this happen to us?" and often develop guilty feelings that they are somehow responsible because of something done or left undone during pregnancy.

They can at least be reassured that they are not guilty of omitting some specific measure for preventing this abnormality, since no such measure is known. It is conceivable that some infection or injury of the mother around the sixth to eighth week of pregnancy when fetal structures are being formed might have some effect in production of cleft palate. But there is much more evidence which implicates hereditary factors. In many cases, if family histories are traced, it is found that an uncle or cousin or grandparent or someone else on one side of the family or the other had a cleft palate. However, if neither the mother nor the father of a cleft palate baby has a cleft palate, there is about a 95 per cent chance that children subsequently born to them will be born with a normal palate.

Cleft lip or palate results from failure of lip and palate structures to fuse properly during fetal development. There are many variations of the deformity. The lip may be cleft only on one side, or on both sides, and the lower part of the nose is involved. The defect may involve the soft palate, or it may involve the hard palate as well, with varying degrees of separation. There may be difficulties in feeding the handicapped young baby, because milk easily "backs up" through the nose, but with patience and special feeding devices this can be overcome.

Correction of the defect requires surgery. Operations may be done in several stages as the child grows older, depending on the surgeon's appraisal of the individual case. Usually the cleft lip is repaired quite early, when the baby is in good general condition and gaining weight. The results usually give a needed boost to the morale of the parents, when the unsightly deformity present at birth is dramatically lessened.

Later closure of the cleft palate, often done in stages, aims to restore structures so that normal speech will be possible. Formation of distinct speech sounds, especially certain consonants, requires complex coordination of muscles and structures of the lips and hard and soft palates and a proper air pathway so the voice does not "escape" in an unintelligible way through the nose.

Defects of the teeth will appear. Dental prostheses may be needed as the child grows older. Speech therapy may be required, not merely to produce intelligible speech but speech that is not so "queer" that playmates will mimic it.

Today, the end results of expert care are often so excellent that it is too bad the parents cannot foresee them at the dreadful moment when they first see their newborn cleft palate baby. It is unfortunately true, however, that the more complicated cases require rather costly teamwork of pediatrician, surgeon, dental specialist and speech therapist. There are a number of "cleft palate clinics" around the country with staffs of specialist teams, and some of the states have programs of assistance in rehabilitation of cleft palate patients. Specific information about community facilities can be given by the doctor who delivers the baby or the pediatrician who assumes its care, and by the government's National Institute of Dental Research in Bethesda, Maryland.

BONES AND MUSCLES AND THEIR DISORDERS

by ADRIAN E. FLATT, M.D.

The Skeleton · Skull, Ribs, and Lower Back · Appendages · The Structure of Bone · Growth and Repair · Red Cells and Minerals

OSTEOMYELITIS

THE SPINE

Low Back Pain · "Disk Trouble" · Chronic Back Strain · Whiplash Injuries

THE SHOULDER

THE ELBOW

THE WRIST AND HAND

THE HIP

THE KNEE

THE FOOT

Foot Strain · Flat Feet · Corrective Foot Exercises

CHILDREN'S FOOT PROBLEMS

Shoes · Adult Foot Problems · Diseases of Bone

SPRAINS, DISLOCATIONS, FRACTURES

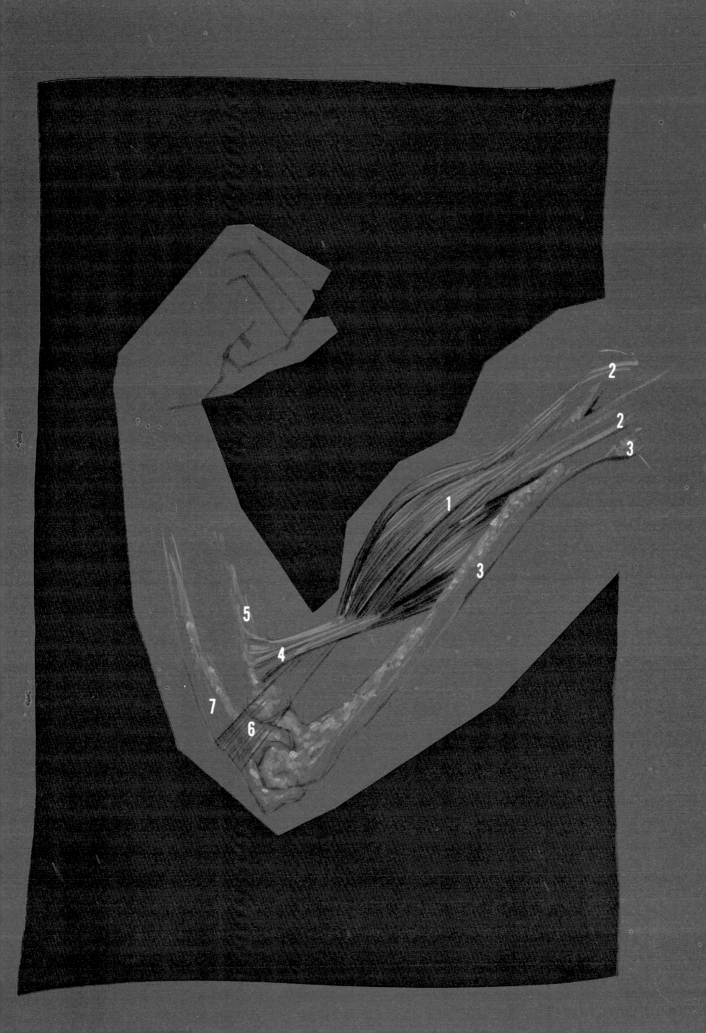

CHAPTER 18

BONES AND MUSCLES AND THEIR DISORDERS

by ADRIAN E. FLATT, M.D.

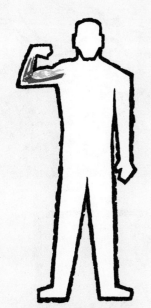

Muscles move body parts by contracting, and in many instances pull against bones that serve as levers. Tendons are fibrous cords at the termination of a muscle that attach it to bone.

The color plate shows the *biceps* muscle (1) which bulges when you flex your arm to show how strong you are. The biceps is connected by *tendons* (2) to shoulder areas where it originates (its name means "two headed"). The *humerus* (3) is the upper arm bone. A *tendon* (4) inserts the biceps into the *radius* (5), one of the forearm bones (the other is the ulna). An accessory *tendon* (6) inserts the muscle within the forearm musculature.

Muscles work in "teams." The biceps on the front of the arm flexes the elbow, and the triceps on the back of the arm extends the forearm; the opposed muscles are "antagonists" in function.

Everybody knows that bones furnish admirable support for the body.

They do more than that. They are busy every instant with vital activities of astonishing variety. They contain blood-forming elements that turn out hundreds of thousands of new red cells every minute. They furnish levers for muscles to pull upon so our movements are not bloblike, like an ameba's. They contain cells which maintain, construct, and repair bone, and others that dissolve and sculpture it. They are warehouses which receive mineral salts for deposit and send them out to the rest of the body in a never-ending flurry of put-and-take transactions. Hardly anything is less lazy than living bone.

Considering the vicissitudes it surmounts in a lifetime, it is not surprising that bone is liable to certain troubles and that people who never see their skeletons are sometimes made uncomfortably aware of them by discomforts, "cricks in the back," dislocations, fractures, and feet that are killing them.

The Skeleton

Bone for bone, the human skeleton is very similar to that of other mammals, except that our upright postures and other aspects that make us human have brought about certain modifications. In broad design, we have a major *(axial) skeleton* and an *appendicular skeleton* to which appendages are attached. Arms and legs are very convenient but not absolutely essential to life. But the axial skeleton which includes the skull, backbone, and ribs is quite indispensable.

The spinal column or backbone is built of a series of blocklike bones, called *vertebrae*, stacked on top of each

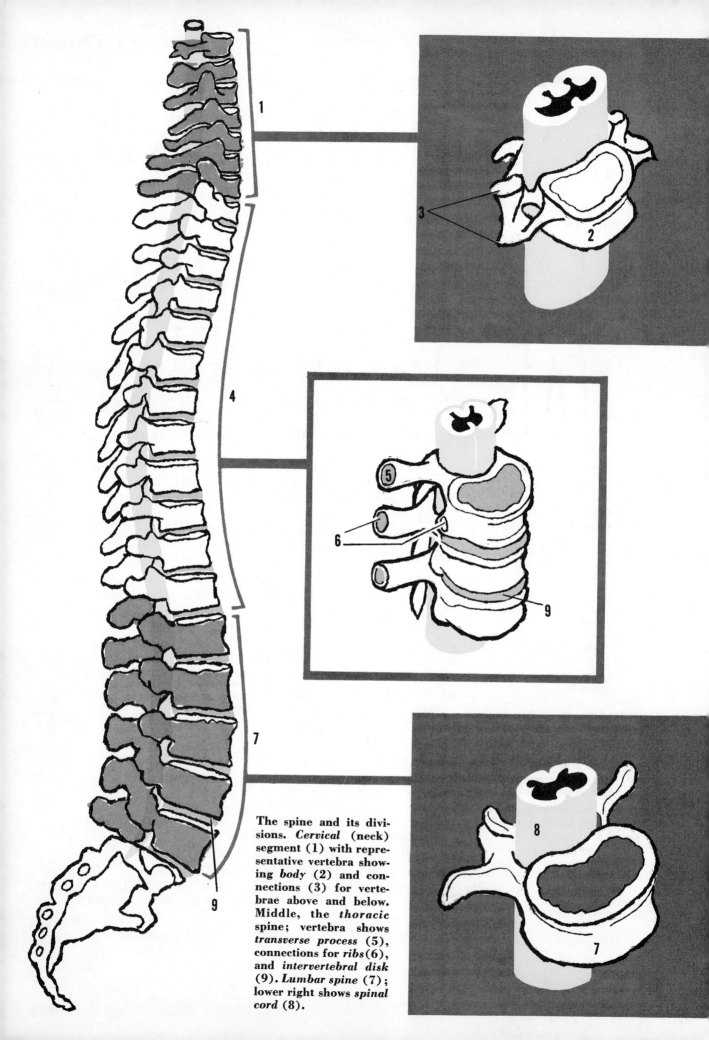

The spine and its divisions. *Cervical* (neck) segment (1) with representative vertebra showing *body* (2) and connections (3) for vertebrae above and below. Middle, the *thoracic* spine; vertebra shows *transverse process* (5), connections for *ribs* (6), and *intervertebral disk* (9). *Lumbar spine* (7); lower right shows *spinal cord* (8).

other. A normal backbone is not straight as a ramrod but has four definite curvatures. A pile of children's blocks stacked in this arrangement would topple over. Fortunately, individual bones of the body are securely bound together and to associated structures by tough bands or ligaments and by tendons that connect muscles to bones. There is also *cartilage* or "gristle", a predecessor of bone, and a sort of subsidiary soft skeleton of connective tissue that pervades the body.

A single vertebra is a flat, roughly circular bone with rearward-projecting knobs (spinous processes) to which muscles are attached. These knobs are what you feel when you run your hand up and down over your backbone. There is a hole in each vertebra which serves as a protective bony canal for the great nerve trunk, the *spinal cord*.

The spine, supported on the pelvic girdle, supports the shoulder girdle, rib cage and skull. Bones are: *cervical vertebrae* (1); *clavicle* (2); *scapula* (3); *sternum* (4); *humerus* (5); *lumbar vertebrae* (6); *ulna* (7); *radius* (8); *carpals* (9); *metacarpals* (10); *phalanges* (11); *femur* (12); *patella* (13); *tibia* (14); *fibula* (15); *metatarsals* (16); *tarsals* (17).

Between the vertebrae are pads of elastic cartilage *(intervertebral disks)* which absorb shocks and permit overlying vertebrae to bend and twist a bit without grating upon each other. Cartilage has a certain amount of springiness and "give" (pinch your external ear or the tip of your nose and you pinch cartilage). It is also slightly compressible and the fluid content of disks slightly reducible, to the extent that perhaps a person at work who is on his feet all day may be a very little shorter at night than when he got up in the morning.

Skull, Ribs, and Lower Back

Doctors have special terms for curves and areas of the spine, although these structures are continuous. The *cervical* or neck region has seven vertebrae, the topmost and tiniest of which has the job

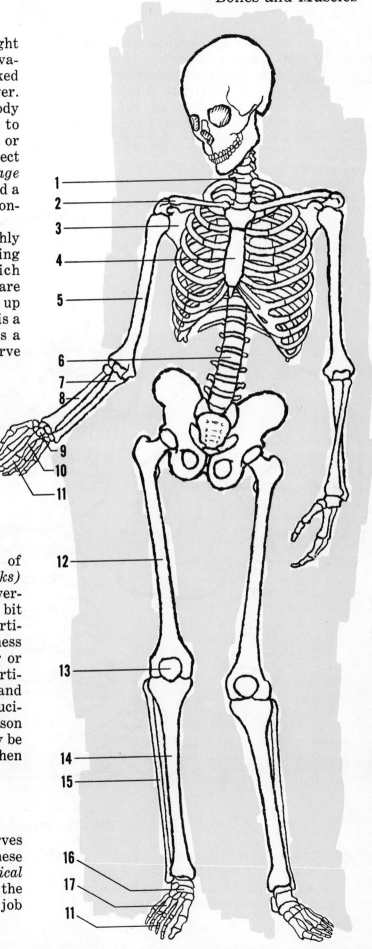

Bones and Muscles

of carrying the head. Below is the *thoracic segment* of 12 vertebrae which carry the ribs, of which the topmost ten are attached in front to the breastbone. Below these at the back are two other pairs which do not have frontal attachments and hence are called *floating ribs*.

Next below the thoracic section is the lumbar area (whence that unpleasant word, lumbago). There are five large *lumbar vertebrae*, and the general region is popularly, or with anguish, called the "small of the back." It is a sort of pivot for rocking movements of the upper part

Bones of the skull in side, front and rear views: *frontal* (1); *sphenoid* (2); *nasal* (3); *zygoma* (4); *maxilla* (5); *parietal* (6); *temporal* (7); *occipital* (8); *mastoid* (9); *mandible* (10).

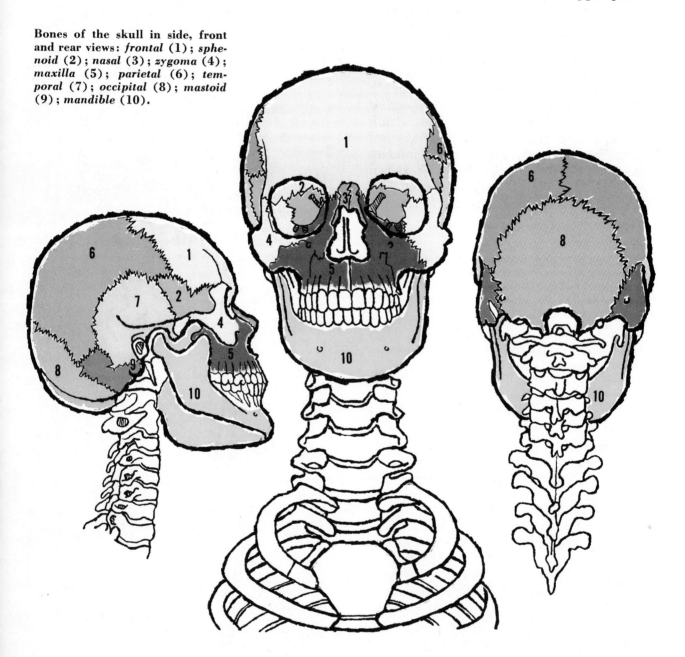

Deviations from the standard pattern of 12 pairs of ribs are not uncommon. Some people have only 11 pairs of ribs (among whom we might include Adam) and some may have 13 pairs by possession of an extra cervical rib at the top.

of the body upon lower parts and like a fulcrum is subject to rather concentrated stresses at times. The prevalence of low back pain around the thoracic-lumbar junction indicates that there is room for improvement in nature's engineering.

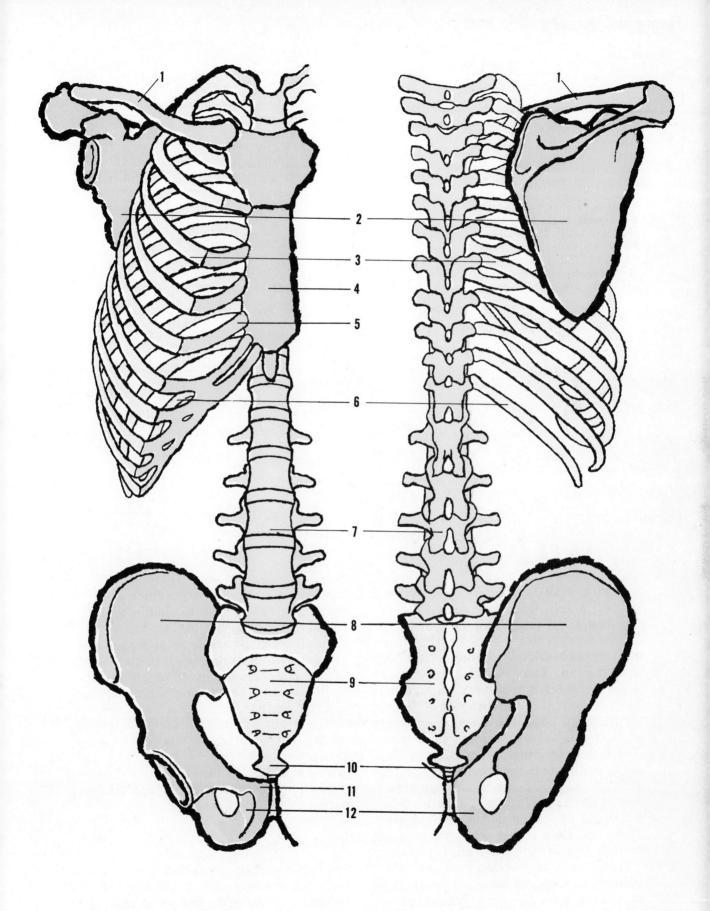

Bones of the axial skeleton in front view, left, and rear view, right: *clavicle* or collarbone
(1); *scapula* or shoulder blade (2); *ribs* (3); breastbone or *sternum* (4); *cartilages* of ribs
(5); *floating ribs* (6); *lumbar vertebrae* (7); *ilium* (8); *sacrum* (9); *coccyx* (10); *pubis*
(11); *ischium* (12).

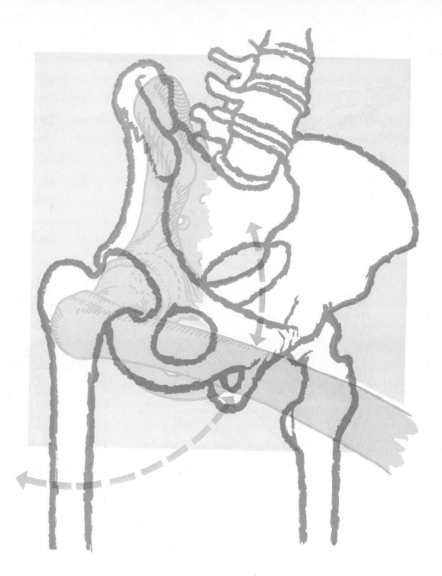

"Ball and socket" joint of the hip permits range of motion, shown in color. The rounded head of the thigh bone (femur) fits into a cup-shaped cavity in the hip bone called the *acetabulum*.

Actually, man brought it upon himself by obstinately walking erect on a spine designed to be slung between four legs.

The lowermost parts of the spine embody bones that we have "lost" by growing up. That is, bones that were separate at birth become fused together. Five "original" vertebrae fuse into a single large bone, the *sacrum*, and four other fused vertebrae form the *coccyx*. The latter, literally and vestigially, is a tailbone that is tucked under the surface. Babies begin life with 33 vertebrae; adults have 26. We "lose" something like 60 bones by fusion as the skeleton matures and reduces our adult complement to 206 bones, with occasional variations.

The skull, perched on top of the spinal column, contains 22 bones (plus six more if one includes the tiny ossicles of the middle ear). The brain cage or *cranium* is composed of eight flat bones, knitted together in irregular suture lines. A newborn baby's skull is quite pliable, and the familiar "soft spots" or *fontanelles* are cranial areas where true bone has not yet formed. Suture lines are points at which bone continues to grow as the skull develops to accommodate the enlarging brain.

The head is almost perfectly balanced on top of the spine, so it is easy to keep it erect without fatigue and to look the whole world in the face. This is a distinctively unique advantage of man's adaptation to upright posture.

Appendages

Another part of the skeleton, concerned with locomotion and manipulation, is integrally related to the axial skeleton. The engineering design is simple in principle if not in execution. The backbone may be likened to a telephone pole which has a crossbar at the top and another near the bottom. The top crosspiece is the *shoulder girdle* and the lower, more massive one the *pelvic girdle*. Appendages — arms and hands, legs and feet — are connected to these structures.

The shoulder girdle consists of two *collarbones (clavicles)* and two *shoulder blades (scapulas)* which at a point of union form a socket in which the arm hangs. The pelvis is composed of three pairs of fused bones. The easiest to recognize is the *ilium* — which has a crest that serves as a handy ledge for balancing packages on the hip — or perhaps the *ischium*, on which we sit. The sacrum connects with the ilia at the back, at the sacro-iliac joints, and pubic bones complete the circle in front.

Joints are cunningly designed structures that permit one bone to glide over another. The hip joint which holds the femur, the upper leg bone which is the longest one in the body, is a deep socket in the pelvis called the *acetabulum*. An analogous socket which holds the upper arm bone, the *humerus*, is called the *glenoid cavity*. Various joints designed like ball-and-socket swivels or door hinges permit different ranges of movement.

We have so many bones, each with its medical name, that it is hardly possible, or even useful, to try to remember them. It's more practicable to refer to the drawing on page 617 if you want to locate certain bone structures in your system or remind yourself that the tibia is the same bone as the shinbone.

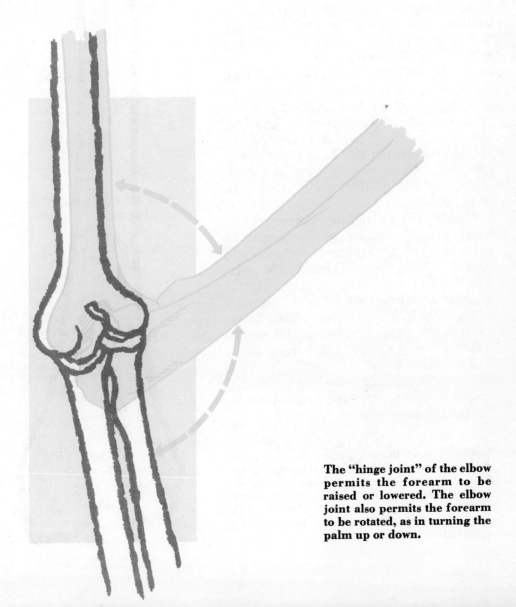

The "hinge joint" of the elbow permits the forearm to be raised or lowered. The elbow joint also permits the forearm to be rotated, as in turning the palm up or down.

The Structure of Bone

A pillar of long bone is much stronger than reinforced concrete, much lighter, much more flexible. Two types of bone work together — *compact* or hard bone, and spongy or *cancellous bone*. Bones are commonly classified as flat, as in the skull, and long and hollow, as in the legs.

A long bone like the femur, between the hip and knee, has a hard, tubular outside and an internal cavity filled with marrow. Flat bones have two layers of compact bone enclosing a spongy middle. The bulging ends of long bones are honeycombed with spongy bone. There appears to be no rhyme or reason to the helter-skelter arrangement of tiny pockets, but the thin walls are actually arranged along stress-lines to give greatest weight-bearing strength.

Disregarding water, bone is about two-thirds mineral and one-third organic matter. The organic matrix is chiefly collagen. Elements are so intimately mixed that if minerals are dissolved out by acids, leaving the organic material, the bone retains its shape but is much too soft to support stresses. Similarly, if the organic matrix is removed by heating, the remaining minerals preserve the original shape but the bone crumbles to ashes at a touch. Whole bone is a community of living cells impregnated with mineral salts.

Nearly all bone surfaces are covered by a tough membrane, the *periosteum*. Bone cells receive nourishment from blood vessels which weave through the periosteum and reach the spongy interior directly or through an intricate network of tiny canals. Nerve fibers follow similar routes; the periosteum mediates sensations of bone pain and pressure.

The *red marrow* of certain bones is the manufacturing site of blood elements. *Yellow marrow* predominantly contains fatty material.

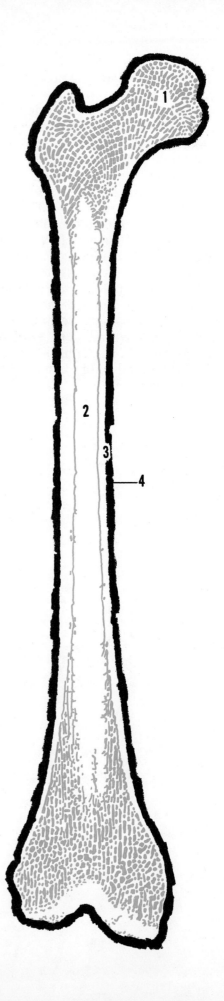

Section through the thigh bone, the longest and strongest bone of the body, showing *spongy bone* (1) with tiny inner walls arranged to give greatest weight-bearing strength; *yellow marrow* (2) in the shaft of the bone; *compact bone* (3); *periosteum* (4), the tough fibrous membrane surrounding bone.

Growth and Repair

Bone grows and repairs itself in very complicated ways. In essence, certain cells secrete the bony matrix and many become imprisoned in it. At the same time, other cells dissolve away bits of bone and help to sculpture materials to the proper shape. This simultaneous bone-building and bone-destroying process goes on elaborately within the bone itself. The ends of long bones of children, sites of active growth, are separated from the main bone by a layer of cartilage. Cartilage does not turn into bone, but is replaced by bone. At about age 20, the cartilaginous growth plate becomes a part of the larger bone. Then the bone grows no longer and the subject no taller.

When a bone is broken, lacerated tissues pour out sticky exudates which stiffen into a bulgy deposit. Little by little, bone-making cells from the periosteum and fractured bone ends penetrate the exudate and replace it with spongy bone which holds the injured parts more firmly in place. This in turn is gradually removed by bone-dissolving cells as spongy bone is slowly replaced by hard bone.

Red Cells and Minerals

The hollow central shafts as well as the ends of the long bones of small children contain red marrow. As the bones mature, the red marrow in the shaft is gradually replaced with yellow marrow, which is mostly composed of fatty material. Red marrow is the site in which red blood cells are manufactured in prodigious numbers, not at a rate of thousands per minute, but millions. These stupendous factories are located in spongy bone, as in the ends of long bones and spongy parts of flat bones of the skull, ribs, pelvis, breastbone and spine.

We need a certain amount of calcium to keep the heart beating, contract muscles, and help blood to clot if necessary. Most of our calcium is stored in the skeleton, in complex combinations with phosphorus and tiny amounts of a few other minerals. But the warehouse is not a mere repository. Its salts are constantly

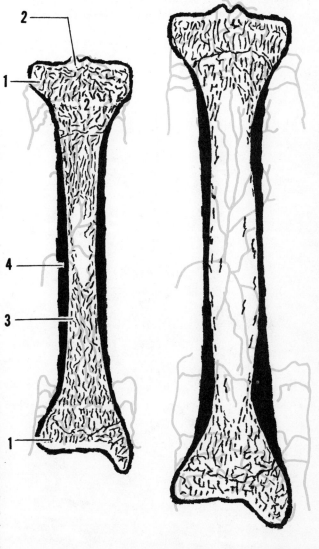

At left below, young developing bone, showing *epiphysis* (1), a piece of bone separated from long bone in early life by *cartilage* (2); *spongy bone* (3) replacing cartilage; *compact bone* (4). At right, union of epiphysis, enlargement of marrow cavity, heavier deposit of compact bone. Blood vessels traverse the periosteum (covering membrane) and networks of canals in the bone matrix.

seeking an equilibrium with the rest of the body that is never attained for long. There is consequently a continuous scurrying of traffic into and out of the skeleton — now, a deposit of calcium received; next, a withdrawal order for calcium to be delivered to the blood supply to spark a heartbeat.

Infection within bone (osteomyelitis) is commonly caused by germs carried in the bloodstream. In children, the infection usually occurs in the long bones, such as those of the knee-joint area shown in the drawing below. Structures shown are the thigh bone or *femur* (1), the shin bone or *tibia* (2), the *joint capsule* (3), *joint cavity* (4), *compact cortical bone* (5). As shown by arrows, *infection* (7) can spread in several directions: toward the joint space and adjoining bone, to the bone-covering membrane, the *periosteum* (8), to the *marrow cavity* (6), or from this cavity to the periosteum and general system.

In short, the concept of bones as dull, inert girders and pillars, as unchanging and uninteresting as concrete, is far removed from the truth. Bone is living tissue that is constantly undergoing changes and being reabsorbed and reconstructed. It may seem rigid, but is remarkably plastic, and any continued pressure can cause bone to be absorbed and to disappear very quickly. The bones of children are especially pliable and usually respond to any measures necessary to correct defects.

OSTEOMYELITIS

Osteomyelitis is an infection of bone resulting from the growth of germs within the bone. It is one of the most important diseases of childhood, but can also occur in adults. In children, the long bones are usually affected; in adults, the infection is more common in the short, flat bones of the spine and pelvis.

In children the infection is caused by organisms such as the staphylococci and less commonly by streptococci or pneumococci. The germs usually reach the bone through the bloodstream from a focus elsewhere in the body. Osteomyelitis can also be caused by direct spread from infected tissues in the vicinity of bone, or as the result of a wound or open fracture.

The first *symptoms* are usually pain and tenderness near a joint. The pain increases rapidly in intensity and jarring of the bone is painful so that children refuse to move the affected limb. The child is obviously ill and the temperature is usually between 102° and 104° F. In the early stages there is usually little or no swelling, and although there is acute tenderness of the bone, the adjacent joint can usually be moved passively without causing additional pain.

These signs and symptoms are usually sufficient to make the diagnosis. It may take ten days before signs of infection show in x-ray films. To wait for x-ray signs to confirm the diagnosis is to wait too long.

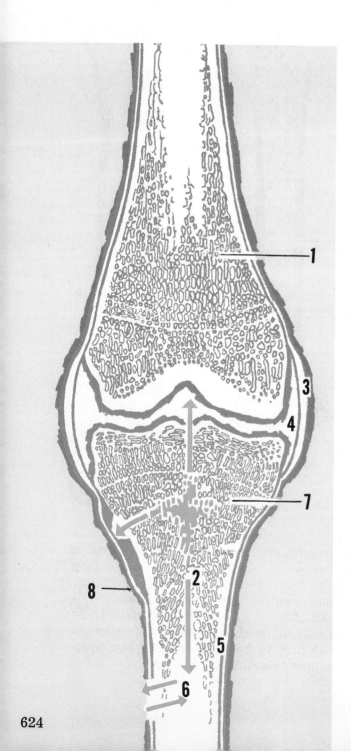

Treatment. A few years ago, acute hematogenous osteomyelitis was a dangerous and crippling disease. Antibiotics have revolutionized the treatment and mortality has been reduced to less than one per cent. However, unless osteomyelitis is treated with adequate doses of antibiotics, the symptoms may be masked, the signs suppressed, and the infection becomes chronic.

Surgery can be postponed as long as there is progressive improvement on antibiotic therapy. But if there are signs of abscess formation, or if local signs do not begin to subside within a day after starting antibiotic treatment, the site of inflammation must be opened for drainage. If pressure from pus is not relieved, large areas of bone will be destroyed. Usually the wound can be closed after all the infected material has been removed, and with immobilization and continued antibiotic therapy, healing should be uneventful.

Cases of acute hematogenous (blood-carried) osteomyelitis which are diagnosed late show extensive local destruction of bone and associated soft tissue abscesses. The abscesses must be evacuated by incision as soon as possible. Unfortunately, extensive infection may not be completely controlled and chronic osteomyelitis with sinuses (suppurating tracts) draining through the skin may be present for many years.

Suppurative arthritis can occur as a secondary result of acute osteomyelitis. The knee joint is usually affected. Fluid from the joint should be aspirated and an antibiotic injected through the same needle into the joint cavity. This treatment will fail if the primary source of infection near the joint is not treated.

Other possible complications of acute osteomyelitis are septicemia ("blood poisoning"), retardation of growth from damage to the epiphyseal cartilage, and development of chronic osteomyelitis.

Chronic osteomyelitis. The chief symptom is usually a discharge of pus from an opening in the skin over the affected bone. The discharge may be continuous or intermittent. Pain is often present and is frequently associated with a "flare" or re-opening of a previously healed discharge channel. The bone feels thickened to the touch and is usually covered by scarred skin showing several open drainage tracts. X-ray shows that the bone is thickened and irregular. Pieces of dead bone or *sequestra* may be seen. It is difficult to remove completely all the pieces of dead bone which are the source of the pus draining through the sinuses. Extensive operations and many months of hospitalization are sometimes necessary.

THE SPINE

Posture. People vary in shape, size, and occupation, and so do their postures. There is no such thing as an identical perfect posture for any and all people. There is a normal range of variation.

One of the key factors in posture is the angle of inclination of the pelvis, the foundation on which the spinal column stands. The hip joint and the position of the feet are other key elements of posture.

The spinal column is a flexible pole with characteristic curves. At birth a baby's spine shows a continuous backward curvature from pelvis to skull. With growth, the spine develops "subcurves" in response to the demand of upright posture. The adult spine shows a forward curvature in the neck region, a backward curvature in the chest area, and a forward curvature in the lower back. Balance is maintained during standing by tilting the pelvis forward. This tilting tends to flatten and broaden out the curves of the spine.

Muscles of the abdomen and spine hold the latter over the body's line of gravity. Movement of the spine is greatest in the lower back and this region is subject to the greatest degenerative changes. Bad posture can result from laziness, poor muscle development, and general debility. However, there is usually a more important local cause for a significant posture defect. Any marked change in the posture of a child or adult deserves a thorough medical checkup to determine the cause.

625

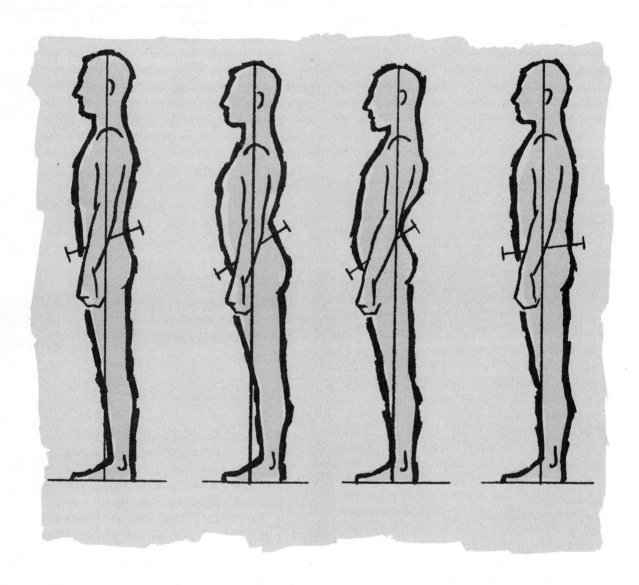

Upright posture is maintained by continuous muscular activity. Poor posture imposes added burdens on bones, ligaments and joints. Normal upright posture and some variations are shown above. The vertical line is the weight-bearing line of the body; the line at the waist indicates the tilt of the pelvis. From left to right, normal posture; lordosis; swayback; flat back. In normal posture, note moderate forward curvature in neck region, backward curvature in chest area, forward curvature in lower back. At the "small of the back," the spine rests upon the first sacral vertebra, a mechanically weak area where many complaints of low back pain, aggravated by poor posture, originate.

Low Back Pain

Pain in the back can be caused by a variety of mechanisms. The main causes are acute injury or degeneration of the joints, ligaments, muscles, or intervertebral disks. Reflex pain can be felt in the back as a result of nerve root irritation. Muscles which are in spasm because of attempts to protect some local injury can also cause secondary pain.

Acute back sprain is usually produced by a sudden bending of the spine, as in a fall or a "snatch lifting" motion. The force is sufficient to tear the ligaments or joint capsules, producing pain and protective muscle spasm. These injuries usually heal in three weeks, if they are protected against further sprains during the healing period. A corset-like support may be necessary during healing.

Chronic back strain is a different condition, in which there is no violent, sudden, precipitating incident, but the structures are subjected to prolonged tension greater than they can resist. Symptoms usually come on gradually and get progressively worse. They are made worse by fatigue, improved by lying down and by physiotherapy.

Treatment is difficult since causes are varied and not always possible to eliminate. The main cause for chronic strain must be discovered and removed if a cure is to be obtained. The prognosis is not always good, particularly if it is not possible to change an occupation which appears to be the main cause of the strain.

Facet syndrome is the name for a condition in which a sudden "catch in the back" virtually fixes the victim in a position from which he cannot move. Usually he is "caught" in a stooped position and cannot straighten from it. The pain is usually poorly localized but does not radiate. Careful manipulations can give dramatic relief, leaving only some soreness which will last for a few days. Bed rest and sedation, however, can give relief in the same length of time without the risks inherent in manipulation. Attacks tend to increase in frequency and duration over the years, until eventually there may be chronic backache. This is particularly likely if the patient continues to perform stooping actions which tend to bring on the attacks.

"Disk Trouble"

The intervertebral disks are semi-cartilaginous buffers or "shock absorbers" between the bony vertebrae. After 20 years of age, it is normal for disks to age and degenerate gradually. Movements through the altered disk change, so that in varied motions of the spine, one vertebra moves on another, producing a forward or backward shift. As degeneration progresses, the symptoms, if any, are likely to change.

Early degeneration of the disk usually does not cause symptoms unless some strain is added. The strain can be slight but prolonged, as in sitting during a long automobile trip without getting out frequently to stretch. There is usually only mild local tenderness in the back and x-rays show nothing abnormal. Treatment should be rest, followed by muscle-strengthening exercises, and education to make the patient aware of avoidable mechanical strains that are unkind to degenerating intervertebral disks.

"Ruptured disk" or *"slipped disk"* is a diagnosis commonly made by neighbors whenever someone has an aching back or sciatica. The terms properly refer only to a specific condition in which the pulpy body at the center of an intervertebral disk (nucleus pulposus) herniates or protrudes through a rent in a surrounding ligament.

In this condition the sciatica is a dull, aching pain which is sufficiently bad to mask the low back pain. It is made worse by coughing, sneezing, or jarring movements. Raising of the straight leg on the painful side is often limited to an angle of 20 to 30 degrees. X-ray films may show nothing abnormal or may show narrowing of the disk space. Sometimes a myelogram (x-ray of the spinal cord after injection of a contrast medium) is necessary to establish the diagnosis and the anatomical level of the disk rupture.

Treatment is usually surgical removal of the portions of the disk which have protruded and a thorough clearance of the degenerated disk space. However, it is wise to try a period of strict bed rest before undergoing surgery, since occasionally the symptoms will steadily improve. In such instances it is probable that the disk is merely bulging and that a free fragment has not protruded.

Spondylolisthesis is the term applied to a spontaneous forward displacement of a lumbar vertebra upon the bone below it. Predisposing factors are a congenital or early developmental defect. Nearly five per cent of spines show such displacement. Spondylolisthesis can exist without any sign of backache and is often discovered accidentally during a routine physical examination.

CHRONIC BACK STRAIN

Helpful measures for "aching backs" not caused by a "slipped disk" or disease:

Sleep on a firm bed; avoid over-stuffed chairs, soft sofas; use straight chairs as much as possible.

Arrange work surfaces (ironing board and bench) to avoid leaning-forward positions that put strain on the "small of the back."

Learn to lift in line of gravity of the body.

Do postural exercises twice a day, such as:

In standing position, contract buttocks and abdomen, head up; hold for five seconds.

Sitting: Clasp arms behind back, bend forward, raise head and bring shoulder blades together, sit erect while pulling backward and downward with hands.

Lie face down, arms at sides, contract buttocks and abdomen, bring shoulder blades together.

When symptoms do occur, they are usually manifested as low lumbar backache with or without accompanying sciatica. Symptoms arise from degenerative changes in the disk. If conservative treatment of symptoms of disk degeneration fails, or if the forward slip of a vertebra is of gross degree, spinal fusion may be necessary.

Symptomless spondylolisthesis should not be made a reason for gross restriction of activities. Many teenagers and young adults lead perfectly normal lives despite their spondylolisthesis.

Scheuermann's disease is a common cause of backache in teenagers. It is sometimes called "adolescent round back." For unknown reasons, certain vertebral bodies undergo changes resulting in more or less wedge-shaped formation. Usually several vertebrae of the back are affected at the same time. In the active stage of the disease there is pain associated with a round back.

The diagnosis is easily made from the history, physical signs, and x-ray findings. This so-called disease is not serious. It is a self-limited condition which lasts about two years. Treatment is mainly symptomatic and usually does not involve more than restriction of activity and back muscle exercises. In severe cases a period of bed rest followed by the wearing of a spinal brace may be necessary.

Scoliosis is a term used to describe a lateral curvature of the spine. There are several types of scoliosis.

Idiopathic scoliosis begins in childhood or adolescence and gets progressively worse until growth ceases. Treatment is unsatisfactory because the cause of the condition is unknown. The deformity is usually worse in the upper back and least in the lumbar region. The earlier the onset, the worse the ultimate curvature.

It is not possible to prevent the deformity from increasing by using exercises or external splints. Several different surgical methods of spinal fusion are employed but no particular method is outstandingly better than another.

Structural scoliosis is secondary to an underlying cause such as muscle weakness after polio or abnormally shaped vertebrae. Usually the only symptom is the visible deformity. In severe cases, spinal fusion is the corrective treatment.

Sciatic scoliosis lasts only as long as some primary painful condition of the spine produces a spasm of muscles to protect the area that hurts. By far the most common primary cause is the protrusion of an intervertebral disk. Abnormal posture occurs quite involuntarily as the body attempts to minimize painful pressure upon a nerve root or, in ordinary language, to "favor" an area that is painful when stretched or moved. The trunk is often tilted well over to one side. Treatment of this form of scoliosis is treatment of the underlying condition, usually a prolapsed disk.

Scoliosis sometimes occurs as a compensation for a sideward tilt of the pelvis, produced by a true short leg, or by an apparent shortening of the leg caused by a hip joint contracture. The spine itself is normal and the scoliosis will disappear when the pelvic tilt is corrected.

Degenerative arthritis of the spine. Degenerative changes occur quite commonly in the intervertebral joints of the upper and lower back and are particularly common in persons who do heavy work. Quite marked degrees of arthritis can exist without causing any symptoms, but if symptoms are triggered by some relatively minor stress they are likely to be persistent. Even without acute aggravation, symptoms will eventually arise in the affected area. Usually there are periodic attacks of discomfort lasting a

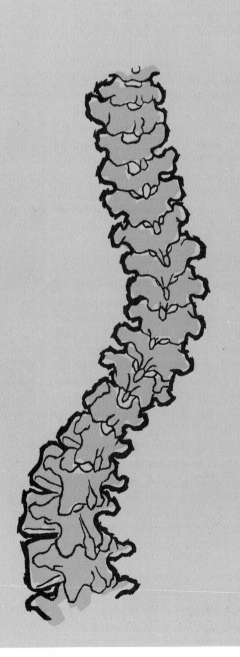
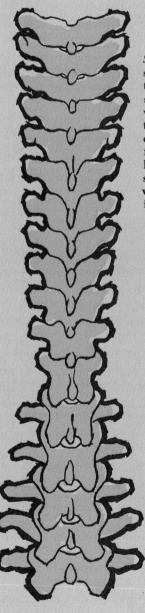

Scoliosis, of which there are several forms, is a lateral curvature of the spine. Such a spine is shown at the left, in comparison with a normal spine. Some functional forms of scoliosis without deformity of bony parts result from defects of posture and can be corrected voluntarily since the spine can "straighten out." Forms which involve structural abnormalities are more difficult to correct.

few weeks, followed by periods of freedom from pain. In mild cases treatment is unnecessary, but in the more severe "low back" cases physiotherapy treatments and some form of supporting garment give good relief.

Torticollis or *"wry-neck"* is a rotational deformity of the cervical vertebrae which causes tilting and turning of the head. The commonest form occurs in infants and is associated with a swelling in muscles of the neck area which is sometimes called a tumor but is definitely not a cancer. In very early cases, gentle manipulation is enough to correct the deformity. In established cases, division of the contracted muscle at its lower end is usually performed.

An uncommon form of adult wry neck is called *spasmodic torticollis*. The cause is not known. This condition does not respond to ordinary therapeutic measures and is often associated with symptoms of mental strain.

Whiplash Injuries

"Whiplash injury" is a phrase which has fallen into disrepute among physicians because it does not describe any specific abnormality or anatomical derangement. It is a general descriptive term such as "dyspepsia" or "lumbago," but unfortunately is still used in courts of law as if it had a specific meaning.

The injury is usually sustained in an automobile accident which causes the head to be thrown forward suddenly and suddenly jerked backward, or vice versa, like cracking a whip. The brunt of the injury is borne at the level of the fifth cervical vertebra where muscles and ligaments can be torn and strained. Occasionally there may be associated bone or nerve damage but this is not common.

The injury is similar to a badly sprained ankle, and treatment is similar. The neck should be protected by a soft felt or sponge rubber collar for two or three weeks. Aspirin, heat, and massage are helpful in relieving symptoms. Occasionally patients have persistent headaches following this injury.

All the symptoms appear to be aggravated by emotional factors and a nervous, tense person generally takes longer to recover than a phlegmatic person.

THE SHOULDER

Pain in the shoulder can be caused by many conditions not originating in the joint itself. For instance, pain may be "referred" from the pleura, the diaphragm, or the pericardium. Shingles, disturbances of the spinal cord in the neck region, and muscular dystrophies can also produce shoulder pain.

Diagnosis is also made difficult because the "shoulder joint" is, in fact, three separate joints acting together. These joints are the *glenohumeral* (the shoulder joint proper), the *acromioclavicular* and the *sternoclavicular joint*. The joints combine to give the remarkably free and full range of movement of the normal shoulder.

Most varieties of arthritis can occur in the shoulder joint, but degenerative arthritis is not common, probably because the joint is not weight-bearing. Most shoulder disabilities are caused by conditions peculiar to the joint.

Supraspinatus syndrome is a term for disorders affecting structures associated with muscle at the "point of the shoulder" region. The typical complaint is pain in the upper arm and shoulder when the arm is raised. The pain occurs in the middle third of the arc described when the arm is raised. There is usually little or no pain during motion on either side of this middle arc of movement. In the normal shoulder there is very little clearance between the undersurface of the *acromion* (the bone at the very tip of the top of the shoulder) and the upper end of the armbone when the arm is partly raised. If there is swelling and tenderness in this narrow space, pain is produced mechanically by pinching of the swollen tissues between the bones.

The most common cause of such shoulder pain is inflammation of the supraspinatus tendon (tendinitis), but it can also be caused by tears of the tendon, injury to bony parts, deposits of calcium within the tendon, or subacromial bursitis. Whatever the cause, the symptoms are the same. The patient has pain in the middle third of the arc both when raising and lowering the arm, and often twists the arm in different ways in attempts to avoid painful movement. In some cases there is agonizing pain, frequently produced by a calcium deposit in the tendon.

Treatment, often unnecessary in mild cases, employs ultrasound or shortwave diathermy and mobilizing exercises which are usually successful. If calcium deposits cause excruciating pain, immediate relief can be given by removing the

Bursitis of the shoulder (subdeltoid or subacromial bursitis). The bursa which lies between the acromion at the end of the collarbone and the "ball" end of the upper armbone is large and extends under neighboring structures. Its inner surface which permits parts to glide freely is smooth and glistening and it is unlikely that a primary bursitis originates here with any frequency. Virtually every case of such bursitis is secondary to a lesion of one of the structures lying in contact with the deep layer of the bursa. Treatment should therefore be directed toward the primary cause which may be single or repeated injury, acute

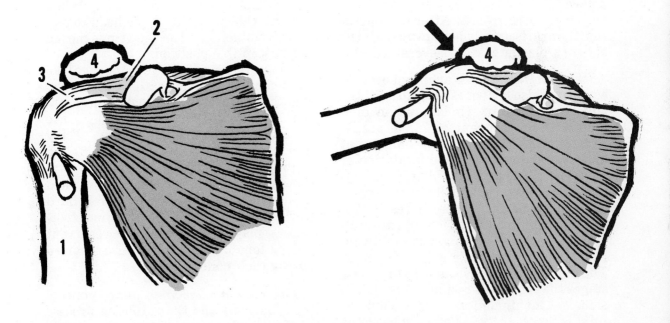

Pain felt when the upper arm is raised to a more or less horizontal position is typical of the *supraspinatus syndrome*, so named for the structures involved. The drawing shows how swollen tissues can be pinched painfully in a narrow space between bones when the arm is raised. At left, structures shown are the upper arm bone or *humerus* (1), the *supraspinatus muscle* (2) and its *tendon* (3), and the *acromion* (4), the bone that forms the point of the shoulder. Little or no pain is felt when the arm hangs down. At right, tissues are pinched when the arm is partly raised.

deposit through an aspiration needle or through a small incision into the tendon. In patients who suffer chronic pain and do not respond to conservative treatment, operation should be considered. The most satisfactory procedure is excision of part of the acromion, removing one of the two bony surfaces which produce the pinching of swollen tissues.

or chronic infection, and other conditions that may produce bursitis-like pain that originates outside of the bursa proper.

Tears in tendons and muscles around joints are common causes of pain. An incomplete tear of the tendinous "cuff" where muscles are attached to bone is one of the causes of the supraspinatus syndrome described above. A *complete* tear greatly hinders the raising of the arm throughout its range of movement. Complete tears are often produced by a relatively minor accident, such as a fall on the outstretched hand. There is immediate pain in the shoulder which worsens during the next few hours and is frequently so great that drugs are necessary for its control. The patient, who is usually over 60 years of age, is unable to raise his arm and there is great tenderness to pressure on the point of the shoulder.

The outlook is good if the tear is repaired surgically within a few days of its occurrence. If operation is unduly delayed it is unlikely that good shoulder movement will return. After the operation the arm is usually held away from the side in a plaster cast for several weeks.

"Frozen shoulder" is an ill-understood condition, also known as pericapsulitis or adhesive capsulitis (inflammation of a membranous sac enclosing a part). Patients with this condition complain of moderate pain and marked limitation of movement. The pain is aching in character and comes on gradually in the shoulder and upper arm. There is restriction of movement in all directions of the joint.

Usually the stiffness gradually disappears, but it may take at least a year. The pain disappears sooner, but in early stages the arm needs rest in a sling. Occasionally, manipulation of the shoulder joint is necessary when all pain has gone and some movement has returned. Manipulation can cause fractures if the bone has been weakened by inactivity and should only be performed by someone skilled in the procedure.

Recurrent dislocation of the shoulder. This is a condition in which repeated dislocations of the glenohumeral joint occur. The re-dislocations usually occur when raising or extending the arm without any great violence. Dislocation can occur when stretching, swimming, putting on a coat, or even brushing the hair. Re-dislocations may be very infrequent or so frequent as to interfere with daily activities. Often the patient is able to reduce

the dislocation himself or with the help of a friend.

The reasons why some primary dislocations of the shoulder heal without further trouble and others go on to repeated dislocations are not fully understood. However, there is no doubt that if a primary dislocation is not properly reduced and adequately immobilized, there is a high risk of recurrent dislocation.

No abnormalities will be found if the shoulder is examined when it is not dislocated. X-rays will not show anything abnormal unless a special medial rotation view is taken. This will usually show a bony defect of the head of the humerus, thought to be produced by "denting" with a sharp margin of the collarbone. When present, this dent allows the head to dislocate completely when the arm is moved to a susceptible position.

There is no effective conservative treatment. If the dislocations occur frequently and are troublesome, an operation should be performed. There are several different procedures, but all try to strengthen the capsule of the joint and slightly limit its range of external rotation. A properly done operation can yield a shoulder that can be used for hard work. There are many professional footballers playing today whose recurrent dislocations of the shoulder were repaired during their college days.

The acromioclavicular joint connects the collarbone and the acromion process of the shoulder blade. Changes in this joint produce pain which is usually localized to the joint. The pain is made worse by excessive use of the joint, particularly for overhead work, such as in painting a ceiling.

Examination of the joint does not show any soft tissue thickening, but bony outgrowth can be felt at the margins. The arm can be raised to a horizontal level without discomfort, but raising it above this level causes pain. X-rays will show narrowing of the joint space and bony outgrowth at margins.

Conservative treatment by diathermy is usually satisfactory. Occasionally, operation is necessary if symptoms are severe and do not respond to treatment. The most satisfactory operation is "decompression" of the joint, either by removal of the acromion or the outer end of the collarbone.

This joint also is prone to *persistent dislocation,* precipitated by trauma. In most cases the displacement is minimal and the symptoms slight. Examination shows that the outer end of the collarbone sticks up beneath the skin. The rest of the shoulder girdle and arm hang down lower than the collarbone. Usually little or no treatment is needed. A sling gives sufficient rest for occasional attacks of discomfort. Operation is rarely necessary, but if performed, the most effective procedure is removal of the outer end of the collarbone.

Sternoclavicular joint. The medial end of the collarbone occasionally dislocates, either permanently, or when the shoulders are braced back. This in-and-out displacement can be troublesome, but does not usually require operative treatment. There is no effective conservative treatment, and if operation is performed, attempts are made to hold the collarbone in its normal place by reconstructing the torn or stretched ligaments.

THE ELBOW

When the arm is held straight by the side, the elbow is bent slightly outward, at an angle of about 10 degrees in men and 15 degrees in women. This is known as the "carrying angle," and if it is greatly increased the resulting deformity is known as "cubitus valgus."

Cubitus valgus usually occurs because of poor union of a fracture of the lower end of the humerus or because local growth has been affected by disease or injury. In itself the deformity is harmless and usually not very noticeable. Function of the arm is not disturbed, but a possible complication which can arise is *ulnar nerve neuritis.*

The ulnar nerve which supplies most of the muscles of the hand passes around the back of the elbow joint and is exposed to direct injury at the point of the elbow commonly known as the "crazy bone." When the carrying angle is greatly increased, the nerve will be bent sharply around the angle and repeated trauma may do damage. Scarring around and within the nerve will produce tingling in the hand and weakness and wasting of small muscles of the hand supplied by the nerve. When symptoms of nerve damage are present, it is wise to have the nerve transposed by an operation which removes it from danger by placing it at the front of the elbow.

The opposite deformity to cubitus valgus is *cubitus varus,* in which the normal carrying angle is reduced or even reversed. The causes of the deformity are the same as those of cubitus valgus. There is usually no disability from this deformity except cosmetic appearance.

Tennis elbow is a name commonly applied to any disorder causing pain on the outer side of the elbow joint. Only in a very few people is it caused by playing tennis. Any activity that requires rotary movements of the forearm and a firm grip of the hand (using a screwdriver, for instance) can cause the symptoms. There is pain and tenderness at the side of the elbow where extensor muscles originate. The pain often radiates down the back of the forearm, and can change into widespread aching in all the forearm muscles, particularly if excessive gripping is involved.

Many mild cases require no treatment, but a variety of conservative measures are available, of which the most common is diathermy combined with massage. Injections of local anesthetics, with or without cortisone derivatives, are also often used. Immobilization in a sling or even a plaster cast is often helpful in early cases. Operation is occasionally necessary in severely disabled patients who have not responded to conservative treatment. Results are not always predictable, but usually the pain disappears after healing has taken place.

The elbow is second only to the knee as a site of *osteochondritis dissecans* (see page 643). It is a condition in which a fragment of cartilage and bone becomes detached, occurring most often in teen-agers. Pain is moderate and movements are usually somewhat limited, but "lock-ing" does not occur until the fragment is completely detached. X-rays will show an area of irregularity in early stages of the condition. In late stages, a cavity and the bony fragment lying free within the joint may be seen.

Conservative treatment which may entail several months of immobilization is used in early cases. If the fragment has separated or is ripe for separation, it must be removed through an incision.

Degenerative arthritis of the elbow is not very common since this is not a weight-bearing joint. When it does occur it is usually secondary to injury or disease of the joint surfaces. Relatively minor stresses, repeated over a period of years, are just as damaging as a major fracture into the joint. For instance, workers using compressed air drills develop quite severe degenerative changes in the elbow joint.

Symptoms are pain and limitation of movement. The joint aches for a consid-erable time after heavy use. In some patients the first abnormal sign is lock-ing of the joint by a loose body.

Massage and diathermy or other forms of heat are useful, particularly if use of the joint can be curtailed. Often, restric-tion of use is sufficient treatment. Opera-tion is rarely needed; loose bodies should be removed, and in exceptional circum-stances the joint can be stiffened in a functional position. An alternative to stiffening of the joint is an operation in which the destroyed surfaces are removed and the joint left movable.

Ruptures of the biceps. This muscle can rupture at either end, but it is extremely uncommon for it to rupture at the "elbow end." The rupture usually occurs to a middle-aged person during lifting or pulling effort, and is only slightly painful. Many men wait months before seeking medical aid. There is little loss of power or interference with cus-tomary work. When using the arm, the muscle fails to harden, and bulges lower

down in the arm than is usual. Operation is seldom necessary but when it is the results are usually good.

THE WRIST AND HAND

"Sprained wrist" is a common lay diagnosis but is almost invariably wrong. The true sprained wrist is very uncom-mon. Symptoms in this area are usually caused by a fracture, a dislocation, or arthritis.

Persistent pain in the wrist following an accident is a serious symptom that needs thorough investigation. X-rays are essential. Fracture of the scaphoid bone below the thumb is quite common and if left untreated can produce crippling arthritis of the wrist long before normal degenerative changes could be expected to occur. Falls on the back of the hand can chip small flakes of bone which can cause troublesome symptoms for weeks.

If such varied causes of symptoms can be excluded, then "sprained wrist" can be safely diagnosed and successfully treated by strapping or temporary immobiliza-tion in a plaster cast.

DeQuervain's disease. A common cause of pain in the thumb side of the wrist is a thickening of the sheaths covering two of the tendons which pass to the thumb. This *stenosing tenovaginitis*, or DeQuer-vain's disease, is most common in women. In general, repetitive actions such as typing, or strenuous actions such as wringing out diapers, produce the symp-toms, which come on gradually. There is pain at the base of the thumb radiating to the nail and up into the forearm. There is usually pain on pressure over the thumb side of the wrist.

Sometimes the condition cures itself if the wrist can be immobilized and precip-itating actions avoided. However, this is often inconvenient and since operation is so simple and satisfactory it is usually advised, if the disability is severe. A simple "unroofing" of the tendon sheath is all that is necessary.

Ganglion of the wrist. A *ganglion* is a cystic swelling which occurs in associa-tion with a joint or tendon sheath. There

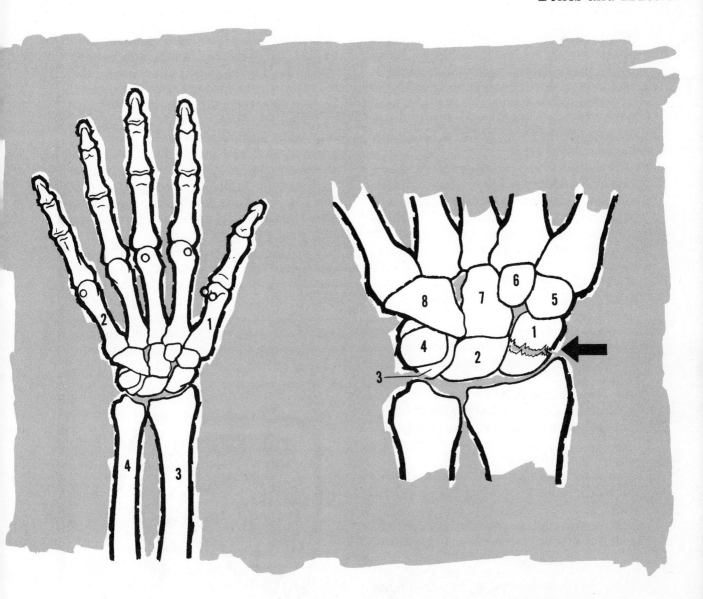

is no completely satisfactory explanation as to how they arise. There is always a connection between the swelling and a joint capsule or tendon sheath, but rarely if ever is there any communication with the cavity of the cyst. Ganglia occur most commonly on the back of the wrist, but can also arise on the palm or fingers.

Usually there are no symptoms except occasional slight discomfort. Since they are harmless, ganglia can safely be left untreated and many will disappear spontaneously. A traditional treatment is to burst them by hitting them with the family Bible. Large ganglia or those which cause pain or pressure symptoms may require excision. This is not always an easy operation since the whole cyst and its root or pedicle must be dissected

What the layman calls a "sprained wrist" is more often than not a fracture, a dislocation, or arthritis. At left above, bones of hand and arm showing *thumb* (1), *little finger* (2), *radius* (3), *ulna* (4). At right, closeup of the eight carpal or wrist bones which are arranged in two rows of four bones each, intricately fitted together. A fracture of the scaphoid bone at the base of the thumb is shown. X-rays are essential to determine the cause of persistent pain in the wrist.

out. Recurrence is uncommon if the whole cyst and pedicle are removed.

Median nerve compression. Pressure on the median nerve where it enters the wrist (the carpal tunnel) is a common cause of discomfort of the hand, especially in women over the age of 40. This big nerve passes along the middle of the arm and forearm and enters the hand at the wrist joint along with all the flexor tendons to the fingers. Thickening of the tendon sheaths and arthritic changes at the wrist tend to reduce the size of the tunnel through which the nerve passes. Since the nerve is softer than the tendons, it will be subjected to considerable pressure with accompanying discomfort.

Symptoms are tingling, discomfort, and even numbness in the thumb, index, and long fingers. If pressure has been present for some time there will be clumsiness in fine movements, dishes may be dropped, and wasting of the thumb muscles may be apparent. Often, patients are especially troubled at night. Shortly after going to sleep they are awakened by intense discomfort in the hand, which does not go away until the hand is exercised. Men can suffer from the same condition, and younger women may notice similar symptoms during late pregnancy, but these symptoms usually disappear after delivery of the baby. Other conditions which can cause similar symptoms must be excluded before the diagnosis is finally confirmed.

Rest occasionally helps, but usually the only satisfactory treatment is an operation which relieves pressure on the nerve. Recovery from the operation is rapid and relief of symptoms occurs overnight.

Degenerative changes at the wrist are quite common because of the frequency with which the joint surfaces are damaged. The symptoms are tenderness around the joint, pain on use, and limitation of movement. Relief can be given in mild cases by resting the wrist with a molded leather or plastic splint. Most patients will not wear splints indefinitely and prefer to have an operation. The only reliable method is an operation for complete stiffening of the wrist.

Degenerative changes of the finger joints are quite common in elderly people and in most cases no treatment is required. The joint at the base of the thumb may be quite seriously affected. Localized pain is produced by movement, the joint is prominent and thickened, and range of motion is reduced. If the symptoms are severe, operation will be necessary.

Dupuytren's contracture is a thickening of tissue (fascia) of the palm which causes the fingers to be pulled down into the palm. It can also occur in the sole of the foot. There is an hereditary predisposition, but the cause is unknown. Changes are more common in the little-finger side of the palm. The condition, more common in men, usually starts as a small nodule opposite the base of the ring finger. As the condition progresses, other nodules may appear and firm bands may spread into the fingers.

All sorts of conservative treatments have been tried ineffectively. The only satisfactory treatment is operative removal. In elderly patients in whom the condition is not progressing, operation is usually not necessary, but the younger the patient and the more extensive the disease, the more is operation justified.

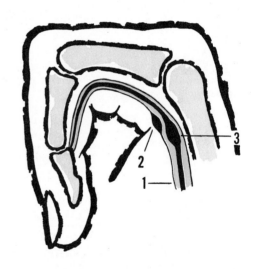

The mechanism of "trigger finger." Structures shown are *tendon sheath* (1), constricted area of sheath (2), and *nodule* (3) of tendon which has difficulty in moving within the sheath when the finger is extended.

Trigger finger is a result of constriction that prevents free movement of tendons in the sheath. The tendons develop a "waist" opposite to the constriction, tend to swell, and the swollen segment often develops into a nodule which has difficulty in entering the sheath when the finger is extended. Usually a snap is heard as the finger bends or extends.

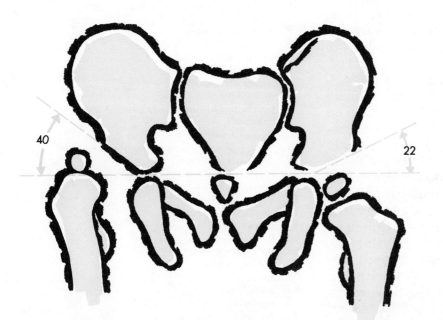

Congenital dislocation of the hip results from abnormal development of the *acetabulum*, the cup-shaped cavity in which the rounded head of the thighbone fits. The normal angle of about 22 degrees between the horizontal and the plane of the upper half of the acetabulum, shown at right side of the drawing, may be increased to 30 to 40 degrees in congenital dislocation of the hip, as seen on the left.

Division of the constriction in the sheath under local anesthesia gives a completely satisfactory result.

Boutonniere deformity, also known as "buttonhole" deformity, results when the central extensor tendon to the base of the middle joint of a finger is cut or ruptured. In the fully developed deformity the middle joint of the finger is flexed and the other two are extended. Immediate treatment should be an operation to reattach the tendon to the bone. Satisfactory treatment is extremely difficult if the deformity is neglected for many weeks after the original injury. In neglected cases it may be necessary to fuse the joint in a better position.

Mallet or baseball finger. This deformity, in which the tip of the finger dips down, is caused by rupture or tearing of a tendon from its insertion. The force to do this is a sudden violent blow on the tip of the finger, as in "miscatching" a baseball. Immobilization of the joint in a plaster cast for about four weeks immediately following injury gives good results. Old injuries or those which have not responded to plaster cast treatment should have surgery to reattach the ruptured tendon to the bone.

THE HIP

The hip is a major weight-bearing joint and is subject to many conditions directly connected with the thrust of body weight. It is a ball-and-socket joint with a very strong capsule surrounding and strengthening it.

Most children with hip troubles are brought to a doctor when parents note some abnormality after the child starts to walk. There is no arbitrarily "correct" time at which a child should start to walk. A hip limp in a very young child is usually caused by congenital dislocation if it is painless, and by acute suppurative arthritis if it is painful.

Congenital dislocation of the hip. This spontaneous dislocation occurs before or shortly after birth as a result of a congenital abnormality of development, usually a flattening of the *acetabulum* (the cup-shaped cavity in which the head of the thighbone rests). Heredity plays a part; a woman with this condition has increased chance of giving birth to a child with the same condition. Girls are affected at least five times more commonly than boys. The congenital dislocation is usually in one rather than both sides of the hip.

The most useful diagnostic signs are (a) limitation of outward motion from the hip, particularly when the infant is lying on the back with the knees bent to 90°, and (b) asymmetry of the "folds" of the leg. The buttock, groin, and thigh folds on the affected side are usually deeper and higher up on the leg than on the normal side. Thigh folds can be asymmetrical in infants who are perfectly normal, but asymmetry of the groin and buttock folds as well is rarely seen except in congenital dislocation of the hip.

Examination of the affected hip often demonstrates a snapping noise caused by the head of the thighbone entering the socket. After the head has snapped into place the hip can be moved within a normal range. X-ray examination usually shows that the bony roof of the socket slopes upward and outward, so that the thighbone "skids" out of place.

The key to successful treatment is early diagnosis. Physical examination alone is not sufficient. An x-ray is essential whenever there is the slightest doubt about the condition of the hip.

Treatment. The basic aim is to place the head of the thighbone in the socket and to retain it there until the structures have had time to develop. Several different methods may be used. Probably the most satisfactory is to reduce the dislocation under general anesthesia and immobilize the leg and hip joint in a plaster cast. Often, after removal of the cast, a bar is attached to the baby's shoes to limit hip movement. In infants with minimal dislocations, a splinting may be sufficient. Operation is occasionally necessary if the hip cannot be reduced by closed manipulation.

If treatment is started within the first six months of life the results will be excellent in nearly every case. The critical time is when walking starts; if treatment has been started by this time the outlook is good. If treatment is delayed until the age of two years or later the prospects for a satisfactory result are not nearly so good. In late neglected cases, reconstructive operations will be necessary and the hip will often show various signs of degenerative arthritis.

MUSCLE CHART →

1. frontalis
2. orbicularis oculi
3. orbicularis oris
4. mylohyoid
5. sternocleidomastoid
6. trapezius
7. deltoideus
8. pectoralis major
9. brachialis
10. triceps brachii
11. biceps brachii
12. obliquus externus
13. rectus abdominus
14. pronator teres
15. brachioradialis
16. flexor carpi radialis
17. flexor carpi ulnaris
18. flexor digitorum sublimis
19. palmaris longus
20. tensor fasciae latae
21. gracilis
22. sartorius
23. vastus lateralis
24. rectus femoris
25. vastus medialis
26. patella (bone)
27. tibialis anterior
28. gastrocnemius
29. extensor digitorum longus
30. flexor digitorum longus pedis
31. tendon of extensor hallucis longus
32. tendon of tibialis posterior
33. temporalis
34. zygomaticus
35. masseter
36. buccinator
37. digastric
38. scalenus medius
39. scalenus anterior
40. scalenus posterior
41. omohyoid
42. sternohyoid
43. subclavius
44. pectoralis minor
45. subscapularis
46. coracobrachialis
47. latissimus dorsi
48. serratus anterior
49. intercostal
50. supinator
51. obliquus internus
52. lumbodorsal fascia
53. flexor pollicis longus
54. flexor digitorum profundus
55. head of femur (bone)
56. obturator internus
57. adductor magnus
58. flexor pollicis brevis
59. adductor brevis
60. adductor longus
61. vastus intermedius
62. quadriceps tendon
63. tibia (bone)
64. peroneus longus
65. peroneus brevis
66. extensor hallucis longus
67. soleus

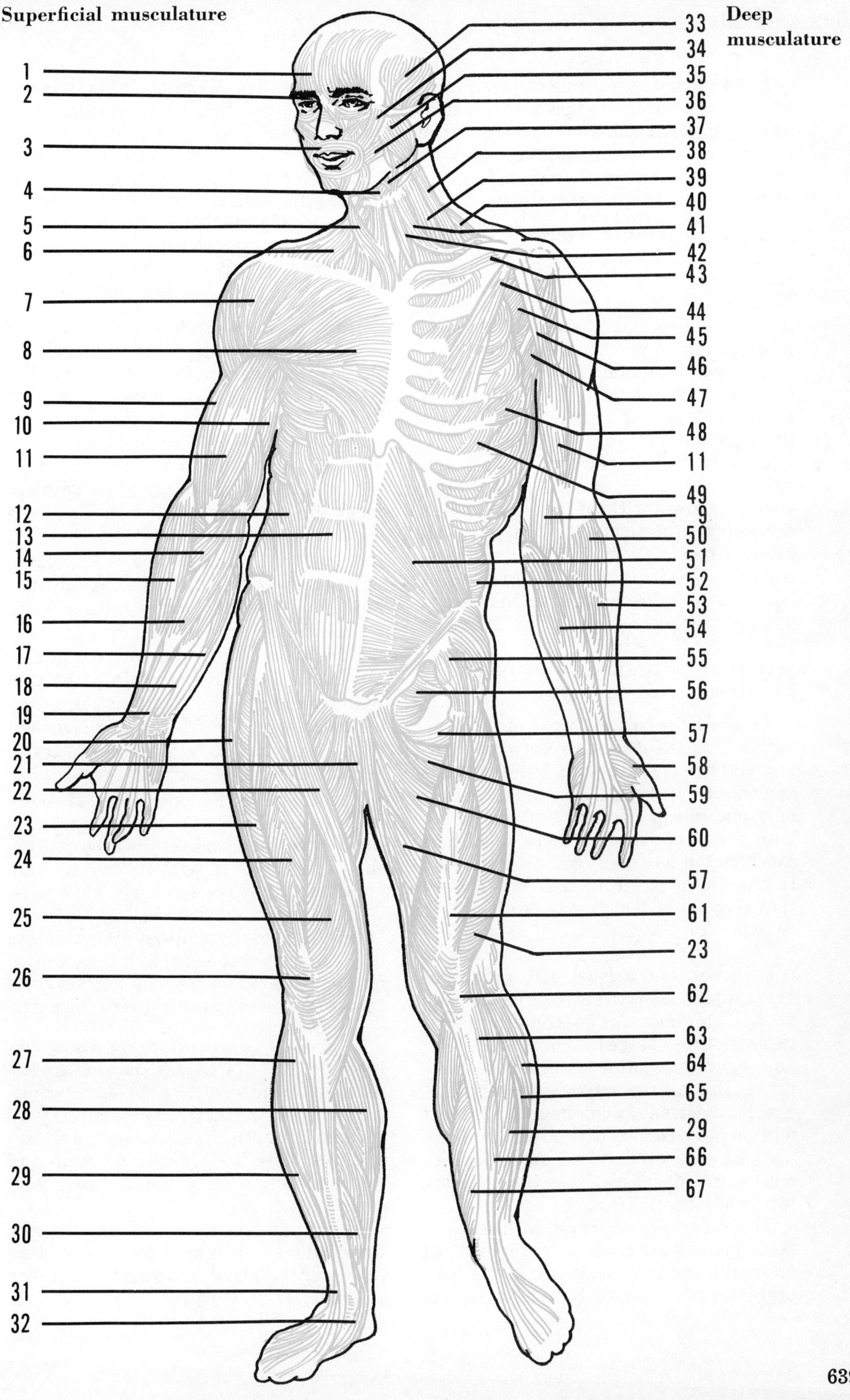
Superficial musculature
Deep musculature
1
2
3
4
5
6
7
8
9
10
11
12
13
14
15
16
17
18
19
20
21
22
23
24
25
26
27
28
29
30
31
32
33
34
35
36
37
38
39
40
41
42
43
44
45
46
47
48
11
49
9
50
51
52
53
54
55
56
57
58
59
60
57
61
23
62
63
64
65
29
66
67

A very small number of children have additional associated abnormalities such as congenital absence of the head of the thighbone. Such abnormal conditions cannot be cured no matter how early diagnosis and treatment is started.

Acute suppurative arthritis. Pyogenic (pus-producing) arthritis of the hip is uncommon, but occurs most frequently in infants and young children. In infants it is usually secondary to infection elsewhere, such as pneumonia, impetigo, or middle ear infection. The baby is obviously sick, has a sudden onset of high fever, holds the hip joint bent and resists its examination.

Usually the infecting organism is sensitive to antibiotics and the proper drug should be given without delay. It is often necessary to aspirate the hip joint because if pus is allowed to build up pressure there will be great destruction of bone. When treatment is started late it is usually necessary to drain the infection surgically. Sometimes the operation is performed too late and the joint cartilage has already been destroyed.

Perthe's disease is now one of the commoner diseases of children between three and eight years of age. It is three times as common in boys as in girls. Usually only one hip is affected, but sometimes both are. The child's general health is excellent but he usually complains of pain in the thigh or groin and has a limp that is so slight that it may be difficult to detect.

The specific cause of the condition is not known, but a local disturbance of blood supply leads to necrosis of the head of the thighbone. The condition goes through three stages — onset, activity, and healing — which may last three years. During the active stage the femoral head softens and deforms and is left with some irregularities after the healing phase is over. These irregularities may lead to degenerative arthritis of the hip joint later in life.

The diagnosis of Perthe's disease is made principally from x-ray pictures. If diagnosis and treatment is late, the femoral head may already have fragmented.

The objective of treatment is to try to prevent the soft femoral head from being squashed and fragmented into a grossly distorted shape. Every attempt to protect the femoral head by limiting weight-bearing through the affected limb should be made. No medicine or other known treatment will accelerate healing, nor is there any way to restore the femoral head to normal after it has been destroyed.

Adolescent "bent hip" or *coxa vara* ("coxa" means "hip joint") is a condition which occurs in later childhood. The rounded top of the thighbone slips from its cartilaginous connection with the rest of the bone and is displaced downward and backward, leaving a "wobbly" part. Usually this is a gradual development, but a fall or injury can cause a sudden displacement. In the past it was thought that all cases were associated with an endocrine disturbance, but it is now known that in many instances the child is of perfectly normal development.

Symptoms usually begin with gradually increasing pain in the hip, associated with a marked limp. Examination shows a characteristic limitation of movement of the hip joint. X-rays are necessary to confirm the diagnosis.

Treatment is by operation. If there is minimal slip of the head, its position can be accepted and retained by nailing the parts together with a "tri-fin" nail. In severe slips, the head will have to be reduced into a normal position before it is held in place by nailing. Manipulation is not always successful in late cases and an open operation may be necessary to restore correct relationships of the parts.

Degenerative arthritis of the hip occurs in later life and causes pain, stiffness, and deformity. In younger people, degenerative arthritis is secondary to congenital or acquired mechanical abnormalities. The basic cause is wear and tear and no medicine can halt or repair this process.

Many patients have such mild symptoms and slight limitations of motion that conservative treatment — minor modifications of work activities, local deep heat, massage and exercises — and possibly an occasional aspirin tablet are all that is necessary.

When symptoms do not respond to these treatments, various operations may be considered. Some that are designed to stiffen the painful hip are usually reserved for younger people with heavy occupations, such as farmers and construction workers. Other operations are designed to retain movement in the hip joint. Some make a false joint by placing a metal cup between the pelvic bone and the head of the thighbone after these bones have been appropriately shaped. This procedure has been used for many years and has yielded excellent results in many cases. Other operations leave the femoral head in place but alter the thrust of body weight through the pelvis. Another common operation is replacement of the femoral head and neck with a metallic prosthesis.

None of the operations are suitable for all cases. Choice depends upon age of the patient, state of disease in the affected

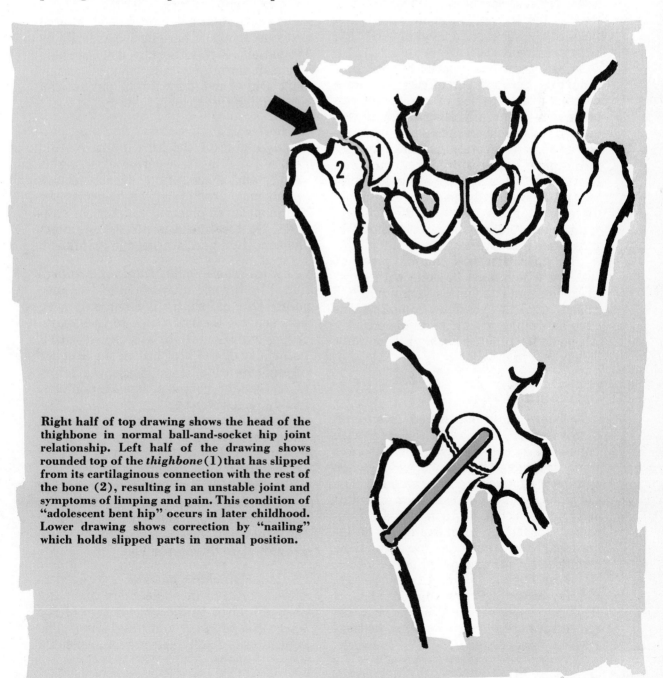

Right half of top drawing shows the head of the thighbone in normal ball-and-socket hip joint relationship. Left half of the drawing shows rounded top of the *thighbone* (1) that has slipped from its cartilaginous connection with the rest of the bone (2), resulting in an unstable joint and symptoms of limping and pain. This condition of "adolescent bent hip" occurs in later childhood. Lower drawing shows correction by "nailing" which holds slipped parts in normal position.

hip, and the condition of the other hip and the spine. Usually there is good relief of pain and restoration of function but it is not possible to give absolute assurance of results in all cases.

Total hip replacement. A relatively new form of hip surgery (low-friction arthroplasty), sometimes called the Charnley operation, after Dr. John Charnley, a British surgeon who developed it, is made possible by use of an acrylic cement which glues prefabricated metal-plastic joint parts to living bone. No screws or pins are used. It is well suited to conditions in which surfaces of the socket and head of the thigh bone are involved.

In selected elderly patients—the procedure is too new for effects in young persons over a period of many years to be known—generally favorable, and frequently dramatic, results have been reported. Many severely handicapped patients have been restored to normal activity, comfort, and excellent gait by the operation. Generally, pain is gone immediately after surgery and the "glued" joint is capable of supporting weight almost immediately.

The operation is a major piece of surgery which must be done with great precision and aseptic techniques to guard against possible complications such as wound infection and dislocation. A search for other, possibly better, joint cements is in progress.

Calcitonin

A "new" hormone called *calcitonin*, discovered in 1962, is associated with bone and calcium metabolism in ways that may have therapeutic value when synthetic supplies become available. The hormone tends to decrease the amount of calcium excreted in urine, and to increase absorption of calcium by the intestines, and thus to preserve bone strength by decreasing mineral losses. The hormone has given excellent results in a few cases of Paget's disease of bone and may be useful in healing of fractures and treatment of bone-wasting diseases such as osteoporosis.

THE KNEE

The knee is the largest joint in the body. It is the hinge in the middle of a long limb and is constantly exposed to injury. Stability of the joint depends primarily on the strength and tone of the *quadriceps* muscles which hold the joint extended. Ligaments of the joint are only of secondary help compared with the muscles, although integrity of the joint at the sides depends on the ligaments.

When the knee joint is affected by accident, operation, or disease, wasting of local muscles occurs. This wasting can be very rapid and can only be countered by many hours of hard active exercise by the patient. Physiotherapy, massage, and drugs do nothing to build up vital muscle bulk. Only hard work by the patient can accomplish this muscle buildup.

Bowlegs *(genu varum)* show an outward bowing of the knee joint. A mild degree followed by a period of straightening, and even slight overcorrection which may produce knock-knees, is the common developmental pattern in children. No treatment is necessary unless the condition persists later in childhood.

Knock-knees *(genu valgum)* are produced by inward angulation of the knee joint. This deformity is commonly seen between the ages of three to five years. It may occasionally be associated with a deformity of the hip. But in the absence of any causative bone disease, the deformity usually corrects itself spontaneously in a few years.

No treatment is necessary in young children, but a shoe wedge is often fitted to the heel. Knock-knee that is present at the age of ten definitely needs treatment by operation, either by removing a wedge from the femur to correct the angulation, or by selectively retarding the growth of the bones so that future growth straightens the legs.

Chondromalacia patellae is a degenerative condition in adolescents or young that is limited to the articulation of the kneecap *(patella)* and thighbone. The condition probably arises from repeated

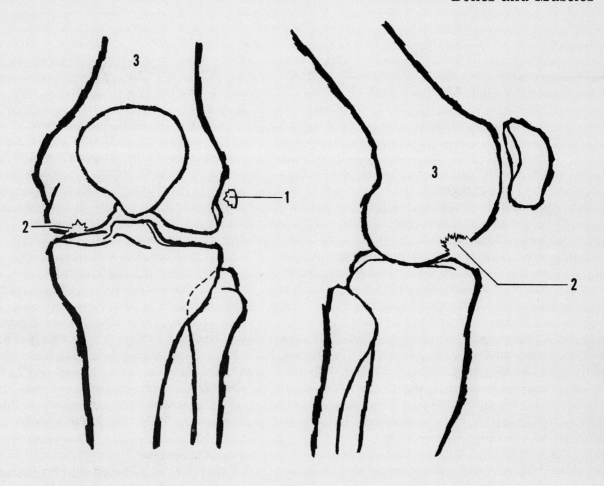

Loose bodies (often called "joint mice") are most frequently found in the knee. One condition that may give rise to loose bodies is *osteochondritis dissecans*, in which, probably because of local disturbance of blood supply, there is death of a small area of bone and its overlying cartilage. A fragment of bone and cartilage may separate and become a loose body in the joint cavity. The drawing shows front and side views of a knee joint with a loose fragment (1) that has separated from a rounded end of the thighbone (3), leaving an excavation (2) that is visible on an x-ray film.

minor injury caused by the kneecap moving on a surface that it does not fit exactly. It is not a true degenerative arthritis, but does predispose to the later development of degenerative changes.

Patients usually complain of pain under the kneecap, slight swelling, "cracking" in the joint during extension, occasional "catching" of the joint, and stiffness after sitting. Late teenage and early adult life is the time when symptoms usually become troublesome; young mothers with much carrying and stairwork to do are often badly affected.

Treatment is difficult but if the diagnosis is made early, firm bandage support, physiotherapy, and restriction of activities is often sufficient. If diagnosis is delayed or symptoms get worse despite treatment, operation is advised. At operation the undersurface of the kneecap is inspected, and if damage is not great, many surgeons will cut away the destroyed areas and leave a smooth undersurface. If damage is severe, there is no alternative to removal of the kneecap.

Osteochondritis dissecans is a fairly common condition occurring in late adolescence in which there is local death of a section of the joint surface of a bone and its overlying cartilage. Eventually the fragment may separate and form a loose body in the joint. The knee joint is most often affected. Injury is probably a predisposing factor.

In early stages the symptoms are vague aching and feelings of weakness in the knee. Symptoms are made worse by exercise and may persist when the knee is at rest. Examination will show wasting of muscles, possibly a slight escape of fluid into the joint, and a full range of motion. X-rays show a well-defined crescent-shaped excavation in the bone substance.

Treatment consists of surgical removal of the fragment if it has separated and is loose in the joint. If it has not separated, the fragment can often be encouraged to revascularize by an operation which drills small holes in the fragment to allow new vessels to grow in from the depths of the bone.

In young patients, the knee can be bandaged, strenuous activities curtailed, and operation avoided. Often a plaster cast is a more satisfactory method of protecting the knee. Weight-bearing is permissible but the cast may have to be worn six months or longer.

Recurrent dislocation of the kneecap. This condition is usually congenital, but is occasionally caused by injury. The congenital form, usually affecting both knees, usually occurs in teenage girls. The dislocation is always sidewise, with the kneecap sliding over the femur when the knee is bent.

The dislocation occurs spontaneously when walking or running, and is often noticed by girls walking up or down stairs at school. There is acute pain in the knee and the victim is unable to extend the joint. Someone else, however, can easily extend the joint passively and the patella slips back into position. X-rays do not usually show any abnormality, but the kneecap may be seen to be at a slightly higher level than usual.

Dislocation of the patella does not always become recurrent, but in most patients it does. Repeated dislocations predispose to later degenerative arthritis. If the patient is seen after the first dislocation, conservative treatment and exercises may prevent further dislocation. If exercise is not effective and the

dislocations recur frequently and cause severe disability, operation to transpose a tendon to realign the kneecap in a more normal position will be necessary.

Torn cartilage. A tear of one of the knee cartilages is quite common in young men, though not so frequent as laymen's diagnoses. A tear occurs when a twisting force passes through a bent or half-bent knee. Sometimes the diagnosis is easy to make because the injury is one that typically produces a tear. Diagnosis requires careful balancing of all the evidence.

There is usually pain in the joint when the tear occurs, and the patient cannot fully straighten his knee or continue what he was doing. Swelling of the knee is noticeable the next day and persists for at least two weeks. The patient often says the knee is "locked," but not in the sense that doctors use the term. The physician thinks of locking as sudden, definite inability to fully extend the knee; unlocking of the joint occurs with equal suddenness.

Treatment is affected by two factors: (a) The torn part is made of cartilage which does not have a blood supply and therefore cannot heal. (b) Weight-bearing through a knee joint which contains a torn cartilage will lead to strain of the knee ligaments, deterioration of the joint, and eventually to degenerative arthritis. Once the diagnosis of a torn cartilage is made, the correct treatment is excision of the cartilage.

Knee ligaments. There are four principal ligaments of the knee joint, one on either side and two inside. These ligaments may be strained or torn in sports and accidents. Injuries to these ligaments can be serious and must be properly treated if disability is to be avoided. For *complete tears* of these ligaments the best treatment is early surgical repair. Moderate sprains can be treated by immobilizing in a plaster cylinder, and minor injuries by wrapping the knee and avoiding strains during healing.

All degrees of ligament injuries will lead to wasting of the quadriceps muscle, and intensive exercises will be necessary to provide future protection for the joint.

Degenerative arthritis occurs more commonly in the knee than any other joint. This is because it is a weight-bearing joint and is exposed to trauma of all sorts. It is particularly common in obese women. The basic cause is wear and tear, but usually some other factor accelerates wear and tear — overweight, previous fracture or disease which has damaged the joint surface, and malalignment between bones of the joint.

The principal symptoms are limitation of movement and gradually increasing pain, often made worse by relatively trivial strains or twists.

Treatment is always started too late, in the sense that structural changes in the joint are irreversible. Although weight reduction helps to alleviate symptoms, it should have been done 20 years previously. Physiotherapy, local heat, massage, and supervised exercise enable patients to carry on for many months in moderate comfort. It is wise to avoid stair walking and walking over uneven ground whenever possible, since these activities impose marked strains through the joint.

Occasionally, operation is justified. If a loose body is present in the joint, its removal often alleviates symptoms. Stiffening of the knee can be done in patients crippled by severe pain and marked flexion deformity, giving complete relief of pain and not too bad a handicap if the opposite knee is not seriously affected.

THE FOOT

A painless, properly functioning foot is essential for well-being of the whole body. Painful or abnormal feet can lead to bad posture, fatigue, headache, muscular cramps, and backache.

The foot contains 26 bones and 33 articulations joined together by over one hundred ligaments. Nineteen muscles provide power and control of the foot. The bones are arranged in two arches — a lengthwise arch and a crosswise arch. The arches are supported by the shape of the bones, the ligaments of the joints, and indirectly by tendons and muscles. The arches have a certain degree of springiness and movement between the bones and elastic supporting structures, essential for proper functioning.

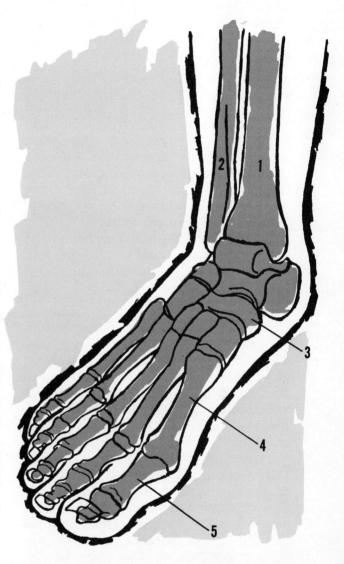

Bones of the foot: *tibia* (1), *fibula* (2), *tarsals* (3), *metatarsals* (4), *phalanges* (5). The bones form a longitudinal arch between the ball of the foot and the heel, as well as a crosswise arch. The intricate arrangement of bones joined by ligaments gives remarkable flexibility and easy rolling shift of body weight. It is not normal for feet to hurt.

The feet support the weight of the body, and act as levers to raise the body and move it forward in walking or running. In normal walking, body weight meets the ground at the heel, moves along the outer border to the ball of the foot, and thence across the line of metatarsal heads (long bones connecting to each toe) and is transferred into the big toe. This rolling, progressive shift of body weight cannot occur in a foot that is rigid. A properly functioning foot alters its shape with every step to accommodate to forces passing through it.

Foot Strain

The arches and supporting structures in the foot can be affected by either acute or chronic strain. *Acute strain* is usually caused by some isolated incident, such as prolonged standing or excessive use, that grossly overtaxes the foot. Symptoms usually respond promptly to rest and strapping of the foot. Unfortunately, the sprained foot, unlike the sprained hand, cannot be placed in a sling and it takes a longer time to heal.

Chronic strain of the foot can be caused by overweight, excessive fatigue, occupational demands, abnormal gait, and faults or diseases within the foot. Most of the symptoms occur in the "hinge" area (midtarsal) between the hindfoot and forefoot, where ligaments have to resist all the weight of the body as it is transmitted to the forefoot.

Treatment, which is usually immediately successful, is provision of a support for the longitudinal arch sufficiently high to halt downward motion before ligaments become strained enough to be painful. Such support does not cure since it does not remove the cause of the original strain of the foot. Every effort should be made to remove the primary cause since it is not good for the foot to become permanently reliant on arch supports. Sometimes the wearing of a permanent support is inevitable because of the difficulty in controlling the primary cause of the difficulty.

Flat Feet

Flat feet are rarely if ever troublesome. Many Olympic athletes have flat feet. However, *flattening feet* are painful and should have treatment. Babies' feet are always flat and it is wrong to diagnose "flat feet" in infants and toddlers before the arch of the foot has had time to develop. Nature provides a big fat pad in all young feet to support the inward side of the foot before muscles and ligaments develop sufficiently to support the longitudinal arch.

Even when a child first begins to stand, the foot is very mobile and flattens on weight-bearing. It is wrong to force these tiny feet into "supporting shoes." Rather, the child should be encouraged to go barefoot to allow muscles and ligaments to develop normal strength. The surface the small barefoot child walks on should not be hard and unyielding, but somewhat resilient, like grass, a thick playpen pad, or cushioned carpet.

True flat foot in children is very uncommon, but when it exists the deformity is usually acquired rather than inherited. Some believe that the deformity can be produced if a baby sleeps on his stomach in a spread-eagled position which puts pressure on the great toe and pushes the feet outward.

Many people tolerate the pain of *flattening feet* for astonishing lengths of time because of a misconception that it is normal for feet to hurt. It is not. Pain of flattening feet is primarily produced by stretching of the ligaments, and in late cases pain can arise in bones that have "fallen" sufficiently to make contact with weight-bearing surfaces.

When the foot is strained it becomes quickly fatigued, weak, and the arch droops when weight is borne. When the foot is raised the arch recovers its normal shape, but in late stages the altered shape becomes fixed and the foot may be permanently flat.

Early treatment props the structures with a resilient "arch support" made of leather, cork, or plastic. It is important that the support be sufficiently mobile to accommodate to the changing shape of the foot during walking. Supports should be used only until the foot no longer hurts. Long-term use of a support means that the foot will become dependent on it and muscles will weaken. Later treatment consists of exercises, sensible footwear, and correct posture which is predominantly important because it is "used" all the time.

Corrective Foot Exercises

Foot-strengthening exercises are excellent in themselves, but too much should not be expected if exercises are done briefly and sporadically, as is often the case. It is particularly difficult to "sell" children on exercises they have no interest in and even resent, and foot troubles, like others, should have the benefit of your doctor's skills.

Dancing is an excellent foot exercise; so is walking barefoot on a suitable surface.

Useful special exercises are:

Pick up marbles with the toes.

In a sitting position with legs slightly bent outward, bend the foot strongly upward.

Walk on the outer borders of the feet.

Walk on tip-toes.

Flattening of the transverse (crosswise) arch occurs almost always in women. The symptom is pain in the instep area (metatarsalgia). Usually the primary cause is weakness in the intrinsic muscles of the foot, and the wearing of high-heeled shoes is responsible for the persistence of symptoms. The ideal treatment is permanent abandonment of high-heeled shoes, but this therapy is almost universally rejected. Symptomatic relief can be given by placing small domed supports within the shoes. When correctly placed, these domes will restore the normal transverse arch and relieve pressure on the metatarsal heads.

Pain radiating into the toes, caused by a small growth on one of the nerves, sometimes resembles the pain of metatarsalgia caused by a fallen transverse arch. This condition can be relieved by surgical removal of the tumor.

CHILDREN'S FOOT PROBLEMS

The greatest difficulty in dealing with the developing foot lies in persuading parents to allow their child's feet to develop unhindered by rigid shoes or so-called corrective orthopedic shoes. The growing foot is intended to move around unshod, thereby allowing full opportunity for muscles and ligaments to develop. True flat feet usually are so uncommon that the diagnosis should be made by a qualified orthopedist rather than a shoe salesman or neighbor.

Pigeon toe, or toe inturning, is very common in the early stages of walking, probably from efforts of the child to improve his balance. At this stage of walking there are often signs of bowlegs, knock-knees, or internal tibial torsion. In the vast majority of cases all these abnormalities are corrected spontaneously as the child develops. Occasionally there are more serious causes such as congenital deformities and those which occur in a spastic child, which need competent medical care for their correction.

Clubfoot. There are two usual forms of clubfoot, congenital *talipes equinovarus* and *calcaneovalgus.* Both deformities respond well to treatment provided it is started shortly after birth. A series of corrective plaster casts will usually restore a normal contour to the foot, although sometimes minor operations may also be necessary to relieve tightness in tendons and ligaments.

It is vital to long-term success that the children be examined at regular intervals to be sure that the correction has been maintained. It is often found that so-called "relapsed" clubfeet have not been followed and checked often enough for any tendency to recurrence of the difficulty to be recognized early.

Web-toes. Webbing (a connecting membrane between digits) is not uncommon. When it occurs between the fingers, correction is necessary, but symptoms rarely develop in webbed toes. There is usually no difficulty in fitting shoes, normal function of the foot is rarely if ever affected, and surgical treatment is usually unnecessary.

Elevated little toe. Occasionally there is an hereditary disposition for the fifth (little) toe to be elevated above the others. There is no disability or discomfort as long as the child goes barefoot, but symptoms develop when attempts are made to force the foot into ordinary shoes. Amputation of the toe is mutilating and a poor solution. Conservative treatment cannot be applied since the basic fault is a deficiency of tissue. When symptoms develop, most satisfactory treatment is an operation designed to lengthen the shortened tissues.

Ballet dancing is often falsely accused of being harmful to growing feet. When properly controlled it is beneficial to the feet, since it produces excellent development of intrinsic muscles of the feet and the calf muscles. This dancing also improves the general tone and posture of the body. Structural changes of the foot can occur only if the amount of dancing is excessive or *if the child goes "up on points" too early.* Ballet dancing should be moderate in amount until about the age of 12 or 13 years, and "points" should certainly not be allowed until the age of 13 years.

Shoes

Except for fashion, the only reason for wearing shoes is to protect the feet from the weather and injury. A shoe does nothing to help the development of the muscles or arches of a normal foot. Barefoot walking is the best possible treatment for growing feet.

Children's shoes. Loose-fitting cloth booties are all that is necessary for infants before they start to walk. When the time comes to fit shoes to a baby's foot, the shoes must conform to the shape of the foot and must be large enough to allow normal movement of the foot within the shoes. The soles and uppers should be of supple leather. Neither arches nor

heels are necessary. It is wrong to force a baby's foot into a miniature adult-style shoe wrongly shaped for infant feet.

Young feet grow at an astonishing rate. The average child outgrows a pair of shoes in three months, and generally needs a larger pair at the end of this time even though the old shoes are not badly worn. Small boys tend to demolish their shoes in three months or, some parents think, three weeks, but girls who are "easy on their shoes" may continue to wear a pair that has become too small. Inspect a child's shoes occasionally to be sure he has not outgrown them.

The most important aspect of shoe fitting is adequate length. There should be a space of one-half to three-fourths of an inch between the end of the big toe and the end of the shoe. The widest width of the shoe should correspond with the widest weight-bearing portion of the foot. Shoes which are too short will gradually cause the toes to flex, and persistence of this position may lead to weakness of intrinsic muscles of the foot and further deformity of the toes.

Tips on shoe fitting. In buying shoes it is a good idea to purchase them in the afternoon, since the foot can increase one size in length during the day, particularly if you have been on them a lot and the day is muggy. When standing in a new pair of shoes, there should be enough room to wiggle your big toe. Walk around in the shoes; if they slip at the heel, try a narrower heel width. A given style of shoe may be wrong for you; a good fit may require a different style. One foot is usually bigger than the other (shoe clerks, trained in human relations, say that one is smaller than the other). The larger foot should be fitted.

Old shoes often give clues to poor fit or gait. Shoes may be worn excessively at one side or the other instead of under the ball of the foot which is the natural weight-bearing fulcrum. The shoe lining may be worn at the toes, indicating a too short shoe, or at the side or back of the heel, indicating a sloppy fit in this area. *Stockings* that are too short can also constrict the feet. When a growing child needs larger shoes he usually needs larger stockings too.

Women have much more foot trouble than men, principally because of the shoes they wear. Pointed shoes cram the toes together and produce pressure symptoms such as corns and calluses. Shoes of this shape force the foot into an abnormal posture which leads to poor distribution of body weight, not infrequently felt as backache. Constant wearing of such shoes may produce distressing deformities that cannot be completely corrected.

A reasonable reason for high heels — to help retain the shoes in stirrups when horseback riding — has been invalid for years. Their survival among women has no relationship to practicality, but is a source of continuous employment to orthopedists. A heel is high if it measures two inches. Any heel of this height or greater will force the full weight of the body onto the metatarsal heads and squeeze the toes into the pointed forepart of the shoe. This crowding will lead to destruction of the transverse arch, produce calluses on the sole of the foot, and varying deformities of the toes. (Calluses on the ball of the foot are not uncommonly mistaken for "plantar warts" which are quite different.)

In young people these deformities are reversible. For example, when pregnant women wear low-heeled shoes their foot symptoms improve and they lose the calluses on the soles of their feet. Women who consistently wear high heels may suffer shortening of the calf muscles to such an extent that walking barefoot or in low heels is extremely uncomfortable. There is nothing medically good that can be said about high heels, and next to nothing that will discourage their use.

Adult Foot Problems

Bunion or *hallux valgus* ("hallux" is the big toe) is a common deformity of the adult female foot, but can also occur in men. The defect is an obvious thickening and swelling of the big joint of the big toe which forces the big toe toward the little toe. There is a protuberance on the inner side of the foot where the "hinge" bends when walking and instead of being straight, the big toe angles toward the little toe.

Bunion is more common in the adolescent foot than is generally recognized because the children rarely complain of pain. If the condition does cause symptoms in young adult life, it is unlikely that splints or "sensible shoes" will do any good or be tolerated by the patient. Sponge rubber pegs between the first and second toes do not force the big toe into a correct position. They are more likely to force the second toe into the same deformity as the big toe.

Once the deformity is established it is self-perpetuating and will get progressively worse if untreated. In elderly people with bunions, surgery is not warranted and shoes should be made to fit the deformed foot. In younger persons there is no real alternative to surgical correction of the causes and results of the deformity. Operations which merely trim the bunion are not usually of lasting benefit since they do not treat the causes which produced the bunion.

Hallux rigidus ("stiff toe"). Pain and stiffness in the big joint of the big toe is quite common in young adults. It is usually produced by repeated minor trauma or a single major accident that overextends the toe with great force. The symptoms usually subside if the joint is protected for a few weeks or months, commonly, by fixing a small steel plate within the sole of the shoe. In a small number of patients the condition persists, and if pain and limitation of toe movement are sufficiently troublesome, relief can be obtained by surgery.

Hammer toe is usually caused by cramping the toes into too small a shoe, although it can be produced by muscle imbalance in a well-shod foot. Usually the clawlike deformity affects the second toe. Symptoms are usually produced by pressure, and may be alleviated by padding. If not, surgery gives excellent relief from the deformity.

Ingrown toenail usually affects the big toe. Commonly, the edge of the nail is driven into soft tissues by the pressure of tight shoes, or a crushing blow may initiate local injury. The forward edge of the nail as well as the side may cut into soft tissue if the nail is trimmed too short. If the area is not infected, the patient may be able to draw the overgrown tissue away from the nail after hot soaks of the foot. Thus the cutting edge of the nail may be freed, and a wisp of cotton placed to cushion the contact area. This should be done daily after the bath until the "corner" of the nail has grown beyond the point where it cuts into flesh.

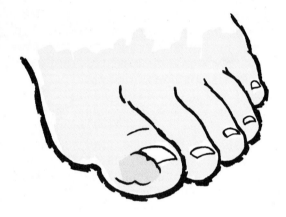

Ingrown toenail commonly results from trimming the nail too short, especially at its corners. This permits the edge of the nail to gouge into soft tissue, causing painful inflammation. Trimming the nail squarely so that corners project slightly beyond soft tissues helps to prevent ingrown toenail.

However, if the condition was caused by tight shoes it will recur unless roomier shoes are worn. When infection is present and there is much overgrowth of granulation tissue, removal of a portion of the nail by simple surgery is usually necessary and successful. To prevent ingrown toenail, the nail should be trimmed squarely, with enough projection at the corners to prevent gouging and possible infection of underlying tissues.

Diseases of Bone

Osteoporosis is a condition of abnormal porousness or "thinning" of bone, due to insufficient production of the protein matrix in which calcium salts are deposited. The most common type is "postmenopausal osteoporosis," occurring in a large proportion of women after a natural or artificial menopause. There may be no symptoms until some local area of fragile bone fractures with slight provocation, such as a crushed vertebra resulting from bending or a relatively minor jolt. "Senile osteoporosis" occurs to some degree in all aging persons. In advanced stages, deformities of the spine resulting from collapsed vertebrae are not uncommon.

Hormonal deficiencies are primarily involved but there are many contributing causes: poor nutrition over a period of many years or poor assimilation although the diet is good; the menopause and aging; prolonged bed rest, immobilization, inactivity; impaired blood supply to bone; various diseases such as forms of rheumatoid arthritis.

Treatment depends upon the stage and nature of the osteoporosis and remedy of underlying factors if possible. Sex hormones are commonly prescribed, and a substantial protein diet, sometimes with minerals to assist calcification, though this requires careful supervision by a physician since excessive mineral intake may harm the kidneys, especially of an immobilized patient. Activity to the extent that it is tolerated is encouraged, with precautions to prevent further fractures. In osteoporosis of the aged, the patient should be regarded as being marked "fragile, handle with care."

Osteomalacia ("softening of the bones") is also called "adult rickets." Bone changes are similar to those of childhood rickets, except that they are more diffuse since there are no special areas of growth in adults. In its simplest form, osteomalacia is a deficiency disease, rare in the United States, but it may also result from impaired absorption of nutrients. Treatment with a high calcium, high phosphorus diet and adequate amounts of Vitamin D usually gives prompt and often dramatic relief from the disease.

Paget's disease (osteitis deformans) is a relatively common bone disease of persons over 40 years of age. It is a chronic process of bone overgrowth, destruction, and new bone formation. In the course of time the involved bone becomes deformed and its architecture disordered. The patients often have arteriosclerosis and impaired blood supply to the bones. The disease is not diffuse but "spotty," with a predilection for bones of the spine, skull, and lower leg. The onset is insidious and patients may not seek medical assistance for many years. The disease may become arrested, or progress slowly. Spontaneous fractures may occur but heal normally. A hearing aid frequently becomes necessary. There is no specific treatment, but irradiation and other effective measures can relieve bone pain if it occurs.

A number of diseases manifested in bone, such as the plasma cell disease, multiple myeloma, involve the reticuloendothelial system (see Chapter 4).

SPRAINS, DISLOCATIONS, FRACTURES

A *sprain* is an injury to a ligament, and a *strain* is an injury to a muscle or its tendon. All joints in the body are held together by ligaments powerful enough to resist all normal forces. When violent force is applied a stretched ligament will tear and a sprain occurs.

Mild sprains do not weaken the joint and usually need only strapping support. The great majority of sprains do well with plaster immobilization. Severe sprains usually produce a complete tear of a major ligament and are best treated by surgical repair of the torn tissues. Sometimes the ligament remains intact and tears away from its bony attachment, even carrying a small piece of bone with it. X-rays will show if the bony fragment is near its original site or if the ligament is curled upon itself. If it is curled it cannot heal satisfactorily and should be repositioned surgically.

A dislocation occurs when the force applied to a joint is greater than that necessary to produce a strain. Dislocations must be *reduced* (returned to proper position), and usually an anesthetic is necessary to relax the spasm in surrounding muscles. Occasionally, manipulation does not succeed, usually because some torn tissue or an adjacent tendon is interposed between the joint surfaces. In such cases an operation may be necessary to achieve the reduction. Following reduction the torn tissues must be given time to heal before allowing movement in the joint; three weeks is usually the minimum time necessary.

A *fracture* is a break in a bone. The strength of bones varies from person to person and at different ages. In elderly people the bones are relatively brittle, in children, more flexible.

The physician who treats fractures is concerned with obtaining the best functional result for the fractured bone. This does not require perfect anatomical juxtaposition. Bone is a living tissue and is perfectly capable of uniting fractured parts that have not been exactly replaced in their original position. Because of this capacity for repair it is possible to treat most fractures by manipulations which place the broken ends sufficiently near for good union to occur. A good blood supply at the fracture site is necessary for repair to occur, and it follows that repair is usually more rapid in children and slower in the elderly.

During healing the fracture area must be protected from excessive movement. Various methods of immobilization are used. The most common is a plaster cast which is easily applied and removed. Some fractures need to be treated in the early days after injury by various methods of *traction* on the limb. A pull can be applied to a limb by adhesive tape stuck to the skin or by a metallic pin placed through an unbroken part of the bone or an adjacent bone. By such means the fracture can be controlled through the healing process and minor adjustments of position of the broken bones can be made.

Some closed fractures which are so grossly unstable that they constantly

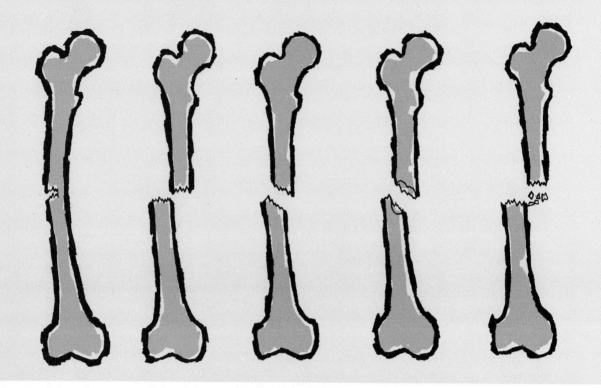

A fracture is a break in a bone, of which there are many different forms, some of which are shown in the drawing. From left to right: a *greenstick* fracture, not uncommon in young children, whose bones are quite flexible and may break only on one side when force is applied; a *transverse* fracture; *oblique* fracture; *spiral* fracture; *comminuted* fracture (crushed into small pieces). A simple or closed fracture occurs without a break in overlying skin; in a compound fracture, broken bone breaks through the skin. Some injuries mistaken for sprains are actually fractures, and x-rays are usually necessary to detect the true situation.

redisplace need to be immobilized internally by some form of metallic fixation. However, operation adds the risks inherent in any operation. Most physicians are conservative in their care of fractures because of the risk of such complications and because few fractures need to be operated upon.

Different names are given to the type of break in the bone, such as *greenstick, transverse, oblique, spiral,* or *comminuted* (see illustration). But all types of breaks are treated by the same general principles: (1) reduction of the fracture into a satisfactory position; (2) maintenance of fracture reduction until healing is sufficient to prevent redisplacement; (3) restoration of normal function to muscles, tendons and joints.

Restoration of function after the fracture has united is a vital part of treatment. It is usual for some joint stiffness and muscle atrophy to be present after the cast has been removed. The stiffness and atrophy are directly proportional to the age of the patient and the length of time of immobilization. It is often hard to decide how soon a cast can be removed from an elderly patient in order to prevent gross stiffness and yet allow the fracture to heal.

Physiotherapy is of great help in the mobilization of a stiffened limb, but active movements and active muscle contractions by the patient are the key to success. Most functional return occurs during the first three or four months. After this period, recovery slows and may not be complete for a year or even longer.

ARTHRITIS AND RHEUMATIC DISEASES

by R. W. LAMONT-HAVERS, M.D.

Non-Articular Rheumatism • Osteoarthritis • Gout

CONNECTIVE TISSUE DISEASES

Rheumatoid Arthritis • Drugs • Diet and Nutrition • Rest and Exercise • Heat • Ankylosing Spondylitis • Psoriatic Arthritis • Systemic Lupus Erythematosus • Progressive Systemic Sclerosis • Polymyositis and Dermatomyositis • Arthritis Due to Infection

LABORATORY TESTS

Misleading Claims

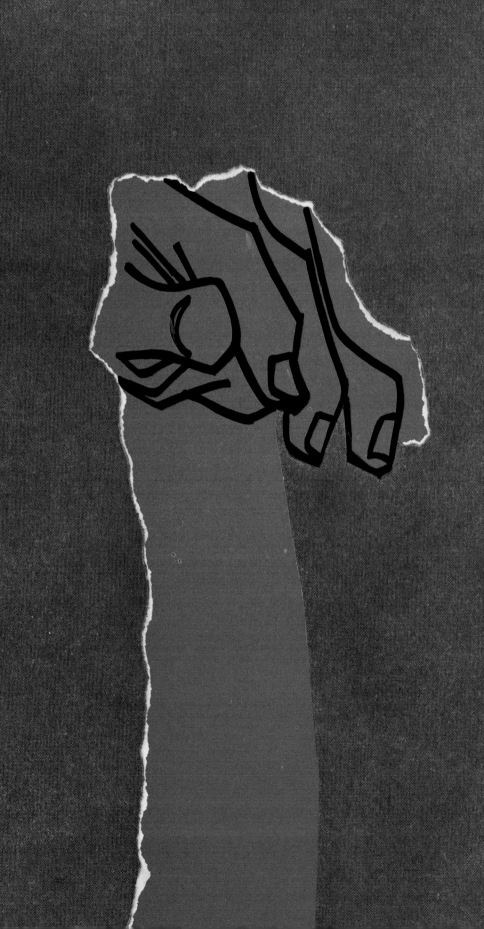

CHAPTER 19

ARTHRITIS AND RHEUMATIC DISEASES

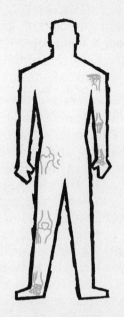

by R. W. LAMONT-HAVERS, M.D.

The terms "arthritis" and "rheumatic disease" are applied to many disorders which affect tissues in and around the joints. Some forms, such as rheumatoid arthritis, are generalized diseases of the entire body with particular manifestations in the joints.

More than 60 different rheumatic diseases are known. Some are relatively mild and some are severe and may cause crippling deformities, symbolized in the color plate. Often, crippling can be minimized or prevented by proper and prompt treatment. The many different forms of arthritis not only vary in severity but in the type of treatment required. Treatment suitable for one form of arthritis may be useless or even harmful in another. Accurate diagnosis by a physician of the particular type of arthritis that is present is the first essential step toward intelligent treatment.

Research in diseases of connective tissue—the weblike substance that glues and binds the body together — is hopefully leading toward better understanding and treatment of arthritis and rheumatic diseases.

A good deal of confusion arises because of the many terms — popular and medical — that are used to describe arthritis and allied diseases.

"Rheumatic diseases" or "rheumatism" are terms used by physicians as a general category of all diseases that cause pain and disability affecting the joints and their supporting structures. The term "rheumatology" is used to describe the study of these diseases.

Arthritis is the term used for conditions arising from involvement of the joints and their immediate surrounding structures by disease. It is also frequently used as a general term to describe rheumatic diseases which primarily attack the joints. Thus, "the patient has some form of arthritis."

Non-articular rheumatism is the term that describes conditions in which the soft tissues of supporting structures are involved — for example, bursitis and fibrositis.

In popular usage these terms are applied much more loosely. "Rheumatism" is often equated with non-articular complaints, usually of a relatively benign nature. "Arthritis" is often used indiscriminately to refer to rheumatic disease as a whole, to a specific disease such as rheumatoid arthritis, and not infrequently to vague complaints which an individual may assume have something to do with his joints or muscles.

There are about 60 conditions which are commonly grouped as rheumatic diseases. Their medical classification presents numerous difficulties, because of complex interrelationships and currently limited knowledge of causes and mechanisms.

For purposes of discussion, however, a grossly simplified classification of the rheumatic diseases is useful. They may be categorized broadly as:

Non-articular rheumatism (fibrositis, bursitis).

Osteoarthritis.

Connective Tissue Diseases.

Gout.

Arthritis due to infection.

Non-Articular Rheumatism

A number of conditions come under this classification, the most common being fibrositis, bursitis, and the painful shoulder syndrome.

Fibrositis is not a distinct disease entity but is a term applied to inflammatory processes occurring in muscles, fascia, ligaments and tendons. The outstanding symptoms are pain, stiffness, and tenderness in the involved area. The most frequent precipitating factor is some sort of injury, acute or chronic. Acute symptoms may follow strenuous or unaccustomed sports activity (for instance, a "charley horse"). Chronic low back strain resulting from poor posture is a well-known cause. Exposure to drafts and chilling may provoke attacks in susceptible persons. Fibrositis often accompanies generalized infections such as influenza and it may be an accompanying manifestation of other rheumatic diseases. **Fibromyositis** implies that muscle tissue is involved.

In most patients, fibrositis is a self-limited, short-term illness which is annoying but not crippling.

Treatment is directed toward removing triggering factors and programs to correct contributory postural defects (frequently difficult because of human laziness). Avoidance of drafts, particularly with air-conditioning, is important for susceptible persons. Treatment includes rest for the affected structures, applications of heat and massage, pain-relievers such as aspirin. The physician may employ other physical medicine techniques such as short-wave or ultrasound

therapy, and if the fibrositis is localized, and particularly if nodules are felt, some physicians may inject a local anesthetic such as a procaine, perhaps mixed with a corticosteroid such as hydrocortisone.

Bursitis is an inflammation of the *bursae*, the small enclosed surfaces which allow ease of motion between structures such as muscles, tendons and surfaces. The cause is primarily injury due to excessive use or abuse of the structures. Local inflammation gives rise to popular descriptions such as "housemaid's knee," in which the bursa in front of the knee becomes inflamed and swollen from too much kneeling, and "coachman's bottom," in which the bursa over the ischial tuberosity (the part of the pelvis on which we sit) is involved. These conditions are not unusual, although the trades from which the names derive have all but vanished.

The involved area becomes painful, tender, hot, red, and swollen if it is close to the skin surface. Treatment consists of rest, applications of heat, and use of analgesics. The physician may give local injections of hydrocortisone or related steroids, and may also prescribe some of the more powerful anti-rheumatic agents in addition to aspirin or other salicylates.

The **painful shoulder syndrome** covers a number of conditions producing pain and limitation of motion about the shoulder. These may arise from local causes such as degeneration and rupture of tissues supporting the shoulder joint, osteoarthritis of this joint, or injury leading to bursitis. Pain and motion-restricting changes around the shoulder may also occur when the primary disease is elsewhere—for example, osteoarthritis of the spine in the neck region, coronary heart disease, and some diseases of the chest. The predominant symptom is severe pain in the shoulder area and inability to raise the arm because of pain and weakness.

Severe cases may proceed to the shoulder-hand syndrome, in which the hand becomes swollen and painful, and the condition may sometimes be confused with rheumatoid arthritis.

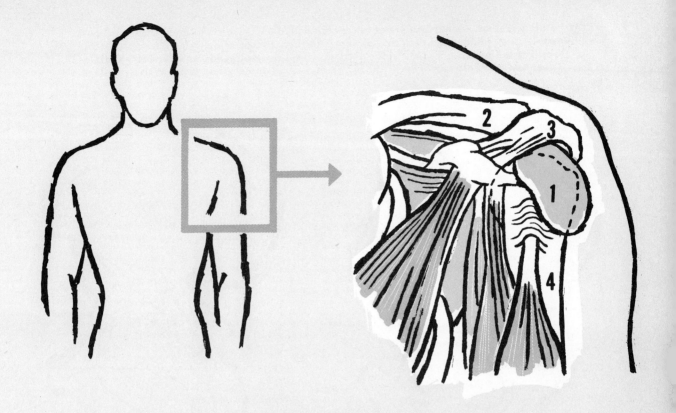

The shoulder is a common site of painful bursitis (subacromial or subdeltoid bursitis). The drawing shows a distended subacromial *bursa* (1), the "lubricating" sac between tissues that must slide over each other. Other structures shown are the *collarbone* (2), *the acromion* (3) at the point of the shoulder, and the *humerus* (4). Slight movements of these bony structures pinch the inflamed bursa and cause excruciating pain.

Therapy usually combines early physiotherapy with a home program of exercises, analgesics, frequently oral anti-inflammatory agents during the acutely painful stage, and local injection of an anesthetic and corticosteroid into the painful area. The vast majority of patients regain the use of their shoulder, although this may take as long as two years and the patient should not become discouraged in the meantime because of apparent slow progress.

X-rays of the painful shoulder frequently reveal calcium deposits. This is a normal body reaction. Such deposits are not infrequently found in unaffected joints of the same or other patients, and can disappear spontaneously. The deposits themselves are usually of little significance but must be considered in individual diagnosis.

(For discussion of the above conditions affecting particular parts of the body, see Chapter 18).

Osteoarthritis ("Degenerative Arthritis")

Changes in the joints due to *osteoarthritis* have been found in the skeletons of early vertebrates, including the dinosaurs and Neanderthal man. Joint changes detectable by x-rays are all but universal in persons in the middle and later years of life. Most people over the age of 50 will show degenerative changes in cartilage of the joints, particularly of

Arthritis and Rheumatism

Some degree of osteoarthritis, not always sufficient to cause symptoms, occurs in most people after middle age. Troublesome osteoarthritis most often affects weight-bearing joints of the hips, knees, and spine. At left below, normal pelvis in side view; at right, "wear and tear" osteoarthritis of the hip joint, with disintegration of protective cartilage.

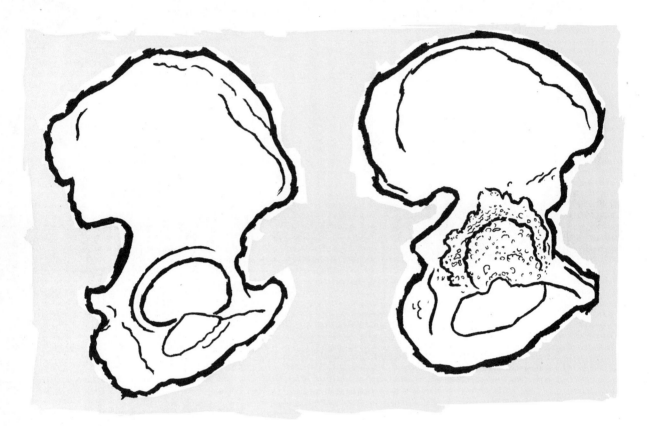

the spine, on x-ray examination. Thus the term "degenerative joint disease," implying a "wear and tear" disorder attendant upon aging, is often used synonymously.

However, only 10 to 15 per cent of people with x-ray-disclosed osteoarthritic changes in the joints have distressing symptoms, and the severity of symptoms is not necessarily correlated with the extent of joint changes. Thus many physicians, particularly in Europe, use the term *osteoarthrosis* to describe symptomless joint changes which have no apparent effect on health or activity. *Osteoarthritis* is descriptive of patients who do have symptoms, regardless of x-ray appearances.

Osteoarthritic changes. The underlying process is a thinning and eventual disappearance of the cartilage which forms the smooth, gliding surface of the joints. This begins insidiously and painlessly (there are no pain receptors in cartilage) as a pitting, flaking, and splintering disintegration of cartilage which covers the ends of the bones, until it may be worn away, the underlying bone exposed, and pain results when "bare bones" are moved against each other.

Throughout life the cartilage undergoes active remodeling to shape it, like a resilient bearing, to joint surfaces. This process may be overstimulated by injury, malformation of a joint (frequently congenital), infection, and may be modified by factors related to age, heredity, and metabolic processes of some obscurity. When the cartilage is shed at an abnormal rate and eventually disappears, underlying bone becomes thickened and bony spurs or projections grow at the margins. This causes pain when opposed bones move. A crude analogy is that of two washboard surfaces grating against each other because an intervening pad of foam rubber (cartilage) is missing.

But osteoarthritic joints do not fuse immovably nor does gross deformity occur. Osteoarthritis is entirely different from, and does not lead to, rheumatoid arthritis (although a rheumatoid arthritis patient may also have osteoarthritis).

Not all joints are equally involved. The ones most commonly affected are those of the knees, hips, and spine. These are joints where there is the greatest shearing action. Symptoms involving the wrist, elbow, and shoulder are rare except as a result of injury.

Heberden's nodes are a manifestation of a common form of osteoarthritis of the hands that occurs almost exclusively in women after the menopause. The nodes, named for the physician who first described them, are knobby, thickened lumps over the end joints of the fingers. Usually the end joint of a single finger enlarges over a period of months or years and the process generally extends to other fingers. These joints are not much exposed to hard wear and tear; the process appears to be sex-linked and hereditary. The affected finger joint may be a little sensitive and reddened when active changes are occurring, but this subsides and leaves no disability other than possible slight clumsiness in delicate finger movements. The main complaint is of unsightliness. Heberden's nodes in themselves should never be taken as an indication that some serious and crippling form of arthritis is at work.

Symptoms. The most usual symptoms of osteoarthritis are stiffness and aching pain which is commonly worse at night or after excessive activity. The morning hours after rest are usually most comfortable. Acute inflammation of the joint is very rare. Pain and stiffness result from exertion and are relieved by rest. However, pain can become quite constant, severe, and disabling, particularly if the hips or knees are affected. Involvement of the spine, particularly of the neck and low back regions, can cause considerable pain and limitation of motion from pressure of bony spurs on nerve roots.

Treatment is directed toward relieving stress and "taking a load off" the affected joints. While obesity does not cause osteoarthritis, many patients are overweight and there is a consequent burden on weight-bearing joints. A program to reduce weight in such instances is important.

There is no way to restore an osteoarthritic joint to its youthful state, but a good deal can be done to lessen further deterioration. Physical therapy with home exercise programs to strengthen muscles and correct the mechanical strains of poor posture is important. Activities should be spaced to allow for periods of rest, and sports, recreation, and walking — relaxing, enjoyable and helpful — should not be so prolonged that stresses on affected joints are continued to the point of fatigue or pain. A cane can be very helpful in decreasing stress on a joint, if the patient's pride permits a sensible aid to comfort.

Applications of *heat* are recommended (see page 665). Simple analgesics are valuable, and stronger ones may at times be prescribed for severe pain. Local injection of hydrocortisone or related compounds into the joint by the physician can frequently give prolonged relief. However, oral corticosteroids are not recommended because of their systemic effects.

Bracing devices for severe spine and knee involvements can be very helpful, and certain surgical procedures, as in severe cases of hip involvement, may be successful. For the great majority of patients, however, osteoarthritis is a mild disorder which may cause some endurable pain and stiffness, which may require some moderation of normal activity, but which rarely causes total disability and does not affect general health.

Gout

This disease, known since antiquity, is due to a defect of body chemistry which leads to the accumulation of *urates* (chalky salts of uric acid) in the body. The kidneys normally excrete uric acid, but in the gout patient they do not do so efficiently and cannot keep excretion in balance with production. Urate crystals tend to be deposited in cartilage. Since cartilage is found at the ends of bones, a sudden acute attack of gout may be manifested as cartoonists have immortalized it: as a "red hot" inflammation of the joint at the base of the big toe. Surrounding skin is tight, shiny, hot, swollen, red, and the area is very painful. Other joints than that of the toe may be involved. In absence of treatment, chronic forms of gout may develop as chalky urates gradually form masses known as "tophi" around joints and in structures composed largely of cartilage, such as the external ear. The deposits are painless, but pain is caused by irritation and inflammation set up around joints.

Gout is most common in men over 30 years of age. Women are not immune, but onset before the menopause is rare. The disease is relatively common, but severe forms like the swollen big toe joint depicted by cartoonists are not, because these are preventable.

Causes. The metabolic defect responsible for gout is almost certainly hereditary. Overproduction of uric acid may be found in close relatives of a patient with gout, although they may not manifest the disease. An abnormally high level of uric acid in the blood does not of itself prove the presence of gout. Certain drugs, including aspirin, can elevate blood uric acid. X-rays are of little diagnostic value in early attacks of gout, but later in the course of the disease will reveal typical joint changes from urate deposits. Examination of fluid drawn from an acutely inflamed joint may reveal uric acid crystals.

The patient's symptoms, uric acid levels, history of attacks of arthritis or kidney disorder or other factors, help to arrive at the correct diagnosis. A drug known as *colchicine,* prepared from roots of the meadow saffron, is remarkably specific in relieving acute gout but no other form of arthritis. A "therapeutic trial" of the drug is frequently used in

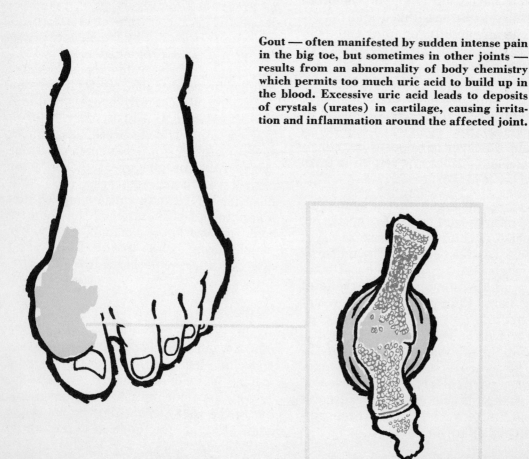

Gout — often manifested by sudden intense pain in the big toe, but sometimes in other joints — results from an abnormality of body chemistry which permits too much uric acid to build up in the blood. Excessive uric acid leads to deposits of crystals (urates) in cartilage, causing irritation and inflammation around the affected joint.

diagnosis. If acute symptoms are relieved by colchicine, the patient has gout; if they are not relieved, some other cause must be sought.

Acute gouty attacks may be provoked by a number of stimuli, not a few of them peculiar to the individual patient. Among these provocations are emotional stresses of various sorts, including marital squabbles; surgery; dietary excesses; and certain drugs such as liver injections. How such different factors pull a trigger on gout in susceptible persons is not fully understood. Extremely high fat diets will cause an increased number of acute attacks of gout. Very few patients normally eat such diets, but, when an obese patient reduces on a low calorie diet, or calorie assimilation is lessened by medical or surgical illnesses, he "lives off his own fat." Under such circumstances, carbohydrate intake should be adequate, and weight reduction should be gradual.

Diet. Contrary to popular opinion that gout is a penalty for high living and over-indulgence in rich foods — an opinion which does not produce much sympathy for the gout victim — there is no good evidence that *severe restriction* of purines, proteins, or alcohol will control the course of the disease. Uric acid, which the gout patient cannot excrete efficiently, is a breakdown product derived from almost every sort of food, so that it is quite impossible to prevent its formation by eliminating this or that foodstuff.

The average gout patient requires little or no restriction in diet. He is advised to avoid foods that are high in purines — liver, kidney, sweetbreads, anchovies, sardines and meat extracts, which contain substances that increase uric acid production. Since such high purine foods are rarely very important to the patient, it is no great deprivation to forego them.

Patients may have individual food idiosyncrasies but these are soon recognized and avoided. Alcoholic beverages can usually be taken in moderation. Patients with severe chronic gout may require a more strict dietary program.

Treatment. Patients with acute attacks of gout are treated with colchicine or phenylbutazone. The initial dose of colchicine sufficient to abate an acute attack quite promptly may cause some diarrhea, nausea and vomiting, but if so the dosage is reduced. Relief is so dramatic that a patient who is in agony from a red hot joint can walk about in a few hours and symptoms are completely gone in 24 to 48 hours. Just how colchicine enacts this chemical magic in gout, but in no other form of arthritis, is an enigma. Phenylbutazone, a quite different drug, is also very effective in relieving acute attacks of gout in most patients. It, too, may cause some side effects that the physician will forewarn the patient about.

Colchicine is frequently used over long periods to prevent recurrence of acute attacks. In such instance the dose is small and may be continued harmlessly and without discomfort for years. Premonitory signs that an acute attack is brewing—slight stiffness of a joint or twinges of pain or other ill-bodings familiar to the patient — indicate that the physician should be notified so that he may prescribe a stepped-up dose of colchicine if he deems it in order.

Despite very effective prevention or control of acute attacks, formation of urate deposits in the body may continue slowly. *Uricosuric* drugs which increase the excretion of uric acid through the kidneys are used to prevent the accumulation of urate deposits in the body. Drugs such as probenecid and sulfapyrazone deplete urate deposits by increasing the excretion of uric acid, but since it may be years, if ever, before such deposits form, the uricosuric drugs are frequently not used until gout has progressed to a chronic state. High fluid intake — say on the order of eight glasses of water a day — is important to assist uric acid "flushing" by the kidneys.

Allopurinol is a newer drug which decreases excess uric acid in a way quite different from the uricosurics. It inhibits an enzyme which produces uric acid from precursor substances, and thus decreases the amount of uric acid in the body, rather than speeding its excretion. This action also helps to prevent the occurrence and recurrence of urate stones and gravel in the urinary tract, a condition to which gout patients are especially liable.

With early medical advice and treatment faithfully followed, the gout patient can be confident that the disease will not cripple him or seriously interfere with his health or accustomed activities.

CONNECTIVE TISSUE DISEASES

A number of the more severe rheumatic diseases are linked by similarities in signs and symptoms. These diseases include such relatively common conditions as rheumatoid arthritis and rheumatic fever, as well as less common diseases such as systemic lupus erythematosus, scleroderma, dermatomyositis, and periarteritis nodosa.

These diseases have in common certain non-specific inflammatory changes of connective tissue which produce local lesions in blood vessels, joints, muscle, skin, heart, and other internal organs. Each rheumatic disease has its typical clinical manifestations which result from the varied distribution and stages of development of these lesions.

Connective tissue serves as the supporting system of the body. Its cells produce the structural elements and matrix of fibrous, bony, and cartilaginous tissues. These not only form a variously tough framework but the matrix supplies lubricating elements of the joint fluids that permit parts to glide smoothly over each other. The predominant substance is collagen, a term formerly synonymous for connective tissue, but now used more specifically to designate connective tissue fibers. "Ground substance" is a sort of cementing material that lies between minute fibers and binds them together. Connective tissue may be regarded as an organ that pervades the entire body and that is subject to diseases of its own or is the "mother site" of diseases which have somewhat similar manifestations as well as clinical differences.

Several names descriptive of this group of diseases reflect the advance of knowledge as well as the limitations of knowledge. They are called "connective tissue diseases" and "collagen diseases," and also "mesenchyme diseases" since all the components of connective tissue arise from the mesoderm, the primary middle germ layer of the embryo.

More recently, the concept of "autoimmune" disease has arisen. This is a rather confusing term to laymen, since it seems to imply that one may be immune to one's self, or have self-immunity. On the contrary, the term means that immunity mechanisms of the body may be so affected or deceived that a person acquires a specific sensitivity to his own tissues, resulting in vascular inflammation and local destruction of tissue. This is very much like an allergic reaction to a foreign protein, except that the substance reacted to is not "foreign" but a constituent of the body — causing a harmful allergic or hypersensitivity reaction to one's self.

There is evidence from studies of blood proteins and precipitation of disease by various sensitivity reactions that an abnormal immune response of the body may be involved. Rheumatic fever, for instance, is associated with a preceding streptococcal infection, but extensive study has failed to implicate a bacterial or virus infection with any of the other connective tissue diseases. A great obstacle to research is the fact that these diseases are only recognized in man. There are a number of relationships of arthritic and rheumatic diseases in experimental animals, but their relevance to human connective tissue diseases is unproved.

Similarity of lesions and symptoms in connective tissue diseases does not imply an identical causative agent or process. Reactions are non-specific, and thus quite different stimuli may provoke a similar response. Research discoveries about any one of these diseases, however, will aid in understanding the others.

Rheumatoid Arthritis

Rheumatoid arthritis is a generalized disease of the body. Its primary manifestations are in the peripheral joints, but there is wide systemic involvement. The disease occurs in every country and climate. About two people out of a hundred in this country have rheumatoid arthritis. But only about ten per cent of these are severely afflicted.

Symptoms. Women are affected three times as frequently as men. Onset of the disease may occur at any age, but most commonly in the years between 20 and 35. Onset may be acute, but is often insidious. Involvement of the joints with fever, loss of appetite and weakness may occur abruptly. More commonly,

signs may stay for a few days, then go away, and recur, and none of them is positive proof of rheumatoid arthritis, but a warning that a physician should be consulted to determine the cause. Symptoms of other disorders may be confusingly similar to arthritis.

Rheumatoid arthritis most often affects the joints of the hands, wrists, knees and feet. Typically, the joint involvement is symmetrical — both hands and both knees. The inflammatory process initially involves the soft tissues of the joint lining and capsule (rheuma-

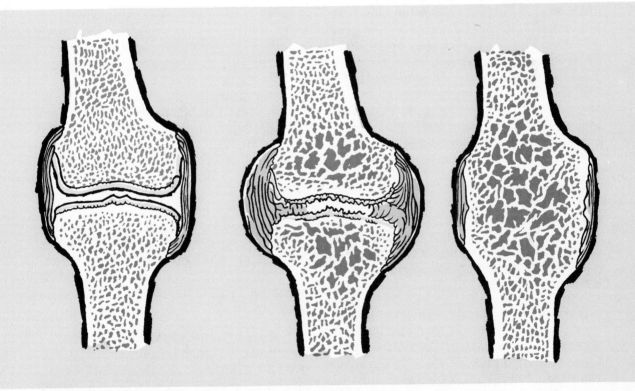

Rheumatoid arthritis has been called "the great crippler," but only about ten per cent of patients are severely afflicted. Drawings of the knee joint, above, show progressive phases of severe rheumatoid arthritis over a period of years. From left to right, inflammation of soft tissues of the joint lining, outpouring of fluids causing swelling; invasion of joint surface with gradual destruction of cartilage; ultimately, in some cases, fusion of bone into a solid mass. Splinting and other measures during active phases of the disease can do much to prevent deformities.

there are vague warning signs that may occur for weeks and months before arthritis sets in.

Early signs may be fatigability, unexplained weight loss, muscular aches and pains, stiffness of joints in the morning that improves as the day goes on. Vague

toid joints often feel warmer than normal). The synovial membrane (joint lining) may produce large amounts of fluid, causing swelling.

Later, the disease may progress to invade the joint surface, with destruction of cartilage, pain on movement, and in some cases, after many years, a fusion of the joint into an inflexible mass of bone. About 15 per cent of rheumatoid arthritis patients develop subcutaneous nodules — hard swellings under the skin, particularly at points of pressure such as the elbows. These are composed of inflammatory fibrous tissue. They may become quite large but do not bother the patient. In a relatively small group of patients with extremely severe disease, the eyes and other sense organs may be involved in the rheumatoid process.

The course of rheumatoid arthritis in an individual patient cannot be predicted with any certainty. The disease apparently may be arrested spontaneously at any stage. Usually it pursues a slow progressive course, interrupted by periods of months, even years, when there is seemingly no activity. In some patients the disease is very mild, causes little if any discomfort, and may be limited to an attack or two. In other patients the disease follows a chronic course for many years before it finally burns itself out.

Diagnosis is based primarily on the history and physical examination of the patient. X-rays can be helpful but may show nothing unusual in the early stage of the disease. Certain laboratory tests, described later, may complement and confirm the clinical diagnosis.

Treatment of rheumatoid arthritis requires the maximum of cooperation and patience on the part of the patient and those who help him. There is no cure for rheumatoid arthritis. Treatment aims to make the patient more comfortable, to modify the disease process by drugs, to maintain and improve muscle and joint function, and sometimes to employ surgery to prevent or overcome deformity.

Drugs

Aspirin (acetylsalicylic acid) in adequate doses is the most widely used, generally effective, safest, and cheapest of all the drugs used in treating the rheumatic diseases. Aspirin is well known as a pain-reliever, but at relatively high doses it also appears to exert an anti-rheumatic effect in ways not well understood (scientists don't yet know exactly how aspirin works).

Patients with rheumatoid arthritis should have an adequate trial of aspirin before other more potent drugs are employed. It is common practice to start with two five-grain aspirin tablets four times a day — i.e., eight tablets a day — and to increase the dosage to the point of intolerance, indicated by ringing in the ears. The daily maintenance dose of aspirin, just below this point of intolerance, is then determined. Many patients are able to take 20 or more aspirin tablets a day for years with safety and with good control of their symptoms, without need of other drugs. This program, however, must be initiated and continued under careful supervision of a physician.

Some patients get stomach distress which generally can be overcome by taking the aspirin with food, or by using aspirin products that are less irritating to the stomach. Aspirin-induced loss of blood through the gastrointestinal tract has been overemphasized. Anemia of such origin has been found to be rare in patients who consume large amounts of aspirin over long periods of time. No matter what other medications are used subsequently, the basic salicylate regimen for rheumatoid arthritis patients is continued.

Gold compounds have been used in the treatment of rheumatoid arthritis for over 30 years and are used quite extensively at present. How they act is not known, but the effect is to modify — not cure — the disease. Gold salts must be given by intramuscular injection since they are ineffective if taken by mouth. A series of approximately 20 weekly injections is given, after which the interval between injections is gradually lengthened to two or three months, more frequently when necessary. It usually requires about six weeks for noticeable improvement to occur. Gold therapy may cause toxic effects, primarily in the skin, blood, and kidneys, in some patients, and the physician makes frequent laboratory examinations of urine and blood to detect early signs of damage to these systems.

Anti-malarial compounds (chloroquine and hydroxychloroquine) have been used in treatment of rheumatoid arthritis for the past decade. Like gold, they seem to exert a modifying effect on the disease, which may become apparent four to six weeks after treatment is started. The drug is usually taken once or twice a day by mouth in tablet form. Very few patients experience any adverse effects, but eye involvement which may be serious may occur in a small proportion of patients. Thus both the patient and the physician must be alert to any early signs of abnormalities of vision.

Phenylbutazone is an effective rheumatic analgesic, the drug of choice in gout and rheumatoid spondylitis, but it is only effective in about 60 per cent of patients with rheumatoid arthritis. The usual dose is 300 mg. per day by mouth; higher doses may be more effective but also more toxic. It takes about three days for benefits to appear. Gastric intolerance is not uncommon and the patient is advised to take the medication with meals. Rarely, toxic effects on the blood may develop, and temporary water retention with swelling of the feet and weight increase may be a problem during the first ten days of therapy.

Adreno-corticosteroids (cortisone and related compounds) can be most useful adjuncts in treatment of carefully selected patients with rheumatoid arthritis. The adrenal glands normally produce hydrocortisone under the stimulus of ACTH from the pituitary gland. A number of steroids which are more potent or effective than the original cortisone, the first synthetic steroid to be used in rheumatoid arthritis, have been produced. These corticosteroids have potent anti-inflammatory effects and can suppress acute inflammatory reactions in rheumatic disease which give rise to heat, pain, redness and swelling. This makes the patient feel better but does not influence the underlying disease process, which remains active.

The same mechanism that is responsible for the beneficial effects of these compounds probably also produces undesirable effects sometimes noted: thinning of the bones, production of peptic ulcers, precipitation of diabetes, psychic effects such as euphoria, and masking of infection. The larger the dose given to suppress inflammation, the more prominent the adverse effects.

Before steroids are employed the patient should have adequate trial of other forms of therapy. Both the patient and physician must weigh the frequently temporary, non-specific relief of symptoms in a potentially progressive disease which can last for years, against the side effects which can cause severe complications.

Nevertheless, steroid therapy has been an important advance, particularly in patients who are not adequately controlled by other treatment and who must continue as active wage-earners and homemakers. For this type of patient, small doses of steroids are given as an adjunct to other therapy, including salicylates.

The former practice of giving large initial doses of steroids and then slowly decreasing the amount is not generally used today. Instead, very small doses divided through the 24 hours are given. This is slowly increased if necessary (usually to not more than two and a half times the initial amount) and decreased if clinical improvement permits. The patient must realize, for his own safety, that *total* suppression of all symptoms by the steroids is neither sought nor desired.

Injection of hydrocortisone or one of the newer derivatives directly into an affected joint may be employed by the physician when only one or two joints are primarily involved. Relief of symptoms by intra-articular injection is usually not as prolonged as in osteoarthritis.

Diet and Nutrition

There is no specific diet for patients with rheumatoid arthritis. No nutritional factor or vitamin has been found to play any part in the cause or treatment of the disease. Vitamin supplements may

may undermine the patient's ability to cope with his disease.

The ability of the patient to consume an adequate and nutritious diet may, however, be impaired by many factors. These include generalized effects of the disease, producing fatigue and loss of appetite, leading to severe weight loss which may be difficult to overcome. Joint deformity, restriction of motion, and pain may cause problems in feeding and preparation of food. Help in overcoming these difficult problems can be obtained through the patient's physician.

Rest and Exercise

These are basic in the treatment of rheumatoid arthritis. Increased rest is mandatory in the active stage of the disease. This may vary from increasing the time spent in bed and adequate rest periods through the day, to sanitarium type care. Even when the disease becomes quiescent the patient should guard against physical fatigue.

Rest for individually involved joints is necessary. For best rest of a joint it should be kept as straight as possible — not flexed or bent, which may seem momentarily more comfortable but tends to increase disability. "Resting splints" to be worn at night or at intervals during the day may be devised, particularly for the fingers, hands or wrists. Knees can be kept straight when resting in bed with footboards and sandbags that prevent the feet from turning out. The use of a cane or crutches should be considered early if joints of the lower limbs are involved; a wheelchair may be advisable.

Rest *does not mean immobilization.* To prevent loss of muscle power and to avoid crippling joint deformity, rest must be accompanied by an active, prescribed exercise program. Simple, effective exercises can be demonstrated by the physician or physical therapist and usually can be carried out at home. (Handbooks for the patient to assist such instructions are available, such as "Home Care in Arthritis" issued by the Arthritis and Rheumatism Foundation).

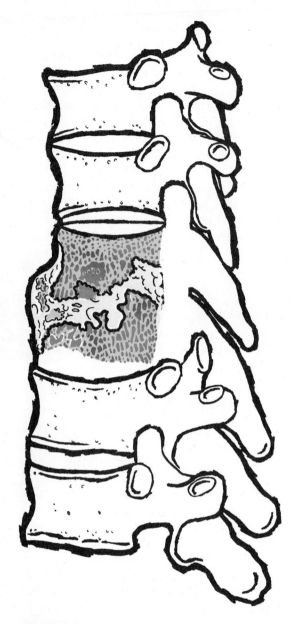

Forms of arthritis caused by infection by specific organisms usually involve only a single joint. Above, cut away section shows arthritis of the spine resulting from infection by tuberculosis germs, associated with tuberculosis elsewhere in the body. Anti-microbial drugs control most forms of arthritis due to infection very effectively, but prompt diagnosis and treatment are necessary to prevent extensive joint destruction.

help the patient's peace of mind but are not necessary for treatment of his arthritis. "Fad" diets should be avoided since at best they are a costly way of obtaining a normal diet, and at worst, by irrational excesses or avoidances,

Important points to remember are that an affected joint should be carried through its *full range of motion* several times each day, and that exercise which produces pain later the same day or the next day should be reduced or stopped but that exercise which is painful only at the time or an hour or two later is beneficial.

Success of an exercise program in strengthening muscles, increasing joint motion and minimizing disability is determined by the persistence and conscientiousness of the patient. Exercises recommended by a physician must become a way of life regardless of the state of activity of the disease.

Heat

Heat is one of the most effective measures for temporary relief of aches and pains of arthritis and rheumatism. It also aids muscles to relax, making exercises more effective.

Care should be taken in applying any form of heat to an acutely inflamed joint, since this may increase pain. In some patients, heat may aggravate symptoms or appear to be of little value; in such situations the physician or physical therapist may advise and demonstrate the use of cold.

There are many ways of applying heat, and the exact method used will depend upon the area involved, the facilities available, and the stage of the disease. Heat therapy is of several types — dry heat, wet heat, and use of counterirritants. In general, heat is applied for 20 minutes a day.

Dry heat is applied by:

An *infra-red tungsten filament lamp* (purchased at a drugstore), an infra-red coil, a household electric heater. These appliances should be kept at least 18 inches from the body.

Bakers, homemade or purchased, using 60-watt electric bulbs in a polished metal frame. These are particularly useful in treatment of the back and lower extremities.

Hot water bottles, bricks, or bags of sand warmed in an oven and wrapped in a blanket.

Electric pads at low heat, with protection of the heated part by a towel to prevent burns.

Paraffin baths using paraffin and mineral oil, prepared in a special container or double boiler. Temperature should not be above 125°F. (see page 29).

Wet heat can be obtained by:

Hot water; when a general bath is used the water should be no more than 102°F. Feet, hands and forearms may be soaked in water of 106°F. In no instance should the soaking be more than 20 minutes.

Hot fomentations are of great value if only one or two joints are painful. These can be given by using a piece of flannel or Turkish towel wrung out of water of 110°F. If such treatments are to be given repeatedly, the use of Hydrocollator steam packs obtainable at a drugstore or surgical supply house is more convenient.

Contrast baths are of particular benefit for hands and feet. The part to be treated is placed alternately in water of 110°F. (for ten minutes) and of 65°F. (for one minute), continuing in the warm water for four minutes and the cold for one minute for a total of 30 minutes, ending in warm water.

Counterirritants may be used in nonarticular rheumatism or osteoarthritis to give a temporary local heating effect. In more acute conditions such as rheumatoid arthritis these should be used rarely and with caution. These preparations consist of various liniments and ointments containing irritant substances which, when applied to the skin, cause a reflex dilation of blood vessels, producing a local feeling of warmth. A common ingredient is methylsalicylate which can be purchased cheaply as oil of wintergreen (caution: toxic if taken by mouth).

Ankylosing Spondylitis

Ankylosing spondylitis (also called *rheumatoid spondylitis* and *Marie-Strumpell disease*) is a progressive disease of the joints of the spine. It primarily affects young men in the third decade of life. The typical initial symptom is low back pain. Examination at this stage may reveal nothing abnormal.

Diagnosis is made primarily by x-rays which show a typical involvement of both sacroiliac joints. Later there is fusion of the small joints of the spine and calcification of the long spinal ligaments, giving the picture of a "bamboo spine."

The disease may become arrested at any stage. In a few patients it may progress slowly until the entire spine from head to pelvis becomes "frozen" or immobile, and chest expansion is impaired by inhibited rib movement. Shoulders and hips may also be affected in some patients, and a few may have involvement of small joints of the limbs in a process typical of rheumatoid arthritis.

The disease is probably related to but is not a form of rheumatoid arthritis as was formerly believed. The test for "rheumatoid factor" is invariably negative. The disease differs from rheumatoid arthritis in its incidence, in that it is almost limited to men, whereas rheumatoid arthritis is most common in women.

Treatment employs analgesic drugs such as aspirin. Phenylbutazone is usually considered the drug of choice in controlling symptoms, and relatively small doses are frequently effective. Adverse reactions to this drug in these patients is rare. Gold therapy is of little or no benefit. X-ray therapy, formerly used to control pain, is not widely employed today.

A program of *posture-correcting exercises* is of great importance, for without its prolonged use the spine will become deformed, leading to severe disability.

Psoriatic Arthritis

Patients with psoriasis may develop a severe, destructive type of arthritis, typically in the fingers and toes. Incidence of rheumatoid arthritis in patients with psoriasis seems to be higher than in the general population. Generally, treatment of psoriatic arthritis is the same as for rheumatoid arthritis except that these afflicted patients should not receive the anti-malarial drugs.

Systemic Lupus Erythematosus

Systemic lupus erythematosus (SLE) is a generalized inflammatory disorder affecting the connective tissues. It is relatively uncommon, although improved diagnostic procedures indicate that SLE may occur more frequently than has been thought. Young adult females are most frequently afflicted. The disorder may be manifested in one or several organ systems — primarily the skin, joints, kidneys, heart, and lungs — at one time.

Joint inflammation, difficult if not impossible to distinguish from rheumatoid arthritis, occurs in most SLE patients. Inflammation of the skin, especially of the face, is common, often with a history of sensitivity to sunlight. Frequently there is a history of pleurisy, anemia is common, and there are various symptoms related to different organs. The red blood cell sedimentation rate is frequently elevated.

Abnormal immunologic reactions in the blood can be demonstrated. The most common of these is the "L. E. cell." These are polymorphonuclear cells which have ingested the nuclei of damaged cells and have a characteristic appearance under a microscope. This phenomenon occurs in preparations studied outside of the body but rarely in the bloodstream itself. L. E. cells are commonly but not invariably found in preparations obtained from SLE patients. A "false positive" reaction to a Wassermann test for syphilis may be one of the early signs of SLE.

SLE was formerly thought to be invariably fatal, but increased knowledge has shown that the disease can exist in a very mild form for many, many years, and that even patients with severe disease can lead relatively normal lives. The extent to which various organs become involved varies a great deal; involvement of the kidneys may be grave.

Treatment is similar to that for rheumatoid arthritis, although gold is not given to patients with SLE. Corticosteroids are used extensively in treating SLE, often with dramatic results. The steroids, which may be lifesaving, are not infrequently used in much larger doses than for rheumatoid arthritis to control the symptoms.

The anti-malarial drugs seem to be particularly effective against the skin manifestations of the disease.

Progressive Systemic Sclerosis

Progressive systemic sclerosis, also called *scleroderma,* is a rare chronic disease in which the connective tissue of the skin and many internal organs is slowly replaced by hard scarlike tissue. The most common symptom is gradually increasing stiffness of the skin, particularly of the face and hands. The skin seems rigid, bound to underlying structures and can't be pinched up easily. This rigidity may interfere with movement of the mouth, eyelids, and other body parts, and, if severe enough, may cause difficulty in swallowing.

Onset of the disease is usually in the fourth to fifth decades, more commonly in women. Generally it progresses slowly over a period of many years.

In treatment, great reliance must be placed upon general aspects of therapy, particularly physical medicine, outlined under rheumatoid arthritis. Gold and anti-malarials are without effect and the corticosteroids are usually of little benefit in treatment.

Polymyositis and Dermatomyositis

Polymyositis refers to an ill-defined group of diseases characterized by weakness and degeneration of muscles, particularly those of the upper parts of the limbs and girdles. When skin changes consisting of eruption and swelling of the face and upper part of the trunk and arms occur, the condition is called *dermatomyositis.* Arthritic or non-articular rheumatic complaints are not uncommon and may be the initial symptoms.

The onset and course of polymyositis may be acute and severe or chronic and indolent. Dermatomyositis tends to be acute, occurs more commonly in children, and in adults is frequently associated with malignant tumors. Diagnosis in early stages is frequently very difficult. Of great diagnostic help are muscle biopsies, muscle enzyme determinations, and studies of muscle electrical potentials.

In general treatment, rest is of prime importance; physical therapy must not be too vigorous. The corticosteroids are the mainstay of therapy. Large doses of selected corticosteroids may have to be given initially, with later reduction to a smaller maintenance level.

Arthritis Due to Infection

Infection of a joint with a pus-forming organism such as the staphylococci requires prompt medical attention to prevent irreversible damage. Such acute infections usually involve a single joint. Swelling, redness, and extreme tenderness develop very rapidly. This type of arthritis may result from infection elsewhere in the body or may follow some injury to the joint.

Treatment is directed at the specific organism causing the infection. Surgical drainage may be necessary in stubborn cases. The joint is immobilized by splints or traction to control pain.

Gonorrheal arthritis, usually affecting only one joint, is always associated with a recent attack of gonorrhea and is not uncommon. Large doses of penicillin are usually very effective in the treatment of this form of arthritis.

Tuberculosis may give rise to a chronic, slowly developing, progressive arthritis, usually involving only one joint and associated with tuberculosis elsewhere in the body. Joints of the spine and knees are most frequently involved. Diagnosis is aided by x-ray, biopsy, and identification of tubercle bacilli by culture or microscopic examination of joint fluid or tissue. Treatment rests primarily on use of the anti-tuberculosis drugs.

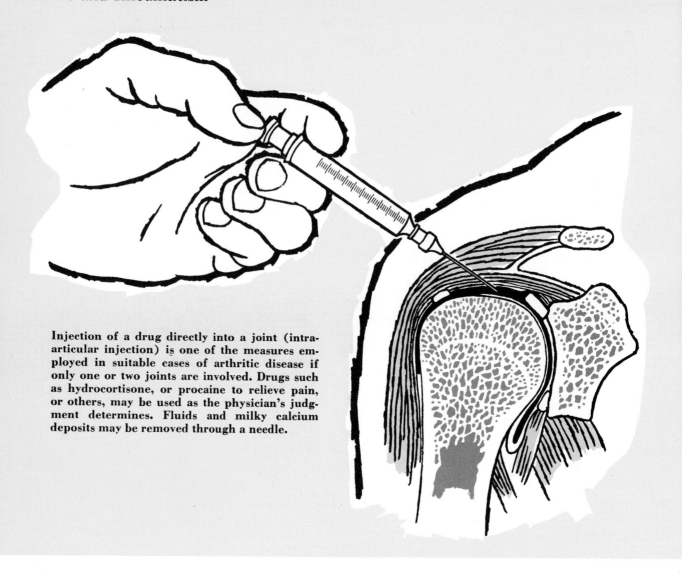

Injection of a drug directly into a joint (intra-articular injection) is one of the measures employed in suitable cases of arthritic disease if only one or two joints are involved. Drugs such as hydrocortisone, or procaine to relieve pain, or others, may be used as the physician's judgment determines. Fluids and milky calcium deposits may be removed through a needle.

Antibiotics and other chemotherapeutic agents have made arthritis due to infection much less of a problem than in the past. This improved outlook, however, implies prompt diagnosis and treatment. Delay can result in extensive joint destruction leading to fusion or severe degenerative joint disease. If the organism is resistant to antibiotics, control of acute infectious arthritis can still be a formidable task.

LABORATORY TESTS

Certain laboratory tests are necessary in diagnosis of rheumatic diseases, in following their course, and in evaluating the effects of therapy.

Routinely at initial examination, and frequently throughout the course of rheumatoid arthritis, white and red blood cell counts, hemoglobin, and the red blood cell sedimentation rate will be determined. Anemia is common in rheumatoid arthritis, and the formed elements of the blood often reflect incipient toxic effects of drugs. The sedimentation rate is an index of the activity of inflammatory lesions of the body.

Urinalysis is necessary not only to determine possible kidney involvement in the connective tissue diseases, but also the toxic effects of medications such as gold.

Tests for the "rheumatoid factor" are performed in rheumatoid arthritis and other connective tissue diseases. It is based on the fact that these diseases, particularly rheumatoid arthritis, give rise to an abnormal protein in the blood. This substance can be detected by using particles coated with a treated normal protein. There are a number of such tests, with names usually derived from the particle used. For instance, a *latex* test employs a polystyrene latex particle; a *bentonite* test uses a special type of clay; a *sensitized sheep cell* test uses specially prepared sheep cells.

The test for rheumatoid factor is positive in a very high percentage of patients with rheumatoid arthritis, but not all. It can also be positive in some other conditions. A negative test is of no diagnostic significance in the determination.

The test for the L. E. cell (lupus erythematosus) is of great value, as are a number of closely allied tests of abnormal antibodies in the blood of patients with SLE and related diseases. Here again such tests are of value if they are positive but not if they are negative. Both the tests for rheumatoid factor and L. E. cell tend to become negative during a complete remission of the disease.

It may be necessary to determine the protein pattern of the serum in the connective tissue diseases. Abnormal relative and absolute amounts of various globulins and albumin are not infrequently found when testing.

Examination of the joint fluid may be important, particularly if only one joint is involved. Tests will consist of culture for microorganisms, microscopic studies for cells and crystals such as uric acid, and tests for the viscosity of the fluid and its ability to form a clot. Biopsy of the joint capsule, either by a special needle or by operation, is sometimes necessary when the diagnosis is in doubt.

X-rays of the joints are necessary not only to establish a diagnosis but to assess the extent of damage. X-ray examination may show nothing abnormal or only soft tissue swelling very early in the course of the disease.

When the rheumatic disease involves other organs such as the kidney, lungs, heart, or eyes, appropriate examinations of these organs must be carried out.

Further descriptions of specific tests and diagnostic procedures, with explanations of purposes and methods, will be found in Chapters 23 and 24.

Misleading Claims

The rheumatic diseases, which commonly inflict pain and have periods of spontaneous remission regardless of what is done, lend themselves admirably to the promotion of questionable products by false and misleading claims. It has been estimated that victims of arthritis spend more than $250,000,000 a year on misrepresented products.

This misrepresentation falls into a number of categories.

Many products are of no value or unproved value. Copper bracelets and similar devices based on a supposed "electrical force," many gadgets with pseudo-scientific rationale, uranium pads, and various vitamin, mineral or herbal preparations, are representative of products that take advantage of human credulity.

Some products do contain an active ingredient, usually a salicylate or form of aspirin, but claims of efficacy may go far beyond the known therapeutic actions and the cost is usually much greater than for ordinary aspirin — a key drug in treatment of rheumatic diseases—which is available cheaply at any drugstore.

Misinformation may be conveyed in books written for the public, not infrequently carrying a physician's byline. Only the advertising of books — not the authenticity of content — is subject to regulation. Some "health" books presenting strange theories or procedures become very popular through effective promotional techniques before regulatory agencies can take action against false or misleading claims. Articles in various media may extol some "magic" cure or treatment and lead innocent sufferers to a tragic loss of money and ultimate disillusionment.

The United States has excellent regulatory agencies to deal with fraud and misrepresentation, but the most powerful weapon against charlatans is education of the consumer. The arthritic patient and the family should know that there are no "secret weapons" against arthritis, that effective measures are known to all reputable physicians and that any new measure of proved effectiveness becomes promptly known to them, and that sensational claims that are heard or read should be judged critically.

Before he buys, the arthritic victim or his family should prudently consider the following points:

Does the advertisement actually say what it appears to say? When read carefully, most advertisements are quite innocuous. If not, this in itself is cause for suspicion of claims.

Are claims put forth in words and pictures reasonable? Many of the visualizations of "unlocking joints" and the like are gross exaggerations that have little relation to reality.

Why is some particular method of therapy presented to the public through media of mass communication, when it has not been presented to or accepted by members of the health professions who are competent to judge it?

The motto of all should be, "Modest doubt is called the beacon of the wise."

ALLERGIES AND HYPERSEN- SITIVITIES

by VINCENT J. DERBES, M.D.

Relationships of Allergy to Immunity · Mechanisms of Allergy · Who Gets Allergies?

ALLERGENS

Inhalant Allergens · Ingestant Allergens · Contactants

DETECTION AND DIAGNOSIS

Skin Tests · Diagnosing Food Allergies

BRONCHIAL ASTHMA

ALLERGIC RHINITIS

Allergic Conjunctivitis

GASTROINTESTINAL ALLERGY

Colic and Allergies · Schoenlein-Henoch Purpura · Indigestion · Urticaria

INSECT ALLERGY

DRUG ALLERGIES

Side Effects · Allergies to Medicines · Cosmetic Allergy

PHYSICAL ALLERGY

Hypersensitivity to Cold · Hypersentitivity to Heat · Hypersensitivity to Light

SPECIFIC TREATMENT

DRUG TREATMENT

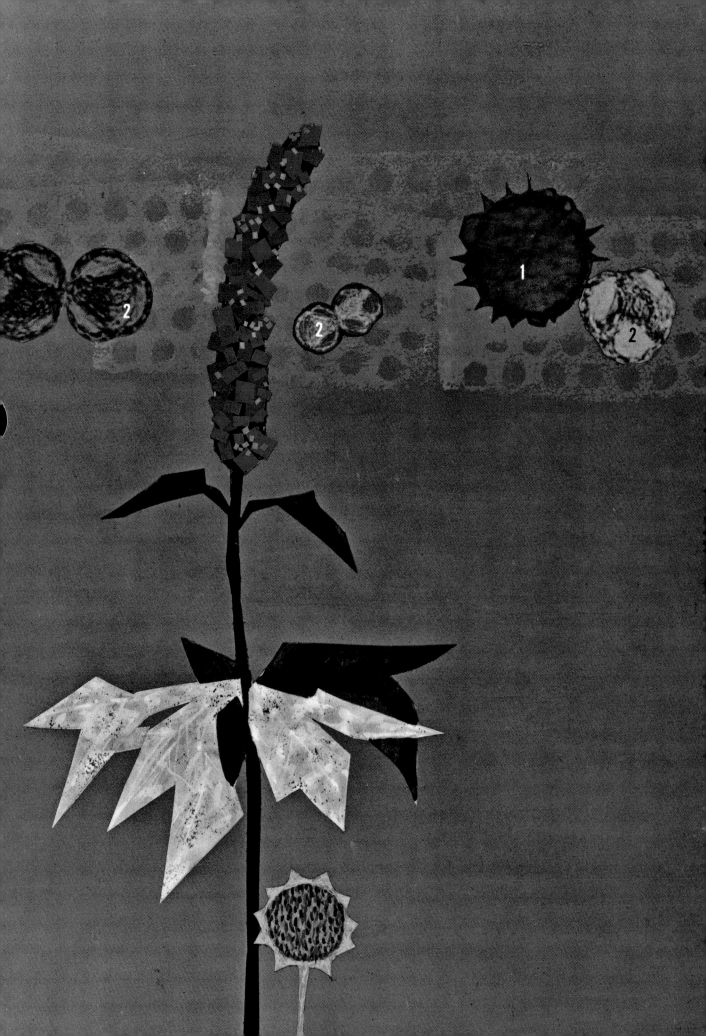

CHAPTER 20

ALLERGIES AND HYPER- SENSITIVITIES

by VINCENT J. DERBES, M.D.

One man sneezes and his nose and eyes water at a certain season of the year. Another man never has such symptoms. One woman wheezes and has difficulty in breathing when a great deal of dust is stirred up in the house. Another woman never does. People who react abnormally to ordinarily harmless substances have allergies. Familiar examples are hay fever, bronchial asthma, allergic conjunctivitis, hives, gastrointestinal allergies, and others which we shall discuss. To people who do not have allergies, the condition may seem trifling and even amusing. But allergies can cause a great deal of discomfort and sometimes are quite serious. Allergies should not be ignored or neglected in hope that they will disappear. We shall see that much can be done to give comfort and prevent matters from becoming worse.

Allergy means an altered capacity to react. The thing to which a person reacts differently is called an *allergen* or *antigen*. An allergen need not be and

generally is not harmful to the vast majority of people. There are hundreds and hundreds of antigens, chiefly foods, dusts, pollens, medicines or other chemicals which cause allergies.

An antibody is a protein molecule which an antigen stimulates the body to make. If the antigen subsequently re-enters the body, the antibody combines with it. This may cause allergic symptoms. Or the process may be protective, like immunization, neutralizing the infectivity of some virus.

A person who is made violently ill by eating some food to which he is allergic will naturally avoid the food and perhaps dislike it intensely. In popular language, "allergy" is sometimes synonymous with "dislike": "I'm allergic to work," "I'm allergic to him or her." Allergy is something far more specific than this. I recall, however, a case where it seemed that a wife had indeed become allergic to her husband. Often when he came home and embraced his wife she felt a tickling in her nose, then sneezed and had difficulty in breathing, and finally broke out with hives. Tensions mounted, until the wife sought medical help. She proved to be

Pollens produced by weeds, flowers, trees and grasses are among the most common causes of allergic reactions. The color plate shows *sunflower* pollen (1) and *ragweed* pollen (2), greatly enlarged.

allergic to horses. The husband had taken to horseback riding, and horse dander in his clothes caused his wife's unromantic reactions. He changed his sport to golf and all was well.

Idiosyncrasy means a reaction peculiar to the individual. *Anaphylaxis* derives from Greek words meaning "removal of protection," and in American usage refers to sudden, life-threatening forms of allergy. In Europe the word is often used synonymously with allergy. *Atopy* is used interchangeably with allergy. An atopen is an allergen, atopic is allergic.

Relationships of Allergy to Immunity

Allergy "acts as if" it were a protective, immunity-giving mechanism gone wildly out of control. It is similar in principle to vaccination which gives immunity to smallpox or polio, but consequences are very different.

When a person is infected by a germ or his cells are in contact with a non-living, non-toxic antigen for the first time, a complex series of events is initiated. Germs invade tissues and chemical substances which stimulate formation of antibodies are set free. In the case of non-living antigens, it is the antigenic material itself which stimulates antibody formation. The time required for antibodies to form is referred to as the incubation period, during which time there are no symptoms.

When antibodies are formed, cells have a specifically acquired capacity to react (for which the word allergy was coined). Specificity means that for each antigen there is one antibody which reacts only on contact with that antigen. However, most substances which cause allergic reactions are complex materials which contain or may contain more than one antigen. Horse serum and milk, for instance, contain several different proteins which may act as antigens.

What happens if a rabbit is injected with a culture of virulent staphylococcus germs? It dies of infection in a day or two. The rabbit's body in effect becomes a culture medium in which the germs appear as individual organisms, not as clumps. Very few are engulfed by white blood cells and there is little or no abscess formation. Competition of the germs for nutritive material needed by the cells, plus toxic materials set free by their growth, causes the animal's death.

Immunization. But suppose that a rabbit receives injections of a culture of the same virulent germs which have been killed by heat. This animal has had experience! It has produced antibodies in response to antigens of the dead germs. Now, if the animal is injected with a culture of the same living germs which kill an unprotected animal, events are quite different. A severe local reaction occurs at the site of injection and an abscess is formed. Few germs appear in the bloodstream and those that do are quickly removed. Germs in the tissues are clumped and most of them are engulfed by white blood cells. The rabbit survives. This is the physical basis of vaccination.

Infection. Similar events occur in an infectious disease process such as syphilis. Within a few hours after syphilis germs enter the body they are widely disseminated but there are no symptoms during the incubation period of several weeks. Thereafter, a chancre develops. Antibodies are now present as is evidenced by the fact that a blood test is positive. The chancre results from tissue reaction to materials formed as a result of union of antigens of syphilis organisms with the newly formed antibody.

The chancre is a local allergic inflammation. If at this time new syphilis germs invade the patient's body, he does not become reinfected. In the chancre area there are myriads of organisms from which toxic materials can be freed by antibody action. In areas where new syphilis organisms gain entrance, antibodies destroy them before they can multiply. Amounts of toxic materials formed are too small to injure cells. The patient has local tissue allergy (chancre), disease (syphilis), and local tissue immunity, all at the same time.

From the foregoing we can see that characteristic features of various infections result from defense mechanisms of our bodies. In the process of competition between the invading organisms and our tissues, we are made ill. Similar events and essentially the same process occur in allergies such as hay fever and bronchial asthma. We see exposure of the body to a non-living antigen, an incubation period during which antibodies are developed, and an allergic reaction following antigen-antibody union.

Allergic diseases may be said to result from deranged immunity machinery. The body goes to the same effort to rid itself of harmless or even nutritious materials as it does to rid itself of severe infections. The effort expended is totally out of proportion to need, like using an elephant gun to kill a mosquito. It is normal for a person to feel a tingling, itching sensation and to sneeze if a small insect gets into the nostrils. But a few microscopic grains of pollen in the nose of a person with hay fever cause explosive bouts of sneezing and grossly excessive outpourings of fluid.

Mechanisms of Allergy

There are two characteristic features of allergic symptoms. Certain body cells become "leaky," or one might say weepy, and pour out fluids. Smooth muscle (the kind concerned with "automatic" actions) contracts. Combination of these effects underline allergic reactions.

The location of an antibody when it unites with an antigen modifies the consequences profoundly. If the antibody is free in the bloodstream *(circulating antibody)*, the antigen is simply neutralized. If the union takes place in or on a cell *(bound, fixed,* or *sessile antibody)*, neutralization may also occur but this is a side issue. Distressing effects may be caused by a disturbance of cells or by release of toxic substances.

Exactly how chemical substances are freed from cells which contain them is not clear. Of these substances, *histamine* is probably most familiar to the public because of extensive use of antihistamine drugs, but a number of other chemicals — serotonin, acetylcholine, a so-called slow-reacting substance, heparin, kinins, and perhaps others — are also involved.

The drawing shows typical characteristics of an allergic reaction in the skin: increased inflow of blood and "leakage" of fluid into spaces between cells. At left, section of normal skin. At right, distended local blood vessels and exudates producing a wheal, a sharply delineated swelling.

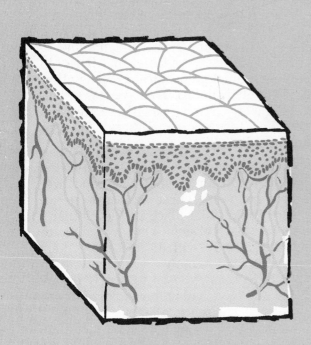
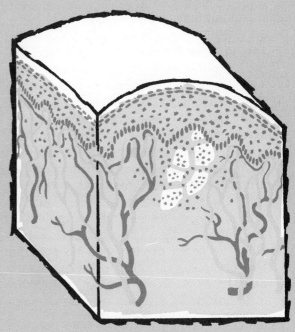

Histamine plays some part in all allergic reactions of the immediate type. It dilates small blood vessels, causing local reddening (erythema) and a central wheal, a raised, sharply delineated swelling caused by excess fluid. Histamine also causes contraction of smooth muscle. Alone or together, these actions may result in symptoms that differ with the nature of the affected "shock organ" — that is, the organ or tissues in which the allergic reaction takes place.

Effects of wheals and swelling, for instance, vary with location. Wheals on the skin are hives. In mucous membranes of the nose, whealing produces stuffiness and if fluids pour out in excess there is a runny nose. Hives in the throat or tongue may interfere with breathing. In bronchial asthma there is swelling of mucous membranes plus contraction of muscle around the bronchioles. The combination constricts air passages and interferes with breathing. Similar changes in the intestines may produce colic and diarrhea. Allergic swellings may produce a type of arthritis. Persistent wheals in the brain may cause unremitting headaches.

Other chemicals. Actions of other chemicals released by cells are not so well worked out. Acetylcholine is interesting because it is the chemical by which important nerves exert their action, and connections with the brain afford a plausible route by which *emotions* may influence, or some would say produce, disease states. Thus far, evidence of acetylcholine's importance is overwhelming in only one allergy: *cholinogenic hives,* a condition seen chiefly in certain red-headed young women when they become overheated from exercise or high temperatures or become emotionally distraught.

Kinins, which may be regarded as miniature proteins, cause pain, whealing, contraction of smooth muscle, and dilation of blood vessels when applied at appropriate sites. They may be responsible for some discomforts of rheumatism or prolongation of attacks of asthma. Drugs such as aspirin which are antagonistic to the kinins relieve rheumatism and often help asthma.

It is to be hoped that research may yield specific knowledge of intricate interactions of these and perhaps other substances, leading to medicines which may block the symptom-producing machinery of allergy.

Who Gets Allergies?

It is difficult to make even a rough estimate of the incidence of allergic diseases. About 10 per cent of the population have frank allergies, usually subacute or chronic; about half give histories of transient episodes. Estimates of the incidence of particular allergic diseases vary greatly. We recently questioned all undergraduate students at Tulane University. Of 4,455 young men and women from all sections of the country, 11.5 per cent had bronchial asthma, 10 per cent had hay fever, and another 15 per cent of these young people had recent episodes of hives or contact dermatitis.

Heredity is an important factor in predisposing people to allergic diseases. But study of heredity in human disease is difficult, nowhere more so than in allergy. Parents and relatives may be unaware of allergic diseases or for various reasons may conceal them. What is inherited is not a specific disease, but a tendency to develop sensitivity. A parent with asthma may have a child with hay fever.

Race has little to do with allergy susceptibility. The opinion is widespread that Negroes are relatively immune to allergic diseases. As Chief of Allergy in a large municipal hospital I can say that this simply is not so. We have few Orientals in New Orleans, but I have seen and treated all of the various allergic diseases in Japanese and Chinese.

Age. Allergy may begin at any age. Even though an incubation period precedes symptoms, first exposure to an antigen may take place in the mother's womb. Most persons who are going to develop allergy will do so before their fortieth year, simply because by then they have been exposed to nearly everything and have had ample opportunity to become sensitized to allergy.

Pregnancy. The effect of pregnancy on allergic disease varies from complete relief to extreme exacerbation. I believe that asthma in particular should be treated during pregnancy because severe attacks may provoke miscarriage. Asthma often worsens at the time of the monthly period. Some women have nasal congestion at this time, and this adds to obstruction already present from allergic rhinitis. Atopic dermatitis often worsens with menstruation or pregnancy.

ALLERGENS
(Substances that trigger allergic reactions)

How do allergens get into the body to provoke reactions? They may be inhaled as dusts or pollens. They may come into contact with the skin. They may be contained in food or drink. We will not attempt to catalogue all possible offenders, but will mention some important ones, together with facts about distribution and mechanisms, which are of value in diagnosis of allergies.

Inhalant Allergens

Pollen granules are formed in enormous numbers in the male sexual organs of plants. Hay fever is the best-known example of an allergic reaction caused by pollen *(pollinosis)*. Plants with brightly colored flowers which attract insects have heavy, sticky pollen which clings to insects and is transported by them to the female flower — the bees and the flowers. Heavy, sticky pollen is not significantly airborne.

Plants which depend on wind pollination produce tremendous amounts of pollen, since only a minute fraction can reach their destination on the female flower. Such pollen is very light and can be carried long distances on air currents. One can get an idea of the prodigious output of pollen from observations made by Dr. A. A. Thommen. A single ragweed plant produces *eight billion* pollen grains per square foot of field surface. If all the ragweed pollen produced in the United States each season were piled together

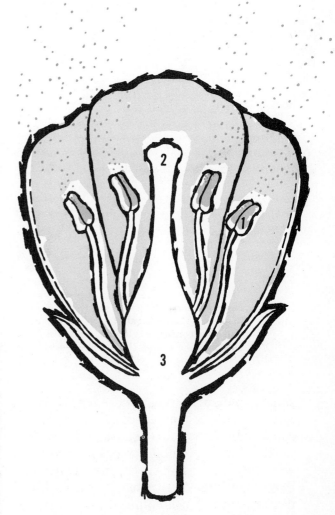

Typical sexual structure of a plant, showing the *anther* (1), the male pollen-producing element. The female element includes the *stigma* (2), which receives the pollen grains, and the *ovary* (3). Plants that depend on wind-borne pollination produce enormous amounts of very light pollen that can be carried over many miles by air currents.

it would form a pyramid as high as a 50-story office building with a base over 1,000 feet in diameter.

Windborne pollen has been found 17,-000 feet in the air and 500 miles at sea. This explains the failure of attempts to eradicate ragweed in Chicago, Denver, Duluth and elsewhere. Even if all ragweed plants were eliminated from a community, copious amounts of pollen

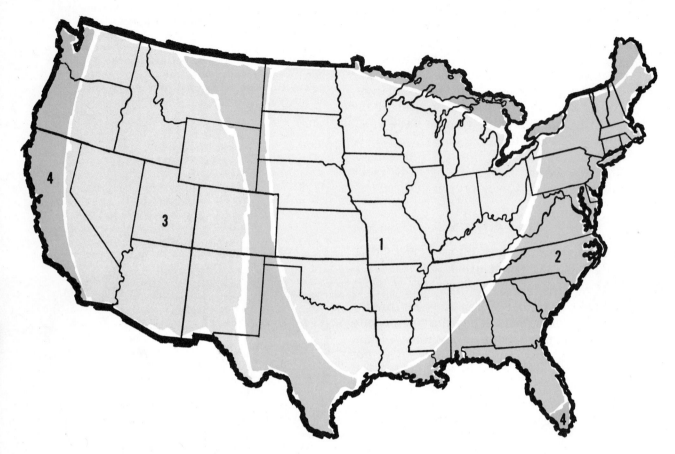

"Hay fever map" showing approximate concentrations of seasonal ragweed pollens. Heaviest concentrations are in the central states area (1), less in area (2), still less in area (3). Best relief is obtained in area (4) which includes the Pacific Coast, extreme southern Florida, and northern Great Lakes and New England regions. Other pollens than those of ragweed and related weeds can cause allergic reactions.

can be blown in from the countryside. Pollen from ornamental flowers may cause hay fever but exposure must be much closer. Rambler roses outside a window and cut flowers within the house have been shown to cause allergy. But flowers in the garden almost never cause hay fever symptoms.

Allergists always question patients as to the *time* when symptoms occur. There are three major pollen seasons:

Early spring:
  Tree pollens

Late spring or early summer:
  Grass pollens

Late summer and fall:
  Weed pollens

Plants do not deliver pollen into the air at a constant steady rate, but in "spurts" during certain periods of the day. A few shed pollen in the afternoon, but more, including ragweed, shed in the morning. More pollen is shed on a sunny day, and a brisk wind stirs more of it into the air and carries it farther.

Pollen counts are made by exposing glass slides covered on one side with sticky material. The slides are exposed to air, protected from wind and rain, for 24 hours, and then the number of granules in a given area are counted under a microscope. Pollens can be identified by shape and size. Grass pollens have a smooth exterior, ragweed pollens a spiny or prickly surface, and others resemble small golf balls.

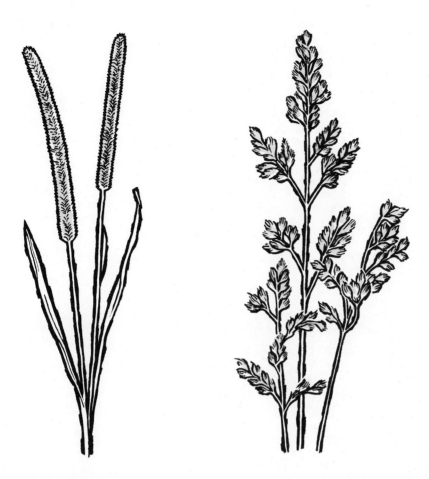

Wind-borne grass pollens are frequent causes of allergic reactions. Two of the most important offenders are *timothy* and *bluegrass*, shown at left and right in the drawing, respectively. Their pollinating season is May and June. Some southern grasses pollinate over more extended periods.

Grasses comprise one of the largest plant families, all wind-pollinated except a few which are self-pollinated. There are perhaps 1100 varieties of grass in the United States, of which about 12 are implicated in hay fever. Throughout the northern states, adjacent Canada, and higher parts of the Appalachian region in the south, *timothy and bluegrass* contribute large amounts of airborne pollen. Pollination of northern grasses begins in late May or early June, depending on latitude, and lasts four to six weeks. In the south and southwest, *Bermuda grass* is the dominant hay fever and asthma grass. Its extreme season is early spring to late fall. Several other grasses are of some local significance as allergens.

Trees. Forest and shade trees of North America are prodigal producers of wind-borne pollen, in contrast to fruit trees and shrubs with colorful blossoms which are insect pollinated. *Oaks* probably cause more early spring symptoms than all other trees, but there is only about one case of oak pollen allergy to 50 of ragweed. *Elm* pollen is sometimes as thickly in the air in central and eastern states as ragweed pollen. *Hickories,* including pecan, walnut, and butternut, shed fairly large quantities of pollen. Greatest exposure is in pecan and walnut-growing areas. Some of the worst hay fever I have seen has been caused by pecan pollen. *Cottonwood* species sometimes cause severe symptoms. *Willow, birch, ash,* and *maple* are of minor importance, but account must be taken of local tree families in allergy testing.

Weeds. The *ragweed* family is the most important group of hay fever and asthma-producing plants. It includes a number of ornamental flowers such as the daisy, coreopsis, dahlia, carnation, and chrysanthemum. Pyrethrum, an important insecticide, is derived from a species of chrysanthemum. Cut flowers of this group and insect sprays containing pyrethrum should not be used in homes of persons allergic to ragweed.

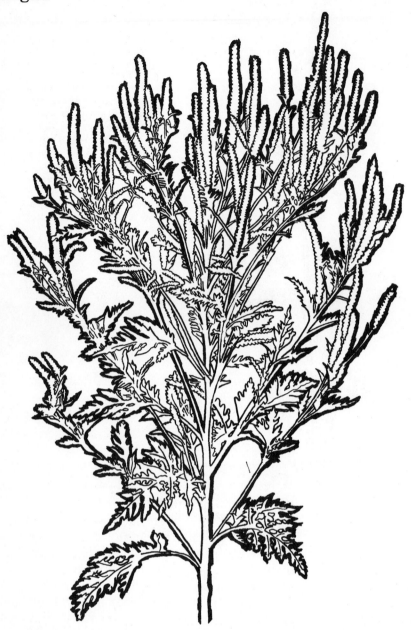

Ragweed is the most important hay fever and asthma-producing plant. August and September are the peak months for ragweed hay fever in most parts of the country. Common ragweed is shown in the drawing. There are also giant and other forms of ragweed, and other plants closely enough related to it to give trouble to ragweed-sensitive persons.

The major ragweeds are *common ragweed, giant ragweed, western* and *southern ragweed, marsh elders,* the *false ragweeds, cocklebur* and *sagebrush,* related *wormwoods,* and *dog fennel.* One or another of these plants is found all over the country and they are sufficiently related that a person who is allergic to one will have some trouble from any of the others.

The *goosefoots* and *carelessweeds* are a closely knit family entirely unrelated to other types of hay fever plants. Important members are *Russian thistle* and *Mexican fireweed;* of lesser consequence are *lamb's quarters* and *redroot pigweed.*

Most of the antigenic species are found in the Missouri River basin, where they are often a more frequent cause of allergy symptoms than local ragweeds. They usually begin to shed airborne pollen about a month before the ragweed season.

Spores. Mushrooms, green bread mold, wheat rust and *corn smut* are examples of fungi which shed buoyant airborne spores. Recognition of fungus spores as an important cause, and a frequent complicating factor, in respiratory allergy is relatively recent. In central agricultural regions of the country mold spores are a more frequent cause of respiratory allergy than animal danders and rank behind pollens and house dust. The fungus species known as *alternaria* contributes the greatest share of airborne spores and is the most important in most parts of the United States. Alternaria was the cause of recurrent potato blights which caused famine in Ireland in the nineteenth century and led to waves of immigration to this country.

Several circumstances suggest fungus allergy. One is that symptoms occur in persons around farms, grain mills and elevators. Another is that hay fever or asthma lasts from early summer to late fall, often a month after the ragweed season is over. Finally, in cases of year-round sensitivity of uncertain cause there is a possibility of fungus allergy.

Hay fever. From May until the first cool snap of fall an unknown allergen appears to be in the air throughout the southern coastal plains area. Large numbers of people react to it with hay fever (nasal obstruction is more prominent than sneezing, itching, or watery discharge). A lesser number have asthmatic symptoms. Evidence suggests that the antigen is one of the airborne fungus spores, probably from a plant parasite.

House dust. The most frequent cause of bronchial asthma and one of the commonest factors in hay fever is house dust. It is a fine grayish powder formed by aging of materials of household articles. It is physically, chemically, and biologically different from materials of mattresses, furniture, rugs, curtains, chests, paper, books and clothing, from which it comes. It is entirely different from street or earth dust. The responsible antigen in house dust is a protein. Allergic symptoms from house dust may be seasonal or perennial. When symptoms are present all year they are usually worse in fall, winter, and spring, particularly in spring and fall. In seasonal cases allergic symptoms appear in cool and cold months and tend to disappear in hot summer months.

Animal danders. All mammals shed their skins, but in bits or flakes seldom larger than a pinhead. This material tends to get trapped in hair and is referred to as scruff, dander, or dandruff. It can cause bronchial asthma, rhinitis, or hives. Of all animal danders, that of the horse is most important. In pre-automobile days, "horse asthma" was common. Many cases are occupational, in farmers, jockeys, stablemen and horseback riders. But susceptible people may react to the odor or dander of horses on a person who has had contact with the animals.

House pets. Numbers of allergic people react to cat or dog hair. All allergists have difficulty in convincing patients that their pets cause their symptoms and persuading them to give them up. For some reason which escapes me, the delusion is widespread that chihuahua dogs in the house will alleviate bronchial asthma. This absurdity may be compared to "prevention" of yellow fever in my father's boyhood in New Orleans by burying a lemon in the front yard.

Dander of rabbits, cows, goats, hogs and other animals rarely causes trouble except when exposure is quite intimate. Wool is generally poorly tolerated by people with atopic dermatitis. In its aging it converts gradually into lint and then into house dust which produces hay fever.

Ingestant Allergens

Sensitivity to foods may produce all the manifestations of allergy, and may be a complicating factor in patients sensitive to inhalants. Attacks of bronchial asthma may be caused by inhaled food antigens, as in bakers or flour millers, but the usual route of invasion is by ingestion.

Methods of detecting foods responsible for individual allergic reactions will be discussed later in this book.

Egg. Albumen or white of egg, and yolk proteins to lesser degree, are common causes of allergy which may be quite severe. Cooking the egg does not denature the protein sufficiently to prevent symptoms except in mildly sensitive persons. Persons allergic to egg should not only avoid it as such, but also the many varieties of foods that contain it.

An incomplete listing of foods containing eggs includes:

salad dressings	frostings
mayonnaise	icings
cream sauces	custards
ice cream	puddings
sherbet	meringues
water ices	waffles
mousses	griddle cakes
most cakes	desserts
cookies	fruit whips
many breads	pancake flours
pastries	candies
French toast	some sausage
muffins	macaroni
pastes	spaghetti
meat jellies	noodles
certain baking	glazing for breads,
powders	buns, pretzels

Eggs are frequently used to clear soups, coffee and wines. Egg batter is used to soak chicken, fritters, and sundry fruits and vegetables before cooking.

Milk is an important allergen, both plain and as an ingredient of a great variety of foods. It causes more symptoms in children than adults and shows a tendency to decreasing potency as age advances. Denaturation of milk by heating or drying decreases its allergenic potency. Commercial cream contains considerable milk and a hypersensitive person should avoid it. There is much less milk protein in butter, perhaps one per cent. Margarines may contain milk protein, hence a milk-sensitive person should use only the types made exclusively with pure vegetable oils. Unless their sensitivity to milk is great, persons may eat reasonable amounts of cheese without symptoms. Milk from goats or other animals, or milk substitutes with a soybean base, may be given to infants intolerant to cow's milk.

Meat. Innumerable kinds of meat are eaten the world over, and frequency of sensitivity depends mainly on frequency with which various kinds are eaten in a given locality. Those of interest to us are *beef, veal, lamb, mutton, pork,* and certain *game*. Pork probably leads the list of animal allergens. Ham and bacon are somewhat denaturized by curing processes. Bacon is further denaturized by frying. Hence, people who cannot eat pork roast may be able to enjoy bacon. Lamb and mutton usually cause less trouble than pork or beef.

Chicken and duck are the most common allergens of the bird family. In general, allergy due to birds is infrequent, but goose, turkey, guinea hen, squab, partridge, pheasant, quail, grouse, and other game birds may sometimes be the cause of these common allergies.

Fish, and especially shellfoods, are potent allergens and may produce severe allergic reactions. One must assume that any kind of edible fish may cause allergy. A short time ago a young boy being tested reacted strongly to trout.

"What happens when you feed him trout?" I asked his mother.

"He has never had it," she said, "because I found out that if I fried it in the kitchen, if he were in a part of the house where he could smell it, he would break out in hives and develop bronchial asthma."

Seafoods are one of the most important groups causing hives and are responsible for much gastrointestinal allergy.

Cereals. Wheat flour is by far the most important offender in this group. It is used in such a variety of ways that complete elimination is almost impossible, and symptoms may persist in a wheat-sensitive patient. *Rice* is an important cereal but has so little tendency to cause allergies that it is a common constituent of trial elimination diets given to allergic patients. *Corn* ranks high as an allergic factor, but corn oil, corn syrup, and corn starch seldom cause trouble. *Rye* may produce the symptoms of asthma.

Vegetables. Almost any vegetable can produce allergic symptoms in sensitive persons. The most common vegetable offenders are legumes (beans, peas, lentils, peanuts), potatoes, tomatoes, and celery. Other vegetables which may cause asthma and other allergic symptoms, though less frequently, are asparagus, beets, Brussels sprouts, cauliflower, cucumber, eggplant, garlic, green peppers, mushrooms, olives, onions, pumpkins, radishes, rhubarb, spinach, squash, sweet potatoes and turnips.

Sensitivity to chocolate is quite common and may cause allergic rhinitis or asthma. Tea occasionally causes trouble, but less so than coffee. Walnuts and other nuts can cause allergy which is sometimes severe.

Allergy to fruits is less frequent than to vegetables. Citrus fruits probably lead the list, but apples may also cause severe symptoms. Strawberries are known as a common cause of hives.

Alcoholic beverages. All types may cause allergic symptoms due to traces of denatured protein of raw materials or substances used in manufacture. Whiskies are made from grains, rum from fermenting molasses derived from sugar cane, malt beverages from cereals. Corn, malt, rye, barley, yeast, fruits, even vegetables, are variously involved in distilling and brewing processes and may evoke symptoms in sensitive people. Wine is a definite offender. Fish glue, egg white, and isinglass are used for clearing beer, wine, and champagne. They are all allergens. Alcoholic beverages (except carbonated) almost always help bronchial asthma and almost always make hives worse in sensitive skin.

Contactants

Acids, strong alkalis, and the like which cause trouble the first time the skin comes in contact with them are *primary irritants*. No one is immune to them and true allergy is not involved. Contact antigens are materials which are harmless to most people but produce allergic symptoms in sensitive skin. Contactants are numerous and of increasing importance.

Persons may develop contact dermatitis from animals or their pelts or leather, but usually the trouble is caused by dyes or materials used in processing. Leather in shoes, gloves and hatbands frequently produces rashes. Wool aggravates dermatitis but is not often the cause. Dermatitis of the hands may follow preparation of fish, meat or fowl dishes.

Plant contactants are of far greater importance than those of animal origin. About two-thirds of people will be allergic to poison ivy or oak after they have touched it once, and most people in this country have done so. Any of the ornamental flowers can sensitize, but the most likely ones are primrose and tulip bulbs. Some weeds, especially ragweed, can cause dermatitis. All of the vegetables can cause contact allergy, as can sawdust of woods used by carpenters and hobbyists.

It is impossible to list all contactant allergens because of the increasing number of synthetic materials, plastics, dyestuffs and chemicals. New offenders are reported almost daily. Paints, insecticides, polishes, waxes, detergents, and other household chemicals cause a certain amount of contact dermatitis. Metals, chiefly nickel and chromium, frequently cause protracted dermatitis but copper, zinc, tin, and the precious metals to a lesser extent, may also be antigenic.

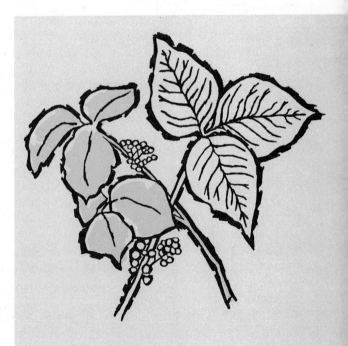

Poison ivy — "leaflets three, leave it be." One's very first contact with poison ivy does not cause any trouble, but later contacts are likely to produce a severe skin eruption in most people. Poison oak and poison sumac contain the same irritating oils as poison ivy.

DETECTION AND DIAGNOSIS

Diagnosis of allergic diseases is generally easy and will be discussed later in considering symptoms of various allergies. Identification of the offending substance is far more difficult and at times taxes the skill of the physician and the patience of the patient to the utmost. It is rather like a detective story in which painstaking work turns up clues which hopefully point the finger of guilt at the responsible antigen.

History. Time of onset (month and year), character (acute or insidious), and probable precipitating factors are important clues. Most patients tend to date onset from their first major episode, but questioning often discloses earlier minor episodes, and time of onset dates from the first symptoms.

Recognition of the month or time of year when symptoms first appeared helps to narrow the search. For example, ragweed allergens are prevalent in late August or September, grasses in May or June, house dusts in colder months when the furnace is on and windows closed. Housewife's eczema may be related to birth of a baby with increased immersion of the hands in water and detergents. Insidious onset suggests gradual sensitization to an everyday allergen of the environment, whereas acute onset suggests the provocative role of something unusual such as a sinus infection, unusual food, new cosmetic or garment, insecticide or rug, or a seasonal pollen. A sudden dermatitis suggests a potent sensitizer such as poison ivy or hair dye.

The terms "daily," "bimonthly," "seasonally," and "continuously" indicate frequency of contact with allergens. Mild episodes as well as major attacks should be noted. This may help to pinpoint the culprit. Examples are the farmer who has mild hay fever daily when feeding his livestock but severe hay fever and asthma when harvesting hay and threshing, or the eczema of a patient which is greatly aggravated by hot water or cold air. Duration of the attack may indicate severity of the allergy or duration of exposure to the allergen, as in the housewife who sneezes a few minutes after making beds, or the victim who has hay fever during an entire pollen season.

Clues. Often the way a patient gets relief from an attack will give a clue to the cause. For example, outdoor exercise or fresh air will help the patient with asthma due to house dust. Hot drinks relieve allergy to cold.

From such clues as the above, attacks can frequently be attributed to pollens, bedding, occupational exposures, or food, in a general way. The next stage is to identify as many specific allergens as possible. Any food believed to produce symptoms should be recorded, as well as any intense dislikes. Dislikes of children are frequently protective and should not be considered whims until so proved.

Inhalants and contactants should be discussed in detail. Common causes of trouble are exposures to vegetation in hunting, fishing, or picnicking. Questions should be asked about sprays and fumes of fresh paint, perfume, disinfectants, formalin, and insecticides, all of which can affect the skin or respiratory tract. What is the effect of face and bath powders, flour, soap flakes, or animals? Is there a room, sofa, chair or bed which causes trouble? Are there any new clothes, furniture, pets or hobbies?

Skin Tests

There are two chief methods of skin testing. One is designed to detect the presence of antibodies which are found in the immediate wheal and flare forms of allergy, for example, hives, hay fever, and asthma. Here a *scratch* or *intracutaneous test* is made. The other type is used for the identification of substances responsible for delayed type allergy, that is, the contact dermatitis group. Here the *patch test* is used.

Scratch tests are usually made on the back or forearm. There are many variations in making scratch tests, but certain fundamentals must be adhered to. The skin is broken in a way that gives a slight oozing of serum but no frank blood.

The disposition of the scratches must correspond to the order of the vials in the testing boards. Each vial contains a separate antigen. For example, if there are seven rows of six vials each in the pollen testing board, the doctor makes seven rows of six scratches on the patient. A different allergen is applied to each scratch. A positive reaction takes place promptly, within 15 or 20 minutes.

In the **intracutaneous test,** a syringe and needle are used to introduce allergens *into* rather than on the skin. These tests are also "read" in 15 to 20 minutes. In either type a positive reaction resembles a mosquito bite, and consists of an itching, irregular shaped wheal surrounded by a pink halo or flare. The wheals persist for an hour or two but rarely may remain for 24 or even 36 hours.

Such tests are most accurate with pollens or inhalant allergens where the reliability is of the order of 95 to 98 per cent. Unfortunately, with foods the reliability is far lower. Errors here are in both directions, i.e., a positive reaction may be given to a food which can be eaten with impunity, or a negative reaction may be present to foods to which the individual is allergic.

In certain instances direct skin testing is not feasible, e.g., in persons with widespread skin disease, or with dermographism (skin writing, a condition in which any injury to the skin, however slight, produces a wheal). Here the *passive transfer* is employed by withdrawing one or two teaspoonsful of blood from the patient's vein, allowing it to clot, and removing the serum. The recipient is usually some member of the family.

One half of the back is marked off checkerboard fashion with a skin marking pencil, and a drop of the serum is introduced into each site. Two to four days later these sites are tested. The uninjected half of the back is used as a control, the same test substances being applied to symmetrical areas.

The patch test when positive duplicates the dermatitis from which the patient is suffering. In the *open* patch test, the material in question is applied to the skin and allowed to remain uncovered. In the *closed* method, which is more widely used, some of the test material is placed on a Band Aid, which in turn is applied to the skin. Reactions are "read" in 48 hours. Patients are told to remove the patches if there is any burning, stinging, itching, or other discomfort.

These tests are quite useful but, as in the case of all tests, must be interpreted with some skill. Even when everything has been done properly, the positive reaction tells only that the individual is allergic to that material. It does not prove that that material is causing the rash in question. As an example, a woman may have a contact dermatitis from hair dye. Yet she will in the majority of cases also give a positive reaction to poison ivy because approximately 70 per cent of Americans are allergic to poison ivy. Not only must the person be allergic to the substance being tested, he must also have come into contact with it prior to the development of the eruption.

Diagnosing Food Allergies

The various methods of skin testing with foods are far less satisfactory than tests with inhalant allergens. Therefore, preliminary to skin testing there should be a detailed discussion concerning the patient's habits and allergic experiences with food. Skin tests are then done, after which the patient is placed on a trial or diagnostic diet which will aid in discovering the food offenders.

This is a temporary diet arranged to relieve symptoms as soon as possible. If the patient becomes symptom free after a week on a given diet, new foods may be added until the symptoms return. The last foods added are again removed, and others substituted. With patience, over a period of some weeks or months, the allergenic foods can be identified by the use of this temporary diet.

Elimination diets. Another approach, when symptoms are present daily, consists of using *elimination diets* of the type described by Rowe. These diets are made up of foods supposedly low in allergenic values.

Alvarez has found that a useful diet is one consisting of nothing but *lamb, rice, butter, sugar, canned pears,* and *water,* these being selected because they are easily prescribed and seldom are offenders. Breakfast consists of a lamb chop with puffed rice (rice flakes, steamed rice, or rice cakes fried in butter). The noon and evening meal will have to consist of the same foods, but their preparation can be varied. No condiments, flavoring, or sauces are used.

If the patient is not sensitive to one of the foods used, relief should be obtained within about 12 hours. If there is no relief, the diet is maintained for another 36 hours. If there is still no relief, it means: (1) the symptoms are not due to foods; or (2) the patient is sensitive to one or more foods in the diet. In the latter case, an entirely new diet of *beef, carrots,* and *string beans* is tried.

Then, if there is no relief from symptoms, the patient may fast for a couple of days. If the symptoms are not relieved, the patient is probably not allergic to foods. Restriction to such an elimination diet for more than two days is unnecessary, as most patients get relief at the end of 12 hours. However, in atopic dermatitis the elimination diet may be necessary for several weeks.

Food diary. If symptoms are intermittent, offending foods may most easily be recognized by the use of a *food diary,* in which everything that is eaten is written down. It is not sufficient to write down a list of the foods in a notebook, for this is difficult to interpret. A record form must be used in which the foods are listed when they are eaten.

The general principle is shown in the accompanying example of a "Sample Food Diary" which, in compact form, identifies the foods eaten by a patient over a period of one month. The chart-like form makes it easier to identify an offending food in association with symptoms that occur when it is ingested, and to exonerate foods that are innocent.

BRONCHIAL ASTHMA

Bronchial asthma is a disease characterized by a wheezing or whistling type of recurrent shortness of breath, associated with an annoying cough. The attack may last from a few hours to weeks or longer. Some unfortunate persons are never free of asthma.

The attack typically comes on during the early morning hours. The patient may have gone to bed feeling perfectly well or may have been aware of certain warning symptoms. An episode of hay fever or sinusitis may have occurred the preceding day. There may have been fatigue for no apparent reason.

The paroxysm starts with wheezing two or three hours after retiring. In the beginning this does not disturb the patient, but may be conspicuously audible at some distance. From a troubled sleep he passes to fitful wakefulness, and as the attack progresses he becomes fully awake and then sits up.

At the peak of the attack the patient presents a distressing sight. He usually sits in a chair, not caring to move or speak. The mouth is open and the expression anxious; the eyes are wide open and the face is pale with slight bluing of the lips. It is such an effort to breathe that beads of perspiration may appear on the forehead, even in cold weather. The muscles which increase the capacity of the chest are strained to the utmost.

Coughing is almost incessant during the attack. The cough is usually nonproductive at first and often precedes the attack. Later sputum is brought up. It usually is thick and tenacious. Generally the character of the sputum changes during the episode, becoming thinner and more readily expectorated as the attack ameliorates.

Vomiting which may follow a severe paroxysm of coughing, especially in children, often relieves the distress. Fever may be present; in the absence of pneumonia it rarely exceeds two or three degrees. More generally the temperature is normal or even subnormal.

SAMPLE FOOD DIARY

DATE:	1	2	3	4	5	6	7	8	9	10	11	12	13	14	15	16	17	18	19	20	21	22	23	24	25	26	27	28	29	30
INDIGESTION OCCURRED:									x							x							x							
FOOD:																														
Coffee	x	x	x	x	x	x	x	x	x	x	x	x	x	x	x	x	x	x	x	x	x	x	x	x	x	x	x	x	x	x
Eggs	x	x	x		x	x	x	x	x			x	x	x	x	x		x	x			x	x	x	x	x		x	x	x
Ham	x	x	x		x					x			x	x			x	x		x	x		x			x	x			
Bacon				x		x	x	x	x			x	x			x	x	x			x			x		x			x	x
Bread	x	x	x	x	x	x	x	x	x	x	x	x	x	x	x	x	x	x	x	x	x	x	x	x	x	x	x	x	x	x
Milk	x	x	x	x	x	x	x	x	x	x	x	x	x	x	x	x	x	x	x	x	x	x	x	x	x	x	x	x	x	x
Beef	x		x	x	x		x		x				x			x			x			x		x					x	
Potato	x			x	x			x		x		x	x	x			x	x			x		x	x	x			x		
Shrimp Remoulade									x							x							x							
Pork		x				x		x		x		x	x						x				x		x					
Chicken									x							x			x			x								
Beans		x				x	x			x				x				x								x	x		x	
Beer			x			x		x				x							x	x						x				x
Fish																x			x					x						
Cauliflower				x															x											
Oyster					x					x									x					x						
Olive									x										x											
Green Salad		x	x			x	x	x		x			x	x			x	x			x			x	x	x		x		
Corn				x		x										x							x				x			
Peaches										x						x												x		

In this instance indigestion consistently followed eating shrimp remoulade on three occasions. Twice indigestion followed ingestion of chicken, but chicken was eaten on two other days without causing trouble. Indigestion developed after eating olive once and not after another time. The other foods, e.g., bread, milk, and so on, although eaten on the same days as the indigestion was manifested, were eaten many times without difficulty, hence are not offenders. Therefore something in the shrimp remoulade is almost certainly the cause of the patient's indigestion. The chicken and olive would be merely suspect. But the prime suspect would be the shrimp remoulade.

The acute attack of asthma either responds promptly to appropriate medication or, in those instances in which no treatment is used, the asthmatic attack usually runs a self limited course.

Status asthmaticus. If the seizures become constant or refractory to treatment, *status asthmaticus* results — intractable asthma that lasts a few days to a week or longer and may end fatally.

As the patient becomes worse, breathing becomes more labored, the oxygen lack and carbon dioxide excess may cause the lips and fingernails to become bluish (*cyanosis*), there is a hacking cough, and often fever which may rise to 103° F. or even higher. The patient may sink into a profound coma or even die.

Status asthmaticus may end then in death due to exhaustion, in recovery in several days or weeks, or in consolidation of portions of the lungs and high fever. In protracted forms, so called right-sided heart failure may occur, a condition which itself is life threatening.

Mistaken "pneumonia." There is a form of asthma which is often erroneously diagnosed as pneumonia. Children especially are apt to retain the secretions of the mucous glands of the smaller bronchial tubes. This mucus may become hardened into plugs, especially, as is often the case, when the child becomes excessively dried out from inadequate

Mechanisms of bronchial asthma. Drawing at left below shows normal lung structures: *bronchiole* (1), *alveolar duct* (2), air cells or *alveoli* (3), *smooth muscle* (4). In an acute asthmatic attack, at right, smooth muscle constricts air passageways in bronchioles, plugs of sticky mucus obstruct smaller bronchioles (5). Spasm of bronchial muscles and/or excessive secretions impedes inflow and, particularly, outflow of air trapped in distended alveoli.

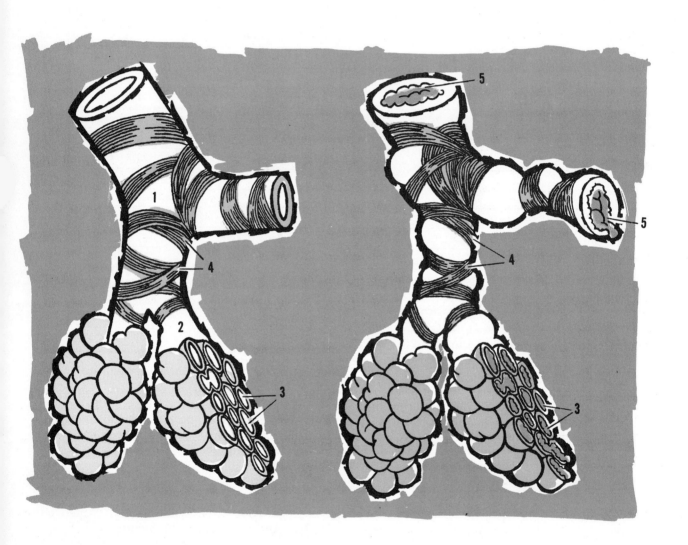

drinking of fluids during the attack, or from vomiting. The area of lung supplied air by these bronchioles collapses. The poor drainage allows infection to set in, with all of the signs and symptoms of pneumonia being present. Allergy should always be considered when a child has repeated bouts of pneumonia.

Forms of asthma. There are two major forms of bronchial asthma. *Extrinsic asthma* is that form in which the offending substance — dust, pollen, food — enters the body from the outside world. *Intrinsic asthma* has its origin from within the body, from such a source, for instance, as a chronic sinusitis.

It is possible for the doctor to differentiate these two types clearly in most instances, but it must not be inferred that these varieties are mutually exclusive. It is not uncommon to see individuals who exhibit combinations of these in varying degree, or who start with one type and later have added to the original variant the characteristics of the second. The separation is by no means an academic one, for the treatment and outlook of the two types vary considerably.

Extrinsic asthma usually starts in childhood or young adulthood in individuals who have a strong family background of allergic disease. Furthermore, they themselves often have other allergic diseases, particularly hay fever or atopic dermatitis. Positive skin tests are the rule, and treatment based on the information derived from these tests is generally successful. Attacks can be anticipated and prevented as the antigen is usually identified. These patients with extrinsic asthma have a good outlook as far as longevity is concerned.

In contrast, *intrinsic asthma* begins, as a rule, after the fortieth year. Positive skin tests are rare; when present, positive-reacting substances cannot be shown to stand in causal relationship to the attack. By the same token, the family incidence is not greater than in the populace as a whole. Again, the concurrence of other allergies is not usual.

Typically, these patients have a history of chronic respiratory infection, usually manifesting itself by cough. This cough becomes progressively worse, and finally symptoms of respiratory distress supervene.

In early cases there are long periods of remissions between attacks, but with the passage of time the remissions become shorter, and the attacks more protracted until finally intractable status asthmaticus results. Many persons with intrinsic asthma are allergic to drugs, chiefly aspirin, and taking them will bring on attacks, but their elimination is followed by only partial relief.

The prognosis here is much worse. The mortality rate for such people is appreciably higher than for other people. The extra mortality from intrinsic asthma is due chiefly to high death rates from respiratory and cardiac conditions.

Diagnosis. The history and clinical picture of bronchial asthma are usually so characteristic that the diagnosis is easily made — often by the patient before he sees the doctor. But occasions arise when there is confusion with other diseases or when other diseases may be mistaken for bronchial asthma.

The presence of other diseases may overshadow the asthmatic picture or vice versa. Important differences in treatment and prognosis of many of these conditions demand that they be ruled out. Difficulty in breathing associated with some type of noisy respiration accounts for the confusion of most of these conditions with asthma.

In childhood, a foreign body in the lung, croup, bronchiolitis, or laryngeal disease present problems in differential diagnosis. In adults, cancer of the lung, heart disease, and emphysema may mimic asthma closely. Sighing respirations (*hyperventilation* syndrome) are very common and may accompany psychoneuroses, but not necessarily so. Stable individuals under unusual circumstances may also present this picture. The patient feels he cannot get air into his chest. In emotional upsets such respirations are more frequent. There is no cough, wheezing, or sputum.

Treatment. As in other allergic diseases, there are three basic methods of treatment: *avoidance* of the offender, *desensitization* if avoidance is not feasible, and *symptomatic* treatment by medicaments. The great majority of asthmatic persons can obtain a considerable degree of relief from symptoms, and many can be cured by modern therapy. Results of desensitization are particularly favorable in children or when the disease has not led to permanent heart or lung damage.

In general, the antihistaminic drugs, so valuable in hay fever and hives, are of lesser importance in asthma. The foremost drugs are adrenalin (epinephrine) and its close relatives. I have not ceased to be impressed with the dramatic benefit which adrenalin so typically affords since my boyhood when I first saw it used in my young brother's case. The family had seen Albert in attacks many times, and we knew that he would suffer for hours. But this was in 1918, and progress was being made!

Our family doctor belonged to the old school, dressed formally, and in fact was somewhat pompous. That evening he came into Albert's room, took out a large gold watch with heavy chain and fob, and placed it on the bedside table. He made his preparations and held the hypodermic syringe up in the air like the baton in a conductor's hand.

"Albert, look at the second hand of my watch. Before it has made one complete circle, you will feel relief," he said.

And so it happened, a miraculous effect, which I have seen repeated many times since. When the epinephrine family fails, recourse is had to cortisone and its relatives.

Various methods of facilitating bringing up sputum, such as expectorants, steam inhalations, and postural drainage may be helpful. In serious cases it may be necessary to hospitalize the patient where supportive measures such as fluid administration by vein can be carried out. Presence of fever indicates infection which is treated as usual.

ALLERGIC RHINITIS
(Hay Fever)

Allergic rhinitis (Greek *"rhinos,"* the nose) is generally characterized by seasonal or perennial sneezing, nasal congestion and blockage, and copious flow of watery mucus from the nose, which usually itches intensely.

Hay fever (pollinosis), the seasonal form, a familiar subject for not-so-funny jokes, is generally induced by wind-borne pollens or fungi.

There are distinct regional patterns, but one may generalize and say that the

spring type is almost always due to *tree pollens* (e.g., oak, elm, maple, pecan, birch, cottonwood). The *summer type* is usually caused by *grass pollens* (e.g., Bermuda, timothy, sweet vernal, orchard, Johnson) or fungus spores (e.g., alternaria, helminthosporium, and hormodendrum, for which there are no common names, as well as wheat and corn rusts and smuts). The *fall type* of hay fever is due to *pollens* of the ragweed family in the Eastern and Central States and to pollens of the chenopod-amaranth family in the Western States.

Symptoms. Every year, and indeed often on the same day, certain persons feel a mild itching of the eyes, a tickling in the nose and throat, and a burning or sore sensation of the mouth. These patients recognize thus that their seasonal attack has started.

During the next few days, as there is increasingly more pollen in the air, the symptoms become increasingly more uncomfortable. There is now a pronounced reddening and swelling of the conjunctiva (the membrane covering the front of the eye), burning feeling in the eyes, and much tearing. On awakening the lids are often glued together by dried mucus secreted during the night.

There is a similar worsening of the catarrhal (head cold-like) signs of the nose and throat membranes. In the mouth the burning and sore sensation persists, but the nose swells to almost or entirely complete blockage; its membranes are intensely inflamed. In place of the earlier mild itching and occasional sneezing, there is now an uncontrollable flow of burning watery fluid with hundreds of sneezing fits. The mucus secretion may be so profuse that 20 or 30 handkerchiefs are soiled daily. The bloodshot eyes are made more uncomfortable by light, which is avoided (*photophobia,* a fear of light). Hay fever may be associated with allergic symptoms of other parts of the respiratory tract such as the larynx (*laryngitis*), trachea (*tracheitis*), the bronchi and bronchioles (*bronchitis, bronchial asthma*). Such a worsening of symptoms is not generally present, but mild air hunger and persistent dry cough are frequent.

In almost all patients there is an associated increase in irritability compared to their normal amount of "nervousness." Their sensitivity to light and sound intensifies. They attempt to protect themselves, for example, by wearing dark glasses, or even by avoiding external exposures, as by bed rest in a quiet, darkened room.

Headache is common, chiefly in the forehead and back of the neck. While usually not intense, its persistence adds to the discomfort. Because much mucus is swallowed, there is often an associated disturbance of the digestive tract. Retching is common, and in some patients, a distinct tendency to vomiting. There may be constipation or diarrhea. Rheumatic joint pains are not rare, and finally many patients complain of itching of the skin or even of dry or weeping eczema during the entire pollen season.

The duration of symptoms corresponds to the flowering period of the plant in question; in the case of trees, generally three weeks; grasses and weeds tend to pollinate six weeks. Multiple sensitivities are common so that a person may successively have periodic symptoms from each of the major groups of offenders with many months of discomfort.

Perennial allergic rhinitis differs from hay fever in that it is not seasonal but runs a continuous course with variations in severity. Symptoms are similar to those of hay fever, but usually less severe. Sneezing may be the only manifestation. Nasal blockage is a prominent feature. The discharge is thin, watery, and often profuse. A high percentage of *eosinophils* (a cell which stains red with the dyestuff eosin) is diagnostic.

Inability to smell *(anosmia)* is much more common than in seasonal hay fever. There is no permanent damage to the olfactory (smelling) nerves, but the passages leading to them are obstructed by swelling of the mucous membranes or by polyps (growths in the mucous membranes of allergic persons, resembling small grapes). As the sense of smell plays a large part in our appreciation of taste, patients often say they cannot taste, somewhat of an exaggeration, for sensing of the primary tastes (sweet, salt, sour, and bitter) is not impaired. There is usually a return to normal function after allergic or drug treatment, although removal of the polyps may be required.

The causative factors of perennial allergic rhinitis are more numerous than those of hay fever. Household dust, foods, and animal danders are the chief offenders. Industrial dusts and vapors are often responsible. Pollens may play a part. Chronic nasal infection, sinusitis, nasal malformation, and polyps are contributory factors to the symptoms.

Diagnosis. The patient often makes his own diagnosis. The finding of numerous eosinophils in the mucus from the nose helps differentiate allergic from other forms of chronic rhinitis. The allergen responsible for the symptoms is to be identified by means of history and skin tests previously described.

Treatment. This includes avoidance of allergens, specific desensitization, antihistamines, and steroid drugs. Nose drops and inhalants are sometimes helpful, but their prolonged use may cause the nasal membranes to become persistently boggy, often long after the particular offender is out of the air.

Allergic Conjunctivitis

Conjunctivitis of an acute or chronic catarrhal form usually is part of a larger allergic syndrome such as hay fever. An acute conjunctivitis often is associated with contact dermatitis of the eyelids which may be caused by overflow of various drugs placed in the eye for treatment. Conjunctivitis may occur alone through direct contact with air-borne substances such as pollens, fungus spores, various dusts, or animal danders. Food allergy has been demonstrated as an occasional cause.

Conjunctivitis caused by infection is discussed on page 568.

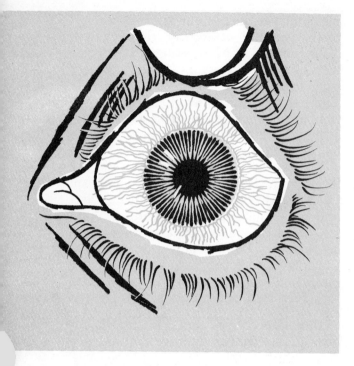

Typical "pink eye" of allergic conjunctivitis associated with hay fever. Vernal conjunctivitis is a variety that appears in the spring and diminishes or disappears in the colder months. There are other non-allergic forms of conjunctivitis caused by infection by bacteria or viruses (see Chapter 16).

Diagnosis. Itching is prominent. Cases associated with hay fever show prominent congestion of the eye vessels, giving a bloodshot appearance (pink eye). The usual allergic tests are employed to identify the offending allergen.

Treatment. Removal from exposure to the cause, when possible, is primary. Otherwise desensitization is attempted. Ophthalmic (eye) adrenocorticoid preparations give prompt relief. Eye washes are soothing. When itching is intense, eye compresses or an ophthalmic anesthetic solution may be employed. If sunlight is offensive to the eyes, dark glasses are mandatory in the treatment.

GASTROINTESTINAL ALLERGY

If the degree of sensitivity is high enough, even the briefest contact of a food with the lips or mouth will produce an allergic response. The most common reactions are itching and burning, leading to swelling or even to hemorrhage into the mucous membranes. In general, the disturbance disappears as soon as contact with the food is ended. The tongue often takes part in the reaction, but the severe swelling, in which the enlarged tongue fills the entire mouth and may even impair breathing, is usually caused by materials brought to the tongue by the blood.

Cold sores or fever blisters on the lips and canker sores in the mouth may be due to food allergy. Fever blisters (herpes simplex) are caused by a specific virus, but there are a number of precipitating factors which cause the lesions to appear, including sunburn and diseases such as head colds, pneumonia, and meningitis. Canker sores are very frequent and are painful out of proportion to their size.

Other causes of *allergic stomatitis* (inflammation of the mouth) include tooth powders and pastes, mouth washes, cosmetics, medicaments, dentures, and other dental material.

Denture stomatitis may be due to ill-fitting plates, but it is not uncommonly due to allergy to the plate itself. This may be tested by applying some of the material from which the plate was made, or the plate itself, to the skin, say of the upper arm. The test substance is held in place with adhesive for 24 or 48 hours. If a positive reaction occurs, some other denture material, similarly tested and found to be nonallergic for the particular patient, should be employed in the making of new dentures.

Digestive symptoms. Antigen-containing foods remain in the stomach long enough for contact-type responses to be common.

Symptoms of *allergic gastritis* (inflammation of the stomach) include a sense of fullness, pressure in the upper abdomen, excess acidity, nausea or vomiting, especially explosive vomiting, shortly after mealtime. Because of spasm of the pylorus (gateway out of the stomach) the food may remain for a number of hours and produce considerable discomfort. The reverse may take place: if the offending food has not been removed by vomiting, the irritated stomach may expel it rapidly into the intestine, which in its turn may also empty rapidly, thereby causing diarrhea.

Anaphylactic shock is the most startling and tempestuous of the responses to allergenic foods. Fortunately, it is exceedingly rare. It consists of a severe acute reaction following ingestion, with nausea, vomiting, diarrhea which is sometimes bloody, violent pains, often hives, collapse of the circulatory system, and even death within minutes or hours.

Colic and Allergies

Colic in infants is extremely common. It is impossible to say what percentage of infants have colic, since a certain amount of fussiness is natural, and crying that might be considered normal in one household might be regarded as intolerable in another. About half of infants up to three months of age seem to have some degree of colic.

The attack usually begins suddenly. The cry is loud and more or less continuous. Recurrent paroxysms may continue for several hours. The face is congested and may be slightly bluish; the abdomen is distended and tense; the legs are drawn up on the abdomen; and the hands are clenched. The attack may end when the infant is completely exhausted, but often there is relief with the passage of feces or gas. Holding the baby upright or permitting him to lie prone across the lap or on a hot water bottle or heating pad is occasionally helpful. Antihistaminic, smooth muscle-relaxing drugs, and sedatives are useful.

Certain infants seem to be peculiarly susceptible to recurrent attacks of colic. The cause is usually not apparent, although it may be associated with swallowed air which has passed into the intestine. Overfeeding may sometimes cause discomfort and distension, but rarely to the degree seen in colic.

Certain foods, especially those of high carbohydrate content, may be responsible for excessive fermentation in the intestines. Food allergy is also a cause of colic, but it is important to realize that other conditions, some of them life-threatening, also can cause colic. The chief of these is intestinal obstruction which usually requires surgery for its relief. The colicky baby should be seen by the pediatrician.

It has recently been pointed out that much colic is due to withdrawal of the mother's hormones at birth. In such instances, administering these has afforded prompt relief. Prevention of attacks should include adequate feeding techniques, including facilitation of belching, the avoidance of underfeeding, and the search for a possible allergenic food in the infant's diet.

Schoenlein-Henoch Purpura

This disease for which there is no common name attacks the skin, the gastrointestinal tract, the joints, and the kidneys. It is by no means rare, and perhaps is increasing in frequency. About one-half of the cases follow an upper respiratory tract infection; about one-fourth are due to food allergy; and in the remaining one-fourth no cause is usually found.

The disease may begin with joint or abdominal pain, followed by a skin rash within hours to a day or two. Sometimes all occur simultaneously, less frequently the rash starts first. There is generally a feeling of malaise and a low grade fever in half of the cases. The skin changes begin as hives. After a varying interval a pink or red spot appears in the hive. When the hive disappears, usually within 24 hours, a purplish spot remains, giving the disease its name. This spot is caused by hemorrhage into the skin and the subsequent changes are those seen in black and blue marks. The skin lesions appear in crops and usually do not itch.

Involvement of the joints, usually of the knees or ankles, is found in about two-thirds of cases. There may be mild pain or swelling or both. Motion may be limited. The joint changes are temporary and do not leave permanent deformity. The kidney is attacked in about half the cases.

If a specific food can be shown to be responsible, the patient should avoid it. When the disease follows an infection, vigorous measures should be used to be sure the streptococcus is eliminated. Cortisone and related drugs are of great value in controlling the tendency to hemorrhage but are less useful in helping the kidney involvement. Relapses are not common unless food allergy is the cause.

Indigestion

Hypersensitiveness to specific foods is a frequent cause of indigestion, but it must not be thought that all or even most food intolerance is on an allergic basis. It is well known that people with gallbladder disease do poorly when they eat high fat meals. Persons with peptic ulcer have their symptoms worsened after highly seasoned foods. Indigestion may also be due to relative indigestibility of foods, such as green apples. Suspicion of an allergic basis of indigestion comes more readily to the patient if he knows that he has a strong family incidence of allergy, or if he suffers from some clearly allergic disease such as hay fever.

Detection of offending foods. Skin tests are so unreliable as to be valueless in many instances. More helpful information can be obtained from elimination diets or food diaries already described, or from a careful, time-consuming history in which the patient is questioned regarding his experience with all the common articles in his diet.

Only by the exercise of certain procedures can we be sure that foods are responsible for the symptoms. There should be an improvement or disappearance within a reasonable time after elimination of the suspected allergen. Similarly, there should be an exacerbation or reappearance of symptoms when the food is again eaten.

One might feel that the diagnosis of gastrointestinal allergy, including allergic indigestion, should be a simple procedure. As a matter of fact, those who have seen persons with gastrointestinal allergies with one or more telltale scars from mistaken surgical diagnosis realize how frequently the symptoms may resemble those of organic disease.

The first requisite in diagnosis is the realization that allergy may be responsible for the given set of symptoms. Following this, appropriate steps as previously described will prevent most of the pitfalls. Treatment here centers about avoidance of offending foods, as desensitization is impracticable. Antihistaminics have a distinct sphere of usefulness here.

Urticaria (Hives, Nettlerash)

Urticaria is familiar to most people because of its frequency. Its diagnosis offers no difficulty to the physician, in contrast to the tedious efforts often required to identify the cause of a particular episode. Usually there is an abrupt appearance of wheals, resembling mosquito bites closely, and varying from the size of a pea to that of the palm of the hand. They may be associated with a mild burning pain, but more generally there is an intense or even intolerable itching.

There may be a few isolated hives, but the rule is for much of the body surface to be covered with wheals. The duration of the individual lesion varies from a few minutes to one or two days, but the attack seldom runs its course in less than a week. Indeed, I have seen many patients in whom hives were continuously present for 10, 15, or even 20 years. Generally the eruption has a whitish color, but it can vary from pink, to rose, to crimson. The surface is smooth, and excoriation of the skin is rare in spite of the intense itching because the eruptions continually change location. The initial burning discomfort is soon transformed into intense itching, which increases particularly at night and leads to paroxysms of uncontrollable scratching.

A characteristic feature of the eruption is the simultaneous presence of fresh and of disappearing lesions. These are not confined to the skin. There is frequent involvement of the lips, the mouth, the tongue, gastrointestinal tract, and the genitourinary system.

Giant hives. The ordinary hive is rather superficial. If, however, the changes are somewhat deeper, it is usual for a larger area to swell, producing *giant hives,* or *angioedema* (Quincke's edema). These do not itch; their importance resides in the fact that their large size may obstruct vital passages.

A number of deaths have resulted from strangulation from giant hives of the tongue or larynx. When the tongue is greatly swollen, curative medicines cannot be swallowed. I know of such a death in which medicine was indeed on hand, but the giant hive developed slowly while the victim slept. He awakened abruptly, found himself unable to talk, but finally got the medicine, which he was unable to get past his enlarged tongue. The horrified family got him into their automobile, but in spite of their haste, he died before they reached the hospital which, ironically, was only five minutes away. Although urticaria is very common, such tragic episodes are rare indeed.

The incidence of hives is such that 15 per cent of individuals have at least one attack. No age group is spared; it is seen in suckling infants as well as the aged. About 60 per cent of cases are seen in the second and third decades of life. Females are afflicted twice as often as males, perhaps because of the increased use of medicines by women for relief of the discomforts associated with menses.

An attack of urticaria, even a severe one, is in the majority of instances a solitary event, not again experienced. But in about one-third of the cases, especially in the middle years, there may be repeated attacks, or the disorder may persist for weeks, months, or even years, continuously or intermittently, with an ever increasing, disturbing influence on physical and emotional well-being.

In contrast to the transient hives of some young people, the chronic form causes great diagnostic and therapeutic problems. Often in spite of the most painstaking efforts the responsible factor is not identified by the allergist.

Causes. The following causes of urticaria are recognized:

1. *Antigens coming from without:*
   Medicaments and cosmetics
   Foods and ingestants
   Inhalants
   Insects, parasites, and worms

2. *Antigens coming from within:*
   Chronic and acute infections
   Internal diseases, especially cancer

3. *Physical factors:*
   Heat, cold, light, pressure, sweating, overexertion, and fatigue.

4. *Nonallergic factors:*
   Insects and plants
   Psychogenic disturbances

Drug antigens. Although hives once were predominantly caused by foodstuffs, the most important cause today is medications. A number of studies indicate that of all instances of urticaria, 30 to 35 percent can be attributed to drugs. But if only acute urticaria is considered, this rises to 53 per cent. The prototype of drug urticaria is *serum sickness* which follows the administration of "foreign" (horse or other animal) serum in the prevention or treatment of tetanus (lockjaw), diphtheria, and so on. The same picture is not rare after other medicines, especially penicillin.

Of particular significance, in addition to the usual signs and symptoms *(hives, joint pains, enlarged lymph nodes, fever)* is the latent period of five to 12 days between taking the drug and developing the allergy. This makes history-taking difficult, and unless the patient is specifically questioned on this point, the historical reconstruction may fail. Such "serum sickness" has also been due to various organ preparations (ovary, testes, pancreas, pituitary), and even to an ordinary aspirin tablet.

The list of drugs which may cause hives is so long that it may be said that there is scarcely one, even the most harmless, which cannot at times cause urticaria. At the head of the list probably would be protein-containing materials such as pollen extracts. In addition to the sensitizing potential of a drug, the method of administration or the frequency of use also play a role. Parodoxical as it seems, antihistamine drugs, of such value in treating urticaria, may at times cause it.

Food antigens. After dinner, I passed a box of candies to my guests.

"That one looks nice. Is it dusted with Brazil nut powder?" one woman asked.

"Leave it alone, Leah!" her husband warned her.

But she ate it. Within minutes, her tongue swelled to the point where it protruded from her mouth, she was unable to swallow her saliva which drooled, her eyes became bloodshot and her face suffused, hives broke out before our eyes.

When the time lapse between eating a food and the appearance of symptoms is short, the cause and effect relationship is quite obvious. But usually the diagnosis of food-caused urticaria is much more difficult.

The ingestion of foods is coupled with the digestive process. The particular food in its original state may not cause allergy, but only after it has been converted to a simpler form by digestion. This may require 12 or more hours. Furthermore, scratch tests for foods often fail for this very reason, namely, that the test material does not correspond to the split products actually causing symptoms. Because each food is split into hundreds of simpler forms, it is impossible to test for all, and we must resort to elimination diets and food diaries. When the food causes trouble prior to digestion, that is when symptoms come on promptly, scratch tests have a high degree of success. But in these instances, the patients have already discovered their allergy. The tests give us most help when they are least needed.

Common food causes of hives. Frequency of various foodstuffs as causes of hives varies with geography, socioeconomic status, and racial origin of the patient. In general, the ordinary nutrients are the commonest antigens. The following list groups foods in an approximate order of importance:

1. Milk and milk products, especially cheese
2. Egg and egg products
3. Fruits (strawberries, gooseberries, pears, bananas, oranges, and other citrus fruits)
4. Vegetables, especially legumes, tomatoes, celery and cabbage
5. Grains, especially wheat, but also rice, oats, and rye
6. Fish, crabs, shrimps, lobsters, clams, and less commonly oysters
7. Meat, primarily pork, but also mutton, beef and fowl
8. Nuts of all sorts
9. Spices, coffee, and chocolate (rarely tea)

Inhalant antigens in general are not of great importance in causing urticaria. Perhaps too little attention is paid to their possible role in eliciting hives. I have repeatedly seen seasonal cases in which pollens could be shown to be causative. About five per cent of bakers and millers have an inhalant urticaria due to flour. Animal danders, house dust, kapok, barn dust, and perfume are occasionally responsible. In contrast to drugs and foods, positive skin tests to inhalants are quite reliable in urticaria.

There are undoubtedly many causes for the itching or nightly urticaria which may appear shortly after going to bed, but bed antigens should be sought for. This is particularly true when nose and throat symptoms, nasal obstruction, and paroxysmal cough are present night after night. In such instances, use of dust-free bedding may produce dramatic results, even without desensitization.

Intestinal parasites. The variable relationships which exist between parasite and host in worm infestations lead to sensitization, in consequence of the absorption of body substances of the worms or of waste products thrown off by them.

The antigenicity of this material is high, only 1/120,000,000 ounce sufficing to sensitize a guinea pig. A high percentage of adults show a positive reaction to worm extracts, yet clinical symptoms are seldom present, presumably because there are no worms in their intestines.

Certain worms in their life cycles pass through our blood or tissues, and these (ascaris, echinococcus, hookworm) often lead to allergic symptoms. The purely intestinal parasites (tapeworm, whipworm) rarely do so. In dracuncula infestations, 40 per cent of patients have a generalized urticaria, and in schistosomiasis the percentage is even higher. Thus the exclusion of worm infestation by stool examination (the naked eye does not suffice; microscopes must be used) is uniformly carried out as part of the diagnostic workup in hives.

A positive skin test to worm extract is not of much help because, especially in echinococcosis, antibodies persist for years after the worms have been expelled. A positive test does not tell us whether worms are present or not, only that the individual is allergic to the worm in question. Finally, a negative test does not mean the individual is not playing host, because every worm infestation does not lead to sensitization. Some persons are infested only with male specimens (ascaris); hence the absence of eggs in their feces does not exclude the presence of worms in their intestines. Other tests must be employed. There are a number of very effective worm-destroying drugs (vermifuges) available today (see Chapter 2).

Occasionally, parasitic or pathogenic protozoa (one-cell microscopic animals) may cause allergic reactions, especially urticaria. These include trichomonas, malarial organisms, amebas, and giardia lamblia (no everyday names for these).

Systemic disease. Urticaria may be present in any acute infection, but it is especially frequent in streptococcic disorders. Hives are not uncommon in acute gastroenteritis ("food poisoning"), either during the active stages or during convalescence. It is the chronic types of infection that are most likely to cause urticaria, and evidence of disease of tonsils, teeth, sinuses, gallbladder, gastrointestinal and urogenital tracts is sought for in the study of longstanding hives. When large numbers of such patients are studied, foci of infection are found in 10 to 20 per cent.

Urticaria, especially of the chronic form, may accompany a number of internal diseases or may be a herald of an unsuspected systemic disorder. This is based on autoantibody formation, in which the patient makes antibodies against some of his own body substances which act as antigens. In my experience this is most apt to occur in malignancies, including particularly a group classified as lymphomas (leukemia, Hodgkin's disease). But urticaria may also be seen in inflammatory or degenerative liver disease, in kidney disorders, in various blood diseases, after x-ray therapy, and during the course of resorption of inflammatory outpouring of fluid or pus in the abdomen or thorax (empyema, pleural effusion).

Psychogenic ("nervous") factors. There can be no doubt of the existence of psychogenic urticaria. Its frequency seems to depend on the point of view and the ability of the investigator. The more carefully the patient is questioned and examined, the less frequently is it necessary for the doctor to say: "Your hives are due to your nerves." Yet there is a clear-cut influence of the nervous system in cholinergic urticaria. In the vast majority of persons who have other varieties of hives, emotional factors can precipitate attacks or even worsen attacks already present but are not themselves the basic cause.

Treatment. References to treatment have been made in considering the different types of hives, but a few more words may be in order. As elsewhere, the basis of control of allergy consists of elimination of the antigen when possible. This is easy when drugs are concerned, less easy for foods or house antigens.

Ubiquitous antigens such as pollens and occupational allergens which cannot be avoided, such as flour, cause the physician to use desensitizing techniques. Internal antigens are removed by antibiotics, or when these fail, by surgery of diseased tissue and by elimination of intestinal parasites. The antihistaminic drugs, ephedrine, and adrenaline, are of considerable value in the symptomatic treatment of hives. ACTH, cortisone, and related medicines are effective, but because of their side effects should be used sparingly, if at all.

INSECT ALLERGY

Many kinds of insects *bite:* mosquitoes, bedbugs, fleas, lice, blackflies, midges, stable flies, deer flies, horse flies, sandflies. Other insects, chiefly such *hymenopterans* as the wasp, honey bee, yellowjacket, and hornet, *sting.* A few species of insects, such as the fire ant, simultaneously *bite and sting.*

Insect Stings

Allergy plays the major role in causing the distressing effects of insect *bites,* and is a substantial component of changes which follow insect *stings.* It is probable that the first allergic disease ever described was that of insect allergy. It occurred in 2461 B.C. when King Menes of Egypt died following a wasp or hornet sting.

No one knows how many severe reactions occur from hymenopteran stings, but the problem is large. Dr. H. M. Parrish made a study of deaths from bites and stings of venomous animals and insects in the United States and analyzed the death certificates of all persons in this country who died from this cause from 1950 through 1954. A totally unexpected finding in this study was the large number of deaths resulting from stings by the hymenopterans, more deaths from these insects than from poisonous snakes. It is probable that these stinging insects cause many more deaths than is realized, because of the tendency to attribute all sudden deaths to heart attacks.

Deaths from bee stings have been reported repeatedly. One concerned a 21-year-old man who had been stung at 18 years by a bee, with immediate intestinal cramps, nausea, vomiting, and diarrhea of four days' duration. At 20 years he was again stung by a bee and became violently ill with similar symptoms. At 21 years he was stung one final time, developed nausea, weakness, coldness, and severe abdominal cramps. He died quickly with terminal convulsions.

The pheidole, a "red ant", is a frequent cause of allergic reactions. The sting is but slightly painful and may pass unperceived. After a few seconds, the victim suddenly feels a burning sensation of generalized heat, quite intense in the palms and soles, eyes, and genitals. There is often apprehension, nausea, and throbbing in the temples.

The victim's face swells grotesquely. The swelling is especially notable at the lips and eyelids, which may be very difficult to keep open. Generalized large hives are seen. There is drooling and reddening of the eyes. Bronchial asthma is frequently present. Symptoms reach their peak in ten minutes, persist four to six hours usually, and there is a gradual return to normal.

I have recently seen an abandoned child who died after being severely chewed by ants. Because the infant was exposed to the elements and without food, possibly for eighteen hours, it cannot be stated that the ant bites and stings were responsible for the death. However, in a patient treated by one of my friends there is little doubt that the death of the child was caused by ant stings. The child died within twenty-nine hours of the time he was stung.

Test precautions. Great caution must be exercised in testing to honeybees, wasps, black and yellow hornets, and yellow jackets. Positive reactions have been produced by fantastically small amounts of material, as little as 0.025 milliliter of a 1:100,000,000 solution, or otherwise simply expressed, by one two-hundredth of a teaspoonful of this highly diluted solution.

Should the test be negative, successively stronger extracts may be employed for testing until a positive reaction is obtained. This last strength is used to start *desensitization*. There is general agreement that even though a person is known to be allergic to only one insect, it is better to desensitize him to the entire group.

Desensitization is highly successful and is urged for all persons allergic to hymenopterans. Of 155 persons who had severe reactions after being stung prior to desensitization, only one had a bad experience on re-exposure after desensitization although all of the group were stung following treatment.

Emergency measures. Persons who are highly allergic to the bee family should carry an emergency kit with them. This kit should contain some 10 mg. isoproterenol tablets for use under the tongue, some adrenalin for use by inhalation, a tourniquet, and tweezers. One of the two medicines should be used at once.

Should the sting occur on the arm or leg, the tourniquet should be applied between the sting site and the body to slow absorption of the venom. The tourniquet should not be so tight as to cut off circulation. The pulse at the wrist or foot should be detectable while the tourniquet is in place. It should be loosened every three to five minutes and discontinued entirely as the symptoms are brought under control.

Honeybees leave their stings and venom sacs attached to the site of the sting. Prompt removal of the sting, carefully so as not to squeeze the venom sac, by scraping motions with a knife blade, finger nail, or tweezers will reduce the amount of venom which enters the sting site. Cold packs applied to the sting site will help control discomfort.

How not to get stung. Dr. Joseph Shaffer, who has studied the problem extensively, points out that bees are more likely to sting on bright, warm days if interfered with while they are busy gathering nectar. They are angry, disappointed, and in a stinging mood after rain has washed nectar from flowers.

Stinging insects are attracted to gaily colored, dark, and rough clothing but take less offense to white clothing with a hard finish. Highly scented hair dressings, perfumes, and other cosmetics should not be used on picnics since they have a tendency to attract bees.

Insect Bites

Sequences in the development of local reactions to insect *bites* are different from reactions to stings.

Initially, nothing is seen to occur, but soon a papule (small elevated lesion) appears, not earlier than 24 hours after the bite. In subsequent bites, the interval between bite and reaction gradually decreases from 24 hours to zero. Coincident with this change in the incubation period an increase in the size of the reaction at first occurs, followed by a gradual decrease, until finally there is no reaction to the bites. This has led some people to believe mistakenly that they are not bitten by mosquitoes.

Predatory insects develop a venom to which the individual may become allergic. The parasites do not secrete poisons, but their bite may induce allergy, and most, if not all, of the results of insect bites are to be explained on this basis.

For the most part, insect bites and stings do not demand or receive much attention. Local applications of lotions such as calamine, cool compresses, or cool baths usually suffice, although the antihistamine drugs have definite value. For more alarming reactions the emergency kit should be used. Desensitization is strongly recommended for all persons who have allergic reactions of a major degree from an insect bite.

DRUG ALLERGIES

The extraordinary development of new drugs in the last 25 years has led to specific treatment hitherto impossible. In my student days, in the early thirties, it was taught that all living protoplasm was so similar that any medicine harmful to a germ would automatically be harmful in some degree to a human being. This was easily seen when we used such things as carbolic acid and tincture of iodine, which were valuable antiseptics but which easily produced tissue damage. But then came the sulfonamide drugs and the antibiotics, which to a doctor of my generation who has seen children die of now curable pneumonia and meningitis, are entitled to their hackneyed title of miracle drugs.

Side Effects

The use of powerful medicines carries with it the possibility of side or untoward reactions. By this is meant undesired or unexpected results attributable to the interaction of the patient and a particular drug.

In order that doctors may free themselves of prejudice in determining that a new medicine really works, a "double blind" system is set up. In this procedure, two groups of patients are matched by age, sex, and severity of disease. One group is given the active drug; the other is given an inert substance, a *placebo*, (from the Latin "I shall please"), usually milk sugar. The drug and the placebo look identical so that neither the doctor nor the patient knows which is which (hence "double blind") until the study is over and drug identity is revealed.

An interesting observation has come from such studies, in many of which I have participated. *Placebos cause side effects in nine to 50 per cent of patients!* Nausea, rapid beating of the heart, excessive sweating, disturbing sensations in the stomach, diarrhea, severe headache, easy fatigue, and drowsiness are "placebo side effects" most commonly complained of.

Nevertheless, reactions of varying types due to drugs are of increasing importance in these studies.

With **overdosage** of a drug, toxic effects occur in direct relation to the total amount of drug in the body. These effects are likely to occur in any patient, provided a threshold level is exceeded.

Absolute overdosage may result from an erroneously given excessive dose. But there are certain drugs, for example digitalis, iodides, and bromides, which tend to accumulate in the body even when they are given in proper dosage. Unless attention is paid to this property, in time toxic levels are reached. My practice in prescribing iodides, for example, is to have the patient take the medicine every day except Sunday, thereby giving an extra day for the body to rid itself of the excess of the medication.

Relative overdosage may be seen in persons in whom all proper precautions are taken. This comes about in two ways. Either they fail to excrete the drug at a usual rate, or they fall into a small group of individuals who have difficulties from quantities harmless to the majority of persons. These last are not allergies; no antibodies are involved. The mechanism lies in the normal variability of people. Just as there is a normal range of intelligence, height, weight, and the like, so is there a range of tolerance to medicines.

The toxic symptoms produced by small quantities of drugs in these hypersensitive patients are the same as the toxic symptoms produced by large quantities in normal persons. Perhaps an example will make this clear. For centuries quinine was given to cure malaria. Anyone who took enough developed ringing in the ears and deafness *(cinchonism)*. In the majority of cases, "enough" consisted of 500 grains. An occasional patient developed cinchonism from five or ten grains. But hives or bronchial asthma would occur, without cinchonism, from small doses of quinine taken by individuals allergic to it.

Another non-allergic form of intolerance to drugs is seen in Negroes, certain of whom lack a particular chemical in some of their red blood cells. If these persons take a sulfonamide drug, the defective cells break down.

Allergies to Medicines

Nonetheless, many people are allergic to medicines. In the case of proteins, e.g., horse serum or insulin, the mechanism is straightforward. The drug itself is antigenic.

A curious modification of the process takes place with nonprotein medicaments. Here the medicines are not antigenic by themselves. They must combine first with one of the body's proteins. The resulting complex of drug and protein now acts as an antigen leading to antibody formation. When next the patient takes the medicine, the previously formed antibodies react with it immediately without the necessity of its combining again with protein. Such substances which can react with antibodies but cannot cause their formation unaided are called *haptenes* and occur in many bacteria as well.

Haptene + body protein → haptene-protein complex

Haptene-protein complex + antibody producing cells → antibody

Haptene + antibody → allergy symptoms.

Symptoms of allergic drug reactions are extraordinarily varied and mimic so many other diseases that they share with syphilis the title of The Great Imitator. The usual allergic diseases may be produced — hay fever, bronchial asthma, hives — but in addition every organ and every tissue in the body may be the site of a drug reaction.

Each organ in the body can react in only a limited number of ways, regardless of the injury. Only the stomach and small intestine are capable of forming a peptic ulcer. No matter how the liver or kidney are damaged, they cannot respond with a peptic ulcer. Thus the clinical picture of drug allergy is not specific for the causative antigen, but rather a kaleidoscopic variety of signs and symptoms are present, depending on the particular organs and tissues taking part in the given reaction.

This does not mean that there are no preferred routes for certain drug allergies. Thus, phenolphthalein (a pink coloring matter used in cake icings and as a laxative) rarely or never produces an exfoliative dermatitis (a severe widespread rash in which the entire skin surface flakes off in scales which are at times the size of leaves), but commonly produces a *fixed drug eruption*.

Fixed eruption. At the turn of the century a young woman consulted Brocq, a famous French doctor. Every month at the time of her monthly period she developed several red, slightly blistered lesions on the abdomen and chest. Each month they reappeared at precisely the same spots, in precisely the same shape. The doctor was not sure of the cause of this fixed eruption, as he called it, but clearly it was related to her menses.

But one day she returned to his office with the eruption present at a time which was not related to her period. He tells us that although his office was full of patients, he was so puzzled that he had them all dismissed so that he could give his entire attention to this problem. Finally after several hours the solution came to him.

The young woman had been taking antipyrine, a pain killer, because of the cramps she experienced each month. On the particular occasion, she had had a severe headache, from which she rarely suffered, and she had taken the antipyrine for relief. Thus the causative factor was not the menses but the medicine.

A fixed drug eruption always returns to the same spot because antibodies are fixed to these skin areas only. When the drug is taken by mouth, although the blood carries it everywhere, only the prepared areas are capable of reacting.

Serum sickness. One of the really great steps forward in control of infectious disease was the discovery that immunity built up could be "borrowed" by someone who needed it urgently. This procedure was first used in diphtheria. Horses were injected (and still are) with the toxin produced by the diphtheria germ. Starting with harmless amounts, ever-increasing quantities are introduced until finally there has been produced a large amount of antitoxin, the antibody which neutralizes toxin. The lives of many children have been saved by this discovery.

But it was soon found that horse serum, or indeed any foreign (rabbit) serum, might produce *serum sickness.* This is an allergic reaction that appears eight to 12 days after serum is injected. Other drugs, notably penicillin, given by needle or by mouth, may produce a syndrome (disease) clinically indistinguishable from serum sickness.

The incidence of serum disease is from five to 90 per cent of individuals receiving foreign serums, depending on the kind and amount given and the route of administration. A large dose is more likely to produce a reaction than a small one. The most severe types follow administration by vein, and the incidence is greater when given in the spinal canal than when given under the skin, or more deeply into muscles. The injected foreign serum, although it consists of highly purified antibodies, is still a protein and as such capable of inducing antibody production. After a sufficient concentration of anti-horse serum antibodies have been built up, these react with the horse serum, thereby producing serum sickness.

Urticaria is the usual skin manifestation. Less frequently the drug-induced rash resembles measles, scarlet fever, or other skin diseases. Fever, which occurs in one-third of patients, either precedes or is coincident with the eruption. It usually is mild and lasts only a day or two; in more severe cases, the temperature may reach 105°F. and last seven to ten days.

Enlargement of lymph nodes (kernels) near the area injected is usual, but all lymph nodes may increase in size. The reason for this is that lymph nodes are important sites of antibody formation. Mild to severe joint involvement, at times with intense pain, often occurs. Not uncommonly, wheals form in the intestine, larynx, and bronchi, with resultant local symptoms.

Diagnosis. A history of serum injection plus the classical signs and symptoms usually makes the diagnosis obvious.

If drug reactions take place while the patient is under treatment for some other condition, they are ordinarily promptly recognized and accurately diagnosed, for it is known what medicines are being taken. Yet a careful history is important, for not all drugs are prescribed by physicians. There is a huge volume of proprietary medicines sold over the counter for self medication. Furthermore, drugs are often added to various toilet articles, soaps, and even foodstuffs as preservatives. The regular or occasional use of these household products seems so harmless to the patient that, unless specifically questioned by the doctor, the identification of the responsible agent will not be made when symptoms occur.

Management. When a medicine comes under suspicion, it should be withheld. If then the symptoms disappear, the medicine may be taken again but in much reduced amount. If this leads to a return of the symptoms, the case is proved. Certain drugs lend themselves to the usual skin test methods, e.g., foreign serum and penicillin, as well as various organ preparations. But the majority of medicaments cannot be so tested, and in point of fact such testing may be hazardous.

If skin testing seems imperative because no substitute drug will work as well as the one under suspicion, it is far better to test by proxy, that is, to use the *passive transfer* technique in which some of the patient's serum is placed in the skin of a nonallergic person. This site can then be tested with entire safety, and as much information can be obtained as if the patient were tested directly.

Cosmetic Allergy

Cosmetic dermatitis, a form of contact dermatitis resulting from applications of various agents to the skin, is discussed in Chapter 5.

Cosmetic allergy is a more all-inclusive term. Cosmetics may cause allergic symptoms in the respiratory tract. Any odor, pleasant or not, can trigger off an attack of hay fever or bronchial asthma, and perfumes in cosmetics are in this category. For a number of years, orris root (apparently a corruption of "iris root") was an important inhalant allergen. The rhizomes (roots) are freed of the bark and dried, in the process acquiring a delicate but distinct odor of violets. Once widely used in the manufacture of cosmetics such as toilet water, face powder, talcum powder, tooth powder, sachets, and cold creams, it is coming into disfavor with cosmetic manufacturers as they become familiar with its dangers.

It is preferable to avoid orris root, and desensitization is seldom necessary. The same statement applies to other cosmetic substances capable of producing allergy of the respiratory tract, such as perfume, rice powder, oatmeal powder, bath salt, hair tonic, soap, skin cream, and various lotions. Persons with respiratory tract allergy should purchase so-called "hypoallergenic" cosmetics which eliminate known allergens from their formulas as much as possible.

Although many minor reactions to cosmetics may be solved by the patient through change of brand, the severe and complicated problems require testing to determine the specific offending allergen.

PHYSICAL ALLERGY

By *physical allergy* is meant the development of allergic symptoms such as bronchial asthma or hives after exposure to physical factors such as heat, cold, or light. Physical allergy may be spontaneous, or secondary to food or drug allergy; it may be entirely hereditary, or it may be an aspect of some systemic disease.

Hypersensitivity to Cold

Cold may cause various allergic reactions. Some years ago, during the winter, a young medical student was drawing blood from a patient's vein, using a syringe he had previously used repeatedly. He took the blood to his cold room, where he found he could not manipulate the syringe. Thinking to clean it, he put it in warm water, but to his surprise, as soon as it warmed up, the plunger moved freely in the barrel. He took the syringe out and allowed it to get cold. Again the

plunger stuck, only to be freed again by heat. This unusual effect was caused by a protein in the patient's blood called a *cryoglobulin* (Greek "cryos" — cold). It dissolves when warm and precipitates out of solution when cold. Such cryoglobulins are found in a number of diseases, the best known being rheumatoid arthritis.

Sensitivity to cold is present in two thirds of people who have these odd proteins in their blood. The changes produced by cold weather include hives, bleeding into the skin (purpura), bleeding into the mucous membranes of the nose and mouth and into the retina. In addition, severe frostbite with tissue death may take place after exposure to degrees of cold which would be harmless to normal persons. These cryoglobulins may be isolated from the blood and introduced into the skin of a normal recipient. For about two weeks the area where the serum was placed will produce hives when chilled.

Another type of sensitivity to cold is seen in syphilis. This is caused by the presence in the blood of another chemical which is capable of rupturing red blood cells. This occurs when such an individual is warmed after exposure to cold. Breakdown of the red cells frees the hemoglobin which is excreted in the urine, thereby changing its color to red or even black. In severe attacks, chills, fever, sweats, abdominal cramps, weakness, backache, and vomiting may precede the passage of red urine. Cold urticaria may be the presenting symptom.

Essential cold urticaria, by far the most common type, develops without the presence of abnormal serum proteins. *Histamine* is known to be responsible for this reaction. The acquired type has a sudden onset and patients are ordinarily able to date precisely the first episode.

For example, I saw a young boy about ten years of age who had had this condition for two years. The mother told me that the boy had been well until the family went on a Fourth of July picnic. There was a tub of iced drinks, and the boy was playing with the ice and eating it copiously, for it was a hot day. He became flushed, developed hives, had difficulty in breathing, and complained of pain in the chest.

The parents were terrified, thinking he had been bitten by a snake or was having a heart attack. Police were quickly on the scene with pulmotor and oxygen. The lad soon recovered, but the picnic was spoiled by the mysterious illness. It later became clear that similar but usually milder attacks were precipitated whenever he was chilled or ate something cold.

Provoking factors include serum sickness, measles, scarlet fever, chickenpox, childbirth, and emotional disturbances. Cold urticaria may occur only after eating certain foods, or when intestinal parasites of the roundworm variety are present, but in the majority of instances no precipitating or underlying causes can be determined.

For the most part, urticaria is limited to areas of exposure, but generalized hives may follow. Should much of the body surface be in contact with cold water, as in swimming or cold showers, generalized urticaria is present together with signs of histamine shock: profound drop in blood pressure, rapid pulse, flushing of the face, and loss of consciousness. Under such circumstances the danger of drowning is obviously great.

Diagnosis is easily confirmed by applying an ice cube to the skin for a few moments. A hive appears, having the exact dimensions of the ice. Although the symptoms of cold urticaria can be controlled effectively with antihistamine drugs, treatment of the basic condition is difficult and indeed usually fails.

Congenital (familial) cold urticaria is a less common inherited condition. Hives are present from birth or shortly thereafter and continue throughout life. Cold air is more effective than cold foods or drinks in bringing on attacks. The famous diarist Pepys had an attack of hives while walking in the park on a cold day in February, 1663.

In all families the condition appears shortly after birth in those affected. The attack is brought on in every case by cold wind or extreme changes in temperature. In addition to the hives, which usually are free of itching in contrast to other varieties, there is a burning sensation, pain and swelling of the joints, and mild fever. Drinking cold fluids has no effect. The members of affected families know what to do. They simply go to bed and bundle up warmly, whereupon they soon recuperate from the attack.

Hypersensitivity to Heat

Just as there is an occupational "cold bronchitis" seen in workers in cold storage plants and ice houses, so also is there a "heat bronchitis," seen in laborers in the hot environments of steel and aluminum mills.

There are documented examples of attacks of bronchial asthma brought on by exposure to heat, but urticaria is far more common. It occurs in two forms: (a) *generalized* (cholinogenic) urticaria produced by heat, exercise, and emotional stress, and (b) *localized* (noncholinogenic) urticaria produced by heat alone and only on the exposed area. The second type is unusually rare and is of little importance. The first is far more common and is of considerable interest to the doctor, in that it represents the one skin disease where the mechanism is known whereby a psychic stimulus can produce a definite lesion in the skin.

"Heat hives." In the generalized type, hives are produced by the heat of a warm room, hot foods, hot weather, clothes, fever, or a hot bath. Emotional stress and exercise produce identical reactions. In some cases a combination of all three, as in jitterbugging or dancing the "Twist," or various competitive sports, may be necessary to bring out lesions.

The wheals are characteristically small, one to two millimeters in diameter, but are surrounded by a large flare. When these merge, large "blush patches" appear, the more striking because of the tendency to this disorder to affect young red-headed women. At times there are only bright red flares.

Any part of the skin may be involved except the palms and soles, although these are often the sites of hives in other forms of urticaria. In about half of these patients in whom there is sufficient release of acetylcholine, such systemic symptoms as abdominal cramps, diarrhea, faintness, sweating, salivation, and headaches usually occur.

Mechanisms. The mechanism was worked out by Grant. If one leg is placed in hot water for 20 to 30 minutes, generalized hives result. The body temperature must be raised 0.2 to 1° F. If before the test the circulation in the veins is cut off by placing a blood pressure cuff on the limb, no wheals appear anywhere until the cuff is released and circulation is restored. This indicates the essential stimulus is transmitted by the blood and not by the nervous system.

Heated blood carried to the brain acts on some central heat-regulating mechanism, stimulating the nervous system to carry impulses to the skin where acetylcholine is released. If in a similar experiment the arterial circulation to one arm is cut off by the blood pressure cuff, bluish spots can be seen beyond the cuff. When the circulation is restored, wheals appear in these bluish areas, indicating that the stimulus is carried to the area by nervous impulses and not by the blood stream.

If acetylcholine is introduced into the skin of one of these patients, it produces transient lesions in an irregular fashion because the acetylcholine is destroyed rapidly by an enzyme. If the enzyme is blocked by a drug, urticaria is produced which persists as long as the drug is still working (ordinarily two or three hours).

Management. Peculiarly enough, anticholinergic drugs are strikingly ineffective, primarily because they do not prevent the release of acetylcholine. These people, who are not more prone to emotional crises than the rest of us, do not produce an abnormal amount of acetylcholine, but they are allergic to it. Antihistamines give partial relief. The treatment of choice is the application of cold or iced water to the hands and arms. This plus rest will abort the episode.

Of great practical importance is the fact that after an attack there is an unresponsive period. After a moderate outbreak this may last for some hours, but after a generalized severe attack produced by warming the legs for an hour, the period of freedom may last for a day or two, rarely longer.

This is of therapeutic value and can be utilized before one goes to a dance or sporting event. One of my beautiful young patients was being courted by three suitors. She used this device so as not to let them know to what extent she reciprocated their ardor. Until, that is, she had made a choice and then proudly used it to show the sincerity of her love.

Hypersensitivity to Light

In spite of man's centuries-old worship of the sun, much damage results from injudicious exposure. Aside from burning the skin, causing crow's feet and cancers, sunlight also produces hypersensitivity reactions which are being seen with increasing frequency.

Solar urticaria is a rare disease. Hives may appear on any part of the body, especially the trunk, arms, and legs, because although these areas are customarily clothed, the face and hands are only one-twentieth as sensitive to light. With sufficient exposure, the victim may have generalized symptoms (malaise) or may even go into collapse. Moderate exposure to sunlight produces urticaria; prolonged exposure may cause dermatitis.

The condition begins suddenly without apparent cause, at any time of life. Women are involved three times more frequently than men, a prevalence also seen in other light sensitivity conditions such as *lupus erythematosus*. Except for cases caused by drugs, the condition persists for years.

Those cases in which sensitivity to invisible ultraviolet light is present may clear up spontaneously. Persons sensitive to visible light have a poorer outlook, and the condition may persist indefinitely without change. Urticaria is also seen in *hydroa vacciniforme, eczema solare,* and *polymorphous light eruptions.* Patients with these conditions usually do not mention the hives, for they are less troublesome than the other symptoms. Wheals can be produced regularly in patients ill with these disease states by light exposure. It is believed that this group of diseases is closely interrelated, the connecting link being a photoallergic mechanism.

Experimentally, exposure to light will produce lesions in any part of the skin surface. Such a wheal is sharply demarcated and lacks the irregular, delicate fingerlike processes which extend from the borders of other varieties of hives. All parts of the visible spectrum, as well as ultraviolet and infrared light, have been found to cause urticaria. The majority of patients are allergic to ultraviolet light, but another clearly defined group has trouble from blue and violet wavelengths.

The allergen is a substance produced in the skin of everyone by the sun's rays, but an allergen against which only certain persons have antibodies. This theory is now universally accepted, chiefly because the phenomenon can be transferred to a normal person by introducing some of the patient's serum into his skin.

Perhaps the most convincing argument consists in irradiating the skin of a normal person. Nothing apparently happens. Then when serum from a light-sensitive person is placed in the irradiated area, a hive promptly appears. Sun exposure at one site may provoke lesions at remote regions because of the union of circulating antigen with antibody fixed in these reaction areas.

The theory might be summarized thus:
normal skin + light → antigen (no visible reaction)
normal skin + antibodies → no visible reaction
normal skin + light + antibodies → hives

Treatment is unsatisfactory, especially when the difficulty resides in the visible portions of the spectrum. Some degree of "hardening" of the skin may be produced by gradually increasing exposures to sunlight, but in general this is of limited value. Sunscreen ointments are effective in preventing light from reaching the skin. The antimalarial drugs (atabrine and chloroquin) are of definite value and presumably act as sunscreens to block light.

Allergy also plays a role in *solar dermatitis* (polymorphic light eruption) which may be defined as an acute or chronic inflammatory reaction to sunlight. The eruption consists of itching areas which are flushed. They may take the form of hives, papules (small, solid elevations on the skin), or small blisters. They appear on exposed parts of the body, usually worsen during the summer, and may disappear during the winter. In regions such as southern Texas where the winters are short, there may be no clearing of the lesions.

As would be expected, the victims are for the most part outdoor workers such as farmers, engineers, surveyors, postmen, oil field workers, and stockmen. In many persons who drive a car constantly in their work, the eruption is often limited to the left side of the face and neck. In indoor workers, the use of fluorescent lighting has been thought to provoke the eruption as well as prolong it.

SPECIFIC TREATMENT

Avoidance

Elimination of the allergen is the treatment of choice when possible. This may require change of diet, occupation, or residence; withdrawal of a drug; or removal of a household pet, or certain articles of furniture, cosmetics or clothing. Some geographic areas, free of many allergens common in others, serve as havens for afflicted individuals. Pollen can be avoided by leaving one's community and going where the offender is not found. A convenient source of such information is the book *Regional Allergy* by Oren Durham and Max Samter. Various air-conditioning devices help in reducing exposure to pollen grains by filtering them from the air.

It is unfortunately true that campaigns designed to eliminate various grasses and weeds have failed. Thus Chicago embarked in 1932 on a three year campaign to eradicate ragweed. After considerable expense, it was found that the pollen counts were higher than they were in the years preceding the campaign. Even had the eradication of ragweed been complete in Chicago, when it is considered that ragweed is carried into the city from a radius of at least 75 miles, the futility of local efforts may be realized.

Although complete avoidance of house dust cannot be attained, measures can reduce its amount. This may be done with varying degrees of vigor, but I feel that the minimum involves replacement of pillows and mattress with nonallergenic materials such as foam rubber, or encasing them in dust proof rubber-lined or plastic envelopes. Another measure is complete avoidance of wool blankets, down quilts, and chenille bedspreads.

Desensitization

Most people do well if they are *desensitized*. There are various ways of going about this. *Coseasonal desensitization*, which is perhaps the least effective, is employed when the patient first presents himself to the physician during the pollen season. It will help about 40 per cent of patients. The technique consists of giving small amounts of pollen extract daily.

Preseasonal desensitization is used when the patient consults the physician six weeks or more prior to the expected onset of the pollen season. It affords relief to about 80 per cent of patients. This method of treatment requires about 20 injections of gradually increasing amounts of pollen extract.

The *perennial method* is best, but many patients prefer to forget their disease when their symptoms have disappeared. It consists of giving one injection a month throughout the year, at the top level built up by the preseasonal method.

In recent years, *depot methods* have come into increasing use. These "one shot" schemes seem to have about the same efficacy as the multiple injections. The fundamental difference is that watery solutions are used for conventional desensitization, and an oily emulsion for the depot methods. The procedure may prove to be a tremendous clinical advance, but it is still considered experimental at this time.

House dust is probably the most important single cause of bronchial asthma and perennial allergic rhinitis. Desensitization is quite effective, and as in the case of pollen allergy, involves giving increasingly larger doses of dust extract.

Reactions

It is a rare patient who does not experience a *local* reaction during the course of desensitization. These resemble hives or angioedema and vary from pinhead size to involvement of the whole arm. It indicates that increase in dosage is being made too rapidly, but otherwise is not of significance.

The *generalized* reactions vary from malaise to severe anaphylaxis or even death. The most common ones are widespread urticaria and cough. Sterile abscesses have been reported from the depot method of treatment.

DRUG TREATMENT
(Non-Specific)

Epinephrine (adrenalin) is the most potent bronchodilating drug available and the most important medication for management of the acute paroxysm of bronchial asthma. It is also quite useful in treating hives. It may be given by injection or by inhalation, but not orally.

In contrast, related drugs such as ephedrine or propadrine can be taken by mouth in pill, tablet, or liquid form. These drugs act directly on the tissues involved in the allergic reaction.

The antihistaminic drugs act by competing with histamine. They are of greatest use in hives, in gastrointestinal allergy, and in relieving itching. They can be taken orally, and many ingenious methods have been devised to prolong their action.

Cortisone, its relatives, and ACTH all act alike. They have an extraordinary ability to reverse inflammation, including allergic inflammation. They are used topically, by mouth, by injection, and by inhalation. Any and all allergic symptoms can be controlled by them.

Prolonged use carries a distinct hazard; among the possible undesirable results are peptic ulcer formation, worsening of diabetes or tuberculosis, mental disturbance, and predisposition to fracture of bones. *All these effects are reversible and disappear when the medicament is withdrawn.* They are least likely to cause trouble when applied to the skin or mucous membranes. The consensus today is that these agents should be used with discrimination, but when called upon they rarely fail.

EMOTIONAL AND MENTAL ILLNESS

by ROBERT FELIX, M.D., and MORTON HUNT

WHAT IS MENTAL ILLNESS?

Prevalence • Definitions • Symptoms • Warning Signs

TYPES OF MENTAL AND EMOTIONAL ILLNESS

Minor Maladjustments • Character Disorders • Pyschosomatic Diseases • Neuroses • Psychoses • Mental Retardation

TREATMENTS

Is Treatment Necessary? • Psychotherapies • Physical Therapies • Drugs • Social Treatment • Hospital Treatment • Choosing a Therapist

SOURCES OF HELP

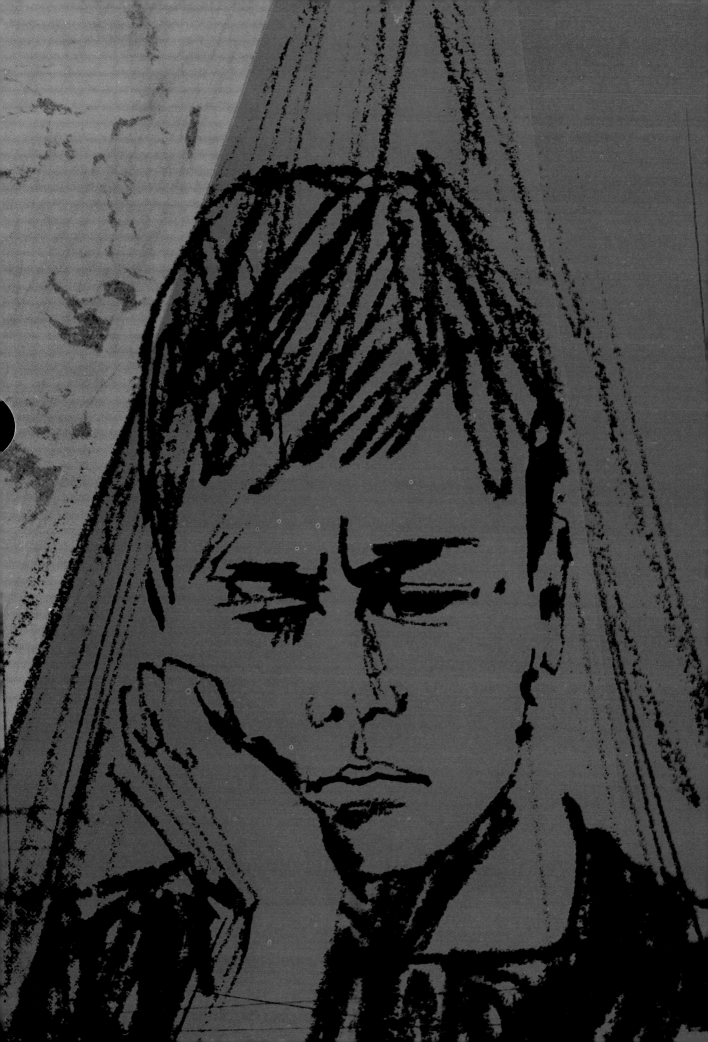

EMOTIONAL AND MENTAL ILLNESSES

by ROBERT FELIX, M.D. and MORTON HUNT

What Is an Emotional or Mental Illness?

Emotional and mental illnesses very often pose a special problem for both layman and doctor — that of deciding whether a given set of abnormal feelings and behavior do or do not constitute a disease. There is no bacillus to put under a microscope, no suppurating lesion, no fever reading, to act as irrefutable evidence of the existence of sickness. There is only a distortion of human emotions and actions. Yet the borderline between what is distorted and what is normal is not fixed by science; it varies from society to society, and even within our own culture it has been rapidly changing in recent decades.

Overtly disturbed behavior is, of course, easy to recognize, but psychological disorders of lesser degrees of severity were long accepted as normal, though today they are coming to be re-evaluated and labelled "sick".

In most of the past, the strange conduct or the personal misery of the eccentric, the hermit, the religious fanatic, the timid soul, the Don Juan, and the village fool, among others, were thought to lie within the bounds of normality. Changing social standards and the growth of psychology into a science are, however, leading us to classify these as psychological ailments capable of being diagnosed and, in many cases, relieved or cured.

Practitioners of mental healing today, therefore, are concerned not only with the grossly disturbed patient, but with delinquent children, unwed mothers, alcoholics, persistent marriers-and-divorcers, job-hoppers, and numerous others. Some laymen still regard such persons as self-indulgent "weaklings," but professionals see these mentally ill persons as victims of a broad range of psychological disorders, unable to end their troubles simply by an act of will or the decision to "do right".

Prevalence. In this modern view of the subject, a considerable number of people have psychological disorders. Using various surveys, the Joint Commission on Mental Illness and Health recently estimated that nearly 20,000,000 Americans (one out of every ten persons) suffer from either a minor or a major form of psychological difficulty. The larger part of these, to be sure, are minor and noncrippling; all but 717,000 of the 20,000,000 affected persons are able to remain outside mental hospitals, in the body of society. But the cost to these many millions, in terms of misery, frustration, and the wastage of their lives, is incalculable.

Because the popular acceptance of psychiatry is very recent, many people still are frightened or angered by any statement that their own failures or dissatisfactions might be the products of an emotional illness. The same people, however, willingly call the common cold, or an ingrown toenail, or a simple rash, a form of disease, and take steps to get rid of it. When they are able to think and act as rationally about emotional and mental illnesses—sometimes including quite minor ones — they will have gone a long way toward making their distorted lives both happier and healthier.

Definitions and symptoms. Yet there still exists no generally accepted definition the professional can offer to guide the layman as to the precise meanings of "normal" or "abnormal", "emotionally healthy" or "emotionally ill." Freud, when asked what a normal person should be able to do, replied, "He should be able to love and to work."

Contemporary psychologists and psychiatrists have added somewhat to his reply: the normal person should also be able to play, to see the people and things around him without distortion, to live relatively free from pain, and to obtain a good deal of satisfaction from life.

In contrast, the emotionally or mentally ill person may (1) feel undue or lasting distress, (2) suffer some "limitation of function" — that is, be unable to work as well as his abilities warrant, or unable to live with, and love, other people adequately, (3) unjustly misinterpret or misunderstand the words and actions of people around him, seeing, for instance, hostility where there really is friendliness or at least neutrality, and (4) be unable to take joy in play, and satisfaction from his accomplishments.

Warning Signs. Many of these criteria are hard for the layman to judge, but they often produce specific and very recognizable symptoms.

Among the more common ones — the presence of which should act as warning signs — are phenomena such as these:

Waves of severe anxiety not attributable to any realistic threat.

Sexual disorders such as impotence and frigidity, promiscuity, and perversion.

Inability to hold onto a job.

Self-destructive acts, including heavy drinking, persistent gambling, and risky or daring deeds.

Recurrent nightmares.

Unreasonable fears of foods, germs, or vehicles.

Unjustified feelings of persecution.

Apathy, and fatigue for which there is no physical cause.

Temper tantrums and rages.

Suicidal thoughts or actions and so on.

No one of these symptoms is adequate evidence, for the layman, of the existence of any one special kind of psychological disorder.

The interplay of forces is very complex, and only the expert can diagnose the condition. But the layman who is familiar with these major warning signals can at least recognize when he, or someone in his family, needs professional examination and diagnosis, and treatment.

Man long thought it was his lot to suffer on earth from emotional and mental distress.

Today we believe that it may be man's lot to fall prey to such conditions, but that he need not passively endure them.

Major Types of Emotional and Mental Illnesses

No one method of classifying psychological disorders is currently accepted by all schools of thought, and some contemporary psychiatrists — notably Dr. Karl Menninger — even deplore the use of standard diagnostic terms on the grounds that they are inadequate to explain the varied and complex human being. Still, a majority of therapists and researchers find the grouping of symptoms and mechanisms essential, in order to bring some order out of the chaos.

The following sixpoint categorization represents a median viewpoint in the psychiatric profession. The reader is warned that these categories do not have rigid bounds, but overlap very considerably. When psychiatrists differ about a patient, it is often more a matter of their terminology than of a basic difference of opinion as to the faulty mechanisms and the recommended treatment.

1. *Minor Maladjustments.* A number of authorities use this term to refer to a group of non-critical emotional disorders affecting work, marriage, or money. Difficulties in these three areas can, of course, signify very serious mental disorder. Most of the time, however, such difficulties originate in low-level, noncrippling emotional disorders of the sort with which people in previous centuries lived all their lives, neither hoping nor expecting to get relief.

The emotional outbursts and loneliness of Beethoven, the spells of depression that attacked Lincoln, the excessive shyness of Lewis Carroll, may all be typical of personal difficulties of this type—maladjustments productive of pain, and moderately hurtful to at least some part of the pattern of life, though not crippling to the rest of it. Indeed, people with minor maladjustments may — as in the cases just cited — be outstandingly productive, and contribute greatly to society, while remaining personally miserable or unhappy much of the time.

The term "minor maladjustments" may sound reassuring, but a person suffering from such a disorder may be sleepless, angry, discouraged, or miserable in any one of a number of other ways. His illness is, however, minor in the sense that he is not afflicted with gross symptoms such as paralysis without a physical cause, hallucinations, strange fears and compulsions, weird ideas, or the like.

He may simply be chronically dissatisfied with his work — no matter what he tries — or unable to decide which girl to marry, or unable to make a go of marriage, or unable to live within his budget, and so on. He not only lives with more than the usual amount of discontent, but cannot seem to solve his problems by himself. The healthy person, on the contrary, meets many of the same problems, but manages to solve them by himself and to wrest a fair measure of satisfaction from this imperfect life.

2. *Character Disorders.* More harmful than the minor maladjustments, both to society and to the individual, are those illnesses called character disorders, behavior disorders, character neuroses, or psychopathic personality (all four terms meaning roughly the same thing).

The person with a character disorder behaves very much like a wilful child or or an uncivilized primitive. He acts impulsively, selfishly, and often destructively, without regard for the society around him and without any particular anxiety or guilt about his actions. He is sane; his lack of anxiety stems not from serious mental disorder, but from a faulty or immature development of his conscience (technically, his "superego"), that part of the personality which embodies the parental and societal codes. Such people have sometimes been categorized as "moral morons."

A character disorder of a minor sort may result in an inability to care about doing one's work well, expressed in frequent absenteeism for trivial reasons. A character disorder of a more serious sort may be expressed in cheating, stealing, sexual promiscuity, alcoholism, perversion, or drug addiction — none of these things being indulged in as analgesics to dull emotional pain, as is true in many other kinds of emotional disorder, but simply because the psychopath himself sees and feels no reason why he shouldn't try them if he wishes, though he knows they are abhorrent to society.

In some cases, it is not at all clear whether one can classify character disorder as an emotional illness. In many slums, for instance, there is a widespread rejection of middle-class American values. The children growing up in such an environment accept and internalize that rejection.

Sometimes, too, the morals of a cultural sub-group run counter to the morals of the majority. Violence for example, is an accepted characteristic of young manhood among certain lower-economic immigrant groups, and only a philosopher could decide whether the gang-fighting, car-stealing, promiscuity and drunkenness of such young men are symptoms of emotional illness, or of emotionally normal but *socially* deviant attitudes. At any rate, it is clear enough that antisocial, selfish, impulsive, immature, or criminal behavior, *in an otherwise psychologically well person who has been reared according to accepted American codes*, is indicative of a species of serious psychopathic emotional illness.

3. *Psychosomatic Diseases.*

This group of ailments is closely related to, and often overlaps, the *neuroses*. Certain fears, angers, guilt feelings, and so on, the sources of which are deeply rooted and usually unknown to their victims, express themselves in the form of physical diseases. Psychosomatic illnesses are not imaginary, like the diseases of the hypochondriac; they are real and visible, but their origin usually is emotional rather than organic.

Among the illnesses which may be, though are not always, to some degree emotional in origin, are chronic diarrhea or constipation, colitis, stomach ulcers, and other digestive disorders; frequent and persistent headaches, insomnia, and fatigue; skin rashes, mouth ulcers, asthma, and chronic colds; irregular heartbeat, anginal heart pain, and poor circulation; and many others.

The particular psychosomatic illness a patient develops often has a symbolic significance. The gasping and wheezing of an asthmatic, in the midst of an anxiety-provoked attack, is not unlike the wailing and sobbing of a frightened child trying to summon his mother. Similarly, the immature adult with stomach troubles, who requires special feeding and attention by his wife, may unconsciously be forcing her to give him a kind of mothering that he never grew up enough to do without.

It is essential to remember, though, that many cases of asthma, stomach trouble, and the like are of purely physical origin. One must not arbitrarily assume such illnesses to be neurotic, but seek professional diagnosis.

A competent physician can determine to what extent any given disease has a physical basis or not. Even if it has significant emotional components and is therefore recognized to be psychosomatic, its symptoms can be ameliorated somewhat by physical means. But full recovery is far more likely to require a combination of psychological and physical forms of treatment, or important changes in the life circumstances of the patient.

4. *Neuroses.*

These ailments are, in many ways, similar to the minor maladjustments, but far more severe and handicapping. The handicaps are not necessarily physical, since only a certain proportion of neurotics develop psychosomatic diseases or present primarily physical symptoms. Rather, they are emotional, since neurosis makes one *feel* terrible much of the time, thereby hampering efforts to work, love, and pursue a normal life.

To understand how a neurotic feels, one need only recall his own embarrassment or anxiety at the first dance he went to, or his feeling of panic after some near-accident on the highway, or his impotent rage after being unfairly bawled out by his boss. Such feelings, multiplied greatly in strength, exist within neurotics — not just for moments or hours, but week after week and year after year.

Some neurotics are plagued by nameless fears and feelings of imminent doom. Some cannot stand the slightest disorder in their surrounding, and are fanatically neat or hygienic. Some, whether hungry or not, overeat until they become grossly obese. Some imagine themselves sick or dying, and haunt the doctor's office. Some cannot make any decisions, even about simple everyday matters. Some are continually haunted by nameless, unidentifiable anxiety.

In a general way, we can explain a neurosis as a *defensive reaction* of the personality to serious threat, just as fever, edema, vomiting, and the like are defensive measures taken by the body against certain threats to itself.

The psychic threat may, for instance, be a conflict between opposing desires, in which the clash produces such alarming feelings of guilt or expectations of punishment that the personality defensively hides or resolves the conflict through a development of pathological symptoms.

Puritanically reared persons, caught between conflicting desires to be sinless and to enjoy pleasures of the flesh, may end the inner struggle by becoming impotent or frigid — a solution which is neurotic because it "solves" the problem at the cost of severe personal handicap. The child reared by a domineering parent, and caught in adulthood between conflicting desires to succeed and to be meek and submissive, may solve his inner conflict by "accidentally" failing each time he is near success. The wronged husband or businessman, caught between the desire not to commit a violent or hateful act, may "choose" paralysis, or amnesia, or a heart ailment, or become so preoccupied with trifles that he has no time to pursue and punish the enemy.

5. *Psychoses.* The illnesses thus far described may, from time to time, require hospitalization, but the great majority of people suffering from them are able to remain in the world and to get along, even though imperfectly. But with the *psychoses*, we are in the realm of serious mental illness which more frequently is so disabling, or so disturbing to the patient or society, as to require treatment in a hospital for a period of time.

A psychotic may, for instance, be so depressed as to refuse food altogether or to attempt suicide. He may be so confused that he fails to recognize relatives and friends, and is not even sure of his own identity. He may hear voices, see apparitions, imagine himself in contact with God, and actually act upon what his "voices" tell him to do. He may be prey to uncontrollable spasms of laughter, senseless rages, or total apathy.

As a result of such symptoms, about half of all psychotic persons in this country, or about half a million people, are currently patients in state, federal, and private mental institutions. Probably another half million psychotics are borderline cases, and get along on their own or are cared for at home by their families.

Although a psychosis is an illness of the mind, it can be produced either by psychological or physical causes.

In a little over half of all hospitalized psychotics, the mental illness seems to have primarily psychological causes — i.e., internal emotional tensions and conflicts, acted upon and aggravated by external pressures such as deprivation or tragedy. They suffer from diseases whose names have become familiar to almost everyone — *schizophrenia, involutional psychosis, manic-depressive psychosis,* and others.

The other half of the hospitalized psychotics are victims of "organic psychoses," or serious mental illnesses which have primarily physical causes. Brain tumors, hardening of the brain arteries due to age, and damage to brain tissues from alcoholism, drug addiction, or injuries, all cause serious mental malfunctioning with symptoms which are often rather similar to those of the functional (psychologically caused) psychoses. Physical and mental tests enable psychiatrists to distinguish between the two and prescribe treatment accordingly.

6. *Mental Retardation.* This category, also known as *mental deficiency, mental subnormality,* and *feeblemindedness,* includes many quite different conditions. All of them cause the development of the mind to be slowed and halted before adolescence, leaving the victim below average in mental powers. Such persons are classified as either "profoundly," "severely," "moderately," or "mildly" retarded.

The *profoundly* retarded have IQ's under 20, and the *severely* retarded have IQ's from 20 to 35. The estimated 60,000 to 90,000 persons in these categories in the United States are clearly unable to take care of themselves, and need constant care and supervision in order to survive; accordingly, nearly all of them are in mental institutions.

The *moderately* retarded have IQ's between 35 and 50, number some 300,000 to 350,000. Generally, given an adequately protected environment, they can learn to take care of themselves and to do semi-productive work. Many of them are therefore able to live with their families.

The *mildly* retarded, whose IQ's range from 50 to 70 or even sometimes a little higher, and who number about five million, are hard to distinguish from normal persons until school highlights their learning limitations. Without special attention, many of them become problem members of society — frequently unemployed, frequently in trouble. With timely supervision, guidance, and training, however, most of them could be — and many are — completely assimilated into the life of the community.

Causes of mental retardation are numerous but, for the most part, not yet clearly identified. Currently it is possible to identify precise causes in only one-quarter or fewer of the cases, these usually involving organic pathology which has resulted in profound or severe retardation.

Among the many diseases or conditions which cause gross brain damage are certain infections or poisons in the mother's system during pregnancy, such as syphilis, German measles, or overdoses of powerful drugs; a variety of hereditary disorders involving freak genes which cause abnormal metabolism and development; and injuries to the brain at birth or during childhood.

While some of these disorders are beyond present remedy, medical science has been learning to overcome others of them by prevention (as is true of German measles) or early treatment (transfusions for infants with Rh blood factor incompatibility, dietary changes to overcome faulty body chemistry in such diseases as *phenylketonuria* or *galactosemia*).

But for the great majority of individuals who are only moderately or mildly retarded, individual and specific causes cannot now be assigned. Nevertheless, statistical studies are giving researchers today some idea of the general factors at work.

Some of the mildly retarded are undoubtedly the result of genetic and hereditary factors. They are one end of the curve of distribution of abilities, the other end being the highly gifted. A second general factor consists of faulty prenatal care and poor nutrition, which affect the brain in ways which elude present identification.

The most significant factors among the vast mass of the mildly retarded, however, seem to be adverse social, economic, and cultural conditions, for the incidence of retardation is strikingly higher among the deprived classes of every race than among the more advantaged. A number of educational experiments with ostensibly retarded children from slum areas seem to show that a major cause of retardation may be the lack of learning opportunities and mental stimuli. Such deprivation seems to stunt young people intellectually during their development.

THE TREATMENTS

With emotional and mental illnesses, as with physical ones, the most important questions to decide are whether or not the particular condition requires treatment, and if so, what type or types.

A bruise or a common cold will get better thanks to the body's own reparative processes, and in most cases satisfactory recovery takes place without professional attention. In the same way, many of the sorrows, anxieties, and nervous disabilities we suffer from are minor and self-terminated, or are basic to the human condition and are not significantly changed by treatment. The grief caused by the death of a loved person, the anxiety caused by the prospect of a major operation, are usually normal, and usually self-terminating. The loss of zest that comes with aging, and the fear of death, may be sorrows of life itself which are usually inescapable.

Is Treatment Necessary? Each person must therefore decide — with professional help, whenever needed — whether a given emotional or mental disorder in himself or a member of his family is serious enough to require treatment, or could be eliminated by treatment. It would be both unrealistic and unfair to urge all people to seek treatment for every psychological disorder. Only about 2,000,000 people are currently receiving any kind of psychiatric or psychological therapy. This is probably only one-tenth of all those with some form of psychological disorder, and were the other nine tenths suddenly to seek treatment, the situation would become utterly chaotic.

Moreover, surveys made here and in England show that a majority of neurotic symptoms recede or disappear of their own accord within a few years from the time of onset. Finally, some conditions which do not go away by themselves may be imperfections not really requiring removal. Stinginess, slovenliness, or a domineering or bullying nature, may be tolerable, even if not desirable.

In a sense, therefore, it is for the affected individual to decide whether he wants to be changed, or to continue as he is. Yet a decision made by one's self may be an uninformed decision, based on insufficient evidence and made the more erroneous by the distortions of the emotional disorder itself. It is folly to avoid the doctor until a cancer has metastasized; it is folly to allow an emotional disorder to progress until it produces nervous breakdown.

Even though the data indicate that many untreated nervous conditions get better by themselves, other data indicate that many of them grow worse and become catastrophic. When there is therapeutic intervention, however, about two-thirds of persons treated by psychological methods show distinct improvement or cure.

The clearest evidence in favor of active treatment comes from mental hospitals. Several generations ago, when psychotics were locked up in hospitals and given next to no therapy, a great many of them grew worse and worse, becoming virtual vegetables. Today, with combined somatic and psychological therapies being given them as soon as they arrive, four-fifths of newly admitted patients at the better mental hospitals can be released within half a year as cured or at least improved enough to get along in society.

Making such a crucial decision, except where the problem is very obviously quite minor, requires the diagnostic help of a highly trained professional — usually a psychiatrist, although the highly qualified psychologists and social workers on the staffs of mental health clinics and family service agencies can do quite competent preliminary diagnostic work where physical ailments are not involved in the emotional or mental disease.

The Psychotherapies

"*Psychotherapy*" is the general term for psychological methods of treatment of emotional and mental illnesses. Actually, the word refers to several different kinds of treatment, and it would be more accurate to speak of "the psychotherapies." With a few exceptions, the psychotherapies do not involve the use of drugs, operations, shock treatments, or other physical therapies, though these may be used in conjunction with psychotherapy as a combined form of treatment.

Psychotherapies themselves involve treatment through *words* and *concepts* exchanged by patient and therapist; these may be spoken in the form of discussions, advice, self-searching, and so on. The result may vary from a kind of mental first-aid, in which the patient is reassured and given good advice, to a comprehensive, profound remodeling of personality and feelings. The many types of psychotherapy can generally be grouped under three headings:

(a) *Surface psychotherapy.* This term covers treatments of a simple, superficial type, not probing further than the conscious part of the mind, and not making any changes in the personality. Such therapy is a type of emergency repair, like the checking of bleeding. In a great many cases, it takes only this much help to enable a stunned, or depressed, or panic-stricken, but basically healthy, person to take hold of himself again and deal with his problems on his own.

Such psychotherapy consists of face-to-face discussions between the patient and the psychotherapist, who may have been trained as a social worker, a psychologist, or a psychiatrist (a physician trained in psychiatry). Indeed, a great deal of uncomplicated psychotherapy, consisting of sympathetic noncritical listening, while a distraught person talks out his worries or spills out his angers, can be performed by a family doctor or minister.

Deep psychotherapy, however, should be performed only by highly trained experts who are fully prepared to deal with their own feelings and reactions in the presence of emotional disturbance.

Surface psychotherapies include *ventilation* (the blowing off of steam or talking out of worries), *reassurance, direct advice,* and *support and encouragement.* These terms, all familiar in our language, make surface psychotherapy sound deceptively easy.

The patient's problems, his worries, his emotional attitudes, may cause him to accept advice eagerly or to reject it in anger, to benefit from support and reassurance or to lean upon the therapist like a crutch. Furthermore, just as the diagnosis of infections and the prescribing of antibiotics looks simple, but is fraught with risk, so is the diagnosis of emotional disorder and the use of surface psychotherapy full of danger to both patient and the unskilled practitioner.

Most physicians would prefer to see psychotherapy either done by doctors, or supervised by doctors, as is true of treatment performed in the 1,600 mental health clinics throughout the nation, which handle a caseload of about 650,000 persons per year. Yet it is also beyond question that a great volume of excellent casework — an estimated 700,000 persons per year — is being done by non-physician therapists, without medical supervision, at the 300 family service agencies throughout America. In addition to therapists working in these agency and clinical set-ups, all species of psychotherapists working in private practice also use the surface psychotherapies just described.

(b) *Reparative psychotherapy.* When the therapist tries to get the patient to see deeper than his everyday thoughts about his problems, becoming aware of some of the inner forces that underlie his difficulties and feelings, treatment becomes more involved and prolonged, but more likely to achieve valuable changes.

In these forms of therapy, the patient is encouraged to speak freely and at considerable length about his emotions, his experiences, his problems, and his hopes. The trained therapist, listening very intently, is able to recognize the unspoken or unconscious processes underlying the actual words. A patient may, for instance, claim he loves his parents, yet despite a good-natured and affectionate way of talking about them, may mention only complaints against them. The therapist may recognize that there is much hostile feeling involved, and can judge how much of this the patient needs to recognize in order to make progress.

Using his knowledge of the patient's inner emotional processes, the therapist guides the discussion toward the crucial issues, offers careful but pertinent interpretations to give the patient a certain amount of insight (recognition of his own inner conflicts and traits), and may even suggest specific changes in his work, his surroundings, and his habits which will ease his tensions or offer outlet for his drives. In short, reparative psychotherapy is often a combination of insight, plus direction by the therapist.

The reparative psychotherapies can be performed by some, but not all, social workers, and by psychologists and psychiatrists, some of whom have had special training as psychoanalysts. Many marital problems, child-rearing problems, and work difficulties — the minor maladjustments—respond well to reparative psychotherapy, and even neuroses of a not-too-severe nature may benefit greatly from it. A patient with a severe neurosis, however, needs still more intensive psychotherapy (see *Reconstructive psychotherapy,* below), while a patient with a psychosomatic disease may require medical treatment, and it may be necessary that he be seen by a physician other than a psychiatrist. Every patient with a *psychosis* should be seen by a psychiatrist, and some of these patients will require medical treatment as well.

(c) *Reconstructive psychotherapy.* In contrast to support, or repair, some forms of psychotherapy aim to get the patient to uncover even his deepest-hidden conflicts, hidden distortions of thought, and forgotten emotional wounds, and through examining them with the therapist, reconstruct his personality along more nearly normal and healthful lines.

Classic Freudian psychoanalysis is only one of the techniques that fall into this category. Others include such forms of deep psychotherapy as "analytically oriented psychotherapy," "ego analysis," "existential analysis," and the varied methods of analysis used by followers of Harry Stack Sullivan, Karen Horney, Carl Jung, and other off-shoots from traditional Freudian methods.

Nearly all psychiatrists agree that neither conscious thinking about one's problem, nor even insight into one's conflicts, can yield major changes in the personality. To do so requires an emotional re-education — a bit-by-bit reconditioning of the patient's reactions to people, thoughts, and situations.

A woman who is frigid in the marital bed may achieve insight enough to know that her coldness is the result of, say, a conflict between her puritanical upbringing and her desire for a normal relationship. But this insight does not automatically cause her to feel normal desire or to achieve satisfaction. An irrational response is not conquered by simply admitting that it is irrational. The multiple connections of the mind have to be rewired, so to speak, through hundreds of hours of therapeutic rethinking and refeeling.

Little wonder, then, that deep psychotherapies such as psychoanalysis may be protracted and sometimes difficult. The unconscious material, for one thing, must be painstakingly sought through free association (speaking whatever comes to mind), recounting and examining dreams for their clues to the secrets of the unconscious, continual analysis of the patient's own changing feelings about the therapist himself (since the therapist comes to stand for all sorts of persons who have been important in the patient's life), and the like.

Precisely because psychoanalysis deals with the shadowed, hidden, and often unpleasant aspects of our lives, it is over-praised by its friends and over-criticised by its foes, has collected an entire mythology, and attracts both brilliant therapists and quacks. It achieves few complete cures (one study indicates that perhaps a fifth of all patients are thoroughly reconstructed), but many major improvements (two-thirds or more of the patients in several studies got major benefits from treatment).

Who is qualified to help? In some states, deep psychotherapy can be practiced by almost anyone who chooses to call himself a therapist. The would-be patient should check closely into the qualifications of a psychotherapist before beginning treatment.

Your family physician or your county medical society can be of assistance in helping you find a physician qualified to do deep psychotherapy, or you can, by yourself, consult the *Directory of Medical Specialists* at a library, to get the names of qualified psychiatrists in your area. Most of those psychiatrists who have been trained to do psychoanalysis will have gone to any one of 19 training institutes affiliated with the American Psychoanalytic Association. A list of those institutes can be found in the Association's publications.

In addition, *Action for Mental Health* — the final report of the Joint Commission on Mental Illness and Health to Congress — stated that "a narrow enforcement of a psychiatric conviction that 'nobody should do psychotherapy except psychiatrists' would effectively deny its benefits by patients now receiving it from non-medical therapists".

Accordingly, the Joint Commission recommended that psychotherapy continue to be practiced by non-medical persons with special training and competence.

These would include primarily psychologists, but also some social workers with appropriate training. A partial list of recognized institutes training non-medical analysts can be obtained from the Council of Psychoanalytic Psychotherapists, c/o Jacob Nussbaum, Ph.D., 315 Central Park West, New York, N. Y.

Somatic (Physical) Therapies

Somatic or physical forms of treatment are used primarily in the case of psychosis, alcoholism, and mental retardation, but only rarely in the case of neurosis. Somatic therapy may be required for either one of two quite different reasons.

First, where there is a special physical condition creating a psychological impairment, a physical therapy may yield a direct benefit. Thus, the confusion, stupor, or even rage resulting from a brain tumor may disappear when the tumor is operatively removed. The delusions and hallucinations resulting from a chronic toxic condition such as alcoholism may disappear when the patient is "dried out."

The forgetfulness, ill humor, and general lassitude often seen in senile psychotics, who have impairment of brain tissues due to age, are often overcome in good part by an energetic program of physical therapy and retraining in motor skills. Certain types of mental retardation are minimized or offset by chemotherapies which help compensate for the lopsided hormone production of a defective body, or by diet control to overcome metabolic deficiencies which have been causing an accumulation of poisonous products in the body and brain.

The *second* reason for somatic therapy is that in the functional (primarily psychological) psychoses, though there may be no demonstrable physical cause for the disease, certain influences exerted upon the body seem to calm the excited mind, or dissipate clouds and visions. In recent decades these therapies have included *barbiturates,* the *"wet pack"* (a heavy, wet, snugly wrapped sheet), *insulin shock, electric shock,* and *lobotomy.* For reasons not clearly understood, these measures have calmed some excited patients, roused others out of depressions, and helped others lay aside wild delusions or visions.

Drug therapies. Since 1955, however, the tranquilizing drugs — primarily chlorpromazine and reserpine, and their many relatives — have pushed most of the other somatic therapies into the background. The tranquilizers greatly reduce disturbed, abusive, dangerous, or confused behavior in a large percentage of newly admitted psychotics, and are useful to a somewhat lesser extent with psychotics of long standing.

The drugs do not, of themselves, "cure" mental illnesses, but via undiscovered chemical pathways they manage to dampen the intensity of feelings of fear and anger, and to reduce the impact of hallucinations and delusions. With this help, the mind is enabled to rebuild its defenses, repair the shattered ego, and reach out once again to outsiders. Such healing does not, of course, correct the internal weakness and conflicts which underlay the breakdown. But with those conflicts back under control, the patient may get along well in the outside world, for anywhere from months to decades, depending on the emotional forces which his life brings to bear upon him.

Lithium

Classic manic-depressive psychosis is manifested by patients who swing from moods of extreme euphoria—tireless excitement, scene-making, wild schemes, sleeplessness—to deep depression. Antidepressant drugs are useful in managing the "down" phase. Large doses of tranquilizers can take the edge off excitement but often at the price of dulled, drugged, strait-jacketed feelings. A drug which seems to strike at the core of the illness, by alleviating symptoms without impairment of alertness or memory, is lithium carbonate.

Lithium is a metallic element; its salts are relatively simple (and unpatentable). Lithium got a bad name a quarter of a century ago when its use as a common salt substitute resulted in numerous poisonings and a ban on its sale. It is still a potentially toxic agent, but its striking effects have led to its release for medical use in the manic or "high" phase of manic-depressive illness.

In general, daily doses of lithium carbonate greatly improve the condition of about 80 per cent of hyperexcited patients in one or two weeks, more or less irrespective of age or duration of the disorder. Whether or not continued doses can prevent manic outbursts and cyclic mood swings is not fully established, but there is evidence of prophylactic value.

Close medical supervision of lithium therapy is imperative. The drug is especially hazardous for patients who have severe heart or kidney disease or who require low-sodium diets or use of diuretics. The physician must make frequent determinations of lithium concentration in the blood to establish dosage, and regular but less frequent determinations thereafter. Some patients who are predisposed to thyroid disease may develop goiter on lithium therapy, but this is usually controllable by medication.

Depression. Most people have occasional bouts of "the blues" or periods of low spirits from which they generally rebound rather quickly. Depressive illness is different, serious, and not uncommon in clinical practice. The patient characteristically has feelings of utter hopelessness, worthlessness, and despair for the future, for which there can often be found plausible reasons that actually have little bearing on his illness. Drugs have attained a useful role in treatment of depressive illness in the past decade. The most widely prescribed anti-depressants are tricyclic drugs (such as imipramine) and monoamine-oxidase inhibitors. The drugs act slowly. Recognition and close medical supervision of true depressive illness are important.—D.G.C.

Social Treatment

Both *psychological* and *physical* therapies, as described above, deal with the patient as a solo entity. But mental illness is as much a matter of interference with inter-personal relationships as it is with inner mental functioning. The third approach, therefore — which is used not in place of, but in addition to, the first two — consists of building around the patient a network of reassuring and satisfying *social* contacts.

Most typically, this method is used within mental hospitals and residential treatment centers for juvenile delinquents and youthful psychotics. The persons involved with the patients are staff members (including nurses, attendants or psychiatric aides, and doctors), volunteer workers, hospital employees, and fellow patients. The therapeutic activities may include anything from games and dances to reassuring group therapy discussions and paid employment.

Social treatment is designed to give the patient many comforting, satisfying experiences with other human beings, both to restore his faith in them and to rebuild his concept of himself as a useful and likeable human being. Like tranquilizers or shock treatment, these experiences enable him to discount and lay aside the harmful thoughts about himself and other people that had been ruling him.

In a hospital where tranquilizers have given the patients enough emotional control to be allowed to move about freely from building to building, social treatment functions most effectively. Indeed, the entire hospital becomes a therapeutic atmosphere, its whole milieu becoming useful to the patient. The name "milieu therapy" is an effort to indicate this total utilization of all the patient's experience toward helping him get better.

Hospital treatment for psychotics, the mentally retarded, the more seriously neurotic, and for alcoholics or drug addicts, is offered by the 300-odd state hospitals throughout the country. Unfortunately, only about one-fifth of these hospitals are able to apply modern therapeutic methods. The rest, understaffed and underbudgeted, do little more than keep their patients under control, fed, clothed, and sheltered.

State mental hospitals are inexpensive (they charge anywhere from nothing to a maximum of about $200 a month, depending on ability to pay), and care for the great majority of the hospitalized mentally ill in the United States.

Over 700 community general hospitals have by now established psychiatric wards or beds, and accept patients on a short-term basis. Those who can be sufficiently helped in a month or two are kept, those who need longer care are referred to state or private hospitals. The community hospitals are a good deal more expensive than state hospitals, but most patients pay only a part of the average $35-per-day cost, the rest coming from community funds. To an increasing extent, part of these costs is being covered by Blue Cross, Blue Shield and other insurance programs.

There are also about 300 small private mental hospitals in the United States, some of which represent the best facilities available, in terms of staffing, comfort, individual attention, and number of therapies used. They are, of course, expensive, ranging from several hundred to $2,000 a month. Despite having relatively few beds, they take care of 14 per cent of all first admissions to mental hospitals each year.

Finally, throughout the nation there are some 1,600 mental health clinics (out-patient clinics), serving about 650,-000 non-hospitalized people each year. Most of these are persons with character disorders and neurotics, receiving psychotherapy. Some, however, are borderline or "ambulatory" psychotics who get not only psychotherapy but tranquilizing drugs and even, in some of these clinics, shock treatments. The clinics do not, however, maintain beds.

Biological Factors

The hypothesis that some forms of psychotic illness for which there is no recognizable organic basis express physico-chemical rather than purely environmental factors is a challenge to investigators, for if specific biochemical differences between the ill and the not-ill can be identified, design of drugs to correct imbalances is theoretically possible. Every person is biochemically unique, possessing (or lacking) some enzyme systems which differ subtly from those of others. Since such systems are inherited, a few researchers have begun to study the genetic aspects of forms of mental illness. The task is difficult, for genes and environment interact in complex ways, but a considerable degree of progress is being made.

No particular gene or biochemical pathway has been identified as a "cause" of schizophrenia, but the association of genetic factors has been confirmed quite decisively. It has long been known that schizophrenia tends to run in families. A child of schizophrenic parents is some 15 times more likely to develop the disorder than a child of non-schizophrenic parents. Classic manic-depressive psychosis, with swings from hyperexcitement to depression, often has distinctive family histories. One institutional study indicates that the disorder is transmitted in an X-linked (female chromosome) fashion and is probably associated with the gene for color blindness.

"Super-males" with an extra male chromosome (XYY) have been associated with violence and proneness to sex-linked crime, although most known XYY men don't commit any crimes. Large-scale studies are difficult because chromosome analysis is time-consuming.

As yet there is no practical outcome of such genetic investigations, but continuing studies should lead to better understanding of mechanisms of mental illness and perhaps to better measures of prevention and treatment. —D.G.C.

Choosing a Treatment and a Therapist

As already pointed out, the choice of treatment or no treatment — at least in the case of the minor emotional ailments — is more or less up to the patient, though he may need professional advice in making his decision. Assuming a person does want relief from emotional distress, he faces a second decision: what type of treatment, and how prolonged, does he need?

In many early cases of emotional illness, where symptoms are not severe and not deeply ingrained as a pattern of behavior, great help can be obtained in a few sessions of psychotherapy for relatively little cost (sessions run anywhere from a few dollars in clinics to $25 in private practice).

For deeper-seated difficulties, deeper-reaching (reparative) psychotherapy may be needed. It will cost about the same amount per hour, but often requires many more hours. Finally, psychoanalysis, costing $20 to $25 per hour on the average, in private practice, may take a number of months or even years, at several hours per week.

In the case of more serious disorders, including the psychoses and mental retardation, the choice is somewhat narrower. If the patient can be maintained at home, it is often better for him to stay with his family. Yet sometimes the presence of a borderline psychotic or a retarded child may produce emotional disorder in other family members.

A psychiatrist's opinion on such a decision is almost essential. If the decision is in favor of institutionalization, the second question is whether to apply to a state, community, or private hospital. This is a matter of economics and of a realistic appraisal of the patient's chances of recovering.

Sources of help. In the making of any of the above decisions, professional advice, examination, and diagnosis may be called for. As already indicated, the family doctor is a primary resource, though only a limited number of family doctors are presently capable of making detailed psychiatric diagnoses. But those who are not will know competent psychiatrists to whom to refer their patients. So will the local medical society.

Psychiatrists working in a clinical, low-cost setting can be found in mental health clinics, which can be located in the classified phone book under "Mental Health Association of [Your County]." Mental health clinics, moreover, have additional personnel, besides psychiatrists, who can make preliminary diagnoses, with referral to psychiatrists in the clinic or in private practice, where needed.

The same functions of preliminary diagnosis, casework, or clinical referral to outside psychiatrists where needed, are performed by family service agencies, which can be found in the classified directory under "Family Service Association of America—Accredited Agencies." All the family agencies, incidentally, maintain lists of qualified psychotherapists and psychiatrists in their own area for the benefit of those who primarily seek referral rather than treatment within the agency.

Other sources of names are the national organizations of qualified therapists. These include the American Association of Marriage Counselors, 27 Woodcliff Drive, Madison, New Jersey; The National Association of Social Workers, 2 Park Avenue, New York, New York; and the American Psychological Association, 1333 16th Street, NW, Washington, D. C. As for the American Psychiatric Association and the American Psychoanalytic Association, it is not necessary to write them directly, since their membership lists are available in major libraries.

Locating a Hospital

.To locate the right mental hospital for the patient in your family, call your local *county medical society, family service agency,* or *mental health clinic.* Your *family physician* may also have some special knowledge in this area. In an emergency, where the patient's behavior is suicidal, homicidal, violent or hysterical, call your doctor first. If necessary, he can arrange for an emergency admission to a hospital. If he is not available, call your local medical society; it will help you find a doctor to perform these functions.

What Shakespeare wrote of death could as well be written of psychiatric treatment, as far as many people are concerned: it is fear that makes us "rather bear those ills we have / Than fly to others that we know not of." But the time has come to lay aside that fear. The majority of people treated by any legitimate psychological or somatic therapy, for any kind of emotional or mental disorder, now are benefited or completely cured — the sooner the treatment being started, the better the chances for swift and complete recovery.

CHAPTER 22

YOUR OPERATION

by JAMES GRAHAM, M.D.

HOSPITAL PROCEDURES

Preparation • Anesthesia • Recovery
• Children's Surgery

OPERATIONS

Stomach • Intestines • Gallbladder •
Female Organs • Hernia • Lungs •
Heart • Genitourinary Tract • Ear •
Head and Neck • Breast • Nervous
System • Eyes • Orthopedic Surgery
• Plastic Surgery

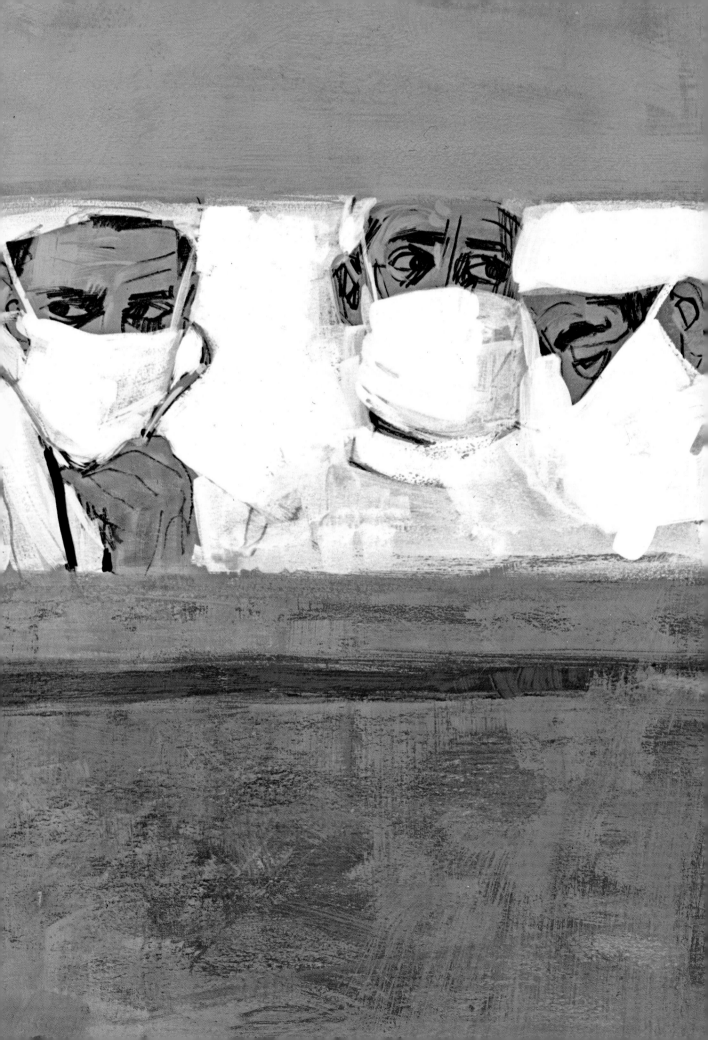

CHAPTER 22

YOUR OPERATION

by JAMES GRAHAM, M.D.

Every morning, 50,000 Americans wiggle out of bed for a stretcher ride down hospital corridors to an operating room. Here each of these finds himself alone, without relatives or friends, in what appears to be a strange wonderland of different sights, sounds, odors, tastes and feelings. Soon, however, one recognizes his doctor and probably also the anesthetist who talked with him the day before, and the patient realizes that he is the right person in the right place.

If you should find yourself among the 50,000 some morning, you won't be the only one trying to make sense out of the routine. Routine it is, and has to be, for surgery is a precision operation and always a serious one, geared to a tolerance of no mistakes. There is no room for emotion in the usual sense—friendliness, yes; kindliness bounded by disciplined strictness; compassion suppressed in minds preoccupied with the primary task — but not emotion.

Pre-operative preparations. Let's take a stomach operation as an example of the routines you go through before reaching the operating room. The day before surgery your doctor orders a *liquid supper,* an *enema,* a *sleeping capsule, preparation of skin, no breakfast* the next morning, a *stomach tube,* and an *injection* (shot in the arm).

The liquid supper insures that your stomach and intestine will be empty the next morning. Because this is a stomach operation, a stomach tube will be put in your nose to drain out the natural digestive fluid that forms in your stomach through the night. This is a thin tube of soft plastic that passes through your nose and down to the stomach. It is connected to a suction bottle that draws liquid and gas from the stomach by vacuum.

Any residue of food you ate before the liquid supper will be taken care of by an enema which flushes out the lower intestine and rectum.

The surgeon wants the stomach to be empty in case there should be vomiting. This would be dangerous in a sleeping person because the vomitus might well up in the throat into the windpipe.

The sleeping capsule helps put you in a relaxed state and along with the "shot in the arm" the next morning paves the way for the anesthetic. Less anesthetic gas is required for a relaxed patient, and the less required the better.

The skin of the operative area is cleansed with detergents and antiseptics and then shaved. With stomach operations, this extends from the middle of the chest to the hips, but of course the incision won't extend over the whole area.

Routines. Lots of things will happen to you as a matter of routine. This is because all of the doctors as a staff decide that, in the interests of safety, certain tests must be made on all patients, no matter what the reason for their admission to the hospital.

A technician will take a specimen of blood from your finger and a specimen of urine will be collected. These will be analyzed in the laboratory before morning. Other tests that are not routine will be made when ordered by your doctor because of your particular problem.

All of this routine has been worked out very carefully. These procedures are not just old customs that the hospital staff follows unthinkingly. They are the checks and safety factors that integrate the complexities of modern surgery.

If you are to have a general anesthetic, you will be put to sleep in the operating room. There is no need to worry about not being fully asleep before the operation begins. The anesthetist checks for anesthesia just like the pilot checks his motors before he heads the plane down the runway. Some 10,000,000 anesthetics are given each year in this country.

How long will the operation take? People often judge the seriousness of an operation by the time it takes, but seriousness is not related to the time required. A very grave operation may take but a short time, whereas several hours may be needed for a slow-moving procedure of much less gravity.

Although isolation of the operating suite from the general public adds mystery to the proceedings, mystery is not the intent. Sterility is the reason. Bacteria and germs must be kept out, hence the scrubbing, the changing of clothes and the putting on of gowns, gloves and masks. Street shoes are not allowed in the inner rooms; either the shoes are changed or they are covered with canvas overshoes. Only surgical personnel are permitted in the operating rooms. This is why the patient must go in alone. Mother and Dad may be convinced that little Johnny could be spared a fearsome experience by their presence, but maintenance of sterility for Johnny's operation demands that parents be excluded.

The surgical team. Who are the people of surgery? Probably you don't even recognize them in the halls of the hospital because you met them behind masks and gowns. Despite this, they are ordinary people just like you, doing the things you do and liking the things you like. You can be assured they are not indifferent.

First there is the *surgeon*. Although he is the important figure, he does not work alone. He is the head of a team that performs your operation. A second doctor acts as first *assistant*. Two *"scrub nurses"* handle the instruments in the operating field. A *"circulating nurse"* moves in and out of the room as a liaison between the operative field and the central sterilizing supply. In the sterilizing rooms there are *surgical technicians* and *surgical aides*. At the head of the table is the *anesthetist*.

Of longest training and discipline is the surgeon. His work is scrutinized by the medical audit committee of the staff. Technicians and aides have been through special courses and trained on the job. The anesthetist may be a doctor with specialized training in anesthesia, or a nurse who has finished at both regular nursing school and anesthesia school.

These are the team; trained, disciplined, stimulated by the intricacies of their work; on the overall, quite understanding of the trials of their fellow men. These are the people who perform the operations we shall examine later.

Recovery. After the operation you are still in a deep sleep. Lifted from the operating table, you are wheeled to the recovery department where you will get special attention. There is an experienced nurse here for every one or two patients. Each bed is in a small area partitioned on two sides but opened on the end to face the nurses' station. This keeps you under minute-to-minute observation.

Each patient stays in the recovery department until he has pretty well wakened. This may mean an hour or several hours. As soon as you swallow when there is something in your mouth, or cough when there is something in your throat, or make some kind of motion or sound when anything hurts you, you will be ready to return to your room. The nurse will know that your blood pressure is stable, that your pulse is strong and that your breathing is natural.

If special attention is required for a longer period you will go to "Intensive Care". The set-up here is pretty much like that in the recovery department. The idea is to keep the ratio of one or two patients per nurse to allow constant observation and attention. The stay in intensive care may be for a day or several days.

Post-operative care. Naturally an operative wound would hurt if nothing were done to relieve pain, but there are medicines for this. Until your stomach is ready to accept food, the medicine will be given in your arm. Because pain medicines have a tendency to depress body functions, excessive doses slow down the recovery process. But if you hurt, say so. Don't suffer pain without letting the nurse know about it. Sleeping medicine will be given to you to assist in relaxing under the unusual circumstances of a hospital, the bodily discomfort, restricted motion, new sounds, interruptions, other people in the room, but you should not expect to be drugged to sleep every night from the time of your operation until you are ready to go home.

Deep breathing is very important after surgery. When the lungs do not expand fully, the small air sacs at the edges of the lungs remain collapsed like the folds at the ends of an accordion and the folds may stick stogether. This could set the stage for pneumonia. Because you are dry, the mucus in the air passages becomes sticky and it clings to the bronchial tubes. For this reason it has to be coughed out.

Simple measures used to overcome the tendency to shallow breathing include moving about in bed, from side to side, or up to a sitting position. Other means are ready when these simple measures don't work well enough.

Moisture is restored to the bronchial tubes by breathing oxygen that comes bubbling through a solution. There are machines, operating by oxygen pressure and fitted with a breathing mask, that can make you cough forcibly and yet without pain. Another machine can make you breathe deeply to fill up the air sacs, again without hurting.

Emptying the bladder may be difficult for a patient in bed, because the control muscle of the bladder may not relax. When the bladder wall becomes stretched, the force for expelling urine is weakened. This situation is relieved by passing a small soft rubber tube into the bladder.

Intravenous feedings. If you cannot take food or drink, you still must be nourished. The common method is to let a nourishing liquid drip through a hollow needle placed in a vein in your arm. The nourishing element in the liquid may be sugar or mixtures of proteins and fats. Other chemical compounds are sometimes added, depending upon the requirements. These liquid feedings in the vein are called *intravenouses*. They are run in slowly to prevent overloading of the circulation and to allow a good mixture with the blood. In addition to nourishment, you are getting fluid which is necessary to vital functions. The human machine must have water to humidify or air-condition the air in the lungs, to discharge heat through the skin as perspiration, and to eliminate waste chemicals.

Bowel movements will be irregular and sluggish after your operation because you are out of your usual routine and are not physically active. In addition, you may be trying to have a bowel movement lying down instead of sitting up. Bowel activity is checked daily on your record so don't worry about the nursing staff forgetting your bowels. In due time you will be given an enema or a mild laxative.

Since the muscle wall of the intestine is weak after surgery, even normally swallowed air is not pushed along. Thus air builds up in some sections causing gas pockets. Because of this some liquids that produce more gas than others will be forbidden.

There are no hard and fast rules about the time for getting out of bed because the condition of each patient and the operation are so variable. When you are given the green light, go ahead and move. Motion prevents complications of surgery by improving breathing, circulation, urination, bowel movement, and general muscular tone of the patient.

The fewer visitors the better, except for long term patients who are not seriously ill. Acutely ill patients who will be home shortly need only the immediate family, and this means those who live in the same house. A get-well card will do more good than a visit. Illness is a time for privacy.

The *skin sutures* in your wound may be removed before you leave the hospital or the surgeon may prefer to delay this. This is not the ordeal many patients think it is going to be. The skin sutures are not holding you together, because this is the job of other sutures placed in the depths of the wound. Only the skin sutures are removed. They are just loops of thread that come free when clipped. If nothing further were done after clipping, the sutures would fall out in due time.

You will be given instructions on what you can eat and what you can do before you go home. If you have questions about wearing a support, going up and down steps, going outside, lifting, driving a car, taking a bath or washing your hair, be sure you have the answers before you leave the hospital.

STOMACH OPERATIONS

Although most stomach operations are for ulcers or tumors, other troubles also call for surgery. One such trouble is *hernia of the diaphragm*. Here the stomach is dislocated into the chest cavity through a hole in the diaphragm. In the operation for correction of this condition, the stomach is returned to its natural location in the abdomen and the hernia hole is repaired.

Just the opposite is the case when the surgeon has to put the stomach up into the chest cavity after fashioning it into a tube to replace an esophagus that has been removed. The stomach is sometimes opened out onto the skin surface of the abdomen so that feedings can be put into it directly. This is called a *gastrostomy*. A fairly common operation in infants corrects an overdeveloped stomach outlet muscle that won't let food through. The outlet muscle is cut across.

Ulcers

Although ulcers are referred to so often as stomach ulcers, most of them are not in the stomach but are located in the duodenum. Some ulcers cannot be healed by medicine and diet and therefore they must be handled by surgery. The conditions that make surgery necessary in ulcer cases are:

1. *Bleeding.* The ulcer erodes deeply enough into the stomach or duodenal wall to cut into a blood vessel.
2. *Perforation.* The ulcer erodes deeply enough to open a hole. It bursts.
3. *Obstructions.* The dense scar tissue around the ulcer twists and angulates, damming up the outlet of the stomach.
4. *Intractability.* Despite strict observance of dietary regulation, the ulcer will not heal.
5. *Location in the stomach.* An unhealed ulcer located in the stomach cannot be distinguished from a cancer of the stomach. Ulcers in the duodenum do not present this problem. Disappearance of an ulcer of the stomach should be demonstrated by x-ray examination after several weeks of treatment, or the condition should be corrected by an operation.

Surgical operations for ulcer accomplish one of the following objectives:

1. Removing the ulcer.
2. Removing the lower part of the stomach.
3. By-passing food stream.
4. Enlarging the stomach outlet.
5. Cutting the stomach nerves.

In a normal person, the *vagus nerves* energize the stomach glands when food is taken. The glands secrete digesting fluid for about two hours; then the mechanism is shut off. The stomach outlet muscle opens at intervals to let the mixture of food and stomach fluid out into the intestine. This goes on for about four hours. During the night when no food is taken the stomach is at rest.

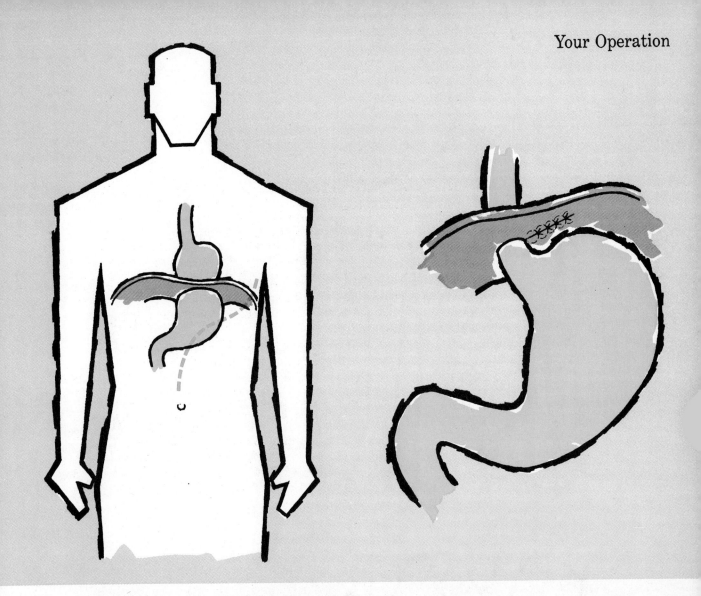

The diaphragm, the great muscle which separates the chest from the abdomen, has several openings which permit vital structures to pass through it. The gullet or esophagus passes through a normal "hole" in the diaphragm as it enters the stomach. This area may "rupture" or enlarge, permitting a pouch of the stomach (and even a bit of intestine in some cases) to protrude through the hernial opening into the chest cavity, as shown diagrammatically in the drawing at left above. Hernia of the diaphragm is repaired by returning the stomach to its normal location and closing the abnormal hole in the diaphragm. One of several routes of incision is shown in dotted lines in the figure.

In the person who has an ulcer, the vagus nerves energize the stomach glands continuously, day and night. Because of this the stomach lining is in continuous contact with digestive fluid, which is acid. Likewise, the sensitive lining of the duodenum just beyond the outlet of the stomach is bathed by discharging jets of acid stomach fluid day and night. It is this continuous contact with acid secretion that brings about ulceration of the stomach and duodenum.

Removing the ulcer. The area of the stomach that contains an ulcer is re-moved by cutting out a pie-shaped wedge of the stomach wall. An immediate "frozen section" examination of the tissue by a pathologist determines whether there is cancer. If no cancer is present, the edges are sewed together. This is called a wedge resection. Most often, however, even though the tissue is shown to be non-cancerous, the operation is carried further by one of the methods described below.

Removing the lower part of the stomach. The normal acid of the digestive fluid is produced in response to a

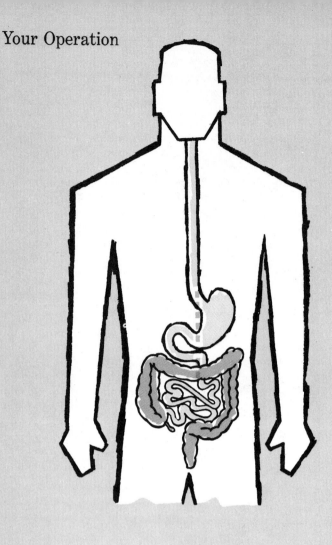

Diagram at left shows normal relationships of structures of the digestive tract; colored dotted line indicates one of the incisions a surgeon may choose to enter the abdomen. Flexibility of organs permits the surgeon to make a variety of new "plumbing connections," depending upon the nature of the patient's disease. At left below, stomach ulcer in lower portion of stomach to be removed (1). One way of connecting the healthy upper part of the stomach to a loop of intestine is shown at right below. The upper half of the stomach (1) is joined (*anastamosed*) to a loop of the jejunum (3), the part of the small intestine that begins beyond the duodenum, and the duodenum (2) is closed. Removal of the lower part of the stomach (gastric resection) is frequently done to reduce excessive acid secretion associated with ulcers.

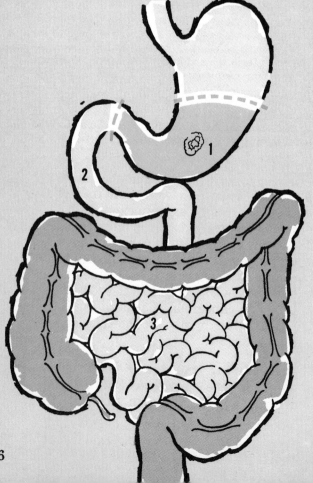

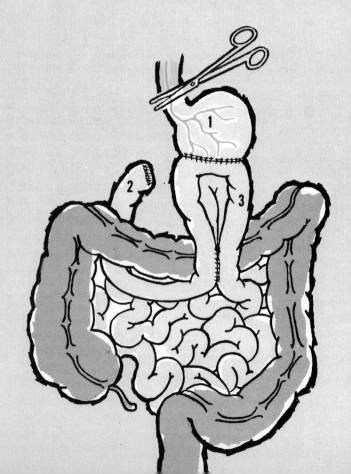

hormone released in the lower half of the stomach. In cases of ulcer the acid is produced in excessive amounts. Therefore, this section is removed. In this type of operation the ulcer itself may or may not be removed. Even though the ulcer is not removed, the area will heal promptly because acid exposure has been limited. This operation is called *gastric resection*.

By-passing the food stream. This operation is used for duodenal ulcers when obstruction of the stomach outlet is the chief problem. In these cases the stomach is joined to a loop of intestine a little farther along than the duodenum, allowing food to go directly into the new loop and to by-pass the duodenum. This is called *gastroenterostomy*.

Enlarging the opening. This is an operation that corrects obstruction at the outlet of the stomach, an obstruction caused by twisting scar tissue. This operation is a permanent enlargement that refashions the gateway out of the stomach; it is called *pyloroplasty*.

Cutting the stomach nerves. The excessive volume of acid stomach fluid is reduced sufficiently to permit ulcer healing by cutting these nerves that energize the stomach gland. This is a *vagotomy*. Cutting of these nerves is often combined with gastroenterostomy or pyloroplasty, either of which will allow the stomach to empty faster.

After-events. Nothing is needed to replace the portions of the stomach and duodenum that have been removed. The digestive process is still essentially the same. Stomach fluid, now without the excess of acid, still acts upon food as it did before. Bile and pancreatic fluids still mix with food as they did previously.

After some operations, such as the resections, the size of the stomach is reduced, but this reduction in size is not noticeable ordinarily after about six months. After this time, partly because of stretching of the remaining stomach and partly because of adjustment, the diminished size is not noticed.

Diet after a stomach operation will vary from one patient to the next. Although a severe diet is not necessary, still one should be careful about eating habits. Restrictions are lifted gradually and progressively.

While the adage "once an ulcer, always an ulcer" is not necessarily true, it is true that persons with certain types of body makeup must exercise caution in respect to foods, stimulants and nervous tension. Nervous tension may play a larger role than irritating foods and it has been said humorously that "it is not what you eat that causes an ulcer, it's what eats you". This means control probably for a lifetime, not necessarily medicine for a lifetime, but reasonable control of diet, stimulants, and emotional irritations. Tobacco and liquor should be avoided.

Although it is probable that ulcers do not cause cancer, it is sometimes difficult to tell by testing before the operation whether the diseased area is ulcerous or cancerous. This is particularly true with the stomach. For this reason it is often considered safer to operate in the case of stomach ulcer. Should the condition prove to be cancer, the likelihood of removing it at an early and favorable stage is increased.

Cancers are not the only tumors of the stomach. Benign tumors also occur here. Operations for cancer of the stomach are more extensive than those for ulcer or for benign tumors. With cancer the surgeon aims at removing every part of the stomach to which cancer cells might spread even though he cannot see or feel any spread.

INTESTINAL OPERATIONS

Diseased parts of the intestine usually must be removed, generally the sooner the better, for nourishment and elimination can be disturbed very quickly. Furthermore, an accurate diagnosis of the nature of intestinal disease is often impossible, short of direct observation by the surgeon or by analysis of the removed specimen.

Only rarely is the entire length of intestinal tube involved by a disease. Ordinarily it is just a section. When your garden hose is faulty, it isn't the whole length of the hose, just a section of it. The defect might be repaired, but more often the better solution will be just to cut out the bad part. Sometimes it is necessary to remove only a short segment of a few inches. At other times a section of several feet must be taken.

The removal of sections of the intestinal tube is better understood if one pictures the intestine as hanging from

wedge. The freshly cut ends and their blood vessels come to a fit as the sides of the wedge are sewed together.

Various diseases that affect the intestine bring the patient to surgery because the disease does one of the following things: it makes the intestine *bleed*; it *obstructs* the intestine; it causes the intestine to *telescope* into itself; it *weakens*

At left below, a diseased section of small bowel in process of being cut out. Pairs of clamps are applied to healthy bowel at either side of the diseased area. The surgeon cuts across the healthy bowel sections between the clamps that enclose them, and at the same time cuts a pie-shaped wedge from the mesentery (dotted lines). The mesentery is an apronlike sheet of tissue from which the intestines hang, as from the hem of a skirt. At right, the diseased section has been removed and the healthy ends of the bowel are being sewn together (end-to-end anastamosis).

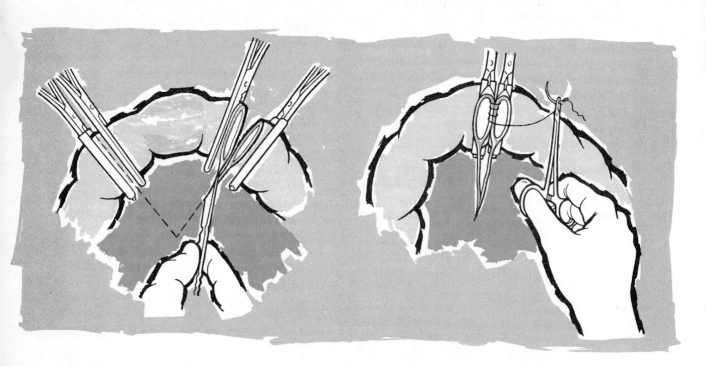

the backbone by an apronlike skirt called the *mesentery*. Although the intestine is quite long, over 20 feet, the attachment of its apron is gathered into about four inches, and thus the intestinal tube hangs at the hem of its mesentery, pretty much like the hem of a pleated and flowing skirt. Blood vessels to and from the intestinal tube fan out from the waist of the mesentery to the intestinal tube at the hem. When a part of the intestine is removed, a pie-shaped piece of the mesenteric skirt is taken with it. The blood vessels of the diseased part are in this

the intestinal wall to the bursting point; it *strangulates* the intestine by twisting it; it causes an *infection* in the segment of intestine.

The passageway through the intestine can be blocked either by plugging or by squeezing or by kinking. Very few objects that can get into the intestine are large enough to plug it, although some things can, such as an enormous gallstone that breaks out of the gallbladder, a hair ball that forms in the stomach, or a tumor that grows on a stalk. Objects that might be swallowed accidentally, such as a pin, a fish or meat bone or a broken tooth, will not plug the intestine. They may cause inflammation or perforation but they will not directly plug the tube. A cancer squeezes by growing around the intestine like a napkin-ring. Kinking is caused most often by adhesions that interfere with free motion of the normally moving coils and thereby cause angulation, twisting, knotting or locking and consequently obstruction.

Telescoping is called *intussusception*. In this condition the intestinal tube is telescoped into itself. The sleeve of your coat will telescope into itself, if when removing the coat, the cuff of the sleeve is caught at the wrist. A ball-like tumor hanging by a stalk and partially plugging the intestine will make the muscle of the intestinal wall work so hard that it will telescope itself over the tumor.

Disease may erode an area in the intestinal wall, thinning it to the breaking point, like rust eroding the bottom of a pan. As pressure builds up, the tube bursts or perforates at the weak spot. This, of course, allows intestinal fluid to spill out into the abdominal cavity, irritating the sensitive lining membrane.

Bleeding will occur if disease erodes the blood vessels in the intestinal wall but the blood will come out with the bowel movements.

If the mesentery of the intestine becomes twisted the blood vessels are also twisted and blocked. Without a supply of blood, the section of intestine dies. This is called *gangrene* and the twisting of the mesentery that chokes the blood vessels is called *strangulation*.

The disease in the intestine may be of an inflammatory nature and is called an infection. The intestine is red and swollen, like a boil or abscess, and the swelling may be severe enough to cause an obstruction.

Although the diseases of the intestine differ in their natures, they produce similar effects like bleeding, obstruction, strangulation. It is the *nature of the disease* that the surgeon must bear in mind when he makes his incision to repair the defect, or to bypass it or to cut it away. It is the nature of the disease that determines how much of the intestine must be removed, how much of the mesentery must be taken with it and how the healthy parts will be put together again.

A hole caused by an injury might lend itself to simple patching, the hole in an eroded cancerous part requires removal of an extensive area of intestine and mesentery, a hole in the swollen and infected tissues of a badly inflamed appendix might permit nothing more than drainage of the abdominal cavity because the manipulations of cutting and sewing would spread the infection.

Tumors. If the surgeon discovers a tumor, he determines by analysis at the time of surgery whether it is cancerous or benign. A long section of intestine must be removed for cancer and with this a large and deep pie-shaped wedge of mesenteric apron. The purpose is to remove all of the primary drainage filters, called lymph nodes, that drain the affected part of the intestine through the mesentery. Only a short section of intestine is removed and very little mesentery if the tumor is benign. The cells of benign tumors do not wander away from the immediate area and therefore the removal of parts is not so extensive.

Appendicitis. When the appendix becomes inflamed, it swells and a spot in the wall of this small hollow tube becomes thin by erosion and the tube may burst, allowing pus to escape into the abdominal cavity. The broad lacelike curtain of fat tissues that hangs from the colon and is called the *omentum*, sticks to the appendix, gathering around it and sealing it into a corner or pocket.

The operation for appendicitis is carried out as soon as the diagnosis can be proved. If the appendix has already burst and an abscess has been formed around it, the surgeon may find it preferable to drain the abscess and leave the appendix for removal at a later date, usually four to eight weeks. The appendix is often removed when the abdomen has been opened for another operation. The decision will depend upon the location of the incision and the gravity of the primary operation.

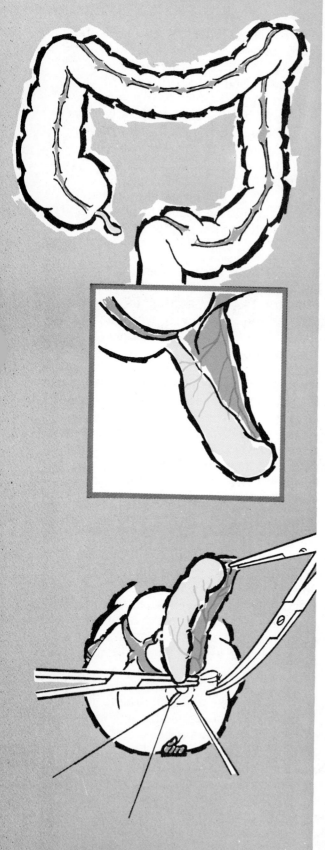

Diverticula are pouchlike protrusions through weak spots in the intestinal tube, usually found in the colon. An inflamed *diverticulum* may burst and thus open up a passageway from the intestine into the abdominal cavity, the final result being peritonitis or an internal abscess. If a diverticulum has burst and formed an abscess, an emergency operation may be necessary for drainage only. Drainage means that a tunnel is made from the abscess to the skin outside. A rubber tube is placed in the tunnel to keep it open for drainage. If the section of intestine affected by diverticula is not badly inflamed, the section may be removed and the cut-ends joined together. It is sometimes necessary to do this in stages, that is, over a course of two or three operations, using a *colostomy* to by-pass the bowel movement away from the recently joined ends of the intestine until healing has taken place.

There is a type of *diverticulitis* that occurs in a single pouchlike tube that hangs from the lower part of the small intestine. The diverticulum is a defect present at birth. When this diverticulum becomes inflamed, the reaction is swift and severe and the symptoms of the patient are very much like those of appendicitis. When it is necessary to remove a *Meckel's diverticulum*, which this is called, usually the coil of intestine containing the diverticulum and measuring several inches in length is removed.

Ileitis. A slow form of inflammation that affects the ileum, which is the lower part of the small intestine, is called *ileitis*. Sometimes the portion of intestine with ileitis is removed and at times the diseased area is by-passed so that the intestinal stream does not flow through it. In this resting condition the ileum can heal. The bypass is inside the body and does not open to the outside. It is permanent.

Appendectomy — removal of an inflamed appendix. Top drawing, appendix in normal location, attached to cecum. Middle drawing, blood supply from membrane that holds down the appendix. Bottom: blood supply is clamped and tied, clamp placed across potential stump, and purse-string suture applied, preparatory to amputation. Following the cut, the stump is cauterized.

Mesenteric thrombosis is a condition in which the arteries to the intestine passing through the mesentery become caked with blood clots that are called thrombi. The mesenteric arteries are said to be thrombosed, hence the name. Losing its blood supply, the intestinal wall becomes gangrenous and will burst. The defects of this condition are so severe that the patient collapses into a state of shock and will die if the thrombosed section of intestine cannot be removed quickly.

Defects in the intestinal arteries are demonstrated by x-ray examinations made when shadow solutions are injected into the abdominal arterial system. For this kind of testing a fine plastic tube is threaded into a thigh artery and up the mainline artery (the aorta) to the level of the navel. The injected shadow solution mixes with blood in the intestinal arteries to show their outlines clearly on the x-ray films.

Ulcerative colitis affects the entire colon, causing sores or ulcers inside the tube. The entire length of colon is thick and stiff like a garden hose. Almost all of the colon must be removed for ulcerative colitis and this removal will usually

Sections of the intestine may be re-routed or used as "spare parts" to perform unusual functions in unusual instances of disease. Below, a portion of the colon (large bowel) replaces and partially serves the functions of a stomach. At left, stomach with cancer (1); dotted lines (4, 5) show where cuts are made for removal of stomach (total gastrectomy); normal position of transverse colon (2). At right, section of transverse colon (3) serving as "stomach"; ascending (6) and descending colon (7) are joined end to end.

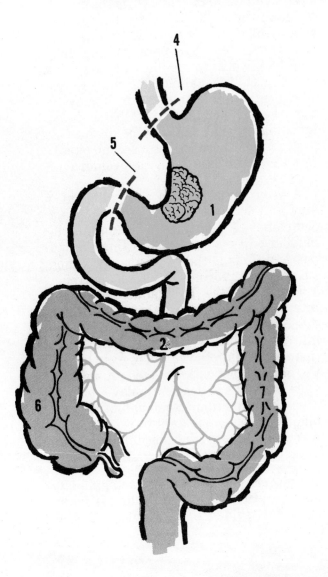
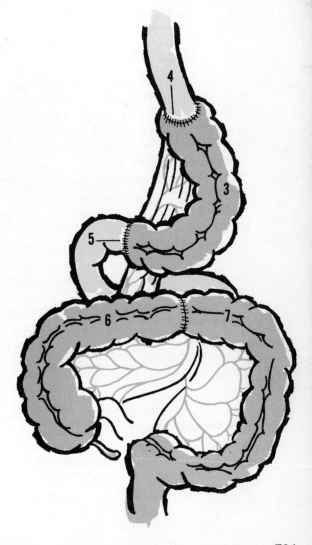

include the rectum because the ulceration is most severe in this area. Since the entire colon and rectum are removed, bowel movements must be diverted out onto the abdominal skin through an opening that is called an *ileostomy*.

Long sections of the first half of the *small intestine* may be removed without noticeable effect on digestion, but the loss of a lengthy section of the second half may interfere with the absorption of fat or iron or some vitamins. A drop in weight or anemia may appear several weeks or months after removal of this part of the small intestine and medicine will have to be taken to counteract this.

Either the right half or left half of the *colon* may be removed without a great change in the bowel movements. The colon has the job of taking water out of the liquid intestinal material after it leaves the small intestine. When more extensive sections of the colon must be removed, the usual amount of water absorbed in the colon will be lost in part in the bowel movements. These therefore may be loose.

Colostomy. When it is necessary to remove the rectum, usually for cancerous tumors, the lower colon is cut across and is diverted like a detour through an artificial hole made in the skin of the abdomen. A special apparatus is placed over the opening to assist in the bowel movements. This is called a *colostomy*.

A temporary colostomy may be needed to protect a surgical suture line that reconstructs the lower colon or rectum. This puts the intestine at rest for healing. At the end of this time the colostomy is closed and normal bowel movements through the rectum are resumed. Temporary colostomies may be lifesaving for gunshot wounds and the tearing wounds of serious highway accidents.

The intestinal operations may be performed in stages. The first step in correcting a tumor of the colon that is obstructing the passage may be a temporary colostomy. Bowel movement is passed through a colostomy from the section of intestine containing the tumor. In the second step the tumor area is removed. As a third step the colostomy is closed, thus restoring the normal operation of the intestine and rectum.

GALLBLADDER OPERATIONS

If you should turn up with **gallstones** the probability is your doctor will advise removal of the gallbladder. There is not much point to removing just the stones because the stones are formed in the gallbladder and if the gallbladder will do this once, it will do it again. The general rule is that anyone in average physical condition under age 60 had better get rid of gallstones, and this means losing the gallbladder.

A stone slips from the gallbladder into the duct that leads from it to the main bile duct. The main duct runs from the liver to the intestine. The gallbladder is a reservoir off to the side. Once the duct is blocked, the gallbladder swells and becomes inflamed because bile cannot get out. If the blockage persists, the gallbladder swells to double its size, pus forms, and the gallbladder may burst. When infection is this severe it may be that the gallbladder cannot be removed immediately, but can only be drained to the outside. There will be a second operation at a later date for actual removal of the diseased gallbladder.

A stone imbedded in the gallbladder duct may block it only partially, but not completely. From time to time the gallbladder will swell because of this blocked passage. This is the condition for which surgery is performed most frequently.

Removing the gallbladder does not interfere with digestion because the job it was doing is taken over by the cells that line the bile ducts inside the liver. In most instances this job was taken over before the gallbladder was removed; it was not working and had ceased to play a part in digestive function. Removal of a gallbladder has no important physical significance, and there is no special restriction of diet subsequent to its removal.

Surgical procedures. In each gallbladder operation the main bile duct is examined for evidence of stones. If such

The outline figure shows the location of the liver and the gallbladder which hangs from its under surface. Dotted line is one of the incisions a surgeon may choose to reach the gallbladder area. A cutaway view of the gallbladder with stones blocking its duct is shown at right below. Bottom drawing shows top of gallbladder incised and stones being removed (cholecystostomy). More commonly, a diseased gallbladder is completely removed (cholecystectomy) because of the risk that inflammation and formation of stones may recur if it is left in place.

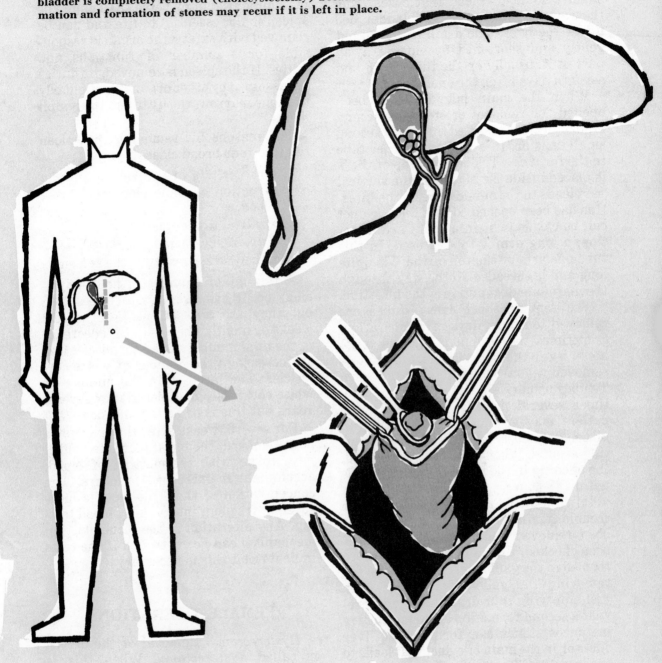

evidence is present, the duct is opened and cleaned out all the way to its termination in the intestine. This is called *choledochostomy*.

If there is no evidence of stones in the main duct, it is not opened. This determination may be made by x-ray examination on the operating table. Sometimes it is necessary to open the intestine to

dislodge a stone imbedded at the termination of the main bile duct. This is called *duodenostomy*. In this procedure the main bile duct can be cleaned out in both forward and backward directions.

A drain is used after most gallbladder operations. A soft rubber tube inserted leads down to the space that was formerly occupied by the gallbladder. The purpose is to drain away serum and a small amount of blood that oozes from the raw surface of the gallbladder bed under the liver. The drain is drawn out gently and shortened by cutting away part of it, usually on the third, fifth and seventh days after the operation.

When the main bile duct has been opened for removal of stones, a second kind of drain is inserted through a second small incision. It is a hollow rubber tube in the form of a T. The short top of the T is placed inside the bile duct; the vertical part leads to the outside. When the intestine has been opened so that the bile duct can be cleaned out in a backward direction, a long arm T-tube is used. In this tube one arm of the top of the T is quite long and is threaded all the way through the main bile duct and into the intestine.

The regular short arm T-tubes are removed ten to 12 days after operation. Sometimes the patient is allowed to go home with the tube in place and it is removed at a later date. Long arm T-tubes usually are left in longer, sometimes several months. Here again the patient may go home with the tube in place. This does not interfere with getting around. When T-tubes are removed, the opening in the bile duct usually heals within 48 hours.

It is unlikely that stones will cause trouble again once the gallbladder has been removed and the bile ducts have been checked. Virtually all gallstones are formed in the gallbladder. The reason for removing the gallbladder rather than just emptying it or draining it is to prevent a second formation of stones. In rare instances stones can form in the liver ducts or in the main bile duct that leads to the intestine. This can happen even after the gallbladder has been removed.

SPLEEN OPERATIONS

The *spleen* is located high in the left upper part of the abdomen, almost to the back. The outer free surface of the spleen is just about the size of the surgeon's hand. Enormous amounts of blood are pumped through the spleen, coming in through an intricate branching system of arterial pipes and leaving through a matching system of veins. Although the spleen is not essential to life and can be removed with safety, the organ is responsible for a number of functions and duties. If the spleen is removed, its duties are assumed by other organs, particularly the bone marrow, the liver and the lymph nodes.

The reasons for removing the spleen fall into four broad classes:

1. *Overactivity* of the spleen and destruction of some elements of the blood.
2. *Injuries* to the spleen.
3. *Tumors*, cysts and abscesses.
4. Other *rare diseases* of the spleen.

A few minor changes in body physiology occur after removal of the spleen but they are not serious. For several weeks or months there will be a decrease in the total number of red corpuscles and an increase in the number of white corpuscles. The increase in the number of white corpuscles may persist for several years but this is of no significance.

For several weeks after the spleen has been removed, the blood platelets, which have to do with the clotting of blood, accumulate in increased numbers. The concentration of these platelets is measured at frequent intervals by blood testing. Any alteration in the blood clotting mechanism can be controlled if the tests indicate that this is necessary.

FEMALE OPERATIONS

Hysterectomy. Removal of the uterus is called *hysterectomy*. When this is necessary, the surgeon chooses between one of two general methods, removal through an incision in the *abdomen* or removal through the *vagina*.

If the uterus is quite large or is distorted by tumor formations, it will be removed through the abdomen. If previous trouble has caused adhesions that bind the uterus to other organs, the abdominal operation will be selected. When the chief trouble is *prolapsing*, or falling, of the womb, the vaginal method is more suitable. The idea that vaginal hysterectomy does not require an incision is erroneous. There is, of course, an incision but it is made deep in the vagina in an area that is not normally visible and that is relatively painless when compared to the muscular abdominal wall.

Vaginal hysterectomy. Removal through the vagina makes for less disturbance during the postoperative days. The main supports and blood vessels that must be severed are much closer to the location of the vaginal incision and this means that fewer organs have to be moved out of the way. Thus, with less handling and manipulation of other organs, particularly the intestines, bloating and gas pains are not so annoying.

The vaginal method permits a more advantageous repair of the stretched and sagging muscles that support the vagina, the bladder and the rectum. This is an important consideration because hysterectomy is performed so frequently on women who have passed the child-bearing period and who have begun to experience difficulty with bladder and rectal muscles. Although a repair of these muscles and ligaments works out very nicely in connection with abdominal hysterectomy, the necessity for incisions in two areas makes this method a little cumbersome in comparison with the more direct vaginal method. The choice of the surgeon in a particular case will depend upon the nature of the trouble.

Abdominal hysterectomy. The course of events in abdominal hysterectomy is much the same as outlined under abdominal operations in general. The preparation before the operation and the postoperative days are about the same. Hospitalization is a matter of some seven to ten days.

With either type of operation, vaginal or abdominal, the entire uterus is almost always removed. The uterus, shaped like a pear, has two parts; the wide part is the *body* and the narrow tapered part is the cervix. The larger body portion rests on the bottom of the abdominal cavity and the cervix protrudes through into the vagina. The cervix thus forms the

opening of the womb to the outside. As the surgeon sees it in the depth of the vagina, it looks like the top of a pear with the stem pulled out. The two parts of the uterus that are so vulnerable to cancer are the interior lining and the opening in the cervix.

Years ago the entire uterus was not removed. It was cut across at its neck, or cervix, leaving as a stump the cervix which protruded into the vagina. Modern technique and instruments make removal of the cervical stump easier. Like removing a tree, it used to be that the tree was cut across at the level of the ground, leaving the stump. With modern tree equipment the stump is detached from its roots and removed. Similarly, in present day surgery the "entire uterus" is most often removed. With the cervix gone a woman does not have to bother further about what is commonly referred to as the "cancer test" during routine examinations of the female organs.

When the uterus is removed, the attachments of the tubes and ovaries to the uterus are severed and these structures are left in place. If there is evidence of disease or abnormality they are removed in part, or entirely. In older women the surgeon may consider it advisable to remove the tubes and ovaries along with hysterectomy even though there is no evidence of disease in these organs.

The ovaries are removed sometimes because of tumors or because of large fluid-filled cavities called *cysts*. This is accomplished through an abdominal incision. When an ovary is removed, its tube that leads to the uterus is removed along with it because tubes and ovaries are closely attached to each other. In addition, a tube serves no purpose when its ovary is absent.

Either tumors or cysts of the ovaries may be of small size, no bigger than a walnut, or they may grow to enormous size, larger than a person's head. It may be surprising to learn that a tumor or cyst bigger than a grapefruit may give rise to no symptoms and may remain undetected until discovered at a routine examination by a physician.

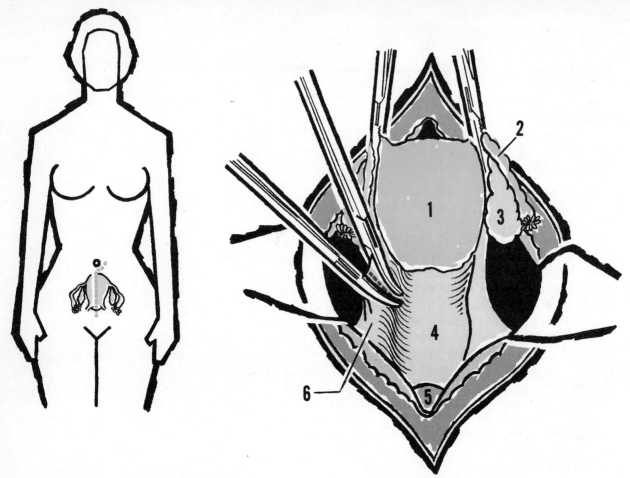

Outline figure shows location of uterus, tubes, and ovaries, with midline incision below navel which the surgeon may use in performing an abdominal hysterectomy. This drawing and companion drawings on opposite page show stages of a complete hysterectomy with removal of tubes and ovaries (the latter structures need not always be removed). Drawing at right above shows clamps across the suspending broad ligament (6) which is dissected along body of uterus (1) to below cervix (4) where amputation is done. Other structures are Fallopian tube (2), ovary (3), bladder (5).

Cystocele and rectocele. Supporting muscles of the bladder and rectum sometimes sag and lose their tone. Then there is interference either with urination or with the passage of bowel movements, or with both. The sagging bladder is called a *cystocele*, the sagging rectum a *rectocele*. Either or both may be corrected by an operation that shortens and tightens the supporting muscles. These surgical procedures may be carried out in combination with hysterectomy or independently. The uterus is removed so that its supporting ligaments can be used to support the bladder and rectum. The surgeon will base his decision upon the nature and extent of the trouble and the age and physical condition of the patient. These operations are performed through the vaginal area and do not require an abdominal incision.

"D & C." A very common minor operation is known as *dilation and curettage*, or "D & C" for short. A *curet* is a kind of scraper or spoon.

The canal opening into the uterus through the cervix is stretched or dilated to allow the insertion of a long, thin-handled scoop that scrapes out the inside lining of the uterus. This is done for a variety of reasons; for example, to obtain tissue for laboratory analysis in cases of abnormal bleeding, to remove small fleshy growths called *polyps*, or to remove remnants of tissue that will not come away naturally after a miscarriage. This minor operation is performed under

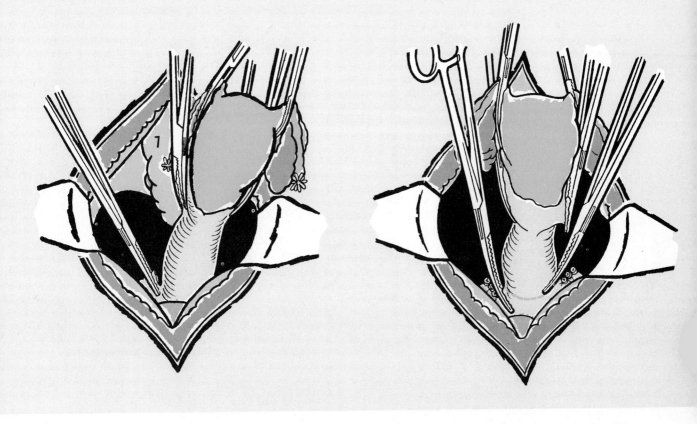

At left above, dissection of broad ligament carried to point of amputation. Blood vessels of this highly vascular structure have been tied off all along the route of dissection. Separation is done on both sides. The rectum (7) can be seen behind the freed uterus. At right, the vagina is cut across and sewed shut just where it is attached to the uterus. In this way the length of the vagina is not disturbed.

general anesthesia and requires but a few days hospitalization.

Cervical erosion. Surgery may be necessary for a condition known as erosion of the cervix. This is a rough spot in the membrane lining the opening in the cervix, looking much like a child's skinned knee. A piece of this area may have to be removed for analysis in the laboratory, or the entire cervical opening may have be be cored out. If the "Pap smear" test for cancer made during a routine physical examination is reported from the laboratory to be "suspicious," a biopsy of the cervix will be necessary to clear up the diagnosis. Radium, x-ray, and cobalt irradiation are generally preferred over surgery in treatment of cancer of the cervix.

HERNIA OPERATIONS

A ***hernia,*** also called a *rupture,* is a bulge of the lining membrane of the abdominal cavity through a weak spot in the muscles. These muscles, together with the skin, form a casing for the abdomen. The lining membrane is thin and stretchable just like the membrane you have seen in a fish or chicken cavity. A gap develops in the muscle casing, the muscle fibers separate, and any increase of abdominal pressure brought on by coughing, lifting, or straining will push the lining membrane through the gap, separating the muscles still further. Remember the old tires that developed a "balloon" on the side? Air pressure inside found a weak spot in the casing and pushed the inner tube through it.

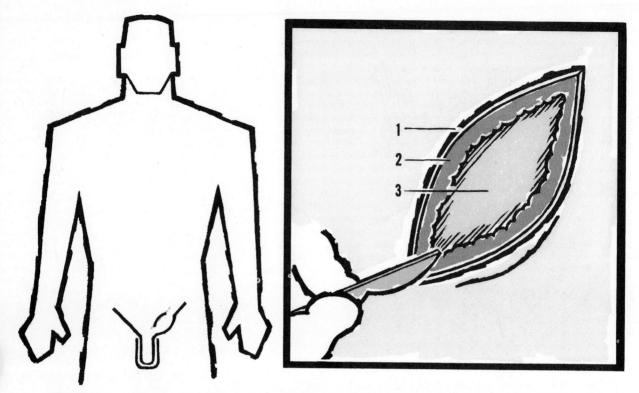

Figure shows bulge in left groin and line of incision for repair of an indirect inguinal hernia. This drawing and companion drawings on opposite page show stages of surgical correction. In males, the spermatic cord from the testicle enters the body through an opening in muscle (external ring), runs along a sort of groove through muscular structures (inguinal canal), and passes into the abdominal cavity through another "doorway," the internal ring. Protrusion of a pouch of abdominal contents through this weak area is a hernia or "rupture." At right, drawing shows incision through skin (1), fatty layer (2), and exposure of fascia (3), which connects muscles with parts they move.

There are several weak areas in the abdominal muscles, the groin being the weakest in both men and women. In men, the cord which carries the pipeline from the testicle up into the abdominal cavity occupies a passageway, called the "canal", between the several layers of the abdominal muscles in the groin. In women, the suspending ligament of the womb runs out of the abdominal cavity and through a similar canal, to its attachment at the front of the pelvis bone. These natural passageways through the muscles are weak spots. Another passage subject to hernia is below the groin where the large blood vessels to the thigh leave the abdominal cavity. Muscles may become weak around the incisions of previous operations. The navel is another weak spot.

Once the lining membrane has popped out through the muscles, it will remain stretched and will protrude as a bag or pouch. This is called the *hernia sac*.

Whenever the hernia patient stands, the intestine slips out of the abdomen into the sac and the bulge is visible. When the patient reclines, the intestine will fall back into the abdominal cavity and the bulge will disappear; the sac collapses. Thus a hernia bulges when the patient stands and collapses when he reclines.

As long as the bulge disappears with reclining, the hernia is said to be *reducible*. Here the intestine slips readily in and out of the sac. If the hernia does not disappear when the patient lies down, it is called *incarcerated*. It is caught. The intestine, slipping into the sac, may twist, and if it does this it will swell to such an extent that it cannot slip back even in the reclining position.

The real danger of a hernia is *strangulation*. When the intestine is trapped in the pouch, it will swell so tightly that its blood vessels become choked and blood cannot flow through them. The intestine

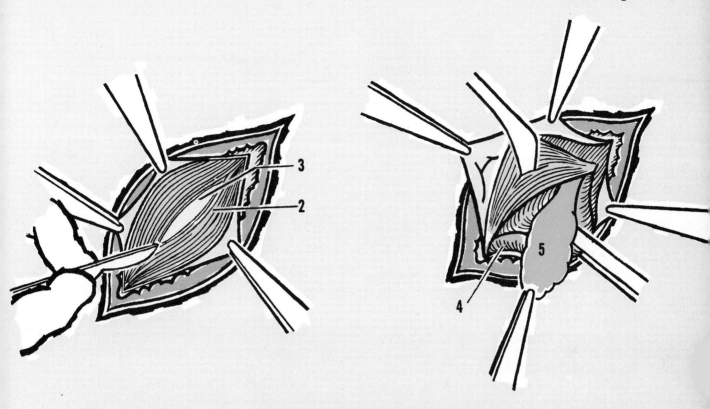

Above: Drawing at left shows knife cutting and separating muscle fibers (2), to expose the hernia sac and spermatic cord. Hernia lies under bulging membranous layer (3). At right, the spermatic cord (4) is seen under the exposed hernia (5), which is protruding through the same "muscle door" through which the spermatic cord enters the abdomen.

Below, left: After the hernia sac (5) is opened, inspected, and emptied, the stump is sutured (arrow). Stump slips back through internal ring which intestine herniated through. Poupart's ligament (6) is a strong anchor for fine wires placed across inner muscle layers. These are drawn together to close opening. At right, layers are sutured to form new reinforced canal for spermatic cord (4). Outer fibrous layers will be drawn together over cord by fine sutures.

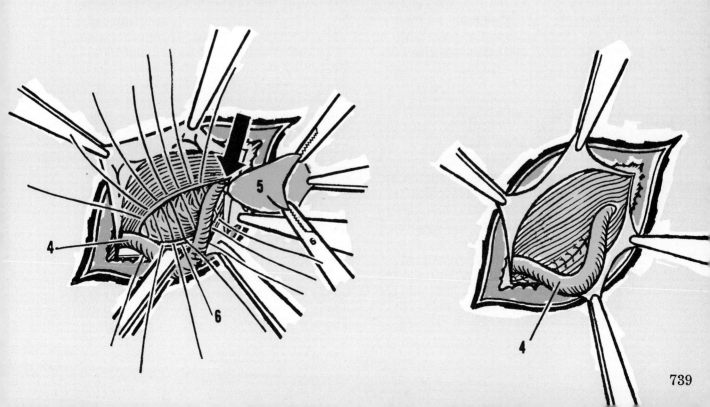

becomes gangrenous, dead. The hernia is then painful and swollen. Strangulation is a real emergency, always requiring immediate operation for removal of the gangrenous intestine.

Hernia repair. When a hernia is repaired by operation, the sac is removed completely and the stretch in the lining membrane is pulled together by stitching. The muscle and fibrous layers are rearranged by overlapping and then drawn up snugly around the cord. A new canal is formed for the cord and the back wall of the canal, which was previously weak, is now reinforced. When the muscles are of poor quality and are thin and frayed, a screen or mesh of fine, non-irritating wire or plastic is sewn in as an extra supporting layer. The screen is very flexible and cannot be noticed by the patient no matter what movements he makes.

After a healing period of six weeks the newly reconstructed groin is of normal strength. There is no further need to curtail activities or lifting.

You should not expect to get another hernia. The fact that you had a hernia does not indicate that there is anything wrong with your muscles in general, to make you subject to more hernias. It is natural in many people to feel that because they have once had a hernia operation they must curtail their activities. There is no reason for cutting down your normal activities nor for worry about another rupture. The possibility of a new hernia breaking out in the same place usually is very slight.

LUNG OPERATIONS

During lung operations the chest cavity, of course, is opened. This exposes the lungs to the pressure of outside air, whereas normally they are sealed in a vacuum in the chest cavity. Opening the chest breaks the vacuum like opening a can of vacuum-packed coffee.

It is the vacuum that allows the alternate up and down movements of ribs and diaphragm to act as a bellows on the lungs, inflating and deflating them. Since the lungs are elastic, they would remain collapsed like a deflated balloon if it were not for the vacuum drawing them out and expanding them to the size of the chest cavity. During surgery there must be a substitute for bellows vacuum.

So long as the lungs can be made to suck in air and blow it out again, gas exchange will go on. To accomplish this the lungs are assisted by a substitute bellows arrangement. The anesthetist inserts an *intratracheal breathing tube* into the windpipe (trachea), and then connects this tube to a rubber bag that is filled with oxygen and anesthetic gas. Each time the rubber bag is squeezed the lungs are inflated with gas from the bag. The lung cells then exchange oxygen for carbon dioxide. When the bag is let go, the elastic recoil of the lungs pushes carbon dioxide gas out through the tube to the bag and the bag expands.

As a further refinement, the intratracheal tube can be inserted still further to fit into either the right or left main bronchial tube. This allows one lung to be inflated and deflated for breathing while the other lung remains collapsed. Sometimes the surgeon can work better on a collapsed lung. The collapsed lung can be inflated by rearranging the intratracheal tube.

When the operation within the chest cavity has been completed, the anesthetist inflates the lungs to full capacity by squeezing the rubber gas bag. He keeps the lungs in this expanded condition until the ribs have been drawn together and the muscles and skin have been closed tightly by stitches. A long rubber tube is brought out from the inside of the chest cavity through a hole in the skin and is connected to a glass bottle on the floor. The bottle contains about an inch and a half of water and the tube coming from the chest cavity is securely anchored under the water.

Each time when the lungs are inflated to full capacity by the anesthetist's air bag, a little air is pushed out through the tube and bubbles up under the water in the bottle on the floor. No air can go back in because the end of the tube is sealed by the water. In this manner, the vacuum inside the chest cavity is re-established. The air tube to the bottle on the floor is left in place for several days. By the end of this time the surface of the lung has becomed sealed to the lining of the chest cavity and from this point on will not collapse nor will the vacuum be broken. At this time the chest tube is removed.

Removing Sections of the Lung

A person can get along with only one good lung, and this is fortunate, because some patients are faced with the removal of an entire lung. The major loss in this event is that of reserve breathing capacity. This is the reserve we use for running, climbing, heavy exercise and exertion. To go about our usual routines we use only a small part of full lung capacity. These usual things the person with one lung can do.

Another fortunate circumstance is that so many lung diseases are confined to just a section of one lung and are not scattered throughout both lungs. Because of this the surgeon gets rid of disease by removing only one or two subdivisions of one lung.

All of this comes about because each lung, right and left, is divided into separate units, like the petals of a flower. The lung units are called *lobes*. Although the clefts between the lobes are not so deep as those between the flower's petals, the independence of a lobe is just as great as that of a petal. The surgeon can, so to speak, pick off one lobe without disturbing the others.

Still more wonderful is the fact that each lobe is subdivided further into smaller independent units. These units, called *segments*, and varying from two to five in a lobe, are not visibly separated from each other but are partitioned off like apartments in an apartment building, their walls back to back but still separate. Each segment has an independent supply line through its own blood vessels and an independent air duct system through its own bronchial tube, coming off the main line.

When the surgeon must remove a whole lung, he works close up against the heart, disconnecting the main inlet arteries and the outlet veins to the diseased lung. The main bronchial tube is then cut across right at its take-off from the windpipe. The open cuts across these structures are sealed by suturing. This operation is called *pneumonectomy*, removal of a lung.

When only a lobe is to be taken out, the blood vessels and the bronchial tube to that lobe are isolated and severed. This is a *lobectomy*. The same principle is used for the removal of one or more segments, but this time the blood vessels and the bronchial tube are severed farther out along the line. Segment removal is known as *segmental resection*.

It's like tree pruning; cut the tree off at the trunk and the tree dies, but trim off a main limb, a branch, a branchlet or a twig and the tree survives, with less and less disturbance the farther out the trimming is done.

HEART OPERATIONS

If blood flow is stopped for more than a few minutes, death occurs. A substitute pump is necessary to maintain blood flow when the heart has to be stopped and opened for repairs. The patient's blood is bypassed through the substitute pump. The pipe and valve connections between the lungs and heart are so short and complex that a bypass around the heart calls for a bypass around *both* the heart and the lungs. A combination of a pump with an artificial lung, called a *heart-lung machine*, is used for this purpose. (See diagram, page 107).

When you call the plumber to fix a valve in the bathtub faucet, he first shuts off the water inlet in the basement. Then he can work on the plumbing without spilling out all the water. In heart and blood vessel surgery we call this "cross-clamping," shutting off the pipes. The main blood vessels are clamped.

Open heart surgery. When the plumber repairs the water tank on the toilet, he shuts off the pipes, drains out the water and opens the tank. This is "open tank plumbing." The inside of the tank is dry and open to full view and the mechanism is shut off. In *open heart surgery*, the surgeon cross-clamps the pipes, opens up the heart for a full view of the inside, and stops the heart mechanism.

A heart-lung machine is made up of a pumping system and an artificial lung that "breathes" oxygen into the blood. Plastic tubes are connected to the vein system to carry blood out of the body, through the machine, and then back to the main artery, thus bypassing the heart and the lungs. Blood is pumped through the machine as a thin film over wide screens in a container rich in oxygen. Blood cells pick up oxygen from the enriched atmosphere of oxygen.

Hypothermia. Not all surgery on the heart is "open heart." Some heart operations that require an actual opening in the heart for only very short periods can be performed without passing the blood through the heart-lung machine. The brain can take two periods of five minutes each without any oxygen-filled blood coming to it if the body temperature is lowered to 30 degrees centigrade. At this low temperature the brain needs less oxygen. The technique of lowering body temperature is called *hypothermia,* sometimes referred to incorrectly as freezing.

Heart action can be stopped temporarily by putting ice water or sterile "slush" in the sac (pericardium) that encloses the heart. Lowering the temperature of the heart muscle decreases the oxygen requirement of the muscle.

Heart operations correct:

1. *Defects in the main blood vessels.* These are the vessels that connect directly to the heart. They are the big conduits that carry blood to and from the big pump itself.
2. *Defects in the valves,* the flood gates between the chambers of the heart and at the main outlets from the heart.
3. *Defects in the partitioned walls,* the walls that separate the chambers from each other.

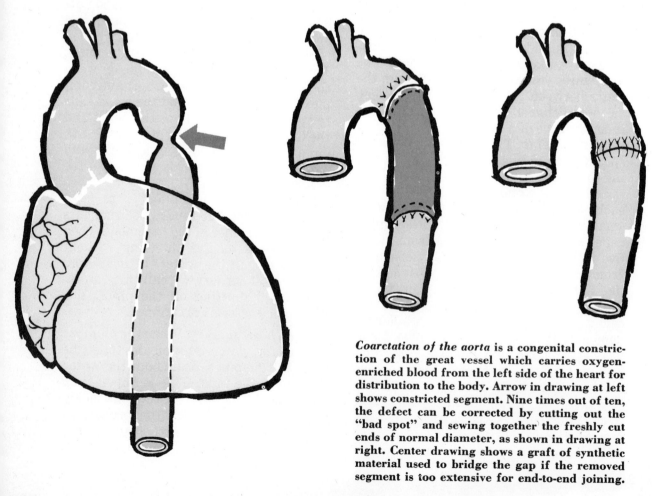

Coarctation of the aorta is a congenital constriction of the great vessel which carries oxygen-enriched blood from the left side of the heart for distribution to the body. Arrow in drawing at left shows constricted segment. Nine times out of ten, the defect can be corrected by cutting out the "bad spot" and sewing together the freshly cut ends of normal diameter, as shown in drawing at right. Center drawing shows a graft of synthetic material used to bridge the gap if the removed segment is too extensive for end-to-end joining.

Coarctation of the Aorta

The aorta is the primary conduit leading out from the heart, the vessel that carries blood full of oxygen to the main circulatory pathways. Some infants are born with a narrow section in this big pipe, a section that varies usually from a quarter inch to an inch and a half in length. This is a *coarctation* and it looks like the narrowed section in the casing between two link sausages.

Because of the short length of this faulty section and because the blood vessels have a surprising elasticity, the narrow part is cut out like a bad spot in a hose, and most often the freshly cut ends of normal diameter are joined together directly by sutures. If the coarctation is longer and there is not much "give" in the aorta, a length of plastic tube is sutured in place as a graft.

To accomplish this operation the aorta is squeezed shut, cross-clamped, upstream and downstream from the coarctation, during the period of cutting and rejoining the pipe. Since the narrow section is downstream from the brain take-off pipe, the cross clamps do not interfere with the flow of blood to the brain. The other organs can stand longer periods of shut-off. If it appears that the time required for making the repair will be unusually lengthy, a plastic tube is connected to the aorta above and below the working area and blood is bypassed around it to all the downstream organs of the body.

Patent Ductus

The *ductus* is a short blood vessel, about one-fourth inch in length and diameter, that bypasses blood away from a baby's lungs during its life in the mother's womb. The baby's blood in the womb gets oxygen from the mother and not from the baby's lungs. As soon as the infant is born and its own lungs begin to work, the ductus closes, shrinking away in time to a small cord.

If the ductus fails to close after birth, some of the oxygenated blood goes through the ductus and back through the lungs again. This adds an extra load on the lungs and heart. This is called a *patent* (open) *ductus*. To correct this defect the ductus is cut across and the two ends are sutured shut. If the pressure in the lung circuit is too high, the condition cannot be corrected. The operation for the correction of this defect is not "open heart" and does not require a bypass through the heart-lung machine.

Pulmonary Stenosis

Another malformation that is present at birth is *pulmonary stenosis*. "Stenosis" means "narrowing." Here the channel that carries stale venous blood that is leaving the heart and is on its way to the lungs is too narrow. Blood cannot get through the opening fast enough and is dammed back in the heart. This throws a strain on the heart wall. The problem is handled in several different ways, depending upon how severely the channel is narrowed.

The channel can be slit in several places and then stretched; usually it will remain stretched to a good size. The slits are made by a long, narrow-handled knife with folded blades at the end. The blades can be opened out like umbrella stays. The knife is punched through the wall of the heart and guided into the narrowed pulmonary valve channel. When it is in the proper position, the switch blades are opened. The stretcher works pretty much the same way, with folding arms that spread out on the same umbrella stay principle to expand the freshly cut channel.

In some cases the valve and the channel must be opened to full view so that the cutting and stretching can be done under direct vision. The time required for the actual cutting and stretching is usually less than ten minutes and for this reason the operation, when done this way, can be performed without a bypass heart-lung machine. The flow of blood is stopped by cross-clamping the main blood vessels. The patient's body is cooled by hypothermia.

Sometimes the defect in the valve and in the pulmonary channels is so severe that the heart chamber must be opened

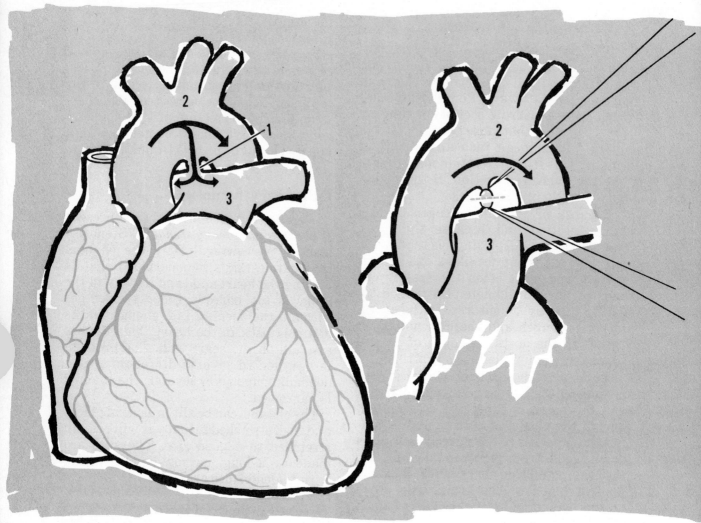

The *ductus arteriosus* is a short tube which bypasses blood from a baby's lungs before birth. Normally the tube closes after birth. If it does not, the *patent* (open) *ductus* (1), shown in drawing at left above, permits some of the oxygen-enriched blood from the *aorta* (2) to mix with blood in the *pulmonary artery* (3), putting extra work on lungs and heart. At right, surgical repair: ductus is cut at dotted line and the ends are closed; this disconnects an abnormal bypass and keeps blood flow (arrow) entirely within the aorta.

up for full and complete vision of the valve and the channel area. Under these severe circumstances the operation is "open heart" and a heart-lung machine is used for bypassing the blood around the heart and lungs.

The Mitral Valve

The *mitral valve* is the floodgate between the two chambers on the left side of the heart. Disease, particularly rheumatic fever, attacks this valve more often than any of the other valves. The valve becomes so scarred and twisted that it will not open wide enough to let blood through at a normal speed. This is *mitral stenosis*. On the other hand disease may so affect the valve that it becomes flabby and stretches to a diameter that is so great the valve flaps cannot close tightly. When the valve is supposed to be in the closed position to hold blood in the chamber, the blood leaks out. This is called *mitral insufficiency*.

Mitral stenosis is corrected by one of two methods, either by replacing the valve with a plastic substitute or by splitting the tightened and strictured valve ring to open up its channel.

Sometimes the valve flaps are so stiffened by scar formation that they can be split apart by the surgeon's finger which is pushed gently but forcibly into the valve opening. The surgeon inserts his index finger into the valve through a small incision in the heart. This operation is called *commissurotomy* because the commissures or natural indentations between the valve flaps are split apart. This is a closed heart operation.

Mitral insufficiency, likewise, can be corrected by replacing the stretched and leaking valve with a plastic substitute. Or the flaps can be adjusted by "taking a tuck" in them with a permanent suture or by grafting on a small piece of heart sac membrane.

The *aortic valve,* located at the heart exit into the inch-wide aorta (outlet artery), also is subject to excessive tightening (stenosis) or leaking (insufficiency). The prime causes are rheumatic fever in young people and arteriosclerosis in older patients.

A severely malfunctioning aortic valve is removed by cutting out completely and is replaced by a plastic substitute in an open heart operation.

Septal Defects

The partition walls between the heart chambers are known as *septa* and the defects in these walls are called *septal defects.* A septal defect is an abnormal hole in a wall. These are congenital malformations present at birth. The hole in the wall between two chambers allows oxygenated blood in the left side of the heart to leak into the right side and recirculate through the lungs. This is a strain on both heart and lungs. If this defect occurs in combination with pulmonary stenosis, the leak is from right side to left side. In this case, venous blood (blue) is recirculated in the body and the patient becomes "blue" with exertion.

Small defects can be closed by suturing, larger ones are covered with a graft of plastic material. Several different methods are used, either closed heart or open heart. The method chosen will depend upon which septum is involved, the size of the hole between the two chambers and its position in the septum.

Combination Defects

In general, heart abnormalities are due either to faulty formation of the heart before birth and are called *congenital* defects, or they are the result of disease later on and are then called *acquired* defects. Only the more common defects are described here. A heart may be faulty in more than one way; for example, a septal defect may be combined with a faulty valve channel or an abnormal placement of an intake or outlet blood vessel. A person with a congenital heart defect may be stricken with rheumatic fever so that a valve, faulty at birth, becomes additionally defective as a result of disease. In such instances of congenital heart defect the repair requires a combination of surgical procedures.

Coronary Sclerosis

The small blood vessels that lead back from the aorta to the muscle in the heart wall, the *coronary arteries,* may become hardened and clogged. The linings of these vessels can be scraped out in the operation known as *endarterectomy.* These operations obviously are performed on older people.

GENITOURINARY SURGERY

Prostate Surgery

The **prostate gland** is a small chestnut-size organ, straddling the urethral tube that leads from the bladder through the penis in the male to the outside. Since the channel for urine passes through the prostate, like a tunnel through the side of a mountain, it is understandable that enlargement of the organ will impinge upon the channel and obstruct the flow of urine. Back pressure of urine from the bladder up to the kidneys damages the kidneys to the extent that they cannot eliminate waste products of the body and thus there occurs a kind of poisoning from these waste products called *uremia.* The obstruction at the bladder outlet must be relieved.

Slender telescopic operating instruments can be inserted through the penis into the bladder, permitting a direct look

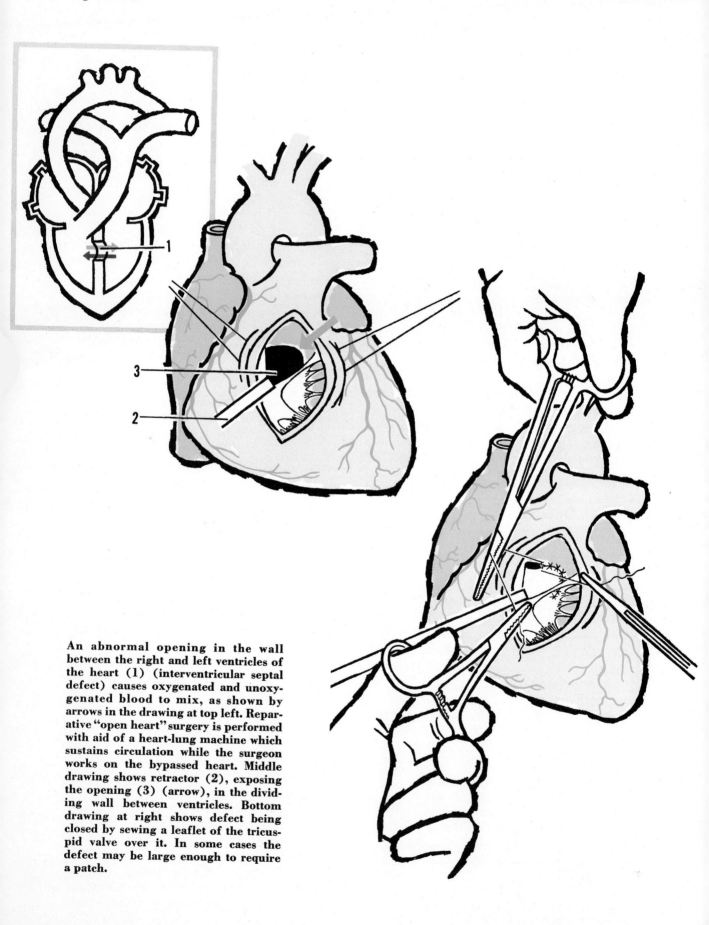

An abnormal opening in the wall between the right and left ventricles of the heart (1) (interventricular septal defect) causes oxygenated and unoxygenated blood to mix, as shown by arrows in the drawing at top left. Reparative "open heart" surgery is performed with aid of a heart-lung machine which sustains circulation while the surgeon works on the bypassed heart. Middle drawing shows retractor (2), exposing the opening (3) (arrow), in the dividing wall between ventricles. Bottom drawing at right shows defect being closed by sewing a leaflet of the tricuspid valve over it. In some cases the defect may be large enough to require a patch.

at the interior to determine the nature and extent of the poisonous obstruction caused by the prostate gland.

"Open" and "closed" procedures. There are four kinds of prostate operations. Three of these operations are called "open procedures", because they are performed through an incision made either in the lower abdomen or between the legs. There is one closed operation accomplished through the penis with the slender telescopic viewing instruments.

In *suprapubic prostatectomy* the bladder is opened and the surgeon introduces his hand into it. His index finger is inserted into the outlet of the bladder and is pushed forward into the section of the urethra that is surrounded by the prostate gland. The lining of the urethra is then split by the index finger and the prostate tissue peeled from its capsule.

Retropubic prostatectomy is very similar, but the bladder is not opened. The capsule of the prostate gland, a thin fibrous sheath, is split below the bladder and then the prostate tissue is peeled out with a finger or is cut out with scissors.

Perineal prostatectomy, the third of the open operations, is carried out through an incision between the legs. It permits the most complete removal, not only of the prostate and its capsule, which remains in the other operations, but also of surrounding structures. This operation is used more often for cancer of the prostate gland.

The closed operation is called *transurethral prostatectomy.* The slender tube-like operative instrument is inserted through the urethra into the bladder and the entire area of obstruction is viewed from inside the bladder. A wire loop, moved back and forth by a lever mechanism, acts as a cutting instrument by connection with special electric currents. By this means the prostatic tissue is removed piece by piece.

KIDNEY AND BLADDER STONES

Kidney stones are fairly common. *Bladder stones* on the other hand are rather rare, being limited for the most part to older persons. Most of the stones are found within the urine reservoir of the kidney, a kind of collecting bag off its side. The stone may remain there or it may slip out of the kidney reservoir and become engaged within the thin muscular tube (ureter) that conducts urine from the kidney to the bladder. When the ureter becomes obstructed, urine accumulates in the kidney reservoir to such a degree that the kidney itself becomes swollen and stretched. Obstruction to the flow of urine at any level in the urinary tract brings infection.

If infection can be prevented and if the obstruction to the outflow of urine is not severe, the patient, under supervision of his physician, may wait for a while for the stone to pass. If on the other hand infection sets in, or if the obstruction builds up enough pressure in the kidney to keep urine from filtering through it, surgery will be necessary. Complete obstruction continued for several weeks will cause damage to the kidney.

There are closed and open operations for removing stones. Small stones within the lower end of the ureter may be removed with what is called a "stone basket," a thin catheter with a loop at its tip. A cystoscopic viewing instrument is passed into the bladder through the penis and the catheter is inserted through the instrument and up the ureter. If the catheter loop can be made to engage the stone, the stone is withdrawn into the bladder. Once in the bladder the stone can be washed out through the cystoscopic instrument.

Sometimes the stone cannot be engaged by the loop, in which event the ureter is stretched by one or more catheters. This maneuver may allow the stone to pass into the bladder from which it can be removed with ease. Stones that are wedged in the ureter often must be removed by an open operation. The nature and location of the incision will depend of course upon the location and size of the stone.

The slit made in the ureter for removing the stone is closed by sutures placed very loosely to avoid scar formation and

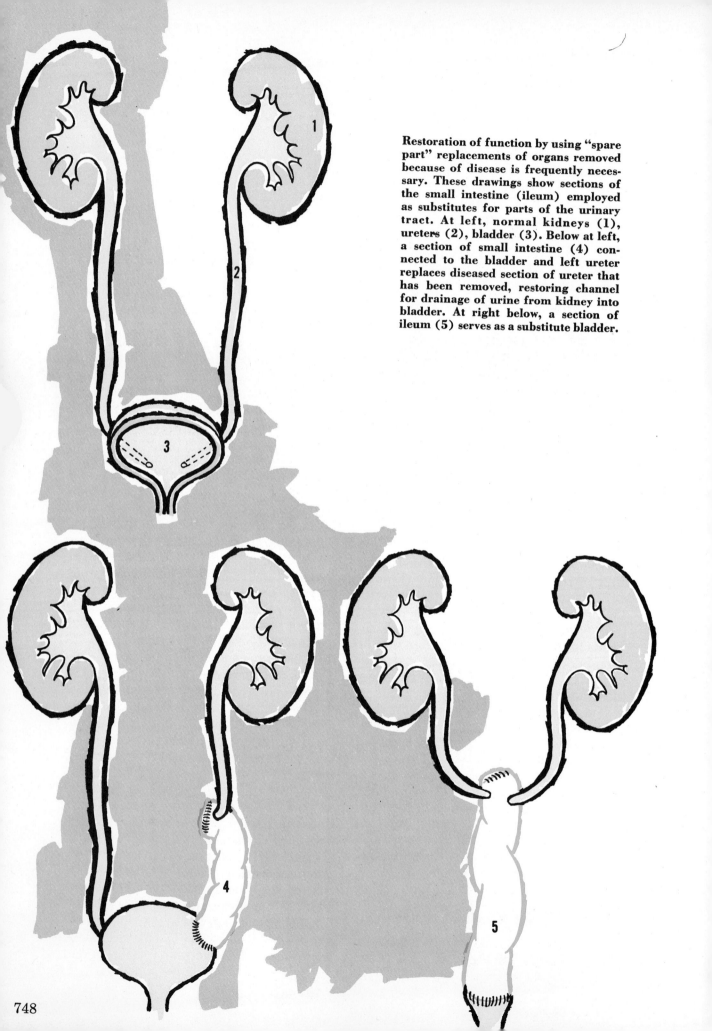

Restoration of function by using "spare part" replacements of organs removed because of disease is frequently necessary. These drawings show sections of the small intestine (ileum) employed as substitutes for parts of the urinary tract. At left, normal kidneys (1), ureters (2), bladder (3). Below at left, a section of small intestine (4) connected to the bladder and left ureter replaces diseased section of ureter that has been removed, restoring channel for drainage of urine from kidney into bladder. At right below, a section of ileum (5) serves as a substitute bladder.

narrowing of the slender ureter. Therefore after stone operations a drain is passed from the ureter to the outside because it is anticipated that there will be some leakage for several days.

Stones of considerable size remain in the collecting bag of the kidney for a long time, often without causing symptoms to make the patient aware of their presence. Such stones are too big to pass down into the ureter and therefore they cause no obstruction to the flow of urine. Eventually, however, infection or bleeding occur and the stone is discovered, but the kidney harboring the stone may have been damaged to such a degree by this time that it will be necessary for the surgeon to remove the kidney. This is done through an incision in the flank and the whole kidney is removed. The surgeon of course determines by examination that the other kidney is healthy and capable alone of carrying the load of eliminating waste from the body.

Stones in the urinary bladder, rare today, are removed by opening the bladder through an incision in the lower abdomen. Small stones can be removed through the normal channel of the urethra by cystoscopic instruments that are equipped with small crushing devices at their tips. These instruments crush the stones into tiny pieces that can be washed out through the cystoscope.

Cancer may appear at almost any place in the urinary tract, the kidney, the ureter, the bladder, the prostate and in other structures of the urinary system. Most often the organ must be removed. A diseased member of any of the organs that come in pairs, such as the kidneys, can be removed without impairing body functions if remaining organ is healthy. When it becomes necessary to remove the urinary bladder, a substitute bladder is formed from a section of intestine, and the ureters that bring urine down from the kidneys are transposed into the new bladder. This type of bladder opens directly to the outside and is without muscular control of the patient. It is necessary to use a plastic container that adheres to the skin.

TONSILLECTOMY

Tonsillectomy is not a minor operation. It is therefore undertaken only when the seriousness of recurrent attacks of tonsillitis clearly indicates that the patient would be better off without his tonsils. The operation is done in the hospital where safety devices and precautionary measures are available. Children are put to sleep under a general anesthetic; occasionally tonsils are removed from adults under local anesthesia.

Over the years, instruments for tonsillectomy and methods of anesthesia for this operation have been refined. Years ago only the tops of the tonsils were lopped off in hurried and sometimes rather bloody operations, even at times without a full anesthetic.

Anesthetic methods of today allow for protection of the opening into the windpipe by inserting tubes through the nose or mouth and directly into the windpipe. These tubes allow oxygen and anesthetic gases to enter the lungs and at the same time block off the normal entrance into the windpipe from the throat. Any blood or mucus from the field of operation in the back of the throat is therefore prevented from entering the windpipe. There are other methods for accomplishing this same purpose, particularly with the aid of instruments that suck in like vacuum cleaners to keep the entrance to the windpipe clear at all times.

These developments in anesthesia permit a meticulous and careful dissection and removal of the tonsils with no element of hurry.

Sometimes, however, despite the most meticulous technique and despite all precautionary measures, *bleeding* will occur after the operation. This may be within a few hours or as long as ten days later. Most often such bleeding is caused by a collection of clotted blood in one spot of the operated area. If this is the case, the hemorrhage is stopped by merely washing out the blood clots. Sometimes bleeding is persistent and the child may even have to undergo a second anesthetic for control of the bleeding point. It's like a nosebleed, though; it stops or it gets

Your Operation

Various methods of removing the tonsils employ special instruments. The surgeon employs techniques suited to his developed skills, experience, and needs of patients. The dissection and wire-snare method of tonsillectomy is shown in the drawings. At left below, dissector separates tonsil (grasped by forceps) from attachments in which it is imbedded. At right, snare is applied to base of tonsil after main body is freed from attachments. Loop of snare is drawn tighter and tighter through tissue until tonsil is out.

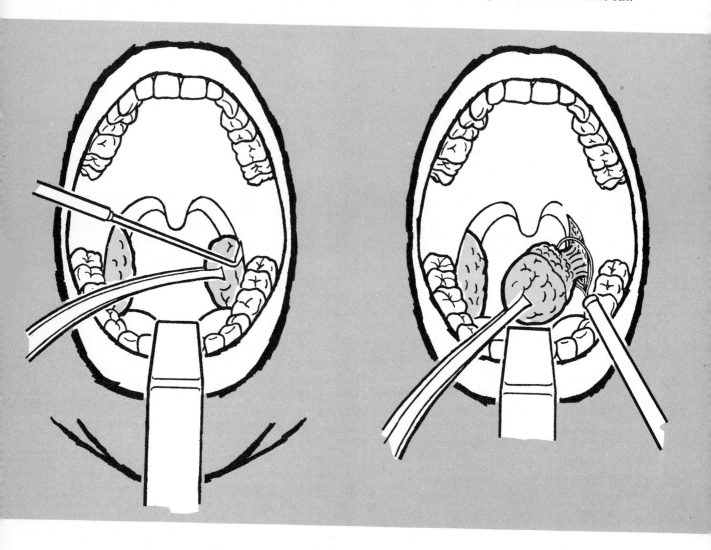

stopped. Parents of course are always instructed to notify the surgeon if there is the slightest bleeding after the child has been returned to his home.

The patient's throat will probably be quite sore for a day or two, but it is usually completely healed in about a week.

Adenoids are of about the same type of tissue as the tonsils. They are located high in the back of the throat and at the back end of the nose cavity. They become infected along with the tonsils and it is for this reason that the adenoids and tonsils are removed at the same time, not always but usually. Adenoids are removed with ingenious and delicate instruments that slide into the upper cavity of the throat behind the nose and their mechanisms are manipulated by the surgeon's fingers with small levers. If a child were to see an *adenotome* he might imagine it as an earth-excavating scoop attached to the end of a crane, all in miniature.

SURGERY OF HEAD AND NECK

Tumors

The complexity of the face, jaws, nose, voice box and the neck is such that tumors arising here involve several organs or organ systems at the same time. When they are brought under treatment in their early stages, surgical removal is simpler because fewer organs and structures are involved. Fear of disfigurement caused by surgical removal causes many people to delay unnecessarily. If the tumor is benign, and so many are, delay will necessitate removal of more tissue than would have been necessary. If the tumor is malignant, and some are, the patient who procrastinates is battling heavy odds that the tumor will be fatal.

Small tumors of the voice box, for example, can be eliminated nine times out of ten by the removal of a small amount of tissue. The same tumor, on the other hand, allowed to grow and expand and involve other portions of the throat, will require a far more extensive removal of tissue with much less chance for cure. Because they are brought to the patient's attention in their early stages, tumors of the head and neck carry a better chance for cure if treated in these early stages than the other, more hidden, tumors in deeper regions of the body. When extensive removal of tissue is required for far-advanced tumors, synthetic prostheses are used to mask the removed areas. The fabrication of these prostheses has developed into a fine art to the extent that it is hard to distinguish the artificial from natural.

Techniques have been developed not only to restore appearance but to substitute for function. The patient whose voice box has been removed for cancer of the larynx, for example, can be taught a type of speech that will be quite satisfactory for normal communication.

Thyroid Operations

Partial or complete surgery of the *thyroid gland* frequently is necessary because of goiters, although all goiters do not have to be removed.

It is seldom that the entire thyroid gland is removed. Whenever possible enough thyroid tissue is left to supply the body with natural thyroid chemical, called thyroid hormone. Sometimes almost all of the gland is diseased. In this case the surgeon recognizes that the small amount of good tissue he will leave will not be adequate. However, he must make a choice between healthy and diseased thyroid gland tissues.

Thyroid operations require an incision in the neck. This runs across the lower part of the neck in a gently curved fashion. The thin straplike muscles of the neck are separated to bring the gland into view and the diseased areas are removed. The thin scar from the wound is, of course, in a prominent place and this makes it somewhat annoying. Like all scars, it remains reddened for 6 to 12 months and this adds to the prominence. After this time the scar fades and is less conspicuous. In men it is usually below the collar line of the shirt. Women sometimes cover it with a necklace.

Recovery from the operation is usually quite rapid. Pain in thyroid wounds is much less than that in abdominal or chest wounds. Breathing and swallowing are almost never bothered to the extent patients expect. The stitches are usually removed within several days. Most often there is a drain to let excess serum out of the depths of the operative area. A thin serum accumulates in the wound rather frequently. This may be bothersome but it is not painful and the nuisance rarely persists for more than a week or two.

It is possible that another tumor may develop in the remaining healthy thyroid tissue at a later date. This does not happen commonly; it is consoling to know that operations made on the thyroid gland a second time are quite unusual and third operations are quite rare.

Operations for removal of what is known as a *toxic goiter* are unusual in this generation. Antithyroid medicines and radioactive isotopes are now available for control of the symptoms of overactivity or toxicity developing from overactivity and excess formation of the

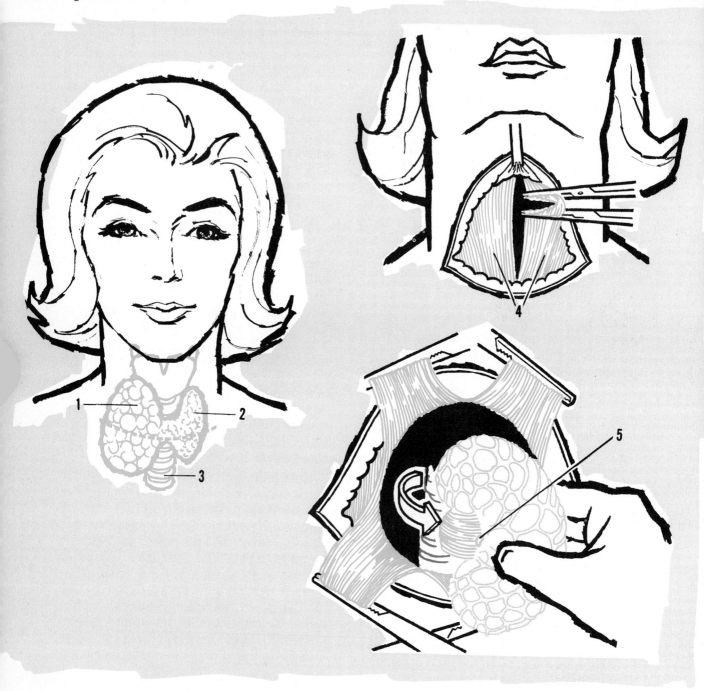

Many goiters respond to medical treatment. Serious pressure, deformity, malignancy, may make surgical removal necessary or desirable. Whenever possible a portion of the thyroid gland is left to supply the body with thyroid hormone. Drawing at top above shows abnormally enlarged right lobe of thyroid gland (1), with lobe of normal size (2) for comparison, and trachea (3). Broken-dash line shows curved incision to enter area. Upper right drawing shows sectioning of strap muscles (4) which lie over gland. Drawing at lower right shows goiter being rotated to expose grain-size parathyroid glands (5) imbedded in the thyroid. These are essential to calcium metabolism and are not removed when the goiter is resected.

thyroid hormone. Sometimes, however, these medicines do not control the over-active gland and it must be removed.

Cancers, of course, can develop in the thyroid gland. They are relatively rare but it is because of the possibility of development of cancerous tumors that the lumps in the thyroid gland are carefully watched by the physician. Every lump that is removed is analyzed. If it should happen that cancer is present, the operation becomes more extensive and is followed by x-ray treatments.

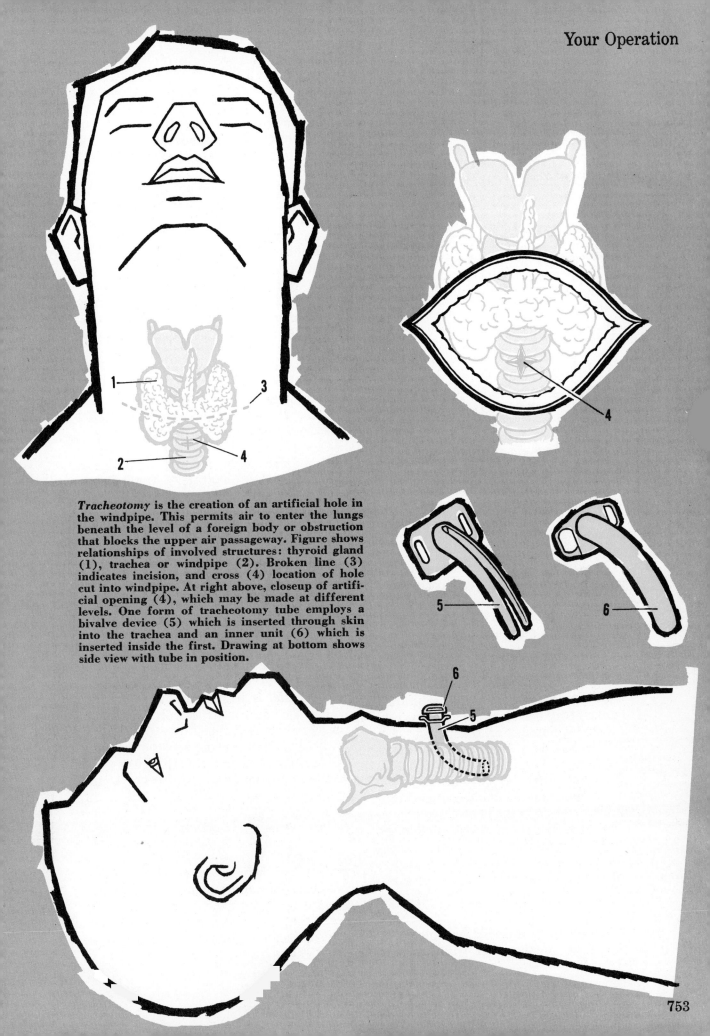

Tracheotomy is the creation of an artificial hole in the windpipe. This permits air to enter the lungs beneath the level of a foreign body or obstruction that blocks the upper air passageway. Figure shows relationships of involved structures: thyroid gland (1), trachea or windpipe (2). Broken line (3) indicates incision, and cross (4) location of hole cut into windpipe. At right above, closeup of artificial opening (4), which may be made at different levels. One form of tracheotomy tube employs a bivalve device (5) which is inserted through skin into the trachea and an inner unit (6) which is inserted inside the first. Drawing at bottom shows side view with tube in position.

Tracheotomy

Blockage of the upper air passages by foreign objects is relieved by *tracheotomy*. This means putting a temporary hole in the front of the windpipe just below the Adam's apple so that an obstruction higher up can be bypassed. A silver breathing tube is placed in this opening to allow air to enter the windpipe directly. Small soft tubes can also be passed through the silver breathing tube and down into the windpipe and bronchial tubes to draw out obstructing secretions.

An incision is made in the front of the neck and after pushing the muscles and other tissues aside, the windpipe is opened and the tube is inserted. When the tube is put in the windpipe for this purpose it is temporary. So long as the tube is in place it is kept clean and open. This is done by the patient himself as quickly as he is able to learn how to do this under instructions from the nursing staff. After a tracheotomy tube has been removed and the wound has healed the voice will be as normal as it was before and there will be only a small scar in the front of the neck.

When the structures of the larynx and voice box must be removed because of benign or malignant tumors, a tracheotomy tube is placed in the windpipe and here it remains permanently.

SURGERY ON THE EAR

The development of surgical techniques for correcting ear troubles has brought relief for a number of frustrating disabilities that were accepted as practically incurable years ago. These troubles include loss of hearing, chronic discharge of pus from the ear, sudden attacks of dizziness, noises in the head.

The usual ear infection is located in the middle ear. It may erode through the roof of the middle ear to make its way into the mastoid bone and through this bone into the skull cavity to cause meningitis or abscess of the brain.

Hearing loss is caused by trouble in the conducting mechanism that crosses through the middle ear or by trouble in the inner hearing nerve. If either your radio, or the audio on your television set is not working, it is likely that the trouble will be located in one of the three areas — in the loud speaker, or in the electronic tubes, or in the conducting wires that connect the loud speaker and tubes. If you can't hear, it is likely that your trouble will be located in the eardrum, or in the hearing cells of the inner nerve, or in the conducting bones that connect the drum to the ear nerve.

Most often a defective conducting mechanism, drum or bones, can be corrected by surgery, but a damaged nerve cannot be restored. With the help of sensitive tests the surgeon can estimate the outcome of surgery; good, poor or no hearing, fair hearing with the use of a hearing aid, improvement of the benefits already obtained by a hearing aid.

One form of dizziness is associated with a defect in the balance nerve of the inner ear. Sudden attacks of disabling instability and dizziness are characteristic of a condition called *Meniere's disease*. Most people who suffer from dizziness do not have Meniere's disease.

Some **head noises** are caused by a hardening condition of the third and most inner of the small conducting bones in the middle ear. This bone, shaped like a stirrup, and called the *stapes*, touches against a membrane which when vibrated sets up motions in the fluid around the inner ear nerve. The condition is called *otosclerosis*. It begins as a hearing loss which becomes progressively worse. As the attachment of the stapes to the membrane becomes hardened, the hearing nerve is irritated and it is this that sends impulses to the brain. Since the sound impulses are abnormal due to irritation, they are interpreted as noise such as ringing, roaring, buzzing.

Myringoplasty

This is the name of an operation for repairing a hole in the ear drum. A small graft of skin or vein is used to seal the hole. This closes the middle ear from the outside and prevents ear infection. In a good many cases hearing is improved.

The operation is performed through the ear canal with local anesthesia. A hospital period of several days is necessary. Healing is complete in about six weeks, at which time hearing improvement is noticeable.

Myringotomy is a relatively simple surgical incision of the eardrum.

Tympanoplasty

Tympanum is the Latin word for the middle ear. Tympanoplasty is the name for an operation in which the middle ear, including its roof in the mastoid bone, is completely cleaned out, revised and restored. All infection is eradicated. This type of operation is necessary when both the eardrum and the conducting bones are diseased. The extent of the surgery will depend upon how much normal structure is left after all of the infection has been cleaned out. The destroyed parts of eardrum and the ear bones will have to be replaced by skin or vein grafts and by plastic or wire substitutes.

The operation can be performed through the ear canal under local anesthesia, or if the infection is severe an incision behind the ear may be necessary and this will require a general anesthetic. The improvement in hearing is noticeable within eight weeks. The hospital stay is less than a week. Infection may be so severe that two operations will be required. At the first session all of the infection is cleaned out and at the second session the eardrum and the bones are reconstructed with substitutes.

Mastoidectomy

This is the oldest of the ear operations. Years ago, acute inflammation of the mastoid bone was a fairly common complication of ear trouble. To relieve this condition the surgeon exposed the mastoid bone through an incision behind the ear and chiseled a cavity into the bone to allow pus to drain out. In time the acute infection subsided, but the chronically infected ear remained. Acute mastoiditis is seen only rarely today.

Chronic mastoiditis, on the other hand, is common today. The chronic infection in the mastoid and middle ear should be cleaned out because of the potential danger of abscess of the brain. All infection here must be eradicated before any of the reconstructive operations for restoration of hearing can be accomplished.

Fenestration

In this operation the mastoid bone is opened and the "balance canals" of the inner ear are laid bare. A tiny hole, called a *fenestrum,* is made in one of the balance tubes. A paper-thin piece of skin taken from the ear canal is then placed over this hole. This allows sound waves from the air to vibrate the piece of skin at the small opening and in turn the fluid in the balance tube will transmit sound vibrations to the hearing nerve.

This was the first of the modern ear operations and was designed for otosclerosis. Its purpose was to bypass the hardened stapes that was stuck to the membrane that normally vibrated the fluid of the hearing nerve. For the most part, the fenestration operation has been replaced by the stapes operation. Fenestration is reserved for persons who are born without an outside ear or ear canal or for those who have had extensive destruction of the bone around the hearing nerve, the result of infection.

Stapes Operation

The stapes is removed and the membrane upon which it rests comes along with it. A small bit of vein is grafted over the opening and a section of wire or plastic material is positioned to bridge the gap between the membrane and the bone next to the stapes. This restores the conducting mechanism.

If the stapes surgery is not successful, hearing may be about the same as it was before. It is possible that it might be worse but this does not happen often. In some instances, fortunately not many, head noises can be worse than they were before. Because of the possibility of a poor result, the ear with the greater hearing defect is usually operated upon first.

Surgery for Meniere's Disease

Formerly only the most severe and disabling forms of this disease were treated surgically because the operation for relief of these sudden dizzy attacks required destruction of the hearing nerve. Until micro-surgical instruments were developed it was impossible to separate the hearing and balance filaments in the main nerve, where many filaments are carried as the wires in a telephone cable. Now that these can be separated it is possible to clip only the balance filaments. It is possible also to use selective ultrasonic beams for destruction of the balance filaments without damaging the sensitive hearing filaments.

Instruments for Ear Surgery

Intricate and delicate ear operations are done under an operating microscope and with micro-instruments of hardened steel. The drills are similar to those the dentist uses. The tiny bones are reshaped and replaced in a small cavity not much larger than the cavity the dentist works in when he designs the gold inlay for a tooth. The patience required is similar to that of the New England fisherman constructing the four-masted ship inside a long narrow-necked bottle.

BREAST OPERATIONS

A lump in the breast could mean cancer, so the surgeon must prove that the lump is not cancer.

This means a "biopsy"; the lump is removed and analyzed in the pathology laboratory. The usual practice is to remove the lump in the operating room with the patient asleep; most often the analysis is made right then by "frozen section". The removed specimen is quick-frozen, sectioned on a machine into tiny slices a thousandth of an inch thick, stained, mounted on little glass slides and analyzed under the microscope by the pathologist. This takes about ten minutes.

If the analysis shows no cancer, the small wound is sutured and the patient is home the next day. The net result, a small scar on the breast and no lump.

If the analysis shows cancer, the breast must be removed and this is done immediately. The extent of the operation varies from removal of only the breast tissue to removal of the underlying muscles and all of the tissues under the armpit, along with the breast. Usually the more extensive operation is performed because the drainage paths from the breast run through the muscles and to the armpit. In instances where it is deemed necessary, both breasts are removed.

Post-surgical measures. What happens after breast surgery? Usually there are x-ray treatments. These sterilize, so to speak, a further area around the breast. There are exercises. These bring about a re-education of the adjoining muscles to give strength to the shoulder and arm. Within months shoulder motion is free and strong. Bowling, golf, tennis, swimming are resumed. Then there are fittings and adjustments to make the artificial form fill out your dresses as they should. The texture and mobility of these forms will relieve many of your anxieties.

The recovery period after breast operations is usually surprisingly short and the emotional adjustment is always more rapid than has been anticipated by the patient and the relatives.

Benign lumps. If the lump isn't cancer, what is it? Most of them are milk ducts that have become blocked and then filled to stretching by a fluid made by the breast cells. The tube-shaped duct stretches out into a ball shape. In this manner it becomes a cavity filled with fluid and is called a *cyst*. Every woman has hundreds of pinhead-size cysts in the breasts, the natural result of the swelling and activity of the breasts that occurs before each menstrual period. It is only the larger cysts that show as lumps. Sometimes a hollow needle is put into a cyst to draw out the fluid and collapse the cavity.

The lump may be a non-cancerous tumor, a growth that is enclosed in a capsule and that is not capable of getting into the blood stream and spreading. In this case, only the fluid-filled lump is removed, not the breast.

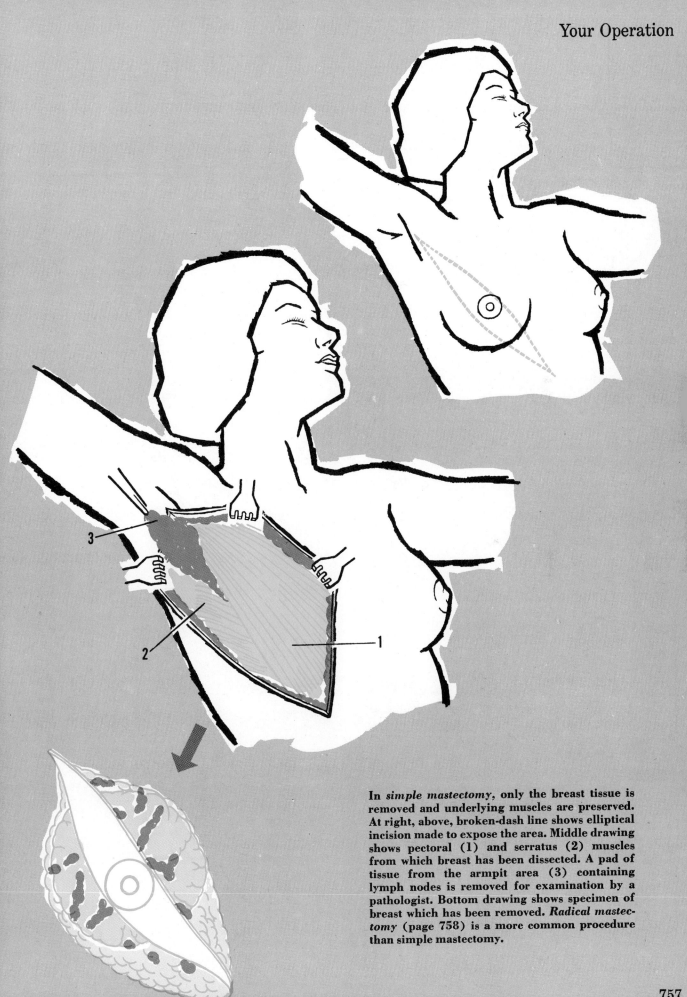

In *simple mastectomy*, only the breast tissue is removed and underlying muscles are preserved. At right, above, broken-dash line shows elliptical incision made to expose the area. Middle drawing shows pectoral (1) and serratus (2) muscles from which breast has been dissected. A pad of tissue from the armpit area (3) containing lymph nodes is removed for examination by a pathologist. Bottom drawing shows specimen of breast which has been removed. *Radical mastectomy* (page 758) is a more common procedure than simple mastectomy.

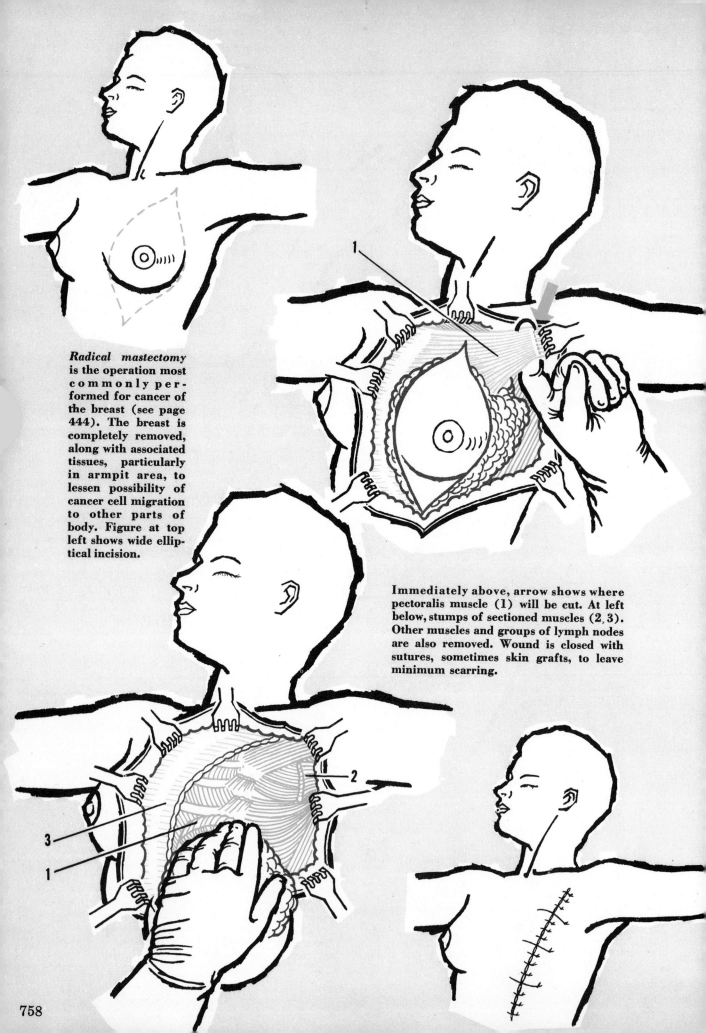

Radical mastectomy is the operation most commonly performed for cancer of the breast (see page 444). The breast is completely removed, along with associated tissues, particularly in armpit area, to lessen possibility of cancer cell migration to other parts of body. Figure at top left shows wide elliptical incision.

Immediately above, arrow shows where pectoralis muscle (1) will be cut. At left below, stumps of sectioned muscles (2,3). Other muscles and groups of lymph nodes are also removed. Wound is closed with sutures, sometimes skin grafts, to leave minimum scarring.

NEUROSURGERY

Craniotomy

Instruments called *trephines,* used for boring holes into the skull cavity, are among the remains of the most ancient civilizations. Archeologists have uncovered trephined skulls in almost all areas of the world. The skull was opened to let out fluid or blood that accumulated under pressure in the covering cap of the brain. There is no doubt that the method was effective in controlling the convulsions and coma of head injuries, or for removing splinters of fractured skull bones, but its use generally for fits, insanity, and demons left the patient with a hole in his head and very little improvement.

Under more refined circumstances and with the help of diagnostic x-ray and laboratory techniques, holes are bored in the skull today in modern operating rooms. These are called *burr holes.* A plug of bone comes away and is taken out like the testing plug in a watermelon. Burr holes are required most frequently for the head injuries of automobile and machinery accidents. A burr hole may vary from a half inch to an inch in diameter and frequently the opening may be enlarged with a strong-jawed biting forceps that nips away quarter-inch sections of bone around the hole.

Brain surgery. For more extensive operations on the brain a larger opening, called a *flap,* is necessary. The word *craniotomy* is reserved for this larger and more complicated opening into the skull cavity. Several burr holes are made at intervals and the bone between the holes is sawed through, using either a hand operated instrument that looks like a heavy roughened wire, or a circular electric saw that operates from a motor like the dentist's drill.

The bone plugs or bone flaps may or may not be replaced by the surgeon, depending upon the condition of the bone and upon the location of the operating site in the skull. A metal or fabric mesh may be used to cover the opening in the bone. More often, however, the heavy muscle and scalp tissues that make up the flap will be sufficient and actually more satisfactory as a cover.

"Electric knife." Bleeding from the numerous tiny blood vessels that carry an abundant supply of blood to the scalp and to the brain cap is controlled by an electric current that is applied to the severed blood vessels through a needle-tipped instrument that is called an "electric knife." The current jumping from the needle tip seals the opening in the blood vessel by baking it. By altering the electric current supplied to the instrument the baking action is changed to a cutting action. Thus, the needle can be used as a knife for cutting and hence its name, "electric knife."

The operative field of the exposed brain is flushed frequently with a diluted salt solution which is sprayed over the brain tissue and then drained out through a narrow tube attached to an electric suction pump.

Brain tissue is handled delicately with damp cotton pads attached to the ends of forceps. Anesthesia for brain surgery is most often general, that is, the patient is asleep. Some operations are performed under local anesthesia. Pain nerves are in the scalp and coverings only.

Varieties of brain operations. Operations have been devised for a variety of troubles that affect the brain. In serious head injuries the skull must be opened for removal of bone splinters and blood clots and for the removal of brain tissue that has been damaged.

Tears in the brain capsule are repaired to protect underlying brain tissue.

Tumors are removed by "shelling them out" when they are enclosed in a capsule, or by directly cutting through brain tissue when there is no capsule around the tumor. Some areas in the brain are said to be "silent", meaning that the cells in these areas serve the physical and mental processes to such a minor degree that their loss is not a major one.

Defects in the fluid canals inside the brain may be restored or the canals may be rerouted. Special nerve filament pathways in the brain are sometimes severed purposely to reduce abnormal impulses

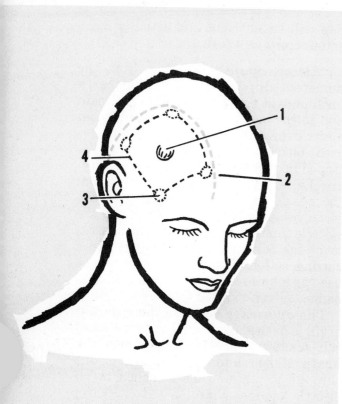

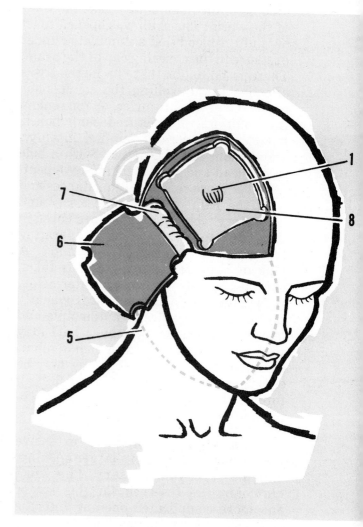

muscles, two and three inches in diameter, lying on each side of these vertebral tips are peeled back from the surfaces of the vertebrae. The portion of a vertebra that extends backward to form the back

Brain surgery involves *craniotomy* (excision of part of the skull). Above, drawing shows surgical approach for removal of a meningioma (1), a tumor in membranes that envelop the brain. Broken-dash line (2) is incision through skin of scalp; dotted circles (3) are burr holes bored through bone; these are connected with saw cuts (4). At right, reflected skin flap (dotted line, 5); bone flap (6) reflected, exposing tumor (1) and dura (8), outermost brain membrane. Temporal muscle (7) acts as hinge for bone flap.

that cause convulsions, palsy or pain. Ingenious locating devices are combined with special x-ray equipment to pinpoint the seat of trouble.

Spinal Cord Operations

The *spinal cord*, extending from the base of the skull to the lower back, may be exposed for surgery at any point along its course. The approach to the cord is through the back, the incision placed in a vertical direction over the tips of the spinal vertebrae, which are the bony projections you can feel up and down the center of your back. The huge strap

wall of the spinal canal is called the *lamina*. Since it is the laminae that are removed when the spinal cord must be exposed, the operation is called *laminectomy*. The laminae of two or three vertebrae are nipped away with strong but slender biting forceps. This opens up the spinal canal which measures about an inch in diameter. The covering of the spinal cord is cut open to bring the cord into full view.

It is this type of operative approach that is used for tumors of the spinal cord,

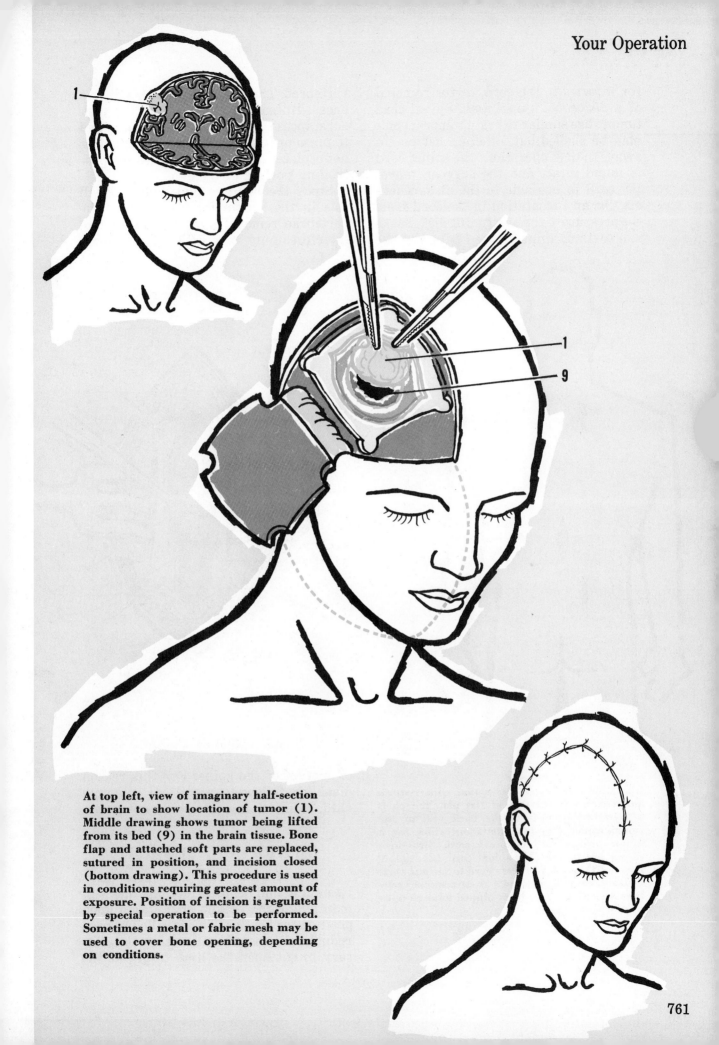

At top left, view of imaginary half-section of brain to show location of tumor (1). Middle drawing shows tumor being lifted from its bed (9) in the brain tissue. Bone flap and attached soft parts are replaced, sutured in position, and incision closed (bottom drawing). This procedure is used in conditions requiring greatest amount of exposure. Position of incision is regulated by special operation to be performed. Sometimes a metal or fabric mesh may be used to cover bone opening, depending on conditions.

for *injuries* to the cord, or for removal of a *dislocated spinal disk*. Spinal cord tumors are similar to brain tumors; some may be shelled out, others must be cut away. In disk operations the spinal cord is found intact and the surgeon moves the cord to one side to the disk. There may be an indentation in the cord from the pressure of the protruding disk. Disks are soft cushions located between the vertebrae. The capsule in which a disk is encased breaks open, allowing the disk substances to protrude into the canal and to press upon the cord. The surgeon does not replace the disk, he removes the protruding portion of it.

Since the laminae play only a small role in the supporting function of the vertebrae, removal of one or two laminae interferes only very little with support

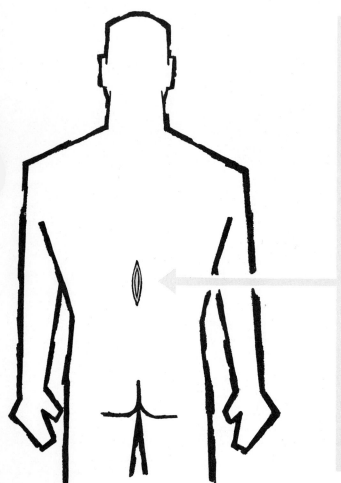

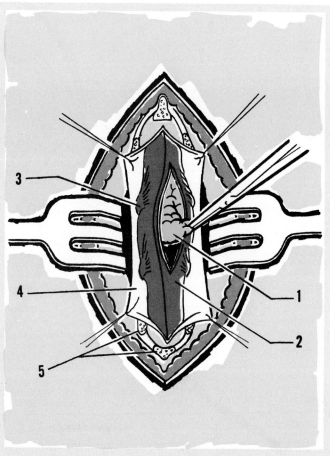

Operations to expose the spinal cord require *laminectomy* — excision of flat platelike parts of vertebrae that form the back wall of the spinal canal. Drawing shows operation for a tumor arising in the spinal cord. Structures shown are tumor (1), spinal cord (2), spinal nerves (3) which run from cord to various parts of body, covering of cord (4), and spinal vertebrae (5) which have been nipped away to open up the spinal canal.

or motion of the spine. For this reason disability following operations on spinal cord, laminectomy, is usually not long.

ORTHOPEDIC SURGERY

A *bone fracture* can be reduced (set) by pulling and bending motions that will manipulate the broken ends into a good position for healing. This is called "closed reduction", closed because it is not necessary to cut open the limb to get at the bone ends directly. X-rays may show beforehand that a closed reduction will not work, either because the bone is splintered into many pieces or because the break is on a slant. Splintered or slanted ends will slip away from each other. On the other hand, the x-rays might indicate that a closed reduction is worth a try.

If the ends cannot be positioned properly, or if they will not hold position, an operation is necessary to open the fracture to full view to "reduce" it with bone levers and bone clamps and then fasten the fitted ends together ("open reduction") with some fastening device.

Devices. All kinds of devices are used to fasten broken bones — pins, nails of many sorts, wires, metal plates, and even long rods that extend the entire length of the bone through the marrow canal. All of these are made of special alloy metals that ordinarily will not irritate body tissues. Sometimes there will be irritation of the bone and the muscle, even to the extent that the appliance will have to be removed before the bone has had a chance to heal. Some of these metal devices remain in the bone permanently, some are removed after healing is complete.

The use of appliances fixed into the bone to heal a fracture is called "internal fixation". This may be all the support that is needed, but more often a cast is put around the limb for additional external fixation. Metal pins can be punctured through the skin and into the bone under x-ray guidance to secure internal fixation without making an incision to expose the fracture to view. This is "internal fixation combined with closed reduction".

The time required for fracture healing, called "union" of the bone, will vary with the size of the bone, the extent of splintering, and whether the bone bears any of the body's weight, as is the case with bones of the spine, the pelvis and the lower limbs.

Occasionally a fracture, whether set by closed reduction or by open reduction, may not heal. This will happen if the broken ends become hard and calloused without knitting to each other. In this case, an operation will be necessary to open the fracture for removal of the hard callous. At the same time, bone chips are put around the fracture to stimulate knitting, or a solid piece of bone shaped like a stick is grafted into the bone across the break. Bone used for the stimulation of knitting is obtained usually from the hospital's bone bank.

Compound fractures demand special surgical attention because of contamination of the exposed marrow of the bone by dirt and bacteria that get in through the torn skin and muscle. This calls for immediate surgery to clean out the wound and it may require actual removal of some muscle and skin tissue, if dirt has been ground into it. If the wound can be cleaned satisfactorily, the fracture may be reduced at this time. If the surgeon judges the contamination to be too severe, he will pack the wound with gauze and place the limb in a cast, holding off on the actual reduction of the fracture for as long as a week, during which time any contaminants in the wound will drain out into the gauze packs. As soon as the wound is clean, the fracture can be reduced and secured in place by whatever means are necessary.

Fractures of the Femur

The upper end of the thigh bone, the *femur,* is a common location for fractures among people in their 60's and 70's. This common fracture is sometimes referred to as a fracture of the hip, but this is not a good name for it because the pelvis bone, which is a part of the hip joint, is not usually broken in these people. The fracture is a bad one because it won't knit unless the bone ends are held still by some method for as long as three to six months. Any method that keeps an elderly patient in bed for this length of time may lead to pneumonia, bladder infection, pressure sores and death. This was the case years ago when these fractures were held in place by weights over the end of the bed or by plaster casts.

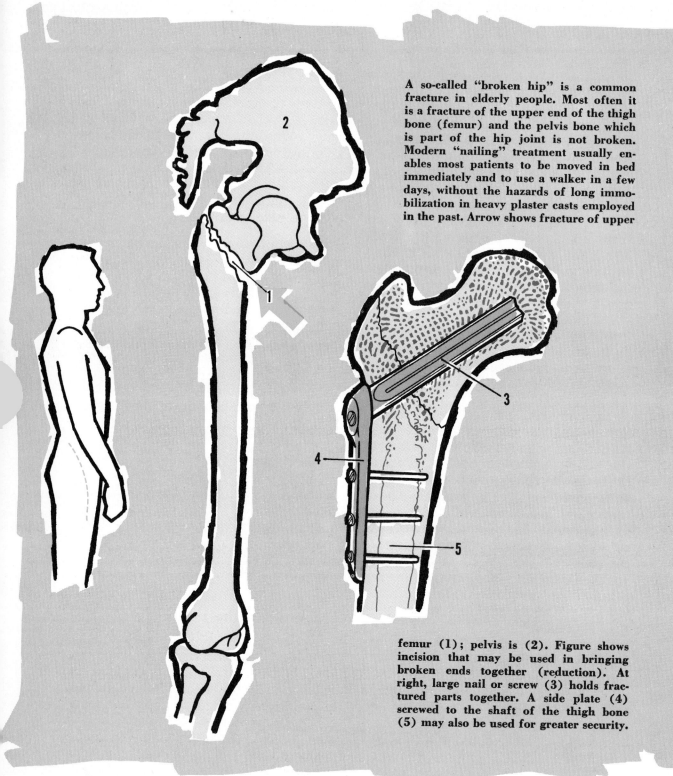

A so-called "broken hip" is a common fracture in elderly people. Most often it is a fracture of the upper end of the thigh bone (femur) and the pelvis bone which is part of the hip joint is not broken. Modern "nailing" treatment usually enables most patients to be moved in bed immediately and to use a walker in a few days, without the hazards of long immobilization in heavy plaster casts employed in the past. Arrow shows fracture of upper

femur (1); pelvis is (2). Figure shows incision that may be used in bringing broken ends together (reduction). At right, large nail or screw (3) holds fractured parts together. A side plate (4) screwed to the shaft of the thigh bone (5) may also be used for greater security.

Unless the patient is in a practically dying condition, an operation will give him his best chance for survival and restoration to walking. The fractured ends are reduced into a good position under anesthesia and the bone is secured by large nails or screws and possibly also by a plate that is attached to the long end of the bone. With the bone secure, the patient can be moved about in bed immediately and within a short time he can be helped to a chair and to a walker.

The higher in the bone, the worse the fracture, because the ball-like head at the top end of the bone is nourished by only a small artery that is usually torn with the fracture. If the head of the bone should die after fracture, it might have to be replaced at a later date by a metallic ball anchored to the bone.

Arthroplasty. If the ball-shaped head of the thigh bone (femur) has been shattered or if it has become disintegrated as a result of disease, it can be replaced with a metal ball. The ball is attached to a stem that the surgeon can seat into the hollow marrow canal of the shaft of the thigh bone. The operation is called *arthroplasty.* The same operation—with variations—is used for reconstruction of a painful hip joint that has been ravaged and stiffened by arthritis. Hip arthroplasty is a very serious operation and is reserved for patients who are in fairly good physical condition.

Smooth surfaces can be fashioned for smaller joints—elbow, fingers—that are stiff and motionless. The roughened cartilage at the ends of the bones is removed and the bone ends that form the joint are covered with a piece of the membrane that encloses the outer thigh muscle.

Amputations

The artistry and mechanical genius of today's prostheses have brought a new world of rehabilitation to patients who are faced with amputation of a limb. Any such ingenious replacement that overcomes a frustrating physical loss deserves the name *prosthesis* and we should say "prosthesis", we should not say "artificial limb" or "peg-leg". The moving fingers and hands of a prosthesis can thread needles, hammer a nail, or quiet a baby; these ankle and knee joints can dance or hike; these feet can stand at a lathe all day.

When forced to amputate, the surgeon considers the wide variety of available prostheses as they relate to his patient's age, training, occupation and pattern of life. This is necessary because the site, or level, of amputation and the manner of shaping the bones and muscles of the limb, bear directly on the different types of prostheses the patient will be using. Some prostheses require special rearrangements of the muscle bundles in the limb for their most effective use. This is called a *cineplastic amputation.* The con-

dition of the blood vessels is a major factor in determining the site and type of amputation.

The time required for adjustment, both physically and emotionally, to amputation and to the prosthesis will again depend upon the patient's particular problem. Help is always available through private sources and through public Rehabilitation Agencies. Re-training, education in physical adeptness and financial assistance are open to the amputee.

Amputations are necessary for a number of reasons. Limbs are sometimes mangled and damaged beyond all possible restoration in highway accidents, by explosions, or in mishaps with heavy machinery. It is the younger people who are involved more frequently in accidents. Farm machinery is particularly dangerous if it is not used with great caution. Hardened blood vessels, especially in diabetic patients, not infrequently become clogged, shutting off the supply of blood to the limb with the result that a foot and part of the leg become gangrenous (dead). Cancerous growths do not attack the limbs often but when they do, their removal may require the sacrifice of greater part, or all, of a limb.

Amputations are necessary more frequently in the lower than in the upper limbs. Amputation through the foot and behind the toes may require only a rubber shoe filler and a small bar on the sole of the shoe. Only rarely can the surgeon choose amputation through the instep. If this is possible, a partly filled orthopedic shoe will serve satisfactorily.

Amputations through the ankles or heel bones are difficult to fit. Fitting of a prosthesis for an amputation through either the ankle or heel bone is generally more difficult and therefore less satisfactory than the fitting for an amputation made horizontally just at the top of the ankle bone. The patient usually adjusts quite readily to a filled-in leather boot-lacing in front and extending almost to the knee. Above the ankle, a prosthesis will fit best at a point about six inches below the knee. If this much bone cannot be saved below the knee, an amputation above the knee will be preferable for the mechanical fitting of a comfortable and well-functioning leg.

Finger amputations are designed to save as much working finger length as possible and this is especially true with the thumb. To conserve bone length in the fingers, grafts of skin padded with fat tissue are taken from other areas of the body to cover the tips of the bones. Otherwise, extra bone would have to be removed to allow the skin of the finger to cover the bone end. If the finger is irreparably damaged as far back as the hand knuckle, the knuckle is better removed. If the fifth finger is lost, its knuckle is conspicuous and gets in the way. Removal of the knuckle makes for a better looking and a better working hand. If the index finger should be lost, removal of the knuckle allows the thumb to work more closely with the middle finger and here again the loss of the finger is much less conspicuous. The same principle applies to the knuckles of the other fingers.

For amputations within the forearm and the arm there are numerous surgical techniques for shaping the bones into levers covered with skin and working like big fingers, or for construction of muscle and tendon pulleys over skin tunnels. The human levers and pulleys manipulate the intricate mechanical devices of the prostheses.

RECTAL OPERATIONS

Crypts, papillas and fistulas. Pockets (crypts) and mounds (papillas) are natural structures just inside the rectum. They are part and parcel with the pleats and folds that are gathered in the rectal membrane by the pursestring muscle that closes the rectum. They cause trouble when inflamed and swollen. Infection in a crypt spreads through the rectal wall and burrows in the soft flesh about the anus to form an abscess. When the abscess breaks through to the skin an inch or two distant from the natural opening, a tunnel remains as an abnormal passageway from the rectum. This is referred to as a *fistula*.

Whether surgery for a fistula will be simple or involved will depend upon the contour of the tunnel and upon whether it runs a straight course to the outside or has ramifications and more than one opening. All tissue over the fistula is cut away, even a part of the muscle. If muscle loss may be large, the operation can be performed in two stages, that is, there may be two operations to preserve the circular pattern and pursestring function of the muscle.

Rectal polyps. These are soft fleshy growths that are encountered frequently during proctoscopic examination. A piece of the polyp is taken for examination—biopsy—and the growth is removed, either by snipping it away with a scissorlike instrument or with an electric needle. This is done through the proctoscope. The patient is not always confined to the hospital. An anesthetic is not required.

Pilonidal cyst. This birth defect is a small cavity in the fat over the tailbone. When swollen from inflammation, it may have a depth of one and a half inches. A short tunnel leads to a sometimes invisible opening in the skin.

When infected, a cyst may have to be lanced to let out the pus. Later, the cavity must be removed, usually by cutting away all of the tissue around the cyst and down to the covering of the tailbone (coccyx). The gaping trough-like hole that remains after removal of the cavity may be sewn shut or it may be left open to heal gradually from the bottom. If the slower healing course is chosen by the surgeon, a matter of six weeks may be involved in the process. However, the wound needs only a covering that can be slipped inside the underclothing. Within two weeks the patient may be back at work. Once this is so, either showering or tub bathing will be safe.

Cancer. An operation for rectal cancer may or may not require an opening in the side for bowel movements (colostomy, see page 732). If all of the rectum must be removed, including the muscle—a very small percentage of all colon and rectal cancers—this will be because the

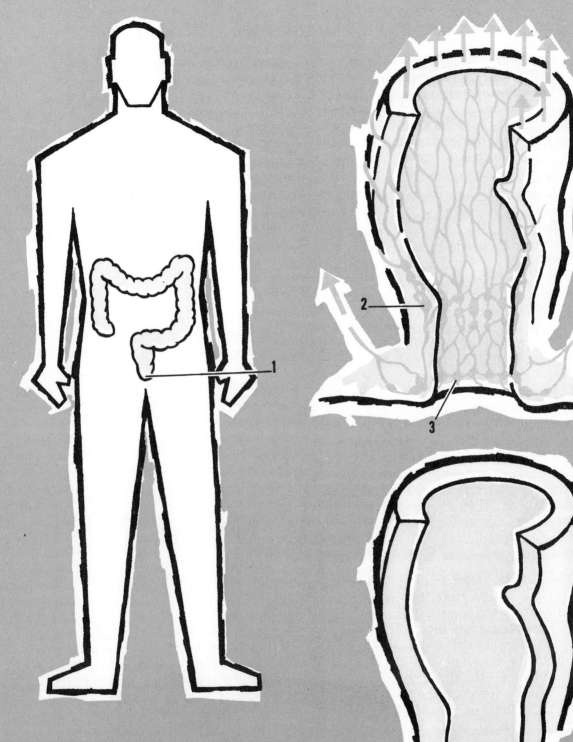

Hemorrhoids are varicose (swollen, knotted) veins in and around the rectal opening (1). Drawing at upper right shows pattern of veins around lower rectum and opening: internal hemorrhoidal plexus (2) which may develop into internal hemorrhoids (in canal above pursestring muscle of opening), and external plexus of veins (3). External hemorrhoids arise in skin around opening outside of pursestring muscle. At lower right, a thrombosed (clotted) external hemorrhoid (4) protruding from rectal opening.

malignant growth lies within several inches of the muscle at the natural anal opening. Otherwise, the involved part of the rectum can be removed through an incision in the abdomen and the cut ends of the colon and rectum sewn together. Thus, the muscle at the anus will be preserved so that bowel movements can take place in the normal fashion.

Hemorrhoids, also called piles, are varicose veins in and around the rectal opening. "Varicose" means permanently stretched in both length and breadth.

With each bowel movement, the rectum is stretched open to let the stool come through. A straining effort to force the stool will, of course, increase the stretching force. The membrane, the muscle wall of the canal and the veins imbedded in it are all stretched in this process. After the stool has passed through, all of these parts recoil to natural size, and the circular purse-string muscle of the canal tightens to close the opening. The canal is about an inch in length and stretches to a diameter of one and one-half inches.

The thin walls of the veins do not tolerate this repeated stretching as well as the membrane and the muscles. If the veins are weaker than normal, and this is the case in many people, they will be stretched permanently to become hemorrhoids.

How hemorrhoids develop. Veins dilate to the extent that they bulge and actually at times hang out of the opening. Once the process has set in, it can only get worse because the stool as it is forced through the canal pushes the bulging veins outward, stretching them still further. Usually there will be three, but no more than four, of these bulging veins formed into clusters. In time the membrane that covers the veins becomes thinned and stretched.

Larger, hanging clusters of hemorrhoids lose their elasticity and then they are unable to recoil back inside the opening after the stool has passed through. Now, when the pursestring muscle closes, the hemorrhoids are squeezed half way in and half way out. Patients with hanging *prolapsed* hemorrhoids find it necessary to push them back into the canal after a bowel movement. Such hemorrhoids are also called *protruding piles.*

When subjected to the pushing force of the stool, the thinned membrane over the hemorrhoids is easily torn. Blood leaks out of the veins and they are then said to be *bleeding hemorrhoids.* With rare exceptions, bleeding occurs only with bowel movements. Usually the bleeding is not great and it stops within a few minutes after the bowel movement.

The circulation of blood in these tortuous hemorrhoidal veins becomes stagnant and the blood in them is subject to clotting. When a clot, often called a thrombus, forms, the hemorrhoid is called a clotted or *thrombosed hemorrhoid.*

Pain comes in "attacks" that last ordinarily no longer than a few days. After this there is a quiet and comfortable spell that may last for months before there is another attack. The painful attacks arise from swelling that is occasioned by prolonged squeezing of prolapsed hemorrhoids that have not been pushed back in after a bowel movement.

Types. Hemorrhoids are classified as *internal* or *external,* or as combined internal and external. These listings have to do with the location of the bulkier portion of the hemorrhoidal mass of veins in relation to the tightening pursestring that is called the rectal *sphincter* muscle. Those that are situated well up inside the canal and further in than the sphincter muscle are internal hemorrhoids. External hemorrhoids actually are in the skin around the opening and are outside of the sphincter muscle. Although hemorrhoids may be solely external or solely internal, in most instances the stretched veins run the whole length of the canal, including the entrance and the exit. These are referred to as combined internal-external hemorrhoids.

Hemorrhoids will not become cancerous nor will they cause cancer. However, since bleeding from the rectum is one of the signs of rectal cancer, bleeding that supposedly comes from hemorrhoids must be investigated to make certain the hemorrhoids are the sole cause of the bleeding. But here again this does not make one safe for the rest of his life. If bleeding continues, it will have to be checked frequently, as often as every six months, for a cancer may develop, quite apart from the hemorrhoids, and hide behind the bleeding that is assumed to be hemorrhoidal bleeding.

the varicose veins are removed. They are cut away along with the stretched membrane over them. For each hemorrhoidal cluster, a double incision in the form of an ellipse is made the full length of the rectal canal to include both the internal and the external portions of each hemorrhoid. There may be as many as four incisions along the length of the canal.

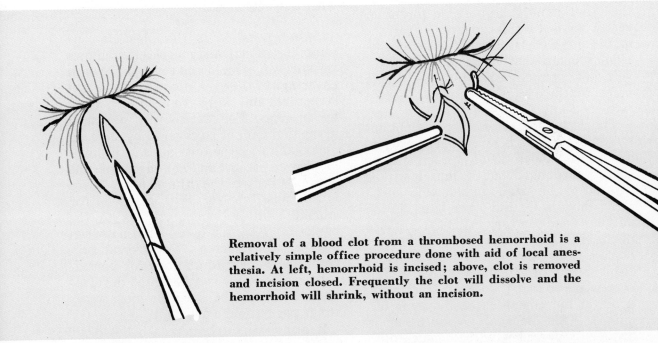

Removal of a blood clot from a thrombosed hemorrhoid is a relatively simple office procedure done with aid of local anesthesia. At left, hemorrhoid is incised; above, clot is removed and incision closed. Frequently the clot will dissolve and the hemorrhoid will shrink, without an incision.

Rectal examinations are made with an instrument called a *proctoscope*. This is a tube open at one end and equipped at the other end with an electric light and a magnifying view window through which the surgeon can see the interior of the rectum. The instrument, handled gently and well lubricated, can be inserted into the rectum with no pain.

Large hemorrhoids that are giving trouble from bleeding or pain should be removed. Only rarely does this call for emergency action. The operation can be arranged for a convenient time.

Removal of hemorrhoids is called *hemorrhoidectomy*. It is performed in the hospital and most often under a general or a spinal anesthetic. From three to six days hospitalization will be sufficient in most cases. In a hemorrhoid operation,

A clotted, or thrombosed, hemorrhoid may be relieved by a small incision through which the clot is removed. This is accomplished with the help of a local anesthetic and hospitalization is not required. Most often an incision is not necessary because the clot will dissolve on its own and the hemorrhoid will shrink.

Patients are generally apprehensive about the first bowel movement after a rectal operation, but they are almost universally surprised when the actual experience proves far less uncomfortable than anticipated. As a general rule, the bowels will move on the third or fourth postoperative day with the assistance of mineral oil or some other soft and lubricating laxative that is started on the first or second day after operation. Sitz baths (sitting in warm water) are used two or three times daily and they are initiated again on about the second postoperative day. If a bowel action is not forthcoming by the fourth day, several ounces of warm oil are inserted in the rectum as an oil enema. This usually brings on a reasonably comfortable bowel movement for the patient.

Recurrence. A patient who has had a hemorrhoidectomy may wonder whether he can get hemorrhoids again. The answer is that he probably won't but on the other hand it is possible for other rectal veins to enlarge even after the main veins have been removed surgically. Hemorrhoids that have been removed will not form again. However, other veins in the rectal canal may become stretched and varicosed.

The rectal sphincter muscle is not cut to any extent in a hemorrhoid operation. Therefore under usual circumstances there is no danger that the muscle will be injured to the extent that it will not be tight enough. On the other hand, if the surgery has been very extensive because of the extremely large size of the hemorrhoids, it is possible for scar tissue to form through the canal and thus stiffen the muscle so that it does not stretch for a bowel movement as easily as it did before. This unusual complication is ordinarily overcome without much difficulty by dilating the rectum.

PLASTIC SURGERY

Plastic surgery is concerned with remodeling and restoring. It revises parts of the body that have been malformed in the growing process before birth or it restores parts that have been deformed or destroyed by injury and disease. The name does not imply that synthetic plastic materials are used.

Although plastic methods and principles govern more than half the things surgeons do, the name "plastic surgery" is used ordinarily for operations on areas that are visible. A cleft lip in a newborn baby is closed by plastic surgery. A limb crippled by rigid and binding scars is returned to function. Disfiguring and incapacitating injuries to structures of the face are actually sculptured into proper alignment for healing.

A severe burn may destroy all of the skin in and about an arm pit, leaving a thick mass of scar tissue that fuses the arm to the chest and prevents any motion in the shoulder. Arm motion is restored by removing the scar to allow the arm to swing out freely and up over the head. In this extended position the large denuded area of the chest and underarm is covered with a sheet of skin.

Skin grafts. It is the plasticity, or pliability, of skin and muscles that allows the surgeon to mold and reshape the skin coverings of the eyes, nose and lips when structures and skin have been torn away by injuries. For extensively damaged areas that cannot be covered by shifting and realigning the torn flaps, skin must be moved from another area of the patient's body to the injured area. There is no substitute for skin. Methods for storing skin in banks, similar to the banks for blood or bone, have not been generally satisfactory. Transfer of skin from one person to another for permanent replacement is still in the developmental stage. The surgeon must rearrange the patient's own skin.

Healthy skin can be detached, lifted out and fitted into a raw area just like sod is taken from a field and transferred to bare ground. This is called *free grafting*. The graft is completely free from its attachment and derives its nourishment from the raw surface on which it is laid. There is no nourishment from the edges. The outer layers of skin can thrive on this kind of nourishment, absorbed from the raw surface, but the deeper skin layers do not do so well.

The outer layers therefore are split away from the deep layers with an electrically driven razor-sharp blade. This is a *split graft* and is in contrast to a *full thickness graft*. The depth of the split graft will vary but it will average about ten thousands of an inch. The sheet of outer skin is transplanted and a new outer skin will sprout up quickly from the deep layers which are still in place and intact. Thus, the outer layers are skimmed off in a solid sheet about the depth of a bad floor burn in a basketball game, and the deeper layers grow a new cover in about the time it takes a floor burn to heal.

A whole sheet of split skin, removed by the grafting instrument, can be laid in the denuded area as a single sheet shaped to size, or it can be cut into small pieces the size of a postage stamp. The latter are called *stamp grafts*. The instrument can cut sheets three inches wide and as long as six to eight inches. Stamp grafts are advantageous for the larger raw areas of burns, because they can be spaced at half inch intervals. The edges of the grafts, still taking nourishment from the undersurface, will grow out at their edges to meet each other.

Small full thickness pieces of skin can be free grafted, but larger sizes must be attached by a *pedicle* through which intact blood vessels can bring nourishment to the raised flap of skin. This is known as *pedicle grafting*.

For **pedicle grafts** the skin is elevated as a broad flap joined to the body by a pedicle. If the flap can be raised in such a fashion that its pedicle is adjacent to the area to be covered, it can be fitted by rotating its pedicle. Neither the flap nor the pedicle can be on a stretch; extreme twisting or tension will choke off the blood supply in the pedicle.

If the distance between the donor site and the bare area is too great for a rotating pedicle, a longer skin flap is raised and fashioned into a tube, but attached at both ends by pedicles. After a rest period of several weeks during which the blood vessels in the pedicles grow larger, the pedicle farthest from the bare area is cut across. The tube is then rotated to bring the cut pedicle to the site for grafting to the skin.

Sculpturing and reshaping the face and neck require intricate realignments of the bones that frame the face and jaws. This phase is combined with muscle transplants and skin grafts. Delicate facial bones, shattered in highway accidents, or removed along with tumors, can be reconstructed with wires and splints that are fabricated from synthetic materials. Flaps of muscle are used in the reconstruction of vacant spaces left by destroyed or removed bone.

EYE SURGERY

Cataract Operations

In a *cataract operation* the lens of the eye is removed because it has become hardened and opaque to the extent that light rays can't get through. It's the difference between clear glass and milk glass. Although there are many varieties of cataracts, occurring at all ages, the most frequent form is seen in persons over 50 years of age, usually in both eyes with one forming more rapidly than the other.

In years past surgery was delayed until the cataract "ripened". This meant that the hardening process had finally involved the entire lens and loosened it from its capsule. In this condition the lens could be separated from its capsule without leaving bits of cataract that would later become opaque and again block the light rays. The ripening process might come about in a few months or it might take years.

It is current practice to remove the lens as soon as useful vision has deteriorated to the point that the patient cannot carry on with his usual occupations. Modern techniques insure that all of the lens substance will come away. Even with this trend toward earlier operation, extraction of the lens from the first eye is delayed as long as there is still good vision in the better eye. The reason for this is that there would be a refracting difference between the operated eye, now without a lens, and the unoperated eye, so long as this eye retained good vision. The good eye, being the stronger of the two, would dominate and take over all of the seeing.

There is no emergency about the usual cataract operation. The cataract is a mechanical impediment and not a disease that will spread to other parts.

Cataract operations are performed under local anesthesia. A half circle inci-

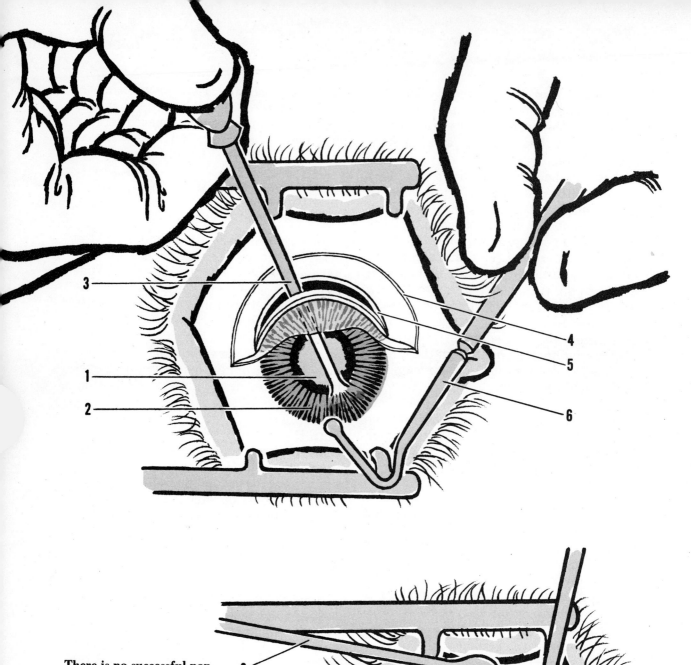

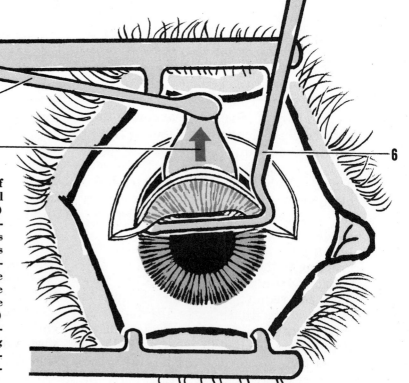

There is no successful nonsurgical treatment for cataract. In cataract surgery, the lens of the eye, with its opacities that obstruct vision, is removed through an incision in the upper perimeter of the eyeball. One method of removal employs an instrument (erysiphake) shaped like a small spoon and a suction cup on the end to grasp the lens and pull it out. Top drawing shows surgeon freeing lens (1) from attachments under iris (2) with erysiphake (3). Incision has been made in the conjunctiva (4), and limbus (5) where cornea and sclera (white of the eye) come together. Hook (6) exerts delicate pressure. At right, lens (1) being pulled out by erysiphake (3) in direction of arrow, aided by external pressure of hook (6).

sion is made in the white portion of the eye above the clear cornea. The upper half of the cornea and the upper half of the colored rim around the pupil, the iris, are cut open at their edges. This gives access to the lens which is drawn out by a small cup-shaped instrument that holds onto the lens by a vacuum suction. The incision is then closed by suturing.

Detached retina

The retina, likened to photographic film at the back of a camera, is normally held against the blood vessel layer next to it in the wall of the eyeball by pressure within the eyeball fluid. The retina becomes detached when a crack in the retina allows eyeball fluid to seep between the layers. With no contact between the layers there is no vision.

Eight of every ten patients who are treated for detachment are benefited, although frequently the retina may be jarred loose again and require further treatment.

Anesthesia for surgery is local, by surface application and by injection of an anesthetic solution behind the eyeball. A hollow needle is inserted into the eye to drain out the fluid between the retina and choroid layers. Then the contact is sealed with a freezing rod, or a laser beam or an electric needle.

Another, and successful, surgical method for this condition buckles the outer layer of the eyeball in the detached area and thus pushes the choroid blood vessel layer against the retina. The buckling suture remains in the outer coat of the eyeball permanently.

Corneal Scars

If the *cornea* is scarred in its central portion from a scratch or infection, light rays will be blocked from the lens, like putting a finger in front of the lens of a camera. The scarred portion can be removed and replaced with the cornea of a donor eye. If the scar does not extend the entire depth of the cornea, the outer layers can be removed down to clear cornea and replaced by a cornea graft of the same thickness. It is also possible to replace the full thickness of the cornea if the scar is this deep. The defective cornea is bored out and removed as a plug in a single piece. A plug of the full thickness of cornea is bored out of a donor eye with the same instrument. The graft cornea of the same size and shape is fitted exactly into the hole and is sutured in place.

It is possible also to let vision images into the eye without removing the scarred cornea. This is done by removing a portion of the iris at the edge of the pupil. The iris is opened at its lower inner edge. The effectiveness of this operation can be estimated ahead of time by paralyzing the iris with a drug. This allows the pupil to open up widely behind the scar to let in the image outside the edge of the scar.

Eye Muscle Operations

Disturbances of the coordinated action of the eyeball muscles are corrected by operations that change the position and the length of the muscles. Usually this will amount to relocating or altering one or two muscles of one eye or perhaps both eyes, depending upon the nature of the trouble.

Although the limitless eye motions used for seeing and expressing, even staring and rolling, might seem beyond analysis, still only six basic movements are possible because each eye has only six muscles. For each coordinated movement of the eyes, several muscles of each eye pull at the same time, but each muscle has its particular field to cover.

The eyeball is a globe seated in a bony socket. The muscles are all attached at the back of the bony socket and reach around the globe to be inserted in front about three-eighths of an inch from the top, bottom and sides of the cornea. Four of these muscles (rectus) run a straight course around the globe. Two of them come in at an angle (obliques). The muscles of the two eyes are controlled by the coordination center in the brain so that the proper muscles for the left and right eyes move at the same time.

After a determination has been made of the basic one or two directions that are

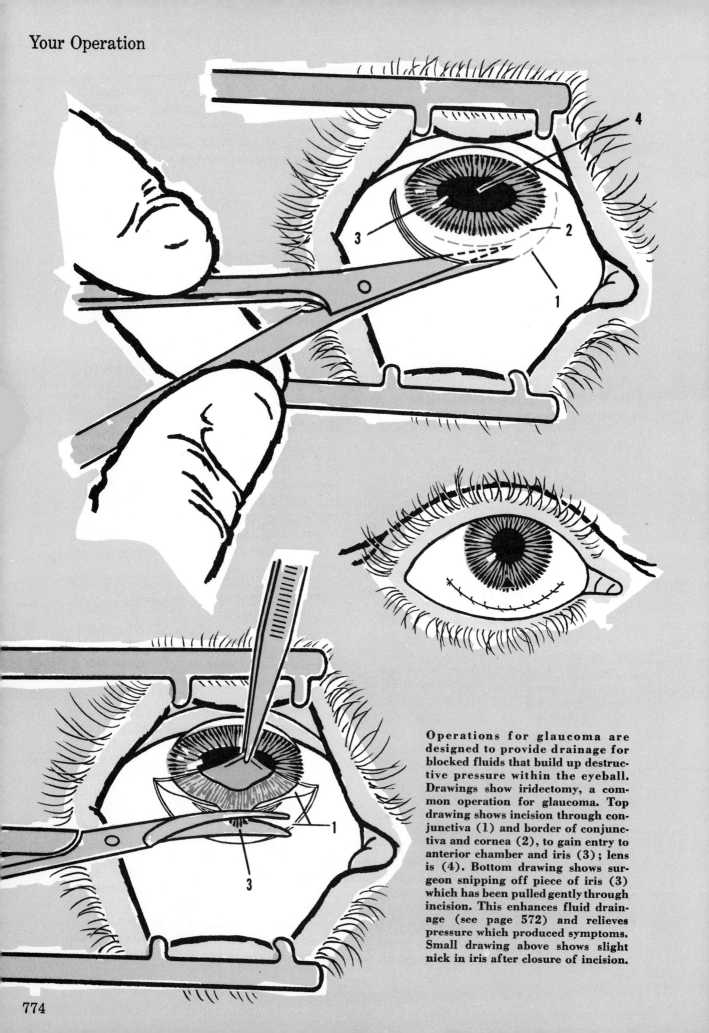

Operations for glaucoma are designed to provide drainage for blocked fluids that build up destructive pressure within the eyeball. Drawings show iridectomy, a common operation for glaucoma. Top drawing shows incision through conjunctiva (1) and border of conjunctiva and cornea (2), to gain entry to anterior chamber and iris (3); lens is (4). Bottom drawing shows surgeon snipping off piece of iris (3) which has been pulled gently through incision. This enhances fluid drainage (see page 572) and relieves pressure which produced symptoms. Small drawing above shows slight nick in iris after closure of incision.

out of balance, the surgeon can make a correction by altering the one or two muscles concerned in each eye. Frequently only one eye is out of balance.

One can envision the six eye muscles in terms of tautness as though they were rubber bands reaching around from a central point at the back of the socket to separated points on the front of the eyeball. A weak muscle is compared to a loose rubber band, attached too far back on the ball and therefore not taut enough. A muscle pulling too strongly is likened to a rubber band attached too far forward and therefore too taut. Either situation prevents good teamwork.

This, then, is about the way the operations go. A strong overacting muscle is detached from its position on the front of the eyeball and is reattached several sixteenths of an inch farther back. This is called *recession* or retroplacement of a muscle. A weak or understretched muscle is advanced by relocating its attachment farther forward. Sometimes the correction in tautness is made by cutting out a short piece of the muscle and then sewing the two cut ends together. This is a *resection*. Still another method tucks a muscle by sewing a fold into its length.

Glaucoma

Glaucoma is a condition of increased pressure within the eyeball. Although it is possible to control this pressure by drugs that open up the natural drainage channels from the eyeball, drugs may not work. Then the situation demands surgical drainage. If the pressure is increasing rapidly and cannot be brought under control by drugs, an emergency operation is necessary.

Operations for control of glaucoma are many and varied. The simplest is called *iridectomy*. It is performed in early cases if there is rapid and severe blockage of the drainage channels. A piece of the iris is cut loose to deepen the drainage channels by correcting the forward ballooning and swelling of the iris.

Sometimes, in long standing cases that show damage to the filtering sponge-like tissue of the outflow channels, a filtering operation is used. This form of operation is chosen when the field of vision has been reduced by damage to the optic nerve and when medicines have failed. The object is to promote drainage through the tough outer coat of the eye by drilling a small hole through it. This is called *sclerectomy*. Aqueous humor, draining through the hole into the subconjunctival space, is absorbed into the blood vessels as the pressure builds up. The drill hole is covered by the conjunctiva, which is the membranous veil that lines the eyelids and covers the white sclera.

Sometimes a piece of iris is cut in a fashion that will allow it to be drawn into the sclerectomy hole, where it functions as a wick. The wick keeps the hole from scarring and thus helps keep the hole open. This is *iridencleisis*. The tags of iris, drawn through the hole, are covered by conjunctiva to seal over any communication with the outside.

ORGAN TRANSPLANTATION

One's chances for having an organ transplantation are remote, simply because the total number of such operations is quite limited. Transplants of less than a whole organ, of course, are commonplace—skin grafts, bone grafts, corneal transplants. But surgical operations for transfer of entire and intact organs are rare by comparison.

First of all, the supply of transplantable organs runs far behind the number of patients who need them. Why? Removing healthy organs from willing donors is risky. Kidneys and spleens can be taken from living persons.

As for "cadaver" organs—kidney, heart, lung, and pancreas—consent by grieved relatives for removing organs from a recently deceased person is not easily obtained within the short time allowable—an hour. Nor are proper facilities generally available on short notice for the speedy and surgically satisfactory removal of organs from any deceased persons.

Lastly, rejection of a "new" organ by the sick patient's body (the recipient) presents a difficult and, for the most part, an unsolved problem.

Even the ethical aspects of transplantation are still debated. Which patients have the highest priority? When does death really take place?

Kidneys. Most successful and most numerous of the organ transplantations are kidneys, more than 2,500 of them between 1954 and 1970, and with the chance for success better than even. Most successful are kidney transplants between identical twins where there is practically no chance for rejection. Then, in order, are brother and sister and parent to child. Last in line are kidneys from deceased persons.

Eight thousand young adults and children—in the United States alone—die each year from kidney diseases. Half of these victims have healthy organs except for their kidneys. Thus, 4,000 patients annually are potential candidates for kidney transplantation. The supply of this many "new" kidneys, either from living donors or from deceased persons, is a problem.

There is no emergency about kidney transplantation insofar as the patient sick with kidney disease is concerned. Such patients with kidney failure can be maintained—and will be able to work—indefinitely by kidney *dialysis* (kidney machine) with out-patient treatments two or three times weekly. Arrangements for transplanting a living kidney can be scheduled for a time that is generally suitable to the patient, the donor, and the surgical team. By contrast, transplantation of a *deceased* person's kidney must be arranged for quickly—within an hour. Storage of organs for transplantation at a later date has not been satisfactory.

The operation. A kidney transplantation operation moves along swiftly once everything needed for surgery has been readied. Three connections are necessary in hooking up the "new" kidney—a single artery for the entrance of *mainline* blood into and through a kidney's screening and filtering system, a matching vein to return filtered—"clear"—blood to the circulation, and finally, the kidney tube (ureter) that drains the solution of filtered wastes (urine) to the urinary bladder for discharge from the body through the urethra.

The new kidney does not have to occupy one of the natural kidney positions in the small of the back on each side of the spine. The transplant is placed in the lowermost part of the abdominal cavity (the pelvis) to the right of the urinary bladder. Usually the donor's left kidney is taken for the transplant because the left kidney is more accessible surgically. The open end of the new kidney's intake artery is joined to an opening made in the side of the stout artery that leads to the recipient's right thigh and leg (iliac) artery. The kidney's vein is attached to the main vein returning from the thigh (iliac vein). The ureter (exit tube from the new kidney) is joined to an opening made in the right side of the recipient's bladder. All of these connections are made by suturing with fine silk thread.

Urine passes from the newly transplanted kidney within ten to fifteen minutes after the artery and vein connections have been completed, even before the kidney has been joined to the bladder.

The sick patient's diseased kidneys are removed a week or more before the transplantation. Elimination of waste from the blood is accomplished by dialysis on a kidney machine until the time of the transplantation operation. The dialysis machine can also be used to assist the new kidney if necessary. The recipient needs only one kidney.

Heart transplantation is reserved for patients who are beyond all hope of treatment with medicines. Unfortunately, in such patients, other organs have deteriorated because of the heart's failure to maintain an adequate circulation of blood through them. This is especially true of the lungs. Thus, of the 150 persons (up to 1971) who had received transplanted hearts, only a third had lived for more than six months. A few of these had survived for a full year. The Cape Town dentist, Doctor Blaiberg, first to receive a heart transplant, lived 594 days. Rejection is the prime cause for failure.

It is difficult to estimate the number of persons who could benefit from heart transplantation. The annual death toll from coronary heart disease in the United States is about half a million persons.

Everything must be in readiness for a heart transplantation because the operation is performed on an emergency basis immediately after the death of the donor —a person who died as the result of injury or from a brain tumor and, hence, has generally healthy organs.

Almost all of the patient's diseased heart is removed. The back walls of the patient's right and left intake chambers (the *atria*) are left in place because the six veins that drain into the heart open through the walls of these chambers. Thus, only two sutured connections are made—the two chamber walls—to accommodate six vein connections. There remain only two more blood vessel hookups, both arterial, one with the pulmonary artery to the lungs and the other with the aorta which is the main trunk line for circulation to the body in general.

A transplanted heart may start beating on its own or an electric shock may be necessary to stimulate its muscle. The sewing time on the heart itself—two atria and two arteries—may be less than thirty minutes. A heart-lung machine is used to maintain a supply of oxygen and blood circulation, the same as in open heart surgery.

The problems beginning immediately after surgery are wound healing and control of infection, both of which are natural functions of the body that are weakened by the medications used to stave off rejection.

Liver. More than one hundred livers have been transplanted, but here again rejection has been a major stumbling block. Few of the recipients of new livers have lived for more than a year.

Among the 4,000 possible candidates yearly for liver transplantation (United States) are infants with a malformed or absent bile drainage system, children and young persons whose livers have been ravaged by infection, cirrhosis (not alcoholic), abscesses, cysts, or special liver tumors called hepatomas. The liver is responsible for numerous functions.

Liver transplants are performed on an emergency basis—within minutes after a deceased accident victim's liver becomes available, because a removed liver deteriorates rapidly. As a part of the emergency procedure the recipient's diseased liver is removed and the "new" one connected almost simultaneously, for there are *no* "liver machines" to maintain a patient deprived of his liver.

Liver connections are complex, with oxygenated arterial blood and "waste" venous blood from the intestines flowing to the liver, and with "decontaminated" but oxygen-exhausted venous blood flowing out of the liver to the *vena cava*— only three inches from the right heart intake chamber. Bile flowing out of the transplanted liver is routed to the intestine, either directly by way of the main (common) bile duct or roundabout through the gallbladder.

Other organs. Spleens, responsible for several blood conversion functions, have been successfully transplanted into the lower part of the abdomen like kidneys— connected with the *iliac* blood vessels. The new spleens supply substances that clot blood for bleeders (hemophiliacs) or supply leukemia victims with *antibodies* that reduce the production of white blood corpuscles. The pancreas has been transplanted a dozen times to overcome diabetes. There has been one six-month survival (1970). Lungs have been transferred on more than twenty occasions with at least one patient surviving more than a full year. Just about every major organ in the body, with the exception of the brain, has been transplanted with at least one short-term survivor.

Rejection remains a major problem. The capability of rejecting a *foreign* substance is a characteristic of all living tissues and organisms. Although this capability is a defense against bacteria and viruses and foreign substances such as steel, glass, splinters, or dirt and gravel, it is also the defense mechanism that makes successful transplants next to impossible. The major defenders are the white blood corpuscles and chemical substances called antibodies. Various methods such as radiation with x-rays and injections of cortisone-like substances and anti-white blood corpuscle serum have been used to hold these defense mechanisms in check.

Another approach has been to match tissues and cells in the fashion of blood typing and matching. In this manner, certain groups of donors of organs, whether living or deceased, are found to have "compatibility" with similar groups of recipients.

ANESTHESIA

After your doctor has explained what is wrong and what ought to be done, the thought of taking an anesthetic will cross your mind. If you are like most people, chances are your ideas and experience are limited to second and third hand stories and consequently you have some pretty grim ideas on the subject.

In past centuries it *was* pretty grim. Before the days of ether, patients for surgery were merely stupefied with alcoholic concoctions. Even with ether the idea was to render a patient unconscious as quickly as possible and then rush through the operation with all possible speed. The choices besides ether were chloroform or nitrous oxide (laughing gas). The essence of surgery was speed because this kept the anesthetic time to a minimum and reduced the chance for poisoning the brain, liver or kidneys.

Modern anesthesia is a complex science that employs a number of drugs, with each serving one or more purposes. Today, the term anesthesia includes four separate components, and "going to sleep," which pertains to the patient's *mental* state, is only one of them. The other three components have to do with *pain sensation, muscle relaxation,* and *paralysis of the reflexes.*

Herein lies the big change in anesthesia, the use of several different drugs at the same time. Each drug is used in the amount necessary to control one of the components of an overall anesthetic mixture. It's like balancing volume, tone, brightness and shadow components on a TV set to get the particular reception best suited to you.

Unconsciousness is held in a safe range by using one drug for control of the mental state and separate drugs for control of the other components. Sodium Pentothal given in an arm puts one to sleep quickly and naturally. However, in its safe range this drug will not obliterate pain sensation nor will it paralyze the muscles into the state of relaxation required for many operations. Pentothal may even stimulate reflexes rather than depress them, and this could create difficulties. This drug therefore is used only in amounts that will block out consciousness, and at that stage other drugs are used to bring about a complete anesthetic balance.

Another type of drug is succinylcholine, which does not produce unconsciousness but is highly effective for relaxing the muscles into a state of temporary paralysis. This drug allows the larynx muscles to open widely so that a breathing tube can be slipped easily into the windpipe of the patient.

A variety of inhalation or gas anesthetics can be used to block pain sensation, and also to produce unconsciousness, though more slowly than Pentothal. Among them are Cyclopropane, Fluothane, Penthrane, ether and nitrous oxide. They are used to block pain sensation after Pentothal has brought on unconsciousness. Spinal anesthesia is excellent for handling pain, muscle relaxation, and the reflex components, but it has no effect on the mental state.

Anesthesia includes more than anesthetic agents. Blood transfusions, nourishing fluids, supportive and corrective drugs are administered and controlled by the anesthesiologist. Discriminating attention to all these factors makes it possible for a patient with a medical as well as a surgical illness to be operated on with complete safety.

Anesthesia may be classed as *general,* in which consciousness is lost; *spinal,* in which nerves are blocked at their exit from the spinal cord; and *regional,* in which the nerves entering the field of operation are blocked.

Spinal anesthesia. Patients seem to have many misconceptions about spinal anesthesia and it is important that they be set straight about this very effective form of pain relief.

The spinal cord ends in the back at about the level occupied by the navel in front. It is encased in a tube that extends all the way to the tailbone. The covering layers of the tube are called the *meninges.* Spinal fluid circulates in the tube between the cord and the meninges. The picture is that of a flower stem inserted part way into a narrow bud vase full of water.

A needle is inserted between the vertebrae to pierce the meninges below the level of the cord. The anesthetic solution is then injected into the tube and mixes with the spinal fluid, which in turn bathes the nerve roots of the spinal cord. The level of anesthesia depends on the amount of anesthetic solution, the position of the patient, and the speed of injection. Anesthesia lasts for from one to several hours, again depending upon the type of anesthetic drug.

Spinal anesthesia does not involve "sticking" the spine. The needle is introduced between the vertebral bones. The spinal cord is not punctured by the needle because the cord is located above the site of puncture. It is the fluid-filled tube that is pierced, about like piercing a vein in the arm for taking a blood test.

The anesthesiologist checks the patient's general condition during the operation by means of continuous monitoring devices. Among them are instruments for continuous electrocardiographic tracing of the heart action, stethoscopes that can be slipped down the gullet and into the stomach for continuous listening, thermometers that record continuously, and instruments that keep a constant record of the oxygen saturation in the blood.

The anesthesiologist and surgeon consider every aspect of a particular patient's condition and medical history in choosing the most suitable anesthetic or anesthetics.

SURGERY ON CHILDREN

Children accept surgery and hospital routines on faith and trust which reflects the conversations and actions of their parents. Anxious parents should guard against any display of their worries.

A child's intellect does not demand any detail of anatomy and physiology. Most of the child's curiosity will be satisfied secondhand through the parents. The doctor's explanation to the child is best given in the parents' presence, thus giving the child a point of reference for further inquiries. The simplest explanations are best, relating chiefly to the need for correcting an abnormality. Timing is also very important. Discussions far in advance of the time for hospital admission may cause anxiety.

Actually children are more curious about the hospital environment and if this aspect of the operation is emphasized, an interesting experience can relegate pain and discomfort to the background. The Pediatric Department of a hospital is a children's world where all the attention is directed toward them: eating in bed, riding in wheelchairs, wearing pajamas all day. All of the adults are nurses and doctors who seem to have the confidence and admiration of mother and father.

Children can tolerate pain and discomfort even better than adults, so long as there is affection and kindness, but they have a hard time bringing themselves around to it. More so than adults, they are procrastinators when it comes to pain. They will try to persuade anybody that anything uncomfortable would be less so if it were put off until just a little later. Their natural optimism leads them to believe that if something unpleasant is postponed, things will take care of themselves in the vague future. After an unpleasant experience has passed, such as a blood test or removal of adhesive tape, they appreciate the gentle firmness that got things done right away and quickly. Their memories of discomfort are usually short when there is affection, kindness and dispatch.

Infants and children come through surgery and anesthesia exceedingly well in comparison with adults. They require special attention in respect to fluid volumes for they dehydrate and overhydrate quickly. Their air passages are narrow in comparison with those of adults and their cough reflexes are relatively weak. Special attention to the airways brings them through safely.

Children are sensitive to infections but they also respond quite readily to antibiotics.

Age is not a deterrent to surgery. Even premature infants, weighing only four or five pounds, stand up very well under extensive surgical procedures that must be done immediately if they are to survive. A tiny infant's heart is remarkably stout.

CHAPTER 23

X-RAYS
AND YOU

by TED F. LEIGH, M.D.

RADIOLOGY

DIAGNOSTIC
EXAMINATIONS

Body Section • Bones • Skull and Brain
• Lungs and Chest • Colon •
Gallbladder • G.I. Series • Heart •
Kidneys • Pregnancy • Sinuses • Spine

THERAPY

X-rays • Gamma Rays • Radioactive
Isotopes • Effects of Radiation •
Safety

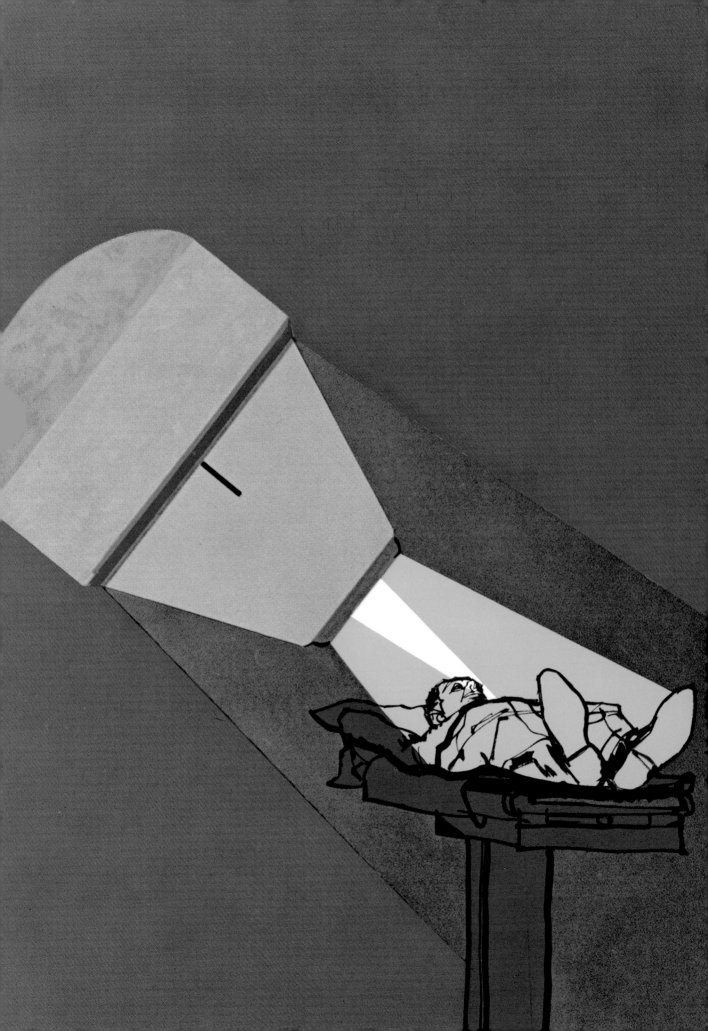

CHAPTER 23

X-RAYS AND YOU

by TED F. LEIGH, M.D.

Your doctor has made an appointment with a radiologist for you or some family member, and you may be wondering what is in store. This chapter will try to tell you about many of the diagnostic and therapeutic procedures that a radiologist follows, and what this means to you.

But, first, you may want to know just what radiology and radiologists are. Why is your doctor sending you to him? How can he help your doctor to help you?

Radiology (pronounced, raid-ee-AHL-oh-gee) is that branch of medicine which uses certain forms of radiant energy to diagnose and treat disease. Radiant energy includes x-rays, radium and man-made radioactive substances known as *isotopes* (ICE-oh-topes). A term used in connection with x-rays is "ionizing radiation." In terms of chemistry and physics, it means radiation which gives off an electrified particle called an *ion* (I-on) when a molecule of a gas looses an electron by the action of the rays.

The sun's ordinary rays are not ionizing, but rays produced beyond the earth's atmosphere, called cosmic rays, are. All radiation used in dentistry and medicine is *ionizing radiation.* So is radiation from nuclear testing fall-out and background radiation from the earth, rocks, certain building materials, TV sets, luminous markers, watch dials.

As a medical specialty, radiology is young in years when compared with the full sweep of medical history. In 1895 a German scientist, Wilhelm Conrad Roentgen, discovered x-rays. A few years later, in 1899, Pierre and Marie Curie isolated the chemical element radium. From these two discoveries radiology was born.

A *radiologist* (raid-ee-AHL-oh-jist) is a physician, a doctor of medicine, who is intimately concerned with your well-being and health. He has the same basic medical education as all physicians. After he becomes a doctor he spends three or more years of hospital training to become a specialist. During this time he attends lectures, demonstrations and receives personal instructions in the actual doing and using of radiologic techniques and equipment under the guidance of professors and experienced radiologists. He also learns what diseases respond favorably to radiation treatment, those that respond only occasionally, and those that do not respond at all.

When this special preparation for his career has been completed, the young radiologist looks back on nearly 15 years of work in universities, medical schools and hospitals. Then, and not until then, may he present himself as a candidate for examination by the American Board of Radiology to get his certificate as a specialist. Today in the United States there are about 6,000 specialists in radiology. (*page 783).

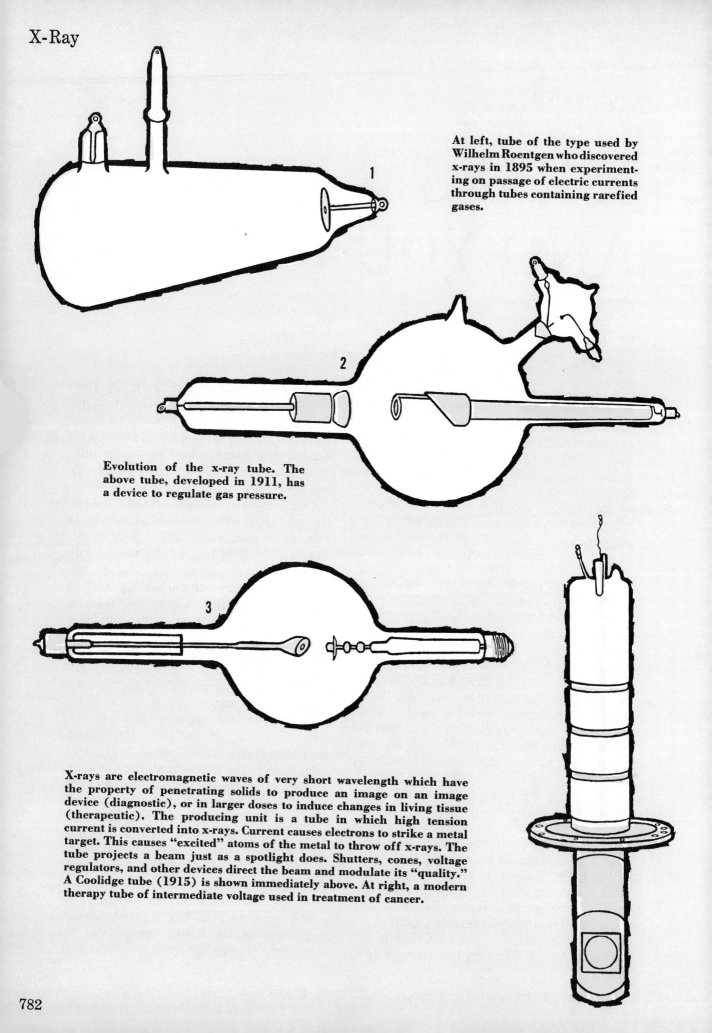

At left, tube of the type used by Wilhelm Roentgen who discovered x-rays in 1895 when experimenting on passage of electric currents through tubes containing rarefied gases.

Evolution of the x-ray tube. The above tube, developed in 1911, has a device to regulate gas pressure.

X-rays are electromagnetic waves of very short wavelength which have the property of penetrating solids to produce an image on an image device (diagnostic), or in larger doses to induce changes in living tissue (therapeutic). The producing unit is a tube in which high tension current is converted into x-rays. Current causes electrons to strike a metal target. This causes "excited" atoms of the metal to throw off x-rays. The tube projects a beam just as a spotlight does. Shutters, cones, voltage regulators, and other devices direct the beam and modulate its "quality." A Coolidge tube (1915) is shown immediately above. At right, a modern therapy tube of intermediate voltage used in treatment of cancer.

The radiologist can help your doctor help you by obtaining a more accurate diagnosis of many disorders through the use of x-rays so that your doctor may then be able to judge more accurately the type of treatment to give you. The differing appearances on an x-ray film between normal and abnormal conditions is sometimes so slight that only a highly trained and experienced specialist can find them. The competent radiologist can help you directly by treatment of many conditions, including certain forms of cancer, that are responsive to x-rays, radium and radioactive isotopes.

Diagnosis. Let's discuss first the radiologist's contributions in diagnosis.

Accurate diagnosis is most important. Surgical or medical treatment, no matter how brilliantly done, is useless if directed against the wrong condition. Therefore, the diagnosis has to be right.

Suppose you are sick.

The key to your recovery is an accurate diagnosis. Somewhere in your doctor's study of your illness, it is likely that an x-ray examination will be required. Shall you have any doctor or commercial technician just "take an x-ray" or shall you have a thorough x-ray examination by a qualified radiologist? A competent x-ray examination is not just "taking a picture." It is the careful study of your inner structures by a doctor who is trained to use x-rays as his special instrument.

Nearly every organ in the human body may be explored by x-rays. This means that in every field of medicine the x-ray examination is a most valuable diagnostic contribution. As a result, the radiologist might be referred to as the "detective" in the fight against sickness. In trained hands all these examinations

* The American Board of Radiology is one of the National Qualifying Specialty Boards. The Board examines the candidates to see if their training has been satisfactory. Members of the Board are outstanding professors and practicing radiologists. When the doctor passes the rigorous examinations given by the Board of Radiology he becomes qualified as one of the following specialists: *Radiologist*: Qualified in the use of x-rays, radium and radioactive substances for diagnosis and treatment. *Roentgenologist* (RENT-gen-ahl-ohjist): Qualified in the use of x-rays alone for diagnosis and treatment.

are safe. (Radiation hazards will be discussed in detail later in the chapter.)

Because you have been referred to the radiologist by your doctor, who wants to consult with him after you have had your x-ray examination, the radiologist is called a "consulting physician" by his fellow M. D.'s. He is a doctor's doctor.

Preparations for examination. You may fret and wonder about certain necessary requirements for a radiological examination, but all the requirements are necessary to obtain clear x-ray films free from confusing shadows.

The table you may lie on will not be padded because the pad might cast a shadow on the finished film. All hairpins, earrings, and even false teeth have to be removed for examination of the head. A special gown usually is provided for examination because jewelry, buttons, safety pins and belts will cast shadows on the film which might either hide a disease process or appear as a shadow suggestive of some disease process.

Before some types of examinations the radiologist will ask the patient not to eat or drink for a certain number of hours, again to avoid misleading shadows. Various tablets and liquids will be given the patient for different examinations, and enemas are required in others. (These will be explained later in descriptions of specific examinations.)

The patient may be placed on a table which can be tilted so that the radiologist can examine him in different positions. In most instances it is necessary to get different views of a body structure on x-ray film to better comprehend the patient's difficulties.

In a *fluoroscopic* examination the radiologist probably will wear a special apron and gloves to protect him from the radiation that he works with every day. He may appear in the examination room wearing red goggles; they are to adapt his eyes to the dark and he will have worn them for about 20 minutes before he starts your examination.

When a simple *radiograph* (x-ray film) is needed you may be prepared for the examination by an x-ray technician; and under the radiologist's direction, the technician may take the x-ray and develop it. But the technician is not qualified for any film interpretation and does not attempt any.

Now, let's look at what some specific x-ray examinations by a radiologist will mean for you or your family.

DIAGNOSTIC EXAMINATIONS

Body section radiography. (Doctors also refer to this by such names as *tomography, laminography* and *planigraphy.*) With this method the radiologist uses special equipment to produce films that look blurred and almost as though a mistake has been made. But it hasn't. Actually, it is a film taken of a layer or section of the body. The section is about half an inch in thickness. Those portions of the body above and below the section are blurred and indistinct while only the structures in the desired section are recorded in sharp detail.

Why is body section radiography necessary? Because it is sometimes difficult to locate lesions in places like the lungs and bones because they are hidden by other structures lying above or below them. But by taking "sectional films" at different levels it is possible to find these conditions. This type of body section radiography is useful at times in just about every part of the body.

Bone Injury. Probably you are familiar with the appearance of bones and joints on an x-ray film. If there is a bad "break" it is easy for anyone to see. However, fractures occur from minor injuries more often than many of us realize, so it isn't smart to ignore a "trivial" injury when your doctor advises an x-ray examination.

Many times it is necessary to take radiographs from various angles to detect a fracture. At the same time, it may be necessary to x-ray the opposite arm or foot to be certain that small "extra" bones are not a little "chip" fracture. In some of the newer ways of setting difficult bones, such as pinning a fractured hip with metal pins, x-ray

equipment is taken right into the operating room and the position of the bones and the pins is checked at each step in the procedure.

It also takes training and experience to tell the difference between certain types of bone tumors and changes in bones that take place in other disorders. Arthritis, infections and growth problems provide x-ray clues which usually take a specialist to interpret and understand. Tuberculosis, for example, may show changes in an x-ray examination long before the symptoms indicate that such a lesion is present. Many conditions may masquerade as others for a long time, only to be proved correctly by the radiologic examination.

Skull and Brain: X-ray examinations of the head and brain are in widespread use today for many different types of neurological disorders. There are several ways in which these examinations may be done. First, the radiologist will usually make radiographs of the skull to study whatever changes may have taken place in the bones and other structures.

If these are changes from the normal it may indicate that an abnormal object is occupying space within the skull, or that some other abnormality is present. It could be a collection of fluid or a growing tumor. To identify it further, another diagnostic procedure known as an *air-contrast study* can be done. This is performed by replacing some of the fluid with air in the space around and in the brain.

Following this, radiographs are then made and by studying the changes in the position and shape of the air spaces it is frequently possible to locate and identify a tumor, cyst or inflammatory process. Sometimes the radiologist wants to see the blood vessels in the skull and he can do this in an examination called *cerebral angiography* (ce-REE-bral an-gee-AH-gra-fee). By injecting opaque material into the blood stream leading into the head, he can then take radiographs of the now-visualized blood vessels. If there is any change from the normal in these vessels, such as clogging, or displacement, or abnormal connections, it can be seen by the practiced eye of the radiologist. With the information gained from these procedures, the defect may be corrected.

Breast. The recognition of small tumors in the breast has always been difficult and uncertain. Recently, however, techniques for better-visualizing the soft tissues in the breast have been greatly improved by a procedure called *mammography* (mam-AH-gra-fee). In this procedure, several views are taken of both breasts, and these radiographs are studied. When a lesion is present, the radiologist can frequently spot it, and determine with a high degree of accuracy whether it is malignant or benign (cancerous or not). Mammography is not a substitute for the clinical examination of the breast, nor does it replace the need for taking a biopsy of a lump in the breast.

Bronchial Tubes. In an examination called *bronchography* (bronc-AH-gra-fee), some iodized oil is injected into the lungs through a tube which has been inserted into the lungs through the windpipe. The x-rays cannot penetrate the iodine compound very well, and therefore the iodine-filled bronchial tubes stand out on the radiograph for the radiologist to see clearly. This type of examination can determine whether the bronchial tubes are shut off, displaced by tumors or cysts, or enlarged.

Chest. Today everyone knows that the yearly x-ray examination of the chest by a radiologist is one of the best means of discovering tuberculosis, lung cancer, and other serious conditions. Fortunately, most of us have normal lungs and we do not have to be worried. The examination is purely a protective measure to insure our continued good health. If anything is found, it will be picked up in an early — and hopefully curable — stage.

Children. All the ordinary x-ray procedures apply just as much to your children as they do to you. But there are other procedures that apply especially to children. Many of these are to find out whether a child's bones are developing as they should. Underdeveloped or badly formed bones can mean a number of things (rickets, for example). Faulty bone development can also mean various kinds of glandular disturbances.

With the aid of x-rays, physicians now know exactly what a child's skeleton should look like at each age. Certain diseases are found only in children. For instance, a common cause of rectal bleeding among infants less than two years of age is "telescoping of the intestine," called *intussusception*. It can be seen by radiologic examination.

Respiratory distress in a newborn is an alarming symptom, and its cause must be determined quickly. A chest examination will frequently disclose the reason for the distress. Obstruction in the intestinal tract gives tell-tale signs on an examination of the abdomen. Not only will the films show the obstruction, but to the practiced eye of the radiologist, the location in the intestinal tract as well. X-ray examinations also are important in the diagnosis of "blue babies" and children with congenital heart defects.

Colon. In these examinations all fecal material has to be eliminated. Some patients require more cleansing than others. But it usually means castor oil in the afternoon before the examination, and one or more enemas the morning of the study. A light diet for lunch the day before the examination is advisable, followed by clear fluids that evening and the following morning, to eliminate the bulk.

The examination begins with still another necessary and important enema; this time a *barium* (BEAR-ee-um) solution is put into the colon so that the radiologist can see it and take films. The barium mixture will be carefully and slowly run into the colon while the radiologist watches it under the fluoroscope. When the colon is filled, radiographs will be made with the patient in various positions to show details of all the loops of the bowel.

The patient then evacuates the barium and returns for a film which will record the detail of the lining of the bowel. Sometimes the radiologist may want to inflate the colon after the barium has been expelled. Then air is blown gently into the colon to demonstrate the lining of the bowel in more detail.

Fluoroscopy. The patient stands behind a fluoroscope and the radiologist sits in front and moves the screen up and down the patient's body to see the inner functioning of the body as it is actually taking place. At the same time he is doing this he can take "spot" films when he sees something suspicious. He can also take moving pictures so that later he can go back over the film and "see" again the workings of the patient's system.

Motion pictures during fluoroscopy are recent developments and have enabled the radiologist to eliminate some repetition in fluoroscopic examinations, thus cutting down on the radiation exposure for the patient and himself.

Gallbladder. The radiologist may first have a radiograph made of the gallbladder area to see if he can detect gallstones that are surrounded by a ring of calcium or contain a central deposit of calcium within them. X-rays cannot penetrate the calcium very well, so the stones appear as white rings or balls on the x-ray film.

Most people, however, do not have this type of gallstone. It is necessary for these persons to swallow some iodized tablets the day before the examination. These tablets will dissolve in the stomach and then pass into the small intestine. Here the iodine compound is absorbed, taken by the blood stream to the liver, and excreted into the gallbladder along with the bile. The gallbladder now will "show up" on the x-ray film, and non-calcified gallstones which previously could not be seen are now visible, surrounded by the much denser iodine material.

Most patients feel no discomfort from the tablets, but a few are slightly nauseated; some have mild intestinal cramps; and some occasionally have a transient diarrhea. The tablets, however, have to be taken or the radiologist cannot see the gallbladder on the films.

If you are the patient, you may also be asked to omit fats from your diet before this examination. This is because fat causes the gallbladder to contract and to empty. This could expel the iodine from the gallbladder and again it could not be seen on the x-ray film. Before this examination you will be given tea and fruit juices to drink.

Occasionally, the gallbladder doesn't fill with the chemical swallowed by the patient. When this occurs, it usually means that the lining of the gallbladder is diseased or a bile duct is stopped up by a gallstone. The failure of the chemical to appear in the gallbladder is just as important in diagnosing the nature of gallbladder disease as is the actual discovery of gallstones.

If your gallbladder is functioning properly, the dye you took the day before will make your gallbladder stand out on the x-ray film. If the gallbladder shows that it can store bile normally, the next thing to see is if it can release it as needed. So the radiologist will ask you to eat something rich, like an egg or a glass of cream, and after a while he will take more radiographs. The fatty food makes the gallbladder contract and expel the dye-laden bile into the intestine. If this doesn't happen or happens slowly or partially, it may indicate gallbladder disease.

G. I. Series. G. I. stands for gastrointestinal, and in this examination the esophagus (or gullet), stomach, and duodenum (the small intestine just beyond the stomach) are examined. The study is called a "series" because a large number of films, as well as fluoroscopy, are required (see *fluoroscopy*).

For this examination the stomach must be empty. The patient must not eat any food or drink any fluids for eight hours before the examination; this is because material in the stomach can cast misleading shadows on the x-ray film. This is why you usually report to the hospital department or doctor's office early in the morning for this examination.

When the examination begins, you'll be given a barium "milkshake" made of barium sulfate that has a chalky, not too unpleasant taste. Barium is also opaque to x-rays and appears white on the x-ray films. As the barium fills the esophagus, stomach, and duodenum, the radiologist will examine them for ulcer, cancer, obstruction, and other conditions. During this examination he will probably make "spot" films or motion pictures to have a permanent record of what he sees through the fluoroscope. Additional films will be made at the end of the examination. All of these pictures can be studied after you have gone home.

With improved techniques, small lesions that 25 years ago might have gone unnoticed can be seen. But even yet the radiologist in some instances cannot determine whether a lesion which he sees in the stomach, for instance, is benign or malignant. In doubtful cases your doctor may suggest certain drugs and a diet, and then reschedule an examination with the radiologist. If healing has been slow or not at all, surgery may be indicated.

Sometimes it is necessary to examine the entire small intestine by x-ray. In this examination, x-rays of the abdomen are taken at regular intervals (usually every half hour) as the barium progresses through this long tube. When the barium reaches the large intestine, the examination is terminated. Then, by a study of the films, the radiologist can determine whether or not anything is wrong.

Heart. To a trained and practiced eye many types of heart trouble can be spotted by telltale signs in the heart and in the lungs as well. Under the fluoroscope and in films the individual chambers of the heart (there are four of them) can be studied for their size and function.

Some types of heart trouble are *congenital* — that is, the patient is born with defects in the heart chambers and valves — other types are *acquired*, like those that result from high blood pressure, hardening of the arteries, and blocks in the coronary arteries (the arteries that supply the heart muscle).

Many types of heart trouble, both congenital and acquired, cause changes in the large blood vessels and in the lungs, and many of these can be spotted on x-ray examinations of the chest. Sometimes these changes can be seen on the x-ray film and at fluoroscopy before they can be picked up by a history or physical examination of the patient.

Sometimes it is necessary to study the heart, lungs and blood vessels by injection of opaque materials into the blood stream or heart. When this is done, motion pictures or large films in rapid sequence can be made and studied to see what the patient's trouble may be.

In practically all types of heart conditions, the x-ray examination of the patient gives valuable clues as to the type of illness which is present.

Kidneys. The urinary tract can be studied in several different ways. Sometimes it is examined by placing dye directly in the bladder and the mouth of the kidney through the little tubes called the ureters, and then radiographs are made. Another type of examination calls for a dye to be injected into one of the veins of the arm. Because the kidney's job is to pick certain waste products out of the blood and eliminate them through the urine, the kidney picks the dye out of the blood and passes it down to the bladder through the ureters. And while the dye is going through the urinary tract the radiologist makes radiographs.

This examination will help to tell him how your kidneys and bladder are functioning and whether they are the proper size and shape. These radiographs can also tell him if the ureters are functioning correctly, whether there are any stones in the kidneys, and whether the bladder empties promptly and completely.

Pregnancy. Radiologic examination of a woman during pregnancy is done only when special indications require it; it should not be done routinely But if there are special reasons (the baby may not be in a normal position, or there may be more than one baby, or perhaps more exact pelvic measurements are needed), then radiographs and the radiologist can give the doctor the information.

It is important that a woman tell her doctor or dentist about her pregnancy in the early part of pregnancy if x-ray examinations are contemplated. Doctors prefer not to expose the fetus to radiation in early months of its growth.

Sinuses. Parts of the head frequently x-rayed, aside from the teeth, are the sinuses. They are the small hollow sections inside your skull that are connected with your nose by tiny openings. There are two above your eyes; one on each side of your nose; and some behind and between your eyes. Sinuses normally are full of air, but if your nose is badly stopped up the infection may back up through those tiny openings into your sinuses. They may get inflamed and swollen and even filled with pus, and if they do, will probably show up by abnormal changes on your x-ray films. So if your physician wants to find out more about your sinuses, he may suggest that you have them x-rayed.

Spine. If you have a pain in your back which shoots into a leg, your lower spine may be examined by taking films in front and side views. But if this fails to give the answer to your problem, you may be given a *myelographic* (MY-eh-low-graf-ic) examination.

This is used to detect a "slipped" (or ruptured) intervertebral disk. In this procedure the patient is placed on an x-ray table and an oil containing opaque iodine is put into the spinal canal. The patient is rocked up and down while the radiologist, using a fluoroscope, watches the oil as it passes through the spinal canal over the disks. If one is ruptured the oil will be stopped or forced to flow around the offending fragment. The radiologist can demonstrate this to the surgeon who can them remove the piece of broken disk that is pressing on a nerve. (A disk is the pad of fibrous tissue which serves as a cushion between the vertebrae.) Tumors of the spinal cord are fairly rare but this examination can pinpoint them if they are present.

TREATMENT

Now let's turn to therapy and see what the radiologist does for his patients in this part of his medical specialty.

Sometimes the same radiologist will do diagnostic work and give radiation therapy, too. Other times a radiologist will limit his practice to either diagnostic work or therapy.

What equipment and what kind of radiation is used for therapy?

Treatments are usually given by conventional x-rays, the gamma rays, and man-made radioactive isotopes.

X-Rays. Of all the forms of radiant energy used for treatment, the most common are the x-rays. These x-rays range from those produced by 40,000 volts of electricity to those produced by millions. The multi-million volt machines, and the large cobalt "bomb" (see *Radioactive Isotopes*), have an advantage for some locations of cancer, but actually the skill of the radiologist is more important than the voltage. The x-rays produced by the lower voltages are used to treat diseases and tumors on the surface of the skin. The higher volt x-rays are directed against conditions located below the surface of the skin and deep in the body.

Gamma Rays (Radium). Gamma rays are the powerful penetrating rays given off by radium. They are used in the treatment of malignant tumors and produce the same changes as do the high voltage x-ray machines and the cobalt bomb. Radium is one of the most valuable agents available in the treatment of cancer of the female organs. Depending on the condition being treated, very small amounts of radium having high intensity can be put in tiny hollow tubes which can be placed inside various cavities in the body. At other times radium is sealed in hollow needles of different sizes. They can be inserted directly into tumors.

Radium also can be placed in flat applicators called "plaques." These can be laid on the surface of growths, and have beneficial effects similar to those which are placed in deeper areas of the body.

As radium decays or breaks down, it gives off a gas called *radon*. This gas can be put into tiny, hollow seeds of gold which are then inserted directly in the tumor where they have their therapeutic effect. These are called *radon seeds*.

Radioactive Isotopes. These are substances which have been made radioactive

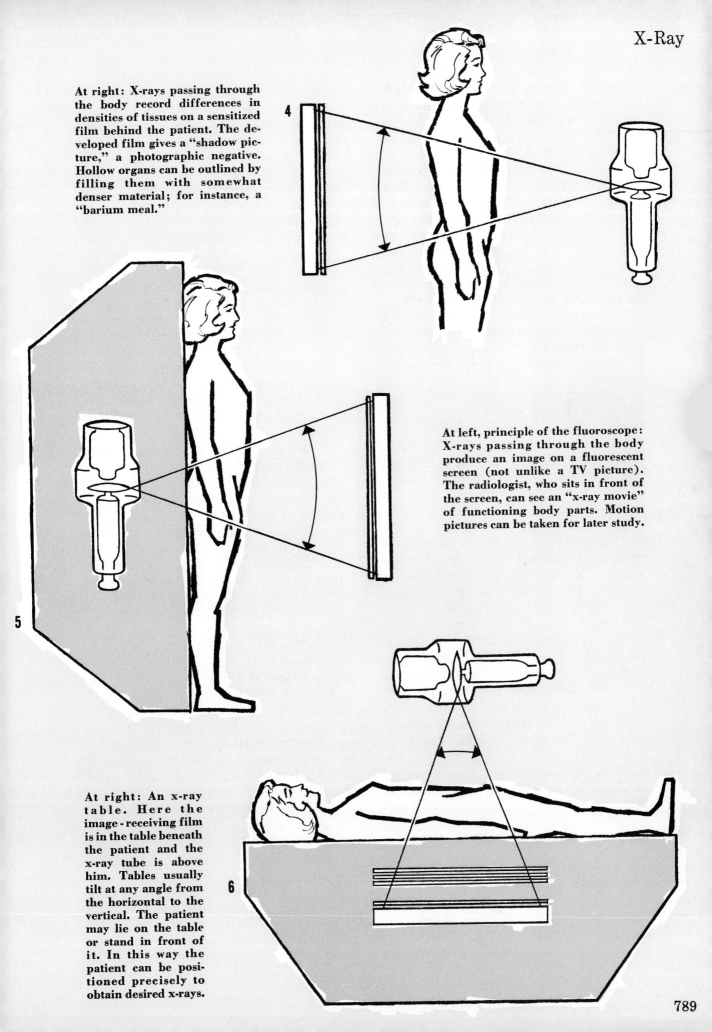

4

At right: X-rays passing through the body record differences in densities of tissues on a sensitized film behind the patient. The developed film gives a "shadow picture," a photographic negative. Hollow organs can be outlined by filling them with somewhat denser material; for instance, a "barium meal."

5

At left, principle of the fluoroscope: X-rays passing through the body produce an image on a fluorescent screen (not unlike a TV picture). The radiologist, who sits in front of the screen, can see an "x-ray movie" of functioning body parts. Motion pictures can be taken for later study.

At right: An x-ray table. Here the image-receiving film is in the table beneath the patient and the x-ray tube is above him. Tables usually tilt at any angle from the horizontal to the vertical. The patient may lie on the table or stand in front of it. In this way the patient can be positioned precisely to obtain desired x-rays.

6

by being "bombarded" in atomic piles. All elements have stable or radioactive isotopes. Numbers distinguish one from another and indicate the mass of the isotope. Radioactive isotopes include cobalt 60, iodine 131, phosphorus 32, iron 59, gold 198, strontium 90, and many others.

Some of these "atomic medicines" give off gamma rays similar to the rays emitted by radium and are used for the same purposes. Cobalt 60, for instance, can be placed in the cobalt "bomb" and its rays used for the treatment of growths deep in the body in the same way as high-voltage x-ray machines. Cobalt 60 may also be made into a very thin wire and used as "needles" for direct placement in tumors or body cavities, like radium needles.

Radioactive gold emits "beta" rays which penetrate only very short distances — fractions of an inch at the most. A solution of radioactive gold may be injected into such body cavities as the chest and abdomen, where it can be used to control fluid formation occurring in cancer patients.

The most widely used of the radioactive isotopes is iodine 131. It is employed not only in minute doses as a "tracer chemical" to test the activity of the thyroid gland, but also in the treatment of patients with thyroid diseases.

An interesting characteristic of all the atomic medicines is that they are radioactive for varying periods. Some last for just a few hours, others for months, and some are radioactive for years. For example, cobalt 60 loses one half of its strength in five years; cesium 137 in 33 years; and iodine 131 in eight days.

Although isotopes are useful in treatment of certain diseases, they also play an important part in diagnosis of disease. With isotopes we can measure the function of almost all organs of the body, and make a "map" of many of these.

What changes take place during radiation therapy?

To begin with, the cells in the body which are diseased and causing the trouble are the target for these rays. The abnormal cells are more sensitive to x-rays and gamma rays than normal cells and are destroyed, while the normal cells are only temporarily damaged. It is this difference in reaction to the rays that makes it possible for the normal or "healthy" cells to get well and to grow into the place of the destroyed cells. These profound chemical and electrical changes take place within the microscopic cells and in the spaces between them.

Do radiation treatments cure?

Yes, in many instances they do. They also control. Suppose you are undergoing treatment by x-rays for a painful shoulder, shingles, or a similar benign illness. The x-ray tube from which the x-ray beam comes is centered over the affected area and the machine turned on. The treatment may be repeated a number of times, depending on how quickly the condition clears up.

Patients with *thyrotoxicosis* (an overactive thyroid gland) often are treated to an "atomic cocktail" by the radiologist. The "cocktail" is a carefully determined amount of radioactive iodine. The thyroid gland takes up iodine. When radioactive, this iodine gives off a continuous stream of beta and gamma rays. These rays slow down the overactive thyroid cells and the gland returns to its normal working condition.

Suppose someone you know has a cancerous growth. If his trouble has been discovered in the early stages he has a good chance of being cured. First, the radiologist will learn the patient's history by talking with the patient and his referring doctor. He also will do his own examination of the patient. Then he will review the report on the tissue, or actually go over the microscope analysis of the small bit of tissue which has been taken from the growth (the biopsy) with the pathologist.

He then develops the plan of radiation treatment best suited for the patient. He maps out a schedule of treatment fitting the radiation to the particular growth. He must decide how many treatments given within a certain number of days will deliver the amount of radiation necessary to destroy or control the growth. In many instances, by using many small treatments, it is possible to bombard the growth and the area around it with a large dose of radiation without permanently damaging the healthy tissues. This allows them to recover with the least discomfort to the patient.

What do radiation treatments feel like?

There is no sensation during the time the x-rays or gamma rays are being administered. After two or three weeks of therapy the patient may notice that his skin appears to be sunburned over the treated area. Actually, his "sunburn" is very similar to that which develops from over-exposure to the sun. This reaction in the skin is part of the treatment and will gradually disappear. Perhaps at the same time the patient may also complain of nausea and loss of pep. This is called "radiation sickness." Fortunately, most patients do not experience this condition. If it does occur, it can be readily controlled. In any event, it will disappear as soon as the series of treatments are over.

Is radiation safe?

The answer leads to other questions: Are surgical operations safe? Is the administration of sulfa drugs safe? Is the injection of cortisone safe?

Yes, they are all safe, but they all can be hazardous in the hands of the inexperienced and the untrained. Each has a proper role in the fight against disease and, when employed by trained specialists, all are "safe." Each is used in the effort to keep you and your family in good health, yet there is always a risk in every form of treatment.

The major risk of excessive exposure to radiation is the genetic risk (the possible mutation of genes which pass on hereditary traits) and radiation exposure to the reproductive organs — both in diagnostic procedures and in treatment — should always be kept to a minimum. Genetic injury, once incurred, is permanent — it doesn't necessarily hurt the person x-rayed for diagnosis or for treatment, but it may possibly cause injury to his unborn child or its descendants. Thus, most careful consideration is

given to x-ray examinations or treatment for anyone in the child-bearing age. Over that age, persons have no need to be uneasy about any kind or number of radiological procedures performed by a qualified physician.

The hazards of diagnostic radiation are so small as to be insignificant when performed by a qualified doctor. The hazards of radiation therapy are extremely small in the less serious diseases. When compared with the gain from the treatment of cancer, for example, the risk becomes trifling in the hands of the experienced radiologist. In recent years modifications have been made in the indiscriminate use of x-rays.

For instance, as the initial screening procedure for tuberculosis in infants and children and in prenatal programs, the tuberculin test now is preferable to large scale x-ray screening programs. It is usually unnecessary to perform x-ray examinations in those who show negative reactions. For those who show positive reactions there should be no hesitancy about seeking an x-ray examination because the hazards of tuberculosis far outweigh whatever tiny future hazard might occur from the x-ray procedure.

X-ray therapy for benign conditions (conditions which are not cancerous) has been reviewed and, in many cases, abandoned. Therapy for presumed enlargement of the thymus has been almost completely abandoned. For such conditions as acne, eczema, fungus infections and other diseases of the skin, bursitis, peritendonitis, and arthritis, if another treatment gives comparable results, then in most cases other treatment is employed. On the other hand, in conditions like distinguishing hemangiomas of the face in infants, x-rays can save the child much emotional upheaval and this fact outweighs the small hazard involved in possible future genetic damage. And in older patients past childbearing age there seems to be little or no damage in treating such conditions as acute bursitis with x-rays.

Fluoroscopy of the chest, which once was frequently done as a routine examination even though no symptoms were present, now is strongly discouraged by the radiologist unless he thinks it is warranted by symptoms.

Shoe fluoroscopes, which even in this enlightened day are sometimes used for the "correct fitting of shoes," are condemned as a hazard by the American Medical Association and the American College of Radiology. Many of these machines deliver far more radiation than they are supposed to. Persons exposed to some of these machines could, and frequently do, receive a large dose of radiation in the process of buying a single pair of shoes.

Just as bad are some machines, never used by radiologists, which deliver a dangerously large dose of radiation over the whole body.

Radiologists, who by their long training and experience are aware of the hazards as well as the tremendous benefits of medical radiation, continuously have their machines checked and calibrated (adjusted for accuracy in output) by radiation physicists, to be sure the x-rays are being delivered in the proper quantity and quality.

Cones and diaphragms, which regulate the size of an x-ray beam, are used on the machines to guide the beam to the spot where it is needed — and only to that spot. Aluminum filters eliminate radiation which is unnecessary for radiographic examinations. Faster film has enabled the radiologist to cut down on the exposure time. To safeguard persons who are around radiation every day, protective devices are used. Lead, which absorbs most x-rays, is used in doors, control booths, floors and ceilings; this keeps radiation from escaping into nearby rooms and exposing persons in these areas.

An image intensifier added to fluoroscopic machines enables the radiologist to see the body's inner structures more clearly with less radiation. Medical specialists, too, by conferring with the radiologist, not only make sure each examination and treatment is necessary; they also make sure they are getting the right kind of examination they want the first time, thereby cutting down on unnecessary examinations that do not help them confirm a diagnosis.

Natural radiation. For many generations, even before the discovery of x-rays and radium or the first explosion of an atomic bomb, mankind has been exposed to cosmic and gamma rays from natural radioactive sources. Some experts have estimated that a person taking a sun bath in a mountain resort is subject to as much radiation exposure to his reproductive organs from natural causes as he would be from having his wrist x-rayed. Natural background radiation comes from the earth, bricks in housing, cosmic rays, and from our own bodies, which contain radioactive chemicals in tiny but unavoidable amounts.

The atomic bomb fallout has added to this but not enough to reach a level which alarms qualified scientists. Other manmade radiation includes medical and dental, occupational, and miscellaneous items such as radioactive luminous markers, personal and household effects with slight radioactivity.

But with all this radiation people still are growing bigger, living longer and are healthier than previous generations.

Radiation of any kind is not a plaything for persons without specialized knowledge of its uses and abuses. But used by medical specialists, x-rays and other forms of radiation can be vital in immeasurably safeguarding your health or, possibly, even your life.

LABORATORY TESTS

by THOMAS M. PEERY, M.D.

PURPOSE OF TESTS

SCREENING TESTS

TESTS TO DIAGNOSE DISEASE

TESTS TO GUIDE TREATMENT

ROLE OF PATHOLOGIST

DEFINITIONS OF TESTS
AND PROCEDURES

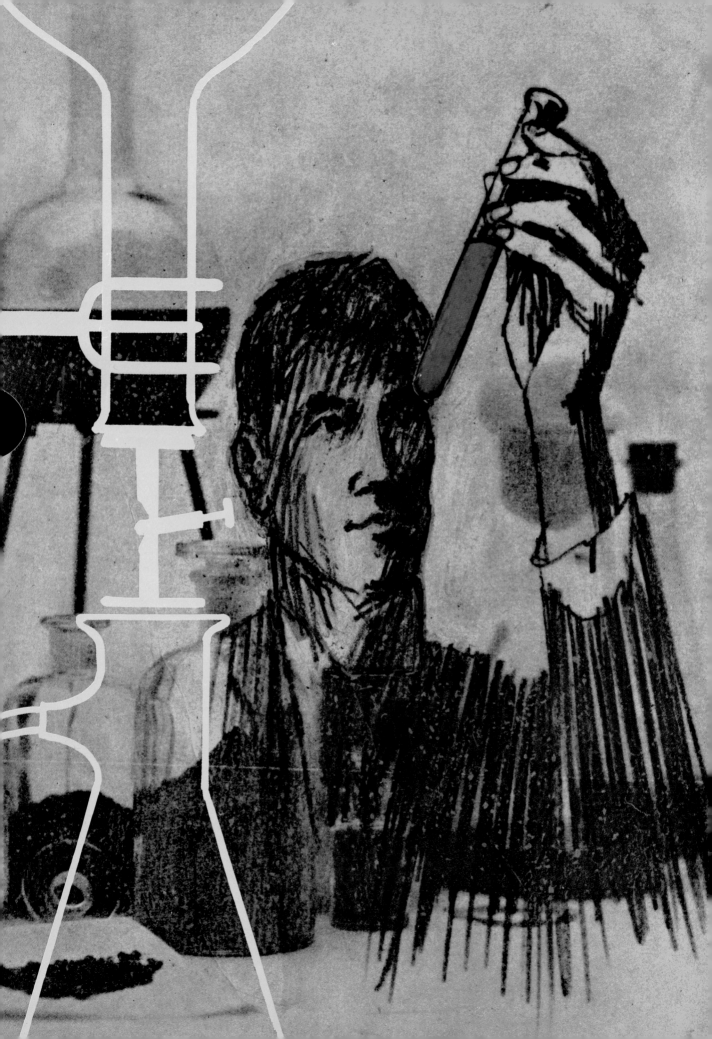

CHAPTER 24

LABORATORY TESTS

by THOMAS M. PEERY, M. D.

Newspaper item:... "*Senator*......
*entered the hospital last evening.
His office emphasized that the Senator is not ill, but that he was undergoing a series of laboratory tests as
a part of a routine checkup.*" ...

Why laboratory tests? Are they a necessary part of the "routine checkup"?
Can't the doctor find out all he needs to
know in his regular office examination?

The truth of the matter is that the
regular office examination is not very
informative in the earliest stages of
many diseases. Most of the organs are
located deep in the body, so inaccessible
to ordinary examination as to make it
very difficult for the doctor. The automobile mechanic, by comparison, has a much
easier task when you take your car to
him. He can remove the distributor cap
and inspect the points, take the spark
plugs out and measure the spark gap, or
pull a wheel and check the bearings. The
doctor can't even raise the hood or cut off
the motor for his examination!

All testing procedures in medicine —
x-rays, blood counts, chemical analyses,
electrocardiographs, skin tests and microscopic examinations, to name a few—
are designed to enable the doctor to learn
more about his patient than is evident
externally, and to discover hidden diagnostic signs. The physical examination
reveals only those signs which are manifest to the physician through his senses
— things he can see, hear, feel or smell.
X-rays permit the doctor to observe the
form and movements of internal organs
and parts. Clinical pathology tests let him
study their chemical make-up and function in minute detail.

Laboratory tests are used by the medical profession in three different ways: to
safeguard health, to *diagnose disease*,
and to *guide treatment*.

Tests to Safeguard Health

For more than a generation the staff
of the health department laboratory has
worked to promote the public health. This
they have done by testing drinking water
for evidence of bacterial contamination,
by analyzing milk and other dairy products for purity and nutritive value, by
checking food handlers for evidence of
communicable disease, and the like.

More recently, the clinical pathologist
in his laboratory has developed techniques for evaluating the personal health
of the individual. By testing apparently
healthy individuals at regular intervals
he has learned to detect disturbances
of function before organ disease has
occurred. Modification of diet or habits
may then correct the functional disturbance before actual illness develops.

The diseases that may be prevented
by these means are the chronic diseases,
slow in onset and dangerous when undetected, especially those which tend to

appear in middle age and to cause prolonged illness and death.

The physician must give careful thought to the selection of laboratory tests to be used in the health examination. In general the tests which are most useful are "screening tests" which provide a broad survey or profile of the various organ systems, especially those systems which are most apt to be affected by chronic diseases. If one of these tests yields an abnormal result, the physician then extends the examination in order to pinpoint the diagnosis.

Recommended tests will differ somewhat for different individuals, depending upon their history of familial diseases, prior illnesses, occupational or environmental hazards, social contacts, diet, habit, age and sex. Since most persons undergoing annual physical examinations are mature adults, certain tests are commonly used for all, and to this group are added other tests that are appropriate for the specific individual.

There are a great many tests which may be employed with benefit in health maintenance, but considerations of cost, convenience and safety to the patient tend to reduce the list to those procedures most likely to yield useful information.

Ideally, patients should be in a baseline state at the time their specimens are collected for laboratory examinations, since certain blood chemical studies may be influenced by food intake and physical activity. If specimens are always taken before breakfast and after a good night's sleep, the results will reflect the true basal state and can be compared to normal values.

By regular annual repetition of the whole series of laboratory tests, it is sometimes possible to recognize a beginning functional disturbance, even before the test result is definitely abnormal. Thus if a man in his middle thirties has shown consistently a blood cholesterol of 175-200, and then in his forties his cholesterol values rise to 250, it would seem wise to give consideration to this change in spite of the fact that the new value is still not definitely abnormal.

In the following section are listed certain tests and procedures that are commonly used as part of the annual physical examination. For a brief explanation of the various tests, see definitions at the end of this chapter.

SCREENING TESTS FOR HEALTH EVALUATION, BY ORGAN SYSTEMS

Heart and blood vessels:
  EKG, cholesterol
Lungs and bronchi: chest x-rays
Stomach and duodenum:
  gastric analyis
Colon and rectum: stool exam
Liver and gallbladder:
  bilirubin, transaminase
Kidneys and urinary bladder:
  urinalysis, urea nitrogen
Female reproductive system:
  cervical cytology ("Pap smear")
Endocrines and metabolism:
  glucose (sugar), PBI
Blood: hemoglobin or hematocrit;
  white cell count
Eyes: tonometry
Bones and joints: calcium, alkaline
  phosphatase, uric acid.

To these procedures can be added certain tests having no particular relationship to organ systems: VDRL test for syphilis, and the sedimentation rate. No tests are suggested for the nervous system; spinal fluid examination is not recommended as a part of the annual health evaluation, and no other tests are considered suitable.

Tests to Diagnose Disease

When a patient goes to his doctor because of illness, his symptoms — cough, weakness, fever, or weight loss — give the doctor a clue as to what the trouble is. The investigation is then directed toward running down this clue. The modern doctor ordinarily does not treat symptoms without attempting to learn their cause. Thus, when headache is severe and persistent, it is not enough to give a headache remedy; the cause of the headache must be sought, and treatment must be directed at that cause.

Screening tests like those used in health evaluation are ordinarily not satisfactory in such a case. Instead, the questioning must be much more detailed and the examinations and laboratory tests must survey specifically those parts of the body and those diseases which may cause the symptoms in question.

Diagnostic laboratory tests are based upon a number of different principles.

In *infectious diseases*, the tests ordinarily depend upon finding and identifying the germs which cause the particular disease.

In *diseases of the blood*, the tests are based upon direct microscopic examination of the blood cells and counting the different types of cells in a measured quantity of blood, in either case comparing the results with the normal.

In *cancer*, the diagnostic procedure is based upon microscopic examination of a bit of tissue removed from a suspicious lump or ulcer.

In other instances the tests are based upon the assumption that each organ in the body has a certain job to do, and that if the organ is healthy it will do that job; these tests require specimens that can in some way reflect organ function.

The range of laboratory tests that may be used to diagnose disease is almost without limits. Some can be carried out in the physician's own office while others require the special facilities of the clinical pathologist's laboratory. No list of tests can be considered final, complete or authoritative. New tests are added every year, and old tests fall into disfavor.

The following list of tests, grouped by organ systems and by diseases, covers most of the commonly used clinical pathology tests and some of the procedures used in radiology and other fields.

References to particular tests appear in many chapters of this book, in discussions of functions and disorders. Definitions (page 799) may aid in understanding the methods and purposes of tests that may be ordered for individual patients.

LABORATORY TESTS TO DIAGNOSE DISEASE, BY ORGAN SYSTEMS

Heart and Blood Vessels

rheumatic fever: anti-streptolysin O; sedimentation rate; EKG; chest x-rays.

bacterial endocarditis: blood culture; EKG; chest x-rays.

coronary thrombosis: EKG; transaminase.

Lungs and Bronchi

tuberculosis: sputum exam; chest x-rays.

pneumonia: sputum exam; chest x-rays.

cancer: sputum cytology; chest x-rays; bronchoscopic exam and biopsy.

Stomach and Duodenum

ulcer: gastric analysis; GI series (x-rays).

cancer: gastric analysis; gastric cytology; GI series (x-rays).

Colon and Rectum

colitis: stool exam; barium enema (x-rays).

cancer: barium enema (x-rays); proctoscopic exam and biopsy.

worms: stool exam.

Liver and Gallbladder

cirrhosis: proteins; BSP; cephalin flocculation; needle biopsy of liver; transaminase; cholesterol; ammonia.

jaundice: same as for cirrhosis.

cholecystitis: gallbladder x-rays; duodenal drainage.

Pancreas

pancreatitis: amylase; lipase; calcium.

cystic fibrosis: sweat test; stool exam.

Kidneys and Urinary Bladder

nephritis: urinalysis, urea nitrogen, NPN or creatinine; PSP; needle biopsy of kidney.

stone: urinalysis; KUB (x-rays); cystoscopy; calcium; uric acid.

infection of kidneys (pyelonephritis)

or *bladder* (cystitis): urinalysis;
urine culture.
cancer: urine cytology; KUB
(x-rays); cystoscopic exam with
biopsy.

Male Reproductive System

urethritis: urethral smear.
prostatitis: prostatic smear.
prostate cancer: acid phosphatase;
needle biopsy of prostate.
infertility: sperm exam.

Female Reproductive System

pregnancy: chorionic gonadotropin.
infertility: hormone studies;
endometrial biopsy.
uterine cancer: "D and C" and cervical
biopsy.
breast cancer: nipple cytology;
breast biopsy.

Endocrines and Metabolism

diabetes mellitus: urinalysis; glucose
(sugar); glucose tolerance; CO_2.
thyroid diseases: PBI; T_3; BMR;
cholesterol; iodine uptake.
adrenal diseases: hormone studies;
Thorn test; sodium; chlorides;
catecholamines.
parathyroid diseases: calcium;
phosphorus; bone x-rays; KUB
(x-rays).
pituitary diseases: hormone studies;
glucose tolerance; skull x-rays.
acidosis and alkalosis: pH; CO_2;
potassium; chlorides.
phenylketonuria: diaper test; Guthrie
test.

Blood

anemia: red cell count; hemoglobin;
hematocrit; iron; gastric analysis;
hemoglobin C and S; bone marrow
exam.
leukemia: white cell count;
differential; bone marrow exam;
platelet count.
purpura: coagulation time; platelet
count; prothrombin time; partial
thromboplastin time; tourniquet
test.
infectious mononucleosis ("mono"):
see *Lymph Nodes and Spleen.*
malaria: thick and thin smear.

erythroblastosis: Rh on baby and
mother; bilirubin; Coombs' test.
infection: white cell count;
differential; sedimentation rate;
blood culture.

Lymph Nodes and Spleen

infectious mononucleosis ("mono"):
white cell count; differential;
heterophile antibody test.
Hodgkin's disease: chest x-rays;
white cell count; differential; lymph
node biopsy.
sarcoid: proteins; calcium; lymph
node biopsy.
leukemia: see *Blood.*

Nervous System

meningitis, polio, encephalitis: spinal
fluid exam.
tumor: spinal fluid exam;
pneumoencephalogram (x-rays);
arteriogram (x-rays); EEG.
multiple sclerosis: spinal fluid exam.
stroke: spinal fluid exam.

Bones and Joints

fracture from minimal injury: bone
x-rays; calcium; alkaline
phosphatase.
arthritis: sedimentation rate; LE
prep; proteins; uric acid; synovial
fluid exam; bone x-rays.
cancer: bone x-rays; alkaline
phosphatase.
rheumatic fever: see *Heart and Blood
Vessels.*

Infectious Diseases

typhoid fever: blood culture; stool
culture; urine culture;
agglutination tests (Widal).
brucellosis: agglutination tests;
blood culture; skin tests.
diphtheria, strep throat: throat
culture.
whooping cough: cough plate.
rheumatic fever: see *Heart and Blood
Vessels.*
meningitis and polio: spinal fluid
exam.
syphilis: dark field; Wassermann;
Kahn; VDRL; TPI; spinal fluid
exam.
virus: virus isolation; neutralization
test; complement fixation test.

Tests to Guide Treatment

In one sense, all laboratory tests are used as a guide to treatment, since they promote accurate diagnosis. In this section, however, reference is made to the use of laboratory tests to select the type of treatment to be used, to determine how much treatment is required, to confirm that the desired effect is being obtained, and to avoid harmful side effects of treatment. The need for tests of this type is greatest in those chronic diseases where treatment must be continued for a long time, perhaps for life.

Tests of antibiotic efficacy. In a dangerous *infection* such as meningitis, it is extremely important to obtain an optimum therapeutic effect without delay. Since meningitis may be due to different bacteria, and each of these may respond differently or not at all to the various antibiotic drugs, it is common practice to test the various antibiotic drugs directly against the bacteria that are present in the particular case. This can be done in the following way:

Spinal fluid from the patient is mixed with melted agar in a sterile dish and the warm mixture is allowed to cool and solidify. Tiny paper disks, each of which has been impregnated with a different antibiotic, are dropped onto the surface of the agar and the dish is set aside for several hours in an incubator. The bacteria that were present in the patient's spinal fluid begin to multiply and form "colonies" in the medium, except that where they are in contact with the paper disks their growth may be modified by the antibiotic.

If all bacterial growth is suppressed about the paper disk saturated with tetracycline, but growth is abundant about the disk saturated with penicillin, it is clear that tetracycline is a better drug than penicillin to use in the treatment of this particular patient with meningitis. The test is a combination of *spinal fluid culture* and *antibiotic sensitivity.*

Dosage regulation. Probably the oldest use of laboratory tests to regulate drug dosage is in the *diabetic patient.* Some diabetics have a different requirement of insulin from day to day, depending upon appetite, diet, exercise, colds and the like. If the regular dose of insulin is sufficient, the urine test for glucose will be negative. If it is insufficient, the test may give a green, yellow or red color, depending upon the amount of glucose present. The doctor teaches the patient how to test his own urine and to regulate the dose of insulin depending upon the color of the urine test. From time to time the diabetic patient must also have a glucose test on blood, so as to avoid overdosage of insulin.

The following are other examples of the use of laboratory tests to guide treatment. After an attack of *coronary thrombosis,* many patients are given drugs to reduce the clotting tendency of their blood. The effect must be precisely controlled by coagulation tests, since overdose of the drug could cause a tendency to hemorrhage.

X-rays, radium and drugs used in the treatment of cancer sometimes destroy blood cells as well as cancer cells; occasional counts must be taken of white cells, red cells and platelets to make sure that this harmful effect is avoided. Some drugs used in the treatment of high blood pressure produce in some patients a condition resembling a special form of sensitivity disease known as *lupus erythematosus;* special blood examinations ("LE prep") can anticipate this effect.

Transfusions. Of life-saving importance in certain diseases is the use of *blood transfusions.* However, different people have different types of blood and it would be extremely dangerous to give a patient blood of a type different from his own. To detect these types and determine compatibility between donor's and recipient's blood, blood group and Rh tests must be carried out meticulously.

Similar tests (blood group and Rh) are of importance in determining whether the blood of an unborn baby is compatible with that of its mother. If incompatibility is present, it may be necessary to give the baby an "exchange transfusion" immediately after birth.

Frozen section. The surgeon often calls upon the pathologist to help him decide whether a lump in the breast should be simply removed or whether the whole breast and the nearby lymph nodes should also be removed. This test, known as the "frozen section," is performed while the patient is under anesthesia.

The surgeon removes the lump and passes it to the pathologist who freezes a portion of it in a jet of carbon dioxide gas. Once frozen, a very thin slice or section is cut, stained with a dye, mounted on a glass slide and examined under the microscope. If cancer is present, as determined by the pathologist, the surgeon will normally remove the entire breast and related tissue so as to "get around" the cancer. If the pathologist determines that the lump is benign, the surgeon ordinarily does not remove the remainder of the breast.

Role of the Pathologist and Medical Technologist

Modern medicine depends heavily upon the pathologist to bring the advances of the research laboratory, in biochemistry, microbiology, immunology, physiology, and the other experimental sciences, into the office and hospital. The pathologist has been described as "the doctor the patient never sees."

Few physicians will make a final diagnosis of tuberculosis, cancer, diabetes or pernicious anemia without laboratory confirmation from the pathologist. He and his skilled staff of medical technologists are qualified by training and experience to provide clinical laboratory services of dependable quality. This is important because laboratory procedures that are not subject to quality control and careful professional scrutiny are apt to mislead.

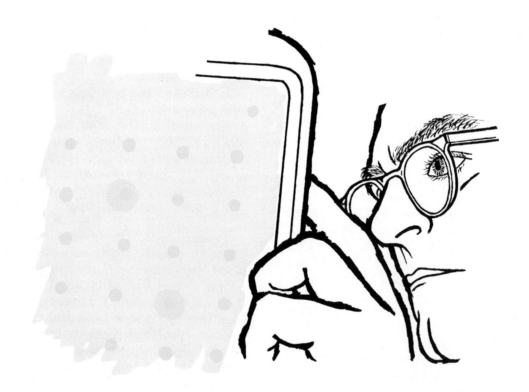

Guthrie test for *phenylketonuria* (PKU). Affected babies cannot metabolize a common element of protein foods, phenylalanine. Excessive phenylalanine in baby's blood indicates PKU. Paper disks containing samples of babies' blood are placed on surface coated with special nutrient and culture of bacteria. Bacteria used in test multiply only if blood disks contain phenylalanine. Most of disks shown being inspected at right are normal. But blood disk of one baby is surrounded by halo of multiplying bacteria, indicating that phenylalanine is present and baby has PKU. Special foods reduce phenylalanine in baby's diet, lessen threat of mental retardation from damage to developing nervous system.

DEFINITIONS OF CERTAIN LABORATORY TESTS AND MEDICAL PROCEDURES

acid phosphatase: an enzyme test on blood; for diagnosis of prostate cancer.

agglutination tests: antibody tests on blood; for the diagnosis of typhoid fever, brucellosis and certain other infectious diseases.

alkaline phosphatase: an enzyme test on blood; used as a screening test in bone disease, and for diagnosis in obstructive jaundice.

ammonia: a chemical test on blood; used as a guide to treatment in severe liver disease.

amylase: an enzyme test on blood; for diagnosis in acute pancreatitis.

antibiotic sensitivity: a bacteriologic test on blood, urine and sputum; to determine the most suitable antibiotic in a specific case.

anti-streptolysin O: an antibody test on blood; used in cases of suspected rheumatic fever.

arteriogram: an x-ray test after injecting "dye"; for the diagnosis of brain tumors.

barium enema: an x-ray test after rectal injection of barium; for diagnosis in cancer and other diseases of the colon and rectum.

bilirubin: a chemical test on blood; used as a screening test and also for diagnosis of certain blood and liver diseases.

biopsy: a tissue test, usually used in cases of suspected cancer.

blood culture: a bacteriologic test on blood; for the diagnosis of fevers.

blood group and Rh: an antibody test on blood; used to select suitable blood for transfusions, and in pregnancy to evaluate the possibility of blood disease in the baby.

BMR: basal metabolic rate, a breathing test for the diagnosis of thyroid diseases and certain other metabolic abnormalities.

bone marrow exam: a microscopic test on cellular material obtained by needle; used to diagnose leukemia, anemia, and certain other diseases of the blood.

bone x-rays: an x-ray test for diagnosis in all types of bone disease: fractures, cancer and cyst.

breast biopsy: a tissue test, used in cases of suspected breast cancer.

bronchoscopic exam and biopsy: a surgical procedure combined with a tissue test, used in cases of suspected lung cancer.

BSP: bromsulphthalein, a chemical measure of liver function; an injection is given, and some time later a blood specimen is taken for analysis.

calcium: a chemical test on blood; used as a screening test and also for the diagnosis of bone diseases and certain parathyroid, kidney and pancreatic diseases.

catecholamines: a chemical test on blood or urine; used for diagnosis in tumors of the adrenal gland.

cephalin flocculation: a test for abnormal proteins, done on blood; used in the diagnosis of liver diseases.

cervical biopsy: a tissue test, used in cases of suspected cancer of the uterine cervix.

cervical cytology ("Pap smear"): microscopic test of fluid obtained from the uterine cervix, smeared on a glass slide after the method of Papanicolaou; a screening test for cervix cancer.

chest x-rays: an x-ray test for screening and for diagnosis of diseases of the heart, lungs and ribs.

chlorides: a chemical test on blood, sometimes on urine; used for the diagnosis of certain metabolic diseases and as a guide to treatment.

cholesterol: a chemical test on blood; used in screening for heart disease, and also for the diagnosis of certain metabolic diseases.

chorionic gonadotropin: a biological test on blood or urine; for the diagnosis of pregnancy.

coagulation time: a clotting test on blood; used for diagnosis in cases having a tendency to hemorrhage, and also as a guide to treatment in patients receiving anticoagulant drugs.

CO_2: a chemical test on blood; used as

a guide to treatment in various conditions of acidosis and alkalosis.

complement fixation tests: antibody tests on blood; used for the diagnosis of syphilis and certain virus and bacterial infections.

Coombs' test: an antibody test on blood; used in selecting blood suitable for transfusion, and in the diagnosis of certain anemias.

cough plate: a bacteriologic test in which the patient coughs in a sterile plate; for the diagnosis of whooping cough.

creatinine: a chemical test on blood; a measure of kidney function.

cystoscopic exam with biopsy: a surgical procedure combined with a tissue test, used in cases of suspected bladder cancer.

cystoscopy: a procedure for inspecting the lining of the urinary bladder through tube inserted via the urethra.

cytology: the study of cells; the term is often applied to the microscopic screening test for cancer first developed by Papanicolaou.

D and C: a surgical procedure on the uterus; used to obtain a tissue specimen in cases of suspected uterine cancer.

dark field: a microscopic test for the diagnosis of syphilis in its earliest stage; serum from the ulcer is used.

diaper test: a simple chemical test, done on a baby's wet diaper; a screening test for phenylketonuria.

differential: a microscopic test done on a blood smear; used for diagnosis of leukemia and certain infections.

duodenal drainage: an intestinal specimen is obtained via a swallowed tube and examined, for diagnosis of gallbladder and pancreas diseases.

EEG: electroencephalogram — an electrical test based on "brain waves"; used in the neurological exam.

EKG: electrocardiogram — an electrical test used both as a screening test for heart disease, and as a diagnostic test in heart disease.

endometrial biopsy: a tissue test on the uterus, used in the study of infertility, and also for the diagnosis of cancer of the uterus.

frozen section: a rapid tissue test, usually done during a surgical operation, for the diagnosis of suspected cancer.

gallbladder x-rays: an x-ray test after taking "dye," for diagnosis of gallstones and gallbladder diseases.

gastric analysis: a specimen of stomach juice is obtained by stomach tube and examined chemically and microscopically as a screening test for ulcer and cancer.

gastric cytology: microscopic examination of stomach juice in cases of suspected stomach cancer.

GI series (x-ray): a series of gastrointestinal x-ray tests after swallowing barium; used for the diagnosis of suspected ulcer and cancer of stomach and duodenum.

glucose (sugar): a chemical test, either on blood or urine, used as a screening test and also for the diagnosis of diabetes mellitus and other metabolic diseases, and as a guide to treatment.

glucose tolerance: a series of chemical tests for blood glucose after taking glucose by mouth; a test for early diabetes and other metabolic diseases.

Guthrie test: a combined chemical and bacteriologic test on urine; used as a screening test for phenylketonuria.

hematocrit: a mechanical test on blood; used as a screening procedure, and for the diagnosis of anemia and also as a guide to treatment.

hemoglobin: a chemical test on blood; used as a screening procedure and as a guide to treatment in anemia.

hemoglobin C and S: an electrophoretic test on blood; for diagnosis of sickle cell anemia and related blood diseases.

heterophile antibody test: an antibody test on blood; used for diagnosis of infectious mononucleosis ("mono").

hormone studies: a broad group of tests, some chemical and some biological, usually done on urine; used in the diagnosis of endocrine and metabolic disorders.

iodine uptake: a radioisotope test for diagnosis of thyroid diseases; done after taking a dose of radioactive iodine.

iron: a chemical test for diagnosis of

anemia, using a blood specimen.

Kahn: an antibody test on blood; used for diagnosis of syphilis.

KUB (x-rays): a kidney-urinary-bladder x-ray test after administration of "dye," for diagnosis of cancer and other diseases of kidney and bladder.

"L E prep": lupus erythematosus preparation, a microscopic test of a blood preparation, for diagnosis of lupus erythematosus.

leukocytes: see *white blood count.*

lipase: an enzyme test on blood; for diagnosis of acute pancreatitis.

lymph node biopsy: a tissue test, used in cases of suspected cancer of the lymph nodes.

needle biopsy of kidney: a tissue test for diagnosis of kidney diseases, using as a specimen a bit of kidney tissue obtained through a long needle.

needle biopsy of liver: a tissue test for diagnosis of liver diseases, particularly cirrhosis.

needle biopsy of prostate: a tissue test, used in cases of suspected cancer of the prostate.

neutralization test: a combined antibody and biologic test for diagnosis of virus infections; blood is used.

nipple cytology: a microscopic test of nipple secretion; a screening test in cases of suspected breast cancer.

NPN: non-protein-nitrogen, a chemical measure of kidney function; blood is used.

"Pap smear": see *cervical cytology.*

partial thromboplastin time: a clotting test on blood; used as a screening procedure in patients having a tendency to hemorrhage.

PBI: protein-bound iodine, a chemical test used for screening, and also for the diagnosis of thyroid diseases; blood is used.

pH: an electrical test used as a guide to treatment in patients with acidosis or alkalosis; blood is used.

phosphorus: a chemical test on blood; used in diagnosis of certain diseases of the kidney and of metabolism.

platelet count: a microscopic test on blood; used in the diagnosis of patients having a tendency to hemorrhage.

pneumoencephalogram: a combined neurological and x-ray procedure after air injection; for the diagnosis and localization of brain tumors.

potassium: a chemical test on blood; used as a guide to treatment in patients with such symptoms as vomiting, diarrhea and intestinal obstruction.

proctoscopic exam and biopsy: a medical procedure combined with a tissue test, used in patients with suspected cancer of the rectum.

prostatic smear: a microscopic test for diagnosis of infection of the prostate gland; the specimen is obtained by prostatic massage.

proteins: a chemical or electrophoretic test on blood; used for diagnosis in diseases of the liver, lymph nodes and bone marrow.

prothrombin time: a clotting test on blood; used in patients having a tendency to hemorrhage, in liver diseases, and also as a guide to treatment in patients receiving certain anticoagulant drugs.

PSP: phenolsulphonphthalein, a chemical test on urine; used as a measure of kidney function following the injection of a "dye."

red cell count: a microscopic or electronic test for diagnosis of anemia; blood is used.

Rh: an antibody test on blood; used in transfusion studies, and in pregnancy to evaluate the possibility of blood disease in the baby.

sedimentation rate: a mechanical test on blood; used as a general screening procedure.

skin tests: sensitivity tests using the patient's skin; for identification of substances to which the patient is allergic, and to detect evidence of prior infection in tuberculosis and brucellosis.

skull x-rays: x-ray tests to diagnose fractures, pituitary tumors and bone disease in the skull.

sodium: a chemical test on blood; used as a guide to treatment in patients with vomiting, diarrhea and intestinal obstruction.

sperm exam: a microscopic test of fertility in the male.

spinal fluid culture: a bacteriologic test for diagnosis of meningitis; specimen is obtained by lumbar puncture needle.

spinal fluid exam: various chemical, microscopic and bacteriologic tests on spinal fluid; used for diagnosis of such ailments as meningitis, poliomyelitis and brain tumor.

sputum cytology: a microscopic test of sputum in cases of suspected lung cancer.

sputum exam: various chemical, microscopic and bacteriologic tests on sputum; used for diagnosis of lung disease, especially tuberculosis, pneumonia, cancer and abscess.

stool culture: a bacteriologic test on feces; used for diagnosis of typhoid fever, bacillary dysentery and other intestinal infections.

stool exam: a series of microscopic, bacteriologic and chemical tests on feces; used as a screening test and for diagnosis of stomach and intestinal disease, including worms, amebas, ulcer and cancer.

sugar: see *glucose.*

sweat test: a chemical test on sweat; used for the diagnosis of cystic disease of the pancreas.

synovial fluid exam: a series of chemical, physical, microscopic and bacteriologic tests for the diagnosis of gout and other forms of arthritis; joint fluid, removed by needle, is the specimen.

T₃: a radioisotope test on blood; used both as a screening test and for diagnosis in thyroid disease.

thick and thin smear: a microscopic test, using blood smears of different degrees of thickness, for diagnosis of malaria.

Thorn test: a microscopic test on blood after hormone injection; used as a measure of function of the adrenal glands.

throat culture: a bacteriologic test for diagnosis of such throat infections as diphtheria and streptococcus.

throat smear: a bacteriologic screening test in throat infections; a cotton swab is rubbed across the throat.

tonometry: an ophthalmological test of eyeball tension, used as a screening procedure and for the diagnosis of glaucoma.

TPI: treponema pallidum immobilization, an antibody test on blood; used for the confirmation of a diagnosis of syphilis.

transaminase: an enzyme test on blood; used as a screening procedure for liver disease, and for the diagnosis of coronary thrombosis, liver diseases, etc.

tubeless gastric: a chemical test done on the urine after administration of "Diagnex"; the test gives information similar to that obtained by gastric analysis.

urea nitrogen: a chemical test on blood; a measure of kidney function.

urethral smear: a bacteriologic test in cases of suspected gonorrhea.

uric acid: a chemical test on blood; used as a screening procedure and also in the diagnosis of gout.

urinalysis: a series of chemical, microscopic and physical tests on urine; used as a screening test and also for diagnosis of diseases of the kidneys and bladder; diabetes.

urine culture: a bacteriologic test for diagnosis of infections of the urinary tract.

urine cytology: a microscopic test used in cases of suspected cancer of the kidneys or bladder.

uterine cytology: a microscopic test used as a screening procedure for uterine cancer.

VDRL: the Venereal Disease Research Laboratory screening test for syphilis; blood is used.

virus isolation: bacteriologic and biologic tests for the diagnosis of virus infections, spinal fluid, bronchial washings, and may be used as specimens.

Wassermann: an antibody test for the diagnosis of syphilis; blood is used.

white cell count: microscopic or electronic test for the enumeration of leukocytes in blood; used as a screening procedure and for the diagnosis of infections and leukemia.

Widal: an antibody test for diagnosis of typhoid fever; blood is the specimen.

MEDICAL GENETICS

CONGENITAL OR HEREDITARY?

INHERITANCE OF TRAITS

GENETIC BLUEPRINTS

CHROMOSOMES

DNA—RNA

WHERE TO SEEK HELP

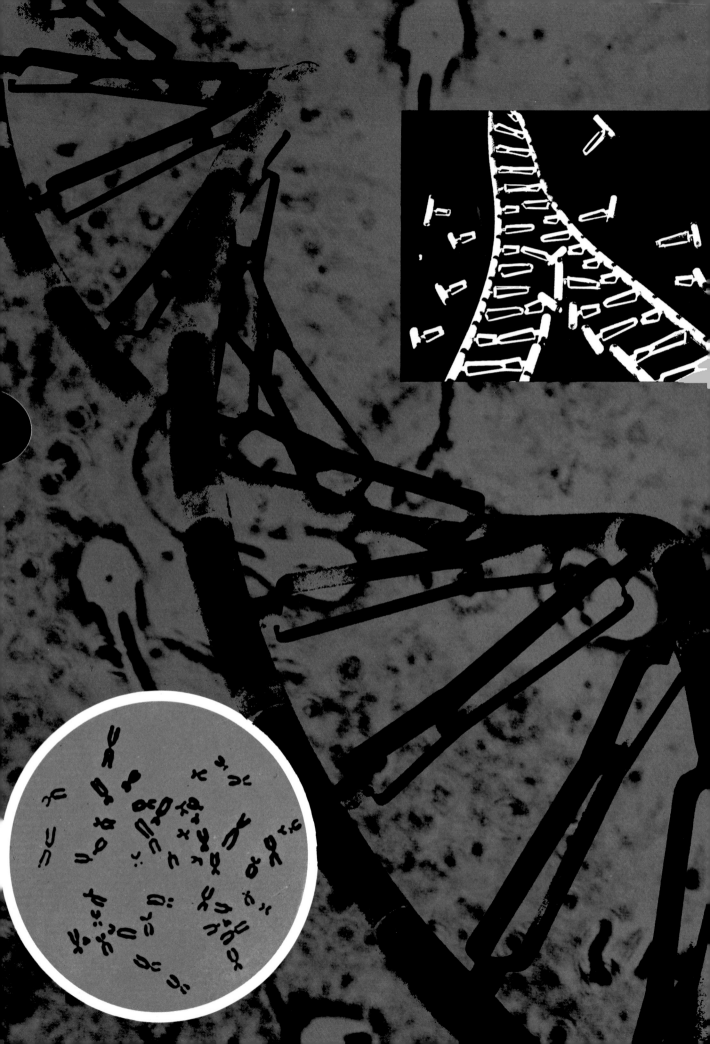

MEDICAL GENETICS

Every parent wonders prenatally, "will the baby be normal?" Usually the baby turns out to be 100 per cent perfect in the eyes of the parents, although an expert might detect a trifling, harmless, or easily correctible imperfection that is of little consequence.

Very few prospective parents or couples contemplating marriage have the slightest reason to undergo exhaustive tests and genetic studies to assess the liabilities of offspring. However, there is reasonable cause for concern if a defective infant has already been born to a couple, or if a demonstrably hereditary trait recurs in direct blood lines.

If hidden fears are brought to light by asking questions, one's physician or obstetrician can give answers that are often comforting. He can assure the non-hemophiliac brother of a hemophiliac that he himself cannot transmit the disease, or assure a couple that cerebral palsy is not hereditary. Diagnosis and treatment of the most frequent forms of congenital disease are within his area of competence. He can refer the small number of patients who need special help to genetic counselors and specialists who embrace many scientific disciplines.

The young science of medical genetics continues to take tremendous strides. About 1600 hereditary disorders—too rare and too many to be enumerated—are now known. Probably most diseases have a genetic component, if all the facts were known, but there are still great gaps in knowledge. Medical geneticists cannot give hard-and-fast answers to every problem. Sometimes, answers are immensely consoling; sometimes, qualified; often, risks can be stated only in rather cold terms of mathematical odds.

Congenital or Hereditary?

A congenital abnormality is one that is present at birth. It is not necessarily hereditary—that is, transmitted by germ cells of the parents.

Accidental birth defects are not inherited and will almost certainly not be repeated in subsequent offspring. Among the causes of such accidents are infections of the mother with German measles or toxoplasmosis, or her exposure to drugs, toxins, or radiation, which may harmfully alter the environment of the fetus in the womb at a critical stage of development.

Truly *hereditary* birth defects are transmitted by parental germ cells; mathematical odds for or against repetition can usually be stated.

Some birth defects are thought to result from extremely complex interac-

The chemistry of heredity. Background: "spiral ladder" design of DNA molecule; thousands of bases ("rungs") link with sugar-phosphate chains. In square: down-the-middle split of DNA into complementary halves which replicate original molecule. In circle: chromosomes which contain DNA.

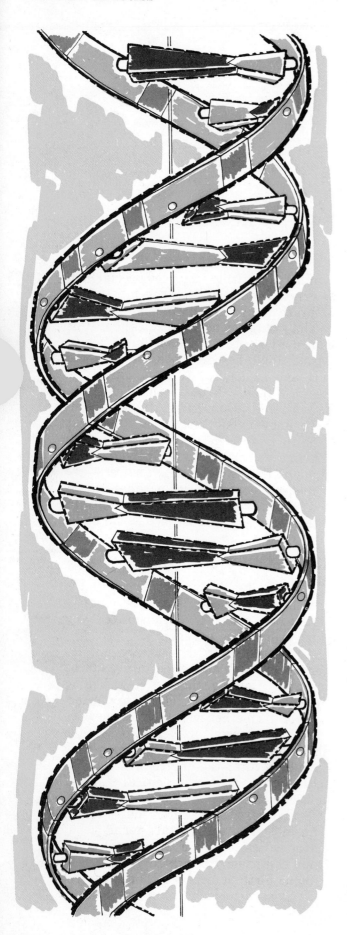

tions of genes and environment. The more complex the genetics of a particular defect (cleft palate, heart abnormalities) the less likely it is to be repeated in offspring. Parents of a baby with a cleft palate can be told that odds are 20 to one against repetition—a 5 per cent risk, about the same as the defect-risk of the general baby population.

A number of diseases are not inherited as such, but have an hereditary component—probably a subtle susceptibility which may be provoked by multiple factors. Diabetes tends to recur in families, but a potential diabetic may never develop the frank disease if he keeps his weight down. Women with close female relatives who had breast cancer are three times more likely to develop the disease than the average woman. Pernicious anemia patients inherit a predisposition to premature degeneration of stomach membranes, and psoriasis patients a tendency to excessively rapid turnover of epidermal cells. Some day, medical genetics may play a great role in preventive medicine by informing us early of hereditary vulnerabilities against which medical defenses may be built.

Genetic Blueprints

All the directions for the structure and functioning of our bodies are contained in our *chromosomes*, which contain DNA, which contains our *genes*. These are molecules and parts of molecules; heredity is a chemical phenomenon.

Chromosomes are threadlike particles in the nucleus of every cell which, when stained and prepared, can be seen under a microscope. Human beings normally have 46 chromosomes, arranged in 23 pairs. One in each pair comes from the mother, one from the father.

Heredity is encoded in DNA (deoxyribonucleic acid) within the chromo-

At left, the mighty "double helix" of DNA (deoxyribonucleic acid) which contains the genetic code. The long molecule is shaped something like a spiral stairway. The sides or rails are chains of sugar (ribose) and phosphate molecules; the steps or rungs are built of four bases (thymine, cytosine, adenine, guanine) repeated thousands of times in different sequences.

somes. Long DNA molecules consist of two intertwining chains coiled around a common axis, something like spiral ladders, with thousands of connecting "rungs" or steps. The rungs are built of four rather simple chemical units, repeated thousands upon thousands of times in different sequences along the length of the chain.

A *gene* is a very small cluster of chemical units which constitute the rungs and sides of a tiny portion of the long DNA molecule. A gene or gene combination is a unit of heredity, specifying some particular trait, such as whether an organism will have blue or brown eyes; and, collectively, whether an organism will have the organs and functions of a mouse or a man.

How can an infinitesimal group of molecules have such omnipotence? The "one gene, one enzyme" concept holds that a gene directs the assembly of an enzyme, or catalyst, essential for some body process. If a gene is defective, its associated enzyme is defective or lack-

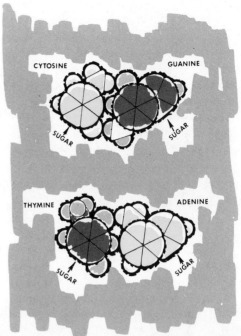

Scheme of a gene: pairs of DNA bases in the structure of the molecule. A gene is thought to be a tiny segment of DNA in which a cluster of several base pairs activates a process of heredity, singly or in conjunction with other genes.

ing. The effect may be harmless and inapparent; on the other hand, it may impose a major derangement of some physiological process.

Gene-containing DNA imprints the genetic code upon a slightly different nucleic acid (RNA, ribonucleic acid). Forms of RNA direct the cell to manufacture specific enzymes and other proteins by linking scores and hundreds of amino-acid building blocks (some 20 different ones) in inviolable sequences. A seemingly insignificant error—a "wrong" amino-acid or two in a chain of many hundreds—may have far-flung effects. Sickle cell anemia is a classic instance of molecular disease. The hemoglobin of sickle cell patients contains only a couple of "wrong" amino acids, but that is quite enough to establish a very serious disease.

Inheritance of Traits

One of the 23 pairs of human chromosomes is a sex chromosome, designated XX in the female and XY in the male. The other 22 pairs are called autosomes. Sexual reproduction makes human vari-

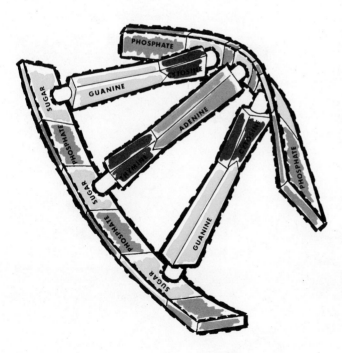

Closeup segment of the DNA "ladder." Guanine always links with cytosine, thymine with adenine, to form "rungs" or bases attached to sugar-phosphate chains, but there are different sequences of bases encoded with genetic information.

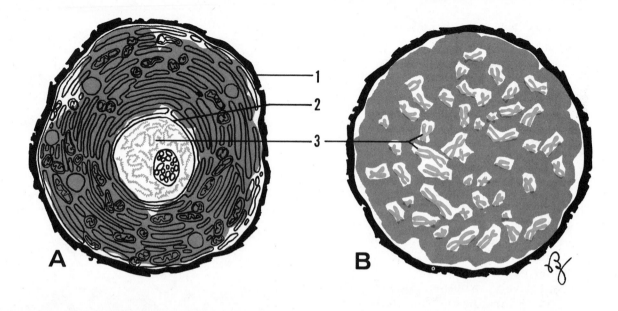

← CHROMOSOMES

Drawings A and B show: 1, cell wall; 2, nucleus; 3, chromosomes. Delicate filaments (A) contract, segment, form "arms" during a stage of cell division (B). The "package" of chromosomes characteristic of a particular organism is called the *karyotype*. The normal karyotype of human beings contains 23 pairs of chromosomes. For purposes of study and systematic identification, researchers usually arrange the pairs according to descending order of size and position of the *centromere*, the constriction between "arms." The 23rd pair of chromosomes determines sex. It contains either a large X chromosome and a small Y chromosome (male) or two X chromosomes (female). Drawings C through F show normal and abnormal human chromosome patterns. (C), normal male karyotype. (D), normal female karyotype. (E), abnormality characteristic of *mongolism*; chromosome 21 is not a normal pair but a triplet (*trisomy*). (F), abnormal chromosome with part of a long arm missing (*Philadelphia chromosome*), found in a high percentage of patients with chronic myelogenous leukemia.

ation possible by drawing upon the unique traits of parents in random ways. Sex determination, for instance, is a matter of chance: whether an X- or Y-carrying sperm fertilizes an egg. If a male X unites with a maternal X (the female sex chromosome is always XX), the offspring will be female; if a male Y unites with a maternal X, the offspring (XY) will be male. If you predict a boy or a girl, you have a 50 per cent chance of being right—or wrong. So it is that genetic counselors must often state the chance that a given trait will recur in terms of mathematical odds.

Two or more genes may work together to modify a given trait, and there are other complexities and unknowns. But in common genetic language, hereditary traits are "recessive" or "dominant."

One might think of a recessive gene as "weak," unable to generate its specific enzyme, or too little of it. But if it is paired with a normal gene, the latter takes over the job and no abnormal symptoms appear. However, if two recessive genes unite, one from each parent—a "double dose"—the trait appears

in offspring. If only one parent has a recessive gene, he or she is a carrier, but offspring will be normal. A dominant trait is transmitted by a gene "dose" from only one parent, which overrides the effects of a normal matching gene from the other parent.

Most inherited metabolic diseases are transmitted recessively. The most common are cystic fibrosis and sickle cell trait. Dominant hereditary disorders are quite rare (for instance, Huntington's chorea, and a form of dwarfism). Conditions such as hemophilia and color blindness are linked to the sex chromosome, usually transmitted through the mother who is a carrier but does not have the condition herself.

Relatives in a family with recessive disorders should know that both parents of an affected child are almost invariably normal, but both are carriers of the trait. Neither is more "to blame" than the other.

Relatives in a family with a history of a dominant hereditary disorder should know that only the affected members can transmit the disease to their children. Unaffected members cannot.

What the odds mean. If a child has a recessively transmitted disease, chances that a subsequent child of the same parents will have the disease are 1 in 4— that is, a 75 per cent chance that the next child will *not* be affected. In two-child families, if one child has a recessive disorder, the second child will be normal in 86 per cent of instances. If a disorder is dominantly transmitted, there is a 50 per cent chance that offspring will be affected—about the same chance as boy or girl determination.

A statement of odds is not overly reassuring but gives a basis for hard decisions. Whatever the odds, it is quite possible that a given hereditary defect will appear in *none* of the children of a couple, or in *all* of them. If a coin is tossed and comes down heads, chances that the next toss will come down tails are not increased—still 50-50. Each toss is a whole new ball game. So with parenthood, an adventure not without risks but with commensurate rewards.

Diagnosis and Counsel

If supposed hereditary diseases or birth defects are a cause for worry, the first step is accurate diagnosis, which often need go no further than the family physician. Rare and complex hereditary conditions require careful detective work, detailed knowledge of genetics, and exacting discrimination—there are, for example, several forms of hereditary deafness and muscular dystrophy.

Several kinds of tests and studies—rapidly increasing in number and sophistication—help greatly to identify defective fetuses, often quite early in pregnancy, and to establish the facts as a sound basis for counsel.

Amniocentesis is the withdrawal, through a hollow needle inserted into the mother's womb, of a sample of amniotic fluid in which the fetus "swims." The fluid contains fetal cells, which can be grown in culture, and other products, which are studied for chromosomal or chemical abnormalities that may indicate the presence of certain birth de-

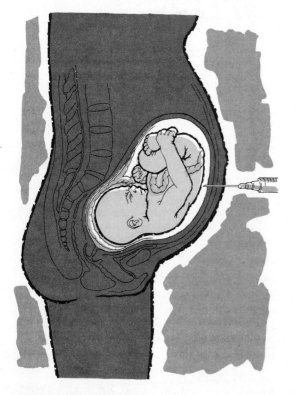

Amniocentesis: needle withdraws amniotic fluid which surrounds fetus and contains cells and products that yield genetic information.

fects (about 40 genetic diseases can now be diagnosed in this way).

Although considered to be safe in competent hands, amniocentesis is not trivially resorted to. It is invaluable if there is substantial risk of abnormality, as in a woman who has previously borne a child with genetic disease, and many specialists feel that it is indicated if the mother is of advanced maternal age (over 35 years) because older women have much greater risk of giving birth to a mongoloid infant. The favored time for amniocentesis is around the sixteenth week of pregnancy. Analysis takes about two weeks.

Sex of the fetus is readily determined by amniocentesis, and sometimes this determination alone is immensely heartening. Hemophilia is a genetic disease manifested only by males. If the fetus is found to be female, the baby will not have hemophilia.

Chromosome studies. A number of birth defects can be diagnosed by identifying abnormalities of structure or number of chromosomes. Many such defects are not hereditary but "developmental" or environmental, which is to say, "something" happens to disturb the fusion of normal parental chromosomes in the fertilized egg.

The most common chromosomal birth defect diagnosable by amniocentesis cell studies is *mongolism*. The affected child has somewhat oriental features, mental retardation, abnormalities of many systems of the body. The child carries an extra chromosome (No. 21), caused by a defect in separation of chromosomes called *nondisjunction*. The parents practically always have normal chromosomes, so the defect is not truly hereditary. Chances that a subsequent child will be normal are quite good except that there is a striking association between mongolism and the relatively advanced age of the mother.

A different, quite rare form of mongolism, which affects infants of young as well as older mothers, also has a distinctive chromosome abnormality: one pair of chromosomes carries an extra part from another chromosome (*transloca-*

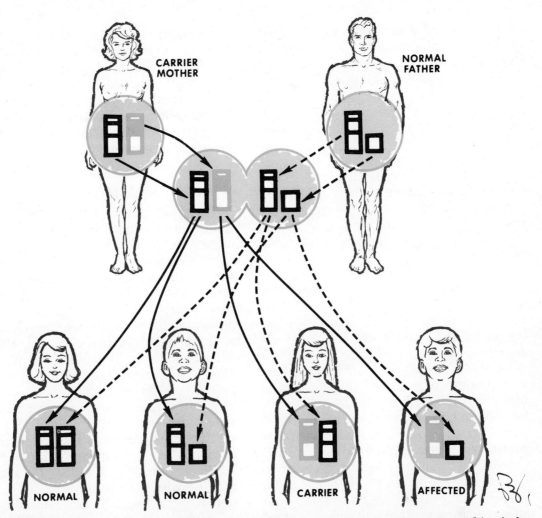

How sex-linked trait of classic hemophilia is transmitted by carrier mother. Rectangles within circles represent X (female) chromosomes; hemophiliac chromosome shown with black center. Squares are Y (male) chromosomes. A normal X chromosome negates the effect of a hemophiliac X chromosome in female carriers, who do not manifest the disease although they can transmit it. The Y chromosome gives no protection to males who receive a hemophiliac chromosome from a carrier mother. Genetic pedigrees trace heritable disorders farther back in family tree.

tion). This form of mongolism is hereditary. One of the parents carries the defect but is not affected by it. If the mother is a carrier there is a 50 per cent chance that her children will be mongoloid. Differences in two seemingly identical diseases underline the importance of fine discrimination when undertaking genetic studies.

Pedigrees. Accurate interpretation of genetic factors may require that facts be obtained by pedigree studies—painstaking investigation of the health histories of blood relatives through parents, siblings, cousins, aunts, grandparents and beyond. Pedigrees can give insight into patterns of inheritance of a trait and give a basis for prediction. It is vital, of course, that this information be accurate. This is not always easy if relatives live at great distances or if vital statistics records in their communities are sketchy. Many pedigree studies are done by researchers in genetic aspects of disease and often are not strictly necessary in a family situation.

Treatment

A very few genetic disorders are treatable to a fairly satisfactory degree. Modifications of diet, if begun early, may prevent mental retardation in instances of galactosemia and phenylketonuria. Cystic fibrosis may respond to pancreatic enzymes and mist inhalations. Distressing symptoms of various disorders can often be relieved. But there is no useful treatment and presently no cure for most diseases in which the underlying defect is hidden in the genes.

If tests reveal that a fetus is seriously defective, the parents have a choice, strictly their own, of terminating pregnancy or of having an infant that will be abnormal in ways that are determined by the disease.

If chances that some serious genetic condition will recur can only be stated mathematically, say one chance in four, the risks are real but not so overwhelming as to be totally unacceptable to every couple.

Genetic diseases vary in implications and handicaps. Many developmental birth defects, such as heart abnormalities, have no known genetic basis. Not a few worries about supposed hereditary taints arise from misconceptions. Medical counsel can bring the facts to light.

There is reason to hope that genetic disease may some day be treated and actually cured by "gene therapy." Intensive research in genetic manipulation is exploring some astonishing possibilities: use of harmless viruses to carry correct genetic information into cells; taking samples of a sick person's cells, transferring correct genetic information to the cells, growing them in tissue culture and returning them to the donor; transferring whole chromosomes by cell fusion. Such possibilities sound like far-out science fiction, but serious investigators pursue them.

Where to Seek Help

The first source of help in matters of inherited disorders is the family physician who, if he recognizes that special skills are needed, can refer patients to reliable laboratory and counseling centers. Some services are evaluation centers where a team of specialists determines an infant's medical problem and recommends treatment in consultation with the family physician and the parents. Another type of service is a birth defects treatment center, usually established in a teaching hospital or in affiliation with the medical school of a university. Few communities are far away from laboratory and counseling services in large towns and cities. Persons or families who wish to know where genetic counseling is available can request a free list of such services in the United States and Canada from the medical department of The National Foundation-March of Dimes, P. O. Box 2000, White Plains, New York 10602.

CHAPTER 26

CANCER

Its Nature ... Varieties ... Causes ...

The Many Pathways of Research

Throughout this book the authors have discussed cancer in relation to their medical specialties, since treatment is different in different forms of cancer and in individual patients. The present chapter concerns general aspects of cancer and the current basis for massive research programs which give hope that fundamental knowledge will lead to better measures of treatment, prevention, and control than we now have.

Defenses Against Cancer

Cancer is not inevitably fatal if it is promptly recognized and treated. Better than one out of three cancer patients survives five years or longer and many are permanently cured. Prospects of successful treatment of some forms of cancer are excellent; for some other forms, the outlook is less heartening. Although cancer may exist for some time before it is detected or causes symptoms, authorities generally agree that early discovery and treatment enhance the prospects of cure. No little responsibility rests upon us as individuals to be aware of signals which may (or may not) warn of cancer, and not to procrastinate in going to one's physician. Any of the following symptoms, if it persists for two weeks or more, calls for prompt attention by you and investigation by a doctor:

Unusual bleeding or discharge.
A lump or thickening in the breast or elsewhere.

A sore that does not heal.
Change in bowel or bladder habits.
Hoarseness or cough.
Indigestion or difficulty in swallowing.
Change in size or color of a wart or mole.

Regular physical examinations are important in personal defense. For women, these include "Pap" tests and breast examination. If anything suspicious is discovered, a tissue specimen (biopsy) may be taken, and specific tests and x-rays may be ordered. Sometimes an exploratory operation is deemed necessary to determine the nature and extent of a patient's condition.

Many tumors and abnormal growths are *benign* (non-cancerous), though not necessarily harmless. Cancer is said to be *malignant* because of its life-threatening capacity to spread to distant parts of the body (*metastasis*), to press upon and invade nearby organs, and to drain vital resources of the body. We usually think of cancer as a localized solid tumor, but it can be manifested in non-solid structures, as in leukemia.

Treatment. There are three recognized, effective forms of cancer treatment: (1) *surgery*, removal of all or as much as possible of a cancer, and often of lymphatic structures through which it might spread; (2) x-ray and other controlled forms of *radiation* to destroy malignant cells; and (3) *chemotherapy*, treatment with drugs.

Choice of treatment demands expert medical evaluation of a particular form of cancer in a particular patient. Some cancers are radio-sensitive and shrink miraculously under x-rays; other forms are not benefited at all. Treatments may be combined or given in sequence; for instance, radiation or chemotherapy before or after surgery. A few forms of cancer (e.g., breast and prostate) are said to be hormone-dependent and antagonistic hormones may play a part in treatment. Generally, doctors do not expect that drugs alone will cure cancer, but drugs often give remissions of many months or years during which the patient is substantially free of symptoms.

Detection of *pre-cancerous* abnormalities, which in the course of time may develop into actual cancer, is one of the great benefits of regular medical checkups and alertness to symptoms. Many potentially cancerous abnormalities are readily recognized by doctors. Prompt treatment may well prevent cancer from ever developing.

Unorthodox treatments. Some persons who have cancer, or think they have, turn in hope or desperation to unorthodox treatments—more bluntly, quackery. Rarely do such treatments do physical harm. The tragedy is that precious time is lost during which recognized treatment might possibly bring the disease under control.

Older forms of quackery tend to disappear as they become discredited, but newer forms arise from time to time to be vigorously promoted by advocates. Self-defense requires some awareness of the hallmarks of quackery:

The treatment, if a medicine, is of secret composition, or a potpourri of "natural" substances or indeterminate chemicals. The treatment may be given by a mysterious machine which jiggles electric dials or glows strangely. It is alleged that "organized medicine" and governmental agencies will not give the product a fair trial. Testimonials from "cured patients" generally lack proof that the patient actually had cancer. It is implied that doctors wish to suppress any cancer cure because it would deprive them of patients and profits. The treatment usually has to be bootlegged or obtained at a private clinic which has no ties with orthodox medicine.

There are no useful treatments for cancer which are not known to or not used by reputable doctors.

What is Cancer?

Cancer is not a single disease but a group of several hundred diseases with a common characteristic: uncontrolled, invasive growth at the expense of normal body systems. "Something" transforms a living cell into a cancer cell, reduces its control over orderly growth and function, and transmits this abnormality to succeeding cell generations.

Many factors are associated with the occurrence of cancer: radiation, sunlight, chronic irritation, aging, genetics, inhalation or ingestion of innumerable kinds of chemicals. But the basic cause of cancer is unknown. However, the site where the cause acts is, many investigators feel, quite well pinpointed by circumstantial but persuasive evidence. A cancer cell's heredity, its genetic control of orderly function, is drastically changed. This must involve a chemical change in the genes and nucleic acids of the cell, which control life processes (see Chapter 25).

What makes a living cell cancerous and keeps it that way? More and more, our heredity-controlling molecules—nucleic acids—are prime targets of cancer research. Investigators seek knowledge of the complex chemistry of tumor induction—alterations of molecules—by which radiation, chemicals, viruses and unknown factors may incite cancer. From such knowledge there may come preventives and cures that are presently unknown.

Viruses

There is no conclusive proof that viruses cause human cancers, but few scientists seriously doubt that they can. Numerous animal cancers are known to be caused by viruses, and there is no known biological reason why man should be uniquely immune.

Viruses have their own genetic codes for transmitting hereditary traits. They contain the same classes of nucleic acids (DNA or RNA) as other forms of life. Their genetic machinery is enclosed in a protein coat which plays a part in causing familiar viral *infections* (see page 53). Hypothetical ways in which viruses may cause cancer are mysteriously different from the ways in which we "catch" common viral diseases.

One hypothesis is that a virus inserts some of its genetic material into the nucleic acids of a normal living cell. This changes the heredity of the cell, like a "bad" gene which gives distorted directions for some life process. The viral material "sickens" the cell's nucleic acids so that daughter cells inherit a trait of wild proliferation at the expense of normal cells—a characteristic of cancer.

Enormous difficulties confront investigators. The cancer-causing viral "gene" may lie latent for a long time until, or if, other factors trigger it into action. The viral part may be so fractionated or so transformed that it is nearly impossible for investigators to recognize it as having originated in a virus.

Vaccines. If certain viruses are identified as causes of cancer, preventive vaccines become theoretically possible. It is highly unlikely that we will ever have a single vaccine to prevent all forms of cancer. Prospects for individual vaccines to prevent a few forms of cancer are better but achievement is probably several decades away. An obstacle to future development of vaccines, which must be proved to be safe and effective, is the fact that neither society nor the consciences of scientists permit human trials of proved cancer-causing agents.

Immunity to Cancer

Probably we all produce a few cancer cells every day but never know it. The body recognizes the cells as abnormal and destroys them. Such is the immunological theory of cancer defense.

So-called immune systems defend the body against foreign agents by recognizing things that are not "self" and destroying them. We are most familiar with immunizing procedures such as vaccination, but defense systems are constantly alert to crack down on anything foreign that gets into the body. Cancer cells are presumably different enough from normal cells to be recognized as "foreign" and rejected before they can gain a foothold.

At least there is considerable evidence that immunity is somehow involved in cancer. Patients who receive organ transplants are given drugs which suppress their immune systems, to improve the chances that the transplant will not be recognized and rejected as a foreign body. Such patients have a somewhat increased risk of later developing cancer. Many cancer patients have definite impairment of immune responses, although whether this is a cause or a result of cancer is not known.

Researchers are studying the surfaces of cells, where most immunological events initiate, and looking into cancer cells for antigens which could be latent chemical fingerprints of long-vanished viruses.

Toward Better Therapies

Research pathways take unexpected turns and new directions. One can only make informed guesses about possible cancer cures and preventives that lie in the future.

If specific chemical events that induce cells to become cancerous are discovered, antagonistic chemicals to turn them off are conceivable. Little is known about constitutional differences of different kinds of cells—of the lung, uterus, bowel, etc.—which imply chemical differences in forms of cancer. If understood, the differences may lead to highly selective treatments which affect specific tissues rather than the whole body.

If our genes worked incessantly to carry out every order they contain, the result would be chaos—mob rule instead of teamwork. Monstrous overgrowth, not unlike cancer, would ensue if our genes were not inactive most of the time. Fortunately, cells have mysterious control units, probably chemical, which are sensitive to external conditions and give "feedback" orders that regulate gene activity. "Repressor" molecules that turn off gene activities have been identified in living cells. A repressor chemical that could stop the action of a malignant gene would indeed be a cure for cancer.

So-called "genetic engineering" has a wildly futuristic sound. The concept is that human genes, and hence heredity, may be alterable by inserting "correct" genetic information into living cells, perhaps with the transport help of harmless viruses. Much speculation along this and related lines concerns management of genetic diseases, discussed in the preceding chapter, but ultimate discoveries would be just as relevant to cancer if, as many investigators believe, cancer is basically a disease of DNA.

What causes surveillance mechanisms of the body to drop their guard so that stray cancer cells "leak" through immune defenses and become established? Immunologists may find ways of stimulating natural immunity to cancer which possibly, if not probably, exists in healthy people.

All of the above suggests an answer to the often-asked question, "Why can't a nation that can put a man on the moon find a cure for cancer?" It is incomparably more difficult to find a cancer cure than to rocket to the moon. We have less knowledge of the infinitely small than of the cosmically vast. Cancer, no less than life itself, is founded in the incessant transactions of atoms and molecules that conduct the business of living cells.

It has been estimated that one ten-trillionth of an ounce of DNA in a fertilized egg can be coded for genetic information that would fill 50 sets of a 24-volume encyclopedia. Scientists have barely got beyond the first page of the first set, but they are closing in.

CHAPTER 27

DRUG USE AND ABUSE

Modern drugs prescribed by doctors can produce enormously beneficial results, totally unavailable to grandfather's generation. Over-the-counter drugs bought without a prescription are useful in many minor conditions. Many sorts of drugs are readily obtained in our society. Unfortunately, unquestioned benefits of properly used drugs are endangered by widespread attitudes that medicines can magically overcome the ordinary stresses of life, that "there's a harmless pill for every problem." This false, indeed unhealthful, notion can lead to overmedication, resort to using pills to feel different than we do, habituation, and even to the very serious problems of drug addiction.

In a culture replete with casual "pill poppers," it is important that society and we as individuals develop profound respect for all drugs and chemicals and that we take our medicine exactly as directed. No drug that is useful at all is totally safe for all persons in all doses at all times. The safety of non-prescription drugs is predicated on the assumption that they will be taken exactly as specified on the label or package insert. Look at the label of a prescription drug. It names the one and only person for whom the medicine is intended, gives directions for taking, and often names the drug and strength of dosage, a practice recommended by the American Medical Association's Council on Drugs. "Follow directions exactly" is the beginning of

wisdom. (Classes of drugs most commonly prescribed are discussed in the ENCYCLOPEDIA OF MEDICAL TERMS).

Unless for treatment of chronic conditions, prescription drugs should be discarded after recovery from an illness. Drugs can deteriorate, and a stockpile of old drugs tempts one to self-prescribe for an undiagnosed condition. Don't hoard drugs. Keep current drugs in a medicine cabinet, apart from cosmetics and toothbrushes. Don't keep pills in handbags or on kitchen shelves where curious children can get at them. Teach children not to take medicines except those you give them because other kinds of pretty pills might make them very sick. Remember that children tend to model their drug-taking behavior after that of parents. Set an example in the home that can help protect the child as he grows up.

Dangerous Drugs

Any drug is dangerous if taken in excess. Some are dangerous if taken along with other drugs that a physician may not know his patient is taking unless he is told. But for present discussion, dangerous drugs will be considered to be those distributed in a vast illegal drug traffic which endangers the health and indeed the lives of innumerable addicts or drug-dependent persons.

One should first know the facts about drug abuse, although the causes and consequences are not yet fully understood.

The following facts are furnished by the National Clearing House for Drug Abuse Information, a division of the National Institute of Mental Health, the focal point for Federal information concerning drug abuse.

Marihuana ("pot" or "grass") is dried material from the Indian hemp plant, resembling coarse tobacco in appearance. A resin produced by the plant contains the active ingredient. Marihuana is usually smoked in cigarette form or in a pipe. It smells like burning rope. Most marihuana available in the U. S. is quite mild, mixed with seeds, stalks and leaves of low resin content. *Hashish*, about six times stronger than ordinary marihuana, is a concentrated resin of the plant that has been compressed into a mass from which portions are broken off for smoking in a pipe.

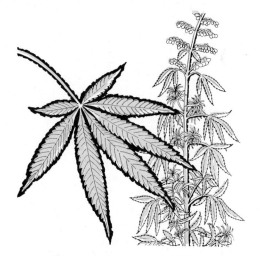

Marihuana leaf and plant.

Immediate physical effects of marihuana include reddening of the eyes, increased heart rate, and cough due to irritating effects of the smoke. Mood effects vary. Time may seem extended, sounds and colors intensified. There may be a false feeling that one is thinking more keenly. Some experimenters get very little reaction, some find the effects unpleasant. The user may be relaxed, happy, silly, talkative, or may withdraw into himself.

Marihuana does not cause physical dependency, hence is not addicting. Chronic users may become psychologically dependent on it, as a way of avoiding normal life stresses and problems. It has no known aphrodisiac property. Nothing in marihuana itself produces a need to use other and stronger drugs. Most marihuana smokers do not progress to heroin. However, a person who is predisposed to abuse a drug, in an environment where many drugs are readily obtainable, is likely to have an emotional need to seek out other kinds of drugs and to try them repetitively.

Young people are usually introduced to marihuana by 'friends' in their group who use and furnish the drug. Not all people who experiment with marihuana are alienated or disturbed, but "potheads" who use large amounts every day are likely to be.

'Hard' Narcotics

Narcotics relieve pain and induce sleep. Opiate narcotics are morphine, heroin, opium, and codeine, derived from opium. Several synthetic narcotics have morphine-like action. Narcotics are highly addicting; severe withdrawal symptoms ensue if accustomed doses are stopped. Experimenters who think "it can't happen to me" easily become "hooked" and require larger and larger doses of the drug to satisfy their "habits" or to avert painful symptoms.

The preferred drug of narcotics addicts is *heroin*, a white powder about six times more powerful than morphine. It is wholly illegal, and has no medical use in the U. S. A heroin addict usually injects a solution of the drug into a vein or under the skin, although the powder can also be sniffed through the nose. The typical reaction to a dose is reduction of tension, a brief "high" period, followed by near-stuporous inactivity.

Acute symptoms associated with heroin are sniffling, flushing, drowsiness, constipation, and contracted pupils. Abscesses, needle marks, and tracks along leg and arm veins are generally detectable. The addict's health deteriorates; death from an overdose is always a threat; injection of contaminated material can cause serious illness. Statistics indicate that an addict's life span is shortened by 15 to 20 years.

Hallucinogens

Hallucinogens (also called "psychedelics") are drugs capable of producing bizarre mental reactions—"visions," hallucinations, weird distortions of sensation, thinking, self-awareness and emotion. The most potent hallucinogen is LSD (lysergic acid diethylamide); some of the others are mescaline, peyote, and psilocybin.

LSD, often called "acid," is so potent that one ounce suffices for half a million doses. The drug can be taken in pill or capsule form but minute amounts are often dropped onto sugar cubes or almost any food. Immediate physical effects are enlarged pupils, flushed face, chilliness, sometimes increased heart rate. Mental effects somewhat resemble symptoms of schizophrenia, a severe mental illness. Often there is an *illusion* that one gains fantastic insights into one's personality and behavior. An LSD user may have a "good trip" with pleasant imagery and emotions or a "bad trip" with terrifying imagery and an emotional state of dread and horror.

LSD is not an addicting drug; it does not cause physical dependence. But it can cause panic reactions which lead to real hazards of suicide or accidental death. Heavy users sometimes develop subtle or pronounced signs of organic brain changes. It is not known whether such changes persist or whether they are reversible if LSD is discontinued.

Sedatives

"Downers" and **"goofballs"** are terms used by drug-abusers for sedatives and sleeping pills that have important medical uses. The largest group of sedatives is the *barbiturates,* which commonly have names ending in "-al"; for example *secobarbital.* Many family medicine cabinets contain barbiturates prescribed by physicians. Non-barbiturate sedatives, such as chloral hydrate, glutethimide and many others, have the same potential for danger, if misused, as the barbiturates.

Drug-cultists who go on barbiturate "jags" for thrills, or persons whose excessive use of the drugs creates tolerance and need for increasingly large doses, are seriously threatened. Barbiturate addiction is as real and hazardous as narcotic addiction. Heavy doses produce, not sedation, but restlessness, excitement, even delirium. Barbiturate addicts under the influence act like drunks; speech is slurred, gait unsteady, judgment impaired. In extreme cases, wild aggressive behavior, hallucinations, and delusions of persecution may develop.

Death may result from overdose or sudden withdrawal of barbiturates for a person who is a regular heavy user. Sudden withdrawal can be more dangerous than heroin withdrawal and is an acute medical emergency requiring hospitalization and intensive care. The help of a physician is necessary to break the "sedative habit."

Alcohol and sleeping pills are deadly in combination. The two drugs intensify each other's actions, so that less than lethal doses of alcohol and sleeping pills may be fatal if taken together.

Stimulants

"Uppers" and **"pep pills"** are slang expressions for stimulating drugs which increase alertness, reduce hunger and provide a feeling of well-being. The most widely prescribed stimulants are several forms of amphetamines, usually taken in tablet or capsule form. Large amounts of amphetamines "escape" into illegal traffic and are misused by persons who seek thrills or become dependent on them. Large and frequent doses can produce such pleasant effects—and such dread of severe fatigue and depression which follow if the drug is discontinued—that drug dependence can be established in a few weeks.

Amphetamines tend to increase the heart rate, raise blood pressure, produce palpitation and rapid breathing, dilate the pupils, and cause dry mouth, sweating and headache. Sporadic users may occasionally take amphetamines to stay awake, drive long hours, or cram for an examination. This type of abuse rarely leads to difficulties, but it may. Serious hazards threaten "spree" abusers who use amphetamines repeatedly for "kicks." Especially dangerous to themselves and others are "speed freaks" who inject amphetamine solutions into their veins to get an ecstatic "high." Under the influence of heavy doses the individual may become overactive, irritable, talkative, suspicious, sometimes violent, in combinations that can lead to belligerent or homicidal behavior.

Persons "hooked" on amphetamines are difficult to rehabilitate; treatment may require close support of family and friends plus medical help, and sometimes hospitalization.

Cocaine ("snow") is a violent stimulant that produces intense euphoria which the addict repeats as often as he can. Chronic use leads to delusions, hallucinations, wild behavior and mental disturbances which often explode into anti-social conduct.

Alcohol

A common drug subject to widespread abuse—one which young people often cite as more dangerous than marihuana—is beverage alcohol. Occasional or social drinkers (the great majority) control their intake reasonably well and are not necessarily alcoholic even though their consumption may be quite impressive. It is difficult to characterize an alcoholic except in generalities: a person whose job, responsibilities, income, are ruinously undermined by excessive drinking; who turns compulsively to drink to anesthetize problems; whose family and social life is disastrously sundered by drinking.

Some alcoholics are episodic drinkers who go on several sprees a year with intervening periods of sobriety. Others increase their drinking gradually and continually and merge into alcoholism insidiously. It is popularly believed that alcoholics are somehow allergic to or peculiarly poisoned by alcohol, but no definitive differences in body chemistries of alcoholics and non-alcoholics are known. There are apparent cultural factors; alcoholism is more prevalent in some ethnic groups and occurs in some families more often than in others.

The cure for alcoholism is abstention, which obviously requires great motivation on the part of the alcoholic. Chances of success are reasonably good if the alcoholic is not too old and has emotional support of family and friends, not so good if he has been drinking to excess for many years, is lonely most of the day and night, has nobody who depends on him (or her) and nobody who cares.

Medical treatments play a part in control of alcoholism (and are absolutely essential in management of acute alcoholism and delirium tremens). Aversion therapy makes use of a nauseant drug administered before the patient takes a drink; the ensuing upheaval is associated by him with a beverage which never acted that way before and which he begins to take unkindly to. Another drug, *disulfuram*, produces such a terrifying bodily reaction to alcohol that the patient doesn't dare to take a drink while he knows the drug is lying in wait in his system. Psychoanalysis is of little use in controlling alcoholism, but group psychotherapies are quite effective. The best known group, with a record of success as good or better than other ways of dealing with alcoholism, is Alcoholics Anonymous, composed of alcoholics who give aid, understanding and fellowship to group members. Local chapters of Alcoholics Anonymous in all cities and many small communities are listed in telephone directories.

Sniffing

Some youngsters, even 10-year-olds, sniff the vapors of volatile substances from plastic bags or directly from aerosol cans. They expect to get a feeling of exhilaration. They get symptoms resembling acute drunkenness—slurred speech, double vision, unsteadiness, drowsiness. They may also get temporary blindness, damage to bone marrow, kidneys, liver, brain and lungs, and sudden death.

Substances favored by sniffers—airplane glue, varnish, paint thinners, cleaning and lighter fluids, gasoline, spray-paint, refrigerants, spot removers, benzine, any vaporous substance they can experiment with—are not intended for inhalation. Some of these substances are immediately dangerous and some are cumulatively toxic when repeatedly used. Sudden death has resulted from paralysis of breathing following inhalation of freezing sprays, and from inhalation of some substances that act rapidly and irreversibly so there is no escape.

Drugs and Our Children

There is no certain way of recognizing a person who is abusing drugs. He may look quite normal. Some signs, however, may alert parents to the possibility that a member of the family is misusing drugs: inability to hold a job or stay in school, needle marks in arms or legs, abandonment of old friends, association with strange companions, disappearance of drugs from the home medicine cabinet, spending much time in a locked bathroom, dropping previous interests, unusual activity around hangouts, using the jargon of addicts, spending large amounts of money.

Not everybody who experiments with drugs becomes physically or psychologically dependent on them. Sharp distinctions cannot be drawn, but authorities cite certain traits that are fairly common in addiction-prone persons who may adopt drugs as a way of life. Many have feelings of personal inadequacy and hopelessness and seek easy chemical solutions to problems of work, striving, and human relations which they cannot grapple with realistically. Delinquency and use of "hard" drugs go hand in hand; most narcotic addicts were delinquent prior to taking drugs.

Drug addicts associate with addicts. Novices are usually introduced to drugs by friends or acquaintances. In an environment in which many kinds of illegal drugs are available, the temptation to experiment and not "chicken out" with one's social group is great.

What if parents discover that a youngster is seriously involved with drugs? Harsh denunciation and punitive attitudes don't get far. Ideally, parents should have factual information about drugs (inaccurate information is worse than none) and be able to talk out problems with firmness but not hostility. Some youngsters feel, sometimes rightly, that parents can't understand or "level" with them. Other lines of communication can be tapped in most communities: the family doctor, a clergyman, school counselors, community mental health centers which have drug-abuse units. A physician can generally assure patients that discussion of drug abuse problems will be kept confidential. Practically all enforcement agencies cooperate with the person who wants help.

Detailed, continually updated information about drug abuse can be obtained from the National Clearing House for Drug Abuse Information, P. O. Box 1080, Washington, D. C. 20013.

Emergency Telephone Numbers

		Address	Telephone
Doctor	Office	_____	_____
	Home	_____	_____
Pediatrician	Office	_____	_____
	Home	_____	_____
Hospital		_____	_____
Ambulance		_____	_____
Poison Control Center		_____	_____
Fire Dept.		_____	_____
Police		_____	_____

At places of work

Husband	_____	_____
Wife	_____	_____

Relatives and others

_____ _____

_____ _____

_____ _____

_____ _____

_____ _____

_____ _____

CHAPTER 28

FIRST AID AND YOUR FAMILY

by DONALD G. COOLEY

FIRST RULES FOR FIRST AID

WHAT YOU NEED TO HAVE ON HAND

ARTIFICIAL RESPIRATION

BLEEDING

SHOCK

BROKEN BONES

BANDAGES AND BANDAGING

TRANSPORTING THE INJURED

WOUNDS, CUTS, AND BRUISES

SPRAINS, STRAINS, AND DISLOCATIONS

BURNS

POISONS

BITES AND STINGS

EYES

FOREIGN BODIES

FREEZING INJURIES

HEAT ILLNESSES

UNCONSCIOUSNESS

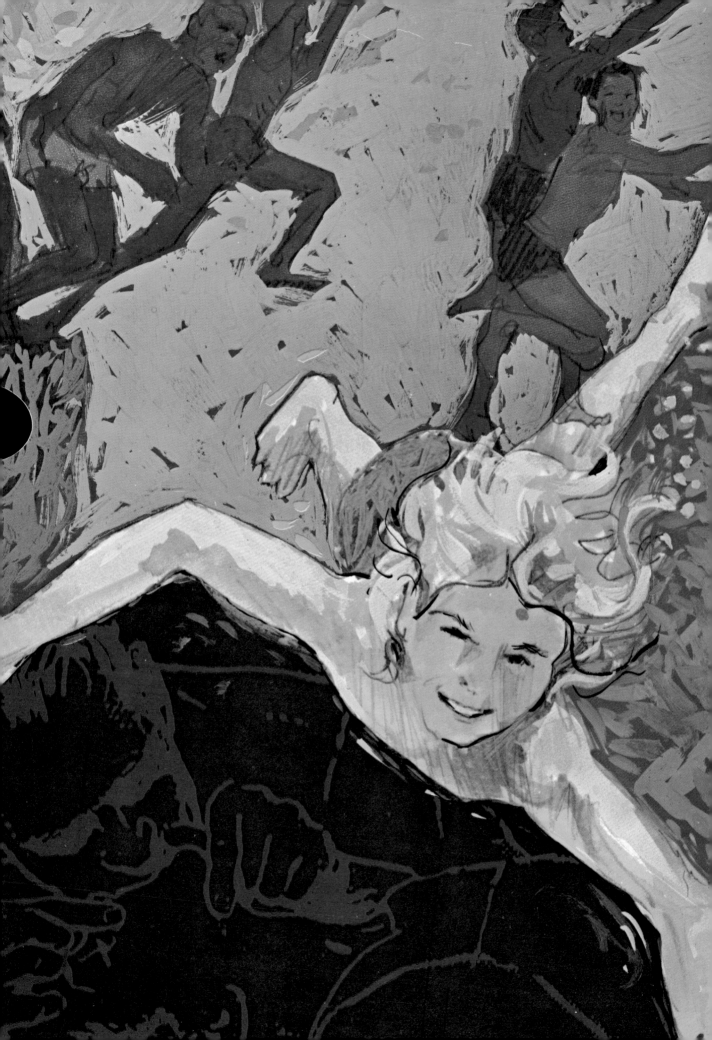

CHAPTER 28

FIRST AID FOR YOUR FAMILY

by DONALD G. COOLEY

First aid is *first* aid — what to do before the doctor comes. It is never a substitute for medical help. First aid is the means by which an informed layman can take lifesaving measures in emergencies and avoid doing harm.

Many first aid measures are quite simple and do not require "split-second speed" in their application. Haste without knowing what one is doing can be worse than doing nothing at all. At other times, *immediate* informed action is essential to save a life or prevent serious complications or aftereffects; action which can only be taken by someone who is on the scene at the moment when minutes are vital.

The first aid measures described in this chapter are up to date and reflect current concepts and practices appropriate in specific circumstances. It is wise to learn about first aid *before* emergencies happen so you will be prepared to give help safely and beneficially when necessary. At least one member of the family should take a first aid course such as the training given by the American Red Cross and other agencies.

Information given in this chapter is terse, concise, stripped to essentials for immediate application when time is important. Index at right locates topics quickly. Many subjects are discussed in more detail in other chapters of this book (see General Index).

FIRST AID INDEX

First Rules for First Aid 822

What You Need to Have on Hand. . .822

Artificial Respiration 823

Bleeding 830

Shock 834

Broken Bones 835

Bandages and Bandaging. 841

Transporting the Injured 846

Wounds, Cuts, and Bruises. 847

Sprains, Strains, and Dislocations. .850

Burns 852

Poisons 853

Bites and Stings 858

Eyes 861

Foreign Bodies 863

Freezing Injuries 864

Heat Illnesses 864

Unconsciousness 865

FIRST AID RULES FOR SERIOUS EMERGENCIES

If Patient Has Stopped Breathing:

Give immediate *mouth to mouth resuscitation* (see page 824).

Make sure that *air passages are open* in *any* unconscious or injured patient. Turn head to one side if nose and mouth are filled with fluid, blood, vomit. Wipe out with finger or handkerchief. Pull tongue forward if it has slipped back to plug throat.

If Bleeding Is Serious:

Apply *pressure* directly over wound until bleeding stops.

Press *hard* with your hand against gauze, wadded cloth, clean handkerchief placed over wound. Use heel of bare hand in emergency. Keep pressing steadily; do not dab. If wound is in leg or arm, elevate limb above level of body and support with pillow or padding. *Do not* elevate injured part if bones are broken.

Do *not* apply tourniquet unless all other measures to stop bleeding fail.

Prevent Shock

Cover patient, keep him *comfortably* warm, not hot or sweaty.

If he can swallow, give warm fluids or "shock solution" — 1 teaspoonful of salt, ½ teaspoon of baking soda, dissolved in 1 quart of water. Give by spoonful.

Do *not* give person in shock anything by mouth if he is unconscious, half-conscious, vomiting, or if he has an abdominal wound.

Do Not Move Victim

Never move patient from scene of accident while waiting for medical help, unless absolutely necessary. Keep him lying flat on back on level surface. Do not lift head, do not help him to sit or stand, do not bundle him into sitting position in back seat of car. Always keep in mind that hasty dragging, pulling, can cause broken bones to cut nerves irreparably. Splinting should be done at the site of the accident. See *Transporting the injured* (page 846).

WHAT YOU NEED TO HAVE ON HAND

Home first-aid supplies (can be bought as unit at drugstore) should be kept in a special container or shelf, separate from other home medical supplies, should not contain poisons, and should never be locked with a key!

Always keep supplies in same place and return materials after use. Replace missing or depleted items promptly. Check condition of supplies regularly. If sterile packages have been broken, replace with fresh units.

Basic supplies mentioned in this chapter will suffice for immediate care of most injuries. You may add other items, but don't clutter the first-aid kit.

Home First-Aid Supplies

Sterile gauze compresses and pads, individually packaged, 2, 3, and 4 inches square.

Sealed roller gauze bandages, 1, 2, and 3 inches wide (elastic crepe bandages are easiest to apply).

Adhesive strip bandages with gauze pads, assorted sizes.

Adhesive tape.

Sterile absorbent cotton.

Large triangular bandages: laundered and ironed muslin, sheeting, about 40 inches square, cut diagonally to make 2 bandages.

Clean sheets, pillowcases, handkerchiefs can be made relatively sterile by ironing just before use.

Equipment

Scissors, rounded ends; tweezers; card of safety pins.

Medicines and Materials

Tube of petroleum jelly or package of impregnated gauze.

Table salt (or salt tablets).

Baking soda.

Aromatic spirits of ammonia (stimulant; dose: ½ teaspoonful in ½ glass of water).

Mineral or olive oil ("sweet oil"), sterile.

Universal antidote for poisons (buy from druggist).

Auto First-Aid Kit

Road accidents may cause injuries too large to be covered by a small gauze compress.

Large bandages may be needed for slings, burns, splinting. Improvised materials may not be available at the roadside. Carry these essentials in car in metal or plastic box, or impervious plastic bag. Antiseptics are not necessary if victim will soon receive medical care.

6 sterile gauze compresses or pads about 6 inches square.

Sealed gauze compresses in smaller sizes.

3 or more rolls of sterile gauze bandages, 2-inch width and wider.

6 or more triangular bandages (see *home first-aid supplies*).

Absorbent cotton.

Petroleum jelly, tube.

Scissors.

Safety pins.

Travelers' Medical Supplies

If you plan to travel in foreign countries, or to camp or work in regions remote from a doctor or hospital, ask your physician about medical supplies you should carry with you. Thermometers used in foreign countries are usually marked in the centigrade scale unfamiliar to most Americans. You may wish to take along a familiar Fahrenheit thermometer. If you wear glasses, take along an extra pair. Also be sure to carry your lens prescription.

Home Medicine Cabinet

Common household remedies, as well as drugs prescribed by a physician, should be stored separately from toothpaste, shaving cream, and other simple items of daily use. Even the simple home medicines which are quite harmless if properly used may be toxic if taken in huge overdosage. If there are children around the house, home medicines should be kept under lock and key in a cabinet of their own, or at least should be dependably inaccessible to youngsters. In addition to first-aid supplies and medicines for personal use, the following items are useful to have on hand in readiness for emergency: *Clinical thermometers, oral and rectal; ice bag; hot water bottle; eye cup; paper cups; flashlight; tongue depressors; cotton-tipped applicators; rubbing alcohol; milk of magnesia; calamine.*

For a Safe Medicine Cabinet

Do not take medicine in the dark or without reading label — if label is lost, discard bottle . . . Throw out all prescription drugs left over from past illnesses . . . Give a prescription drug only to the patient for whom the physician ordered it . . . Date all drug supplies when you buy them . . . Mark all poisons; seal lid with tape, run pin through cork, put sandpaper strip on bottle . . . Dispose of old drugs safely — best done by pouring down sink — so that they are not accessible to children and pets.

ARTIFICIAL RESPIRATION

If a person has stopped breathing *from any cause*, start artificial respiration at once. Seconds count! The most efficient and practical way to save a life is to blow your breath into the victim's lungs — like inflating a balloon, letting out the pressure, inflating again. You can do this without help or equipment. A child can save the life of an adult with this method.

If foreign matter is visible in the victim's mouth, wipe it out quickly with your fingers or cloth wrapped around your fingers.

For an adult, blow vigorously at a rate of about 12 breaths per minute. For a

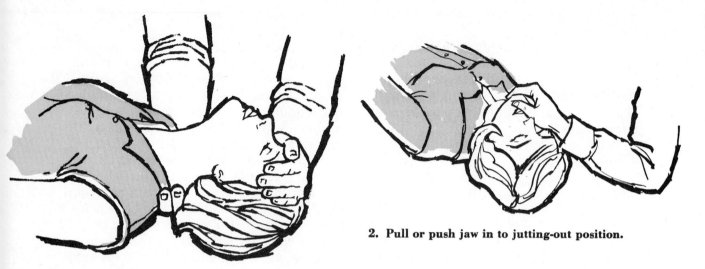

1. Tilt victim's head back so chin points upward.

2. Pull or push jaw in to jutting-out position.

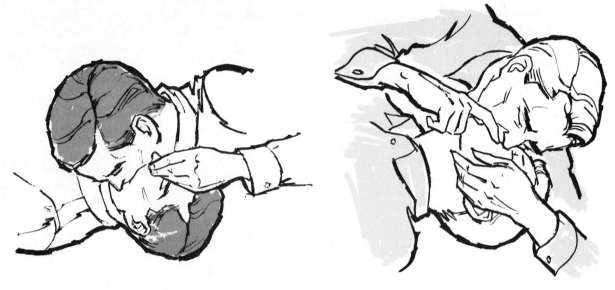

3. Open your mouth wide, place it tightly over victim's mouth. Pinch victim's nostrils shut.

OR close the victim's mouth and place your mouth over the nose.

OR close nostrils with pressure of your cheek.

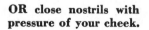

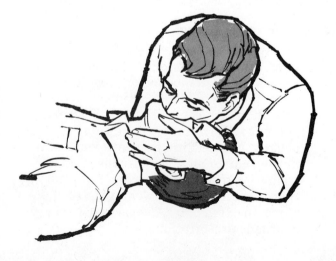

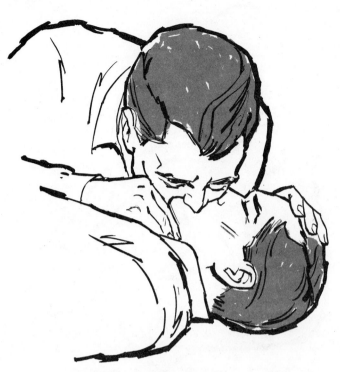

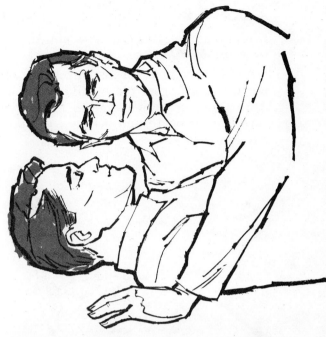

5. Remove your mouth, turn your head to the side, listen for outflow of air from victim's lungs.

4. Blow into victim's mouth or nose, about 12 breaths per minute for adult.

child, take relatively shallow breaths at a rate of about 20 per minute.

If you are not getting air exchange (expansion of victim's chest, return outflow when you remove your mouth), re-check head and jaw positions; make sure mouth and throat are clear.

If you still do not get air exchange, turn victim on his side and give several sharp blows between shoulder blades in hope of dislodging foreign matter. Again sweep fingers through mouth to remove foreign matter. A handkerchief or cloth may be placed over the victim's mouth or nose if the rescuer wishes to avoid direct contact. Several layers of cloth will not greatly affect air exchange.

Start artificial respiration immediately and continue until doctor arrives or you are positive life is gone. It is the victim's only hope of life while rescuers with equipment are on the way.

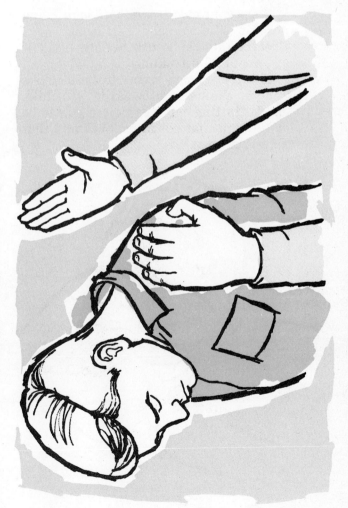

Several sharp pats between shoulder blades may dislodge foreign matter from victim's throat.

Artificial Respiration

Infants and Small Children — Mouth to Mouth Technique

1. Clean visible foreign matter from mouth with finger; place child on back; use fingers of both hands to lift lower jaw from beneath and behind so it juts out (as with adults).

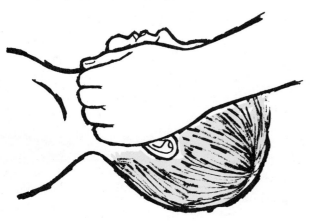

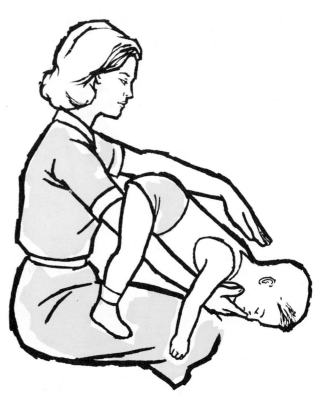

Place your mouth over *both mouth and nose* of child to make "leakproof" seal. Breathe into child with shallow puffs of air, about 20 per minute.

If air exchange seems to be blocked, and you cannot breathe easily into child, check "jutting out" position of jaw to be sure tongue has not fallen back and that airway is open.

2. *If* air passages are still blocked, suspend child by ankles — or — hold child head-down over one of your arms and give several sharp pats between shoulder blades to help dislodge obstructing matter from air passages.

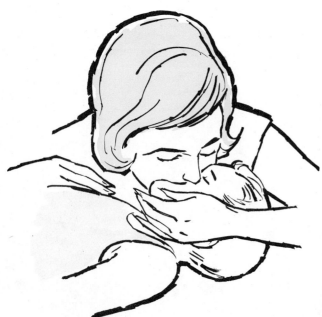

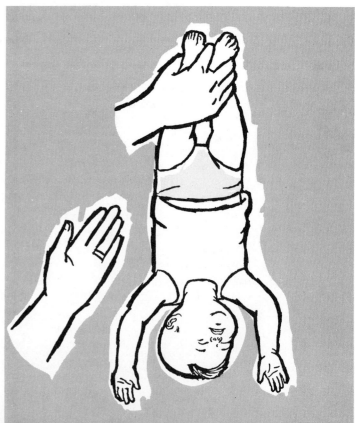

Continue artificial respiration until the victim begins to breathe for himself or until a physician pronounces the victim dead. Time your efforts to breathe into the victim to coincide with the victim's first attempt to breathe for himself.

Normally, recovery is rapid except in *electric shock,* and *drug* or *carbon monoxide* poisoning, which may require artificial respiration for long periods.

Back Pressure-Arm Lift Resuscitation

Other resuscitation measures do not move so much air as direct mouth to mouth, are less efficient, more exhausting to the rescuer, but first-aiders should have an alternative, such as the Back Pressure-Arm Lift method. This method can be used only if victim has no arm injury. Wipe visible foreign matter from victim's mouth with finger or cloth wrapped around finger.

1. Place victim face down, bend his elbows, place his hands one upon the other. Turn his head to one side, extend as far as possible so chin juts out.

2. Kneel at victim's head. Place your hands on flat of his back so your palms lie just below an imaginary line between his armpits.

3. Rock forward until your arms are nearly vertical, with weight of upper part of your body exerting steady even pressure downward on your hands.

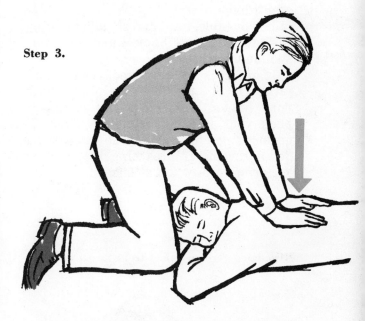

Step 3.

4. Immediately draw the victim's arms up and toward you. Lift enough to feel resistance and tension at his shoulders. Then lower his arms to ground. Repeat about 12 times per minute. Check mouth frequently for obstruction.

A Chest Pressure-Arm Lift method is also taught by the Red Cross. Check with your local unit.

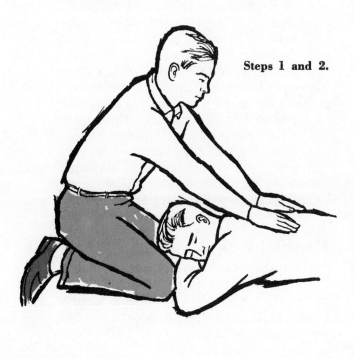

Steps 1 and 2.

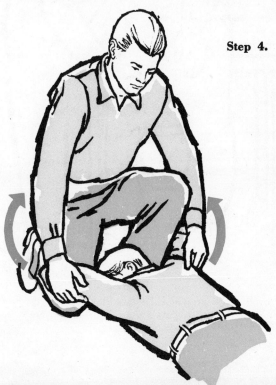

Step 4.

Choking from Foreign Object in Windpipe or Throat

If a child, hold up by heels and slap back hard between shoulder blades. If an adult, have him lie face down over edge of bed or table, head and shoulders hanging down. Slap back hard between shoulder blades.

If object is not dislodged, rush to hospital. Do not try to grasp object with your fingers unless you can obviously hook your fingers around it. There is great danger of pushing object farther down throat. If breathing stops, start *artificial respiration* at once.

Dislodging foreign object from throat of adult.

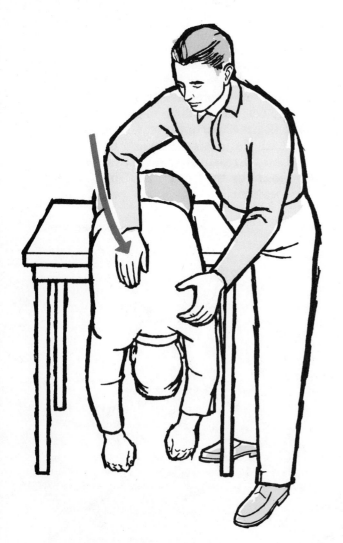

Drowning

Begin *artificial respiration* the instant a near-drowned person is landed. Do not waste time trying to "empty water out of the lungs" by jackknifing or rolling on a barrel. Turn victim's head to side, clean foreign material from mouth, so stomach contents can clear. Begin artificial respiration. Continue without interruption until help comes. Check to see that tongue is clear and airway open at all times. Keep victim warm.

Gas Poisoning (Carbon Monoxide Poisoning)

Get victim into fresh air. Protect *yourself* in entering gas-filled area. A wet cloth over your nose does not protect you. Tie a rope around yourself so someone can pull you out if you fall.

If the victim's breathing has stopped or is irregular, give artificial respiration continuously. Send for oxygen device from local police, fire department, or ambulance service. Give continuous artificial respiration until trained operator with oxygen arrives.

> ### *Prevent Asphyxiation Tragedies*
> Children put small objects into their mouths and sometimes "inhale" them. Keep beans, peanuts, fruit pits, buttons, pins, beads, coins out of reach of small children. Permit no toy smaller than child's fist. Check toys for parts such as doll's eyes that may come loose and be taken into the windpipe ... Never leave a small child alone in a bathtub for a second ... Have gas heaters, ranges, appliances, home furnaces checked regularly by trained servicemen. Never run car engine with garage door closed. Have car exhaust system checked periodically.

Electric Shock

First, shut off current or remove victim from contact (extreme caution — see directions) then give immediate prolonged artificial respiration until you can get someone to help.

Electric shock: whenever possible, turn off current before attempting rescue. If necessary to break victim's contact with live wire, rescuer must insulate himself from earth and victim with DRY non-metallic, non-conducting materials — board, rope, thick newspapers, rubber car mat. Anything DAMP is dangerous.

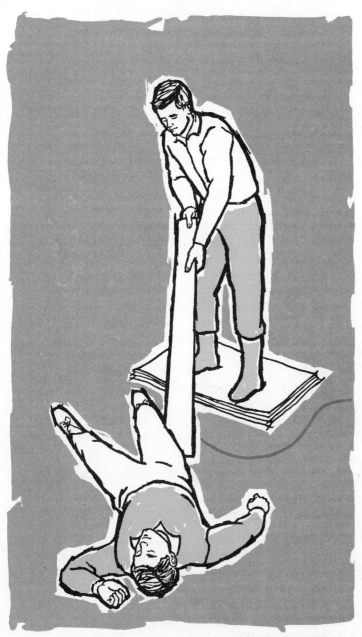

Serious electric shock paralyzes breathing centers, causes unconsciousness. Ordinary house current can cause fatal shock under some circumstances.

Don't touch victim until current is turned off or victim is free of contact with current — you may be risking your life by electrocution.

If indoors, or if switch is near, turn off current at switch.

If outdoors (live wires, no switch) have someone phone electric company to turn off current, but don't wait for this. If victim's muscular contractions have thrown him free of current he may be touched at once. Otherwise, proceed with *extreme caution.*

Insulate yourself from the earth and the victim with *dry* nonconducting materials, such as a long length of dry rope, rubber car mat or cloth. But remember that very few materials are bone-dry, and that you are risking your life.

Never Use Anything Metallic, Wet, or Damp

It may be simplest to pull wire away from victim, as below:

Stand on *dry* newspapers, *dry* board, *dry* rubber floor mat of car, *dry* folded coat.

Use *dry* stick, *dry* board, *dry* rolled newspapers or floor mat to pull or push wire from contact with victim.

If victim lies on wire he may be pushed from it with a *dry* board. Or he may be pulled away with a *dry* rope. Insulate your hands with *dry* gloves, cloth, newspapers. If your hand is insulated you may with *caution* grasp a *dry* part of the patient's clothing and drag him away (do not touch shoes; nails may conduct).

After contact is broken, give immediate *artificial respiration* and continue until help arrives. If victim's body stiffened, do not assume that he cannot be revived. Breathing centers paralyzed by electric shock take a long time to recover — victims have recovered after eight hours of artificial respiration. Don't get discouraged and give up.

Lightning

Use the same first aid as for electric shock except that victims may be touched immediately and artificial respiration can begin at once.

To avoid danger from lightning, seek lowest point, ditch, depression; avoid isolated trees. One of safest places to be in a lightning storm is inside a car.

Have all switches and appliances in locations that can't be touched from bath, shower, sink . . . Never have electrical appliances where they can fall into water, tub, sink . . . Don't touch anything electrical while standing on wet floors or in puddles . . . Touch nothing electrical if your hands are wet . . . Have electrical equipment permanently grounded . . . Remove fuse before making electrical repairs . . . Replace all frayed electric cords. Children chewing on frayed wires can get frightful mouth burns or fatal shock. Cover unused wall sockets with protective plates, seal with adhesive tape, or use inexpensive blank plugs, so children can't push nails or hairpins into opening and receive serious or fatal shock . . . Never touch a dangling wire: may be charged by crossing power line farther back. Call utility company if wire is down in yard; keep children away . . . Don't use metal ladders in proximity to electricity (may be grounded if touch live wires — short circuits) . . . If your car should run into live wire, touch no metal, stay in car until help arrives.

BLEEDING

Serious Bleeding from Wounds, Injuries

Deep cuts, severed blood vessels, spurting or oozing blood: press clean cloth firmly against wound.

Remove enough clothing to see wound clearly. Cover wound with sterile compress and apply *firm hand pressure* directly over wound. Exert firm, steady pressure, not intermittent. Press with finger, hand, or heel of hand until bleeding stops.

Use clean materials, such as sterile gauze, folded clean handkerchiefs, freshly laundered or ironed towels, strips from sheets to cover bleeding point.

If no sterile items are available, do not hesitate to use clothing, soiled materials, or bare hand to stanch flow of blood by pressure. Blood loss is more dangerous than immediate risk of infection.

Bleeding from Legs, Arms

If wound is in arm or leg, *elevate* limb, support with pillows or similar padding. Raise bleeding part above level of body. *Do not* elevate limb if bones are broken or fracture is suspected.

Think first of pressure in severe bleeding wound. Direct finger or hand pressure is the safest and most rapid measure to stop bleeding. Firm sustained pressure and elevation of arm or leg will usually control most bleeding.

Pressure Dressing

When bleeding stops, apply *pressure dressing*. Put gauze compress or folded layers of clean cloth over bleeding point (do not use fluffy absorbent cotton in direct contact with wound). Press compress with fingers and apply suitable bandage to fix dressing in place. Preferably, use gauze compress bandage: strip of cloth with thick layer of gauze in center and tails for wrapping and tying. Many bleeding wounds can be controlled by *pressure dressings alone*.

Bandage must not be *too tight*. Wound area may swell. Inspect occasionally. If edge of bandage cuts into flesh it is too tight; loosen it a little. Otherwise, do not disturb or remove bandage after it has been applied. If blood oozes into bandage, cover with another protective folded layer of bandaging material.

General Measures

Do *not* apply salves, ointments, or any medicines to deep wounds, unless told to by doctor. Covering wound with sterile gauze or clean cloth protects against further contamination.

Do *not* try to cleanse a deep or seriously bleeding wound (bleeding cleanses it internally) unless medical help is long delayed or there is gross contamination.

If essential, cleanse skin around wound with clean (tap or boiled) water stirred with soap to make sudsy solution. Scrub your hands first with soap and water.

Cover wound and small area of surrounding skin with sterile gauze. Dip a tuft of sterile absorbent cotton into soapy solution, apply gently to exposed skin, stroking *away* from wound.

Use fresh cotton tuft for each stroke. Greases and oils may be removed by kerosene, naphtha, rubbing alcohol. Always wash *away* from wound. *Keep patient lying down.*

Suspect Shock

Some degree of *shock* is imminent in all cases of serious bleeding. Have shock victim lie flat on back. Cover patient, keep him comfortable, not overheated. Loosen tight clothing. Cut clothing away if necessary, to avoid twisting, turning, or manipulating patient. *If patient is conscious,* not vomiting, give saline mixture made by dissolving 1 teaspoonful of table salt and ½ teaspoonful of baking soda in 1 quart of water.

Give in small sips as tolerated by patient. Do not give *stimulants*. Do not give anything by mouth if patient has *abdominal wound or if internal bleeding* is suspected.

Pressure Points to Stop Bleeding

In all serious bleeding, *first* try *manual pressure* directly upon wound, *pressure bandage,* and *elevation of limb.*

These are most *rapid* and *safe* measures which control most cases of serious bleeding and need no special training. If bleeding does not stop, or resumes after pressure bandage is applied, press with fingers or hand against proper *pressure point of body where blood vessels pass over bone.*

Pressure at these points shuts off blood like clamping a rubber hose. But *do not waste time* in a serious emergency trying to locate pressure points unless you know about them from first-aid training (ask your Red Cross chapter about instruction courses).

If *immediate* application of pressure against compress directly over wound does not stop violent flow of blood, or if bleeding resumes, exert finger or hand pressure at these points:

Bleeding from Head Above Eye Level
Press with finger against head just in front of the ear (shown below).

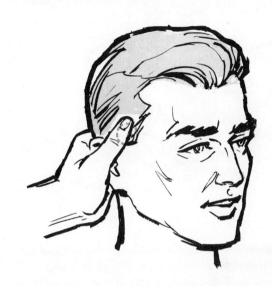

Bleeding Below Eye and Above Jawbone
Press fingers against notch in jawbone which is about one inch in front of the angle of the jaw (shown below).

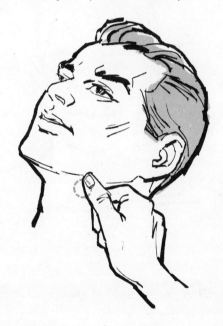

Bleeding from Neck, Mouth, Throat
Place thumb against back of neck, fingers on side of neck below Adam's apple in depression at *side* of windpipe. Press fingers *toward* thumb.

First Aid

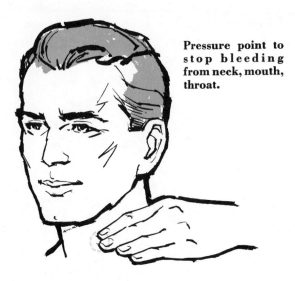

Pressure point to stop bleeding from neck, mouth, throat.

Forearm bleeding: Pressure pad inside elbow, tighten forearm against pad, bind.

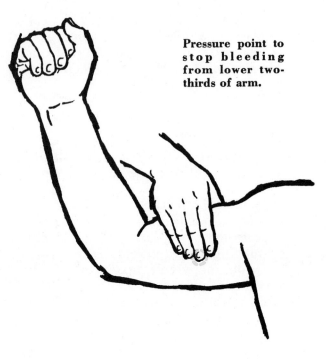

Pressure point to stop bleeding from lower two-thirds of arm.

Bleeding from Armpit, Shoulder, Upper Arm

Place fingers or thumb in hollow behind patient's collarbone, press against upper surface of first rib (shown below).

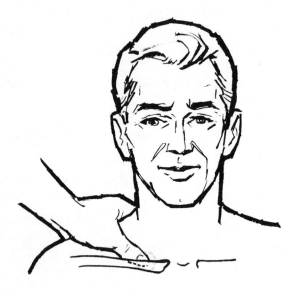

Bleeding from Foot, Leg, Thigh

Place heel of hand in middle of depression on inner side of thigh, just below fold of groin, press down against bone (shown below).

Bleeding below knee: Pressure pad in back of patient's knee, tighten lower leg against pad, bind.

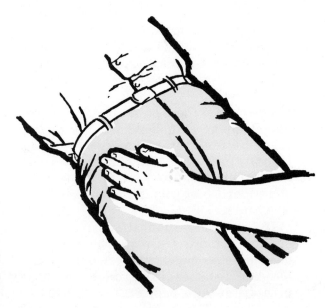

Bleeding from Hand, Forearm, Lower Two-Thirds of Arm

Press against arm bone halfway between armpit and elbow, thumb inside arm, fingers outside.

Bleeding from palm of hand: Place thick pad covered with sterile gauze in palm, close fingers over it, bandage into patient's closed fist.

Tourniquet for Life-Threatening Bleeding

A tourniquet is a dangerous instrument. It is a constricting band around a limb which shuts off blood to points beyond it. Tissues die (gangrene) if deprived of blood too long.

A tourniquet is of value as a first-aid tool *only when there is partial or complete amputation of a body part* — at risk of a limb to save a life. There must always be unbroken skin between the bleeding wound and the tourniquet.

Massive Bleeding from Arm or Leg

General *position* of tourniquet: *Between wound and heart*.

For *arm* bleeding: about hand's width below armpit.

For *leg* or *thigh* bleeding: about a hand's width below groin.

Place tourniquet as close to wound as possible (to save more of limb if amputation becomes necessary) but not at edge or directly over wound.

Tourniquet Materials

Any fairly wide band (about 2 inches) long enough to go twice around limb with ends left for tying. Belt, stocking, scarf, strip torn from clothing or cut from inner tube in emergency — many first-aid kits contain tourniquet that buckles. Do *not* use wire, rope, cord, which cut into flesh, except in dire emergency.

How to Apply Tourniquet

Wrap band twice around limb, tie half knot, place stick over knot, tie tight knot over stick. Twist stick to tighten *just enough to stop blood flow*. Tie free end of tightened stick with another bandage to hold in position. (Shown at right).

Do not loosen or remove tourniquet once it has been carefully applied. Fatal blood loss may result from intermittent loosening. Get as soon as possible to a doctor.

Leave tourniquet in plain sight. *Do not hide* with bandage, clothing. Mark *"TK"* on patient's forehead with lipstick, charred match. Note *time* when applied.

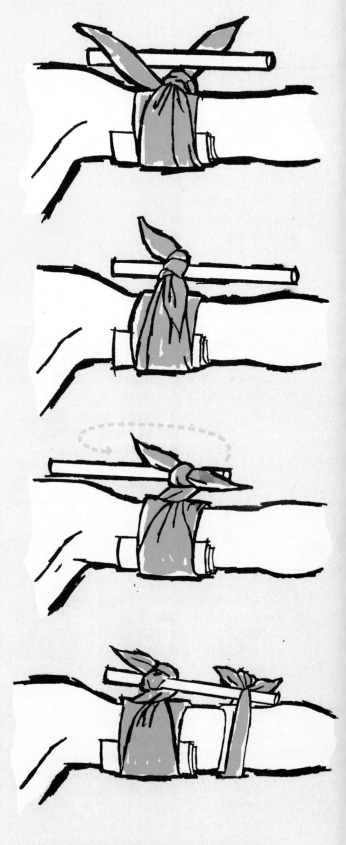

Drawings show successive steps in applying and securing tourniquet. Remember that tourniquets can be dangerous; see text at left; apply only if absolutely necessary.

Internal Bleeding

Injuries may cause *internal* bleeding, with or without outward signs of blood loss. *Suspect* internal bleeding after any severe blow, blunt or crushing injury to abdomen, chest, torso.

Some signs of internal bleeding:

From *stomach:* vomited material looks like large coffee grounds.

From *upper intestines:* stools contain dark tarry material (partly digested blood).

From *lower intestines:* bright red blood in stools.

From *chest, lungs:* coughed-up blood is bright red, frothy.

Some injuries give only *general* signs in internal hemorrhage: *restlessness, anxiety, thirst, pallor, weakness, rapid but weak pulse.* Suspect internal bleeding; get doctor at once.

Keep patient warm, quiet, lying on back, head turned to one side if vomiting or coughing. Keep breathing passages clear of obstruction. Patient with bleeding from lung may not be able to breathe if lying flat — if so, prop high enough so he can breathe.

Nosebleed

Quickest way to stop nosebleeds: Pinch nose between thumb and forefinger for 10 to 15 minutes.

Another way: Put pad of cotton, tissue, or soft cloth under upper lip. Press against nose firmly with forefinger laid along lip.

If bleeding persists, plug nostril *gently* with small strip of loosely rolled gauze. Push backward *(not* upward) into nostril no farther than little finger can push it. Leave strip of gauze dangling for easy removal.

Do not blow nose for several hours after bleeding has stopped. Most nosebleeds stop by themselves and are not serious. If nosebleeding persists or recurs, consult a doctor.

SHOCK

Every serious accident, burn, poisoning, injury is virtually always accompanied by some degree of *shock*, perhaps mild, but often serious, and fatal if shock becomes irreversible. Shock is caused by bodily reactions which slow or stop the circulatory mechanisms, and symptoms are essentially those of insufficient blood supply to vital organs.

After giving immediate lifesaving first aid — stopping bleeding, making sure patient's breathing passageways are open, giving artificial resuscitation if necessary — always think of shock before taking other time-consuming first-aid steps. *Expect* shock to develop after any serious injury. Take preventive steps *before* the doctor arrives to take over.

Signs of Shock

Weakness
Rapid but weak pulse
Pale face
Skin cold, clammy with perspiration of forehead, palms; patient may have chills
Thirst
Nausea
Shallow, irregular breathing
Blood pressure very low (late sign)

Immediate First Aid to Lessen Shock

First deal with any immediate life-threatening emergency that the injury requires.

1. Have patient lie flat, head level with or lower than rest of body (unless he has head injury, in which case, elevate head slightly. Caution: see *broken neck).*

Equivalent of head-lowering, to help flow of blood to heart and brain, is most easily accomplished by elevating legs to height of 12 to 18 inches, if nature of injury permits.

2. Cover patient, protect him from cold ground, air, loss of body heat. Keep him warm but not too warm — just on the warm side of chilling. The object of this is not to heat the patient but to keep him from cooling.

3. Do not let patient see injury. Reassure him. Handle very gently. Pain increases shock.

4. If patient is conscious, not vomiting, does not have abdominal injury, give *shock solution:* 1 teaspoonful of table salt, ½ teaspoonful of baking soda, dissolved in 1 quart of water. Measure proportions carefully.

Give patient all he will drink.

If available, a cup of strong black coffee or tea is helpful.

Get doctor as soon as possible. Patient should be in better condition when doctor arrives if you take above steps promptly.

BROKEN BONES

Suspect broken bones if:

Victim can't move injured part.
Part is deformed, wrong shape.
Pain when trying to move.
Lack of feeling when touched.
Swelling and blueness of skin.

If in doubt, treat as a fracture.

A *simple* fracture exists under unbroken skin and may not be obvious. A *compound* fracture shows bone protruding from the skin, or an open wound at the fracture site; frequently there is severe bleeding from the wound.

General Principles of First Aid For Fractures

Great harm can be done if patient is moved hastily, pulled, bundled into back seat of car, allowed to stand, sit up, or move injured part. A fracture itself almost never is an emergency that requires great speed in treatment. Unless essential for safety, *do not move* or disturb patient while waiting for doctor or ambulance.

If victim *must* be moved from great danger, pull at legs or armpits along axis of body.

Examine first for other injuries. Stop serious bleeding by hand pressure on gauze dressing over wound.

Check mouth, throat for possible obstruction of breathing. Keep airway open. Give artificial respiration if needed.

If necessary, cut away clothing with great care not to disturb injured part.

Keep patient warm, lying down.

Do not put pillow under head if neck is injured but block head with padding to prevent neck movement.

If medical help will be delayed and patient must be transported:

Do not try to set bones.

Always apply *splints* before moving or transporting patient.

Splint the patient where he lies.

Apply clean dressing and bandage (no antiseptic) if bone protrudes through skin or skin is broken.

See *Transporting the injured.*

Splinting Materials

The purpose of a splint is to give the broken part constant support, immobilize it, prevent bone ends from grinding together. Almost anything that is rigid enough will serve in an emergency — boards, sticks, rifle barrel, umbrella, cane, jack handle, tightly rolled magazine or floor mat. The splint must be long enough to extend above and below adjacent joints to prevent motion. Hard objects must be well *padded* with cotton, cloth, soft materials, before placing in contact with injured part.

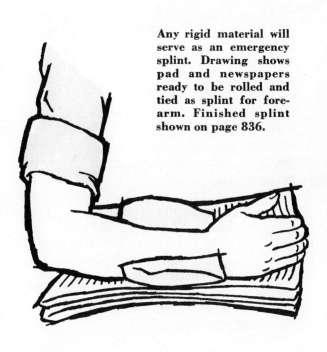

Any rigid material will serve as an emergency splint. Drawing shows pad and newspapers ready to be rolled and tied as splint for forearm. Finished splint shown on page 836.

Broken Arms or Legs

Forearm or Wrist

Have patient lie on back. *Gently* place forearm across chest, right angle to upper arm, palm flat on chest. Prepare 2 padded splints: an inside splint from elbow to palm, an outside splint from elbow to back of fingers. Tie splint in place with 2 bandages, one above, one below the fracture. Adjust necktie sling to hold finger tips 3 or 4 inches above level of elbow unless forearm is more comfortable at a different level.

Newspaper splint: cover fracture site with thick gauze bandage, roll folded newspaper over it; tie.

If splint unavailable, bind arm firmly to side with cloth strips around chest. Support with sling.

In arm fractures: Watch patient's finger tips. If they become blue or swollen, loosen splint slightly. Remove rings, bracelets, wrist watches or other objects which would be hard to get off should arm and fingers swell.

If fingers turn blue, loosen splint.

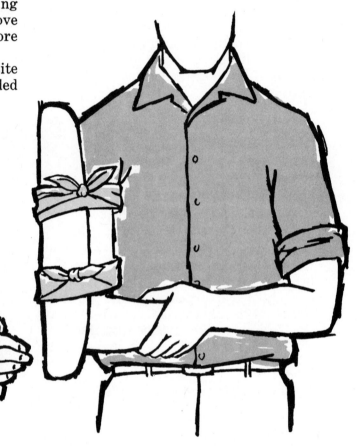

Make splint longer than bone it supports.

Upper Arm (Elbow to Shoulder)

Place arm gently at side in as natural position as possible, forearm at right angles lying across chest, palm side in. Make splint longer than bone it supports. Place 1 padded splint outside arm, from slightly below elbow to slightly above shoulder. Tie with two cloth strips, one above, one below fracture site. Support forearm with necktie sling. Bandage upper arm to body with towel or cloth passed around splint and chest, tied under opposite arm.

Elbow

If elbow is bent, do not try to straighten it. Put arm in sling and bind it firmly to body.

If arm and elbow are straight, leave that way. Put a single padded splint on inside of the arm, from finger tips nearly to the armpit. Tie securely above and below (not over) the elbow. Caution: Splint must not protrude into armpit with such force as to cut off blood supply.

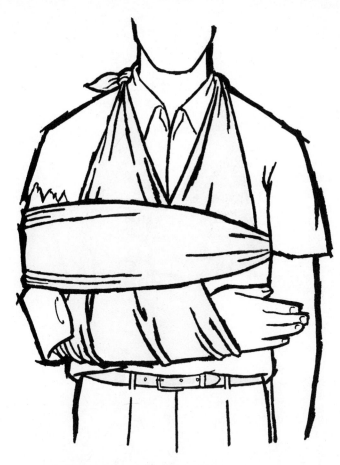

Necktie sling supports splinted upper arm or forearm. Bandage tied around chest as shown minimizes jolting movements.

Broken Leg (Lower Leg, Knee to Ankle)

Caution! Jagged bones may break through skin or cut blood vessels if roughly handled. Use care.

Remove shoe gently; cut laces, leather. Grasp foot firmly and pull slowly to straighten leg and foot to normal position. If working alone, tie feet together after leg is in normal position. Otherwise, hold leg in position while assistant prepares splints.

Pillow splint: Slide folded blanket, robe, or firm pillow under injured leg — lift leg no more than necessary, while supporting broken bones. Tie pillow splint around leg in five places. Use stick or any rigid object for added stiffness.

Board splints: Two padded splints, boards about 4 inches high, reaching from just above knee to just beyond heel. Pad especially well at ankle. Put a splint on each side of leg; tie as shown.

If no splints available, put blanket, folded towels, soft cloth between patient's legs and tie injured leg to sound leg (but *not* if break is near ankle).

Broken Thigh (Upper Leg, Hip)

Very serious. Treat for shock. Get doctor as soon as possible. Injured leg may be shortened, foot flops, victim can't raise heel from ground when lying with knees flat. But there may be no deformity, injury may look like a bruise. When in doubt, treat as fracture. Put one hand under heel, other over instep, steady the limb and pull gently into normal position. If working alone, tie feet together temporarily.

Prepare 7 broad long bandages or cloth strips. Use small stick to push them under hollows beneath knees and back.

Use two board splints, 4 to 6 inches wide, well padded. Outer splint should reach from armpit to heel, inner splint from crotch to heel and tie.

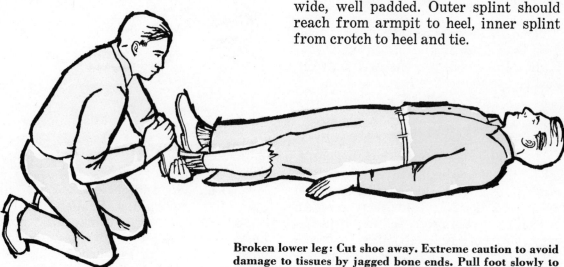

Broken lower leg: Cut shoe away. Extreme caution to avoid damage to tissues by jagged bone ends. Pull foot slowly to straighten leg. Splinting procedures shown on page 838.

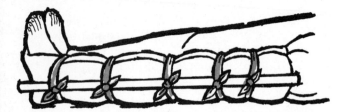

Pillow splint tied around broken lower leg in five places; stick or other rigid object gives stiffness.

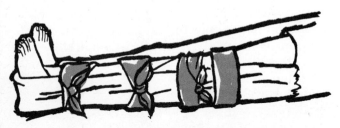

Two board splints on either side of leg; pad well between boards and leg; tie as shown.

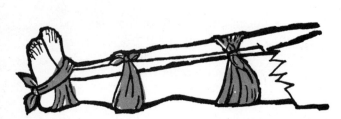

If no splints available, tie injured leg to good leg with padding between (e.g., rolled blanket).

If no inner splint available, put padding between legs and tie legs together. If no splints available, pad well between legs to use uninjured leg as a splint.

If toes become bluish, swollen, loosen splint slightly.

Broken Kneecap

Straighten leg gently, rest leg on 4-inch-wide board splint underneath leg. Pad splint, extra padding under knee and ankle and tie. Leave kneecap exposed. Watch for swelling; loosen ties if necessary. Caution: if knee joint fractured, or if you're in doubt, do not try to straighten patient's leg.

Broken Ankle

Pillow splint or rolled blanket extending well beyond heel. Tie as shown.

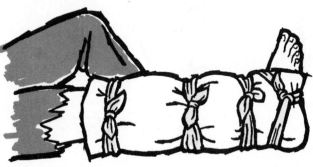

Broken Foot or Toes

Place padded splint under sole of foot and tie, but not too tightly.

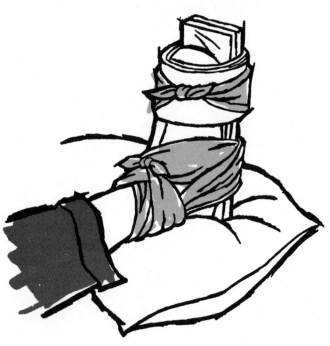

Trunk Fractures

Ribs

Broken rib indications: Pain on breathing or coughing. Shallow breathing to lessen pain. Patient may hold hand over break to limit chest motion when he breathes. Put broad pad over break. Put broad cloth strip around chest, tie single knot over pad. Tighten second knot. Tie two similar bandages in place, to give firm support. Broken ribs should not be bandaged with great force and tightness because of danger of rib end puncturing lung.

Alternative: Make a tight chest binder from pillowcase, sheet strip, any large cloth. Wrap tightly around chest when patient exhales; fasten the chest binder securely with safety pins.

Caution! If patient coughs up bloody froth or bright red blood (lung puncture) *do not* apply tight bandages. Get medical aid immediately. Give first aid for *shock* until doctor takes over.

Hand Fractures

Padded splint under palm, from near elbow to beyond finger tips. Tie.

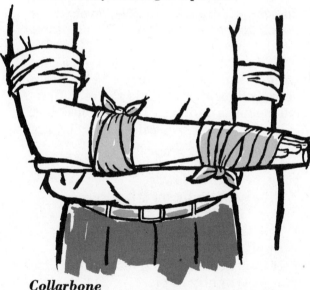

Collarbone

Indications: Fractured ends usually can be felt by passing fingers over curved bone above top ribs. Patient usually

cannot raise arm above shoulder. The injured shoulder will be lower than the other when arms hang.

Put arm in triangular bandage sling, finger tips exposed, adjust height to most comfortable position. Tie arm to body with towel or cloth over sling.

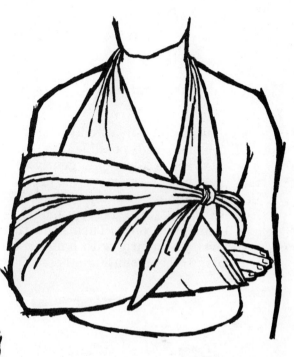

Pelvis

Serious! Broken bones of pelvis (basin-shaped structure between spine and lower limbs) may damage important organs. Car accidents, squeezing, crushing hip injuries may fracture pelvis. Signs: great pain in pelvic region; possible difficulty in urination. If in doubt, treat as fracture. Extreme care in handling person with fractured pelvis!

Broken pelvis: Bandage ankles, knees together; work broad bandage under hips and tie if absolutely necessary to transport victim.

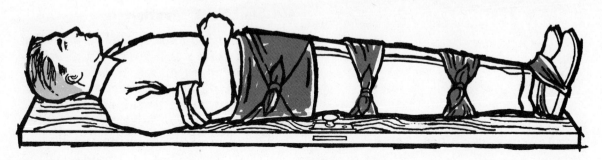

Don't move patient if medical help is on way. Keep him lying down. Bandage ankles and knees together, legs straight or knees bent, whichever is most comfortable to patient.

If patient must be moved, slide broad bandage under hollow of back, work under hips, tie snugly but not tightly or fasten with safety pins. Transport patient face up on board or stretcher (see *Transporting the injured*).

Head and Face Fractures

Jaw (Lower)

Jaw usually sags; saliva trickles; teeth out of line or loosened; possible bleeding from mouth. Raise lower jaw gently to normal position, support with broad bandage under chin tied at top of head.

If patient vomits, bleeds from mouth, *remove* bandage at once. Turn head to side, support jaw gently with hand, replace bandage when vomiting stops.

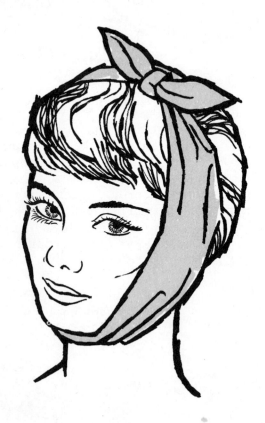

Bandage for jaw fracture; remove at once if patient vomits or bleeds from mouth.

Nose

Don't splint a broken nose. Gauze may be inserted into nostrils if not forced in upward direction, but pushed gently straight back. If there is bleeding, press sides of nose together between thumb and index finger for several minutes. Press cold cloths over nose. Have patient hold head back slightly, breathe through mouth. Apply sterile dressing if open wound. Get prompt medical attention for patient to prevent deformity.

Skull (Fracture, Concussion)

Assume that any severe blow to the head, whether or not the patient is "knocked out," is a skull fracture or concussion (bruise of the brain). *Any person who has suffered head injury should be kept quiet and be seen by a doctor as soon as possible,* even if he seems to have "recovered." Symptoms may be delayed.

Immediate First Aid: Keep patient lying down, warm; do not let him sit up or walk. Keeping quiet is the only first-aid means of reducing internal bleeding.

If face is *flushed,* raise head slightly with pillow or pad.

If face is *pale,* keep head on level with body, or slightly lower.

Give *nothing* by mouth.

Turn head to side, so secretions can escape from mouth.

Apply cold cloths to head.

If scalp is bleeding, bandage gauze compress lightly in place — do *not* press hard on skull bruise or depressed area (may drive bone fragments into brain).

If necessary, transport in lying-down position, head supported by pads at sides to prevent any jarring.

Get doctor as soon as possible.

Broken Neck or Back

Utter tragedy can result if a victim of spinal injury is moved by well-intentioned but uninformed persons. Slight movement of head or back may sever nerves and cause paralysis or death. What you *don't* do the first few minutes is more important than what you do.

DO NOT move or lift patient from where he lies until medical help arrives.

DO NOT bend or twist his head or body in any direction.

DO NOT put pillow under his head or give drink of water or a cigarette.

DO NOT pull him out if he is imprisoned in wrecked car, unless danger of fire — wait for medical help.

DO NOT jackknife him into back seat of a car and rush to hospital — first see *Transporting the injured.*

What to Do:

Suspect a broken back or neck and treat it as a fracture if the patient has had a bad fall, a "whiplash" neck injury, a crushing or impact injury, or, in fact, has taken part in any accident in which the back or neck is bent or struck.

If patient is conscious, ask him to move hands and fingers. If he cannot, suspect neck fracture. If he cannot move feet and toes, suspect back fracture. He may complain of pain in neck or back. There may be no other sign. Consider circumstances of injury.

Summon the doctor and an ambulance at once. While waiting for the doctor and ambulance, keep the patient warm and covered; do not move him, lift him, or allow any person to do so.

If patient *must* be transported to the doctor, see *Transporting the injured.*

Prevent broken bones. Good housekeeping — nothing to fall down, to trip over; dry, clean floors. Carpet slippery floors; anchor small rugs by placing rubber sheet underneath. Good light everywhere; no dark cluttered stairways. Rubber mat in bathtub. Handrails where needed. Don't use furniture for stepladder. Position ladders securely; check rungs. Screen windows securely. Sprinkle icy walks with ashes or sand. Replace ragged carpets. Smooth rough thresholds. See that children's toys are picked up. Check house for objects that might be tripped over: footstools; chairs with spraddly legs.

BANDAGES AND BANDAGING

In an emergency, do not try to apply bandages in complex, precise, professional ways unless you have had special training. The first-aider's bandages will be replaced by a doctor. Elastic bandages, types which conform to body contours, adhesive compresses, help to make bandaging simpler.

1. First, apply sterile gauze compress big enough to cover wound. Apply bandage over compress.

2. Bind firmly but *not* too tightly — just enough pressure to stop flow of blood. Wound may swell and make bandage so tight as to shut off circulation. Watch for swelling, blueness, edge of bandage cutting into flesh — warnings to loosen the patient's bandage.

Materials

Sterile packaged materials in many sizes, including the largest, should be parts of every first-aid kit: roller gauze bandages (can be folded to make compresses), adhesive bandages, bandage compresses, sterile gauze compresses (get some large sizes), cotton rolls (never use fluffy cotton bandage in direct contact with bleeding wound).

Freshly laundered and ironed sheets, handkerchiefs, napkins, pillowcases, towels make suitable improvised dressings. In emergency, use cleanest cloth available.

Triangular bandage: Very useful. Make from muslin, sheet, clean cloth, about 40 inches square; cut diagonally to make two bandages. *Fold* to make strong, long bandages (cravat bandage) of desired width.

Universal protective dressing: Pending medical aid, serves to cover and protect limb wounds, as splint in fractures, pressure treatment of burns.

Layer of sterile gauze (covering compress if open wound). Then, 1-inch layer absorbent cotton.

Wrap with several layers of muslin or clean cloth.

Cover with waterproof plastic film, such as film used for food wrapping.

COMMON BANDAGES

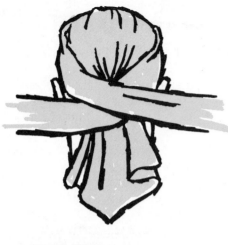

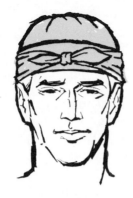

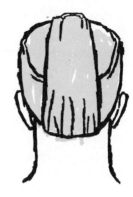

SCALP, FOREHEAD: Tie triangular bandage as shown; "tail" secured with safety pin.

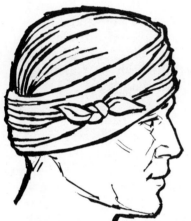

EAR, HEAD: Tie cravat bandage over a compress covering wound.

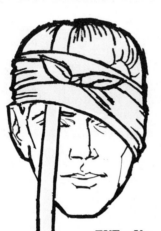

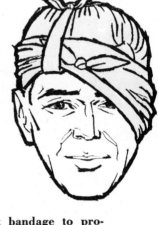

EYE: Use cravat bandage to protect injured eye; snug but not tight.

INJURED PALM: (1) Wrap cravat around hand, leaving thumb out. (2) Carry lower end of bandage back of hand around base of thumb. (3) Wrap remaining ends of bandage around hand and fingers; tie.

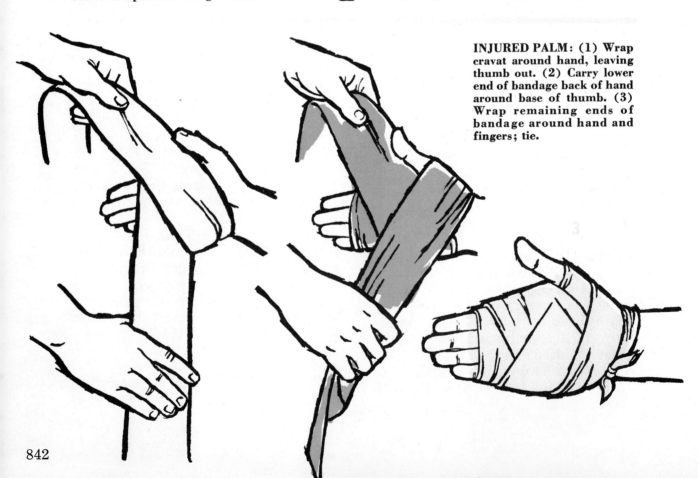

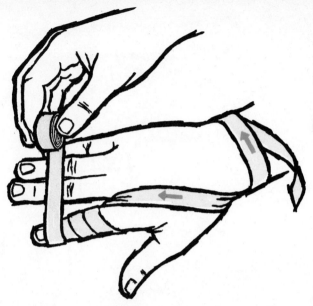

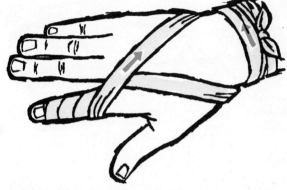

FINGER BANDAGE: First anchor one end of gauze at wrist. Wrap bandage in spiral down finger, then back to wrist; tie at wrist.

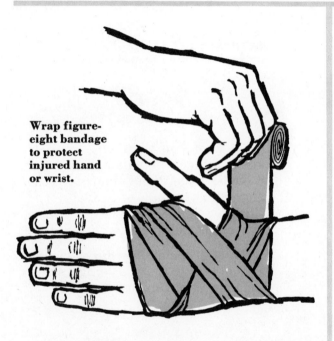

Wrap figure-eight bandage to protect injured hand or wrist.

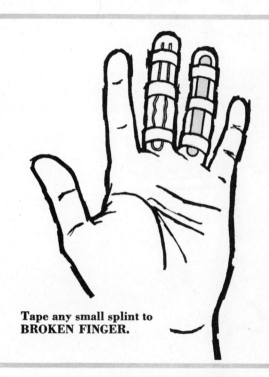

Tape any small splint to **BROKEN FINGER.**

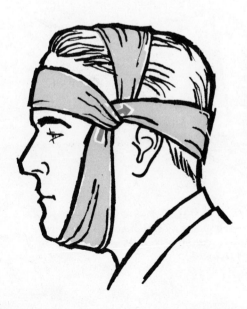

CHEEK OR EAR BANDAGE: Start with middle of bandage over compress at wound. Cross ends at opposite side of the head, tie over the compress.

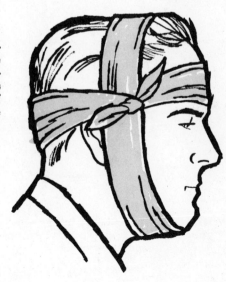

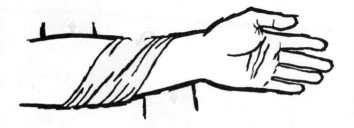

FOREARM: Start spiral bandage on small part of injured limb.

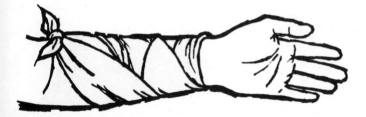

Wrap spiral bandage as far up injured limb as needed.

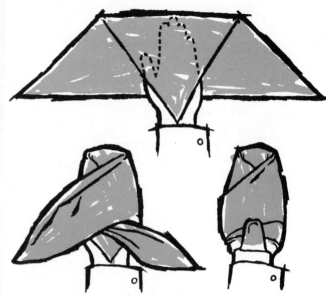

HAND OR FOOT BANDAGE: Use triangular bandage, wrap around as shown, tie.

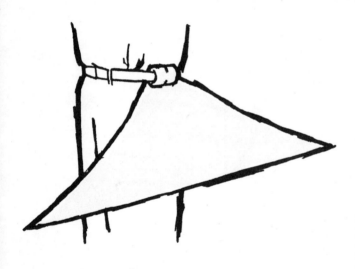

To *hold compress* on elbow or knee, use cravat bandage at least 8 inches wide. Bend elbow to right angle. Place middle of bandage over elbow; continue ends around limb above and below elbow; tie.

To *stop palm bleeding*, clench wad of gauze between fingers, tie bandage over fist.

HIP OR GROIN: Cover injury with large triangular bandage. Tuck top of bandage under a belt. Tie bottom ends around leg.

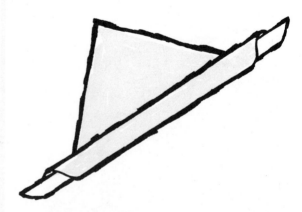

TORSO BANDAGE: Begin by rolling large base of triangular bandage up part way. Complete as shown in top drawing on opposite page.

Torso Bandage

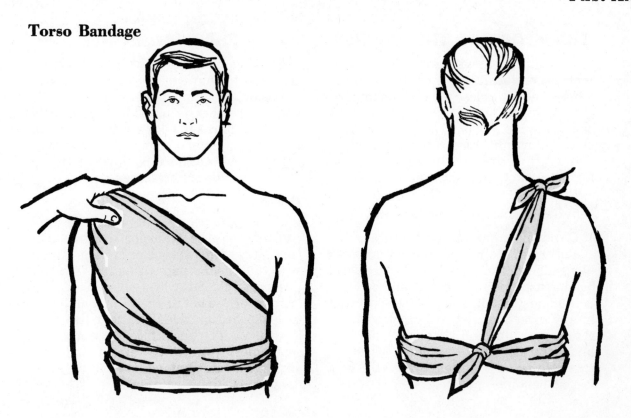

Tie rolled part of triangular bandage (shown on preceding page) at waist. Put point of triangle over shoulder. Adjust to cover wound. Tie extra cloth to top; tie free end at back of waist.

Arm Sling

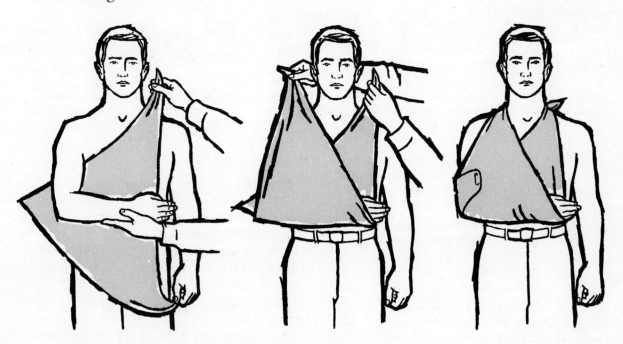

Use triangular bandage to make arm sling. Tie behind neck, but be sure knot isn't directly over spine. Pin corner at elbow. If forearm is injured, elevate hand slightly above level of elbow.

TRANSPORTING THE INJURED

If medical help will soon arrive, do not move a seriously injured person from where he lies unless absolutely imperative for his safety. Haste is rarely necessary, may do grave damage. Take first steps in first aid (page 822) while help is on way. If victim *must* be transported, do any necessary splinting where he lies.

Moving Broken Neck Victim

Do not move before medical aid arrives.

Put rigid "stretcher" such as door alongside victim. One person kneels at head, grasps victim's head firmly between both hands, steadies it so it does not twist in any direction. Helpers grasp victim's clothing at hips and shoulders and *slide* him carefully onto stretcher. *Move his entire body* as if patient were stiff as a log, no bending anywhere.

Moving Broken Back Victim

Treat same as for broken neck except that pad to conform to shape of natural curve or "hollow" of back is needed if board stretcher is used. It is relatively easy to put broken back victim *face down* on a blanket, and transport. Keep the broken back victim face down if transferred to ordinary stretcher.

Vehicle

If *ambulance* is not available and patient *must* be transported some distance, try to get a truck or station wagon with flat floor; pad will ease jolts. If passenger car must be used, remove rear cushion or use board or padding material to make bed on which patient lies full-length. Don't "jackknife" patient into seat unless you are certain his injuries are slight. Jolts, bumps, sudden stops are dangerous; drive cautiously.

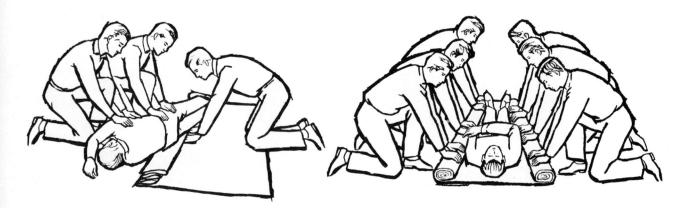

Blanket stretcher (not for victims of broken neck or back). Push rolled edge of blanket under victim's back, turn him onto blanket. Roll both edges of blanket toward victim to give firm carrying support.

If broken neck victim is lying on face, or crumpled: One person kneels and grasps victim's head at jaw angles, exerts traction so head does not turn or move. Then a helper gently straightens and supports legs. One or two other helpers gently turn body onto stretcher — head and neck turning in unison.

Put rolled cloth, sweater, pads around sides of head to prevent rolling. No pillow under head. Fold victim's arms, tie body to board stretcher.

If not sure whether victim has broken neck or broken back, treat as broken neck.

Blanket Stretcher

For patients (*except* broken neck or back) who must be lifted or carried in lying down position. If broken bones, *splint* before moving. Blanket with edges rolled (or rug, or other stout fabric) is usually simplest stretcher to improvise, for *carrying* or *lifting* patient.

Tuck folded blanket edge against patient. Turn him slightly away, very carefully push blanket under him as far as possible. Turn him back to center of blanket, pull edge through.

Roll both edges of blanket toward patient in center. Rolled edges give firm grasp for carrying or lifting. Two bearers at each side, preferably three.

Carrying Without A Stretcher

When victim need not be carried in lying down position. Consider nature of injury. *Never* use these for broken neck or broken back patient.

Three persons kneel, slide hands under victim's body, lift him to their knees in unison, then rise to their feet while turning victim toward their chests. Work as a unit, co-ordinate movements.

If you must work alone, put one arm under victim's knees, other arm around his back, lean back slightly, lift victim to carrying position.

WOUNDS, CUTS, AND BRUISES

Immediate first aid for major wounds: stop *bleeding*, combat *shock*, keep breathing passages clear of obstruction, and give *artificial respiration* if necessary. Suspect *broken bones*. Keep victim warm and covered. Do not move him unless absolutely necessary (see *Transporting the injured*). Elevate wounded limb unless fractured. Give no stimulants until bleeding stops. Cover wound with sterile dressing or clean cloth and get doctor at once. Do not use antiseptics unless told to by doctor. See specific headings.

Abdominal Injuries

"Closed" wounds of abdomen (no break in skin) are easily overlooked. Suspect if victim has suffered severe blow, fall, or crushing injury of abdomen. May be internal bleeding. Little can be done until surgeon explores. Keep patient warm, lying on back. Give nothing by mouth, not even water. Get doctor at once.

"Open" wound of abdomen — deep wound, cut, stab, shot. Sterile dressing or clean cloth over wound to draw edges together, stop bleeding, give protection. May be internal bleeding. Get doctor at once. Keep patient lying flat on back, warm. See *puncture wounds*.

Protruding Intestines

Exposed intestines *must not be allowed to dry out*. This could be fatal. Cover immediately with large sterile dressing and bandage (or clean cloth in emergency) which *must be kept constantly moist*. Use warm salt water to moisten, preferably, boiled water with 1 teaspoonful of salt to pint. In emergency, use cleanest water you can get; intestines must not dry for an instant. Do not try to put intestines back in place. Give nothing by mouth. Keep patient warm, on back, knees bent with rolled blanket or coat under knees. Get doctor at once.

Abrasions

(Skinned Knee, Scraped Elbow)

Scraped skin surface bleeds or oozes blood. If coarse bits of dirt are in wound, pick out with small tweezers sterilized by passing through match or gas flame. Rub gently with bar of plain mild soap under running water, or wash lavishly with soap and water and clean cloth or pieces of sterile gauze or cotton (fresh piece for each swabbing). Rinse under running tap water. Cover with sterile dressing or adhesive bandage. If dirt is ground into wound, see doctor.

Blisters

Water Blisters; Blood Blisters

Caused by pinching, rubbing, or chafing skin. If blister is small, unbroken, not likely to be injured: wash gently with soap and water, cover with sterile gauze or adhesive compress; leave alone until fluids are absorbed naturally.

A large blister is likely to be broken or to rupture spontaneously. Anticipate this by opening blister. Sterilize needle by holding in flame. Puncture edge of blister at two points. Press with sterile gauze to force out fluid. Cover with sterile dressing or adhesive bandage. Do *not* open blisters caused by major burns.

If blistered skin has been rubbed off, exposing raw surface: Clean with warm soap and water and sterile cotton swabs. Cover with sterile dressing. Watch for signs of infection (spreading redness, radiating red lines, pus). At first signs, contact doctor as soon as possible.

Bruises

(Contusions)

Caused by blows or falls that break small vessels under skin without breaking surface. Injury is first red, then discolored ("black eye" is typical bruise). Minor bruises need little first aid. *Caution:* internal bleeding may accompany bruises of abdomen; other severe bruises may involve broken bones — see doctor. If skin is broken, treat as open wound.

For minor bruises, immediate treatment to relieve pain and limit discoloration is application of cold — ice bags, cloths wrung out of very cold water. *After* a day or so, heat may be applied. Your doctor may think it helpful to try newer enzyme treatments which may reduce swollen discolorations quite rapidly.

Chest Wounds

("Sucking" Injuries)

Crushing blows, punctures, stabs, gunshot wounds may create an opening from lungs to outside air. Air may enter and blow out of the wound with "sucking" or hissing sounds. Froth or bubbles may be seen. Stop up this opening *immediately.* Put your hands at each side of wound, push together as victim exhales, to plug the opening. Cover wound with compress and bandage to make airtight, bind firmly. Have victim lie down but keep his shoulders slightly raised, supported with pads, torso turned toward injured side. Get doctor at once.

Give nothing by mouth. Do not attempt to lessen shock by elevating feet, if doing so makes breathing more difficult.

Cuts and Scratches

If Small, Minor:

Wash the area well with a mild soap and a clean cloth or with cotton swabs that have been dipped into warm soapy water (city tap water is safe to use).

Rinse under running water from faucet or poured from pitcher.

Cover with adhesive bandage or sterile gauze held by adhesive tape.

If Deep, Extensive:

Don't apply medicines.

Control bleeding by hand pressure over gauze pad, clean cloth or handkerchief, until doctor arrives. Tie bandage over sterile dressing if help is delayed.

If skin around wound is grossly dirty, and patient is far from medical help, clean gently with soap and water after bleeding stops, washing *away* from wound. Other dirt such as grease may be removed by naphtha, kerosene (never motor fuel — contains lead) or rubbing alcohol.

Deep cuts may need stitches to minimize scars — always get medical aid.

Gunshot Wounds

Control bleeding, think of fractures; treat like other wounds. Don't probe, or put antiseptics into wound. Also see *puncture wounds.*

Puncture Wounds

Penetrating, Perforating Injuries

Inflicted by relatively small objects driven under skin, sometimes deeply, or entirely through body, leaving entrance and exit wounds (perforating wounds). Examples: stepping on nail; bullets or shot; wood, glass, or metal splinters; particles driven by firecrackers, firearms or other types of explosions.

A small puncture wound may be washed with soap and water, rinsed under running water. Cover with dressing or adhesive bandage. But the entrance point of a puncture wound is usually small, bleeds little. It cannot be cleaned in depth. It is useless to try to force antiseptics into the wound. Do not attempt it.

Treat like other wounds according to immediate emergency (shock, fracture). *Encourage* bleeding to "wash out" wound from inside, by gentle pressure around its edges, if you are sure this will not cause further injury to the wound.

Always see doctor for treatment of puncture wounds. There is danger of tetanus (lockjaw) from organisms which may be carried into the body. (See tetanus immunization, page 42).

Never remove a projecting object such as a rod or wood splinter that is deeply buried in the body. It may be plugging injured vessels. Removal may cause serious or fatal bleeding.

Splinters

How to remove small splinters, thorns, near surface of skin: Wash with soapy water. Sterilize large needle, knife blade or tweezers by holding in open flame. Press needle against skin near point of splinter. Scrape and dig gently to push splinter out. Loosened splinter may be grasped at end by tweezers and pulled out at same angle it entered flesh. "Milk" surrounding flesh to encourage bleeding. Cover with sterile compress. If imbedded, see doctor.

Prevent Cuts, Scratches, Penetrating Injuries

Teach children not to run with or throw sharp objects . . . Don't leave cutlery or sharp-edged tools lying around — keep in separate storage compartments . . . Keep home workshop power tools disconnected — lock switches, power supply, so children can't turn on . . . If guns are kept in house, keep them locked up, unloaded . . . Keep a clean yard, free of bottles, cans, broken glass, boards, nails, wire.

Fishhook in Flesh

If accident occurs far from aid, and if fishhook is not imbedded in critical area such as face or near eye, remove as follows:

Press down on shank of hook until barbed end pushes through the skin and is free (a slight incision at point where tip emerges makes it easier). Cut off barbed end with pliers, clippers. Remove shaft of hook. Wash wound with soap

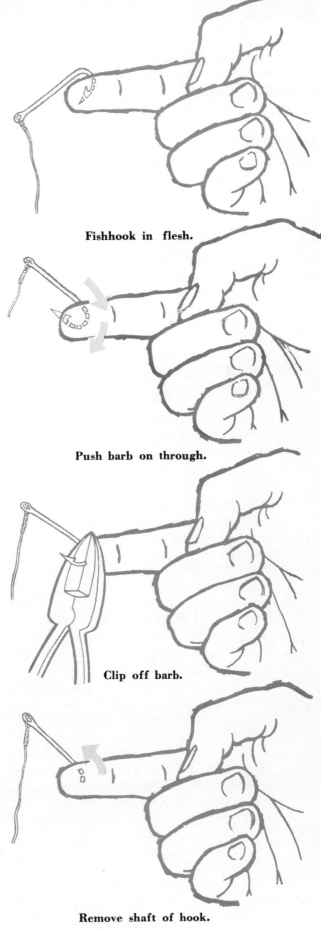

Fishhook in flesh.

Push barb on through.

Clip off barb.

Remove shaft of hook.

and water, encourage bleeding, cover with dressing or adhesive bandage, see doctor as soon as possible.

If hook is in critical area or has caused much damage, cover wound with sterile dressing, protect with soft bandaging, see doctor as soon as possible. All puncture wounds should be seen by doctor because of danger of tetanus.

SPRAINS, STRAINS, AND DISLOCATIONS

Sprains

A sprain results from tearing ligaments which hold bones together at joints. It may be hard to distinguish between a sprain and a fracture—both may result from same injury. If any doubt, handle as fracture (see *Broken bones*). X-rays may be necessary to determine if fracture exists. Many injuries assumed to be sprains by laymen are actually strains.

Symptoms of sprain:

Pain in joint, increases on movement. Tenderness to touch.

Rapid swelling.

Black and blue discoloration (may not appear for several hours).

Immediate Aid:

Send for doctor.

Relieve pain by resting joint. Movement may be dangerous.

Elevate sprained joint higher than rest of body, so it gets less blood. Give support — pillow, padded clothing.

Bandage to prevent unnecessary motion if patient has to walk. Loosen the bandage if swelling increases.

For first few hours after injury, apply ice bag or cold compresses. This contracts vessels, minimizes swelling, eases pain. *After* a day or so, if doctor is not available, change to *hot* compresses. Do not apply heat immediately after the injury.

Sprained Ankle

If injury occurs far from help or it is absolutely essential for a sprained ankle to bear weight, a snug ankle bandage

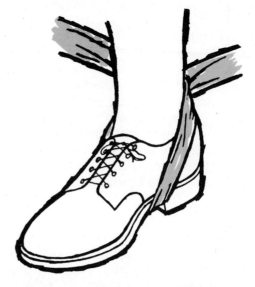

SPRAINED ANKLE: Place middle of bandage under shoe in front of heel.

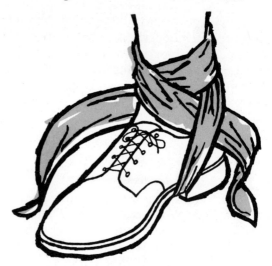

Cross ends at back of heel and in front, over instep.

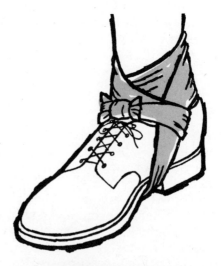

Loop each end under rear of bandage; tie over instep.

gives support for walking. *Never* walk with a sprained ankle (might be broken) unless in serious emergency.

Leave shoe on, loosen laces. Place long bandage under shoe in front of heel. Bring bandage ends behind and above heel, cross, bring forward and cross over instep. Tuck ends under loops formed by first step of bandaging, on each side of foot. Pull ends together, tie over instep.

Strains

A strain is caused by overstretching or "pulling" muscles or tendons. Back strain ("crick in the back") is common. Symptoms:

Sharp pain or "stitch" at time of injury.

Stiffness and soreness get worse in a few hours.

Pain on movement.

How to Help:

Put injured part at rest. Sit or lie in most comfortable position.

Apply heat in any form — hot water bottle, lamp, heating pad.

Give gentle massage with warm rubbing alcohol or witch hazel. Rub toward the heart.

If pain eases sufficiently, rub more forcefully, knead gently, to help loosen stiffened muscles.

See doctor if back strain is severe. Frequently back strains need strapping.

Dislocations

A blow, fall, sudden twisting may force a bone out of place at a joint, causing a *dislocation*. Indications:

Joint looks out of shape compared to similar joint.

Swelling, usually rapid.

Pain and tenderness at site.

Patient can't move joint or motion is limited.

Patient may be in *shock*.

Immediate First Aid:

Send for doctor.

Do not try to straighten out joint or force bone back in place (except jaw, finger, toe dislocations; see below).

Suspect that bones *may* be fractured. In general, handle as if part were fractured (see *Broken bones*).

Put patient in comfortable position. Keep weight off injured part. Give gentle support to injured part.

Apply ice bag or cloths wrung out of very cold water to injured part, to ease pain and minimize swelling.

Finger or Toe Dislocation

Grasp with one hand on each side of dislocated joint. Slowly pull free end of finger or toe in a straight line until it snaps in place. Do not use great force. If one or two attempts fail, wait for doctor. Do not try to reduce large joint at base of

Prevent Back Strain

Low back strain is most often caused by improper lifting technique, or attempting to lift objects that are too heavy. The most important lifting rule is never to let the lower back arch forward. Do not bend over stiff-legged to lift object from floor — place your feet close to object, crouch with back straight, feet flat on floor; grasp object firmly; lift slowly using thigh muscles.

Don't lean over projection such as radiator to lift stuck window. Don't reach to pick up something when one arm is loaded with baby or packages. Get help if object to be lifted is heavy. Don't lift if footing is insecure — a slip or twist may wrench your back.

Sudden, quick lifting of heavy objects is dangerous, especially if you are unaccustomed to it. Do not keep on trying to lift an object if you feel a slight discomfort in your back. Take frequent rests if repeated lifting of heavy objects must be made.

thumb or great toe joint. Don't pull dislocated finger or toe if an open wound is near the dislocated joint. Dress the wound and get medical aid.

Jaw Dislocation

In an emergency a first-aider may try to correct a dislocated jaw. Symptoms: Lower jaw sags down, patient cannot close mouth.

Wrap your thumbs with cloth to protect them. Face patient, put your thumbs in his mouth on lower back teeth, your fingers under his chin. Press firmly down and back with your thumbs, upward with your fingers under his chin. Get your thumbs out fast to prevent injury when jaw snaps back in place.

BURNS

Minor Burns

Skin reddened, unbroken, no blisters, small area.

Hold immediately under cold running water for several minutes until no pain is felt when part is removed. Or, immerse in container of clean cool water or even milk.

Cleanse with plain white soap and water.

For mild burns of moderate size: Apply a paste of wet baking soda. Or gauze, impregnated with petroleum jelly, sold in sterile packets. Or a mild burn ointment. Ointments should be used *only* on minor burns.

Cover with sterile bandage.

Immediate exclusion of air gives greatest pain relief of burns.

Major Burns

Blisters, skin broken, any burn covering about 10 per cent of total skin area.

Immediate step whenever possible: Wrap patient carefully in blanket or sheet and get to hospital at once.

If first step is not possible:

Immerse burned part (leg, arm) in *warm*, not hot, water. If burn is extensive or involves trunk, thighs, large skin areas, put patient (clothes and all) into bathtub full of warm running water.

This excludes air from burn and helps prevent shock. Stir some baking soda into the water.

Remove clothing carefully. Use scissors to *cut around cloth* that sticks to burned skin. *Never* pull clothing that adheres to skin. Leave it. Leave all foreign particles except large ones that come off easily. Keep patient supported in tub until the doctor comes.

If immersion of burned part is not possible, or patient has to be removed from tub, have him lie on bed on freshly laundered sheet. Cover with dry dressings made as thick as possible.

Wrap patient in fresh clean sheet, and cover with blanket to keep him *comfortably* warm while waiting for doctor.

Important Don'ts

Do not open large blisters.

Do not apply antiseptics.

Do not apply greases, ointments, butter, dressings that are not sterile, fluffy cotton, or any materials the doctor will find hard to remove.

Combat Shock

Immediate fluid replacement helps to prevent *shock*, a major threat of severe burns.

Thirst is a sign of impending shock. Give fluids unless patient is unconscious or vomiting. Give this saline *shock solution:*

1 teaspoon salt; ½ teaspoon baking soda dissolved in 1 quart water. Do not give fluids too rapidly (may produce vomiting). Give about one cupful of this solution every hour.

Bandaging

Bad burns are susceptible to *infection*. Immediate first-aid purpose of bandaging is to hold the dressings in place, exclude air, protect against dirt, germs. Leave more elaborate bandaging to doctor. Prevent raw, burned skin surfaces—

between fingers, toes, or under arms — from sticking together by separating surfaces with moistened strips of clean cloth. Cover with sterile bandage until doctor can take over.

Extensive Burns

Whether superficial or deep, burns which cover any large area such as chest, back, or a complete upper extremity are always major burns. So are burns of face and hands (other than the most trivial) which may leave scars or deformities. Medically, burns that cover any nine per cent of the body surface are extensive. Give immediate first aid as described below; get prompt medical help.

Chemical Burns

Of Body from Strong Acids, Alkalis, Corrosive Fluids

Drench burn continuously with lavish amounts of clean water. If possible, rush immediately under bathroom shower, turn on forcefully, strip clothing under running shower. If there is delay, corrosive liquid has dried, do not irrigate; summon doctor quickly.

Powder Burns

Fireworks, Cap Pistols

Unless skin is lacerated, torn (see *Wounds, cuts, and bruises),* cleanse gently with bland white soap, water. Cover with dry dressing.

Greatest danger from most powder burns is not the burn itself but tiny puncture wounds of powder particles which may drive *tetanus* organisms deeply into the skin. All children and adults should have tetanus toxoid inoculations which give protection against the disease.

POISONS

Swallowed Poisons

Call doctor at once, or prepare to rush patient to nearest hospital if no doctor is available, but first give *immediate* first aid. Don't lose time seeking specific poison antidote. Use simple measures immediately available.

If Patient is Conscious:

First, *before* telephoning doctor, *dilute* the poison by giving large amounts of fluids. The fluids may cause vomiting, which should be encouraged. May be more effective than waiting for the doctor's more efficient stomach pump.

Important

Head Lowered for Drainage

If patient vomits, put in prone position, head turned and lowered over bed edge, to prevent inhaling vomited material. If a child, hold face downward on your lap, head hanging over. Induce vomiting by tickling back of throat or putting your finger in throat.

Do not induce vomiting if patient has

Prevent Burn Tragedies

Keep handles of pots, frying pans turned in on kitchen range. Don't put hot tea, coffee, liquids on a tablecloth or scarf hanging over side of a table — child may pull or run into cloth and tip over steaming liquids. Never leave small child alone in bathtub; he may turn *hot water faucet* and get a bad scald. Place child in tub facing faucet so he won't back into hot metal. Keep tubs, pails, pans of hot water off floor where children may run or trip.

Don't hold child in your lap while you drink or pass hot beverages. Cover hot pipes, radiators. Keep matches, cigarette lighters out of reach until child is old enough to be taught safe use and dangers. Never leave children alone around a bonfire, outdoor grill, fireplace, glowing coals or open flame. Remember that Christmas trees dry out in the house and are highly inflammable. Never throw water on a grease or oven fire—smother with salt or soda.

swallowed *lye* or corrosive acids or alkalies (may be burns around face or mouth); or *kerosene, gasoline,* or *turpentine.*

Emetics

To Induce Vomiting

If patient does not vomit, proceed to *dilute* the poison and *wash out* the stomach by giving *large amounts of fluids* which have emetic (vomiting-inducing) effects. *Speed* is important and it is better to give patient *warm milk or water* than to lose time hunting for materials to mix a more potent emetic. It is easier to induce vomiting when stomach is full. Try again after giving fluids.

Give Glass of Milk Immediately

Give several glasses of emetic fluids such as:

Warm tap water.

Warm salt water (1 teaspoon salt to glass).

Warm mustard water (1 teaspoon dry mustard to glass).

Keep giving fluids until vomited liquid is as clear as when swallowed. *Do not* force liquids on a semiconscious patient.

After the stomach is emptied, a large dose of *Epsom salts* is usually good for almost any kind of poison.

Do Not Rely on Antidotes Alone

Always call the doctor. Then give antidote which helps to counteract the poison. If you do not know what the patient has swallowed, a "universal antidote" is a useful emergency measure.

A *universal antidote* for unknown poisons can be bought at drugstores, kept on hand for emergencies. It consists of:

Pulverized charcoal (activated charcoal) — 2 tablespoons.

Tannic acid — 1 tablespoon.

Magnesium oxide — 1 tablespoon.

Mix in ½ glass water; give to patient.

General Antidotes

A similar "homemade" *universal antidote* can be made as follows:

Finely crushed burnt toast — give 2 tablespoons to patient.

Very strong tea — 1 tablespoon.

Milk of magnesia — 1 tablespoon.

Mix in ½ glass of water; give to patient.

The label of the bottle or package from which the poison has come may list a *specific antidote.* Give this *if immediately available* but do not waste time — it is always safe to give a *universal antidote.*

Antidote for Unknown Poisons

Other *quick household antidotes* which help to dilute, absorb, and counteract many kinds of poisons include:

A glass of milk.

Two or three raw egg whites beaten into a glass of water.

Starch or flour made into a thin "soup" with water.

(*Do not* give patient milk, oily or fatty substances in cases of suspected *phosphorus* poisoning.)

Save the bottle, box, or container from which the patient obtained the poison. Save unconsumed portion of the suspected liquid, tablet, powder, or particle. Save labels giving brand names and name of manufacturer. If a drug overdose, save *prescription number and name of pharmacist.* Show to doctor or take with you to hospital so the *poison can be identified* and emergency treatment beyond the range of simple first aid can be begun.

Keep Warm, Keep Breathing

If the suspected poisoning victim is unconscious, semicomatose, shows signs of shock or difficulty in breathing:

Keep air passages open. Keep patient in prone (on stomach) position with head low, turned to one side. Wipe mucous secretions from mouth with handkerchief or finger. Keep tongue from falling back and blocking air passage. Lift nape of neck, put your hand under jaw, pull jaw forward and upward to extend neck and tilt head backward.

Watch for slowed or stopped breathing. If breathing stops, give immediate *mouth to mouth resuscitation* (see page 824).

Keep patient warm, covered. Do not give stimulants.

QUICK-USE CHART

OF COMMON POISON ANTIDOTES

Some poisoning symptoms are immediate, dramatic, and acute; others may be rather long-delayed. Homes, plants, and offices contain hundreds of necessary and indispensable materials which may be mildly or seriously toxic if swallowed. Young children put things into their mouths while exploring the world and are particularly liable to poisoning from large overdoses of simple household remedies and prescription drugs, which are beneficial and harmless when properly used. Always call doctor if poisoning is suspected. Do not wait for symptoms to appear. Give *immediate* first aid. Give fluids. It is safe to give a dose of *universal antidote* immediately, and a *quick glass of milk* almost always does good.

Combined ingredients of *universal antidote* act against common poisons in the same general way as more concentrated and specific antidotes. *If the cause of the poisoning is known,* and first aid has been given, specific steps may be taken while *medical aid is on the way.*

The following chart gives additional first-aid instructions and lists helpful antidotes for some common causes of poisoning. Continue these steps until medical aid is available.

Alkalis, Caustic

Lye, Ammonia, Drainpipe Cleaners, Quicklime, Washing Soda

Do not force vomiting.

Give acid fruit juices, such as juice of 4 lemons in pint of water.

Or, slightly diluted vinegar.

Follow with two or three raw egg whites in water.

Or, glass or two of milk.

Or, salad oil, cooking oil, melted butter.

Acids, Strong

Battery Acid, Sulfuric, Nitric, Hydrochloric

Do not force vomiting.

Teacupful of milk of magnesia

Or, 2 tablespoons of baking soda in pint of water.

Then, raw egg whites in water.

Or, glass or two of milk.

Or, salad oil, any vegetable oil, about ¼ glass.

Carbolic Acid

Phenol (Ingredient of Common Disinfectants), Creosol, Creosol Disinfectants

Give soapsuds immediately.

Or, give Epsom salts (2 tablespoons to pint of water).

Then, large amounts lukewarm water (do not give any strong emetic).

Also, give thin "soup" of flour or cornstarch in water.

Or, raw egg whites in water.

Do not give alcoholic drinks.

Iodine

Flour or cornstarch in water; bread; large amounts of starchy substances.

Follow with emetic; induce vomiting.

Repeat starch and emetic until returned material has no blue color.

Petroleum Distillates

Kerosene, Gasoline, Benzine, Naphtha, Lighter Fluid, Inflammable Cleaning Fluids

Do not force vomiting (danger of aspiration pneumonia).

Give half-cup of mineral oil.

Stimulant; strong coffee, tea.

Keep warm, combat shock.

Artificial respiration if necessary.

Salicylate Drug Overdose

Aspirin, Headache and Cold Pills, Oil of Wintergreen

Induce vomiting unless it has occurred.

Give *universal antidote.*

Or, *weak* baking soda solution (1 teaspoon to pint).

Strong coffee.

"Sleep Drug" Overdose

Barbiturates, Sedatives, Opiates, Codeine, Morphine, Paregoric

If conscious, give emetic, induce vomiting.

Strong black coffee.

Keep patient awake — slap face with wet towel, walk him about, but do not exhaust him.

Artificial respiration if necessary.

Wood Alcohol

Rubbing Alcohol, Denatured Alcohol, Methanol

Emetic; induce vomiting.

Give tablespoon of baking soda in quart of warm water.

Repeat emetic, soda solution.

Follow with glass of milk, containing teaspoon of baking soda.

Food Poisoning

Do not assume that all severe intestinal upsets which occur after eating are due to food poisoning. Appendicitis, other illnesses may cause similar symptoms.

Suspect food poisoning if more than one person becomes ill after eating the same foods which were improperly prepared or spoiled.

The most common forms of food poisoning are infections caused by *bacteria* or their toxins in contaminated foods. Symptoms may be very mild, last only a few hours, or very severe with urgent need of medical aid. Most bacterial food poisonings are caused by *staphylococci* (germ family that causes boils and abscesses) or *salmonella* organisms.

Staphylococcal food poisoning may cause symptoms almost immediately, commonly within 2 to 4 hours after eating. Symptoms of *salmonella* poisoning usually are longer delayed—from 6 hours after eating to a day or even two days later. Recovery commonly takes longer; chills, fever; can be serious; get doctor.

If These Symptoms Occur, Call Doctor:

Abdominal pain and distress.

Abdomen is always *soft,* never rigid or board-like.

Nausea and vomiting.

Cramps.

Diarrhea.

Chills or fever, prostration (salmonella poisoning).

Prevent Poisoning Tragedies

Be aware that many essential household articles are potentially toxic if accidentally swallowed or misused: disinfectants, lye, ammonia, flammable and noninflammable cleaning fluids, insecticides, bleaches, rat poisons, moth balls, kerosene, gasoline, turpentine, paint thinners, household remedies and prescription drugs in overdosage.

If there are small children in the house, keep such articles *on a high shelf* well out of reach, or preferably in a *locked cabinet. Never* put such things into a soft drink bottle, or container associated with food—a sip can be swallowed before it can be spit out.

Never put anything on food shelves except food. Keep drugs and home remedies, even "harmless" ones, locked up.

Do not leave pills in a *handbag* or low *drawer;* children love to rummage.

Never tell a child that a pill is candy or "tastes like candy."

Never take a medicine until you have *read the label.* If label is gone or illegible, discard bottle.

Important Don'ts

Do not give laxatives, cathartics, or *anything* by mouth as long as there is persistent nausea and vomiting.

First aid:

Put patient to bed, keep warm.

After nausea and vomiting subside, give large quantities of luke warm water, fluids.

If no diarrhea, salt-water enemas (1 teaspoon of salt to quart of water) may be given to patient.

Botulinus Poisoning

Caused by powerful toxins of organisms which may be in *improperly home-canned foods,* especially low-acid foods. Commercially canned foods and home-canned foods canned by the pressure method are safe. Boiling of home-canned foods for 30 minutes before eating usually insures safety.

Recognize Symptoms and Call Doctor at Once

These symptoms commonly begin 18 to 24 hours after eating the food but *may* not appear for several days:

Great fatigue.

May be no nausea or vomiting.

Predominant nervous system symptoms:

Dizziness.

Headache.

Disturbances of vision, blurring, double vision.

Difficulty in breathing, swallowing, and speaking.

Muscular weakness.

Temperature may be subnormal.

Mushroom Poisoning

Put patient to bed in quiet room; *very serious!*

Call doctor immediately.

No test can prove unknown mushrooms to be safe and edible. Avoid *all* wild mushrooms.

The following symptoms of mushroom poisoning may appear within a few minutes to 2 or 3 hours after eating, or within 8 to 15 hours, depending upon the variety of fungus:

Abdominal pain.

Diarrhea.

Dizziness.

Derangement of vision.

Cold sweating.

Cramps in arms or legs.

First Aid:

Give large dose of Epsom salts. *Call doctor* at once or take patient to hospital.

Prevent Food Poisoning

Insanitary food handling, lack of refrigeration, keeping foods at room temperature or warmer for several hours, underlie most cases of food poisoning. Food handlers with cut fingers, colds, and boils may introduce germs which can multiply rapidly in *foods that are not thoroughly cooked or are heated very little,* such as salads, meringues, salad dressings, creamed dishes, custard-fillings, cold cuts.

Refrigeration retards growth of germs. If no refrigeration available, consume foods *soon after preparation;* discard *leftovers* that have stood exposed to room or outdoor air and warmth for hours. On *picnics, car trips, camping trips,* keep food in portable icebox. On *vacations,* only raw (unpasteurized) milk may be obtainable. You can *pasteurize milk* by bringing it to a rolling boil, plunging pan into ice cubes for rapid cooling (has slightly "cooked" flavor). A better way, if you have a thermometer and double boiler, is as follows:

Bring water to boil in bottom half of double boiler.

Put milk in top half of boiler (over boiling water), insert thermometer into milk, stir milk until thermometer registers 160 degrees. Hold at that temperature for 15 seconds.

Cool milk by placing container in ice cubes, or changes of cold water. Keep stirring milk until temperature drops to 50 degrees.

Weed and Plant Poisoning

Leaves, roots, berries, seeds and other parts of many weeds, wild plants, and garden plants (foxglove, monkshood, rhubarb *leaves*, lilies, others) may be toxic if eaten. *Teach* children not to eat strange berries, fruits or plant parts; avoid them yourself. *Symptoms* of plant poisoning vary; usually include abdominal pain, cramps, nausea, vomiting (may be juice stains around mouth).

Immediate Treatment

Induce vomiting immediately if it has not occurred.

Give large amounts of fluids, milk if available.

Give dose of Epsom salts.

Give *universal antidote*.

Save specimen of plant or part thought to have caused poisoning; show to doctor.

BITES AND STINGS

Snake Bite

Venomous and Nonvenomous

Venomous snakes of the United States are pit vipers (rattlers, copperheads, moccasins), except for the rare coral snake of Southern regions.

The "bite" of a venomous snake usually leaves *two* small puncture marks.

There may be *one* puncture mark if the snake struck at an angle, or sometimes three or four puncture marks. The "bite" is really a hypodermic injection through hollow fangs which deposit venom. Smaller teeth behind the fangs may cause rows of scratches in addition to the larger puncture marks.

Swelling may obscure the puncture marks. Pain at the site of most venomous bites is immediate and intense.

Nonpoisonous snake bite usually leaves two U-shaped rows of fine tooth marks, as shown. There is little pain or swelling.

The bite of a coral snake closely resembles those of nonvenomous snakes. A coral snake bite usually is accompanied by very little pain.

For *nonpoisonous* snake bite, cleanse with plain soap and water, cover with sterile dressing; see doctor.

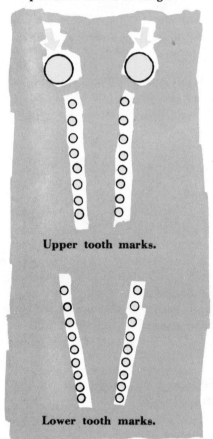

VENOMOUS SNAKEBITE — arrows show puncture marks of fangs.

Upper tooth marks.

Lower tooth marks.

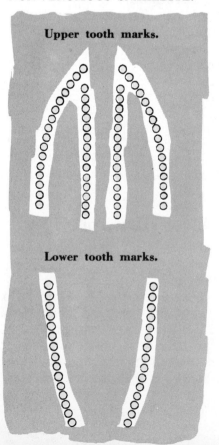

NON-VENOMOUS SNAKEBITE.

Upper tooth marks.

Lower tooth marks.

Poisonous Snake Bite

The only specific measure for venomous snake bite is injection of antivenin as soon as possible to neutralize the venom. "Snake-bite kits" containing antivenin, instruments, instructions, can be bought at drugstores, sometimes rented on returnable basis by campers and outdoorsmen from pharmacies in "snake country." First-aiders can give antivenin injections — *the sooner the better* — although it is best to have a doctor do it.

If antivenin is not on hand: immobilize the victim. Have him lie down, keep quiet, no walking or muscular action that can be avoided. *Do not give whiskey or stimulants.* Ice water, cold cloths, may ease pain but do not stop spread of venom. *Carry* the victim — on stretcher if possible, or on one's back with bitten part hanging down — to nearest doctor or source of help where physician with antivenin can be summoned *urgently.* If there is no possibility of getting medical aid, use the incision-suction method.

Incision-Suction Method

For centuries the only recognized (or available) method of treating venomous snake bite was by incision, suction, and tourniquet, thought to remove venom or slow its absorption. Many physicians use this first-aid method, and the armed forces recommend it.

The standard incision-suction technique consists of: a constricting band (loosened every quarter-hour) between wound and body; cuts to induce bleeding at site of bite and swollen edges; suction through these cuts by mouth or suction cup. (Caution: Venom may be absorbed if there are breaks in tissues of the mouth).

Do not apply tourniquet tightly. Its purpose is to slow blood flow, not stop it.

Make the cuts no deeper than ⅜-inch, and even more shallow on hands to avoid cutting nerves. Apply a pressure bandage if an artery is cut accidentally.

Transportation

When snake bite victim must be moved, keep him lying down if possible.

Make an emergency stretcher from two shirts, two poles.

When one bearer must transport victim, bitten part should hang lower than rest of victim's body. If bite is on upper half of body, bearer should carry victim over shoulder.

Victim with bite on lower half of body should be carried upright on bearer's back. When no antivenin is available, and medical aid is hours away, immediately use the incision-suction method, in hope of removing some of the venom.

Insect Bites

Pain and Itch Relief

Apply ice or wet dressings; hold under cold water. Make a paste of baking soda moistened with water, cover burn or sting site. Apply diluted household ammonia to bite and surrounding skin. Calamine lotion and rubbing alcohol or lotions containing alcohol help to relieve itching. Do not scratch an insect bite. Scratching may result in infection.

Tick Bites

Don't Touch With Bare Fingers!

Some ticks spread diseases such as Rocky Mountain spotted fever, tularemia, and relapsing fever. A tick often can be felt before it starts to burrow under the skin, but after it begins to suck it usually cannot be felt. Examine skin and clothing after a day in tick-infested country.

The head of a tick tenaciously resists removal from skin. Don't try to remove ticks with unprotected fingers or allow crushed parts or juices to contact the skin. It may help to make ticks "let go" if you:

Coat them with nail polish, petroleum jelly, or grease. Smother them with kerosene, turpentine, or gasoline. Remove them carefully with tweezers.

Afterwards, wash site thoroughly with soap and water.

Wear high shoes with trouser ends tied around tops, when hiking in tick country.

Stings:

Bee, Wasp, Hornet, Yellow Jacket — Get the Stinger Out!

Cold packs containing baking soda are a good home remedy for relief of local discomfort from stings of bees and related insects. Ice cubes, ice bags, give most comfort.

If you upset a nest of insects, and suffer a "massive dose" of many separate stings, get into a tepid tub bath with a package or more of baking soda stirred into it.

Bees often leave their "stinger" in the center of the sting. The stinging apparatus can be seen as a tiny dark object. It continues to pump venom into the wound after the bee is gone. *Remove the stinger* with an outward scraping motion of a fingernail. *Do not* pinch the stinger between two fingernails or grasp with tweezers. That forces more venom out.

A few people become so extremely sensitized to insect venom that a sting may cause a serious, even fatal, allergy-like reaction. They should seek medical aid, such as desensitization procedures and emergency steps to take if stung. They may advised to carry an emergency kit containing a drug for prompt injection (see pages 696-97).

Spider Bite

Two common American spiders can inflict serious bites—the small brown (recluse) spider and the black widow. The latter is a coal-black spider with a pea-size abdomen marked with a reddish hourglass design.

The black widow's bite causes intense pain, muscle spasm, weak pulse. The pain moves gradually from the wound and concentrates in the abdomen. The brown spider's bite may not be immediately painful but, if not treated, tissue breaks down in the area of the wound.

Get to a doctor immediately. Save spider for identification, if possible. Meantime, wash wound with soapsuds and apply baking soda compress, give black coffee as a stimulant, watch for signs of *shock*.

Dog Bites, Cat Bites

Other Animal Bites

Immediate first-aid treatment of animal bites is the same as for other common wounds, except for possibility of rabies (see *rabies*, page 58). Bite injuries range from barely perceptible tooth marks to severe injuries to be treated as major wounds.

Most bites inflicted by dogs, cats, squirrels, rats, mice, and small animals are local soft tissue injuries and immediate first aid aims to prevent infection and promote healing:

1. Cleanse wound thoroughly with soap and water. Preferably, wash under running water with liberal soaping. Paint with antiseptic.

2. Cover the bite wound with a sterile dressing and bandage.

3. See doctor. *Always* see doctor if bite, no matter how trivial, is on face, head, or neck areas.

Human Bites

A human bite may be a real bite or it may be inflicted by teeth that stop the blow of a fist. The human mouth commonly contains varied and virulent bacteria and serious undermining, spreading infections often follow human bite wounds.

Give first aid, as for animal bites, then have a doctor take over.

Rabies or Hydrophobia

Rabies is a fatal disease which may be transmitted by the saliva of "mad dogs" and infected animals such as cats, squirrels, skunks, foxes, bats, and others.

Most bites are inflicted by healthy animals. An animal that snaps at anything, attacks without provocation, behaves peculiarly or "acts sick," may have rabies.

If bitten, do not become panic-stricken nor fail to take sensible precautions. Give first aid; *have doctor inspect wound;* follow his advice.

Rabies can be prevented by Pasteur treatments (a series of a dozen or more injections) begun after the bite is suffered. Such treatment can be avoided if the biting animal is kept under observation for a couple of weeks and if it is perfectly healthy at the end of that time. If the animal has been killed, or dies, laboratory examination of its head can usually determine whether it was "mad."

The slow incubation period of rabies usually affords enough time for observation or laboratory tests so that Pasteur treatments need not be started unless tests are positive. Treatments may be started immediately in case of bites of head, neck, shoulders, and hands, but are stopped if the animal proves not to be rabid. If nothing is known about the biting animal, Pasteur treatments may have to be given (depending upon circumstances of the bite) as insurance against a disease which, once established, is invariably fatal. These treatments are almost always effective, if they are started in time.

The doctor's decision depends in part on information you give him and steps you take at the time of the accident.

Prevent Many Bites and Stings

Teach children not to maul or torment pets or tease stray animals. Many nips are inflicted in justifiable self-defense.

Wear calf-high boots in snake country; watch your step in woods; probe underbrush with a stick before trampling on it (75 per cent of snake bites occur near the ankle, most of the rest in wrist or hand areas).

Tie shut the open ends of sleeves and trouser legs when strolling through tick-infested grasses and weeds. *Bees and stinging insects* are attracted to dark-colored clothing, tweeds, flannels, sweaty clothing, hair oils and perfumes. If "attacked" by a hostile bee, *move slowly*, don't make jerky movements, slap, or run, unless a whole hive is after you.

Wear gloves when cleaning out a garage to protect against possible bite of black widow spider.

What to Do

If An Animal Bites You

Capture and confine the biting animal if possible.

Identify the animal and its owner if it belongs in the neighborhood. If a stray, get accurate description so police or dog catcher can track it down.

Do not kill the animal unless absolutely necessary. Do not shoot through head as this may make laboratory studies difficult.

If animal dies or is killed, preserve its head. Your doctor or local health department will tell you what steps to take. Report animal bites to police or authorities according to local regulations.

EYES

Chemical Burns of Eye

There's only one thing to remember when dangerous chemicals get into the eyes: *wash out the eyes immediately with large amounts of cool water.*

Chemicals continue to burn as long as they remain in the eye.

Immediate flushing out of the chemical minimizes eye damage and may prevent it entirely. Don't waste time trying to find out whether the chemical is an acid or an alkali. It makes no first-aid difference.

Hold head under faucet with eye in running stream of cool water. Stream should have good flushing force but not high pressure. Turn head so stream flows over affected eye *away from* unaffected eye. If both eyes are contaminated with chemicals, direct water on both eyes simultaneously or in quick alternation. Flush the eyes thoroughly *before* you take time to call a doctor.

You can't use too much water. Keep on irrigating the eyes with water for 5 or 10 minutes or until you are very sure that all dangerous chemical material has been washed out. *Remember,* powder particles may be trapped under eyelids. Separate lids gently so water can reach all parts.

If there's no faucet handy, seize any source of water or any bland fluid you can lay hands on quickly — a bottle of milk will serve in an emergency. Put patient on floor, flat on his back, pour water from pitcher, tumbler, any container, into corner of eye (next to nose) so fluid streams over eyeball and under eyelids. Repeat, repeat, repeat!

Or, eye may be held in stream of water bubbling from drinking fountain. Or, eyes may be submerged in bowl of water while patient keeps blinking them.

Massive, thorough, continuous irrigation! Instant first aid may prevent blindness!

After all chemical materials are washed from eyes, call a doctor. What you do in the *first few seconds* and the next few minutes to wash acids or alkalis from eyes is more important than anything the doctor can do later. After thorough irrigation, put a few drops of clean oil into the eye (mineral oil, castor oil, vegetable oil). This helps to prevent eyelids from sticking to eyeball. Cover both eyes with sterile gauze compress and rush to doctor.

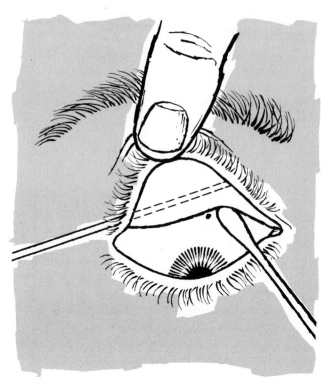

A *non-imbedded* "speck in the eye," seen when upper eyelid is pulled back gently, can be removed with moistened cotton applicator.

Contusions of Eyeball

Hard blows which do not cut or penetrate the eye may "bruise" it internally and can be serious although the injury may not "look bad." Delayed damage may result from slow hemorrhage, injury to internal eye structures. Take no chances if eye has suffered a severe blunt blow. Have prompt examination by an eye physician. Do not depend on first-aid measures alone. *Cold* compresses may be applied. Do *not* use hot compresses.

Foreign Bodies in Eye

It is safe to use simple first-aid measures to remove cinders, eyelashes, or specks which rest loosely on the surface of eyelid or eyeball. Do not attempt to remove imbedded particles that resist simple first-aid procedures. *Never rub or scratch an eye that* "has something in it." This may cause scars, or drive particles farther into the eyeball. Always *wash hands* before touching eyes.

Pull upper eyelid out and down over lower lid, or shut both eyes for a few minutes, to give flow of tears which may wash out the particle.

If this does not work, fill medicine dropper with warm water or boric acid solution, to "flood" eye and flush out foreign body.

If speck is visible (pull lower eyelid gently out and downward for inspection) use *moistened* cotton applicator or corner of clean cotton cloth to lift out speck.

Do not use more vigorous methods to remove particles imbedded in lids or eyes. Cover with sterile gauze compress, held or gently taped in place. Get to doctor immediately.

Foreign Bodies Imbedded in Eye
Penetrating Eye Wounds

All perforating wounds of the eye are serious, no matter how small, need *immediate medical help*. A tiny foreign body buried deep *inside* the eye may leave little outward trace. Do *not* apply oils or ointments. Cover *both* eyes with a sterile compress (to lessen harmful eye movements). Bandage *lightly* in place — no hard pressure. Get to doctor.

Transport victim flat on back on stretcher, if possible.

Some penetrating eye wounds, such as stabs from pointed objects, are obvious and terrifying, but some are not. A tiny piece of steel hurled off from tool grinding or pounding a nail may be lodged in an eye that "looks" normal. Anyone who has "felt something strike the eye" should be examined by a doctor promptly. Glass splinters, sand, transparent sharp particles that become lodged in the eye may not be visible to ordinary observation.

Black Eye

An "ordinary" black eye is a bruise. For *immediate* first aid, apply *pressure* to involved area, preferably with *cold* compresses or cloths wrung out of cold water. This helps to minimize discoloration *if done at once*. A doctor may inject an enzyme which promotes absorption of blood and disappearance of "black-and-blueness" at rapid rate. A severe black eye may involve deeper injury and need more intensive medical attention.

Prevent Eye Tragedies

Think of knives, scissors, needles, and pincushions as if they were deadly poisons to small children. Keep out of reach, off tables from which they may fall, be picked up or run into. Teach children never to play, run with or hurl sharp sticks or objects. Bows and arrows, BB guns, and unsafe toys should be kept from small children. Keep lye, cleansers, acids, household chemicals in a safe place; use carefully, never leave containers open. Hobbyists and do-it-yourselfers: caution with tools which may send metal or wood fragments flying. Wear protective goggles. Ordinary glasses give some protection. In industry, always wear protective goggles if provided.

FOREIGN BODIES

Inhaled, Swallowed, Lodged in Body Orifices

Ear

Children may insert small objects into ear canal. Peas, beans, popcorn swell when wet, are hard to remove.

Do not dig at object with toothpick, hairpin, wire — grave danger of injuring ear canal or eardrum. You may push object further in.

Rarely is there any immediate danger. If object appears loose, gently pull ear lobe backwards and tilt child's head so object can fall out. If this fails, take patient to physician who has instruments to remove foreign body. If object is a bean or seed, a little olive oil or mineral oil can be dropped into the child's ear to lessen the swelling.

Insect in Ear

If insect crawls into ear, turn head to one side and drop in some warm olive oil or mineral oil to suffocate insect. If no oil available, use warm water. The dead insect may float out. If it does not, have a physician remove it.

Nose

Children sometimes slip beans, grains and small objects into nose. No immediate danger, but great harm can be done trying to remove object with crude instruments. Drop olive oil into nostril to soothe tissues and prevent swelling. Patient may blow nose *gently*, never forcibly (*both* nostrils open) after oil is instilled. If this does not dislodge object, take the child to a doctor.

Stomach

Tacks, open safety pins, needles and other small sharp objects are frequently swallowed by children. *Do not* give a laxative. May give child mashed potatoes. Take to doctor. Most foreign objects that reach the stomach pass through the bowel harmlessly, but the doctor may follow progress with a fluoroscope and take steps if it becomes lodged or penetrates tissues. *Never* force a child who has swallowed a sharp object to vomit.

Throat, Windpipe

(See choking, page 838.)

Prevent Foreign Body Accidents

Never give popcorn, candy, nuts or cookies that contain nuts to small children who can't chew them and may inhale them. Don't let small children play with dry beans, peas, buttons, coins, nails, screws. Check stuffed animals and other toys for easily removable small parts which child may remove and swallow or stuff into body openings. Make a habit of closing safety pins every time you use them. Don't hold tacks, pins or nails in your mouth while doing chores, or let children see you doing so. Be sure that all bone fragments are removed from foods to be eaten by small children.

FREEZING INJURIES

Frostbite

Parts of body frozen, white or grayish-yellow, numb. Extremities and face most often frozen.

Do not rub frozen part with snow or anything else. Frozen tissue is fragile, easily damaged.

Do not expose frozen part to intense direct heat of hot stove, radiator, heat lamp.

If outdoors, thaw part by using patient's body or body of another as a warmer — frozen hand under armpit, between thighs; warm hand over frozen ear, nose.

In shelter, immerse frozen part in tepid (not hot) water, temperature about 100 degrees. Or, cover part with warmed — not hot — towels or blankets. See doctor for aftercare. If deeply frozen, serious, get doctor immediately.

Prolonged Exposure to Cold

Chilling of entire body, in degree from mild chilling to numbness, drowsiness, unconsciousness, and death unless rescued.

For mild chill, put patient to bed in a warm room, cover well, give hot drinks.

For serious freezing exposure: Get victim to warm place. If breathing is imperceptible or stopped, give *artificial respiration.*

Rewarm rapidly by immersing in tub of water, 78 to 82 degrees.

Wrap victim in warm blankets; put him to bed.

Give warm drinks.

Get medical help.

HEAT ILLNESSES

Heatstroke, Sunstroke

Grave emergency. Often fatal. Act quickly to cool victim.

Symptoms: Very hot, absolutely dry skin, no sweating. Body temperature very high, 104 up to an incredible 110 degrees. Weakness, dizziness, rapid breathing, nausea, unconsciousness, sometimes mental confusion. Onset is often dramatically sudden.

Cool victim rapidly. Apply ice bag, crushed ice in cloth, or cold cloths to head. If he can't be moved to shelter, drench his clothes with cold water, poured on or sprayed from hose.

Preferably, strip clothing, wrap him in sheet, keep sheet wet with cold water, place electric fans to blow on cold sheet. Keep cold cloths or ice on head.

At same time, *rub his arms and legs* toward the heart through sheet. Continue; important.

Check body temperature every 10 minutes or so, preferably by thermometer, or if necessary by feeling skin.

Keep repeating the cooling procedures until temperature drops to between 101 and 102 degrees. If temperature rises again, repeat cooling procedures.

Summon doctor immediately.

Heat Exhaustion

Patient's skin is pallid, clammy, moist; profuse sweating. Temperature about normal, perhaps slightly lowered or slightly elevated. Nausea likely; scant urine; dizziness. Patient may faint.

Remove patient to circulating air; have him lie down, rest. Loosen clothing. Give sips of slightly salted water (1 teaspoonful of salt to pint). Stimulants: coffee, tea.

If symptoms of heat exhaustion do not pass away readily, call physician.

Heat Cramps

Painful spasms of abdominal, leg or arm muscles. Caused by loss of body salt through profuse, prolonged sweating. Most common in persons who do very hard physical labor in extremely hot surroundings for long periods. Cramps usually respond to firm hand pressure, warm wet towels, hot water bottle. Give sips of slightly salted water.

UNCONSCIOUSNESS

Unconsciousness has many causes. If cause is known, or apparent from quick inspection, treat for the particular emergency: *Sunstroke, poisoning, drowning, choking, electric shock, gas inhalation, concussion, fracture* are common causes.

If cause is not obvious, look quickly for clues: empty bottles, signs of blow, fall or accident, live wires, lip burns (corrosive poison).

Unequal pupils indicate brain injury or skull fracture. *Summon doctor immediately.* Do not assume that victim is drunk even though alcohol or other odors are detected. Look in victim's bag or wallet for card which may say he is a diabetic or subject to other emergencies. *Do not* shake an unconscious person to wake him up.

Never try to give anything by mouth to an unconscious person.

Often a first-aider cannot determine the exact cause of unconsciousness.

What To Do First

If Patient is Unconscious:

If breathing is inadequate or stopped, start artificial respiration at once.

If breathing is adequate, keep patient lying flat on back, warm but not hot, loosen constricting clothing, look for an apparent cause of unconsciousness such as a blow or fall. If the cause is obvious give proper first aid for that condition.

Summon physician, unless unconsciousness is very brief, as in common fainting. A person who has suffered a concussion or brief "knockout" should be seen by a doctor even though recovery of consciousness is prompt.

Apoplexy (Stroke)

Caused by break or seepage from blood vessels within skull — usually in persons over 50 years of age.

Face red, but sometimes pale gray. Strong slow pulse. One eye pupil often larger than the other. One side of body or one limb may be limp, paralyzed; one corner of mouth may droop.

Keep patient quiet, warm but not hot. Apply cold cloths to head. Summon physician immediately. Transport patient in lying position if he must be moved.

Heart Attack

"Heart attack" is a common term for acute coronary disease — usually, a clot in a coronary vessel that supplies blood to the heart muscle. Non-fatal attacks do not commonly cause unconsciousness. Typically, the patient has sudden agonizing pain in the heart region under the breastbone. The pain does not disappear (as the similar pain of angina pectoris does) when he rests for a few minutes. The pain may shoot down the left arm and there may be shortness of breath.

The most important step is to call a doctor who can inject a pain-relieving drug and take charge. An ambulance with oxygen-administering equipment should be summoned to transport the heart attack patient to a hospital.

Immediate first aid measures are limited, but helpful :

Keep the patient lying down, quiet, preferably in bed — any exertion or movement puts extra work on the heart.

The patient may be able to breathe more easily if his back is propped with pillows or other supports.

Keep excited people from crowding around the patient. Speak to him reassuringly to help ease his natural fear which may be quite intense. If there is medicine that has previously been prescribed for anginal attacks, it may be given; otherwise, give nothing by mouth while waiting for the doctor.

Fainting

Most common form of pallid unconsciousness, usually caused by temporary insufficiency of blood supply to brain. Correct by getting head level with or lower than body.

If you feel faint, about to "pass out," lie down if possible. If not, bend forward at waist from sitting position and put head between knees. If you can't lie or sit, kneel on one knee as if tying shoe, to get head lower than the heart.

In a crowded place, if someone feels faint, don't try to walk him out. Bend his head forward between knees until he feels better. Best first aid for fainting : Keep patient lying down, head lowered or legs and hips elevated. Cold water sprinkled on the face helps recovery.

After consciousness is regained, coffee, tea may be given. Recovery should be rapid — five minutes or less. If unconsciousness is prolonged, or fainting fits recur, see physician.

Illustrated
Encyclopedia
of
Medical
Terms

Illustrated Encyclopedia of Medical Terms

Table of Contents

Chapter   *Page*

Words Your Doctor Uses 873

> A clear, easy-to-understand explanation of the
> medical terminology used by doctors to describe
> symptoms, illnesses, parts of the body, and medi-
> cations to their patients.

Encyclopedia of Medical Terms 880

> A complete alphabetical listing of frequently-used
> medical and anatomical words, with brief defini-
> tions, explanations, and Family Medical Guide
> page references.

Words Your Doctor Uses

When we say "I have a pain in a joint," we are using medical language. "Pain" describes a condition and "joint" tells where it hurts. Ordinary English is rich in simple words that express medical and anatomical ideas with admirable clarity. We use such words all the time, and perhaps some of us, if told that we are speaking medical language, would be as astonished as the man who was told by a knowledgeable friend that he had been speaking prose all his life.

Long before they enter medical school, doctors learn everyday English like the rest of us. They know that a bone is a bone before they learn that it is also an *os*. Ordinary English is the language most doctors use in explaining matters to patients, and it is the language they usually expect to hear from patients. We might tell the doctor that we have "arthralgia," a ten-dollar word meaning "pain in a joint." There is little reason to do so, other than to toss around a little erudition or make the doctor suspect that we have been looking at a television ad for pain-relievers.

Any medical term can be translated into simple English. Doctors do it all the time in dealing with patients. But within their profession, technical language is a necessity. Doctors do not use jawbreaking medical terms to confuse the patient or hide the awful truth. They use it primarily for specific, concise professional communication—in medical journals, scientific reports, teaching, textbooks, clinical record keeping. In this they do not differ from other professions and occupations which have specialized language that is not at all secret, but which outsiders may not be privy to. Lawyers have their torts, printers their hellboxes, clergymen their epistemologies, loggers their wanigans, musicians their hemidemisemiquavers.

Specialized medical language, however, is rather exceptional. For one thing, it is enormously larger than other specialized languages. A complete medical dictionary has thousands upon thousands of entries, many of which are rarely referred to even by doctors. For another, medical language applies directly to *us*—our functions, organs, distempers, symptoms, health—and thus its presumed mysteries are of universal self-interest. A medical word we have never heard of or cared about may suddenly have some personal meaning.

Another exceptional thing about technical medical language is its almost total derivation from Greek and Latin. There are a few Arabic intrusions (*alcohol, elixir*) and a few Gallicisms (*tic douloureux*). But Greek and Latin predominate overwhelmingly. This gives medical words an arcane, scholarly, "it's Greek to me" formidability which we hope to show is deceptive. *Patella* is not a superior word for *kneecap*. It is just a different word.

Medical words insinuate themselves easily into the common tongue. Many words, originally quite technical, crop up in ordinary conversation—*antibiotic, Rh factor, hormone, hysterectomy, poliomyelitis, cholesterol, antihistamine, hypodermic, coronary*, and hundreds of others. A good deal of information about medicine (not implying any competence to practice it) is infused into the public mind by magazine and newspaper articles, "health columns," radio and television interviews, shows and novels about the tribulations of doctors, and dissemination of health and research findings by government and local agencies. Animated advertising may even inform us of things that do not exist, such as little hammers beating inside the skull to cause headaches.

Scientific progress continually adds new words to the language. Many of these new words are medical or have medical implications. In the present volume you will find listings under words such as *laser, nuclear medicine, ballistocardiography, tomography, Coxsackie virus, auto-immune diseases, hyperbaric medicine,* and others which did not exist a few years ago. Such words would surely have bewildered Hippocrates.

Indeed, much of the history of medical progress is embodied in words that have come down to us. Primitive ideas and misconceptions are memorialized in some of the most basic medical words. The *tibia* or shinbone got its name from its supposed resemblance to a flute. *Artery* traces back to the idea that the vessels were air-carriers. The *coccyx* or tailbone was named for a bird, the cuckoo. It was supposed to be shaped like a cuckoo's beak, a resemblance nowadays noted only by anatomists, if by them. The *pituitary* gland was thought to be the source of nasal mucus and its name bears the stamp of that humble secretion. A *hypochondriac,* overly fretful of his health, would no doubt worry all the more if told that the word refers to the area under the rib cartilage of the upper abdomen, anciently thought to be the site of melancholy feelings.

Why a Special Language?

One of the virtues of technical language is compactness. "Tonsillectomy" says the same thing as "surgical removal of the tonsils" in fewer words. In a medical discussion of tonsil surgery, it is easier and more kindly to repeat the word "tonsillectomy" than its many-worded equivalent. Specific words take much of the sprawl out of meaningful communication.

A more important virtue of specialized language is precision of meaning. A patient may complain that he has a "stomach-ache." Diagnosis may disclose that he has *gastritis* or *duodenal ulcer* or even something as exotic as a *bezoar.* In fact, the doctor may discover that the ache isn't in the stomach at all. He is conditioned to suspect that some patients believe that the stomach encom-

passes the entire area between the nipples and the pubic bone.

A minor but not to be undervalued virtue of medical language is its wonderful treasury of euphemisms—respectable substitutes for words thought to be tainted by vulgarity. A lady does not *belch;* she may attain the same relief, in impeccable good taste, by genteel *eructation.* Untimely occurrence of *belly-rumbling* is much more embarrassing than a slight touch of *borborygmus.* A stomach-ache may actually be a *belly*-ache or a *gut*-ache. But *belly* is frowned upon in drawing rooms, and *gut*—a wonderfully terse Anglo-Saxon word for bowels—is even more disreputable. In descriptive emergencies, the easily defeated may resort to "tummy-ache," a term so arch as to be coyly vulgar. The more resourceful will seize upon *abdomen,* and can discuss "abdominal discomfort" with aplomb with practically anybody.

Curt Anglo-Saxon words for body parts and functions are not sharpened in meaning by euphemisms but necessary references may well be made more easily. Teaching the medical names of body parts to children tends to make bees-and-flowers instruction more comfortable for all concerned. Nothing makes a supposedly vulgar word more respectable than its equivalent borrowed from a foreign language.

Compound Words

Many medical words, like any new word, have to be looked up in a dictionary. Many of the oldest medical words are those which name body parts, and they must be accepted as arbitrary labels. There is no master design pattern to make us expect that the *jejunum,* the second part of the small intestine, should be called a jejunum. The word descends from a Latin word for "fasting" or "empty," and embodies the mistaken notion that the organ is always empty after death. Who would suspect that? Or who would suspect that mice have something to do with *muscles*? But flex a muscle, look at the moving ripples and bulges—obviously, little mice are running around under your skin, or so it seemed to those who gave us the word *muscle,* from the diminutive form of the Latin word *mus,* a mouse.

But there is a design pattern for hundreds of medical words, generally quite modern words—in fact, new ones of this sort are frequently added to the language. These are compound or put-together words, built of root-words butted together like alphabet blocks. They can be disjointed (or disarticulated) and if we know the root forms we can make a fair guess at the meaning, even if we have never seen the word before. There are hundreds of Greek and Latin roots, but a few dozen of the most common ones are quite enough to give us at least an inkling of the meaning of an unfamiliar medical word. Some root-forms are common in everyday language. The suffix *-itis,* meaning inflammation, is so familiar that words such as *appendicitis* and *tonsillitis* need no translation.

Some compound words are polysyllabic jawbreakers because they contain so much information. Breaking them into their parts cuts them down to size. Take *gastroenterocolostomy. Gastro* pertains to the stomach, *entero* to the intestines, *colo* to the colon, *stomy* to mouth, outlet or entrance. In one word, *gastroenterocolostomy* says "an operation in which a passage is formed between stomach, intestines and colon."

Not all compound medical words are that complicated. Many give the name of a part with a suffix indicating its condition or something that is done to it. Thus, *-ectomy,* a cutting out, preceded by *hyster-,* the womb, gives *hysterectomy,* surgical removal of the uterus.

For exact meaning of a word, consult the glossary. It is possible to make a wrong guess. Nevertheless, familiarity with a few root forms gives a modest amount of assurance and at least robs medical words of their mystery. A Roman speaking of his *genu* is no more mysterious than an American speaking of his *knee.* The list below gives root forms that occur most frequently in medical language. Roots may be prefixes, suffixes, or appear internally in a word. Combining forms may add or omit a vowel to connect syllables smoothly.

ROOTS OF MEDICAL LANGUAGE

a-, an-. Absent, lacking, deficient, without. An*emia,* deficient in blood.

aden-. Pertaining to a gland. Aden*oma* is a tumor of glandlike tissue.

alg-, -algia. Pain. A prefix such as *neur-* tells where the pain is (*neuralgia*).

ambi-. Both.

andro-. Man, male. An andro*gen* is an agent which produces masculinizing effects.

angi-, angio-. Blood or lymph vessel. Angi*itis* is inflammation of a blood vessel.

anti-. Against. An anti*biotic* is "against life"—in the case of a drug, against the life of disease germs.

arthr-. Joint. Arthro*pathy* is disease affecting a joint.

bleph-. Pertaining to the eyelid.

brady-. Slow. Brady*cardia* is slow heart beat.

bronch-, broncho-. Pertaining to the windpipe.

cardi, cardio-. Denoting the heart.

carp-. The wrist.

-cele. Swelling or herniation of a part, as *recto*cele, prolapse of the rectum.

cephal-. Pertaining to the head. *Encephal-,* "within the head," pertains to the brain.

cervi-. A neck.

chol-, chole-. Relating to bile. Chole*sterol* is a substance found in bile.

chon-, chondro-. Cartilage.

costo-, costal. Pertaining to the ribs.

cranio-. Skull. As in crani*otomy*, incision through a skull bone.

cry-, cryo- Icy cold.

cyan-. Blue.

-cyst-. Pertaining to a bladder or sac, normal or abnormal, filled with gas, liquid, or semi-solid material. The root appears in many words concerning the urinary bladder (cysto*cele*, cyst*itis*).

-cyt-, cyto-. Cell. *Leuko*cytes are white blood cells.

dia-. Through.

dent-, dento-. Pertaining to a tooth or teeth; from the Latin.

-derm, derma-. Skin.

-dynia. Condition of pain, usually with a prefix identifying the affected part.

dys-. Difficult, bad. This prefix occurs in large numbers of medical words, since it is attachable to any organ or process that isn't functioning as well as it should.

-ectomy. A cutting out; surgical removal. Denotes any operation in which all or part of a named organ is cut out of the body.

endo-. Within, inside of, internal. The endo*metrium* is the lining membrane of the uterus.

-enter-, entero-. Pertaining to the intestines. Gastro*enter*itis is an inflammation of the intestines as well as the stomach.

eryth-, erythro-. Redness. Eryth*ema* is indicated by redness of the skin (including a deep blush). An erythro*cyte* is a red blood cell.

eu-. Well and good. A eu*thyroid* person has a thyroid gland that couldn't be working better. A eu*phoric* one has a tremendous sense of wellbeing.

gastr-, gastro-. Pertaining to the stomach.

-gen-. Producing, begetting, *gen*erating.

glossa-. Pertaining to the tongue.

gnatho-. Pertaining to the jaw. *Micro*gnathia means abnormal smallness of the jaw.

-gogue. Eliciting a flow. A *chole*gogue stimulates the flow of bile.

gyn-, gyne-. Woman, female. Gyne*cology* literally means the study and knowledge of woman, a daringly ambitious enterprise, but useful in its common meaning: the medical specialty concerned with diseases of women.

-gram, -graph. These roots refer to writing, inscribing. They appear in the names of many instruments which record bodily functions on graphs or charts. The *-graph* is the instrument that does the recording; the *-gram* is the record itself. An *electrocardio*graph records the activities of the heart; an *electrocardio*gram is the record.

hem-, hemato-, -em-. Pertaining to blood. Hemat*uria* means blood in the urine. When the roots occur internally in a word, the "h" is often dropped for the sake of pronunciation, leaving *-em-* to denote blood, as in anox*em*ia (deficiency of oxygen in the blood).

hemi-. Half. The prefix is plain enough in hemi*plegia*, "half paralysis," affecting one side of the body. It's not so plain in *migraine* (one-sided headache), a word which shows how language changes through the centuries. The original word was *hemicrania*, "half-head."

hepar-, hepat-. Pertaining to the liver.

hyal-. Glassy.

hyper-. Over, above, increased. The usual implication is overactivity or excessive production, as in hyper*thyroidism*.

hypo-. Under, below; less, decreased. The two different meanings of this common prefix can be tricky. *Hypodermic* might reasonably be interpreted to mean that some unfortunate patient has too little skin. The actual meaning is *under* or *beneath* the skin, a proper site for an injection. The majority of "hypo" words, however, denote an insufficiency, lessening, reduction from the norm, as in *hypoglycemia,* too little glucose in the blood.

hyster-, hystero-. Denoting the womb. *Hysteria* perpetuates a Greek notion that violent emotional behavior originated in the uterus; when it occurred in men it must have been called something else.

-ia. A suffix indicating "condition," preceded by the name of the conditioned organ or system, as *pneumonia.* A physician wishing to be more specific might call it pneumon*itis,* but a patient, hardly ever.

iatro-. Pertaining to a doctor. A related root, *-iatrist,* denotes a specialist—ped*iatric*ian, obst*etric*ian.

-iasis. Indicates a condition, as *trichini*asis.

idio-. Peculiar to, private, distinctive. As in idio*syncrasy.*

inter-. Between.

intra-. Within.

-itis. Inflammation.

labio-. Pertaining to lips or lip-shaped structures.

leuk-, leuko-. White.

lig-. Binding. A liga*ment* ties two or more bones together.

lipo-. Fat, fatty.

-lith-. Stone, calcification. Lith*iasis* is a condition of stone formation.

mamma-, mast-. Pertaining to the breast. The first root derives from Latin, the second from Greek. *Mamma-* is obvious in *mammal* and *mammary* gland. The *mast-* root is usually limited to terms for diseases, disorders or procedures, as *mastectomy* (excision of the breast) and *mastoidectomy* (hollowing out of bony processes behind the ear). These lookalike words can be confusing. Is there breast tissue behind the ear? No, the root-key in mast-*oid*-ectomy is the three-letter insert "oid," meaning "like" or "resembling." Anatomists who named the bony *mastoid* process thought that its shape resembled a breast.

mega-, megalo-. Large, huge. The prefix *macro-* has the same meaning.

melan-. Black. The root usually refers in some way to cells that produce *melanin,* the dark pigment mobilized by a suntan. But it also endures in *melancholy,* "black bile," a gloomy humor anciently supposed to be the cause of wretchedness.

men-, meno-. Pertaining to menstruation, from a Greek word for "month."

metr-, metro-. Relating to the womb. Endo*metrium* is the lining membrane of the womb.

myelo-. Pertaining to marrow.

my-, myo-. Pertaining to muscle. Myo*cardium* is heart muscle.

nephr-, nephro-. From the Greek for "kidney." Also see *ren-.*

necro-. Deadness.

neur-, neuro-. Denoting nerves.

ocul-, oculo- (Latin) and **ophthalmo-** (Greek). Both roots refer to the eye, "ophth" words more often to diseases.

odont-, odonto-. Pertaining to a tooth or teeth. An ex*odont*ist extracts teeth (*ex-* or *ec-,* "out of," "out from.").

-oid. Like, resembling, Typh*oid* fever resembles typhus fever, or was supposed to when the name was given, but the two diseases are quite different.

olig-, oligo-. Scanty, few, little. Olig*uria* means scanty urination.

-oma. Denotes a tumor, not necessarily a malignant one.

onych-, onycho-. Pertaining to the nails of fingers or toes.

oo-. Denotes an egg. Pronounced oh-oh, not ooh. The combining form *oophor-* denotes an ovary. Oophoro*hyster*ectomy means surgical removal of the uterus and ovaries.

orch-. Pertaining to the testicles. Orchi*dectomy* has the same meaning as castration.

ortho-. Straight, correct, normal. Ortho*psychiatry* is the specialty concerned with "straightening out" behavior disorders.

oro-, os-. Mouth, opening, entrance. From the Latin, which also gives *os* another meaning, to complicate matters. See below.

os-, oste-, osteo-. Pertaining to bone. The Latin *os-* is most often associated with anatomical structures, the Greek *osteo-* with conditions involving bone. Osteo*gen*esis means formation of bone.

-osis. Indicates a condition of production or increase (*leukocyt*osis, abnornormal increase in numbers of white blood cells) or a condition of having parasites or pathogenic agents in the body (*trichin*osis).

-ostomy. Indicates the surgical making of a mouth, opening, or entrance. The opening may be external, as in *colos*tomy, the creation of an artificial outlet of the colon as a substitute for the anus, or internal, as in *gastroentero*stomy, establishment of an artificial "mouth" or opening between stomach and intestine. Compare with *-otomy*.

ot-, oto-. Pertaining to the ear. Oto*rrhea* means a discharge from the ear.

-otomy. Indicates a cutting, a surgical incision (but not the removal of an organ; compare with *-ectomy*). *Myringo*tomy means incision of the eardrum.

pachy-. Thick. A pachy*derm* (not necessarily an elephant) is thick-skinned.

para-. (Greek). Alongside, near, abnormal. As in para*proct*itis, inflammation of tissues near the rectum. A Latin suffix with the same spelling, *-para*, denotes bearing, giving birth, as *multi*para, a woman who has given birth to two or more children.

path-, patho-, pathy-. Feeling, suffering, disease. Patho*gen*ic, producing disease; *entero*pathy, disease of the intestines; patho*logy*, the medical specialty concerned with all aspects of disease. The root appears in the everyday word sym*pathy* ("to feel with").

ped-. A root with two meanings, requiring discrimination. The Latin root pertains to the foot, as in *pedal*. The Greek-derived root signifies children or child, as in ped*odontia*, dental care of children. Interestingly, a *pedagogue* tries to elicit or stimulate a flow (*-gogue*), presumably of learning, from children (*ped-*).

-penia. Scarcity, deficiency, poverty, "starved of." As in *erythro*penia, deficiency in number of red blood cells.

peri-. Denoting around, about, surrounding. Peri*odont*ium is a word for tissues which surround and support the teeth.

phag-, -phagy. Pertaining to eating, ingesting. As in *geo*phagy, dirt eating; *eso*phagus, the gullet; phago*cyte*, a cell capable of engulfing and ingesting foreign particles.

phleb-. Denoting a vein. As in phleb*otomy,* cutting into a vein to let blood; phlebo*thrombosis,* a condition of clotting in a vein.

plast-, -plasia, -plasty. Indicates molding, formation. An objective of *plastic* surgery, as in *mammo*plasty, an operation for correction of sagging breasts.

-plegia. From a Greek word for stroke; paralysis. *Quadri*plegia means paralysis of both legs and arms.

-pnea. Pertaining to breathing. *Dys*pnea is difficult breathing.

pneumo- (Greek) and **pulmo-** (Latin). Both terms pertain to the lungs.

-poiesis. Production, formation. *Hema-topoiesis* means formation of blood.

poly-. Many.

presby-. Old. As in presby*opia,* eye changes associated with aging.

proct-, procto-. Pertaining to the anus or rectum. Procto*plasty,* reparative or reconstructive surgery of the rectum.

psych-, psycho-. Pertaining to the mind, from the Greek word for "soul."

pur-, pus- (Latin) and **pyo-** (Greek). Indicates pus, as in *pur*ulent, sup*pura*tive, *pus*tulent, and pyo*derma,* suppurative disease of the skin.

pyel-, pyelo-. Pertaining to the urine-collecting chamber (pelvis) of the kidney.

pyr-, pyret-. Indicates fever.

-raphy. A suffix indicating a seam, suture, sewing together; usually describes a surgical operation, such as *herni*orrhaphy, a suture operation for hernia.

ren-. Latin for kidney; this root form is usually found in anatomical terms, such as *renal* and *supra*renal. The Greek-derived root, *nephr-,* usually occurs in words describing diseases or procedures. Custom dictates usage. *Nephritis* could as well be called *ren-itis,* but it isn't.

retro-. Backward or behind.

rhag-, rhagia-. Indicates a bursting, breaking forth, discharge from a burst vessel; usually denotes bleeding, as in *hemor*rhage, with an aspect of suddenness.

-rhea. Indicates a flowing, a discharge, as in *oto*rrhea, discharge from the ear.

rhin-, rhino-. Pertaining to the nose.

scler-. Indicates hard, hardness. *Arterio*sclerosis is a condition of hardening of the arteries.

somat-, somato-. Pertaining to the body.

stom-, stomato-. Pertaining to the mouth or a mouth.

supra-. Above, upon.

tachy-. Indicates fast, speedy, as in tachy*cardia,* abnormally rapid heartbeat.

thromb-. Pertaining to a blood clot.

-ur-, ure-, ureo-. Pertaining to urine.

urethr-, urethro-. Relating to the urethra, the canal leading from the bladder for discharge of urine.

veni-, veno-. Relating to the veins.

xanth-. Yellow.

xero-. Indicates dryness, as xero*stomia,* dryness of the mouth.

ENCYCLOPEDIA
OF MEDICAL TERMS

The Encyclopedia is designed for reference with the Better Homes and Gardens Family Medical Guide. Numbers in parentheses refer to pages where a topic is discussed more fully or illustrations are given. SMALL CAPITALS in the text below indicate that the topic can be looked up under its own heading in the Encyclopedia. Also consult the INDEX.

A

Abduction. The moving of a part away from its midline or from the axis of the body; for example, moving the thumb away from the index finger.

ABO. Designates a classic blood group, the one most familiar to people who know their blood type. Blood groups are based on the presence or absence of "factors" or antigens in red blood cells, determined by heredity. Type A blood contains factor A; Type B blood contains factor B; Type AB contains both factors; Type O contains neither. These types are further subdivided by the presence or absence of anti-A or anti-B factors in red cells or serum, and by even more complicated factors.

Abortion. Expulsion of an embryo or fetus from the uterus before it is capable of independent life. *Spontaneous* abortion is a not uncommon event of pregnancy; the lay term is "miscarriage." Some expulsions of an embryo too malformed to live occur so early in pregnancy that they may not be recognized. *Induced* abortions, performed under safe and sterile conditions in a hospital, have long been permissible if reputable physicians agree that the mother's life or health is endangered. *Criminal* abortions ("illegal operations") are often performed under conditions of furtiveness, crudity, and haste which can lead to infection, invalidism, sterility, and sometimes death. Legality of abortion is a matter of state laws, which differ consider-

ably. In recent years, abortion laws have been liberalized in 16 states, in an apparent trend to allow free choice to women. Among the most liberal states in this respect are New York, Kansas, and California which do not impose a waiting period on non-residents.

Abrasion. A scraped skin surface, such as a skinned knee which oozes blood (847).

Abruptio placentae. Premature breaking off of the placenta, accompanied by hemorrhage, near the end of pregnancy. Causes may be mechanical or toxic.

Abscess. A collection of pus within a well-defined space in any part of the body. Treatment is by drainage and overcoming of infection.

Accommodation. Change in curvature of the lens of the eye to bring objects into sharp focus (554).

Accouchement. A French word for childbirth.

Acetabulum. The cup-shaped cavity in the hip bone in which the upper end of the thigh bone rests (620).

Achalasia. Inability to relax a hollow muscular organ; especially, a spasmodic tightening of the lower portion of the esophagus (*cardiospasm*), producing a feeling that swallowed food had lodged itself at the entrance to the stomach (469).

Achilles tendon. The thickest and strongest tendon of the body, extending upward about six inches from the back of the heel. It binds the muscles of the calf of the leg to the heel bone.

Achlorhydria. Absence of free hydrochloric acid from the stomach. The condition is frequently a symptom of pernicious anemia, sometimes of stomach cancer or other diseases, but it may occur in elderly people who are quite healthy.

Acholic. Without bile. Clay-colored *acholic stools* indicate some obstructive or other disorder of the liver or bile ducts.

Achondroplasia. A form of dwarfism; the head and torso are of normal size but arms and legs are very short. The condition results from a congenital defect in the formation of cartilage at the growing ends of long bones which prevents normal lengthening.

Acid and Alkaline foods. There is no reason for a normal person to be in the least concerned about the acidity or alkalinity of foods. Doctors sometimes put patients who have acid kidney stones on a high alkaline ash diet, and patients who have alkaline kidney stones on a high acid ash diet. Persons with peptic ulcer should not drink large amounts of citrus or other acid juices on an empty stomach, because the immediate effect is to increase acidity and irritate the ulcer. But the ultimate effect of most acid juices and of foods which contain organic acids and taste sour is to leave an alkaline ash—that is, their ultimate reactions in the body are alkaline. Almost all fruits and vegetables, although they may taste acid, are alkaline-producing foods. The major acid-producing foods are cereals, meats, eggs and cheese, which don't taste very acid at all. An ordinary mixed diet provides perfectly adequate acid-alkaline ash balance, and even if doesn't, the body has remarkably efficient buffering systems to keep matters in balance.

Foods with alkaline ash:

All fruits except cranberries, plums, prunes, and rhubarb
All vegetables except corn and dried lentils
Milk
Almonds
Brazil nuts
Chestnuts
Coconut
Molasses

Foods with acid ash:

Bread
Cereals
Cranberries, plums, prunes, rhubarb
Bacon
Beef
Cheese
Chicken
Eggs
Fish
Ham
Lamb
Liver
Pork
Veal
Peanut butter
Peanuts
Popcorn
Walnuts
Corn
Lentils

Neutral foods:

Butter
Cornstarch
Cream
Lard
Oils
Sugar
Tapioca
Coffee
Tea

Acid-base balance. Blood is slightly alkaline; it is never acid during life. Mechanisms which maintain this delicate balance are remarkably efficient and do not require continued worry or attention except in presence of disease which a doctor is sure to recognize. Acid-base balance is kept constant by elimination of carbon dioxide from the lungs, excretion of acid by the kidneys (urine is normally acid), and buffer systems of the blood. The chief acid-maker is carbon dioxide which forms carbonic acid when dissolved in water. Sodium bicarbonate constitutes a large alkaline reserve in the blood. Interplay between carbonic acid and bicarbonate keeps the blood exquisitely balanced. *Acidosis* (reduced alkalinity of the blood, but not to the extent that it becomes acid) can result from disturbance of the balancing system by kidney insufficiency, diabetes (349), prolonged diarrhea with loss of bicarbonate, and other conditions that doctors are aware of. Significant acidosis practically never occurs except in diseases which are or should be under treatment. You can get a mild brief acidosis by holding your breath as long as you can, while carbon dioxide accumulates in the lungs; the main sensation is a wild desire to breathe. Strenuous exercise can also produce mild and harmless acidosis because breathing can't quite keep up with carbon dioxide accumulation. Colds and respiratory infections do not cause acidosis nor are such conditions made worse by a vague "acid condition" which is supposedly corrected by taking alkalis to "get on the alkaline side." Excessive intake of antacids or bicarbonate may in fact produce the opposite condition of *alkalosis*—slightly increased alkalinity of the blood. You can induce alkalosis by HYPERVENTILATION; overbreathing forces so much air into the lungs that carbon dioxide is diluted. The same type of alkalosis occurs in MOUNTAIN SICKNESS when overbreathing results from thinness of the air at high altitudes. Alkalosis can also result from prolonged vomiting which removes a large amount of acid from the system.

Acidosis. Decreased alkalinity of the blood and other body fluids. See ACID-BASE BALANCE.

Acid stomach. Burning, gnawing pain in the upper abdomen is often self-attributed to "acid stomach," especially if distress is not continuous. The stomach is naturally acid and a reasonably normal stomach gets along contentedly with its acids. An acid-free stomach is abnormal and possibly belongs to a patient with pernicious anemia. It is possible for stomach contents to become too acid, from slow emptying, oversecretion, or other causes, but analysis of stomach juices is necessary to determine if acid abnormalities are truly involved. Self-diagnosed "acid stomach," encouraged by animated advertising which shows flaming acids dripping onto the cringing mucosa, is often the result of nervous squirming of the stomach, or inflation by gas-producing foods, or irritants, or too much smoking, or food allergy, or gorging, or a dozen causes other than a rain of red-hot acids. If distress persists, see a doctor; it is unwise to take antacids continuously over long periods to subdue symptoms while some possibly serious condition gets a foothold.

Acne rosacea. A chronic disease, entirely unrelated to common acne, resulting from dilation of superficial blood vessels, giving an appearance of constant redness of the flush area of the middle part of the face (184).

Acne vulgaris. Common acne; a skin disorder, most conspicuously affecting the face, with pimples and blackheads as the most obvious lesions. Acne has nothing to do with "bad blood" or bad conduct; it is due to overactivity of oil-secreting glands and hair follicles. It is associated with the increase of sex hormones at puberty, and is in large degree a physiologic condition that most young people pass through on their way to sexual maturity. Acne usually subsides in the twenties, but in the meantime various treatments are beneficial (182). Severe cases particularly should have good medical care in order to avert possible scarring and pitting.

Acromegaly. A disorder of adults due to overproduction of growth hormones by the pituitary gland (317). The word means "giant extremities." There is gross enlargement of the bones and soft parts of the face and hands and feet. The face with its thickened tissues, enlarged jaw, nose, and bony ridges over the eyes, has a characteristic coarse appearance. Height is not increased. However, if the same hormone overproduction occurs in a young person before the growing ends of the bones have closed, he becomes a "pituitary giant" up to eight feet tall.

ACTH. Abbreviation of *adrenocorticotrophic hormone;* a hormone of the pituitary gland which stimulates the adrenal gland to produce cortisone-like hormones (317).

Actinomycosis (*lumpy jaw*). An infectious disease caused by fungi which produce unsightly lumpy, pus-draining abscesses, especially common to the face and jaw (74).

Acupuncture. An ancient Oriental (especially Chinese) system of folk medicine in which needles are inserted into parts of the body and twirled rapidly, to treat disease or induce anesthesia. Traditional acupuncture recognizes 300-odd regions of the body arranged on lines associated with major organs. Theoretically, needles inserted into appropriate sites on appropriate lines restore the ebb and flow of opposing forces (*yin* and *yang;* male and female) to natural rhythms, thus benefiting affected organs. Interest of Western physicians in the theories and mysteries of acupuncture was stimulated by several doctors who visited China and watched major operations in which needling was apparently used successfully as the only form of anesthesia. A few experiments with acupuncture in the U. S. (modified, in some instances, by attaching a source of electric current to needles instead of twirling them) suggest that the procedure might have limited value for anesthesia in some circumstances. Whether acupuncture is a temporary fad, how much of its anesthetizing effects are attributable to auto-hypnosis, and whether it is really practical, are undetermined. Hypnosis itself can produce anesthesia, but few doctors use it because of time required for preparation and induction, and alternatives are always at hand, as with acupuncture. A plausible if unproved explanation of how acupuncture may ease pain is that needles may "close gates" along nerve pathways and thus prevent transmission of pain sensations to the brain. A disadvantage of acupuncture in major surgery is that, while it may ease pain, it does not—unlike conventional anesthetics—produce muscle relaxation which is important in surgical procedures.

Adams-Stokes syndrome. Giddiness, fainting, sometimes convulsions, resulting from slowed heart action caused by heart block (110).

Addison's disease. A chronic disease characterized by weakness, easy fatigability, skin pigmentation, low blood pressure and other symptoms (331). The underlying cause is atrophy or disease of the outer layer of the adrenal gland.

Adduction. The moving of a part toward another or toward the axis of the body: for example, moving the thumb toward the index finger. The opposite of ABDUCTION.

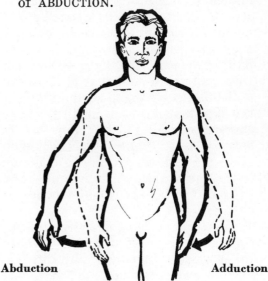

Abduction   Adduction

Adenoviruses. A group of viruses responsible for respiratory infections like the common cold (55), viral conjunctivitis, intestinal infections, and latent infections which may cause some swelling of tonsils, adenoids, and other glandular tissue, especially in children. There are more than 30 different types of adenoviruses. The organisms are widespread and sometimes give rise to epidemics of considerable extent. Most people have been infected by them. Except in small infants, adenovirus infections are rarely serious. They generally run their course in a week or less. Vaccines have been developed but their use is largely limited to military establishments where conditions are favorable for epidemics among young men in barracks.

Adhesions. Abnormal sticking together of tissues which should slip or slide freely over each other. Diseases may produce adhesions: in the chest cavity as a result of pleurisy, in injured joints restricted in movement, in other areas of inflammation. Adhesions in the abdominal and pelvic cavities may occur after surgical operations, particularly if pus has spilled from a ruptured abscess. It is not always or often desirable to do further surgery to free the adhesions unless they threaten to obstruct the bowel.

Adhesive tape removal. Ripping adhesive tape from the skin can be less ouchful if the patient is removed from the tape instead of the tape from the patient. Try it this way: Pick up a corner of the tape, lift it gently, and with fingers of the other hand press the skin that is just beneath the tape slowly away from it. In this way only a small area of skin is peeled down from the tape at a time, in contrast to the entire area which is pulled and lifted if the tape is rudely ripped.

Adipose tissue. Fatty connective tissue; commonly, the part of the body where fat is stored. Usually, "adiposity" is a polite way of saying "too fat."

Adiposis dolorosa. See DERCUM'S DISEASE.

Adolescence. The period of years between the beginning of puberty, when the reproductive organs become functionally active, and maturity.

Adolescent bent hip. A condition of older children resulting from disconnection of the upper end of the thighbone from its normal hip joint attachments, producing a wobbly, painful hip and limping (640).

Adrenalin. Proprietary name for *epinephrine*, the hormone produced by the inner portion or medulla of the adrenal gland (330).

Aerobic. Living or functioning in air or free oxygen.

Aero-otitis media. Inflammation of the middle ear caused by differences in air pressure within the chamber and outside of it. Also called "flyer's ear," since rapid changes of air pressure with changes in altitude tend to produce it. Normally, air pressure is equalized on both sides of the eardrum by the entrance or escape of air through the Eustachian tube which runs from the middle ear to the throat (595). This pressure-valve adjustment is what makes the ears "pop" during rapid ascent or descent of an elevator in a high building. Swallowing usually helps to "massage" a little air into or out of the tube. Infections or obstructions may block the free passage of air through the tube.

African sleeping sickness. A disease with a high fatality rate caused by organisms that get into the blood through the bites of tsetse flies indigenous to parts of Africa (73). It is not the same as sleepiness associated with some forms of encephalitis.

Afterbirth. The placenta and membranes discharged from the uterus a few minutes after the birth of a baby.

After-image. A visual image which remains for a few seconds after the eyes are closed or light has ceased to stimulate. An after-image can be produced by looking at a bright light or bright objects for a few seconds, then closing the eyes, or turning them on a dark surface, or fixing your gaze on a bright sheet of white paper. An image of the object will slowly float into view, become more distinct, and gradually fade away. After-images are either "positive" or "negative." A positive after-image shows the object in its correct shade of black or white or color. A negative after-image reverses dark and light parts and, if the object was colored, shows the complementary instead of the original color; for instance, a red object produces a green after-image.

Agammaglobulinemia. Blood deficiency of GAMMA GLOBULIN, protein molecules which produce protective antibodies against infections. The deficiency leaves the patient extremely susceptible to repeated infections. The condition may be congenital or acquired. The congenital form has an hereditary basis; it is a complex defect of IMMUNITY mechanisms of the body, manifested as undue susceptibility to repeated infections in infancy. It is important to avoid exposure of an affected infant to infections, as far as possible; to treat acute infections with antibiotics; to give regular monthly injections of gamma globulin.

Agranulocytosis. An acute, rare, frequently fatal illness associated with extreme reduction or complete absence of granular white blood cells (142) from the bone marrow. Absence of cells which protect against infection results in weakness, rapid onset of high fever, sore throat, prostration, ulcerations of the mouth and mucous membranes. The disease may arise from unknown causes, but usually it can be traced to some chemical or drug which injures the bone marrow; the agent may be a widely used valuable substance which is harmless to most people but to which the patient is peculiarly sensitive (174). Treatment aims to combat infection while the bone marrow becomes normal.

Air embolism. Plugging of blood vessels by air bubbles carried in the bloodstream, fatal if large numbers of bubbles reach the heart. Air can enter the bloodstream by accidental injection or through wounds of the neck. Air embolism is also a hazard of SCUBA DIVING; holding the breath while ascending from even relatively shallow depths may cause rupture of a part of the lung, forcing air bubbles into pulmonary veins and thence to arteries nourishing the brain.

Air-swallowing (*aerophagia*). The habit, usually unconscious, of swallowing excessive amounts of air. The gas may escape via an embarrassing belch, or lead to FLATULENCE, or may from entrapment cause diversified distentions and twinges of the gut. A small amount of air is naturally swallowed with food or drink or conversation, but excessive intake may be promoted by gulping, chewing with the lips parted, swigging fluids from a narrow-necked bottle, talking while eating, chewing gum, smoking, and nervous swallowing. More often than not the air-swallower hasn't the slightest idea that he is indulging in pneumatic excesses, and he is usually able to overcome the habit if it is called to his surprised attention unless there is some neurotic basis for it.

Air travel. The Aerospace Medical Association and the American Medical Association agree that flying is not harmful to most ill patients and is the most desirable form of travel for those who have certain types of illnesses. This presupposes the availability of oxygen or medication that a particular patient may require, and evaluation by a doctor of some conditions such as severe anemia or recent eye surgery which may increase the hazard. Infants over six days old travel well by air. A very general rule is that "if a person is able to walk 100 yards and to climb 12 steps without manifesting symptoms, flight in pressurized aircraft is permissible."

Alastrim. A mild form of smallpox. See VARIOLA MINOR.

Albuminuria. Presence in the urine of albumin, a protein like egg white (293). The kidneys do not normally excrete albumin, which is a useful substance, and albuminuria suggests damage to the filtering apparatus, but this is not necessarily the case.

Aldosteronism (primary). A remediable form of high blood pressure (116); weakness, headaches, and other symptoms (332), due to excessive production of aldosterone, a hormone produced by the cortex of the adrenal gland. The hormone is a powerful regulator of salt and water balances. Excesses cause retention of sodium and loss of potassium. If the excess is caused by an adrenal gland tumor, its removal is indicated. All the manifestations of primary aldosteronism can be reversed in a few weeks by oral doses of an antagonistic drug, spironolactone.

Alkaline ash diet. A diet consisting mainly of fruits, vegetables and potatoes, with only small amounts of meat and cereals, sometimes prescribed for patients who have kidney disease or kidney stones of the uric acid type. Alkaline environment has been found to deter the formation of acid stones.

Alkalosis. Increased alkalinity of the blood. See ACID-BASE BALANCE.

Alkaptonuria. A rare hereditary disorder in which the body is unable to produce enzymes for proper utilization of certain AMINO ACIDS of protein foods. Byproducts of incomplete metabolism cause the urine to turn dark brown or black on long standing. The disorder

does not affect life expectancy but in later life leads to discoloration of cartilage and possibly to a severe form of arthritis.

Allergy. An altered capacity to react distressfully to specific substances which cause no symptoms in most people (671); a general term for all kinds of hypersensitivities. "Atopy" is a general synonym for allergy.

Allopurinol. A drug which reduces the body's production of uric acid, used in treatment of GOUT.

Alopecia. Baldness; loss of head hair. Some types of hair loss are temporary, some are irreversible (196). Neither hair "tonics" nor any other medical measure known to dermatologists (not a few of whom have nude scalps) can overcome male pattern baldness. This type of baldness affects men who have a genetic predisposition, who produce adequate amounts of male hormone, and who have attained sufficient age (they do not become bald before puberty). New surgical techniques for transplanting hairs from an area of lush growth to the bare scalp have had some success but are not widely popular. The technique consists of punching plugs of skin containing four or five hairs out of the back of the neck and inserting them into the scalp in hope that they will take root and spread like plugs of zoysia grass. In time, after transplants of scores of tufts (about $5 per tuft), the plugs may grow into presentable confluence.

Altitude sickness. See MOUNTAIN SICKNESS.

Alveolus. A sac or chamber; a saclike dilation at the end of a passage; especially, an air cell of the lung (212), the bony socket of a tooth, or a honeycomb cell of the stomach.

Amaurotic familial idiocy (*Tay-Sachs disease*). An hereditary disease occurring in Jewish children, manifested early in infancy, characterized by muscle weakness, progressive helplessness, and blindness ("amaurosis" means blindness). A characteristic bright cherry spot can be seen at the back of the infant's eye with an ophthalmoscope. No known treatment can reverse the condition and life expectancy is short. Certain related diseases which occur later in life do not have a racial incidence.

Amblyopia. Dimness of vision without any organic lesion of the eye. Amblyopia may result from various toxins, or an eye, such as the "lazy" eye of a cross-eyed child, may lose its vision from long disuse (566).

Amebiasis. Amebic dysentery (71).

Amenorrhea. The abnormal absence of menstruation (338).

Amino acids. Building blocks of PROTEIN. There are about 20 important amino acids. An amino acid molecule has an acid group of atoms at one end and an amino (nitrogen-containing) group at the other. In between are carbon units with different side chains which give each amino acid its individuality. The acid end of an amino acid links with the amino end of another, a sort of chemical hook-and-eye arrangement. In this way amino acids form short chains (peptides) or large, complex molecules containing many hundreds of different amino acids in exact sequences (protein). Eight amino acids are called "essential" because the body cannot synthesize them and they must be obtained ready-made from protein foods (493, 503). The amino acids of protein foods are separated by digestion and go into a general pool from which the body takes the ones it needs to synthesize its own personal proteins; thus an amino acid which we may have obtained from a pork chop may become a part of a fingernail, skin, hair, of a hormone such as insulin, or of an enzyme that activates some vital chemical process.

Amnion. The innermost of the fetal membranes, forming the BAG OF WATERS which surrounds and protects the embryo (377).

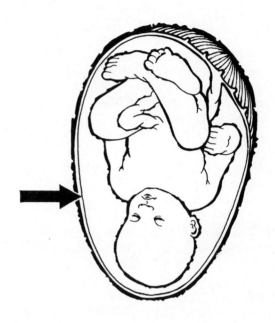

Arrow points to amnion

Amyloidosis. Abnormal masses of fibrous protein infiltrating various organs; primary or secondary to chronic diseases; treatment depends on underlying disease. Diagnosed by biopsy.

Amyotonia. Lack of muscle tone; a congenital form in infants is characterized by small undeveloped muscles and weakness of the limbs and trunk.

Amyotrophic lateral sclerosis. Progressive paralysis and wasting of muscles on both sides of the body; sometimes called "Lou Gehrig's disease" (264).

Anabolic steroids. Drugs related to male hormones, sometimes given for anabolic ("upbuilding") action, to stimulate growth, weight gain, strength and appetite. The drugs are more accurately called androgenic-anabolic steroids, since they are related to testosterone and retain some of the male hormone's masculinizing action. Although the masculinizing action has been minimized in some anabolic steroids, the separation is not complete and prolonged use will cause virilization. Testosterone itself has pronounced anabolic action but is not suitable for prolonged use in women and children.

Anabolism. The "building up" aspect of metabolism; constructive processes of body cells which build complex substances from simpler ones. The opposite of CATABOLISM.

Anaerobic. Living or functioning in the absence of free air or free oxygen. TETANUS and GAS GANGRENE organisms are anaerobic.

Such organisms thrive best if deprived of oxygen, as in deep puncture wounds, or cannot survive at all if oxygen is present.

Anaphylaxis. An acute reaction to a substance injected by a doctor or insect or inhaled or swallowed; a "super allergy." Anaphylaxis is an ANTIGEN-ANTIBODY reaction which occurs in seconds or minutes after a foreign substance has entered the body. The immediate, severe, and sometimes fatal reaction is manifested by hives, rhinitis, wheezing, shock, ANGIONEU-ROTIC EDEMA, difficult breathing, in varying combinations and degrees of severity. The most frequent causes of anaphylactic reactions are serums, drugs, and vaccines; next most common are insect stings (696). Skin tests may detect hypersensitivity to a substance but sometimes even the minute amount used in a test may provoke a reaction. If a doctor asks you to wait in his office 15 minutes or so after giving an injection, it's not a waste of time; he has emergency measures at hand if a dangerous reaction occurs. Because accident victims are often given routine injections of tetanus antitoxin or penicillin, persons who know they are sensitive to these substances should carry a warning card along with driver's license and identification papers where a doctor who is a stranger is sure to see it.

Anasarca. Generalized EDEMA.

Androgen. A substance which has masculinizing effects (335).

Android. Resembling a man; male-like.

Anesthesia. Loss of feeling. This can occur from natural processes or accidents; for example, nerve injury, frostbite, hysteria, blood vessel spasms, diseases. Ordinarily the word refers to obliteration of pain by anesthetic drugs, with or without loss of consciousness. There are many kinds of anesthetic drugs and gases, administered by inhalation, infusion or injection (778). Each anesthetic has specific properties, advantages and disadvantages; selection of the best agent or combination for a particular patient requires special knowledge. The safety and relative comfort of modern surgery, and the ability to perform complex prolonged operations without haste, depends no little upon the anesthesia team headed by an anesthesiologist who regulates the depth of anesthesia, chooses the most suitable anesthetics in consultation with surgeons, and keeps close watch on the patient's condition with the aid of a battery of monitoring devices.

Aneurysm. A blood-filled sac like a thin-walled balloon formed by dilation of artery walls; it is susceptible to rupture and hemorrhage (125, 131).

Angiitis. Inflammation of a blood or lymph vessel.

Angina. Any condition characterized by spasmodic attacks with sensations of strangling, pressure or suffocation; for example, *angina pectoris* (91).

Angiogram. X-ray visualization of blood vessels, usually accomplished by injecting a substance which is opaque to x-rays into the bloodstream. X-ray movies or large films taken in rapid succession may give important information about blood vessels in some types of heart trouble (787).

Angioma. A tumor composed of blood vessels; a class of birthmarks.

Angioneurotic edema. Acute local swelling, like giant hives under the skin, frequently a result of food allergy (693). The swelling is most serious if it occurs around the tongue and larynx, threatening suffocation.

Anhidrosis. Abnormal deficiency of sweat production.

Aniseikonia. A condition in which the image of an object as seen by one eye differs in size and shape from that seen by the other eye. The brain compensates for images of unequal size by suppressing one of them, and in time the eye which produces the suppressed image tends to become, for all practical purposes, blind. This type of blindness is called AMBLYOPIA; the affected person is essentially "one-eyed," and if the "good" eye is lost, the other is useless as a "spare tire." A complete eye examination of a child at about the age of three years can do much to prevent this insidious kind of damage from getting a start.

Ankylosis. Stiffening or growing together of a joint; the fusion may be part of a disease process (666) or it may be a deliberate surgical immobilization of a part.

Antacid. A substance that counteracts or neutralizes acidity. Most commonly, an oral substance taken to reduce acidity of gastric juices.

Anthrax (*wool-sorter's disease*). A bacterial disease of herbivorous animals. Spores of the causative organisms sometimes infect persons who have close contact with raw wool, bristles, or hides (47).

Anomaly. Deviation from normal of an organ or part; abnormality of structure or location.

Anorexia. Loss of appetite. *Anorectic drugs,* sometimes prescribed for a short time for persons on reducing diets, tend to suppress appetite. The drugs usually are amphetamines.

Anorexia nervosa. An emotional disturbance manifested by profound aversion to food, leading to extreme emaciation. The typical patient is a young single woman who rejects food in unconscious protection against an adult sex role she has difficulty in adjusting to. Usually she is not particularly concerned about her extreme skinniness and may even insist that she eats a lot. Management of the condition requires explanation, encouragement of eating, possibly hospitalization and psychiatric help.

Anoscope. An instrument for examining the lower part of the rectum by visual inspection; a SPECULUM.

Anoxemia. Deficiency of oxygen in the blood, almost total.

Anoxia. Oxygen deficiency in organs and tissues and disturbance resulting therefrom.

Antibiotics. Chemical substances produced by certain living cells, such as bacteria, yeasts, and molds, that are antagonistic or damaging to certain other living cells, such as disease-producing bacteria. Different antibiotics may kill disease germs or prevent them from growing and multiplying.

Antibody. A protein in the blood, modified by contact with a foreign substance (*antigen*) so that it exerts an antagonizing or neutralizing action against that specific substance. Antibodies are chiefly associated with GAMMA GLOBULIN in the blood and are key elements of IMMUNITY mechanisms of the body. Usually the antibody-antigen reaction is protective. Measles virus is an antigen which stimulates the body to produce measles antibodies, so we don't have measles twice. But antibody-antigen reactions may also be distressing or harmful, as in allergies (671). So-called AUTO-IMMUNE DISEASES presumably result, at least in part, from harmful reactions of antibodies against normal proteins of the patient's own body.

Anticoagulants. Drugs which slow up the clotting process of the blood. Clots forming in blood vessels are potentially deadly (see THROMBOSIS, EMBOLISM). Anticoagulants are useful in reducing the clotting tendency. The doctor's problem is knowing when and when not to use them; administration requires frequent checks of the patient's blood since overdosage can induce hemorrhage. Anticoagulants are commonly given to patients for a few weeks after a heart attack caused by a blood clot in coronary arteries. Specialists generally agree that such short term use of anticoagulants is valuable. There is difference of medical opinion as to whether the drugs should be continued for preventive purposes for many months or years or the remainder of a lifetime. Some studies extending over a 10-year period indicate that the drugs are of little value in preventing subsequent heart attacks, but there is also evidence that selected patients having recurrent clot-formation problems or recurrent heart attacks or mild strokes benefit from the continued supervised administration of anticoagulants.

Anticonvulsants. Drugs which are used primarily to reduce the number and severity of chronic epileptic seizures. The physician's choice of drugs depends upon the type of seizure (276). Treatment must be individualized. Since the drugs must be used for a prolonged period of time, it is important that the patient be told of possible adverse effects and be instructed to report unusual symptoms promptly to his doctor.

Antidiuretic hormone. A hormone produced in brain areas linked with the pituitary gland; it checks the secretion of urine (321).

Antiemetic. A drug or treatment which stops or prevents nausea or vomiting.

Antigen. Any substance which stimulates the production of ANTIBODIES.

Antihistamines. A large family of drugs which block some of the effects of histamine, a normal substance in body cells which plays a part in allergic reactions. Histamine, triggered by an antigen such as ragweed pollen, may escape from local groups of cells and cause symptoms of hay fever. Deliberate injection of histamine causes the walls of capillaries to become so permeable that fluids leak into nearby tissues. This leakage is characteristic of allergies. The effect may be superficial, as in weepy eyes or runny nose, or giant hives, or more deep-set as in dangerous swelling and constriction of the breathing passages.

Antihistamine drugs are most effective in treatment of acute urticaria and seasonal hay fever and generally give good results in subduing allergic tissue swellings (angioneurotic edema). They may often give symptomatic relief of allergic skin disorders and of itching not of allergic origin. The most widely prescribed preventives for motion sickness belong to the antihistamine family; they are effective against symptoms of dizziness, nausea and vomiting and have some sedative action. Although many attacks of bronchial asthma are allergic in origin, antihistamines have only limited value in prevention and treatment of asthma.

The drugs differ one from another in potency, effects, and duration of action; this is weighed by the physician in prescribing a specific drug. Some antihistamines have a pronounced tendency to cause drowsiness; others have very little sedative action. A person taking an antihistamine with somnolent action should reckon with its effects in driving a car. Some nonprescription sleeping pills and insomnia remedies contain small amounts of an antihistamine compound. These may cause some drowsiness but the effect is not uniform, most persons will acquire tolerance to the drug, and antihistamines cannot be considered reliable remedies against insomnia. Because of the depressant action of antihistamines, patients should not drink alcoholic beverages or take barbiturates which in combination may magnify depressant effects.

Anti-Rh serum. Prevention of ERYTHROBLASTOSIS ("Rh disease") is a possibility for the near future. Pregnant women lacking a substance in their red blood cells (Rh factor) may develop ANTIBODIES against their own babies whose blood does possess the factor. These antibodies can cause severe anemia and damage to the unborn child. The risk increases with each pregnancy after the first, which usually is normal because the mother has not yet become sensitized. A preventive measure now being studied intensively in this country and abroad is treatment of the Rh-negative mother with a specially prepared anti-Rh serum after the birth of each Rh-positive baby, to destroy quickly any Rh-positive blood cells of the baby which might have entered into her circulation, thus greatly reducing the chance of her sensitization. Trials of anti-Rh serum in a number of medical centers have been encouraging. Wide use of the serum may in the future eliminate an important cause of stillbirth and serious birth defects.

Antitoxin. A substance which neutralizes a specific bacterial, animal or plant toxin. Most of the antitoxins injected by doctors for treatment or prevention of disease are prepared from serum obtained from a horse or other animal which has been immunized by gradually increased doses of a particular toxin. Harmful reactions may follow injection if a patient is sensitive to the serum component.

Antrum. See MAXILLARY SINUS.

Antivenin. An antitoxin to venom, especially snake venom (399, 859).

Anuria. Total suppression of urine secretion; suggestive of but not confined to kidney damage.

Aorta. The great vessel which arches from the top of the heart and passes down through the chest and abdomen (82). It is the main trunk line of the arterial system.

Aphakia. Absence of the lens of the eye, as after cataract surgery (576).

Aplastic anemia. A grave form of anemia due to progressive failure of the bone marrow to develop new blood cells; it may be triggered by chemicals which poison the cell-producing mechanisms of the marrow (175).

Apnea. Temporary cessation of breathing because of absence of stimulation of the breathing center, as by too much oxygen or too little carbon dioxide.

Apoplexy. A stroke; cerebrovascular accident (CVA); rupture or hemorrhage of vessels into the brain.

Appendicitis. Acute inflammation of the appendix (489, 729). It occurs in all age groups but is most common in children and young persons. Typically, pain is felt in the region of the navel before it moves down to the appendix area in the lower right quarter of the abdomen, but not all cases are typical. The early pain may be mistaken for colic. If a child's severe "stomach ache" persists more than an hour or two, a doctor should be called to diagnose the trouble, which more often than not isn't appendicitis, but if it is, prompt action is important because an inflamed appendix can reach the bursting point in a few hours.

Appetite depressants (*anorexiants*). These are drugs which tend to allay sensations of hunger and to make the early phases of adjusting to a reducing diet somewhat easier. Appetite depressants prescribed by physicians are quite potent and should not be confused with milder and sometimes dubiously effective products that can be bought without a prescription. Medically prescribed appetite depressants are drugs of the amphetamine family or other "sympathomimetic" amines which cause physiologic changes similar to those produced by the sympathetic nervous system (247). It has been suggested that the drugs act upon an "appetite control" center in the brain stem, although this has not been proved. Some of their effects may be due to mood elevation. The drugs should be used only for a short time as adjuncts to a low-calorie diet for overcoming obesity, as temporary "crutches." Permanent weight control requires re-education of eating habits according to individual metabolism.

Aqueous humor. Watery fluid which fills the chamber of the eye in front of the lens (553). Obstruction of drainage builds internal pressures that lead to glaucoma (573).

Arcus senilis. A white ring around the outer edge of the colored portion of the eye, especially in the aged.

Areola. A pigmented ring surrounding a central point; for example, the pigmented area encircling the nipple.

Argyll-Robertson pupil. Excessively contracted pupils of the eye which do not react to light; a symptom of syphilis (48) of the central nervous system.

Ariboflavinosis. Deficiency of riboflavin, also called vitamin B_2, characterized by dryness of the skin, inflamed tongue, tiny blood vessels in the cornea giving a reddened appearance to the eye, and fissures at the angles of the lips (504).

Arrhythmia. Any departure from normal rhythm of the heartbeat (107).

Arteriosclerosis. A thickening and hardening of the walls of arteries and capillaries, leading to a loss of their elasticity. It is not the same condition as ATHEROSCLEROSIS.

HEART-ASSIST PUMP →

Drawing shows principle of device developed by Dr. M. E. DeBakey and associates of Baylor University. Called "paracorporeal" (the pump itself is outside the body), its purpose as shown in the drawing is to by-pass and thus "rest" a diseased left ventricle by performing the ventricle's function of pumping arterial blood to the body. Numbered structures are: 1, axillary artery; 2, left atrium; 3, pump; 4 and 5, pump filling and pumping; 6, right atrium; 7, right ventricle; 8, pulmonary artery; 9, left atrium; 10, left ventricle; 11, aorta; 12 and 13, tubes to and from pump; 14; axillary artery.

Artificial heart. As body structures go, the heart is relatively simple—a four-chambered pumping device. It may some day be replaceable by an artificial heart. But the obstacles are formidable. Thus far, so-called "artificial hearts" used in a few human patients have been "heart assist" devices using compressed air power to augment the pumping force of the patient's own heart. In principle, the devices consist of a rigid outer shell containing elastic chambers which expand and contract rhythmically in response to pulses of compressed air entering through a tube in the chest. Their hopeful role is that of temporary auxiliaries to help hearts with enough reserves to recover if tided over a crisis. But more than a dozen varieties of artificial hearts have been developed, and many more experimental models will undoubtedly come out of current research. Some of the devices do not aim to assist the patient's own heart, but to replace it entirely. In fact, some artificial hearts have totally replaced the hearts of calves and pigs. The animals seem to function just as comfortably as if they had a heart of their own. But after a few hours, two or three days at most, the animals die. Scientists don't know why. Artificial hearts appear to cause mysterious physiologic changes which, if they exist, will have to be overcome if a me-

Drawing A shows pump in place. Arrows show path of blood, purified in the lungs, from the left atrium (2) to pump (3), and from pump to connection with arterial system via axillary artery (1). Tube from base of pump leads to compressed air power source.

A

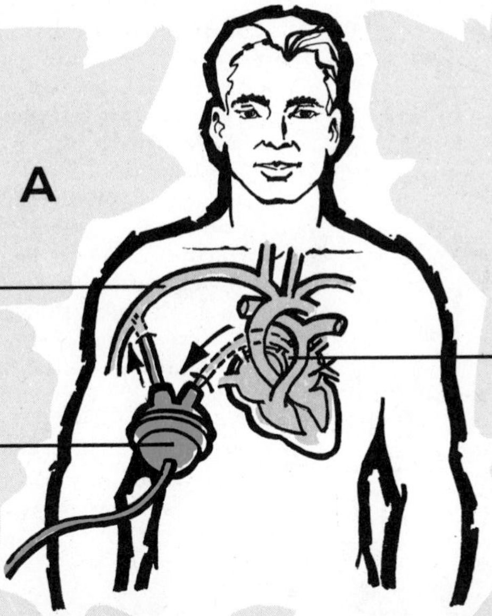

Drawing B. Air suction fills pump (4) with blood (diastole); air pressure (5) pumps blood to arteries (systole). Valves control flow direction.

B

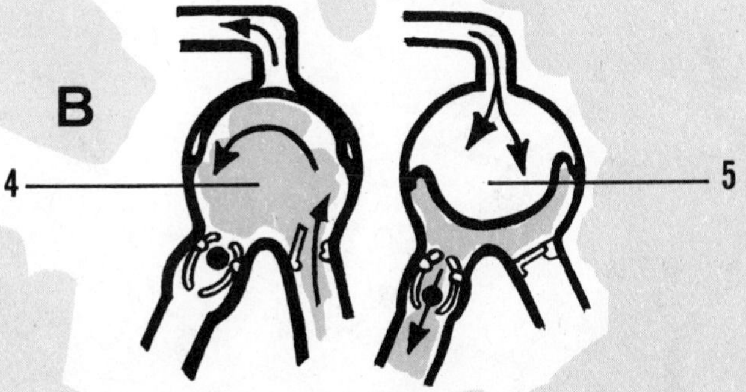

Drawing C, schematic diagram of normal circulation. Drawing D at right shows details: tube (12) connected to left atrium receives oxygenated blood from the lungs which fills pump; tube (13) delivers arterial blood to body, via axillary artery connection (14), when pump compresses by-passing the left side of the heart.

C

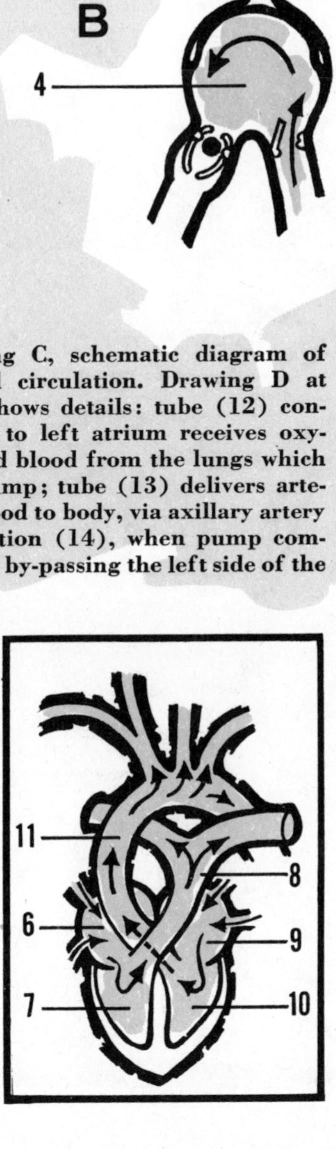

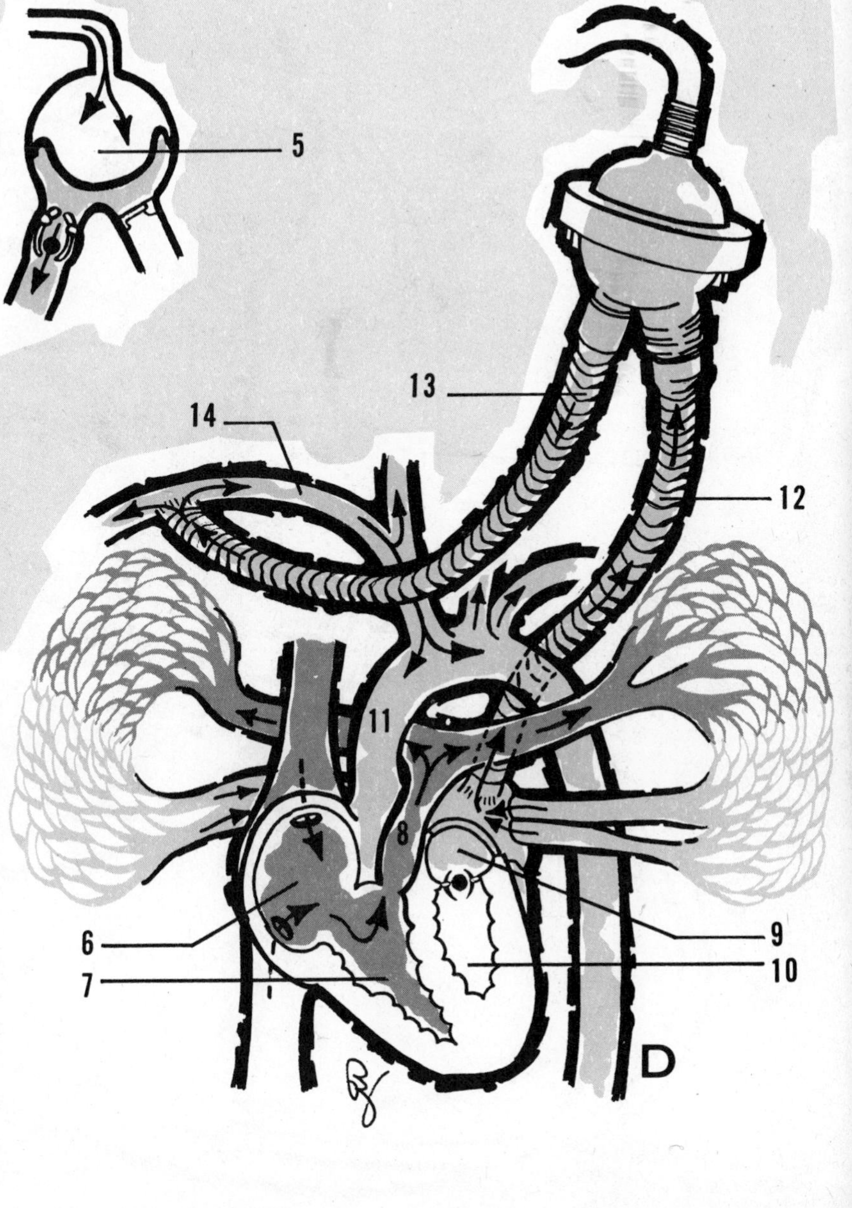

D

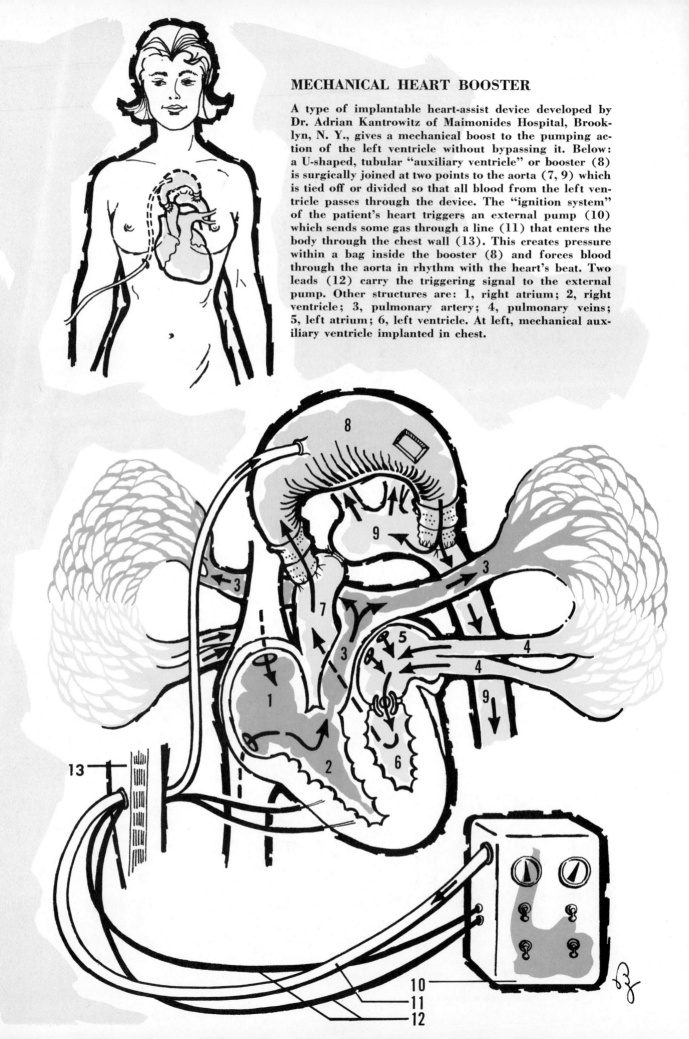

MECHANICAL HEART BOOSTER

A type of implantable heart-assist device developed by Dr. Adrian Kantrowitz of Maimonides Hospital, Brooklyn, N. Y., gives a mechanical boost to the pumping action of the left ventricle without bypassing it. Below: a U-shaped, tubular "auxiliary ventricle" or booster (8) is surgically joined at two points to the aorta (7, 9) which is tied off or divided so that all blood from the left ventricle passes through the device. The "ignition system" of the patient's heart triggers an external pump (10) which sends some gas through a line (11) that enters the body through the chest wall (13). This creates pressure within a bag inside the booster (8) and forces blood through the aorta in rhythm with the heart's beat. Two leads (12) carry the triggering signal to the external pump. Other structures are: 1, right atrium; 2, right ventricle; 3, pulmonary artery; 4, pulmonary veins; 5, left atrium; 6, left ventricle. At left, mechanical auxiliary ventricle implanted in chest.

chanical organ is to serve for many months or years. The ideal artificial heart will have to be light in weight; its vibrations must not be harmful; it must be totally innocuous to surrounding tissues; its power source must be miniaturized and unfailing; and it must not induce blood clotting. The requirements are formidable but not insurmountable, in the opinion of eminent researchers who are tackling the problem whole-heartedly.

Artificial insemination. Mechanical introduction of semen into the vagina or uterus to induce pregnancy. If successful, conception, pregnancy, and childbirth occur in a perfectly normal way. The first recorded attempt at human artificial insemination was performed by the famous English surgeon, John Hunter, in 1799. Artificial insemination is widely employed in animal husbandry, but its availability to couples troubled by *infertility* (340) has largely come about in the past quarter century. Technically, there are two forms of artificial insemination: AIH, in which semen is furnished by the husband, and AID, in which semen is furnished by a donor. Because the husband's infertility is usually the dominant factor, AID is by far the most frequently used method. There are no exact figures on the number of children (popularly called "test tube babies") conceived by artificial insemination, but the number runs into the thousands and some of these children have themselves become parents of one or more offspring.

Artificial kidney. A device, of which there are several types, which diffuses a patient's blood through a membrane outside of the body, to extract wastes and return cleared blood to the circulation (296).

Artificial pneumothorax. Surgical collapse of a lung for therapeutic purposes (221).

Asbestosis. Slowly progressing inflammation of the lungs resulting from in-

halation of fine asbestos fibers (236). It occurs in miners and workers in construction trades exposed to asbestos-containing materials. The lungs cannot get rid of asbestos dusts and normal tissue is replaced by fibrous tissue; the incidence of cancer in persons with asbestosis is high.

Ascariasis. Infestation with species of roundworms which inhabit the small bowel (70).

Ascheim-Zondek test. The "mouse test" to confirm early pregnancy (357). Sex hormones in the urine of a pregnant woman cause blood spots to appear in the ovaries of test animals.

Ascites. Painless accumulation of yellowish fluid in the abdominal cavity, indicative of impaired circulation often related to heart failure, cirrhosis of the liver, malignancy, or kidney disease. Diuretic drugs or sodium and fluid restriction may control this, depending on the underlying disease.

Aspiration. Removal of fluids or gases from a body cavity by suction. Also, inhalation of foreign material, as in aspiration pneumonia, below.

Aspiration pneumonia. A form of pneumonia caused by foreign matter in the lungs. The foreign substance may be inhaled, it may trickle into the windpipe, or it may be forced into the windpipe by gagging, choking spasms, or difficulties of swallowing. Lipoid or "oil" pneumonia is the most common form in infants and elderly persons (237). It can result from oily nose sprays, animal oils, and mineral oils which accumulate in the lungs and remain there. It is best to avoid putting oils into an infant's nose, and to give oily substances such as cod liver oil when the child is in an upright position and can swallow properly.

Asthma. A condition of paroxysmal, difficult, labored, wheezy breathing. See BRONCHIAL ASTHMA and CARDIAC ASTHMA.

Astigmatism. Distortion of vision resulting from imperfect curvature of the cornea or lens of the eye (562). The defect may be so slight that nothing need be done about it, or severe enough to cause eye strain. A rotating chart with parallel vertical and horizontal lines is used in eye tests for astigmatism. The condition is corrected by using a lens that bends the rays of light in only one direction (axis).

Astragalus. The ankle bone.

Ataractics. "Peace of mind" drugs; see TRANQUILIZERS.

Ataxia. Loss of muscle coordination; groups of muscles cannot be brought into concerted action. *Locomotor ataxia,* also called *tabes dorsalis,* usually is a late consequence of syphilis. Degeneration of parts of the spinal cord causes excruciating "lightning pains," staggering gait, disturbances of the eyes, bladder, and other organs.

Atelectasis. A retracted or collapsed state of the lung which leaves all or part of the organ airless. The condition may arise from obstruction of bronchial tubes; gases in the affected part of the lung are gradually absorbed and the area collapses. *Fetal atelectasis* is a condition in which the lungs of an infant do not expand adequately immediately after birth as they normally should (209).

Atherosclerosis. Degeneration of blood vessels caused by a deposit of fatty materials along the lining of the wall of a blood vessel. CHOLESTEROL is one of these fatty materials. Many other factors play a part (86).

Athetosis. A condition usually occurring in children as the result of a brain lesion, characterized by constant slow movements of fingers, toes, or other body parts.

Athletic heart. Changes produced in the heart by normal responses to prolonged strenuous physical exercise. After the athlete relaxes into a sedentary life his heart may somewhat resemble a diseased heart but should be recognized as the normal heart of an ex-athlete. Sudden death is not related to athletic heart.

Atopy. A synonym for allergy (672).

Atresia. Closure or failure of development of a normal opening or channel in the body.

Atrial. Pertaining to the atria or auricles, the blood "receiving chambers" of the heart (78).

Atrophy. Wasting away or shrinking in size of a previously normal organ, tissue or part.

Atypical pneumonia. See PNEUMONIA.

Audiometer. An electrical instrument which emits pure tones that can be made louder or fainter (590). It is used in measuring acuity of hearing for sounds of different frequencies.

Aura. A peculiar premonitory sensation preceding an epileptic seizure (273), recognized by the patient.

Auscultation. Determination of the condition of organs, particularly the heart and lungs, by study of sounds arising from them.

Autoclave. An apparatus for sterilizing instruments by steam under pressure.

Autograft. A piece of tissue taken from one part of a patient's body and transplanted to another part, as in skin grafts to cover raw areas, burns, etc. Autografts "take" because they are not foreign tissues which would ultimately cause the body to cast them off.

Auto-immune diseases. Several diseases of unknown cause may reflect a strange inability of the body to "recognize" itself, so that mechanisms which normally create immunity to foreign invaders somehow establish a specific sensitivity to certain of the body's own tissues, like a "self allergy," with harmful consequences. The concept is complex, relatively new, and mechanisms are not fully understood but are the subject of much current research. Diseases now thought to be caused by auto-immune reactions include *acquired hemolytic anemia* (156) and *thrombocytopenic purpura* (160). Diseases apparently associated with auto-immune responses include *rheumatoid arthritis* (660), *glomerulonephritis* (293), *rheumatic fever* (103), *thyrotoxicosis* (322), *scleroderma* (667), *ulcerative colitis* (490). *Multiple sclerosis* (264) and several other diseases for which no causative agents have been found resemble auto-immune diseases in laboratory studies.

Auto-intoxication. Poisoning by toxins generated within the body; for example, uremic poisoning. To most laymen the word means a vague condition attributed to intestinal toxins resulting from constipation, although no such toxins have been satisfactorily identified and it is probable that distressing symptoms are produced by mechanical pressures.

Avascular. Without blood or lymphatic vessels; the nails, the cornea, and some types of cartilage are avascular.

Avulsion. The forcible tearing away of a part.

Axilla. The armpit.

Axon. A single long fine fiber which conducts impulses away from the body of a nerve cell (242). Most axons are covered with a sheath of whitish material called *myelin;* abnormalities of this covering occur in demyelinating diseases such as multiple sclerosis (263).

Azoospermia. Absence of sperm in the semen.

B

Babinski sign. Upward movement of the big toe and downward movement of other toes when the sole of the foot is stroked; an indication of nervous system disorder (250).

Bacillary dysentery (*Shigellosis*). Acute diarrhea, acquired by person-to-person contact, through eating contaminated food or handling contaminated objects, or through spread of contamination by flies (45). The causative germs are present in the excretions of infected persons. Infection is caused by rod-shaped bacteria called Shigella, of which there are several types of variable virulence. Good sanitary and hygienic practices prevent infections. In infants and small children, bacillary dysentery can cause serious loss of fluids and ELECTROLYTES in a short time; onset of severe diarrhea is cause for calling a doctor promptly.

Bacteremia. The presence of living bacteria in circulating blood.

Bacteria. Tiny, colorless, single-celled organisms of the vegetable kingdom (34). Bacteria can be seen with a good microscope. They are shaped like spheres, rods, spirals and commas. Most bacteria are harmless and even useful to man. Those which cause diseases are *pathogenic* bacteria.

Bagassosis. Chronic inflammation of the lungs caused by inhalation of bagasse, the material left from crushed sugar cane after its juices have been extracted.

Bag of waters. The fluid-filled sac which protects the fetus during gestation. During labor the bag of waters helps to dilate the outlet of the uterus for passage of the baby through the birth canal (379). Usually the bag of waters ruptures at the height of a strong pain and the fluid escapes with a gush, but rupture may occur even before labor pains begin (dry labor).

Baldness. See ALOPECIA.

Ballistocardiograph. An instrument for measuring the "kick" given by the heartbeat to the body (84). It is useful in some aspects of diagnosis.

Bamboo spine. A spine having the jointed appearance of bamboo, deformed by ankylosing spondylitis (666).

Balneotherapy. Bath treatment.

Banti's syndrome. Enlarged spleen and anemia, associated with cirrhosis of the liver and ASCITES (162).

Barber's itch (*tinea sycosis*). A fungus infection of bearded parts of the face, producing reddish patches covered with dry hairs and scales. A more severe condition, *sycosis barbae*, is caused by bacterial infection of follicles of the beard, producing crusts, pimples, and numerous pustules perforated by hairs.

Barbiturates. The type of "sleeping pill" most commonly prescribed by physicians is some form of barbiturate. These constitute a large family of chemical compounds, most of which can be recognized by a name ending in "-al"; for example, *phenobarbital*. Properly used under medical direction, the barbiturates are safe and very effective sedatives and hypnotics. Small daytime doses may be given to reduce restlessness and emotional tension; in such use, the effect is much the same as that of TRANQUILIZERS, except that barbiturates tend to dull alertness and tranquilizers do not or do so to lesser degree. Adequate nighttime doses of barbiturates usually induce sleep within fifteen minutes to half an hour.

Some barbiturates act rapidly but the effects do not last long (three or four hours). These may be prescribed for persons who have a hard time falling asleep but usually stay asleep after they have dropped off. Effects of long-acting barbiturates persist for up to eight hours, and there are forms of intermediate duration, selected by a doctor according to a patient's individual needs. Long-acting forms have some tendency to leave the patient with "barbiturate hangover," a feeling of grogginess and depression the morning after.

The "bad name" of barbiturates derives from gross abuse, quite unrelated to valuable medical uses. Unstable persons may obtain the drugs illicitly and take toxic doses for "kicks." Doses of sufficient size can cause excitement and intoxication somewhat similar to alcoholic intoxication. Gross misuse of barbiturates can result in addiction, with withdrawal symptoms very similar to those of narcotic withdrawal when the drugs are discontinued.

Occasionally, large doses of barbiturates may be taken with suicidal intent. A fatal dose is from ten to twenty times the normal dose. Death from a single ordinary dose of a barbiturate is unknown. The drugs when properly used, even daily for a considerable length of time, are quite safe. Nevertheless, as with all potent drugs, barbiturates should be treated with respect, be used only as directed, be kept in a safe place, and be identified by label or other means to avoid taking them by mistake. Sedatives depress the central nervous system. So does alcohol. A combination of barbiturates and alcohol is especially dangerous. Doses of either, which if taken alone would be well tolerated, can be extremely dangerous if the same doses of the two substances, which intensify each other's depressive actions, are taken close together.

A number of non-barbiturate sleeping pills with a somewhat greater margin of safety than the barbiturates have been developed. However, large doses are toxic and capable of causing stupor, coma, respiratory failure and death.

All of these drugs are sold only on medical prescription. Mild sedatives sold without a prescription do not contain them.

Barium meal. A suspension of insoluble barium sulfate in water, swallowed in preparation for a "G.I. series" (786). The barium has greater density to x-rays than surrounding tissues and thus defines structures clearly.

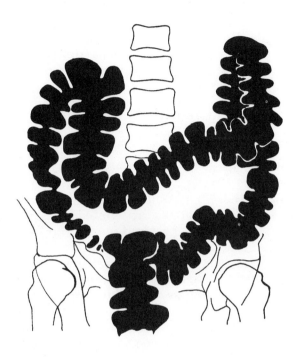

X-ray view of large intestine defined by barium.

Barrel chest. A rounded, bulging, barrel-shaped chest which does not move appreciably with the intake and output of air but is more or less fixed in a position of deep inhalation; characteristic of advanced emphysema (234).

Bartholin glands. Small glands on the floor and sides of the vaginal opening which secrete lubricating mucoid material. The glands are subject to infection and cyst formation.

Basal ganglia. Aggregations of nerve cells in the region of the base of the brain; Parkinson's disease is associated with abnormalities in this area (251).

Basal metabolic rate (*BMR*). A baseline of the minimal rate of energy expenditure for maintaining basal activities such as heart action, breathing, and heat production when the body is at rest; useful in diagnosis of certain diseases, especially those involving the thyroid gland (327).

Baseball finger, also called *mallet finger*. It is a dislocation of the end joint of a finger, which drops down and can't be lifted, due to rupture or tearing of a tendon by a direct blow from a baseball or other object upon the end or back of the finger (636).

Basedow's disease. Hyperthyroidism (322).

BCG. Bacillus of Calmette and Guerin; a vaccine which gives immunity to tuberculosis for a variable time. The vaccine contains strains of live tubercle bacilli grown on ox bile for a long period to reduce their virulence. It is a safe vaccine, extensively used in Europe, but in the U.S. it has been mostly used in persons with special hazards of exposure to tuberculosis, such as doctors, nurses, and members of families of tuberculosis patients. BCG vaccination interferes with the interpretation of tuberculin tests (219), but proponents point out that there are other ways of detecting tuberculous infection.

Bearing down pains. Pains which occur in the second stage of labor (380) when the mother, feeling that something must be expelled, makes powerful contractions of her abdominal muscles in coordination with contractions of the uterus.

Bed cradle. A frame to keep the weight of bedclothing from pressing upon a patient's body (28).

Bedsores (decubitus ulcer). Sores or ulcers resulting from pressures on parts of the body in persons confined to bed for long periods; good nursing care can do much to relieve and prevent them (26).

Bedwetting. Enuresis (400).

Bejel. A non-venereal form of syphilis, transmitted by such means as contaminated eating and drinking utensils, chiefly occurring in the Middle East (50).

Bell's palsy. Paralysis of the facial nerve, usually temporary; it leaves the patient unable to move muscles of the mouth, eye, and forehead on one side of the face (267).

Bence-Jones protein. An abnormal protein in the urine, occurring most often in association with *multiple myeloma* (174). The substance is readily deposited in kidney tubules and leads to impaired kidney function.

Bends. See CAISSON DISEASE.

Benign. Mild; usually the word means that a tumor is not cancerous. Benign tumors are not necessarily harmless; they can cause a wide range of symptoms related to pressure, obstruction, twisting, and excessive production of potent substances such as hormones. Pregnancy has been described rather wryly as a benign self-limited tumor.

Beriberi. A deficiency disease, very rare in this country, chiefly the result of a deficiency of thiamine (vitamin B₁) in the diet (504). *Dry* beriberi chiefly affects the nerves of the extremities; *wet* beriberi is characterized by edema and congestive heart failure.

Berylliosis. Poisoning by beryllium, a metallic element. If beryllium particles are inhaled over a period of time, the lungs are seriously affected (236); growths in the skin occur if the material penetrates the skin.

Bezoar. A solid mass of compacted indigestible material in the stomach or intestines, found occasionally in mentally disturbed persons who swallow rags, rubber, hair, rope, and other inedible materials. Persimmons can produce bezoars. A "hair ball" is called a *trichobezoar.*

B.i.d. Twice a day.

Bile. A yellowish or brownish fluid continuously manufactured in the liver; it is stored and concentrated in the gallbladder and released as needed into the duodenum (461). Bile helps to emulsify and absorb fats and to alkalinize the intestine. It is a complex, bitter-tasting fluid (gall) containing pigments, salts, fatty acids, cholesterol and other materials. Bile salts are sometimes used in medicine to stimulate the secretory activity of the liver.

Bilharziasis. Schistosomiasis (67).

Biliousness. A nondescript word for vague symptoms attributed, usually wrongly, to a fretful liver and maleficent activities of bile. Probably the word survives from ancient times when a "choleric" person was said to have an excess of yellow bile and a "melancholy" person an excess of black bile. Many symptoms, including jaundice, can indeed arise from deviations of bile, but it takes a doctor to determine what's wrong.

Bilirubin. The principal pigment of bile; a reddish substance derived from the breakdown of HEMOGLOBIN. Bilirubin tests are useful in determining the nature of certain blood and liver diseases, in distinguishing different types of jaundice, and in evaluating excessive destruction of blood cells.

Biologic "clocks." Some people can set a "mental clock" to awaken them before an alarm clock goes off. A few are confident enough to dispense with alarm clocks entirely. Many familiar physiologic rhythms recur approximately every 24 hours—sleep, waking, ups and downs of body temperature and heart rate. These are called *circadian rhythms,* from Latin words meaning *"about* a day." There are also multitudes of shorter rhythms, such as brain wave patterns, superimposed upon longer ones. All of these are rather like biologic clocks distributed through the body, ticking away at different speeds, some of their rhythms merging to augment others, some out of phase and dampening others.

Our built-in timepieces are a great challenge to physiologists who are giving a good deal of attention to mechanisms of which very little is known. Some rhythms are undoubtedly affected by external factors—light and darkness, heat and cold—but others appear to be built mysteriously into individual body cells.

Better knowledge of our mysterious internal clocks may have practical applications. The timing of doses of medicine may be significant; test animals are more resistant or susceptible to certain drugs at different phases of their circadian rhythms. Passengers who cross many time zones in jet airplanes suffer lowered mental and physical efficiency for several days, not accountable for by ordinary fatigue. As of now there is no way of re-setting biologic clocks that have lost, or gained, many hours by jet-plane transport, other than to let the body re-set them in its own good time.

Glimpses into physiologic rhythms are tantalizing. Why should the number of certain white blood cells increase when we get up in the morning? Why should malaria parasites be released from a patient's red blood cells most frequently between 6 and 8 a.m.? Why should the peak frequency of epileptic seizures be between 10 and 11 p.m.? One study of 600,000 births showed that the peak frequency of spontaneous onset of labor is 1 a.m. and of births, 3 to 4 a.m. Asthmatic attacks and infarctions of the heart muscle are also most frequent around 3 to 4 a.m. Body temperature and heart rate, low in early morning, increase to a peak between 3 and 6 p.m., whereupon our biologic clocks begin to shut us down for bedtime. Sleep is not a smooth 8-hour rhythm; it has its own clock system which half awakens us periodically and encourages dreams (see SLEEP).

Practical applications of knowledge that all organisms have their peculiar clocks are not extensive. But the U. S. Department of Agriculture has discovered that houseflies and cockroaches are especially vulnerable to insecticides around 4 p.m.

Biopsy. Removal of tissue from the living body for purposes of diagnosis, as in cases of suspected cancer. The tissue specimen may be subjected to biochemical tests; more often, it is set in a paraffin block, cut into very thin slices, stained, and studied under a microscope. If necessary, the procedure can be completed in a few minutes by quick-freezing the tissue. This is frequently done while the patient remains under anesthesia on the operating table and surgeons await the pathologist's verdict as to whether a tumor of the breast or other organ is or is not malignant.

Biotin. One of the 10 recognized vitamins of the B complex. Human deficiency has never been observed under usual conditions.

Birth control. See CONTRACEPTION.

Birth defects. About 2 per cent of live newborn infants have abnormalities recognizable at birth. Some defects such as a slightly twisted toe or a cleft lip are obvious *congenital malformations* (present at birth). Perhaps another 1 to 2 per cent of infants have abnormalities which are not recognizable at birth but which become apparent as they grow older. Many abnormalities are relatively minor, and about 80 per cent of birth defects, including the most serious forms such as congenital malformations of the heart, can be corrected and treated. Better than correction, of course, is prevention of abnormalities. To accomplish this, better knowledge of the causes of birth defects is a prerequisite.

Causes, if not the total mechanisms, of some birth defects are known. Some are hereditary, determined by parental CHROMOSOMES, and genetic counseling is helpful to prospective parents concerned about some real or fancied abnormality that "runs in the family" (see MEDICAL GENETICS). Some defects are *environmental,* quite unrelated to heredity. A disturbance of the environment of the fetus, its womb-nest, distorts its growth. The best-known example of environment-caused abnormalities is infection of the mother with German measles at a critical time of pregnancy. Some abnormalities are believed to be caused by a combination of hereditary and environmental factors, or by an accident at the time of delivery, as in cases of brain damage due to interruption of the oxygen supply to the newborn during delivery.

Time of vulnerability. It is now well established that certain birth defects originate at a critical time of pregnancy; in general, at the time when cells and mere "buds" of the embryo are developing into arms and legs and vital organs. At this time the embryo is peculiarly vulnerable to inimical agents. Before then it is too young; afterward, too old to be seriously affected. See TIMETABLE OF FETAL DEVELOPMENT, page 372.

Blackwater fever. An acute complication of MALARIA, especially in persons who have been treated with quinine. An attack is marked by high fever, shivering, profound anemia; the urine is very dark, hence the name (72).

Black widow spider. A small coal-black spider with a globe-shaped abdomen marked by a reddish design like an hourglass or dumbbell. Its bite is very painful and can be serious if treatment is neglected. (860).

Blastomycosis. A group of diseases caused by yeastlike fungi, variously affecting the skin, lungs, or body as a whole (74).

Bleb. A small blister usually filled with blood or fluid.

Bleeder's disease. HEMOPHILIA (161).

Blepharitis. Inflammation of the eyelids, usually due to bacterial infection; sometimes associated with allergies or seborrhea of the face and scalp.

Blind spot. A small spot on the retina, where the optic nerve enters, which is insensitive to light (555). The blind spot can be recognized by closing one eye, fixing the other on a small black spot, and shifting the gaze of the open eye toward the nose until the spot disappears.

Blood-brain barrier. Some natural body substances, drugs, and chemicals circulating in the blood are unable to reach active brain cells. The apparent blood-brain barrier, serving as a selective traffic officer which permits some substances to "go" and directs others to "stop," is thought by some authorities to consist of a layer of cells around small capillaries in the brain. The barrier is presumably a natural protective mechanism.

Blood tests. Laboratory tests of blood can yield a vast amount of information. The extent of testing depends on what is being looked for. There are many special tests for special purposes. A "routine" blood test does not include unusual procedures, but does include standard studies, for which the following are normal physiologic values:

pH (acid-alkaline ratios; pH 7 is neutral, above 7 is alkaline) 7.35–7.45
Red blood cells (erythrocytes) . . . . . . 4,500,000–5,000,000 per cu. mm.
White blood cells (leukocytes) . . . . 5,000–10,000 per cu. mm.
Polymorphonuclear neutrophils 60–70%
Lymphocytes 25–33%
Monocytes 2–6%
Eosinophils 1–3%
Basophils 0.25–0.5%
Platelets . 200,000–400,000 per cu. mm.
Hemoglobin . . 14–16 Gm. per 100 ml.
Bleeding time . . . . 1–3 minutes
Coagulation time . . . . . . 6–12 minutes

Serum cholesterol ....
......150 to 250 mg. per 100 ml.
Glucose .....80–120 mg. per 100 ml.
Albumin ....3.5–5.5 Gm per 100 ml.
Nonprotein nitrogen ....
.........25–38 mg. per 100 ml.
Urea nitrogen (BUN).............
.. ..8–20 mg. per 100 ml.
Uric acid.......3–5 mg. per 100 ml.
(100 ml. (milliliters) is approximately one-tenth of a quart).

Blue baby. An infant with a congenital heart defect which allows venous and arterial blood to mix, resulting in insufficient oxygen in the blood and a bluish tinge of skin and mucous membranes (97).

Blood poisoning. A general term for the presence of germs or their toxins in circulating blood (38). See BACTEREMIA, SEPTICEMIA, TOXEMIA.

Body build. A general term for variabilities of height, weight, breadth, muscularity, boniness, limb length, etc., characteristic of individuals. Different proportions of bodily components can be measured scientifically; see SOMATOTYPING.

Boeck's sarcoid. See SARCOIDOSIS.

Bone age. An index of physiologic maturity, based on the fairly definite time schedule of development of bone from birth to maturity, independent of chronological age. Bone age is commonly estimated by taking x-rays of a child's hands and wrists and comparing these centers of ossification with standards appropriate to his age. There are normal variations; bone age may be advanced or retarded a year or so without necessarily being abnormal. Advanced bone age may be associated with overactivity of the adrenal or thyroid glands, retarded bone age with deficient thyroid activity or malnutrition. Tall children who reach sexual maturity at an early age usually have advanced bone age; those who have retarded bone age are probable late maturers.

Bone banks. Stored collections of matchstick to pencil-sized pieces of human bone. When transplanted, the dead, sterile bone somehow stimulates the growth of new bone around it, eventually is incorporated into that new bone, and is slowly replaced. In the meantime the graft is a barrier which prevents soft fibrous tissue from filling the hole or defect in the patient's own bone. Bone grafts are used most frequently to correct curvature of the spine in children, and after fractures, if the bone ends fail to unite properly, to assist in mending.

Bone conduction. Bones of the head are natural channels for conduction of sounds to the ears. This can be demonstrated by stopping the ears and touching a vibrating tuning fork to the skull or teeth. Some types of hearing aids, in contact with bone behind the ear, make use of this phenomenon. Bone conduction explains in part why our own voices don't sound exactly the same to us as they do to others.

Bone marrow exam. Microscopic study of bone marrow tissue obtained by needle, used in diagnosing certain diseases of the blood.

Booster shot. Injection of a vaccine or immunizing agent given some time after an original vaccination, to enhance its effectiveness. Immunizations tend to wear off in the course of time; a timely booster shot rejuvenates them. Some primary immunizations are given in two or three spaced injections, several days or weeks apart, to produce maximum immunizing action.

Botulism. A violent form of food poisoning caused by toxins of botulinus organisms in improperly canned foods, especially non-acid foods such as green beans or corn (42), (857).

Bougie. A slender cylindrical instrument introduced into a body orifice to explore or dilate a passage or act as a guide for other instruments.

Boutonniere deformity. Bending of the middle joint of a finger with extension of the other joints, resulting from a cut or rupture of a tendon (637).

Bowlegs (*genu varum*). Outward bowing of the knee joints; common in young children just "getting their feet on the ground," usually requiring no treatment unless bowing persists after five or six years of age (643).

Bowman's capsule. The cup-shaped capsule of a *nephron*, the minute filtering unit of the kidney (283).

Bradycardia. Abnormal slowness of the heartbeat, with a pulse rate of less than 60 per minute.

Brain waves. Minute electric currents of brain cells which, when amplified and transcribed, have the form of undulant, spiked, wavy lines. See ELECTROENCEPHALOGRAPH.

Breakbone fever. Sudden, acute high fever, called "breakbone" for the shattering pain it causes in muscles, bones and joints; also called *dengue* (58).

Breast support. A common source of breast pain, especially if the breasts are unusually large, is a poorly fitted brassiere which supports most of the weight from above by shoulder straps. Correct breast support sustains most of the weight of the breasts from *below*, by the portion of the brassiere which encircles the chest under the breasts; the main function of shoulder straps is to hold the garment in position.

Breath-holding. Crying of infants and small children so furious that they hold their breath until they turn blue or even lose consciousness for a moment. A breath-holding spell can be frightening the first time a parent is confronted with one, but the episode is just a blowoff of temper and anger, and nature has arranged that we can't hold our breath long enough to do serious harm; try it yourself.

Breech delivery. Presentation of an infant's buttocks instead of the head at the outlet of the birth canal (384).

Bright's disease. An old term for several diseases which fall under the general category of *glomerulonephritis* (292); sometimes used as a general term for kidney disease.

Brill-Zinsser disease. A mild form of typhus fever, occurring in persons who had an attack of typhus years before (65).

Bromhidrosis. Foul-smelling perspiration, caused by decomposition of sweat and debris by bacteria.

Bromism. Chronic poisoning from long continued use of bromides; these salts have sedative and sleep-inducing properties and are contained in many prescribed and non-prescription products. Symptoms of chronic bromide intoxication run the gamut from headache, sleepiness, cold hands and feet, worsening of acne, to toxic delirium, disorientation and hallucinations. Bromide salts accumulate in blood and body fluids over a period of continued intake. Treatment consists of stopping all intake of bromides; daily doses of table salt in amounts prescribed by a doctor help to speed their elimination.

Bronchial asthma. The common form of asthma; usually it has an allergic basis (684). Characteristic paroxysms of wheezy labored breathing are due to narrowing of bronchial passages, trapping inhaled air and making it very difficult to exhale.

Bronchial tree. The breathing passages which extend from the windpipe in finer and finer ramifications resembling the branchings of tree roots (211).

Bronchiectasis. Dilation of bronchial tubes, usually a result of pus-producing infections or obstruction by foreign bodies (226).

Bronchitis. Inflammation of the linings of bronchial tubes (224).

Bronchography. The taking of an x-ray film of the lungs after injection of iodized oil (785).

Bronchoscope. A thin tubelike instrument, inserted into the windpipe for purposes of inspecting tissues, withdrawing secretions or tissue samples, administering medicines, or extracting foreign bodies (229).

Bronze diabetes. See HEMOCHROMATOSIS.

Brown spider. A small, shy brown spider (Loxosceles reclusa) which can inflict a serious bite that may not be painful at the time. See SPIDER BITE.

Bornholm disease. See DEVIL'S GRIP.

Brucellosis (*Malta fever, undulant fever*). An infectious disease transmitted from animals to man, most commonly by contact with cattle or consumption of raw milk products (45). Also called *undulant fever*, from the up-and-down shifts of body temperature, down in the morning and up in the afternoon. Recovery from acute brucellosis is usually spontaneous but convalescence may be prolonged. Chronic brucellosis may be unrecognized and hard to diagnose; varied symptoms—obscure fever of long duration, weakness, fatigability, excessive sweating—may puzzlingly resemble those of infectious mononucleosis, tuberculosis, malaria, or rheumatic fever. Positive diagnosis is made by recovery of Brucella organisms from body excretions.

Bruxism. The habit of grinding the teeth (534).

Bubo. An inflamed, swollen lymph node, usually in the groin or armpit, caused by absorption of infective material; most often a concomitant of venereal disease.

Buccal. Pertaining to the cheek.

Buerger's disease. Inflammation of the inner walls of blood vessels with clot formation and interruption of blood supply. The legs, feet, and toes are especially affected. Shutting off of blood supply can lead to GANGRENE and amputation. The cause of the disease is unknown but it chiefly affects young males and is almost never seen in non-smokers. Absolute prohibition of smoking for the rest of the patient's life is an essential part of treatment; resumption of smoking can provoke renewed attacks and gangrene.

Bulimia. Insatiable appetite, requiring enormous meals for satisfaction.

Bulla. A large blister.

Buphthalmos. Enlargement of the eye.

Burkitt's lymphoma. A form of malignant tumor, especially affecting the jaw and facial bones, most frequent in children of central Africa, but also occurring elsewhere. The tumor responds dramatically to therapy. The disease is thought to be caused by a virus (Epstein-Barr) which is also associated with INFECTIOUS MONONUCLEOSIS.

Bursa. A sac between opposing surfaces that slide past each other. It is filled with lubricating fluid, something like the white of an egg, which permits free motion. Inflammation of a bursa causes painful *bursitis* (654), as of the shoulder, elbow, knee, or ankle.

Bunion (*hallux valgus*). Enlargement and thickening of the big joint of the big toe, bending the big toe toward the little toe (649). The deformity gets progressively worse if untreated. Surgical correction is not so simple as it seems, but is indicated for young persons. In older persons, a special shoe made to fit the deformity comfortably may be the most practical solution.

Butterfly suture. A strip of plastic or adhesive tape with a relatively thin "bridge" between wider ends, used to draw together the opposing edges of a minor laceration on a smooth skin surface.

Byssinosis. An occupational disease of textile workers caused by inhalation of dusts produced during certain processing stages in cotton, flax, and hemp mills. Initial symptoms are chest tightness, cough, wheezing, and shortness of breath, which occur predominantly on the first working days after absence from work, as over a weekend. The cause is thought to be a chemical substance in textile dusts which constricts the bronchi and causes asthma-like symptoms.

C

Cachexia. Profound weakness, emaciation, general ill health, resulting from serious disease such as cancer.

Cafe au lait spots. Multiple pigmented patches in the skin, the color of coffee with milk, associated with NEUROFIBROMATOSIS.

Caffeine. A chemical substance contained in tea, coffee, and many cola-type beverages. Caffeine is a powerful stimulant of the central nervous system and tends to increase both mental and physical performance. A great variety of drug preparations contain caffeine, often in combination with other drugs.

Caisson disease. Diver's paralysis; cramping pain in the abdomen, legs and other parts, called "the bends" by divers. Symptoms are caused by nitrogen bubbles in the blood which try to escape in much the same way that a rush of compressed gas escapes when a warm bottle of pop is opened. The nitrogen gets into the blood from air inhaled under pressure, as under water or in caissons or wherever surrounding pressure greatly exceeds that of the atmosphere. Attacks can be prevented by gradual ascent from a deep dive, or treated by putting the patient into a decompression chamber where high pressure is gradually reduced while nitrogen slowly dissipates from body fluids. "The bends" can affect Scuba divers who stay too long under water at depths of 100 feet or so and ascend too rapidly.

Calcaneus. The heel bone.

Calcification. The process by which tissues become hardened by deposits of calcium salts.

Calcium. A mineral element that is an essential constituent of bone and is essential for blood clotting, muscle tone, and nerve function.

Calculus. A stone formed in a duct, cyst, or hollow organ of the body, especially in the gallbladder (479) and kidney (287). Most calculi are composed of mineral salts, often with a mixture of organic matter. The composition of a stone may sometimes give a physician information of value in preventing future stone formation. Stones range in size from "gravel" like specks of sand to stones which fill the entire interior of the kidney. The stuff that stones are made of is somehow extracted and condensed from fluids of the body. Infection and stagnation of fluids play a part in stone formation, but exactly why some people form stones and others do not is not known. Drinking hard water has nothing to do with it. Stones may cause a few symptoms if they stay where they are, but excruciating pain ensues if a stone tries to squeeze through a passage too small for it. *Dental calculus* is tartar that accumulates on teeth (532).

Callus. A patch of hard, thickened skin, usually on the hands or feet; a protective reaction to pressure or friction. A callus is like a corn except that it is more diffuse and has no core, and it tends to disappear spontaneously when the cause is removed. Persons who stand a great deal often develop thick calluses of the heel or ball of the foot. The horny skin may be removed by rubbing with pumice stone, emery board, or a coarse Turkish towel after soaking the foot in hot water. Persistent calluses which cause a great deal of discomfort should have the attention of a podiatrist. "Callus" is also a word for the plastic bony material which exudes from and surrounds broken bone ends and plays a part in the healing of a fracture.

Calorie. A unit of heat. The unit used in measuring body metabolism and the fattening propensities of foods (493) is the "great calorie," the amount of heat necessary to raise the temperature of one kilogram (2.2 pounds) of water one degree Centigrade.

Calyx. One of the several small cuplike chambers which receive urine from kidney tubules and channel it into the funnel-shaped cavity of the kidney which merges with the ureter (284).

Canker sore (*aphthous stomatitis*). Little blisters on membranes of the mouth and cheeks which break and leave open sores. The painful ulcers usually heal spontaneously in a week or so, but attacks may be recurrent. It is no longer thought that canker sores are caused by viruses (the sores may appear at the same time as cold sores or fever blisters which are caused by herpes simplex virus). Scientists at the National Institute of Dental Health have isolated a bacterium which causes canker sores. Persons who have repeated or continuous crops of canker sores may be allergic to some substance in the bacterium's makeup. The organism is sensitive to tetracycline, an antibiotic; oral suspensions of the drug held in the mouth for two minutes and then swallowed (four times daily) shorten the healing time but do not prevent recurrences.

Cannula. A hollow tube for insertion into a body passage or cavity; within the cannula there is usually a *trocar,* a sliding instrument with a pointed tip, designed to puncture a cavity and release fluid, after which the trocar is

withdrawn and fluid drains through the cannula.

Canthus. The angle formed where the eyelids meet at the outer or inner side.

Carbohydrate. The primary fuel of muscular activity, the major source of energy we need for moving, working, acting, living. Carbohydrates occur as sugars and starches, in many complex forms; the starches are converted to sugar in the digestive processes (494). Cereals, vegetables, and fruits are inexpensive carbohydrate foods which are major sources of food for much of the world's population. Carbohydrate is necessary to burn fats efficiently, and it "spares" protein, which can be burned for energy if necessary but is more valuable for other purposes. Cellulose, the indigestible matter in many carbohydrate foods, supplies useful bulk in the intestines. Most of the carbohydrates in the body are stored in the liver and muscles in the form of glycogen (animal starch), but not much more than a half day's needs are held in storage. As the supplies become depleted, hunger pangs remind us that it is time to replenish our energy reserves.

Carbon dioxide snow. Extremely cold snow-like particles (about 100 degrees below zero) formed by rapid evaporation of liquid carbon dioxide. Application of the snow freezes the skin instantly. It is used in treatment of various skin lesions, such as birthmarks (194).

Carbon monoxide. A colorless, odorless gas which is the most frequent cause of fatal poisoning except alcohol. Immediate first aid is imperative (828). Carbon monoxide kills by depriving tissues of oxygen; it combines 200 times more readily than oxygen with HEMOGLOBIN of the red blood cells. The gas is produced by any incompletely burned fuel. Common belief that a fire in a closed space is dangerous because it "burns up all the oxygen" is erroneous; it is dangerous because it emits carbon monoxide. Most of us know that it is dangerous to let a car run in a closed garage even for seconds. It is not so well known that gas can seep into a car in bumper-to-bumper traffic or from a leaky muffler or exhaust pipe. Relatively small amounts of the gas in a car driven with windows closed can dull a driver's senses or cause him to "fall asleep" at the wheel. It is wise to drive with one window at least partly open and to have the exhaust system checked for leaks during routine inspections.

Carbuncle. A deep-seated infection of the skin, like several boils joined together; pus is discharged from a number of points on the tight, reddened skin surface (38).

Carcinogen. Any agent which produces cancer.

Carcinoma. Cancer comprised of epithelial cells, the type that cover the skin and mucous membranes and form the linings of organs. Carcinomas may arise in almost any structure of the body; many forms are curable if proper treatment is begun early.

Cardia. The valve of ringlike muscle at the junction of esophagus and stomach (452).

Cardiac. Pertaining to the heart; a person with heart disease.

Cardiac asthma. Paroxysms of difficult breathing, often occurring at night, characteristic of congestive heart failure (100).

Cardiac catheter. A slender tube which is threaded into a vessel of the arm and pushed into the heart to obtain several kinds of important diagnostic information (88, 93).

Cardiac pacemaker. A device which electrically stimulates the sympathetic nerves to the heart, triggering the "beat" and producing contractions at near the normal rate when the organ itself cannot do so reliably (113).

Cardiospasm. See ACHALASIA.

Cardiovascular. Pertaining to the heart and blood vessels.

Carotid. The principal artery that runs up either side of the neck (123). At approximately the middle of the neck it divides in a Y-formation; one branch continues as the external carotid artery and the other as the internal carotid artery which goes directly to the brain. Some strokes are caused by obstruction of the artery at the crotch of the Y; the structure is close to the surface, readily accessible to a surgeon, and an operation may give dramatic improvement of the patient's symptoms (124). Overstimulation or compression of nerves at the point where the artery divides can cause dizziness and loss of consciousness.

Carpal. Pertaining to the wrist. The *carpal tunnel* through which a large nerve passes from the wrist to the hand may become constricted and cause tingling and numbness of the fingers (635).

Car sickness. See MOTION SICKNESS.

Caries. Decay of bone; the dentist's word for tooth decay (dental caries).

Carotene. A yellow pigment occurring in sweet potatoes, carrots, leaves, yellow vegetables, egg yolk and other foodstuffs. The body converts it into Vitamin A. Excessive intake over a long period of time of carrots or other carotene-rich foods may raise the blood's content of carotene to such an exaggerated level that the skin takes on a yellowish hue, sometimes mistaken for jaundice. This condition, known as *carotenemia*, is harmless but fairly spectacular.

Cartilage. Gristle; white, elastic connective tissue. It is the substance of soft parts in infants which later become bone. It forms part of the skeleton. Pads of cartilage cushion the opposing surfaces of joints; thinning or wearing away of cartilage is associated with some forms of arthritis (656). The stiff but flexible substance of the external ear is cartilage, the most convenient article of cartilage to touch or squeeze. Cartilage does not have a blood supply and if injured cannot heal. Tearing or other injury of cartilage is quite common among athletes. This often requires surgical removal of the cartilage (644).

Caruncle. A small, non-malignant, fleshy growth; a type which causes pain and bleeding (urethral caruncle) occurs at the urinary outlet of women, most frequently at the menopause.

Castration. Removal of the testicles or ovaries. Functional powers of the ovaries can be destroyed by radiation, sometimes necessary in treatment of disease; this is called non-surgical castration.

Casts, *renal.* Castoff particles in sediments of urine, sometimes indicative of latent forms of kidney disease (286). There are three forms of casts, *hyaline* (glassy), *red cell,* and *epithelial,* from which inferences concerning the nature of kidney lesions may be drawn.

Catabolism. The "tearing down" aspect of METABOLISM; the breaking down of complex substances by cells is often accompanied by release of energy. The opposite of ANABOLISM.

Catamenia. Menstruation.

Catarrh. A flowing down; a rather old-fashioned term for inflammation of mucous membranes, especially of the nose and throat, with free-flowing discharge, as in a cold.

Cataract. An opacity of the lens of the eye (576). A cataract is not a foreign substance or something to be peeled off the lens, but a biochemical change in structure. Babies may be born with cataracts and some of these cases are on an hereditary basis. Increasing age, physical injury, chemical injury from certain drugs and industrial chemicals, diabetes and other endocrine diseases, are associated with cataract formation, but the great majority of cataracts seem to be a part of the aging process. The only way to restore useful vision is to remove the lens surgically (771); this permits light waves to enter the eye once again. Of course the light-bending powers and power of ACCOMMODATION of the absent lens are lost. The patient has to wear heavy spectacle lenses to substitute, somewhat inefficiently, for the missing lens. He can see quite well again—a wonderful reprieve from partial or total blindness—but it takes some adjustment and reeducation. Many improvements have been and are being made in cataract glasses but they do not restore normal ease of seeing completely. Contact lenses have been improved and come closer to restoring normal visual function but they are not suitable for everyone. Attempts to insert a permanent plastic lens inside the eye in place of a removed cataractous lens are being made but are still in experimental stages of development.

Catatonia. A phase of schizophrenia in which the patient stands or sits in some awkward fixed position for hours on end and resists all attempts to get him to speak or move.

"Cat cry" syndrome. A peculiar condition of infants who give a cry like that of a cat, because of defective development of the larynx. It is an inherited abnormality, resulting from lack of a short arm on one of the infant's CHROMOSOMES.

Caterpillar dermatitis. Are caterpillars dangerous? Not very, but they can be offensive in more ways than one. Some varieties have tiny hollow hairs containing irritating material. These minute hairs can penetrate the skin and cause an itchy rash, usually mild. The rash may be puzzling because caterpillars are not usually thought of as the source. There may even have been no direct contact with caterpillars. A few mothers have acquired caterpillar dermatitis from contact with invisible hairs trapped in children's clothing. As a general rule, it is prudent to regard caterpillars as untouchable.

Cathartic. A purgative medicine; a substance that increases evacuation of the bowels. Regular use of carthartics is unwise; they can be habit-forming, and do not correct an underlying condition. Cathartics or laxatives should not be used if abdominal pain is present, and powerful cathartics such as castor oil or epsom salts should only be used as a physician directs.

Catheter. A hollow tube for insertion through a narrow canal into a cavity to discharge fluids, especially of the urinary bladder (286). The heart may also be catheterized for diagnostic purposes (98).

Cat scratch disease. An infection characterized by painless swelling of lymph nodes, acquired from a scratch by a cat (64). The offending cat usually shows no sign of disease.

Caul. The head of a baby born with a "caul" is covered with a fetal membrane, the AMNION, which has become detached.

Causalgia. Excruciating, burning pain caused by injury to sensory nerves, especially of the palms and soles; often associated with poor circulation to the part and discoloration, clamminess, and coldness of the skin. Blocking the affected nerves with procaine may give relief.

Cautery. Application of heat or a chemical to destroy tissue. Anciently, a red hot iron was applied to wounds to stop bleeding and infection. Today the most common form is *electrocautery,* in which a wire loop heated by electric current is used to seal bleeding vessels or destroy tissue.

CCU. Initials for Coronary Care Unit or Cardiac Care Unit, a hospital unit with staff and apparatus for constant monitoring and care of heart patients.

Cecum. The blind pouch in which the large bowel begins; the appendix projects from it (489).

Celiac disease. A disorder, believed to have an hereditary basis, in which the small intestine is unable to absorb fat from foods. See MALABSORPTION SYNDROME.

Cellulitis. Diffuse, pussy inflammation of soft, loose connective tissue beneath the skin.

Cementum. The bone-like substance which covers the roots of teeth (522).

Centigrade (C). A thermometer scale, widely used in science and medicine, in which water freezes at 0 degrees C. and boils at 100 degrees C. To convert to Fahrenheit degrees, multiply degrees Centigrade by nine-fifths and add 32. Average body temperature, 98.6 degrees Fahrenheit, is 37 degrees Centigrade.

Centipede bites. Ugly multi-legged creatures of the southern U.S. occasionally "bite," injecting a little venom into a puncture wound. The bitten area may swell, cause burning pain and turn red, but it generally doesn't last long —three or four hours—and there is no danger of serious poisoning. Wet dressings applied to the area are comforting; if pain is very severe, a doctor may give a sedative. Tropical centipedes are bigger, uglier, produce more venom, and their bites may cause vomiting, fever, headache, and inflammation of lymphatic vessels. Innocent visitors to the tropics would do well to shake out their shoes, turn back the bed covers, watch their step, and generally discourage centipedes.

Central nervous system (*CNS*). The brain and nerves of the spinal cord (246). The system is "central" because all of the nerves of the body, except the cranial nerves which connect directly with the brain, enter or leave the spinal cord.

Cephalalgia. A fancy name for headache.

Cephalic. Pertaining to the head. Turning the fetus so that the head presents is called *cephalic version.*

Cerebellum. A specialized part of the brain, about the size of an orange, tucked under the CEREBRUM at the back of the head (249, 265). It is concerned with equilibrium and coordination of movements.

Cerebral palsy. A form of paralysis manifested by jerky, writhing, spastic movements, resulting from damage to brain center controls of muscles (270). Cerebral palsy is not a single disease but a group of syndromes with a common denominator, some form of injury to motor control centers in the brain. It is not always possible to determine the cause of brain damage. It may result from birth injury, from infections of the mother or embryo, from errors of development, and other causes.

Cerebrum. The main part of the brain; the great mass of nerve tissue that occupies the entire upper part of the skull. *Cerebration,* by general human assent, means the most profound sort of thinking. *Cerebral* refers to phenomena that occur in the cerebrum; for example, cerebral hemorrhage.

Cerebrospinal fluid. Clear, colorless fluid that surrounds the spinal cord and is continuous with the same fluid in ventricles of the brain. Examination of cerebrospinal fluid assists in diagnosis of various diseases (such as meningitis, polio, brain tumor) which cause changes in the fluid. The fluid may contain blood, pus and other substances which do not belong there; it may be given chemical, microscopic and bacteriologic tests and may be cultured to determine the presence and identity of germs.

Cerebrovascular accident. A stroke, resulting from interruption of blood supply to the brain (123). The "accident" may be obstruction by a clot of a vessel supplying the brain, or rupture of a vessel with bleeding into brain tissue.

Cerumen. Ear wax (598).

Cervical rib. An extra rib in the cervical or neck region, in addition to the usual 12 on each side. It can be felt as a bony projection at the root of the neck. The spare rib may cause no trouble, but if pressures or other disturbing symptoms develop, it is as dispensable as the appendix.

Cervical effacement. Thinning of the outlet of the uterus preceding the onset of labor (379).

Cervicitis. Inflammation of the neck of the uterus (434).

Cervical erosion. A rough spot in the membrane lining the opening of the cervix, looking much like a child's skinned knee (737).

Cervix. A neck; the word applies to any neck-like or constricted part of the body; especially, the tapering neck of the pear-shaped uterus (428). Also, the neck of the urinary bladder. The seven cervical vertebrae (616) occupy the topmost part of the spine; cervical lymph nodes occur in the neck region.

Cesarean section. Delivery of a baby through an incision in the abdomen and uterus. Legend has it that Julius Caesar was born in this way, but legend is unreliable. The operation in Caesar's time was done only on dead women, and Caesar's mother survived his birth by many years. Julius was a dutiful son who wrote often to his mother during his wars.

Chadwick's sign. A blue discoloration around the entrance to the vagina and on the neck of the uterus; an early indication of pregnancy (359).

Chancre. The primary lesion of syphilis; a hard sore or ulcer at the site where syphilis germs gained entrance to the body.

Chancroid (*soft chancre*). A non-syphilitic venereal disease caused by a specific bacillus, *Hemophilus ducreyi*. Initially a soft sore appears, usually on the genitals. In a few days it breaks down into a painful, pus-discharging ulcer (41).

Chafing. See INTERTRIGO.

Chagas' disease (*American trypanosomiasis*). A disease related to African sleeping sickness, caused by protozoa which enter the body through an insect bite contaminated by the insect's feces (71). The disease is characterized by fever, enlarged lymph nodes, and various complications; it can be fatal but is frequently mild. It occurs in Central and South America.

Chalazion. A painless small tumor or cyst of the eyelid due to an obstructed drainage duct; dammed-up secretions cause the swelling. Hot compresses can be applied, together with an antibacterial medicine if the doctor so directs. If the tumor does not disappear spontaneously, incision and curettage may be necessary.

Charleyhorse. A term most often used by athletes for tenderness and soreness of muscles, commonly of the thigh, incurred by some heroic sports effort. Pain and swelling result from rupture or strain of muscle or tendon fibers. Torn tissues may bleed, producing black-and-blueness or a charleyhorse of another color. Tenderness and stiffness usually disappear in a few days as the affected part is gradually returned to use. The healing process, following the acute stage of injury, may be encouraged by gentle applications of heat, massage, and comforting bandages.

Cheilitis. Inflammation of the lips.

Chemotherapy. Treatment with chemicals which favorably alter the course of disease but do not seriously injure the patient.

Cheyne-Stokes respiration. An abnormal form of breathing in some patients with heart, kidney, or vascular diseases. Intensity of breathing gradually decreases until no breath at all is taken for a few seconds or longer than half a minute. This is followed by increase in breathing and shortage of breath. The pattern occurs in repeated cycles. One of the causes is thought to be a decrease in blood supply to the brain.

Chilblain (*pernio*). An acute or chronic form of cold injury, less severe than frostbite, characterized by inflammation of the skin, itching and swelling, frequently followed by blisters. The immediate cause is exposure to cold, to which some persons have an exaggerated sensitivity; it is advisable for them to stay indoors or wear heavy garments and fleece-lined gloves and overshoes during cold weather. Such persons should begin to wear protective clothing early in the cold season when the environmental temperature drops below 60 degrees.

Chloasma. Discoloration of the skin with yellow-brown spots and patches. The condition is often associated with some endocrine disturbance. Chloasma frequently occurs in pregnancy as a result of increased secretion of a pituitary hormone, MSH (317), which stimulates pigment-producing cells. Hormone production returns to a normal level soon after delivery and the pigmented areas fade, though not always completely.

Chocolate cysts. Cysts of the ovary filled with chocolate-colored material, characteristic of *endometriosis* (437).

Choked disk. See PAPILLEDEMA.

Cholangitis. Inflammation of the bile ducts.

Cholecyst. The gallbladder.

Cholecystitis. Inflammation of the gallbladder. It may occur in acute or chronic forms (479).

Cholelithiasis. Stones in the gallbladder or its ducts (480).

Cholera (*Asiatic*). An epidemic infectious disease with a high fatality rate caused by comma-shaped germs, transmitted in bowel discharges of carriers to food and water. It is characterized by profuse watery diarrhea, cramps, vomiting, prostration, and suppression of urine. The principal mechanism by which cholera weakens and kills is through extreme losses of body fluids and ELECTROLYTES. The disease virtually never occurs in the U. S., but travelers going to regions where cholera outbreaks occur (India, Pakistan, Southeast Asia) should be vaccinated with a cholera vaccine which gives immunity for about six months.

Cholesteatoma. A tumor of the middle ear, like a bag of skin in the wrong place. The first sign may be a scanty discharge from the ear when the tumor liquefies and perforates the drum. The wall of the bag causes erosion of bone which may extend dangerously into neighboring structures. In most cases, surgical removal of the cholesteatoma is considered the best treatment (596).

Cholesterol. A waxy substance resembling fat in its properties, closely related to the sex hormones and Vitamin D. It is present in brain tissue, bile, nerve sheaths, all animal tissue. It regulates the passage of substances through cell walls, keeps us from becoming waterlogged when we bathe, and prevents us from drifting away as a cloud of vapor from evaporation of body water. It is so important to the body that it is manufactured by the liver and other tissues whether we get cholesterol in our diets or not. Despite these virtues, cholesterol has become something of a scare word, blamed for degenerating the walls of arteries and setting the stage for heart attacks. However, most specialists are reluctant to indict cholesterol as the primary, predominant, most vicious villain in heart and blood vessel diseases (89). One reason for cholesterol's bad publicity is that it is easier for doctors to measure than other fatty components of blood serum. Clinically, such measurement is useful as an index of the overall pattern of fatty substances in the blood. The normal range of serum cholesterol is about 125 to 265. It tends to rise in later years, and changes can be caused by variations in thyroid activity, diabetes, kidney insufficiency, and stress. Moderation of fat intake, reduction of overweight if obese, and substitution of polyunsaturated fats for some of the "hard" fats in the diet (89), would appear to be prudent measures in the present state of knowledge.

Chondroma. A tumor with the structure of CARTILAGE, usually benign, but with a tendency to recur after removal.

Chorea. A disease of the nervous system manifested by involuntary, irregular, rapid, jerky movements of muscles of the face, legs, and arms. Its common form (also called *St. Vitus' dance* and *Sydenham's chorea*) is a disease of childhood, often a manifestation of rheumatic fever (104). The jerky movements and facial grimaces subside in a few weeks. Signs of rheumatic disease may never appear, but about half of patients with chorea develop or have rheumatic fever. HUNTINGTON'S CHOREA is an entirely different hereditary disease.

Chorion. The outermost of the fetal membranes (377). The fetal part of the placenta develops from it.

Choroid. The middle coat of the eye, continuous with the iris in front; a thin, pigmented layer composed largely of interlaced blood vessels, vital to the eye's nutrition (553).

Christmas disease. An hereditary "bleeder's disease," having the same symptoms as classic hemophilia but resulting from deficiency of a different blood-clotting factor (162). Named for the family in which it was discovered.

Chromosomes. Threadlike bodies in the nucleus of a cell; they contain the GENES and DNA (see Chapter 25).

Chronic. Long continued ill health as opposed to *acute* illness.

Cilia. Minute hairlike processes of specialized cells which beat rhythmically and keep debris-laden fluids flowing in one direction; for example, out of the lungs. The word also means "eyelashes."

Ciliary body. The part of the eye which suspends the lens and secretes aqueous humor (553).

Circadian rhythms. Cycles and rhythms of body processes that recur approximately every 24 hours; "circadian" means *about* a day." See BIOLOGIC "CLOCKS."

Circumcision. Removal of the foreskin or prepuce.

Cirrhosis of the liver. Chronic, progressive inflammation of the liver, with increase of non-functioning fibrous tissue, distortion of liver cells, enlargement or shriveling of the organ, and various eventual complications and symptoms such as edema, digestive complaints, weight loss, jaundice, bleeding veins of the esophagus (477).

Cisternal puncture. Puncture of a "cistern" at a point beneath the skull in the back of the neck to withdraw CEREBROSPINAL FLUID.

Claudication. Lameness, limping. *Intermittent claudication,* characterized by cramplike pain in the legs which comes on when walking, may be a symptom of obliterative arterial disease (129).

Clavicle. The collarbone (617).

Clavus. A corn.

Cleft lip, -palate. Congenital malformation of structures of the lip, palate, or both, which fail to fuse properly during fetal development (614). The bilateral parts of the lips and palate fuse at about the eighth week of pregnancy. See TIMETABLE OF FETAL DEVELOPMENT (372).

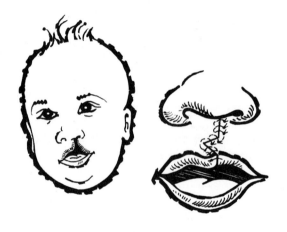

Cleft lip and stage in its repair.

Climacteric. The change of life. See MENOPAUSE and MALE CLIMACTERIC.

Clinical. Pertaining to the bedside; by extension, observation and treatment of patients, results and experience thus gained, as opposed to theoretical, laboratory, or experimental medicine.

Clitoris. The small erectile sex organ of the female situated above the vagina (430); homologue of the penis.

Clofibrate. A drug that lowers fat levels in the blood, prescribed in hope that such lowering may reduce the incidence of heart attacks.

Clonorchis. A chronic Asiatic disease caused by liver flukes transmitted by raw, smoked or pickled fish (67).

Clonic. Spasmodic muscular contractions and relaxations which succeed each other alternately and jerkily. It may be combined with *tonic* contractions which are continuous.

Clubbed fingers. Short, broad, bulbous finger ends with overhanging nails. The condition results from local deficiency of oxygenated blood and almost without exception is associated with abnormalities of the heart and respiratory system such as congenital heart malformations, emphysema, bronchiectasis, chronic diseases of the heart and chest.

Clubfoot (*talipes*). A foot twisted out of shape so that the sole does not rest flat on the floor when standing; there are several types (647). Heredity has little if anything to do with the condition. The principal causative factor is thought to be a fixed position of the fetus in the uterus, maintained for a long period of fetal life; scantiness of amniotic fluid possibly inhibits free movement of the fetus. Pressures of long-maintained fixed posture tend to modify the development of body parts in a mechanical way.

Co-arctation of the aorta. Congenital constriction of the great vessel which carries arterial blood from the heart. The constricted area resembles the narrowed section in the casing between two link sausages (743).

Coagulation time. The time it takes a sample of blood to form a clot, determined by laboratory procedures. This information is useful in treating patients with a tendency to hemorrhage, and as a guide to treatment of patients receiving anticoagulants.

Cobalt bomb. In medicine, not really a bomb but a device employing RADIOISOTOPES of cobalt for powerful irradiation of patients.

Coccidioidomycosis. An infectious disease, most prevalent in the southwestern U. S., caused by inhalation of certain fungi (74). The infection may be so mild that no symptoms occur, but a progressive form can be disabling and serious.

Coccus. A sphere-shaped bacterium. Some types, such as those which cause gonorrhea and pneumonia, occur in pairs; other types form chains; still others cluster in irregular masses like a bunch of grapes (34).

Coccyx. The tailbone (619).

Cochlea. A bony pea-sized structure of the inner ear, shaped like a snail shell, lined with fine hairs and nerve endings which are the essential organs of the sense of hearing (585).

Coenzyme. A partner needed by some enzymes to accomplish a biochemical change. Many vitamins are coenzymes.

Coffee-ground vomit. Dark brown or blackish granular vomited material, somewhat resembling coffee grounds; the color comes from changed blood and indicates bleeding in the upper alimentary tract (396).

Coitus. Sexual intercourse.

Colchicine. A drug prepared from roots of the meadow saffron which is remarkably specific in relieving acute attacks of GOUT (658).

Collagen. Fibers of connective tissue which supports the body; it constitutes 40 per cent of the body's protein. In ways not fully understood, it is associated with rheumatic and other diseases collectively called collagen or connective tissue diseases (660). Collagen fibers vary greatly in structure and function. Some, as in the cornea of the eye, are as transparent as water. Collagen is the cushioning material of cartilage in the joints, the matrix on which minerals are laid down to form bones, the inelastic stuff of tendons which transfer muscle movements over joints, the elastic stuff of skin, a part of webs and struts which hold the body together, a substance which when boiled yields glue or gelatin. Once laid down in the body, collagen is not renewed or replaced. "Old" collagen is less elastic than young collagen. It is related to stiffness of joints and leatheriness of skin with increasing age, and may be a fair index of a person's biological rather than chronological age.

Collapsed lung. Pneumothorax (233).

Colles' fracture. A common fracture of the end of the forearm bone (*radius*) near the wrist joint on the thumb side. It is usually a consequence of falling with an arm thrust out and hand bent backward to break the fall.

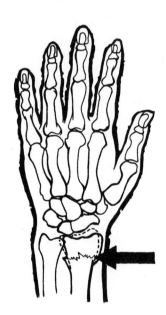

Colles' fracture.

Colloid baths. Soothing baths for excessively dry, sensitive, or itching skin, prepared by adding corn starch, bran, or oatmeal to the bath water (185).

Colloid goiter. Soft, smooth, symmetrical enlargement of the thyroid gland, usually a result of iodine deficiency; "simple goiter" (326).

Colon. The large bowel (459).

Colorado tick fever. Aching, fever, nausea, produced by the bite of a virus-infected woodtick (58). The disease is not limited to Colorado but occurs in all western states where the woodtick is found.

Color blindness. Inability to distinguish colors. There are many types and degrees of color blindness, some so slight that an affected person may never know it. Color blindness does not affect keenness of vision and is no great handicap except in occupations where safety or fine color discrimination is a factor. A color blind man may choose a shirt, necktie, jacket, socks and slacks of violently clashing hues, and think his costume quite sedate, but this does no harm to society and may even win him a good deal of surprised attention. Total color blindness in which everything is seen as shades of gray is extremely rare. The most common type is red-green color blindness, which may range from ability to see only the brightest hues of red and green to inability to see the two colors as other than shades of gray. Injury of the retina or ocular disease may produce color blindness in a person not disposed to it, but this is very rare. Color blindness is almost always inherited; a few women are partially color blind but the condition predominantly affects males. Common red-green color blindness is a sex-linked trait, transmitted to her sons but not her daughters by a mother who herself is not color blind. The inherited defect is in the structure of the CONES, the color-sensitive nerve cells of the retina (556). Nothing can be done to change the defect, although some improvement in discrimination of shades may be attained by training.

Colostomy. A surgically created opening of the colon (artificial anus) in the wall of the abdomen (732). A colostomy may be temporary, to divert intestinal contents while a portion of the colon is healing, or it may be permanent, as is usually the case if a large section of the bowel must be removed because of disease. A *colostomy bag* is a container which covers the artificial opening and receives excretions.

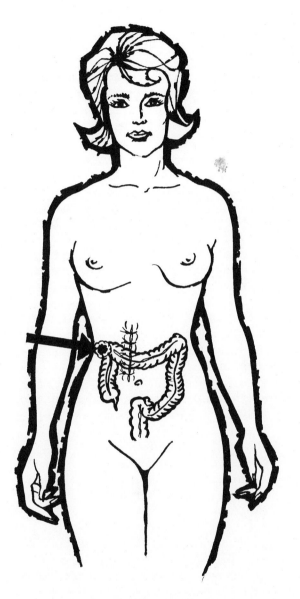

Arrow points to colostomy, outlet through abdomen.

Colostrum. The "first milk" secreted by the mother's breasts shortly after the birth of a child. Colostrum is not "true" milk but a clear or slightly cloudy fluid containing fats and sugars which have a slight laxative effect on the newborn baby. Colostrum also con-

tains IMMUNOGLOBULINS which pass on to the baby some of the immunities acquired by the mother; passive immunity thus transmitted is not long lasting.

Colpotomy. Any surgical cutting of the vagina.

Coma. Unconsciousness so deep that it is impossible or extremely difficult to arouse the patient. Many different conditions are associated with coma: advanced liver and kidney disease, diabetes, poisoning, head blows, tumors, strokes, to mention a few.

Comedo. Blackhead.

Comminuted fracture. One in which the broken bones are crushed into small pieces (652).

Compound fracture. One in which the broken bone breaks through the skin or into an open wound.

Concussion. Violent jarring, shocking, shaking, or the resulting condition. *Concussion of the brain* (840) may result from a fall or violent blow on the head. The injured person may not be "knocked out cold," but may be dizzy, stuporous, nauseated, or he may lose consciousness and have a feeble pulse, cold skin and pallor. Medical help should be sought immediately, even though the person seems to have "recovered" or to be only slightly dazed. A physician treating a concussion may wish to keep the patient under observation, or to make tests, to be sure the skull has not been fractured.

Conduction deafness. Failure of airborne sound waves to be conducted efficiently through and over the external and middle ear structures, so that adequate messages do not reach the nerves of the inner ear (588).

Condyloma. Warty growths on the skin around the anus and external sex organs; usually removed by electrocoagulation (433).

Cones. Specialized cells of the central part of the retina which distinguish colors and are responsible for finely detailed seeing (556).

Congenital malformations. Abnormalities that are present at birth. See BIRTH DEFECTS.

Conization. Reaming out of a cone-shaped piece of tissue by high-frequency current; usually a gynecologic procedure performed on a diseased cervix (737).

Conjunctiva. A thin mucous membrane which covers the insides of the eyelids and is reflected over the front of the eye (568). *Conjunctivitis* is an inflammation of this tissue resulting from infection, allergies, irritation, or inflammation from within the eye itself.

Consanguinity. Blood relationship.

Contact dermatitis. Skin eruption, redness, inflammation, resulting from contact with any of hundreds of commonplace substances in the world around us (185, 681).

Contact lenses. Plastic lenses worn invisibly over the cornea of the eye (563). Meticulous fitting to eye contours is essential. The lenses must have proper sanitary care. Serious complications are rare, minor ones not uncommon. The most painful complication appears to result from wearing the lenses too long. They should not be worn while sleeping, or when the eye is infected, or when there are cold sores on the face (the cold sore virus can infect the eyes dangerously). Flush-fitting contact lenses which cover the white of the eye permit a thin layer of tears to circulate beneath them and have special medical uses as healing aids. Such lenses improve the healing of chemical burns of the cornea, ulcerations, corneal transplants and other conditions. Plastic lenses which absorb moisture have become available; see SOFT CONTACT LENSES.

Contraception. Prevention of conception or impregnation (343).

Contrast medium. A substance which has greater density to x-rays than tissues which are objects of study. Contrast media are given by injection or other means to obtain clearly outlined x-ray or fluoroscopic images of structures being examined.

Contusion. A bruise (848). An experienced mother's prescription for the best treatment of trivial contusions of childhood is, "kiss them."

Cool enema. An enema of cool water with a small amount of baking soda, useful in reducing fever (393).

Cooley's anemia (*thallassemia*). A congenital form of anemia which occurs primarily in people bordering on the Mediterranean Sea or their descendants (158).

Coombs' test. An antibody test on blood, used in determining the compatibility of bloods for transfusion and in diagnosis of certain anemias.

Cor pulmonale. A form of heart disease secondary to chronic disease of the lungs.

Cornea. The curved, transparent tissue over the iris and pupil on the outside of the eye; the "window" of the eye (553).

Corneal transplant. The cornea (553) may become scarred or clouded, obstructing vision as if a curtain were pulled down. If the rest of the eye is in good condition, sight may be restored by transplanting a disk taken from the cornea of a recently deceased person. It is like replacing an opaque pane of glass with a clear, transparent one. The procedure requires a supply of donor eyes, and "eye banks" have been established in many cities to receive and preserve donated eyes, which must be removed promptly after death of the donor. It is futile to donate one's eyes in a will, because of legal delays. Anyone wishing to donate his eyes after death should do so through his physician or an eye bank.

Corns. Horny skin thickenings about the size of peas which occur principally on or between the toes. "Soft corns" between the toes are softened by sweat. The common hard corn has a cone-shaped core which presses on nerves to cause dull discomfort or sharp pain. Corns are caused by continued pressure and friction, as from too tight or ill-fitting shoes and stockings. Pressure can be lessened by wearing softer shoes with ample toe-room and by foam rubber pads and inserts. The hard tissue of a corn usually must be removed occasionally for comfort's sake. Soaking the feet in hot water and paring the surface of the corn with a razor blade often relieves friction and pressure, but there is risk of cuts and infection. Superficial hard tissue may be removed with an emery board, nail file, or pumice stone. The core may be sufficiently loosened by soaking to be lifted out by sterilized tweezers. Corn plasters and medicines usually contain salicylic acid which softens the hard growth. Diabetics should be especially circumspect in care of the feet because of the risk of gangrene (356).

Coronary thrombosis. Commonly called a "heart attack"; a blood clot in coronary arteries that nourish the heart muscle (88, 93).

Corpuscle. Any small round body; the word used to be a synonym for "cell." Technically, a cell has a nucleus; the mature red blood cell does not, and is sometimes called a corpuscle.

Corpus luteum. The "yellow body" which develops from a follicle of the ovary after a ripened egg has been discharged. The yellow body produces progesterone, a hormone which prepares the lining of the uterus to receive a fertilized egg (339). If fertilization occurs, the corpus luteum en-

larges and continues to produce pregnancy-sustaining hormone for several months. If conception does not occur, the corpus luteum shrinks and degenerates.

Cortex. The surface layer of an organ such as the brain, kidney, adrenal gland. The cortex of an organ has different functions from its inner part (medulla); for example, the adrenal cortex produces hormones entirely different from those of its inner part. The thin surface layer of the brain (*cortex cerebri*) consists of gray matter, largely composed of small-bodied nerve cells with rich interconnections, interspersed with larger neurons which send AXONS into underlying white matter.

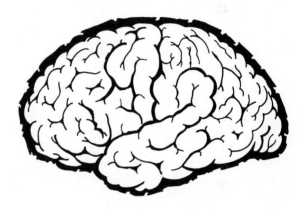

Cortex of the brain.

Corticosteroids. Substances having the properties of hormones secreted by the cortex of the adrenal glands (330). Cortisone, hydrocortisone, prednisone, and many other corticosteroids have important medical uses.

Coryza. An old word for the common cold.

Cosmetic dermatitis. Inflammation of the skin, usually allergic, produced by contact with cosmetic creams, dyes, lotions, perfumes and the like (189).

Cowper's glands. Two small glands of the male which secrete lubricating fluids into the urethra (302).

Cowpox. A disease of cattle so closely related to smallpox, but insignificantly mild in man, that inoculation with vaccine containing cowpox virus has long been the standard method of immunizing against smallpox.

Coxsackie viruses. A family of viruses named for a community in New York whose ill townsfolk furnished excretions from which the viruses were first isolated and identified. A score or more of different Coxsackie viruses cause diseases such as HERPANGINA, DEVIL'S GRIP, and forms of *meningitis* (59).

"Crabs." Infestation by public lice (201).

Cradle cap. Patchy areas of greasy crusts on an infant's scalp, arising from secretions of oil glands (406).

Cranial nerve. A nerve attached directly to the brain, leaving it through a perforation in the skull. There are 12 pairs of cranial nerves, with names that suggest their function or location: transmission of the sense of smell (*olfactory*), sight (*optic*), hearing (*acoustic*); control of movement —of the eyeball (*trochlear*), a muscle of the eyeball (*abducens*), the pupil (*oculomotor*), muscles of the upper throat and taste sensations from the back of the tongue (*glossopharyngeal*), sense of taste, salivary glands and muscles of the face (*facial*), muscles of the larynx and throat (*accessory*), the tongue (*hypoglossal*); sensory nerve of the face and front part of the scalp (*trigeminal*); "wandering" sensory and motor nerve branching to the heart, stomach and esophagus (*vagus*).

Craniotomy. Surgical opening into the skull cavity (759).

Cranium. The skull; the brain-containing part.

Creeping eruption (*larva migrans*). An odd parasitic infection of the skin: thin, red, tortuous lines creep ahead at one end an inch or more a day while fading at the other end. The moving lines mark the progress of larvae burrowing under the skin. The burrowers, often immature forms of cat or dog hookworm, get into people who go barefoot at beaches, children in sandboxes, gardeners, repairmen who work under porches or houses. Freezing the larvae in the skin with an ethyl chloride spray usually stops their migrations cold.

Creeping ulcer. One which creeps slowly outward from its center.

Cremaster. The muscle which retracts the testicle.

Cretin. A child born with impaired function of the thyroid gland (324).

Cross-eye. Eyes that do not work as a team in holding the gaze straight upon an object, because of imbalance of muscles that control movements of the eyeballs (566). An eye that turns in or out in young children may lose its vision completely unless the condition is corrected before it is too late.

Crohn's disease. See REGIONAL ILEITIS.

Croup. Difficult, laborious, raspy breathing and barky coughing of a child. *Spasmodic croup* is more frightening than serious; another type, *laryngotracheobronchitis*, is one of the most serious conditions of infancy and constitutes a medical emergency (406).

Croup tent. An arrangement that confines vapors for inhalation by an infant with croup (29).

Crowning. The stage in childbirth when the crown or top of the infant's head first becomes visible, as wrinkled scalp in the dilated outlet of the womb.

Cryosurgery. Use of extreme cold to destroy or to freeze and later revive tissues. Instruments which apply extreme cold quite precisely to tissues are usually supercooled by liquid ni-

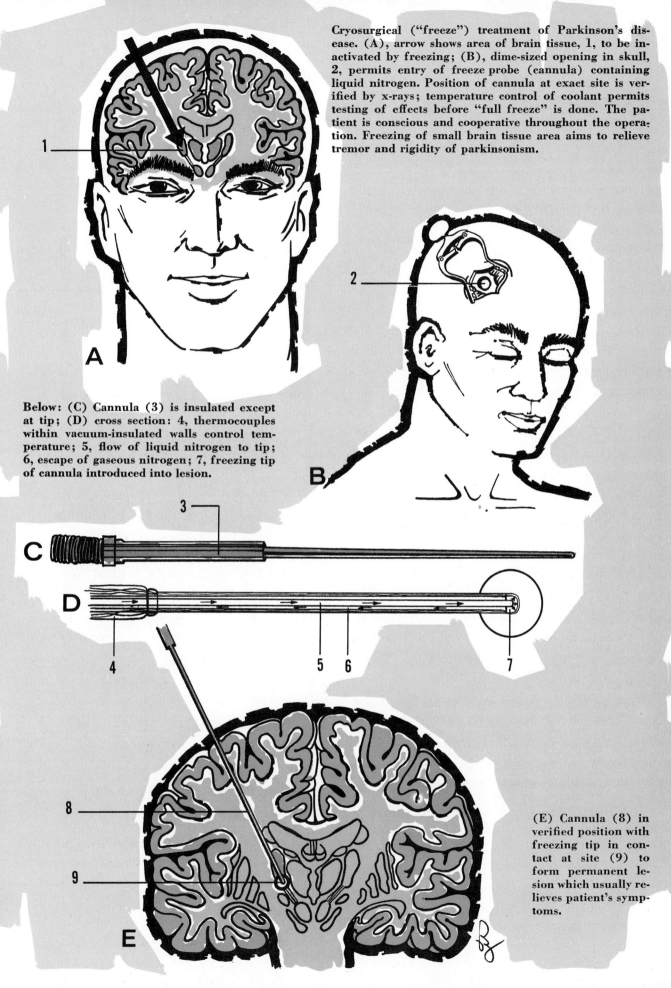

Cryosurgical ("freeze") treatment of Parkinson's disease. (A), arrow shows area of brain tissue, 1, to be inactivated by freezing; (B), dime-sized opening in skull, 2, permits entry of freeze probe (cannula) containing liquid nitrogen. Position of cannula at exact site is verified by x-rays; temperature control of coolant permits testing of effects before "full freeze" is done. The patient is conscious and cooperative throughout the operation. Freezing of small brain tissue area aims to relieve tremor and rigidity of parkinsonism.

Below: (C) Cannula (3) is insulated except at tip; (D) cross section: 4, thermocouples within vacuum-insulated walls control temperature; 5, flow of liquid nitrogen to tip; 6, escape of gaseous nitrogen; 7, freezing tip of cannula introduced into lesion.

(E) Cannula (8) in verified position with freezing tip in contact at site (9) to form permanent lesion which usually relieves patient's symptoms.

trogen. Pioneering cryosurgical work was done in the field of brain surgery, especially in surgical management of *Parkinson's disease* (261). Complete destruction of tissue by super-freezing has been used to relieve benign or malignant obstruction of the *prostate* gland (307). The "freeze treatment" for *gastric ulcer* does not permanently destroy stomach tissue, but tends to decrease acid production; long term benefits are considered disappointing by many specialists. A newer application of cryosurgery (more exactly, cryotherapy, since tissue is not destroyed) is in treatment of *glaucoma* (571). The purpose is to decrease production of fluid in the eye. Cryotherapy is a reserve method if drugs or surgery fail to stop the advance of glaucoma.

Crypt. A cavity, pit, or follicle; as, the natural depressions in the tonsils.

Cryptorchidism. Failure of the testicles to descend into the scrotum during fetal development; the undescended organs remain in the abdominal cavity or groin (311, 337).

Curettage. Scraping out of a body cavity with a spoon-shaped instrument called a *curet.*

Curling's ulcer. An ulcer of the stomach or duodenum associated with severe and extensive skin burns.

Cushing's disease, -syndrome. Disorders resulting from excessive output of certain adrenal gland hormones (332).

Cuspid. A canine tooth (524).

Cuticle. The horny outer layer of skin; the crescent of skin at the base of nails; popularly, the substance of "hangnails."

Cyanosis. A bluish tinge of the skin and mucous membranes resulting from insufficient oxygen in the blood. There are many different causes; for example, congenital heart defects (97), congestive heart failure, emphysema, mountain sickness, respiratory and blood disorders. The lips or beds of the nails may sometimes take on a bluish discoloration without a necessary deficiency of oxygen in the general circulation.

Cyesis. Pregnancy.

Cyst. A normal or abnormal sac with a definite wall, containing liquid or semisolid material. Frequent sites of cysts that may require surgery or other measures are the ovaries, kidneys, skin (wens), the tailbone area (pilonidal cyst) and the breast.

Cystic fibrosis. An inherited disease of the *exocrine* glands which pour secretions into or out of the body rather than into the blood; for example, pancreas, biliary, intestinal and sweat glands. Thick, viscid secretions obstruct or depress the functioning of many different organs and tissues and produce a great variety of symptoms; respiratory distress is prominent (407). Cystic fibrosis was "discovered" in 1938, at which time it was thought to be a disease of the pancreas gland; it is now known that nearly all of the exocrine glands are affected to some degree. The earliest symptom of cystic fibrosis in a newborn infant is MECONIUM ILEUS. Prompt recognition and treatment of cystic fibrosis, with aerosol aids to breathing, postural drainage, digestive enzymes, antibiotics to combat infection, have carried affected infants through critical periods of childhood. The disease is being increasingly recognized in adults who have had it from infancy without knowing it. Specialists think it likely that many patients treated for BRONCHIAL ASTHMA or various chronic lung conditions actually have cystic fibrosis. The disease is transmitted as a recessive trait (the mother and father are carriers but do not have the disease themselves). An abnormal protein in the blood serum of cystic fibrosis patients and of blood-related persons is the possible basis for a test to detect carriers of the trait; if two carriers marry, the chance that each of their children will have cystic fibrosis is one in four.

Cystic kidney. A congenital condition in which the kidneys are filled with bubble-like cysts (290).

Cysticercosis. Infestation of the body with a form of tapeworm, sometimes present in raw beef. Beef should be cooked at least to the rare stage (140 degrees F.) to avoid danger.

Cystinuria. An inherited disease in which cystine, a sulfur-containing amino acid, is excreted in large quantities in the urine. The poorly soluble cystine tends to form recurrent kidney stones (287); alkalinizing the urine and drinking large amounts of water may help to reduce the likelihood of cystine stone formation.

Cystocele. Sagging of the base of the bladder into the vaginal canal (438).

Cystoscope. An instrument for examining the interior of the urinary bladder (288).

Cytology. Scientific study of the structure, elements, and functions of cells.

Cytologic diagnosis. Microscopic study of cells shed by body tissues to detect abnormalities; especially, the presence of cancer cells. The "PAP TEST" for detection of cancer of the cervix is the most widely used cytologic screening test (440), but the technique is applicable to "smears" obtained from the lungs, stomach, bladder and a number of other organs.

Cytoplasm. The substance of a cell outside of its nucleus. Transformations of energy, synthesis of proteins, and uncountable chemical exchanges that keep us alive go on incessantly in the cytoplasm.

D

Dander. Minute skin particles shed by animals. Inhalation of danders is a frequent cause of allergic reactions, the reason why cats make some people weep and sneeze (679).

Dandruff. Fine, whitish, somewhat greasy scales formed upon the scalp (188); the condition is controllable but rarely curable.

Deaf-mutism. Inability to hear and speak. The two disabilities are interrelated. A totally deaf child cannot learn to speak in the normal way because he cannot hear sounds to imitate. Various signs may arouse suspicion of deafness in an infant as young as six months (591). While the child is still young, he can be taught "unnaturally" to speak, by difficult training techniques used in special schools for the deaf.

D & C. Dilation and curettage, a common minor operation on women; the canal of the uterus is dilated and the lining of the uterus scraped with a spoon-shaped instrument called a curet (736).

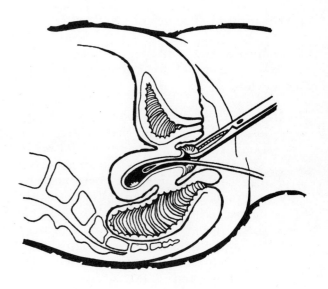

Dilation and curettage.

Debridement. Surgical cleaning of a wound; removal of foreign material and devitalized tissue.

Decalcification. The withdrawal of calcium from the bones where it has been deposited. It may be caused by an inadequate supply of calcium in the diet so that calcium has to be taken from the bones, or it may be caused by hormonal imbalances.

Decibel. The unit of measurement of the loudness of sound, used in tests of hearing (590). A whisper is about "20 decibels loud."

Decidua. That part of the lining of the uterus which is modified during pregnancy and cast off after delivery.

Deciduous teeth. Baby teeth; the teeth which are shed when the permanent teeth erupt.

Decubitus ulcer. A bedsore (26).

Defecation. Passage of feces; evacuation of the bowels.

Deficiency diseases. Those caused by insufficiency of some constituent of the diet, such as vitamins, minerals, protein, fatty acids (503).

Deglutition. The act of swallowing.

Dehiscence. A splitting open, as of a sutured wound that "comes apart at the seams."

Dehydration. Drying out of the body; loss of more water than is taken in. Dehydration may be induced for medical reasons, but often it is an aspect of disease or injury, characterized by dry mucous membranes, fever, scanty urine, tight abdominal skin, possible shock. Treatment, which may present an emergency, requires recognition of underlying circumstances, calculation of water and ELECTROLYTE deficits, and usually replacement of water and salts (sometimes of plasma or blood) by infusion into a vein.

Déjà vu. "Already seen"; an illusion that a present experience has occurred at some previous time.

Delirium. A state of mental confusion, excitement, incoherent talk, restlessness, hallucinations. Delirium may be associated with high fever, poisoning, drug intoxication, infections, and metabolic disturbances. Treatment is directed to the underlying condition while the patient is kept in a quiet room, closely watched to prevent injury. Calming medications may be prescribed. Reassurances by a close member of the family may help significantly to allay fears.

Delirium tremens (*D.T.'s*). A serious, sometimes fatal form of delirium, most often occurring in persons with a long history of alcoholism, but occasionally associated with other poisonings of the brain cells, senile brain changes, and psychoses. The patient has vivid visual hallucinations, often of moving colored animals—he may actually "see" pink elephants—but the hallucinated creatures may be very tiny and frequently he feels as well as sees them crawling over his skin. Anxiety, fear, coarse trembling of the hands, mental confusion, and sleeplessness are other manifestations. Physical restraints may be necessary but skilful attendants can often avoid this. The delirium lasts for a couple of days to a week or more and usually terminates in profound sleep. The patient is often malnourished and run down physically. Appropriate calming medication and large doses of B vitamins are commonly a part of treatment. KORSAKOFF'S PSYCHOSIS may begin as delirium tremens.

Deltoid. Triangular in shape, like the Greek letter *delta;* specifically, the muscle which covers the shoulder joint and extends the arm out from the side.

Dementia. A general term for mental deterioration, usually implying serious impairment of intellect, irrationality, confusion, stupor, "insane" behavior.

Dementia may result from poisons, physical changes in the brain, toxins produced by disease, or psychoses of which the basic cause is unknown.

Dendrites. Fine, branched fibers, somewhat in the pattern of tree roots, which accept and convey incoming impulses to the central body of a nerve cell (242).

Dengue fever. See BREAKBONE FEVER.

Dentalgia. A highflown and superfluous word for toothache.

Dental implants. Replacement of lost teeth, as by re-implantation of a knocked-out tooth (548). The space left by extraction of a decayed molar of a young person may sometimes be filled successfully by transplantation of one of the patient's own immature wisdom teeth. The root of the wisdom tooth does not mature until late adolescence and if it is transplanted before age 18 it may anchor itself permanently in its new position.

Dental plaque. A thin, transparent film that builds up on the teeth. It is made up of material from saliva. The plaques contain bacteria which are thought to be a factor in tooth decay.

Dentin. The ivory-like material, harder and denser than bone, which underlies the enamel of the teeth (522).

Denture. The set of natural teeth; also, a set of artificial teeth; "plates," "false teeth" (539).

Denture stomatitis. Sore mouth due to ill-fitting dentures or allergy to substances in the plates (690).

Depilation. Removal of hair. Permanent removal of unwanted hair is best accomplished by ELECTROLYSIS, which destroys the hair follicle.

Depot desensitization. A "one shot" technique for desensitization to allergies, using oily emulsions (705).

DeQuervain's disease (*stenosing tenovaginitis*). Thickening of sheaths covering tendons of the thumb, resulting in pain at the base of the thumb radiating to the nail and into the forearm (634). Fairly simple surgery corrects the condition, or it may cure itself if the wrist is immobilized.

Dercum's disease (*adiposis dolorosa*). A rare disease of middle-aged and older women. Firm fat nodules, slightly sensitive or exquisitely painful, are distributed over various parts of the body except the face, lower arms and lower legs; overlying skin is red and shiny. There is pronounced muscular weakness and degrees of psychic disturbance. The cause is not known. Non-specific methods of treatment include measures to relieve pain, reduce weight, and combat psychic disturbances that may be associated.

Dermabrasion. A method of removing layers of skin with an abrasive instrument, usually a rapidly rotating wire brush, for cosmetic improvement of scars or blemishes (183).

Dermatitis. Inflammation of the skin; often called eczema (185). Its causes are manifold, its symptoms varied. Chemicals, plants, common household agents, cosmetics, drugs, x-rays, and almost numberless things can produce a dermatitis; allergies to various substances are often involved.

Dermatoglyphics. The study of ridges, whorls, lines and creases which form highly individual patterns of the skin of hands and feet. Readers of detective stories know all about fingerprints for identification; medical uses are new and different. Skin patterns determined by GENES begin to form in the fetus at about the fourth month of pregnancy. Several abnormal patterns, such as a single crease instead of the usual two which run across the top of the palm, are characteristic of infants with congenital diseases. Some disorders such as MONGOLISM and KLINEFELTER'S SYNDROME result from abnormal CHROMOSOMES. Others, such as malformations associated with the mother's infection by German measles, result from unfavorable environment of the fetus at the time when skin patterns as well as organ systems are developing. It is not yet possible to identify specific diseases by abnormal palmprints, but they usually indicate some congenital abnormality. Palmprint studies may give early warning of a congenital disorder, or confirm some suspected condition, such as mongolism, without the need of analyzing chromosomes.

Dermatome. An instrument for cutting thin layers of skin for grafts.

Dermatomyositis. An ill-defined disease of unknown cause, affecting connective tissue structures, manifested principally in the skin and voluntary muscles; characterized by pain and swelling in muscles, weakness, inflammation and swelling of skin of the face, upper trunk, and extremities (667).

Dermatophytes. Fungi which produce blistery, scaly, crusty lesions of the skin; most notoriously, those responsible for *dermatophytosis* or "athlete's foot" (200).

Dermis. The "true skin"; the *corium;* a dense, elastic layer of fibrous tissue underlying the topmost epithelial layers (177).

Dermoid cyst. A congenital cyst (often of the ovary) which contains fragments of skin appendages such as strands of hair, sweat and oil glands, and sometimes cartilage, bone, and teeth, remnants of development.

Dermographia. "Skin writing"; a condition in which a tracing made on the skin by a fingernail or blunt instrument produces a pale streak bordered on each side by a reddened line. The marks disappear after a few minutes. The condition may be associated with URTICARIA but in itself is not injurious to health. Dermographia occurs in persons whose mechanisms for expanding and constricting blood vessels are hypersensitive to any irritation.

Desensitization. Reduction of a person's allergic reaction to a specific substance such as pollen or house dust. Sensitivity is reduced by spaced injections of small amounts of extracts of specific allergens; "hay fever shots" are a familiar example (705).

Desquamation. Shedding of the skin in scales or sheets, as after scarlet fever or severe sunburn.

Detached retina. Separation of the light-receiving layer of the back of the eye from its underlying layer (577-78). In the majority of cases, the detached filmy structure can be "spot-welded" into its proper place by various surgical procedures.

Deviated septum. Diversion from a straight line of the wall that divides the nose into two equal parts, usually a result of injury but sometimes congenital (610). The deformity may not be obvious from the outside. Depending on its nature, a deviated septum may partially obstruct air passages, deflect air currents, and lead to mouth-breathing and very profuse and annoying postnasal drip.

Devil's grip (*Bornholm disease, epidemic pleurodynia*). An infectious disease of sudden onset, produced by COXSACKIE VIRUSES, marked by knifelike pains in the chest or abdomen (59).

Devil's pinches (*purpura simplex*). Bruises or black-and-blue spots caused by bleeding under the skin without apparent cause. The purplish spots range from pinhead size to rather large patches. The condition, which seems to "run in families," seems to be harmless, fortunately, since there is no effective treatment.

Dextrocardia. Congenital transposition of the axis of the heart toward the right side of the chest.

Dextrose (*glucose*). A sugar, often called "blood sugar," since it is an essential constituent of blood, a source of energy, and necessary for combustion of fats. The liver converts dextrose into *glycogen* ("animal starch") and stores it. This reservoir is drawn upon for dextrose, reconverted from glycogen, as energy needs of the body require. Dextrose solutions are often infused into the veins of patients.

Dhobie itch. See JOCKEY ITCH.

Diabetes. The word comes from a Greek term for "syphon," "to flow through," referring to excessive flow of urine and excessive thirst. Used alone, diabetes means *diabetes mellitus* or "sugar diabetes" (349). There are other forms of diabetes, such as *diabetes insipidus* (321), a hormone imbalance causing enormous thirst and compensating urinary outflow, and *bronze diabetes*, associated with HEMOCHROMATOSIS.

Diagnosis. The art and science of identifying a patient's disease, a prerequisite to treatment; fraught with hazard if applied by the untrained in reckless self-diagnosis. Some diagnostic tools are as old as Hippocrates: the patient's history, symptoms, physical signs; thumping and listening, feeling, inspecting, applying all the trained senses. Modern tools project the perceptions of physicians into occult chemical and electrical processes of the body. Instruments amplify and transcribe minute currents of the heart and brain and muscles; "scopes" of many kinds carry educated eyes into caverns of the body; a film of tissue yields secrets to a pathologist; x-rays probe hidden structures; scores of complex tests give clues to what is going on in the infinitesimal world of the body's molecules. The diagnostician gains all possible and necessary information, interprets it, often arrives at a firm diagnosis, but sometimes can only make a tentative diagnosis subject to change by later information and developments.

Dialysis. Separation of substances in solution by passing them through a porous membrane; this is done naturally by the kidney and mechanically by an artificial kidney (295).

Diaper rash. An ammonia burn resulting from breakdown of urine (409).

Diaphragm. The transverse, dome-shaped muscle which separates the chest from the abdomen; the chief muscle of breathing (214). Contraction of the diaphragm expands the chest cage and lungs and air rushes in; relaxation allows the chest cage and lungs to collapse partially, and air is exhaled. A *vaginal diaphragm* is a ringed latex cup which covers the cervix for contraceptive purposes.

Diaphragmatic hernia (*hiatus hernia*). Protrusion of part of the stomach through a weak spot in the DIAPHRAGM (468, 725).

Diarrhea. Abnormal frequency and liquidity of stools (396, 488). In young infants, profuse diarrhea (and vomiting) can cause serious loss of fluids and ELECTROLYTES and the baby should be under care of a physician.

Diastole. The "resting" stage of the heart during which relaxed chambers are filling with blood (80). Diastolic pressure is the lower of the two figures (such as 120/80) by which doctors express blood pressure readings (see SYSTOLE). Diastolic pressure gives the doctor significant information about the condition of blood vessels and the injurious effects of sustained hypertension (116).

Diathermy. Generation of heat in body tissues by passing high-frequency electric currents through them. Resistance of tissues—like the resistance element in an electric toaster—produces the heat, which is very penetrating and can build up to dangerous intensity unless treatment is supervised by an experienced operator. In surgical diathermy, heat is sufficient to destroy tissues or to cut tissues with little or no bleeding.

Diathesis. Inborn, constitutional susceptibility or predisposition to a certain disease or condition.

Digitalis. A drug derived from the foxglove plant which is a powerful stimulant of heart muscle contractions. "Whole" digitalis contains a number of active agents called *glucosides;* some of these, such as *digitoxin,* are prepared pharmaceutically in pure form. *Digitalization* is the procedure of administering digitalis until a desired concentration of the drug is built up in the patient's body, after which maintenance doses suffice. The toxic effect of digitalis is close to the therapeutic effect and expert medical supervision of dosage is necessary.

Diopter. The unit of measurement of the refractive (light-bending) power of a lens, including the lens of the human eye, which has a power of about 10 diopters. Abbreviated as "D" in prescriptions for glasses; +D (plus D) indicates a convex lens for correcting a farsighted person, −D (minus D) a concave lens for correcting a nearsighted person (562).

Diphtheria. An acute contagious disease, once responsible for many deaths of children, but no longer a threat to the child who is properly immunized (418).

Diplegia. Paralysis of like parts on both sides of the body.

Diplopia. "Seeing double"; one object is seen as two. The condition may be temporary or persistent and can be caused by a number of diseases and disorders, including head injuries, alcoholism, and poisoning. The double vision effect is the result of paralysis or improper functioning of muscles that control eyeball movements, or paralysis of one of the nerves controlling action of the eye muscles. Persistent double vision may be the result of a nervous system ailment such as multiple sclerosis, myasthenia gravis, meningitis, tabes dorsalis, or a brain tumor affecting nerves running between the brain and eye muscles. Treatment of persistent diplopia may require surgery, the use of special corrective lenses, or both.

Dipsomania. Compulsion to drink alcoholic beverages to excess.

Dislocation. Displacement of a bone from its normal position in a joint, usually the result of a severe blow, fall, or twisting force; often there is an accompanying sprain (651, 769).

Diuretic. An agent which increases the output of urine; especially, a drug prescribed for this purpose. Along with other treatment, physicians prescribe diuretics for a variety of conditions associated with excessive retention of water; for example, congestive heart failure (102); hypertension (120); premenstrual tension (348); toxemia of pregnancy (375); cirrhosis of the liver (478).

Diverticula. Small pouches like thin-walled balloons opening from a hollow organ. They can occur anywhere along the alimentary tract from the esophagus to the terminus, but the most common site is the colon (488). A person with these superfluous little pockets has *diverticulosis* but may never know it; they may not cause symptoms. It is estimated that 10 per cent of people over 40 years of age have diverticulosis. Chances that existing pockets may become infected, inflamed, or ruptured, resulting in *diverticulitis,* increase with advancing age. Diverticulitis is sometimes called "left-sided appendicitis" because the patient's symptoms are quite similar to those of appendicitis except for reversal of position. Many patients with diverticulitis are well controlled with medical measures. A soft diet with cooked fruits and vegetables and avoidance of irritating foodstuffs such as coarse fibers and seeds is often prescribed to lessen the risk of flareups. Sometimes surgery is necessary to remove a diseased portion of the bowel (730).

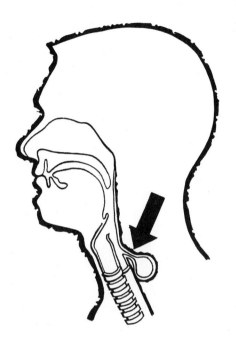

Diverticulum of the esophagus.

Dizygotic. Developed at the same time from two fertilized eggs; fraternal twins (378).

Dizziness. A whirling, head-swimming feeling of unsteadiness and of the world revolving about one (269). The disturbance may be primarily in the inner ear (598A), in nerves serving this area, in reduced blood supply to the brain, in nervous messages from the heart, eyes, or stomach, or in association with many other conditions. An ordinary mild bout of dizziness can usually be abated by sitting or lying down. Dizziness is not always or often a symptom of serious disease but recurrent attacks should be investigated to determine the cause.

DMSO. Dimethyl sulfoxide. A solvent which can penetrate intact skin and carry drugs or chemicals with it. This unique property may prove useful in administering drugs, relieving pain, easing arthritis, but possible therapeutic uses are still under experimental investigation.

Dominant eye. The eye unconsciously preferred in visual tasks such as sighting a rifle (see test, 552).

Dorsum. The back; any part of the body corresponding to the back, as the back of the hand.

Double-blind study. A technique most often used in studying the effects of drugs. Neither the administering physician nor the patient knows whether a given medicine contains an active drug or totally inert ingredients. Presumably this eliminates unconscious bias in knowing that a drug "should" or "should not" have some effect.

Double vision. See DIPLOPIA.

Douche. A stream of water directed against or into a part of the body; used alone, the word usually means *vaginal douche* (432).

Down's syndrome. MONGOLISM.

DPT. Vaccine combining immunizing agents against *diphtheria*, *pertussis* (whooping cough), and *tetanus*, administered in a single injection instead of separate injections for each disease.

Draining ear. Chronic discharge from an ear, a warning that serious infection may erupt at any time (595).

Dreams. See SLEEP.

Dropsy. An old term for EDEMA.

Dry labor. See BAG OF WATERS.

Dry socket. Failure of a protective blood clot to develop in the socket left after extraction of a tooth, or premature loss of a clot, causing pain and delay in healing (542).

Drug addiction. Certain drugs (including alcohol) have an effect on body cells, particularly those of the nervous system, called *tissue tolerance*. Body chemistry is upset and the cells adjust their metabolism to accommodate the drug. The tissues become physically dependent upon the drug to maintain their normal functions.

Over a period of time, increasingly large doses of the drug are necessary to obtain the same original effect and the body, in turn, constantly alters its chemistry to accommodate the larger doses. Eventually the addict is able to tolerate doses of drugs which would be fatal to a non-addict. When an addict suddenly stops using drugs, he experiences severe WITHDRAWAL SYMPTOMS because of physical dependency; he also has psychological dependency. Because "addiction" and "habituation" are often used interchangeably, the World Health Organization has adopted a more general term, "drug dependence," to banish confusion. Dependence is defined as "a state arising from repeated administration of a drug on a periodic or continuous basis." This is subdivided into "dependence of the morphine type," "cocaine type," "barbiturate type," "marihuana type," "amphetamine type," and "alcohol type," applying to all types of drug abuse. (See Chapter 27).

Dry ice. Frozen carbon dioxide or "dry ice" gives off carbon dioxide gas when it sublimes (passes from a solid to a gaseous state without going through a liquid phase). Carbon dioxide gas is not directly poisonous—we exhale it constantly—but in heavy concentrations it can displace oxygen and cause unconsciousness or asphyxiation. This never happens with ordinary amounts of dry ice used to pack a gallon or so of ice cream, but it can occur if a large quantity of dry ice is kept in an occupied confined space without ventilation. Some motorists use dry ice to keep a car cool while driving with windows closed in hot weather. Several accidents have resulted from drivers being made unconscious by this practice. The National Safety Council reports that a 10 per cent concentration of carbon dioxide is sufficient to cause unconsciousness.

Ductus arteriosus. In the fetus, a channel which short-circuits blood from the pulmonary artery to the aorta; normally it closes and ceases to function at birth (99). In certain "blue babies," the channel fails to close. Usually the condition can be corrected by surgery.

Duodenum. The first part of the small intestine; a tubular organ shaped like a horseshoe (455). Here, just beyond the acid stomach, the intestinal environment begins to become alkaline. Highly alkaline bile and digestive juices of the pancreas flow into the duodenum in the general area of its horseshoe bend. *Duodenal ulcer* is the most common type of peptic ulcer (475, 518).

Dupuytren's contracture. Thickening of connective tissue (FASCIA) of the palm of the hand, pulling one or more fingers down into the palm (636).

Dumping syndrome. Symptoms of bloating, diarrhea, vomiting, distress, occurring soon after eating in persons whose stomachs have been partially removed (474).

Dura mater. The outermost membrane of tough connective tissue which covers the brain and spinal cord (265).

D.V.M. Doctor of Veterinary Medicine.

Dyscrasia. Abnormal state, especially of the blood.

Dysentery. Inflammation of the colon with severe diarrhea, abdominal cramps, painful and ineffectual rectal straining; the stools may contain blood and mucus. Chemical poisons and various irritants of the bowel can cause dysentery, but there are two major forms of the disorder: BACILLARY DYSENTERY produced by certain bacteria (45) and AMEBIC DYSENTERY produced by protozoa (71).

Dysfunction. Abnormality or impairment of the normal activities of an organ or bodily process.

Dyslexia. Inability to read efficiently. The child may have simple incapacity to learn, but about 90 per cent of "retarded readers" are children of normal or superior intelligence. The reading difficulty is secondary to emotional, physical, or educational factors. Remedial reading measures are usually successful in this group of children when the specific cause is found and remedied. About one out of ten "reading problem" children has an eye muscle imbalance (566) detectable by an ophthalmologist. Many children with eye muscle imbalances do not have a reading problem; they use their "good" eye and function as one-eyed persons. But some of these children evidently work hard to "fight" eye muscle imbalance and achieve binocular vision; their effort to control the defect is thought to create reading difficulties. In this special group of children, some of whom have been labelled mentally retarded, have failed one or more years of school, and whose reading has not been improved by various forms of training, surgery to correct the eye muscle imbalance has produced prompt improvement in reading skills and comfort. Eye muscle surgery is not recommended as a cureall for all children with reading problems, but is advised when a muscle imbalance, no matter how small, can be elicited, and when no other causative factor can be recognized.

Dyslogia. Impairment of speech.

Dysmenorrhea. Difficult, painful menstruation (431). For helpful exercises, see PAINFUL MENSTRUATION.

Dyspareunia. Painful or difficult sexual intercourse; the cause may be physical, psychic, or both.

Dyspepsia. Disturbed digestion; indigestion. There are several disorders (see MALABSORPTION SYNDROME) in which foods are inadequately digested or assimilated. But the terms "dyspepsia" and "indigestion" are often rather casually applied to symptoms which do not arise primarily from incomplete digestion of food but which originate, or seem to, in the alimentary canal or organs adjacent thereto. Inaccurate use of the word does no harm if it sends one to a physician to find out what the trouble is.

Dyspnea. Difficult breathing, distress, often but not invariably associated with heart or lung disease.

Dystocia. Painful or difficult labor, delivery, childbirth.

Dystrophy. Degeneration, wasting, abnormal development.

Dysuria. Difficult or painful urination.

E

Eaton pneumonia. A form of atypical pneumonia. See PNEUMONIA.

Ecchymosis. Bleeding into the skin and discoloration of skin so produced, as, a black-and-blue bruise which fades from purple to green to yellow as blood trapped in tissues is absorbed.

Echinococcus cyst. Multiple fluid-filled cysts, particularly in the liver or lungs, produced by tapeworm larvae; *hydatid disease* (69).

ECHO viruses. The initials mean "Enteric Cytopathic Human Orphan," the "orphan" indicating that the viruses are not associated with known diseases. The designation has become less appropriate since some of the viruses have been identified as the causative agents of certain diseases (59).

Eclampsia. Convulsions. A serious form occurs in late pregnancy or even during or after delivery; it is an extreme manifestation of *toxemia of pregnancy* (375), often associated with kidney disorders. Early signs of impending eclampsia are practically always evident to the attending physician, in ample time to institute effective preventive measures. Eclampsia is rare in women who receive proper pre-natal care.

Ectopic. In wrong position, out of place; for example, *ectopic pregnancy* (370) in which the embryo is implanted in a Fallopian tube or elsewhere outside of the uterus.

Ectropion. Out-turning of an eyelid, drooping away from the eyeball.

Eczema. Inflammation of the skin (185, 413).

Edema. Excessive accumulation of watery fluid in body cavities and spaces around cells. The fluid produces puffy, boggy swelling of waterlogged tissues. Edema is not a disease but a symptom of little or great significance. The waterlogging may be mild and localized, such as the puffiness around a bruise or a slight swelling of the ankles after standing all day, or it may inflate almost all of the body like a balloon. The underlying cause may be trivial, as in PREMENSTRUAL TENSION, or quite serious. "Pitting edema," the kind which leaves a little pit or depression when pressed, is often associated with heart or kidney disorders. Edema results from some disturbance of mechanisms of fluid exchange in the body, of which there are many causes: allergy, protein deficiency, salt and water retention by the kidneys (see ELECTROLYTES), congestive heart failure, obstruction of lymphatic drainage (see LYMPHEDEMA), inflammation, injury, liver and kidney disease, tumors. Modern diuretic drugs which increase the output of urine and get rid of excess fluid are helpful in management of edema while underlying disease is treated.

Edentulous. Toothless.

EEG. An electroencephalogram; a brain wave tracing or record. See ELECTROENCEPHALOGRAPH.

EENT. Eye, Ear, Nose and Throat.

Effleurage. A stroking movement used in massage.

Effusion. Outpouring of fluid into a body part or tissue.

Ejaculation. Ejection of semen.

EKG. An electrocardiogram. See ELECTROCARDIOGRAPH.

Elective treatment. Postponable treatment, not immediately urgent. *Elective surgery* can be put off until a more convenient or desirable time.

Electric knife. A surgical instrument employing electric current to cut and seal vessels bloodlessly (759).

Electrocardiograph. An instrument which amplifies tiny electric charges in contracting heart muscle and records these on paper in the form of squiggly lines; the written record is an *electrocardiogram* (EKG). Electric impulses are conveyed to the machine from surfaces above several areas of the heart. Skilled interpretation of electrical events within the heart muscle, recorded in an EKG, gives valuable information in the diagnosis of heart disease and in following the progress of a patient after his recovery from a coronary attack (84, 93, 109).

Electroencephalograph. An instrument which amplifies minute electric currents from brain cells and transcribes them by means of an inked arm to a moving strip of paper. This record, called an *electroencephalogram* (EEG), shows aspects of brain activity, popularly called "brain waves," in the form of undulant, spiked, wavy lines (277). Disk electrodes taped to the subject's scalp pick up tiny currents from brain cells near the surface of the skull. The brain has several characteristic rhythms; "brain writings" from different areas of the scalp may vary considerably. Modern electroencephalographs have a score or more channels, each recording changes in electric potential between two electrodes taped to different areas of the scalp. The instrument is useful in diagnosing various disturbances of brain function, such as epilepsy, and is a valuable research tool for investigating the manifold mysteries of the brain. Recent advances in studies of SLEEP and dreams have been greatly aided by the electroencephalograph's ability to identify rhythms characteristic of different and changing levels of consciousness.

Electrolytes. We rarely give the slightest thought to our electrolytes, or need to, but in certain disease states a doctor gives a great deal of attention to electrolyte balances. Electrolytes are dissolved salts or ions in body fluids, analogous to electrolytes in an automobile storage battery. Our electrolytes conduct electric currents; they participate in countless chemical processes of life; they are bearers of electrical energy within our cells; they are in constant motion and exert outward pressure; they are vital regulators of acid-base balance. The principal regulator of water and electrolyte balance is the kidney (284). The major electrolytes are sodium, chlorine, potassium and bicarbonate. Numerous conditions affect or reflect the critical composition of the sea within us: vomiting, diarrhea, kidney or liver disease, congestive heart failure, dehydration, severe burns, diabetes, drug treatments, surgery, edema, to name a few. There may be excessive loss or excessive retention of electrolytes. Sodium (salt) locks considerable amounts of water in the body. This is the rationale for *low-sodium diets* (32), designed to ease waterlogged tissues of their burden. But a gross deficiency of sodium may produce leg cramps and other distresses. Correction of electrolyte deficits or excesses is an important part of management of many ills. Delicate electrolyte imbalances are never a matter of self-diagnosis or self-treatment; they may be of a chronic or emergency nature; they are secondary to disorder which is or should be treated; they are considerations in preparation for surgery, and it is enough to know that physicians are well aware of them.

Electrolysis. Permanent removal of superfluous hair by means of an electric needle which renders the hair follicle incapable of further growth. The word also means decomposition of a salt or chemical compound by means of an electric current.

Electromyography. Tracings of electric currents produced by muscle action, in tests of neurologic disorders (250).

Electroshock. A physical treatment for some forms of mental illness; harmless electric current is passed from temple to temple through the patient's brain, producing unconsciousness (716). The patient has no memory of the shock, but competent supervision is necessary to prevent convulsive injuries or fractures.

Elephantiasis. Gross enlargement of a body part (legs, scrotum) due to fluids in tissue spaces under the skin, dammed back by obstruction of lymphatic drainage channels. See LYMPHEDEMA. The most extreme forms of elephantiasis are seen in persons in tropical countries who suffer from FILARIASIS.

Elimination diets. Menus which start with a few foods that rarely cause allergic reactions, and then add one new food at a time to determine which one a patient reacts to (683).

Embolism. Obstruction of a blood vessel by an EMBOLUS. Consequences vary according to the size of the blocked vessel and the part of the body deprived of blood. The lungs, brain, and heart are frequent sites of embolism. *Pulmonary embolism* which can cause sudden death results from blockage of the pulmonary artery (79) or its large branches. *Fat embolism* results from a crushing injury of bone or fatty tissue which disperses fat into the bloodstream, whence it is disseminated to many organs. Fat embolism is often fatal.

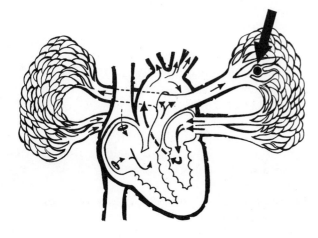

Pulmonary embolism. Embolus in lung (arrow) blocks flow of blood (small arrows).

Embolus. Any foreign substance—a blood clot, fat globule, air bubble, clumps of cells—which is swept along in the bloodstream until it lodges in a vessel and blocks the flow of blood beyond that point (124).

Embryo. The developing human being in the uterus through the third month of pregnancy, after which it is known as a fetus.

Emetic. Productive of vomiting.

Emmenagogue. An agent which stimulates menstrual flow.

Emphysema. Overinflation of air sacs of the lungs or tissues between them with air which cannot readily escape (234). Long-continued pressures stretch and rupture delicate walls of air sacs, reducing the surfaces on which gases are exchanged.

Empyema. Accumulation of pus in a body cavity, especially in the pleural cavity (232).

Encephalitis. Inflammation of the brain. Some forms of encephalitis are caused by viruses (60), others are complications of other diseases or conditions.

Encephalogram. An x-ray of the contents of the skull.

Endarterectomy. Surgical removal of a clot or plaque from the inner wall of an artery (125).

Endarteritis. Inflammation of the innermost layer of an artery.

Endemic. "In the people"; occurring constantly or repeatedly in the same locality.

Endocarditis. Inflammation of the lining of the heart, especially attacking the heart valves (39).

Endocrine. Inpouring, internally secreting; ductless glands which secrete hormones into the circulation (313).

Endodontics. A branch of dentistry concerned with disease and treatment of inner structures of the teeth; pulp, root canal filling, etc. (537).

Endogenous. Originating within or inside the cells or tissues.

Endometriosis. Presence in abnormal locations of fragments of the membrane which lines the cavity of the uterus (436). The displaced tissue "menstruates" where it shouldn't and tends to form "chocolate cysts."

Endoscopy. Visual examination of hollow parts of the body by insertion of a lighted instrument through a natural outlet. There are many types of "scopes" (sigmoidoscope, bronchoscope, cystoscope and others) named for the inspected organs. Some have systems of lenses and auxiliary devices for removing foreign objects or bits of tissue for examination.

Endotoxin. A toxin produced by internal processes of a germ, liberated when the cell of the germ is destroyed.

Enteric coating. A coating of drug tablets which permits them to pass through the acid stomach without dissolving and to liberate their dose in the alkaline intestine.

Enteritis. Inflammation of the intestine, particularly of the small intestine (492).

Enterobiasis. Pinworm infection (71).

Enteroviruses. Viruses, such as polio and ECHO viruses, whose preferred habitat is the intestinal tract.

Enucleation. Removal of the eyeball.

Enuresis. Bedwetting; involuntary discharge of urine (299, 400).

Eosinophils. Certain white blood cells which accept a rose-colored stain called eosin. Large numbers of eosinophils are present in nasal and other secretions during allergic attacks. It is not known for sure whether the eosinophils protect against allergic reactions or accentuate them.

Epidemic. Rapid spread of disease attacking large numbers of people in the same locality at the same time.

Epidemic pleurodynia. See DEVIL'S GRIP.

Epidermis. Popularly, the skin; technically, the outermost part of the skin consisting of four layers without blood vessels (178).

Epididymitis. Inflammation of that part of the semen-conducting duct which lies upon and behind the testicle (311).

Epigastrium. "Upon the stomach"; the upper middle abdomen. A hand stretched across the lower end of the breastbone covers the epigastrium.

Epiglottis. A structure like a hinged lid above the voice box; it opens to admit air and snaps shut like a trapdoor when swallowing to prevent food from going down the windpipe (210).

Epilation. Removal of hair by the roots. See ELECTROLYSIS.

Epilepsy. A nervous disorder of varying severity, marked by recurring explosive "discharge" of electrical activity of brain cells, producing convulsions, loss of consciousness, or brief clouding of consciousness (273).

Epinephrine. The hormone produced by the medulla of the adrenal gland (330). It stimulates heart action, constricts blood vessels, relaxes small bronchial tubes, inhibits smooth muscle, and has many medical uses in allergic and other disorders. Also known as adrenaline.

Epiphysis. The end part of a long bone which in children is separated from the shaft of the bone by a layer of cartilage. As growth progresses, the cartilage layer disappears, the epiphysis is said to have "closed," and the bone does not grow longer. When this process is complete, ultimate height has been attained.

Episiotomy. An incision in the margin of the vulva to enlarge the area through which the baby's head passes in childbirth; the purpose is to prevent or minimize injury to the mother (382).

Epispadias. A malformation of the penis in which the urinary canal remains open on the upper side of the organ (302). The problem is to restore urinary control and then to form a new tube by plastic surgery.

Epistaxis. Nosebleed (834).

Epithelial. Refers to those cells that form the outer layer of the skin, those that line all the portions of the body that have contact with external air (such as the eyes, ears, nose, throat, lungs), and those that are specialized for secretion, as the liver, kidneys, urinary and reproductive tract.

Epitheliomas. Skin tumors of varying malignancy.

Epithelium. Specialized tissue which covers all free surfaces of the body, forms the EPIDERMIS, lines hollow organs, glands, respiratory passages; it does not possess blood vessels.

Epizootic. Epidemic disease in animals.

Eponym. The name of a person applied to a disease, syndrome, or theory which it is presumed he was the first to discover or describe; for example, *Bright's disease, Addison's disease.* This form of honorific has become a little less common since more precise and specific descriptions of disease have been made possible by scientific advances. Physicians generally prefer a scientific name for a condition unless they happen to have been the first to discover it.

Equinovarus. A form of clubfoot (647).

Ergotism. Poisoning with *ergot,* a substance contained in a fungus that grows on rye and other grains. Ergot has powerful constrictive action on small blood vessels; chronic poisoning may produce closure of blood vessels, resulting in gangrene of the extremities. Various ergot drugs and combinations have medical uses, as in prevention of migraine headaches. It is interesting that ergot is closely related chemically to LSD.

Eructation. A belch.

Erysipelas. An acute bacterial infection of the skin and underlying tissue (38).

Erythema. Abnormal redness of the skin. The pattern, intensity, distribution, duration, and appearance of the reddened areas give clues to disease, which may be trifling, or a disease of childhood manifested by a rash, or an allergy or systemic disorder.

Erythroblastosis (*"Rh disease"*). A disease of newborn infants associated with incompatible Rh blood factors of mother and child (376).

Erythrocytes. Red blood cells; elastic, jelly-like disks containing HEMOGLOBIN (140).

Erythrocytosis. A condition of too many red blood cells crowding the circulation; *polycythemia* (153).

Erythropoiesis. The process of red blood cell formation.

Eschar. Sloughed-off tissue produced by a burn or corrosive substance.

Escutcheon. The pattern of pubic hair growth, different in male and female; from the Latin word for "shield."

Esophagoscopy. Direct examination of the esophagus with an *esophagoscope,* a hollow-tubed instrument with a light and lens (463).

Esophagus. The gullet; the muscular tube through which swallowed food is "milked" into the stomach by muscular action (451).

Esophagitis. Inflammation of the lining of the esophagus (467).

Estrogen. A general term for female hormones; technically, that substance which produces changes in the uterus (and psyche) corresponding to activities of the ovaries and endocrine glands (339).

Ethmoid. A sieve-like bone of the upper nose behind the frontal sinus; nerve fibers of the sense of smell pass through perforations in it (604).

Etiology. The study of causes of disease or disorder. "Etiology" is not a word which means "causes," but rather the *study* of causes.

Eunuch. A castrated male; a boy or man whose testicles have been removed. In origin the word means "guardian of the couch." Eunuchs cannot produce SPERMATOZOA or father children, but if only the testes are removed, and this operation is done after sexual maturity, some eunuchs retain a degree of sexual potency. *Eunuchoidism* is a natural condition in which the sex organs are malformed or physiologically inactive (314).

Euphoria. Feeling of well-being; often implies exaggerated elation.

Eustachian tube. A tubular passage about an inch and a half long which leads from the middle ear to the throat (595). Air passing through it equalizes pressures on both sides of the eardrum, enabling the drum to vibrate freely. Infectious material can enter the middle ear through the tube.

Exanthem. A skin eruption or the disease which causes it. *Exanthem subitum* (also called *roseola infantum*) is a disease of childhood; fever comes on suddenly, persists for three or four days, then drops, a skin rash appears, and the child is well (421). The skin eruption of scarlet fever or measles is an exanthem.

Exchange transfusion. Replacement of all of a baby's blood with suitable whole blood of a donor; resorted to in some instances to save the life of a baby with severe blood-destroying anemia resulting from a clash of the mother's and baby's Rh blood factors.

Excision. The act of cutting out.

Excoriation. A scratch mark of the skin, usually deep enough to bleed or become crust-covered, produced by scraping or scratching.

Exfoliation. Peeling or shedding of surface skin in scales or sheets.

Exocrine. Outpouring; glands which do not deliver their secretions to the bloodstream but through ducts and channels to organs and surfaces; for example, sweat glands, oil glands, digestive juices of the pancreas gland. Inherited disabilities of the exocrine glands are the fundamental defects in CYSTIC FIBROSIS.

Exogenous. Originating from outside the cells or tissues.

Exostosis. Projection of a bony growth from the surface of a bone; a bony spur.

Expectorant. A substance that softens or increases bronchial secretions and helps to "bring up" phlegm from the chest.

Exophthalmos. Bulging eyes, "pop eyes," a condition characteristic of thyroid disease (323).

Exstrophy of the bladder. A congenital malformation in which the bladder has no abdominal covering and urine comes out to the surface of the body (299).

Extensor. A muscle which straightens or extends a body part.

External cardiac massage. A first-aid measure to make a stopped heart start to beat, used in conjunction with mouth-to-mouth resuscitation (824); the latter supplies fresh oxygen. With the victim on his back, place the heel of one hand on the lower part of his breastbone (over the heart), and the other hand on top of the first one. Press down with your weight on the breastbone to force blood out of the heart into vessels. Relax the pressure; blood flows into the heart chambers. Repeat at intervals of about one second. Too much pressure can hurt the heart or break ribs; if the patient is a child, pressure of one hand may be sufficient. Ideally, one person gives mouth-to-mouth resuscitation while the other applies external heart massage. If one person must do it all, he can give external massage for half a minute, then mouth-to-mouth breathing for ten seconds or so, and repeat.

Extrasystole. A premature beat of the heart; a contraction that is triggered too soon and is followed by a compensating delay in the next beat (108). The pause between the premature beat and the succeeding one, which is likely to come with a thump, gives a feeling that the heart has skipped a beat. The phenomenon is quite common and almost never serious.

Extravasation. Escape of fluids from a vessel, especially a blood vessel, into surrounding tissues. A black eye looks the way it does because of extravasated blood.

Extrinsic asthma. A form of bronchial asthma in which the provoking substance enters the body from the outside world (686). *Intrinsic asthma* which has its source within the body can co-exist with extrinsic asthma.

Extrinsic factor. Literally, a constituent from outside; medically, the term commonly refers to Vitamin B_{12} which prevents pernicious anemia (150). The vitamin is assimilated from food in conjunction with a substance secreted by the stomach called INTRINSIC FACTOR.

Exudate. Anything that is exuded, oozed, trickled, pushed out. One exudes sweat as well as confidence. Although many exudates are entirely normal, in medical usage the word often refers to pus or other materials of pathologic interest.

Eye bank. See CORNEAL TRANSPLANT.

Eye tooth. A canine tooth (524).

Eye wash. A simple and effective eye wash can be made by adding a level teaspoonful of salt to a pint of boiled water (565).

Eyegrounds. The interior of the eye that can be seen with an OPHTHALMOSCOPE.

F

Face lift. An operation to remove wrinkling caused by loose skin and to tighten fatty tissues which tend to sag in the face and neck with advanc-

ing years. Results vary, depending on the condition of the patient. In time, tissue tends to sag again, but the operation can be repeated. In some cases, improvement may last from five to ten years; in the heavy-faced, improvement tends to be more short-lived. Scarring is not conspicuous, being concealed by hair or crease lines. Face-lift surgery usually takes four to five hours and the patient is hospitalized for three days to a week.

Face presentation. Appearance of the face of the fetus at the outlet of the uterus during delivery, instead of the top of the head, as is normal.

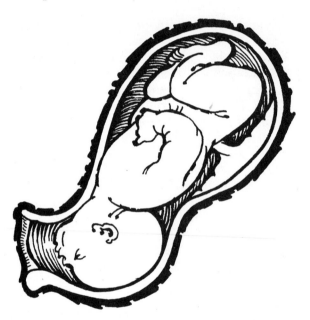

Face presentation.

F.A.C.P. Fellow of the American College of Physicians; a qualified medical specialist.

F.A.C.S. Fellow of the American College of Surgeons; a qualified surgical specialist.

Fahrenheit (F.). The thermometer scale generally used in the United States outside of scientific circles. It marks the freezing point of water at 32 degrees F. and the boiling point at 212 degrees F. See CENTIGRADE.

Fainting (*syncope*). Brief loss of consciousness due to diminished blood supply to the brain. Usually self-corrected; the fainting person droops to the floor and blood flows more easily to the brain. Blood vessels in the abdominal area have immense capacity to hold blood, almost the body's entire blood volume, when fully dilated. Shock or strong emotion may cause these vessels to dilate and fill with so much blood that blood pressure drops and fainting results. Rarely is fainting due to heart trouble. A soldier standing at attention for some time may faint, not from want of military ardor, but because of lack of muscular movement to aid the return flow of blood through veins. Oncoming faint may be prevented by lying down.

Fallen womb. Prolapse of the uterus; sagging of the organ into the lower vagina or occasionally protruding, due to weakness, stretching, or tearing of supporting structures (437).

Fallout. RADIOISOTOPES from nuclear explosions which settle out of the atmosphere.

Fallopian tubes. See OVIDUCTS.

False pregnancy (*pseudocyesis*). Signs and symptoms of pregnancy occurring without conception. The woman herself is usually deceived, and even an able obstetrician may be deceived for a while. The patient is usually a woman with an overpowering, obsessive desire to have a child who through autosuggestion is somehow able to mimic the signs of pregnancy—cessation of menstruation, breast changes, "morning sickness," enlargement of the abdomen at the rate of normal pregnancy—to perfection. Careful examination and tests can determine that no pregnancy exists, but in some instances it is difficult to convince the woman until the expected date of delivery passes unfruitfully.

Fanconi's syndrome. Multiple inherited abnormalities which impair kidney function and progressively depress blood cell formation in the bone marrow (174).

Farmer's lung. An inflammatory disease of the lungs which principally affects agricultural workers exposed to moldy hay, grain, fodder or silage. The disease resembles pneumonia but does not respond to antibiotics as bacterial pneumonias do. Symptoms of chills, fever, cough, headache, and chest tightness are thought to be caused by allergy-like sensitivity to inhaled mold dusts, and may appear a few hours after heavy exposure. Total avoidance of moldy vegetable matter is most important during the illness and after recovery.

Farsightedness (*hyperopia*). A condition in which light from near objects is focused behind rather than upon the retina, usually because the eyeball is too short (562). Close objects are blurred but distant ones are distinct. Farsighted persons may read and do close work with fair success through ACCOMMODATION, but this effort of ciliary muscles (554) can give rise to complaints of "eye strain," "tired eyes," and distaste for tasks of close seeing. With increasing age, the lens of the eye loses flexibility and farsighted people tend to hold their newspapers at arm's length to read them. Glasses for reading, or a reading segment in bifocal glasses, can do much to give comfort and may even minimize the appearance of wrinkles.

Fascia. Tough sheets of connective tissue which give support under the skin, between and around muscles, blood vessels, nerves and internal organs.

Fat embolism. Plugging of a blood vessel by fatty particles carried in the bloodstream; this can occur from crushing injuries of fatty tissue or bone, or injection of oily solutions.

Fatty acid. A compound of carbon, hydrogen, and oxygen which combines with glycerol to make a fat.

Favism. Acute anemia with red blood cell destruction caused by eating fava beans. The condition occurs only in genetically susceptible persons who do not possess an enzyme that is important in red blood cell metabolism. Certain drugs, such as aspirin and sulfas, may produce the same symptoms in susceptible persons. Oddly, absence, of the enzyme seems to give some protection against malaria.

Febrile. Feverish.

Feces. Contents of a bowel movement; the stool. Feces are not simply unabsorbed food residues. The greatest part of the solid matter is made up of materials excreted from blood and cells shed by lining membranes of the intestines; about 10 per cent is bacteria (see INTESTINAL FLORA). Practically all of the protein, fat, and carbohydrate that is eaten is absorbed. Unabsorbed food residues consist largely of indigestible vegetable cellulose, the amount of which varies with the diet. This indigestible "roughage" stimulates activity and secretions of the bowel. Large amounts of undigested food elements in feces are associated with diseases which impair assimilation.

Felon. See PARONYCHIA.

Felty's syndrome. Chronic infectious arthritis with enlargement of the spleen and decreased numbers of certain white blood cells (163).

Femur. The thighbone (617).

Fenestration. An opening (literally, "a window") in a part of the body, or the act of making one. The *fenestration operation* for improving the hearing of persons with OTOSCLEROSIS creates a bony window for passage of sound waves to the inner ear (755).

Fertile period. The period of about one week around the midpoint of the menstrual cycle when conception can occur. The period cannot be pinpointed precisely, but occurs approximately through days 11 to 18 counting from the onset of menstruation (339).

Festination. The taking of hurried short steps to prevent falling, characteristic of *Parkinson's disease* (252).

Fetus. The unborn child after the third month of pregnancy; before that it is called an embryo.

Fever. Abnormally high body temperature. Normally, body temperature varies slightly through the day, is higher in the evening than in the morning, higher internally than at the skin surface, and is increased by such commonplace things as eating and exercising. The most common fevers accompany infections, but disturbances of heat-regulating centers of the brain, as in heat stroke, and other non-infectious conditions can produce fever. Experienced people can often recognize significant fever by the "feel" and look of the patient's hot, dry, flushed skin. Accurate fever-reading, however, requires use of a clinical thermometer (18). Different forms of fever (51) are helpful in diagnosis and following the course of disease. That is why "fever charts" are kept of hospitalized patients, and may be desired by the doctor for patients under home nursing care. Mothers should have a little knowledge about fevers in children (393).

Fever increases the body's rate of metabolism about seven per cent for each degree Fahrenheit of temperature elevation. The heart's ability to contract decreases and it beats more rapidly in an attempt to move more blood to the skin to increase heat loss. Excessively high (*hyperthermic*) fever of 105 degrees F. and more cannot be endured for a long period; the very high fever of SUNSTROKE is so quickly lethal that immediate efforts to bring it down must be made by immersing the patient in an ice bath or applying a stream of cold water to the body. Young children react to the slightest infection with fever, sometimes as high as 104 degrees; the height of the fever does not necessarily parallel the seriousness of the infection. If a doctor cannot be reached promptly, a small child's very high fever can be reduced by an alcohol sponge or cool enema (393).

Whether or not fever is part of nature's treatment to cure infection is an unsettled question. In tissue cultures, temperatures of feverish degree inhibit the multiplication of some viruses. There is some evidence that fever increases the production of IN-TERFERON. But fever-producing organisms in patients survive the temperatures they produce and many authorities doubt that fever has any direct effect on the patient's resistance to infection. All agree, however, that fever is an important guide to the progress of an illness; sometimes it is the only important diagnostic clue.

Fibrillation. Tremor of a muscle, especially the heart muscle. Individual muscle fibers act independently, uncoordinated, out of rhythm, causing rapid, irregular, ineffective heartbeats. The condition may affect the *atria* (106) or *ventricles* (112) of the heart. Defibrillating devices that administer an electric shock are used to restore normal rhythm.

Fibrinogen. A protein manufactured in the liver and distributed into the bloodstream where it acts as a clotting agent when a blood vessel is cut or injured. Fibrinogen combines with another substance, *thrombin*, to yield long, threadlike crystals of *fibrin* which form a mesh to entrap blood corpuscles in a clot.

Fibroids. The word commonly refers to muscle and connective tissue tumors of the uterus (435).

Fibrositis. Inflammation of connective tissue (654); often, combined inflammation of muscle and connective tissue (*fibromyositis*), producing pain, tenderness, and stiffness.

Fibula. The slender bone on the outer aspect of the lower leg (617).

Filariasis. A chronic disease caused by the presence of threadlike worms (*filaria*) in the body (71). The organisms get into the blood through the bites of mosquitoes. The adult worms live in the lymphatic system and cause overgrowth of fibrous tissue which obstructs drainage. Obstructed fluids accumulate in tissue spaces and cause the affected part to swell (LYMPH-EDEMA). The result is some degree of ELEPHANTIASIS. The most extreme forms of the disease occur in long-time residents of tropical countries who are frequently re-infected from mosquito bites.

Fimbria. A fringelike structure; especially, fimbriae of the opening of the OVIDUCTS, close to the ovary (338, 368). The fringelike projections are covered with *cilia*, minute hair-like processes which wave back and forth and set up rhythmic currents in surrounding peritoneal fluid. Their function is to "catch" a mature egg cell released by the ovary and sweep it into the tube which is where fertilization usually occurs. An engineer would consider this method of bridging a small gap to be poorly designed but it has worked pretty well for a good many years.

Fish skin disease. See ICHTHYOSIS.

Fissure. A break or crack in the skin or a membrane, most frequent in the rectal area (403, 490).

Fistula. An abnormal channel between body parts, or leading from a hollow organ to a free surface, which usually discharges fluids or material from an organ. A fistula may be caused by disease, injury, or an abscess which bores an abnormal drainage channel for itself. Many fistulas are named for the body parts they connect; for example, *vesicovaginal* fistula (bladder and vagina). Some fistulas never heal by themselves because of continual infection and surgical correction is necessary to close the abnormal channel.

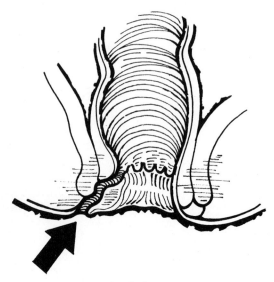

Anal fistula.

Flank. The fleshy outer part of the body between the ribs and hip.

Flash blindness. Visual disturbance resulting from an intense light source, such as an atomic blast.

Flat foot. Ordinarily, if a print of a bare foot on a piece of paper shows that the sole has made flat contact all around, without an open space under the middle inside part of the foot, it is construed as a sign of flat feet caused by "fallen arches." This is not always true. Babies' feet are always flat. Some people have naturally flat feet which are perfectly efficient and comfortable. When feet become *flattened*, and hurt, troubles arise and treatment is necessary (646).

Flatulence. Excessive gas in the stomach or intestines. A normal bowel always contains some gas; balance is maintained by unostentatious gas exchange mechanisms. Excessive "gassiness," vented by belching or passing wind, may result from indiscretions of diet or some disorder of the diges-

tive tract which should be looked into by a physician. Frequently, excessive belching (*eructation* is a more seemly word) is often a consequence of unconscious AIR SWALLOWING.

Fletcherism. A food fad of the late nineteenth century, promoted by Horace Fletcher of Lawrence, Mass., who advocated that each mouthful of food be chewed 50 to 60 times, reducing it to a liquid state before swallowing. Fletcher ultimately went on a one-meal-a-day diet with an alternate day of fasting, spit out all food that did not liquefy after thorough chewing, developed permanent constipation, and his death from chronic bronchitis was speeded by malnutrition.

Flexor. A muscle which bends a limb or part, as in flaunting the biceps.

"Floaters." Cells or strands of tissue which float in the VITREOUS HUMOR and move with movements of the eyeball, casting shadows on the retina (581). The floaters, particularly when seen against a bright background such as open sky, look like moving spots, "clouds," threads and swirls of diverse shapes. Floaters are most prevalent in nearsighted and older persons. Usually they are more annoying than serious, but if very worrisome or exaggerated, an eye examination is indicated.

Floating kidney. A loose, somewhat wandering kidney, abnormally movable from its normal location because of slack attachments and inadequate support from surrounding fat.

Flora (intestinal). Bacteria and other small organisms found in the intestinal contents.

Flukes. Parasitic flatworms, rarely encountered in the U. S., which cause infections of the intestines, liver, and lungs (67).

Fluorides. Salts of fluorine, a gaseous element. The role of fluorides in helping to lessen tooth decay is well known (530). Recent studies have furnished evidence that fluorides contribute importantly to sturdy bones as well as teeth and may play a part in treatment and prevention of *osteoporosis* (650), a condition of abnormal porousness, thinning, and easy fracturing of bone, common in women after the menopause and in old persons. One study of more than a thousand persons over 45 years of age has shown osteoporosis to be much less frequent in those who lived most of their lives in areas of relatively high fluoride content of drinking water than in those who lived in low-fluoride areas. There was also much less hardening of the AORTA in those who lived in high-fluoride areas. It appears that fluoride helps to keep calcium deposited in hard tissues of the body and not in soft tissues. If such action is confirmed, fluorides may assume an important preventive role in osteoporosis and hardening of the arteries, two of the main diseases of aging.

Fluoroscope. A device for viewing x-ray images on a fluorescent screen. The patient stands behind the screen and x-rays passing through the body make structures visible to the radiologist. The digestive tract, heart, lungs and other organs can be viewed in action, and the progress of a BARIUM MEAL can be followed through the alimentary tract.

Flutter. Rapid, fluttery, but rhythmic beats of the heart auricles, resembling fibrillation (109).

Folacin. The name officially selected to replace the term *folic acid*, a vitamin of the B complex. Also known as *pteroylglutamic acid*. It is a bright yellow compound needed in very small amounts in the diet of animals and man. A deficiency results in poor growth, anemia, and other blood-related disorders.

Foley catheter. A tube inserted through the urethra into the bladder for drain-

age of urine; it has a small balloon at the bladder end which is inflated after insertion and which serves to hold the catheter in place (286).

Folic acid. A vitamin important for blood formation.

Folie a deux. Mental disorder communicated from a person who has it to a closely associated person so suggestible that he is persuaded that he has it too.

Follicle. A small sac or cavity which produces secretions or excretions. Hair grows from a follicle linked with sebaceous glands which produce skin oil (180).

Fontanel. The "soft spot" on the top of a baby's head. The area, which is covered by a very tough membrane that is by no means so fragile as some mothers fear, will be filled with bone as the skull grows. It takes anywhere from one to two years for the spot to close.

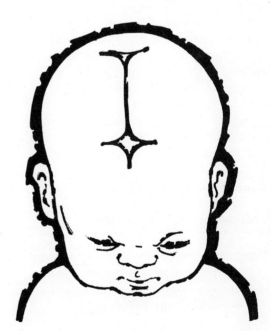

Fontanels ("soft spots") of an infant's head.

Food diary. A complete record of everything that is eaten for a period of time, a guide to detection of food allergies (684).

Food poisoning. Intestinal infection caused by bacteria or their toxins in foods. Many attacks of food poisoning are not recognized for what they are. Even severe attacks with nausea, vomiting, violent diarrhea, perhaps abdominal cramps, fever, and dizziness, may be blamed on "intestinal flu" or a "24-hour virus" unless several people who attended the same banquet or picnic are simultaneously stricken. The most common causes of food poisoning are strains of *salmonella* bacteria (43) which are widespread in the animal kingdom, and *staphylococci,* readily spread by human carriers. An originally slight population of salmonella in pies, eclairs, egg dishes, cakes, custards and salads can multiply enormously if such foods are left to incubate for a short time at room temperatures. Violence of food poisoning symptoms varies with the "dose" of bacteria and with individual susceptibility. Attacks two or three hours after eating suggest that the poisoning was caused by bacterial toxins rather than by live bacteria. Thorough cooking destroys bacteria and some toxins (see BOTULISM) but heat must be sufficiently high, penetrating, and long continued. A large turkey may not be thoroughly cooked because the stuffing acts as a sort of internal insulation. Proper refrigeration and sanitation guard against food poisoning (857).

Foot drop. Drooping of the foot, due to paralysis or injury of muscles or tendons that extend or lift it.

Foot supports. Simple arrangements of bedding or accessories to keep the weight of blankets off a bedridden patient's upturned feet (16).

Foramen. A perforation or opening in a body part. There are many such perforations, especially in bones, to permit passage of blood vessels and nerves. Some are abnormal, such as openings in congenitally malformed hearts of "blue babies" (97).

Forceps. An instrument with two opposing blades and handles, on the general principle of pliers, for grasping, compressing, or holding body parts or surgical materials. *Forceps delivery* is extraction of the fetus from the birth canal with the mechanical aid of OBSTETRIC FORCEPS of special design (383).

Foreskin. The fold of skin covering the head of the penis; the part removed in circumcision.

Formication. Sensation that ants are crawling over the skin.

Fornication. Sexual intercourse of unmarried persons.

Fortify. To add one or more nutrients to a food so that it contains more of the nutrients than was present originally before processing. Milk is often fortified with Vitamin D, margarine with Vitamin A, beverages with Vitamin C, various cereal products with thiamine and riboflavin. Foods with vitamins added to replace lost values are said to be "restored."

Fossa. A pit or trench-like depression in a body part.

Fovea. A pit, cup or depression in a body structure; especially, the *fovea centralis,* a pinhead-sized depression near the center of the retina which is the area of sharpest, most finely detailed seeing (556).

Fraternal twins. Twins of either sex originating from two separate eggs; they are no more closely related genetically than brothers and sisters (378).

Free grafting. Transplantation of a completely detached piece of skin from one part of a patient's body to another (770).

Frenum. A fold of tissue which partially limits the movement of an organ, like a checkrein. A small frenum can be seen as a band of tissue connecting the underside of the tongue with the floor of the mouth.

Frigidity. Sexual coldness in women. There may be some physical cause, but more often the aversion has a psychologic origin which may be difficult to recognize and overcome. Frigidity which occurs after the menopause, in women who have previously had normal sex drive, may respond to judicious hormone treatments (348).

Froelich's syndrome. Excessive fat deposits in the pelvic area and lack of genital development in young males, often with retardation of growth, somnolence, and other symptoms. The condition results from impairment, as by a tumor of the pituitary gland, of functions of the *pituitary* and *hypothalamus* (315). Careful diagnosis is necessary because most obese, genitally underdeveloped adolescent boys do not have this specific disorder.

Frog test. A pregnancy test, employing frogs, which gives a verdict in three to five hours (358).

Frozen section. A piece of tissue removed from the body which is quickly frozen by carbon dioxide spray, sliced, and examined immediately under a microscope. This is most often done when cancer is suspected and the patient is on the operating table, while surgeons await the verdict which will determine the extent of the operation.

Frozen shoulder. Pain, stiffness, and limitation of movement in the shoulder and upper arm (632).

Frozen sperm. SPERMATOZOA frozen at very low temperatures with a small amount of glycerol added "come alive" when thawed and are capable of fertilization. See ARTIFICIAL INSEMINATION and SPERM BANKS.

FSH. Follicle stimulating hormone (317).

Fulguration. Destruction of tissue by electric sparks.

Fulminating. Sudden in onset, explosive, severe, rapid in course.

Functional disease. Disease without any discoverable organic disorder.

Fundus. The part of a hollow organ farthest from its opening; for example, the back part of the eye; the top part of the uterus farthest from its cervical outlet.

Fungi. Low forms of plant life, including molds and yeasts, some of which are capable of causing annoying or serious infection. See the *mycoses* (74) ; *ringworm* (199), *otitis externa* (594) ; *thrush* (417) ; *yeast infections* (434).

Funnel chest (*pectus excavatum*). A congenital deformity in which the breastbone is depressed toward the spine, forming a more or less funnel-shaped cavity. The deformity rarely affects the heart and lungs adversely unless unrelated diseases are present.

Funny bone. It isn't the bone that's funny, but a nerve which tingles crazily when the elbow is banged just

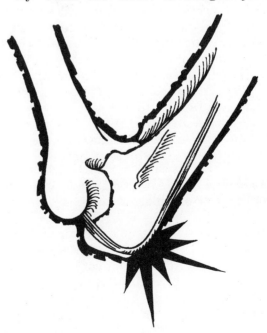

Blow on nerve at elbow causes "funny" tingling.

right. The ulnar nerve which runs down the arm from the shoulder to the hands passes over bones and is quite close to the surface at the inner side of the elbow; a bump there causes the fingers to tingle and feel "funny."

Furuncle. A boil (38).

Fusiform. Spindle-shaped.

Fusion. Union, cohesion, merging together; for example, *spinal fusion*, the uniting of two vertebrae by disease or by surgical procedures to improve some painful condition of the back. Also, the fusion of images from the two eyes for efficient binocular vision.

G

Galactosemia. An hereditary condition of infants who cannot handle milk sugars (*lactose, galactose*) because their bodies lack a necessary enzyme (512). Milk feedings lead to toxic accumulations of galactose in the blood, injuring the lens of the eye, the brain, and kidneys, with formation of cataracts and mental retardation unless all milk and milk products are immediately and stringently removed from the infant's diet. The outlook with strict dietary control is good and children who survive early infancy are often normal. Galactosemia is inherited as a recessive trait (see Chapter 25). If a galactosemic infant is born into a family, the physician will test later offspring of the same parents and institute a galactose-free diet immediately after birth if necessary.

Galactagogue. An agent that promotes the flow of milk.

Gallbladder. The saclike organ underlying the liver in which bile is stored, concentrated, and delivered to the digestive tract as needed (462).

Gallstones. Stones in the gallbladder; they may or may not cause noticeable symptoms (480).

Gallop rhythm. Sounds of the heart resembling the gallop of a horse, indicative of failing heart muscle.

Gamete. A germ cell; an egg or sperm.

Gamma globulin. An IMMUNOGLOBULIN; a protein in the blood which gives immunity to certain diseases through ANTIBODY production. Gamma globulin injections containing specific antibodies are sometimes given in hope of preventing an infection in a person who has been exposed to it, or making it milder. Antibodies which protect against bacterial and viral infections are mostly in gamma globulin circulating in the blood; other closely related immunoglobulins occur in internal and external secretions outside of the blood, as in saliva, tears, nasal, bronchial, and intestinal fluids.

Ganglion (of the wrist). A cyst of a tendon sheath on the back of the wrist, traditionally treated by striking a bursting blow with the family Bible (634). A *ganglion* is also a cluster of nerve cells which serves as a center of nervous influence.

Ganglionic blocking agents. Potent drugs, prescribed for some patients with high blood pressure, which reduce the actions of ganglia (clusters of nerve cells) that transmit impulses which constrict blood vessels and increase pressures. Ganglionic blockers produce the greatest fall in blood pressure when the patient is standing, relatively little change when the patient is lying down. Sometimes a patient who has been lying down may feel faint when he suddenly rises to a sitting position.

Gangrene. Death of tissue due to failure of blood supply to the area. There are many precipitating causes: vascular disease, frostbite, burns, crushing injury, pressure, obstruction of blood vessels, too tight a tourniquet. *Wet gangrene* has an offensive watery discharge and becomes infected so that complications of infection are superimposed upon the gangrene. Amputation of the part may be necessary to save the patient's life. *Dry gangrene* does not become infected but the part becomes shriveled and mummified. Small areas of dry gangrene may sometimes be saved by appropriate treatment, but amputation may be necessary. Diabetics are especially prone to gangrene of the feet and legs and preventive measures are very important (356).

Gargoylism. An hereditary condition characterized by opacities of the cornea, protruding abdomen, large head, short arms and legs, mental deficiency.

Gas endarterectomy. A recent technique for removing a clot from an artery by using a jet of carbon dioxide gas to separate the outer coat of the artery from the inner core containing the clot. Gas pressure is applied by means of a needle inserted into the wall of the artery; the separated inner core is then pulled out and amputated.

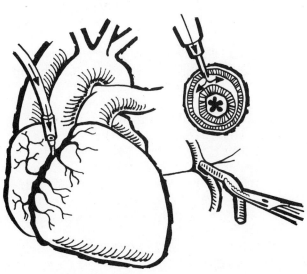

Gas endarterectomy: Gas jet separates clot from inner wall of artery (small drawing, upper right). Loosened clot is withdrawn.

Gas gangrene. An infection of injured tissues with bacilli which produce bubbles of foul-smelling gas given off by the wound (42).

Gastrectomy. Surgical removal of all or part of the stomach.

Gastric analysis. Analysis of stomach juices for acidity, presence of cells, organisms, and other elements. The juice, obtained after the patient has fasted 12 hours, is withdrawn by a syringe connected to a tube passed through the nose into the stomach.

Gastric freezing. A treatment for peptic ulcer; the patient swallows a balloon which is cooled by passing freezing agents through it (473). The treatment gives transient pain relief, stops gastric bleeding, but long-term benefits are questionable and freezing has not superseded conventional medical treatment of ulcer.

Gastric resection. Removal of the lower part of the stomach (727).

Gastritis. Inflammation of the stomach (471).

Gastrocnemius. The long muscle of the inner side of the lower leg which bends the leg and extends the foot.

Gastroenteritis. Inflammation of the stomach and intestine, producing such symptoms as diarrhea, abdominal cramps, nausea, vomiting, fever. There are many causes: infections, food poisoning, parasites, allergies, bacteria, viruses, toxins, to mention a few.

Gastroenterostomy. Joining the stomach to a loop of intestine to bypass the duodenum (727).

Gastrointestinal. Pertaining to the stomach and intestines.

Gastroscope. An instrument which permits the examining physician to see into the inside of the stomach (463).

Gastrostomy. A surgically created outlet of the stomach onto the skin surface of the abdomen (724).

Gaucher's disease. A disorder of LIPID metabolism, transmitted as a recessive trait (see Chapter 25). It is characterized by enlarged spleen and liver, bone and joint pains, brown pigmentation of the skin, due to accumulation of abnormal fat-like substances.

Gavage. Feeding of liquid nutrients into the stomach via a tube.

Genes. The ultimate units in transmission of hereditary characteristics, contained in the CHROMOSOMES.

Genitalia. The reproductive organs.

Genitourinary. Pertaining to genital and urinary organs—kidneys, u r e t e r s, bladder, urethra, prostate, testes— which are interrelated (281).

Geophagia. Dirt-eating. See PICA.

Geographic tongue. Fancied resemblance of the surface of the tongue to a relief map gives this disorder its name. Thickened patches like miniature islands, seas, and continents occur on the tongue and shift positions from day to day. This odd appearance is the only symptom. The cause is not known. The disorder usually occurs in children and adolescents; debilitated persons appear to be more susceptible.

Geotrichosis. An infection caused by species of fungi, affecting mucous membranes of the mouth, lungs, or intestinal tract. Chronic cough is a common symptom. The condition responds well to proper treatment.

Geriatrics. The medical specialty concerned with care of old people.

German measles (*rubella*). A mild viral infection producing a pink rash which spreads all over the body, sometimes with symptoms of headache and slight fever, sometimes with symptoms so slight that the infection passes unnoticed (418). A preventive vaccine and a blood test to determine susceptibility to the disease are available.

Gestation. Pregnancy.

G.I. Gastrointestinal.

Giant hives. Larger, deeper swellings than ordinary superficial hives, life-threatening if air passages are affected (693).

Giantism. Abnormal tallness, most often a result of excessive secretion of GROWTH HORMONE by the pituitary gland before the growing ends of the bones have closed, but other factors may produce excessive height (318). Boys up to six feet six inches tall and girls up to six feet are not considered to be giants; they fall at one extreme of a normal bell-shaped distribution curve of height in the population, with unusually short people who are not dwarfs at the other extreme.

Gibraltar fever. See BRUCELLOSIS.

G. I. series. X-ray films and fluoroscopic observations of the gastrointestinal tract; details are defined by a BARIUM MEAL, opaque to x-rays, swallowed prior to examination (786).

Gingiva. The gum. *Gingivitis,* inflammation of the gums, is the most common form of *periodontal disease* (532).

Gland. A cell or organ which makes and releases hormones or other substances used in the body. *Endocrine* glands secrete their products into the bloodstream; *exocrine* glands, to body surfaces or elsewhere, via ducts or channels (for example, sweat glands).

Glandular fever. INFECTIOUS MONONUCLEOSIS.

Glaucoma. The most common cause of blindness in adults, produced by intensive destructive pressure of fluids inside the eye (571). An acute form may come on suddenly and cause intense pain; a chronic form may cause no symptoms that the patient is aware of although his vision is being insidiously stolen away. Measurement of internal pressures of the eye with a *tonometer* (577) is an important part of an eye examination.

Gleet. Chronic gonorrheal discharge.

Glia. Supporting cells and fibers of nervous tissue, sometimes called "nerve glue." *Glioma* is a tumor of glial tissue, occurring principally in the brain and spinal cord.

Globe. The eyeball.

Globus. A "lump in the throat" which does not disappear on swallowing; also called *globus hystericus* when no disease or organic cause can be discovered (469). The condition, most common in women, is associated with anxiety and tightness or spasm of throat muscles. The feeling may also be caused by a foreign object in the throat, or swelling of lymphoid tissues such as tonsils or adenoids. The complaint if persistent calls for medical examination to rule out possible physical causes.

Glomeruli. "Little balls"; tufted networks of capillaries which bring blood to chambers of the kidney for filtration of wastes (283).

Glomerulonephritis. Acute or chronic inflammation of fine blood vessels of the glomeruli, usually preceded by a streptococcic infection (292).

Glossitis. Inflammation of the tongue.

Glottis. The aperture between the vocal cords, including parts of the voice-box concerned with sound production.

Glucagon. A hormone produced by cells of the pancreas gland, comparable to insulin but opposite in action. Glucagon's function is to correct LOW BLOOD SUGAR levels by stimulating the liver to convert more of its reserves of GLYCOGEN into sugar.

Glue-sniffing. The dangerous, perverted practice of inhaling volatile intoxicating fumes of airplane glues and similar cements, indulged in by some teenagers for "kicks." See Chapter 27.

Glucocorticoids. Cortisone-like hormones of the adrenal gland which influence carbohydrate, protein, and fat metabolism (330).

Glucose tolerance test. A test for early diabetes and other metabolic disorders. It measures the patient's ability to reduce blood sugar levels at a normal rate. After fasting, a blood sugar level is taken as a baseline and the subject is given a measured amount of dissolved sugar to drink. Blood sugar levels are then taken at hourly intervals. Abnormal rise or persistence of blood sugar is indicative of diabetes. The test is used in borderline cases.

Gluteal. Pertaining to the *gluteus* muscles of the buttocks.

Gluten-free diet. A regimen which excludes wheat, rye, oats, and their products from the diet of patients with *celiac disease*. See MALABSORPTION SYNDROME.

Glycerol. Same as glycerin. Serves as the framework of a molecule for attachment of fatty acids to make a fat.

Glycogen. "Animal starch," quite similar to vegetable starch; the form in which carbohydrate is stored in the liver and released as energy needs demand. The liver manufactures glycogen from DEXTROSE (glucose), a sugar, and re-converts glycogen to blood sugar as needed.

Glycogen storage disease. An hereditary disorder of infants; survival beyond the second year of life is rare. The infant lacks certain enzymes necessary for converting glucose to GLYCOGEN and vice versa. This leads to abnormal deposits of glycogen in various tissues of the body, with progressive slowing down of body processes.

Glycosuria. Sugar in the urine.

Goiter. Enlargement of the thyroid gland. There are several types of goiter (322).

Goitrogens. Substances such as are contained in plants of the cabbage family and some other vegetables, which in excessive amounts induce goiter (326).

Gold salts. Rather toxic compounds of gold, used in progressive, crippling *rheumatoid arthritis* (662) with hope of suppressing the active inflammatory disease and decreasing bone and cartilage destruction.

Golf ball hazard. Liquid-center golf balls are made by freezing liquid material into a solid and wrapping windings around it. When the center thaws, it exerts tremendous pressure against its covering. This is good for long drives down the fairway, but not without hazard to curious children who may cut into a nicked old ball to see what is in it. A golf ball can explode in the face when its liquid center is cut.

Gonads. The primary sex glands, ovaries or testes.

Gonioscope. An instrument for studying angles of the eye where fluids drain (561).

Gonorrhea. The most common venereal disease, an infection produced by sphere-shape bacteria (40). Recovery from gonorrhea does not give significant future immunity; re-infection is frequent. Incidence of the disease has increased in recent years.

Gonorrheal arthritis. A specific form of arthritis associated with gonorrhea, responsive to penicillin (667).

Gonorrheal ophthalmia. Blinding eye disease of newborn infants, acquired in passage through the birth canal of a mother who has gonorrhea. Obstetricians are required by law to put drops into the baby's eyes at birth to prevent the infection.

Gooseflesh. Little skin bumps induced by chill or shock, almost but not quite hair-raising. The bumps arise around hair follicles in response to vestigial muscles which attempt to raise the hair but can't quite make it.

Gout. An hereditary disorder of body chemistry resulting in too much uric acid in the blood, with chalk-like deposits of urate crystals (derived from uric acid) in cartilage of the joints and sometimes elsewhere (657).

GP. General practitioner.

Graafian follicles. Tiny, round, transparent "blisters" imbedded in the ovary (339). Each follicle contains an immature egg cell. Under the influence of the follicle-stimulating hormone of the pituitary gland, one of the blisters is stimulated to grow, and its egg matures in preparation for fertilization. The follicle bursts at about the fourteenth day of the menstrual cycle and releases the "ripened" egg; this is called *ovulation*.

Gram-positive, -negative. Classification of bacteria according to whether they do or do not accept a stain named for Hans Gram, a Danish bacteriologist. Different life processes and vulnerabilities of germs are reflected by their Gram-positive or Gram-negative characteristics. For instance, an antimicrobial drug effective against certain Gram-positive germs may be ineffective against Gram-negative ones, or vice versa.

Grand mal. Severe epileptic seizure; convulsions, loss of consciousness, jerking and stiffening of the body (273).

Granulation tissue. Tiny red, rounded, fleshy masses having a soft pebbly surface and granular appearance; the type of tissue that forms in early stages of wound healing. Each granule has new blood vessels and reparative cells. "Proud flesh" is an excessive overgrowth of granulation tissue.

Granulocytes. White blood cells containing granules that become conspicuous when dyed (142). They are manufactured in red marrow of the bones. One of their functions is to digest and destroy invading bacteria.

Granuloma. A tumor, new growth, or chronically inflamed area in which GRANULATION TISSUE is prominent.

Granuloma inguinale. A mildly contagious venereal disease produced by rod-shaped bacteria (41). It is named for the *inguinal* region (groin) where lesions appear.

Gravel. Fine, sandlike particles of the same substance as kidney stones, often eliminated in the urine without anything being noticed.

Graves' disease. Hyperthyroidism, toxic goiter (322).

Gravid. Pregnant. In obstetrician's language, a *gravida* is a pregnant woman; a *primagravida,* one who is pregnant for the first time; a *multigravida,* one who has had several pregnancies.

Greenstick fracture. An incomplete fracture of a long bone, usually in children whose bones are quite pliable (652). The break does not go all the way through the bone, which is splintered on one side only, in much the same way that a green stick splinters on the outside if you hold an end in each hand and bend it inward until it breaks.

Gristle. CARTILAGE.

Grippe. Influenza (55).

Groin. The lowest part of the abdomen where it joins the legs; the groove at this junction. Also called the *inguinal* area, a common site of hernia (738).

Ground substance. Semi-fluid material which fills spaces between connective tissue fibers and cements them together (660).

Growing pains. Pain in a child's legs or arms may be associated with subacute rheumatic fever and the complaint should be investigated by a doctor, but there are other quite harmless causes of what grandma called "growing pains." Non-rheumatic muscle pains at night are quite common in normal healthy children. These pains may possibly be due to normal growth, but more probably are an after-effect of vigorous if not violent playtime activities. The harmless pains usually occur in muscles of the legs and thighs at the end of the day or soon after the child goes to sleep; there is no pain on motion and the child does not limp; he is vague in pointing out where it hurts and is free of pain in the morning.

Growth hormone. A hormone of the anterior pituitary gland which stimulates growth (317).

G.U. Genitourinary.

Guaiac test. A dye test, usually of a stool specimen, for the presence of blood; the specimen takes on a blue color if occult blood is present.

Gullet. The esophagus; the muscular tube through which food passes from mouth to stomach and sometimes vice versa (467).

Gumboil. A swelling of the gum produced by an abscess at the root of a tooth, usually painful.

Gumma. A firm, rubbery mass of tissue resembling GRANULATION TISSUE, occurring almost anywhere in the body but most frequently in the skin, heart, liver or bones. It is a characteristic lesion of late syphilis (48).

Guthrie test. A blood test for *phenylketonuria* (512, 798).

Gynecoid. Resembling a woman; female-like; as, a gynecoid pelvis.

Gynecologist. A physician who specializes in diseases of women.

Gynecomastia. Abnormal enlargement of either or both male breasts. It may result from therapeutic use or unintentional absorption of female hormones, from glandular abnormalities, from drugs such as digitalis, amphetamine, or reserpine, or it may be associated with conditions which have little in common, such as thyroid disease, adrenal or testicular tumors, cirrhosis of the liver. Gynecomastia frequently occurs in perfectly healthy adolescent boys and usually disappears in a few weeks; this form is a transient phase of the body's coming into mature hormonal balance.

H

Hairy tongue. A rare condition which may occur after use of antibiotics, or from unknown causes; intertwining hairlike filaments form black or brownish patches on the tongue. The disease, if it may be called such, is harmless. The hairy patches may disappear quickly or persist for months.

Hallucinogenic drugs. Chemical agents which produce distortions of the mind. See Chapter 27.

Hallux. The big toe.

Hallux valgus. See BUNION.

Hammer toe. A toe which is bent upward like an inverted V and cannot flatten out, usually caused by cramping the toes into too small a shoe (649).

Hamstring. Tendons above the back of the knee. A person crippled by cutting of the hamstring tendons is said to be "hamstrung."

Hand-Schuller-Christian disease. An insidiously developing disease in the first decade of life, manifested by bulging eyes, excessive thirst, deposits of CHOLESTEROL in bones and tissues under the skin (173).

Hansen's disease. See LEPROSY.

Hashimoto's disease. A form of chronic thyroiditis occurring most frequently in middle-aged women (327). It is thought to be an AUTO-IMMUNE DISEASE, sensitization to one's tissues.

Haverhill fever. See RATBITE FEVER.

Hay fever. Pollinosis; an allergic reaction to inhaled pollens, characterized by reddened, weepy eyes, runny nose, sneezing, nasal stuffiness. (688).

Hearing aids. Choice of the right hearing aid requires hearing tests by an ear specialist, since there are many kinds of hearing impairment, improved by different types of instruments (593). The ear specialist will suggest which type of hearing aid is suitable. The decision depends upon the type of hearing loss, its severity, and other factors. The specialist may suggest a brand-name of hearing aid or make general recommendations.

In selecting a hearing aid:

Compare for clarity and quality of sound. Listen to familiar voices with different aids.

Compare how well you understand speech with each of the aids. Listen in noisy places as well as in quiet. Try the aids outdoors a well as indoors.

Compare for comfort and convenience. Controls should be easy to operate. Batteries, parts and minor repairs should be available locally.

Compare costs. A low-priced aid may be just as satisfactory as a high-priced aid, depending on your needs. Does the price include the ear mold, the cord and the receiver and the battery? Ask about the costs of batteries.

Compare extra services. Does the dealer give you a convenient repair and replacement service? Will the dealer help you to learn to use your aid?

Hearing and Speech Centers can make thorough non-medical study of hearing problems. The centers do not have a commercial interest in hearing aids, but they do have the staff and instruments to help you decide whether an aid will be of benefit. The non-medical tests describe how well you hear at different levels of loudness, under different noise conditions and for different speech sounds. Hearing and speech centers will compare how well you hear when using different models and makes of hearing aids. The centers can help you make better use of whatever hearing you have. This is done by lessons in auditory training and lip-reading. You can get a list of Hearing and Speech Centers near you from the Speech and Hearing Service in your State Department of Health or from your State Vocational Rehabilitation Service.

Heart attack. Common term for *coronary thrombosis* (93).

Heartburn. Mild to severe burning sensations in the upper abdomen or beneath the breastbone, usually resulting from backing-up of stomach contents into the esophagus. Heartburn typically occurs after a heavy meal containing fatty foods, often occurs when the patient is lying down, or sitting with feet slightly elevated, as in watching television, and is relieved by sitting up. Occasional heartburn associated with dietary orgies is not uncommon and does not necessarily require treatment. Weight reduction, antacids, diet regulation, and sleeping with the head of the bed elevated are helpful measures. Persistent or severe heartburn, or pain thought to be heartburn, may be associated with disease requiring medical diagnosis. Heartburn is the most common symptom of *hiatus hernia* (468). It is frequent in the middle and later months of pregnancy (362).

Heart-lung machine. A device which infuses oxygen into a patient's venous blood (a lung function) and pumps the freshened blood to the circulation (a heart function). Several types of such devices make open heart surgery feasible (107, 742).

Heart murmurs. Various sorts of soft, swishing sounds murmured by the heart to a physician's discriminating ears. The mere presence of murmurs does not necessarily indicate serious disease. Some murmurs are congenital, some are acquired (as from rheumatic fever), some are functional and of no great significance. Murmurs are heard in many healthy children and adults. The meaning of murmurs, as of all symptoms, must be interpreted by a physician; some indicate a need for tests and studies leading to corrective treatment (409).

Heat cramps. Painful muscle spasms of legs and abdomen resulting from loss of salt through profuse, prolonged sweating (865).

"Heat hives." Wheals and "blush patches" on the skin produced by external warmth or internal warmth (as by vigorous jitterbugging) in sensitive persons, especially red-headed young women (702).

Heatstroke (*sunstroke*). A very serious reaction to exposure to extreme heat. The heat-regulating centers in the brain are paralyzed; the victim's extremely high temperature must be reduced immediately with ice packs or streams of cold water (864).

Heberden's nodes. Knobby lumps at the end joints of a woman's fingers, occurring usually after the menopause (657). The condition is a form of osteoarthritis which does not progress to severe crippling. The classic description by William Heberden, an English physician, is as valid today as when he published his account in 1802: "... little hard knobs, about the size of a small pea, which are frequently seen upon the fingers, particularly a little below the top, near the joint. They have no connection with the gout, being found in persons who never had it; they continue for life; and being hardly ever attended by pain, or disposed to become sores, are rather unsightly than inconvenient, though they must be of some little hindrance to the free use of the fingers."

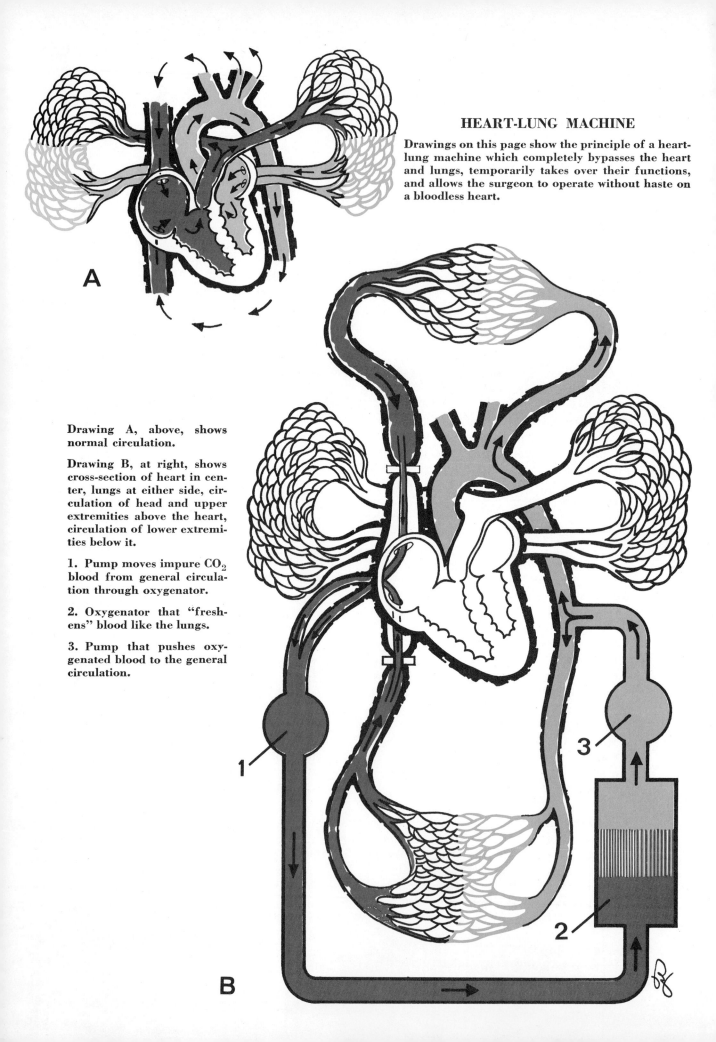

HEART-LUNG MACHINE

Drawings on this page show the principle of a heart-lung machine which completely bypasses the heart and lungs, temporarily takes over their functions, and allows the surgeon to operate without haste on a bloodless heart.

A

Drawing A, above, shows normal circulation.

Drawing B, at right, shows cross-section of heart in center, lungs at either side, circulation of head and upper extremities above the heart, circulation of lower extremities below it.

1. Pump moves impure CO_2 blood from general circulation through oxygenator.

2. Oxygenator that "freshens" blood like the lungs.

3. Pump that pushes oxygenated blood to the general circulation.

B

Helminthiasis. Infestation with *helminths,* parasitic worms (67).

Hemangioma. A red, often elevated birthmark; "strawberry mark." It may or may not be present at birth. Only superficial blood vessels are involved. The mark often disappears of itself after some months, but in some cases, treatment may be required (194, 402).

Hematemesis. Vomiting of blood.

Hematocele. A swelling produced by effusion of blood into a cavity.

Hematocrit. The percentage of red blood cells in whole blood, by volume; a reading is obtained by whirling whole blood in a centrifuge to pack the cells.

Hematoma. A swelling filled with blood which clots to form a solid mass. The blood accumulates from vessels injured by a blow or disease. A *subdural hematoma* is one that occurs under the skull. The "cauliflower ear" of boxers results from a neglected hematoma.

Hematuria. Blood in the urine. *Occult* blood in the urine is not visible but can be detected by tests. Hematuria may occur from relatively harmless causes (for example, prolonged marching, and severe stresses of physical contact sports), but it may portend serious disease and always requires medical investigation (291).

Hemocytometer. A device for counting blood cells.

Hemianopsia. "Half vision"; blindness for one half of the field of vision. One or both eyes may be affected.

Hemiplegia. Paralysis of one side of the body, due to a clot or rupture of a brain artery (stroke, 123), or a lesion or injury of the spinal cord or another part of the nervous system.

Hemochromatosis (*bronze diabetes*). A progressive disease characterized by abnormal deposits of iron in many organs of the body, associated with bronzing of the skin, diabetes, and impaired functioning of the liver and pancreas. Mild forms of the disease with few if any clinical symptoms may require liver biopsy to make the diagnosis. Just why enormous amounts of iron are stored in tissues is not fully understood. It is thought that the patient has an abnormal capacity to absorb iron, rather than lessened ability to excrete it, and that the trait is genetically determined. A key treatment of severe hemochromatosis is frequent bloodletting (PHLEBOTOMY) as often as once a week, to deplete the stores of iron that harm the patient.

Hemodialysis. Separation of waste materials from blood by passage through a semipermeable membrane, especially as performed by an artificial kidney (296).

Hemoglobin. The coloring matter of red blood cells. The molecule contains a protein part (*globin*) joined with an iron-containing pigment, *heme* (from which comes the prefix *hem-* for many medical words denoting some relationship to the blood). *Heme* is the oxygen-carrying portion of hemoglobin. The molecule functions like a pickup truck for oxygen and a dump truck for carbon dioxide. Hemoglobin picks up oxygen in the lungs, holds it loosely, carries it in arterial blood and delivers it as a fuel to cells. In exchange, it picks up carbon dioxide which cells must get rid of and carries it to the lungs where it is dumped and exhaled while a fresh load of oxygen is taken on. Iron is the key element of this remarkable gas-transporting molecule but the protein part is vital too; not all kinds of anemias are benefited by merely taking iron.

Hemolysis. Dissolution, breakdown of red cells with release of HEMOGLOBIN. Red cells are constantly being broken down and replaced; the process balances out in healthy persons (142). Excessive hemolysis may result from chemicals, incompatible transfusions, snake venom, and congenital or acquired conditions leading to hemolytic jaundice and anemia (155).

Hemophilia. Bleeder's disease (161). Hope that hemophilia may be conquered received great impetus in 1967 with development of a concentrated anti-hemophilic protein (*globulin*) which may lead to a dosage form that the patient can inject daily to prevent bleeding episodes.

Hemoptysis. Spitting of blood that originates in the chest.

Hemorrhage. Bleeding. The only normal form of bleeding is menstruation. Otherwise, bleeding is a sign of something wrong, often the major symptom to be dealt with immediately in giving first aid (830). *Arterial bleeding* comes in spurts and jets of bright red blood with each beat of the heart, unless blood wells up into a wound from a deep artery. *Venous bleeding* is indicated by a continuous flow of dark blood. *Capillary bleeding* is a general oozing from a raw surface such as a skinned knee. *Internal bleeding* is to be suspected if the patient has suffered severe blows, crushing, falls, penetrating injuries which may lacerate internal organs. Disease, such as erosion of a peptic ulcer, may cause hemorrhage into closed body cavities, with signs of impending shock (834).

Hemorrhoids (*piles*). Dilated, overstretched, varicose veins in and around the rectal opening. The condition is common, often is tolerated quite well for years, sometimes is temporary, as in pregnancy (363), and frequently responds to medical treatment and improvement of bowel habits (490). Hemorrhoids may shrink of themselves, or get worse. Some are best removed by a common surgical operation, *hemorrhoidectomy* (769).

Hemostat. An instrument which stops bleeding by clamping a blood vessel, or an agent which stops bleeding.

Henoch-Schoenlein purpura. An allergic form of hemorrhage into the skin, beginning with pain in the abdomen and joints. Recovery is usually spontaneous unless the kidneys are affected. The condition may be associated with streptococcal infection or rheumatic fever or food allergy (691).

Hepatitis. Virus-caused inflammation of the liver (60, 418). There are also non-viral forms, such as amebic, alcoholic, toxic, and syphilitic.

Hepatolenticular degeneration. See WILSON'S DISEASE.

Hepatoma. A tumor of the liver (478).

Heredity. Great unravelings of structures in cells which transmit hereditary characteristics from ancestors to progeny have been made in recent years. The "gross stuff" of heredity, the CHROMOSOMES, can be seen under a microscope and have long been known to scientists. The finer, infinitesimal structures of heredity—molecules invisible to man—have only recently yielded some of their age-old secrets. Message-carrying molecules in the chromosomes are called *deoxyribonucleic acid*. See Chapter 25.

Hermaphrodite. A person with the sex organs of both sexes. True hermaphrodites are rare. More common are *pseudohermaphrodites*, examples of *intersex* (310, 333). Such persons, "assigned" to the wrong sex at birth, may in later life be candidates for SEX REVERSAL operations, which do not actually change the basic sex, but give it better expression. Assignment of true sex at birth can be very difficult because of great variation in external and internal structures. Males with HYPOSPADIAS and UNDESCENDED TESTICLES may be assigned a female role; females may be mistaken for males with these abnormalities. Surgical exploration is often necessary in doubtful cases, and it may be possible for surgery to correct the condition, if not completely, at least to a degree of sat-

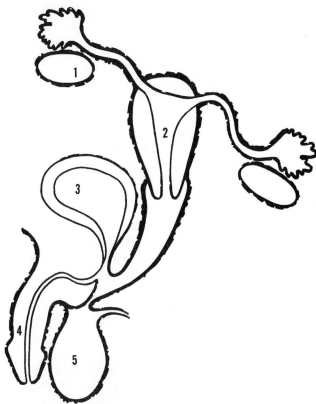

Schematic drawing of true hermaphrodite with organs of both sexes: 1. ovary; 2. uterus; 3. bladder; 4, penis; 5. testicle.

isfactory adjustment. But the varieties of hermaphroditism are far too numerous and complex for any single "rule" of sex assignment. Even the genetic sex may be "wrong." "Girls" with testicular feminization have internal testes and are genetically male, but they have a body of normal female appearance, with a vagina but without a uterus or menstruation; their hormones at puberty are exclusively feminizing and their entire psychic outlook is feminine. Cases of doubtful sex require individual study and technical knowledge. If the sex of an infant is in doubt, appropriate steps, surgical or otherwise, should be taken at an early age, not only that the child may identify with its appropriate sex, but because in some cases an endocrine disturbance detrimental to health may underlie the condition.

Hernia (*rupture*). Protrusion of an organ or part of an organ through a weak spot in tissues which normally contain it. There can be herniations of the brain, lung, or other organs, but the most common herniations are of organs contained by the abdominal wall. A natural weak spot in the groin area, especially in men, who have an opening through which the spermatic cord passes, is the site of *inguinal* hernia, the most common type in both men and women. It is repairable by a common surgical operation (737), as indeed are other forms of hernia (411, 468, 725).

Herniorraphy. Any operation for repair of hernia which includes suturing.

Herpangina. A COXSACKIE VIRUS infection, usually of infants and children, producing fever, sore throat, loss of appetite, sometimes nausea and vomiting (59).

Herpes simplex. The cold sore or fever blister virus (56).

Herpes zoster. See SHINGLES.

Hiatus hernia. DIAPHRAGMATIC HERNIA.

Hiccups (hiccough). The annoyance is known to all; its definition—spasmodic contraction of the DIAPHRAGM and sudden closure of the glottis—is rather formidable. Irritation of nerves that control the diaphragm (213) causes spasm, and the glottis, the chink between the vocal cords, snaps shut, causing a peculiar sound. The hiccup trigger may be an overloaded stomach, trapped gas, something that went down the wrong way, swallowing hot foods or irritants, gulping, or unknown trifling provocations. Virtually all of the popular cures for hiccups (rebreathing from a paper bag, holding the breath as long as possible, taking a dozen swallows of water without stopping to breathe) increase the carbon dioxide content of the lungs and thus help to stabilize the breathing center. Severe hiccups which continue for hours or days may be associated with liver, abdominal, or intestinal disease or lesions of the breathing center; temporary surgical interruption of the phrenic nerve may be necessary to stop incessant spasms.

Hip dislocation, congenital. Spontaneous dislocation of the hip shortly after or before birth (637).

Hippocratic oath. A statement of ethics traditionally demanded of the young physician on entering practice. It contains some anachronisms—mention of freemen and slaves, and apparent ruling out of operations for bladder stone (*lithotomy*) as beneath the dignity of reputable men of medicine. Anciently, through the Middle Ages and beyond, the operation of "cutting for stone" was usually attempted by itinerant operators who acquired some skill through trial and error at the expense of patients. Surgery was necessarily crude and dangerous, devoid of aseptic techniques, reliable anesthesia, and other supports of modern surgery, and mortality was high. If the patient survived, the operator benefited from word-of-mouth advertising; if the patient died, the operator was usually long gone to some other community. But the ethical precepts of the Oath endure. The Oath bears the name of Hippocrates, the famous Greek physician, born about 460 B.C., who is called the "Father of Medicine" for his sound and close observations of patients and diseases which began to give the medical arts a scientific foundation, but whether or not Hippocrates himself wrote the Oath is not known; more likely it is a collective expression of his followers. There are several English translations of the Oath; the wording that follows is best known:

"I swear by Apollo the physician, by Aesculapius, Hygeia, and Panacea, and I take to witness all the gods, all the goddesses, to keep according to my ability and my judgment the following Oath:

"To consider dear to me as my parents him who taught me this art, to live in common with him and if necessary to share my goods with him, to look upon his children as my own brothers, to teach them this art if they so desire without fee or written promise, to impart to my sons and the sons of the master who taught me and the disciples who have enrolled themselves and have agreed to the rules of the profession, but to these alone, the precepts and instruction.

"I will prescribe regimen for the good of my patients according to my ability and my judgment and never do harm to anyone. To please no one will I give a deadly drug, nor give advice which may cause his death. Nor will I give a woman a pessary to procure abortion. But I will preserve the purity of my life and my art. I will not cut for stone, even for patients in whom the disease is manifest. I will leave this operation to be performed by specialists in this art.

"In every house where I come I will enter only for the good of my patients, keeping myself far from all intentional ill-doing and all seduction, and especially from the pleasures of love with women or with men, be they free or slaves. All that may come to my knowledge in the exercise of my profession or outside of my profession or in daily commerce with men, which ought not to be spread abroad, I will keep secret and will never reveal.

"If I keep this oath faithfully, may I enjoy my life and practice my art, respected by all men and in all times, but if I swerve from it or violate it, may the reverse be my lot."

Hirschsprung's disease. See MEGACOLON.

Hirsutism. Abnormal hairiness of body parts not normally hairy (340).

Histamine. A normal chemical of body cells which plays a part in allergic reactions (674).

Histoplasmosis. Systemic infection due to inhalation of dusts containing spores of a species of fungi (75).

Hives. Urticaria (692).

Hoarseness. Generally a trivial (and socially benevolent) symptom resulting from using the voice at the top of the lungs too long; if it persists more than a couple of weeks, a doctor should be consulted to determine the cause which may be trivial or serious (613).

Hookworm. Infestation of the carelessly barefooted who tread upon soils contaminated with eggs of the responsible worm (69).

Hobnail liver. A liver studded with small nodules which somewhat resemble hobnails; characteristic of the most common form of CIRRHOSIS OF THE LIVER (477).

Hodgkin's disease. Malignancy of the lymph nodes (170). The pessimistic view that the disease is incurable (stemming from crude diagnostic methods and primitive radiation equipment of the past) is just not true, in the light of results with intensive high-energy x-rays which give apparently permanent cure to 80 to 90 per cent of patients with only a few lymph nodes affected by the disease.

Hordeolum. A stye (568).

Horseshoe kidney. Kidneys linked at their lower ends by a band of tissue instead of being separate; their shape somewhat resembles a horseshoe (291).

Hot flashes. See MENOPAUSE.

Household pets. The family dog, cat, or other pet is a pleasure-giving member of the household—if the animal is healthy and well cared-for. Most pet-owners realize the importance of having a veterinarian vaccinate an animal against RABIES. Less well known are some of the discomforts, and even serious diseases, which may arise from animals that do not get the veterinary or loving care that they deserve. Puppies and kittens in particular should be de-wormed by a veterinarian to prevent contamination of soil and materials with worm eggs in their excretions. Children and puppies make a pretty intimate team. Ingested eggs of the common dog roundworm can enter the bloodstream and larva

can reach many parts of the body. Mysterious cases of SCABIES, "the itch," have occurred in persons who never dreamed that the family dog carried the mites. Animals may be hosts to ticks which can cause disease. Animals with fur or feathers (even stuffed toy ones) are suspect inhabitants if someone in the family has allergies, even though skin tests may not show sensitivity to a particular animal. Allergic persons have a tendency to become sensitized to danders. Pets that give a lot deserve a lot, and should have veterinary attention if they show any of the following symptoms: Abnormal behavior, sudden viciousness or lethargy; abnormal discharges; abnormal lumps or difficulty in getting up or lying down; loss of appetite, marked weight loss or gain, or excessive water consumption; excessive head shaking, scratching, and biting any part of the body.

Housemaid's knee. Bursitis of the knee joint (654).

Housewife's eczema. A more dignified term than "dishpan hands" for dermatitis associated with soaps, detergents, and water (187).

Humor. Any fluid or semi-fluid of the body; for example, aqueous and vitreous humors of the eye (553). No connection with the ancient humoral theory of disease, which held that sickness results from lamentable disproportions of four body humors—blood, phlegm, yellow bile and black bile—respectively associated with sanguine, phlegmatic, choleric, and melancholic temperaments. Our word "melancholy" literally means "black bile."

Hunner's ulcer. An ulcer of the lining of the urinary bladder, associated with chronic interstitial cystitis (shrinkage of the bladder wall, splitting, decreased capacity).

Huntington's chorea. A rare hereditary disease, appearing in middle life or later; there is progressive deterioration of the nervous system, manifested in jerky, involuntary movements of the arms, legs, and face; personality changes, speech defects, difficulties of walking and swallowing. Profound nervous degeneration ultimately leads to idiocy and death. The disease is transmitted as a dominant trait (see MEDICAL GENETICS). Members of families in which the disease has appeared should have the benefit of genetic counseling; if they are carriers of the defective genes, half of their children, statistically, will have the disease, and for that reason they may choose to forgo parenthood.

Hutchinson's teeth. Widely spaced, narrow-edged upper central incisors with notching at the biting edge; a sign of congenital syphilis, though not always of that origin.

Hyaline membrane disease. A condition of pronounced respiratory distress which affects newborn infants, especially premature infants, at birth, and may be fatal in a day or two. It is the most common cause of death of live-born premature infants. The affected infant can't get enough oxygen because ducts leading to tiny air sacs in the lungs are lined with hyaline (glassy) material, probably derived from the baby's own secretions. Breath is rapid and labored almost from the moment of birth; CYANOSIS appears; the tiny heart works desperately to push enough blood through the lungs. Absence of a substance which reduces surface tensions and normally lines the air sacs seems to be the most important abnormality. Treatment consists of measures to avoid premature delivery if possible, rapid resuscitation at birth of premature infants, care in an incubator and, recently, the forcing of moist oxygen-rich air under pressure into the infant's lungs.

Hydatid disease. Infestation with animal tapeworms which produce clusters of fluid-filled cysts in the lungs and other organs (69).

Hydatidiform mole. A rare complication of early pregnancy, resulting from degeneration of membranes which would normally become a part of the placenta. The mass resembles a bunch of grapes of irregular size.

Hydramnios. An excess of fluid produced by the innermost of the fetal membranes (*amnion*) which forms the BAG OF WATERS that surrounds the fetus. *Acute hydramnios* is rare; it begins during mid-pregnancy and rapidly expands the uterus to enormous size. The condition terminates in spontaneous abortion or abortion induced to save the mother's life. *Chronic hydramnios* is a more common and less threatening form, does not often terminate in miscarriage, but frequently provokes premature labor.

Hydrocele. Swelling of the scrotum from accumulation of fluid in the sac of the membrane that covers the testicle (312). It is painless but weight of the fluid causes a dragging sensation. Usually only one side is involved. The condition may be related to some injury but in most cases the cause is obscure and the testicles function normally. Chronic hydrocele, most frequent in middle-aged men, is relieved by withdrawal of fluid (TAPPING) but the swelling tends to recur.

Hydrocephalus. "Water on the brain"; actually, water *in* the brain—abnormal amounts of CEREBROSPINAL FLUID in brain cavities, exerting destructive pressure on brain substance (272).

Hydronephrosis. Swelling of the cavity of the kidney because of obstruction to outflow of urine, as from a stone, stricture, or tumor, in the kidney itself or in a ureter or within the bladder (297, 298).

Hydrophobia. A common word for RABIES. The literal meaning of the word is "fear of water."

Hydrotherapy. Treatment by means of water.

Hymen. A membranous partition which partially blocks the external orifice of the virginal vagina (430).

Hyperbaric therapy. Treatment by inhalation of oxygen at greater than atmospheric pressure; an auxiliary to other appropriate treatment. The patient, physicians, and nurses occupy a large, long pressure chamber wherein the atmospheric pressure is increased to about three times the sea level pressure. The patient breathes pure oxygen to increase the amount delivered to body cells. The technique has been employed experimentally in treatment of carbon monoxide poisoning, tetanus, and infections caused by bacteria which do not thrive in the presence of oxygen.

Hyperchlorhydria. Excessive hydrochloric acid in gastric juices.

Hypercholesteremia. Excessive amounts of CHOLESTEROL in the blood.

Hyperemesis gravidarum. Vomiting of pregnancy, more severe than simple MORNING SICKNESS which clears up by itself; may require hospitalization.

Hyperhidrosis. Excessive sweating.

Hyperinsulism. A condition of abnormally low blood sugar resulting from an excess of insulin or deficiency of sugar; similar to insulin shock.

Hypernephroma. A malignant tumor of the kidney which occurs primarily in persons over 40 years of age (295).

Hyperopia. Farsightedness.

Hyperplasia. Overgrowth of an organ or tissue from an increase in the number of its cells which are, however, in normal arrangement.

Hypertension. Abnormally high arterial blood pressure (114).

Hypertensive heart disease. A form of heart disease associated with high blood pressure which forces the heart to work harder to pump blood against resistance (85).

Hyperthyroidism (*thyrotoxicosis, toxic goiter.*) Overactivity of the thyroid gland (322).

Hypertrophy. Increase in size of an organ because of overgrowth of cells, without an increase in the number of cells. It is usually a response to increased activity or functional demands; voluntary, as when a robustly exercised muscle increases in size, or involuntary, as when the body enlarges one kidney to compensate for a deficiency of its partner.

Hypnotic. Inducing sleep; a sleeping-pill. BARBITURATES are hypnotics most often prescribed by physicians.

Hypnosis. There is no black magic about medical hypnosis, and its purpose—to assist in treatment of patients—is quite different from the entertaining art of the stage hypnotist. Hypnosis is not a curative treatment, but at times it can be helpful to a physician in undertaking procedures he is qualified to undertake without hypnosis. The American Medical Association recognizes that there is a significant place for hypnosis in modern medical practice. Medical hypnosis first of all requires that the practitioner be trained as a physician. The hypnotic trance itself is harmless but it can be misused by the medically untrained; a headache which can be temporarily "hypnotized away" may result from a low-grade brain tumor. The major medical uses of hypnosis are for relief of pain and anxiety; for example, in childbirth (367), dentistry, psychological preparation for anesthesia and surgery. Hypnosis may reduce the amount of an anesthetic that is needed, and is especially useful when anesthetics and sedatives are for some reason undesirable. Unreasonably high hopes for medical hypnotic miracles are not justified. A physician who occasionally uses hypnosis treats his patients as usual but sometimes uses hypnosis as an adjunct. A principal disadvantage of hypnosis is the amount of time required. It may be difficult to find a physician who employs hypnosis; if found, he is not necessarily more skilled in treatment of disease than physicians who do not. About one physician in 40 or 50 uses hypnosis more or less regularly in his practice. A dozen medical schools now offer courses in hypnosis as a part of medical training.

Hypodermic. Under the skin; commonly refers to hypodermic injection, or the needle which effects it, or to the "shot" itself.

Hypoglycemia. Deficiency of sugar in the blood. *Hypoglycemic shock* due to an overdose of insulin is the same as *insulin shock.*

Hypoovarianism. Inadequate functioning of the ovaries (338).

Hypophysis. The pituitary gland (316).

Hypospadias. A congenital malformation in which the urethra, the urinary outlet, fails to fuse completely, but takes the form of an open trough-like channel on the underside of the penis (303). A similar malformation in the female permits urine to escape into the vagina.

Hypotension. Low blood pressure; sometimes significant, but usually harmless, not warranting treatment or concern, and perhaps even a promise of longevity (122).

Hypothalamus. A part of the "old brain" concerned with primitive functions such as appetite, procreation, sleep, body temperature; closely associated with the pituitary gland (315).

Hypothyroidism. Deficiency of thyroid hormone, leading to a slowing down of mental and physical processes. If the deficiency occurs in an infant before birth, it is known as *cretinism;*

if it occurs in an adult, it is known as *myxedema* (324).

Hysterectomy. Surgical removal of the uterus (443), either through an abdominal incision, or through the vagina, which leaves no abdominal scar (734).

I

Iatrogenic diseases. Those unintentionally induced by words or actions of a physician. A patient may misconstrue a doctor's remark or ominous look and be convinced that he has a grave disease which doesn't exist or is not nearly so grave as he fears. Iatrogenic heart disease is not uncommon; a doctor's casual mention of a murmur or premature beat may send a fearful patient to his rocking chair with iatrogenic invalidism, although he would be much better off if he remained active. A sort of pseudo-iatrogenic disease can be induced by "recognizing" in one's self the horrendous symptoms of exotic maladies described on television or in the press; in such case the obvious cure is to consult a doctor and believe his reassurances. Some iatrogenic disease is unavoidable, the side effects of drugs nevertheless necessary for the patient's welfare.

Icterus. Same as JAUNDICE.

Ichthyosis (*fish skin disease*). Dry, fishlike scaliness of the skin, a congenital abnormality (206). There are two forms of ichthyosis, both of which are hereditary. The commoner form is transmitted as a dominant trait; the other is determined by a sex-linked recessive gene. The latter type affects males only but is tranmitted by apparently normal females. See MEDICAL GENETICS.

Identical twins. Twins, always of the same sex and having the same heredity, developing from a single fertilized egg (378).

Idiopathic. Originating spontaneously from unknown causes, not the result of any other disease; it is peculiar to the individual.

Idiosyncrasy. Peculiar personal capacity to react differently than most people to drugs, foods, or treatment.

Ileitis. Inflammation of the ILEUM (730).

Ileum. The lower portion of the small intestine, a tube about ten feet long in which major processes of digestion and assimilation take place (451). It is continuous with the *jejunum,* a section of the small intestine which lies above it, and joins the colon at the *cecum,* a bulgy, dilated pouch from which the appendix dangles. The *ileocecal valve* at this junction controls the admission of semi-liquid contents into the colon.

Ilium. The broad upper part of the hipbone (619).

"Immediate" dentures. Artificial dentures worn immediately after extraction of the front teeth, the other teeth having been removed previously. While the gums are healing, the denture is prepared and is worn as soon as the front teeth are removed. This saves the patient the embarrassment of being conspicuously toothless for a while (540).

Immunity. Complex body mechanisms which create immunities to disease germs and foreign substances are not at all well understood, but a continuing ferment of research in this area has produced exciting bits of knowledge which may ultimately be relevant to cancer, arthritis, and other diseases which many authorities think may be related to the inability of immunity mechanisms to cast out abnormal cells and substances. The role of the thymus in producing protective ANTIBODIES has only recently been clarified (see THYMUS GLAND). It now seems probable that the human body has two im-

munity systems. The second system has not been pinpointed, and its existence is debated by specialists, but it is known that chickens have two immunity systems. In addition to a thymus, chickens have an organ at the end of the intestinal tract (bursa of Fabricius) which controls antibodies. While researchers are hopefully looking for something comparable in the human appendix, intestines, tonsils, spleen, and other tissues, present methods of immunizing against diseases (418) give certain protection to all except a very few unfortunate persons who have defective immunizing mechanisms (and whose deficiencies have given scientists an invaluable tool for prying out secrets of the mechanisms). There are two kinds of immunity. *Passive immunity* is the kind borrowed from someone else, when a doctor injects GAMMA GLOBULIN or some other substance containing preformed antibodies made by another person or animal, or when a mother's antibodies are transferred to her unborn child. These donated antibodies wear out in a few weeks. *Active immunity* is the kind produced by vaccination or exposure to disease germs; the body is stimulated to produce its own antibodies, continues to do so for a long time, and steps up antibody production when renewed by a booster shot or another contact with germs it "recognizes" immediately.

Immunization. Procedures by which immunities to diseases are produced in a person; especially, by vaccines and toxoids. See IMMUNITY, *active* and *passive.*

Active Immunizing Agents
Diphtheria toxoid
Tetanus toxoid
Pertussis (whooping cough) antigen
Poliomyelitis
Measles
Vaccinia (smallpox)
BCG (tuberculosis)
Yellow fever
Rabies
Typhoid

Influenza
Mumps
Tularemia
Typhus
Rocky Mountain spotted fever
Cholera
Plague
Adenovirus
Rubella

Immunoglobulins. Substances in the blood and in certain body fluids other than blood which build immunities to various diseases; loosely synonymous with ANTIBODIES.

Impacted. Firmly lodged, wedged in place; as, an impacted wisdom tooth, imbedded in the jawbone (526).

Imperforate hymen. Complete closure of the membrane at the opening of the vagina (427).

Implant dentures. Artificial dentures with projecting buttons which snap into metal receptacles implanted in the jawbone, like snap-fasteners of a garment. The purpose is to prevent dentures from wobbling if the gums are too flabby to hold them firmly (539).

Impotence. Incapacity of the male to have a penile erection and perform the sexual act. Impotence is an impediment of delivery rather than of production of SPERMATOZOA; it is not the same as infertility, which may affect perfectly potent males. Anatomical defects, injuries or disorders of the nervous or endocrine systems, and systemic diseases may cause impotence, and the possibility should first be investigated. But the great majority of cases have a psychic basis; the affected male may be impotent with one sexual partner but not with another; emotional factors are varied and complex and counseling or psychiatric help may be required.

Incisors. The four cutting teeth at the front of the jaw, upper and lower (*central incisors*). Each pair is flanked by *lateral incisors* (523).

Incontinence. Inability to restrain feces or urine.

Incubation period. The time between infection with disease organisms and the first appearance of symptoms (418). The period varies for different diseases, as short as a day or two for influenza and as long as 50 days for infectious hepatitis.

Incus. A tiny anvil-shaped bone, the middle bone in the chain of *ossicles* of the middle ear which conduct sounds to the inner ear (584).

Indigestion. A general lay term for abdominal distress with such symptoms as heartburn, bloating, gas, cramping, "fullness" (471).

Indolent. Slow to heal, as an indolent ulcer.

Induction of labor. Artificial stimulation of labor before it starts naturally; accomplished by rupturing the BAG OF WATERS or use of drugs such as *oxytocin* (384).

Indurated. Hardened.

Infant sleep patterns. Newborn infants don't actually sleep most of the time. They sleep about 16 hours out of the 24, and can sleep only about 4 hours at a stretch. One study of newborn infants showed only a gradual decrease in amount of sleep per day over a 16-week period. By the time they were four months of age they slept about 14½ hours a day, while increasing the length of a single sleep period to a little more than eight hours. Waking periods of newborn infants are more frequent from 5 p.m. to 3 a.m. than during the day. Long intervals between feedings may account for nighttime wakefulness. At two to three weeks of age, CIRCADIAN RHYTHMS (24-hour cycles) of sleep and wakefulness begin to develop. At three years of age a child has generally consolidated his sleep time and sleeps about ten hours a night. "Sleep problems" may be aggravated about the fifth year when daytime naps are given up. There is no arbitrary time for giving up afternoon naps, but generally they should be tapered off when a nap delays the onset of sleep in the evening and keeps the child awake after going to bed.

Infantile eczema. An eruptive skin disorder of infancy, frequently due to food sensitivities (413).

Infarct. An area of dead tissue resulting from complete blockage of its blood supply. This frequently occurs in *coronary thrombosis* when a clot in a coronary artery stops the supply of blood to a portion of the heart muscle, producing *myocardial infarction* (93). "Infarction" is easily misspelled or misread as "infraction."

Infectious jaundice. See LEPTOSPIROSIS.

Infectious mononucleosis. An infection thought to be caused by Epstein-Barr (EB) virus which is associated with BURKITT'S LYMPHOMA. The name comes from involvement of *mononucleocytes,* a type of white blood cell. The disease is generally benign (63). Occasionally it may cause temporary and usually harmless liver changes. Some of the fear that infectious mononucleosis is a very serious disease may arise from confusing minor liver changes with the much more serious changes of viral hepatitis. Reports from several college infirmaries indicate that "mono" generally lasts about two weeks; patients with the most acute symptoms require on the average only four days of bed rest, the majority require no bed rest.

Infertility. Barrenness (340).

Inflammation. In origin the word means "to set on fire"—an admirable description. Inflammation is a defensive reaction to all sorts of tissue injury. The names of hundreds of inflammatory processes are designated by the suffix "*-itis,*" preceded by the name of the affected tissue—for example, *appendicitis, arthritis.* The four characteristics of inflammation are reddening, swelling, pain, and heat (in classic medicine, *rubor, tumor, dolor, calor*). Reddening results from increased blood supply to the affected part; white blood cells whose job it is to trap and destroy germs are also increased. Concentration of fluids causes swelling. Increased local metabolism produces heat. Pain is a warning not to abuse the part and to get something done about it. These are signs of reparative processes. They may not suffice in themselves. A doctor is needed if inflammation is at all serious, to find out what is wrong and what to do about it.

Influenza (*grippe, flu*). An acute, highly contagious viral infection tending to occur in epidemics (55). The causative viruses, photographed in an electron microscope, have the look of innocent fluffy cottonballs.

Infusion. Introduction of fluid into a vein.

Ingrown hairs. Curled, corkscrew-like hairs that burrow into the skin particularly affect the bearded area. Shaving may cut such hairs more or less longitudinally, leaving a sharp point which turns upon its master. The ingrown hair may cause inflammation of the follicle, and usual treatment is to pull it out with antiseptic precautions. A better method which also tends to prevent ingrown hairs is recommended by some dermatologists. Brush the affected areas briskly at night with a stiff-bristled nail brush, brushing against the direction of beard growth.

Inguinal. Pertaining to the GROIN. A frequent site of hernia.

Inkblot test (*Rohrschach test*). A test sometimes used by psychologists and psychiatrists. Formalized figures used in the test are weird, splotchy, irregular silhouette patterns of the sort obtained by splashing a drop of ink on a piece of paper and folding the blot in the middle. What a person says he sees depicted in the patterns gives, it is believed by believers, profound information about his state of mind.

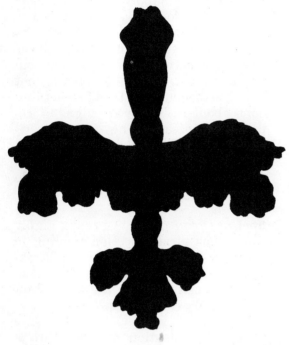

Inkblot; standardized designs are used in tests. What one sees in figure (bird, airplane?) gives clues to thought patterns.

Inoculation. Introduction of a disease agent into the body to produce a very mild form of disease giving immunity; for example, cowpox vaccination for smallpox.

Insemination. Introduction of semen into the vagina, by natural means or by artificial insemination.

In situ. In a normal place.

Inspiration. Inhaling, breathing in.

Inspissated. Thickened, from absorption or evaporation of fluid.

Insufflation. Blowing gas or powder into a body cavity, as the lungs or vagina.

Insulin. A hormone produced by islet cells of the pancreas gland, essential for metabolism. Insulin in treatment

of diabetes (351) must be given by injection, since it is a protein molecule broken down by digestion. Pharmaceutical companies prepare insulin in a number of different forms from animal sources. The structure of insulin was worked out by Frederick Sanger, a British biochemist. Insulin is a rather small protein molecule composed of 51 amino acids in two chains held together by a sulfur-containing link. Human and animal insulins have the same properties but differ in a sequence of three amino acids in one of the chains. Some diabetics become sensitized to insulin from a certain animal source. This complication may be averted, and insulin may be obtained independently of animals, if laboratory methods of synthesizing insulin become practicable. Scientists have already synthesized insulin by laborious mechanical methods, not commercially feasible. Some progress has been made in developing computer-controlled machines to perform synthesizing operations automatically. If "protein-making machines" become practicable for large scale production, a great many substances of medical importance may roll off the assembly lines.

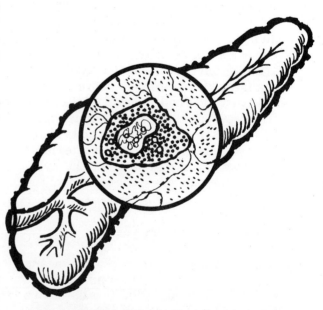

Islet cells of the pancreas gland secrete insulin. Magnified cell in center of circle; tiny black granules indicate insulin production; pancreas gland and ducts shown in background.

Integument. The skin.

Intention tremor. Involuntary trembling triggered or intensified when some voluntary movement is attempted.

Intercostal. Between the ribs.

Interferon. Infection caused by one virus may prevent concurrent infection by a different virus. This phenomenon, called viral interference, has been recognized for a quarter of a century. An apparent mechanism which gives this protection has recently come under intensive study. It is now known that body cells invaded by a virus produce a substance called *interferon* which diffuses out of the cells and into neighboring cells. The cells then become resistant to infection by viruses. Interferon is a complex protein. Its production by the body is a generalized phenomenon occurring when cells are exposed to viruses. Its unique properties suggest that it might be developed into a powerful agent for treatment of viral diseases, but great practical difficulties stand in the way. Interferon is too complex for synthetic manufacture and difficulties of producing large amounts of the pure substance are formidable. Even if large amounts of interferon become available, medical uses may be limited. Interferon must be absorbed into cells to block the multiplication of viruses, and means must be found to get interferon into cells in time to produce a curative or beneficial response. It is possible that some chemical agent (a drug) may be found, which triggers the production of interferon by body cells without exposure to viruses.

Intermenstrual pain. A usually brief attack of moderate to severe cramping pain which some women experience about midway between menstrual periods, coincidental with OVULATION, rupture of an egg-sac of the ovary and release of a mature ovum (339). Primary DYSMENORRHEA never occurs in absence of ovulation; intermenstrual pain of this nature is a rough guide to the time of ovulation and the fertile period. Discovery as long ago as 1940 that ovulation is essential for menstrual cramps, and that administration of estrogen early in the cycle could eliminate the cramps, was an aspect of studies which later led to the development of oral contraceptive pills. For physical exercises which help to relieve menstrual cramps, see PAINFUL MENSTRUATION. The right ovary lies near the appendix and midmenstrual pain in that region may be mistaken for a symptom of appendicitis. A physician can distinguish between intermenstrual pain and appendicitis on the basis of laboratory tests and dates of the menstrual cycle.

Intermittent claudication. Pain in the calf muscles and limping, occurring while walking, due to inadequate blood supply (129).

Intersex. See HERMAPHRODITE.

Intern. A graduate M. D. who serves in a hospital for a year or more, taking care of patients under supervision of the medical staff, preparatory to his being licensed to practice.

Internist. A specialist in internal medicine; that is, diseases of internal organs. Allergy, cardiovascular disease, gastroenterology, and pulmonary disease are subspecialties of internal medicine.

Intertrigo (*chafing*). Redness, abrasion, and maceration of opposing skin surfaces that rub together. Common sites are the armpit, groin, anal region, and beneath the breasts. Moisture and warmth with friction of adjacent skin parts set the stage for chafing, which may be complicated by bacterial or fungus infection. Regular use of a dusting powder and reduction in weight if obese are helpful preventives. Diabetes increases the susceptibility to intertrigo.

Intervertebral disks. Cartilaginous cushions between vertebrae (617, 627).

Intestinal flora. Bacteria which normally inhabit the intestine, do no harm and even some good. Various species of intestinal flora which we have grown accustomed to normally get along together like a happy family. Varieties of intestinal bacteria vary somewhat with diet. Diseases or antibiotics or other circumstances sometimes incapacitate one or more floral species, permitting others to thrive disproportionately from lack of competition; this may cause disturbing symptoms. A few kinds of bacteria may get through the stomach, but most kinds do not survive a bath in highly antiseptic, acid gastric juices. The floral population flourishes increasingly from the stomach downward. Some intestinal bacteria synthesize all the vitamin K we need, some synthesize other B vitamins but not all are well absorbed.

Intestinal juices. Digestive juices secreted by the intestinal walls, in contrast to gastric juices secreted by the stomach and pancreatic juices secreted by the pancreas gland. Intestinal juices contain enzymes which complete the final stages in digestion of protein, fat, and carbohydrate.

Intestine. The digestive tube from the outlet of the stomach to the outlet of the rectum. Although it is a continuous structure, each of the different sections has a different function. See DUODENUM, JEJUNUM, ILEUM, CECUM, COLON, RECTUM.

Intubation. Introduction of a tube into a hollow organ such as the larynx, to keep it open.

Intima. The inner lining of an artery; the innermost of its three coats or layers.

Intracutaneous test. Introduction of allergens into the skin; a positive reaction indicating sensitivity to a test substance will manifest itself in a few minutes in the form of an itching skin eruption somewhat resembling a mosquito bite (683).

Intradermal. Into or within the skin.

Intramuscular. Into or within a muscle. Many drugs are injected into muscles. A doctor's favorite site for intramuscular injection into somebody else is the buttocks.

Intrauterine transfusion. An emergency method of preventing death in the womb of an infant with severe ERYTHROBLASTOSIS, "Rh disease" (376). Appropriate blood is transfused via needle through the mother's abdomen into the peritoneal cavity of the fetus, whence it enters the fetal circulation. This makes it unnecessary to deliver the baby so prematurely that it might not survive or at best would have the additional hazard of premature birth.

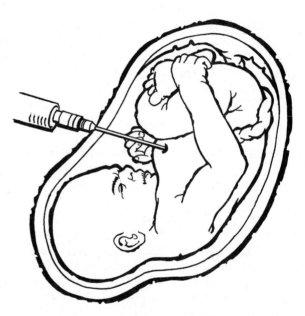

Intrauterine transfusion.

Intrauterine contraceptive devices (IUD, IUCD). Flexible devices of stainless steel, silkworm gut, or plastic, inserted by a physician into the uterus and retained there indefinitely for prevention of conception. Various devices are shaped like a bow, spiral, ring, or loop (345).

Intravenous (*I.V.*). Into or within a vein; as, *intravenous feedings* (723).

Intrinsic asthma. Bronchial asthma which has its origin within the body, from such a source as chronic sinusitis (686).

Intrinsic factor. A substance produced by the stomach for the transport of vitamin B_{12} across membranes into the blood. The fundamental defect in *pernicious anemia* (150) is absence or deficiency of intrinsic factor so that vitamin B_{12}, necessary for normal development of red blood cells, cannot be absorbed from foods. Intrinsic factor is a very elusive substance which has not yet been isolated in a pure state.

Introitus. The entrance to the vagina.

Intussusception. Sliding of a part of the intestine into its hollow interior; "telescoping," like the pushed-in finger of a glove (414, 483).

In vitro. In glass; pertaining to studies done in test tubes or laboratory hardware, outside of the living body. *In vivo* studies are done with living persons or organisms.

Ionizing radiation. The effect of radiation (x-rays, radium, radioisotopes, etc.) is to drive electrons out of atoms; the electrons become attached to other atoms or molecules, forming chemical units called *ions*. Such alteration of the electron patterns of components of living cells, changing their functional capacities, is the basis for the therapeutic use of x-rays (781).

Iontophoresis. Passing medication through the skin by electric current.

Iridectomy. Excision of a piece of the iris to open drainage channels for relief of *glaucoma* (774).

Iris. The circular, pigmented structure of the eye, perforated by the pupil (555). The iris controls the amount of light entering the eye and gives the eyes their color. *Iritis* is an inflammation of the iris (571).

Iron. The essential mineral of HEMOGLOBIN. The body preserves its iron reserves quite tenaciously, constantly re-uses iron salvaged from broken-down red blood cells. The small amount lost each day is easily replaced from the diet, but if reserves are depleted, food alone will not restore them. Infants and children particularly need good sources of iron; milk, which may constitute a large proportion of their diet, is relatively low in iron and a pediatrician's advice about addition of solid foods or possible supplements should be followed. Pregnancy increases a woman's requirements for iron; supplements are usually given.

Chronic blood loss, dietary deficiencies, or disorders of absorption may result in iron-deficiency anemia (149). It is very easy for a physician to determine if iron-deficiency anemia exists in a patient. Unless it does, iron will do nothing to correct fatigue or a possibly serious underlying disease of which fatigue is a symptom. In men, iron-deficiency anemia leads the physician to look for some cause of chronic blood loss, such as bleeding ulcer or hemorrhoids. Women of childbearing age are somewhat more susceptible to iron-deficiency anemia because of monthly blood losses, but the loss normally is very small in terms of iron.

Good food sources of iron:

Whole grain and enriched cereals
Dried beans and peas
Greens
Eggs
Apricots
Meats and Poultry
Liver and organ meats
Prunes and raisins
Molasses
Dried figs and peaches
Bouillon cubes
Brewer's yeast
Wheat germ
Oysters
Nuts

A once important source of iron has all but vanished from American kitchens: iron cooking utensils. Considerable amounts of iron are dissolved into foods, especially acid foods, prepared in iron cookware. An iron cooking pot may not be very handsome but its occasional use can contribute very significantly to a family's iron intake.

Iron lung. Popular name for a machine which expands and contracts the chest, so that a person with paralyzed respiratory muscles can breathe; a respirator.

Iron poisoning. Common "iron pills" or tablets, prescribed for iron-deficiency anemias and very commonly for pregnant women, are dangerous and even deadly to small children who get hold of a bottle and swallow the pills which sometimes have a candy-like appearance. Children have died from swallowing as few as a dozen of the tablets, usually five-grain tablets of ferrous sulfate. Symptoms of poisoning develop in an hour or so, with signs of shock, coma, vomiting, diarrhea. Iron poisoning is an acute emergency requiring immediate medical treatment.

Irradiation, medical. Treatment or diagnosis of disease with x-rays, RADIOISOTOPES, or other sources of IONIZING RADIATION. The body normally contains a certain amount of radioactive potassium and is subject to radiation from rocks and other unavoidable background sources.

Irreducible. Incapable of being put back in normal position; said of a hernia.

Irrigation. Washing out of a cavity.

Irritable colon. Over-reaction of the colon to emotions or other stimuli, without discoverable organic cause (486). Symptoms include cramping pain in the lower abdomen, bloating, "gassiness," distention, abdominal ache.

Ischemia. Local deficiency of blood supply, due to spasm or obstruction of an artery. A frequent concomitant of *coronary heart disease* (85).

Ischium. The bone we sit on (619).

Islet cells. The cells of the pancreas gland which produce INSULIN (481). Also called *islands of Langerhans.*

Isometric exercise. A form of exercise in which a muscle group exerts utmost force without moving a part. No special equipment is needed. Muscles of the abdomen or other parts of the body can be held at maximum tension while sitting or standing; arms can push against the sides of a doorway while standing in the opening; the palms of the hands can strain upward under the kneehole space of a desk while one sits in front of it. Isometric exercise builds strength up to a plateau. After the plateau is reached, increasing frequency of exercise does not increase strength further. Mild effort is useless. Strength increases only if absolutely maximum effort is maintained for at least six seconds.

I.V. Intravenous.

J

Jacksonian seizure. A *focal* epileptic seizure, so called because the spasm or convulsion originates in a local part of the brain and its effects are limited to one part of the body; for example, a twitching arm or leg (274). The patient usually remains conscious.

Jactitation. Extreme restlessness, tossing about in bed.

Japanese encephalitis. A virus-caused infection, occurring in eastern Asia, transmitted by the bites of mosquitoes (60).

Jaundice. Yellowish discoloration of skin and tissues by bile pigments in the blood (476). The skin is usually very itchy and the urine dark yellow or brown. The whites of the eyes have a yellowish tinge; in skin discolorations which might be mistaken for jaundice, the whites of the eyes remain clear. The symptom indicates that something has happened to cause bile pigments to back up into the blood. The underlying abnormality may be in the liver, in bile drainage channels outside the liver, or in the blood itself. *Hemolytic jaundice* is due to increased destruction of red blood cells; the stools are dark. A harmless form of hemolytic anemia occurs in newborn babies, lasts three or four days; the baby has an excess of red cells which are destroyed during the first few days after birth. *Toxic* or *infective jaundice* reflects injury to liver cells by some agent which interferes with their ability to eliminate bile pigment. *Obstructive jaundice* results when bile channels are blocked by disease, inflammation, gallstones, infection, tumors, causing pigments to spill over. In this type of jaundice the discoloration of skin and mucous membranes is intense, the stools clay-colored, the urine deeply colored. Underlying causes of jaundice are numerous. Various laboratory tests help to pinpoint what is wrong.

Jejunal ulcer. A peptic ulcer occurring near the opening between the stomach and jejunum, after a surgical operation to establish a direct connection between the organs (*gastrojejunostomy*).

Jejunum. An arbitrarily designated portion of the small intestine, eight to ten feet long, continuous from the DUODENUM to the ILEUM (451). Absorption of food elements is practically limited to the small intestine. Digestion is accelerated in the jejunum which is the recipient of gruel-like materials from the stomach after thorough mixing with bile and pancreatic juices in the duodenum.

Jellyfish stings. See PORTUGUESE MAN-OF-WAR.

Jet injection. A technique for vaccinating without a needle or the stab thereof. A volume of liquid is suddenly compressed and forced through a very fine orifice at such speed that it penetrates the skin painlessly and delivers a cone-shaped spray of material into tissues under the skin. Various types of jet injectors have been developed; some have reservoirs holding enough material for several hundred "shots." The devices have been used principally for speedy, mass vaccination of large numbers of people.

Jiggers (*chiggers*). Sand fleas; pregnant females of the species bore into the skin, causing intense itching and inflammation.

Joint mice. Small loose fragments of bone that have become separated within a joint, often the knee (643).

Jockey itch (*tinea cruris*). Ringworm of the groin; a fungus infection of the skin of the upper thighs near the genital organs (200). It is caused by the same group of organisms responsible for athlete's foot. Because the symptoms are similar to those of psoriasis and other skin diseases, a physician should be consulted.

Jugular veins. Veins of the side of the neck which drain blood from the head and neck toward the heart. The internal jugular veins are deep-lying; the external ones are near the surface.

K

Kahn test. A blood test for syphilis.

Kala-azar. An infection transmitted by the bites of sandflies, occurring in Mediterranean, tropical, and oriental regions (73). It is characterized by fever, anemia, enlarged spleen, emaciation, and has a high fatality rate if left untreated but responds well to medical treatment.

Kaposi's disease. See XERODERMA PIGMENTOSUM.

Keloids. Irregular ridges, nodules, and cordlike bands of skin like raised scars, at first rubbery and later very dense and hard (206). The growths tend to occur on the site of previous scars. The cause of such effusive growth is not known. Keloids can be removed by surgery but have a tendency to recur.

Keratin. The hard, horny protein which is the chief structural stuff of the outermost layer of the skin, of hair and nails, and in animals lower than man, of claws, horns, hoofs, and feathers.

Keratitis. Painful inflammation of the cornea (573).

Keratoconjunctivitis. Acute inflammation of the cornea and conjunctiva, tending to occur in epidemics, caused by a specific virus.

Keratoconus. Cone-shaped projection of the cornea; vision is impaired by the bending of light waves in distorted ways. Good vision may be restored by contact lenses (563).

Keratoplasty. Surgical procedures on the cornea, such as CORNEAL TRANSPLANT.

Keratosis. Overgrowth of the horny layer of the skin; for example, a wart or callus.

Kerion. Fungus infection of the beard or scalp, producing pustules (199).

Kernicterus. A severe form of JAUNDICE characterized by deposits of bile pigments in parts of the brain and degeneration of nerve cells, occurring in infants with ERYTHROBLASTOSIS.

Ketogenic diet. A diet high in fat relative to carbohydrate, deliberately designed to produce KETOSIS. In the past, ketogenic diets were sometimes used in treatment of epilepsy and urinary tract infections, but since the advent of effective drugs, such diets are rarely resorted to.

Ketosis. A condition produced when more fat is eaten than can be burned completely by the body. The unburned fats produce acid chemical substances called *ketone bodies*. An excess of ketones produces a form of ACIDOSIS to which some diabetics are especially susceptible; acetone derived from incomplete combustion of fats can produce a characteristic vinegary odor to the breath of diabetics with *keto-acidosis* (353).

Kidneys. Paired organs in the small of the back behind the abdominal cavity. Evolution of the kidney permitted primitive creatures of the sea to live on dry land by carrying with them an internal sea quite similar to the sea they took leave of. The kidneys regulate the volume and composition of body fluids, filter out impurities, keep ELECTROLYTES and blood composition in balance, and secrete substances which modify blood pressure. The kidneys are subject to infections, stone formation, tumors, malformations, circulatory and other underlying diseases (281).

Kimmelsteil-Wilson disease. A specific form of kidney disease (sclerosis of structures of the GLOMERULI) associated with diabetes of long duration.

Kinesthesia. "Muscle sense"; we all have it in addition to the standard five senses. It is the sense by which we perceive weight, position, movement, resistance, and rapidly integrate countless muscle-registered stimuli—from a grasped steering wheel, baseball bat, bicycle handlebars, or from muscles that tell us an arm is outstretched or bent without our looking at it.

Kinins. Miniature proteins associated with rheumatism and allergic reactions (674).

Kissing ulcer. One that appears to result from parts that press upon or "kiss" each other.

Klebsiella pneumonia. A type of pneumonia caused by a type of bacteria other than the common pneumococci

(36). It tends to produce chronic lung abscesses.

Klinefelter's syndrome. Undeveloped testes and female characteristics such as breast enlargement in males, due to an abnormality of the sex-determining pair of CHROMOSOMES. A normal female has two X chromosomes (XX), a normal male, an X and a Y (XY). A person with Klinefelter's syndrome has an extra and harmful X chromosome (XXY), triplets instead of a normal pair of chromosomes.

Kline test. A blood test for syphilis.

Knee jerk. The patellar reflex; sudden jerking forward of the lower leg when tapped below the kneecap. A test of the integrity of nerves.

Knock-knees (*genu valgum*). Inward bending of the knees at the joint; in young children it usually corrects itself spontaneously (642).

Knockout drops. Chloral hydrate, a potent hypnotic drug, poured into a victim's drink to cause rapid blackout; a Mickey Finn.

Koplik's spots. Small bluish-white spots on mucous membranes of the cheeks and lips, present shortly before the rash of MEASLES appears.

Korsakoff's psychosis. This severe mental disturbance usually, but not always, follows a bout of DELIRIUM TREMENS which blends into it. The outstanding manifestation is loss of memory for recent events, and falsifications of memory, such as "remembering" things that never happened. The psychosis is associated with chronic alcoholism and chronic malnutrition; treatment is much the same as for delirium tremens. Some patients recover their memories after weeks or months, but some never do.

Kraurosis. Progressive drying and shriveling of the skin, due to atrophy of glands, often accompanied by severe itching; especially, kraurosis of the vulva in elderly women (441).

Krukenberg tumor. Cancer of the ovaries which has spread from the stomach.

Kwashiorkor. A PROTEIN deficiency disease occurring most often in children in subtropical countries who are raised on exclusive cereal diets after weaning. Affected children have pot bellies, apathy, muscular wasting, edema, and fail to grow. It is an extreme form of disease which may occur in lesser degree in persons whose diets are severely curtailed in protein. The basic deficiency is lack of AMINO ACIDS for synthesis of proteins.

Kyphosis. Humpback, backward curvature of the spine. A mild form is "round shoulders." Kyphosis may result from poor posture or from diseases such as rickets, tuberculosis, osteoarthritis, and rheumatoid arthritis, which affect the spine.

L

Labia. Lips or liplike organs. *Labia majora,* folds of skin on either side of the entrance of the vulva; *labia minora,* folds of tissue covered with mucous membrane within the labia majora (430).

Labor. Childbirth. There are three stages: dilation of the cervix; expulsion of the child; expulsion of the placenta (380).

Labyrinth. Intricate passageways, intercommunicating canals; especially, structures of the inner ear (586).

Laceration. A wound caused by tearing of tissue; for example, lacerations of the perineum in childbirth.

Lacrimal. Pertaining to tears, produced by the *lacrimal gland* in the upper outside region of the eye socket (559).

Lactation. Secretion of milk (516). Interacting hormones initiate and sustain this complicated process. The milk-duct system of the breast enlarges during pregnancy under the influence of *estrogen*, an ovarian hormone. Milk-secreting lobules also proliferate under the influence of a different hormone, *progesterone* (444). During labor, OXYTOCIN, a hormone which has the property of "letting down" milk (and of stimulating contractions of the uterus) takes effect. Shortly after the baby is born the breasts secrete COLOSTRUM, which is not true milk but a secretion containing protective antibodies of the mother. True milk appears when *prolactin*, a pituitary gland hormone, acts upon breasts already prepared by estrogen and progesterone. Lactation can be suppressed by giving suitable hormones.

Lactose. A sugar that occurs in milk.

Lactovegetarian. A person who lives on a diet of vegetables, cereals, fruits, and dairy products.

Laennec's cirrhosis. The most common form of cirrhosis of the liver; portal cirrhosis (477).

Laminectomy. Surgery of the wall of the spinal canal to expose underlying structures (760).

Lancet. A short, pointed, double-edged surgical knife, used for *lancing*—that is, cutting open.

Lancinating. A description of sharply cutting, shooting pain.

Lanugo. Fine downy hair on the body of the fetus and on the adult body, except the palms and soles.

Laparotomy. Opening of the abdomen by an incision; a variety of surgical procedures may be used subsequent to the opening.

Larva migrans. See CREEPING ERUPTION.

Laryngectomy. Surgical removal of all or part of the voice box, usually because of cancer. There is a high rate of cure if the cancer is discovered early. The patient is left without vocal cords, but with persistence and encouragement can learn to speak again by "burping" air and manipulating it with muscles of the tongue and mouth. "Laryngectomees," as persons who have lost their voice boxes are called, have formed "Lost Chord Clubs" in many cities to teach and reassure recent laryngectomees that they too can learn to speak again.

Laryngitis. Inflammation of the LARYNX (voice box). Acute laryngitis is often associated with a common cold, infection, or overuse of the voice. The throat is dry, swallowing may be affected, it is not possible to speak above a hoarse whisper if at all. Absolute rest of the voice is an essential part of treatment (613).

Laryngoscope. A hollow metal tube with a light inserted into the throat for examining the LARYNX.

Laryngotracheobronchitis. An acute, very serious, "croupy" condition of children, rapid in onset, requiring immediate medical care (406). The outstanding symptom is extreme difficulty in breathing, due to thick mucus and fluid which can quite rapidly plug the breathing passages.

Larynx. The vocal apparatus, located between the base of the tongue and the windpipe (608). It includes the vocal cords and muscles which modify the vibrations of air passing through them, to produce controlled sounds.

Laser. A remarkable device which gets its name from the initial letters of Light Amplification by Stimulated Emission of Radiation. Essentially, a laser multiplies the triggering energy of a light source, such as the flash of a photographic bulb, into a tremendously powerful emission of parallel light waves of the same wave length,

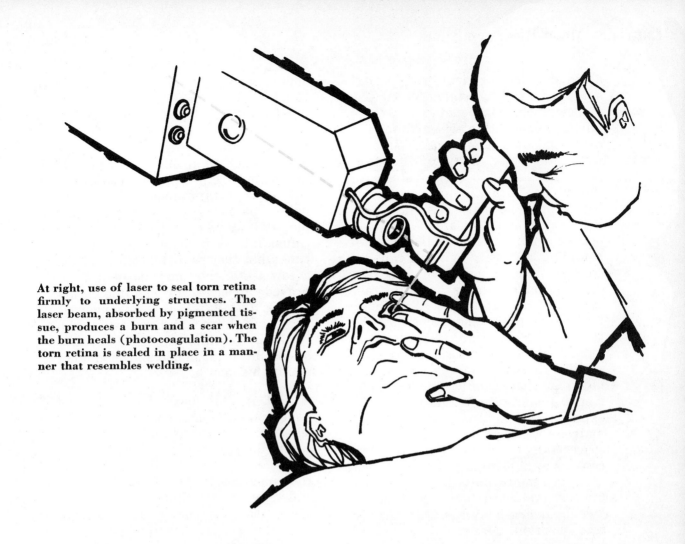

At right, use of laser to seal torn retina firmly to underlying structures. The laser beam, absorbed by pigmented tissue, produces a burn and a scar when the burn heals (photocoagulation). The torn retina is sealed in place in a manner that resembles welding.

Below: torn retina (1) is shown separated from choroid layer (2) to which it normally adheres. Laser beam enters through pupil of eye to make contact with very tiny area of retina.

Magnified representation of "spot welding" effect of laser beam inside eye. Beam at retina (3) causes formation of scar tissue that "welds" retina to choroid (4).

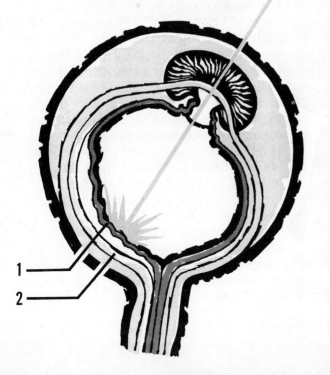

1
2

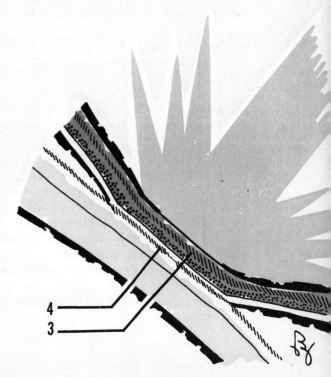

4
3

all in step. The original "ruby laser" employed a ruby crystal about the size of a cigarette, impregnated with chromium atoms, with a reflective mirror at one end and a semi-transparent mirror at the other. Setting off a high-powered flash bulb excites atoms in the crystal to higher energy levels; they drop to normal levels and in doing so excite other atoms, trapped between mirrored ends of the tube, rebounding, intensifying, until an extremely intense burst of coherent (non-diffuse) light is emitted from the semi-transparent end of the tube. For a very brief time, hundredths of thousands of a second, a laser beam is more brilliant than the sun and its parallel rays can be focused on a spot no wider than a millionth of a millimeter. Medical uses of a laser are still experimental and many problems remain to be solved. Laser beams have successfully destroyed pigmented skin cancers in human patients, have been used to remove portwine stains and tattoos, and have been employed to "weld" *detached retinas* (578) firmly into position. Many new types of lasers are being developed.

Laurence-Moon-Biedl syndrome. A genetic disorder of the pituitary gland producing obesity, mental retardation, degeneration of the retina, webbed fingers or toes, and underdevelopment of the genital system.

Lavage. Washing out of a hollow organ such as the stomach or a sinus.

Lead poisoning. Intoxication from absorption of lead or its salts into the body; *plumbism*. Mild lead poisoning may produce no apparent symptoms but the metal can accumulate in the body over a period of time and produce chronic poisoning. Some of the signs of lead poisoning are abdominal pain, constipation, pallor, drowsiness, mental confusion, a "blue line" on the gums. It has been suggested that the use of lead pipes to carry water may have hastened the decline of the Roman empire; continued ingestion of

small amounts of lead may have led to lassitude and mental torpor in the population. Lead poisoning occasionally occurs in young children who nibble on materials containing paints with a lead base. Insidious lead poisoning is not rare in children who live in old, poorly maintained houses with flaking paint and plaster. Infants explore the world by putting all sorts of things into their mouths. Around the time when they begin to walk and have a few teeth, they may develop a depraved appetite for non-food substances (see PICA). It is a dangerous habit which should be sternly corrected by teaching the child as early as possible what should and should not go into his mouth.

L. E. cell. A white blood cell which has undergone changes characteristic of *lupus erythematosus* and related diseases (669).

Left-handedness. When a left-handed child appears in a right-handed family there may be some consternation. "Lefties" suffer unjustly in a right-handed world. Words originating from the left, such as "sinister" and "gauche," have denigrating meanings, while those originating from the right, such as "dexterous," are complimentary. Perhaps it is such considerations that lead some parents to force a naturally left-handed child to favor his right hand. The consensus of authorities is that if a child wants to use his left hand, let him. Some things we learn to do with either the right or left hand because it's most convenient. A left-handed person shakes hands with his right hand because that's the way the world shakes. A right-handed person holds a telephone receiver with his left hand (and uses his left ear) to leave his right hand free for writing. We are left- or right-eyed as well as handed; it's easy to determine one's dominant eye (552). Teachers and parents never make any effort to change eye dominance. If handedness is to some extent hereditary, the mode of transmission has not been elucidated. Some investigators think that a left-handed person is the mirror-image of his right-handed twin who was not able to survive the early stages of cell division.

Left-sided appendicitis. See DIVERTICULA.

Leishmaniasis. A parasitic disease transmitted by sandflies; it has several forms (73).

Leprosy (*Hansen's disease*). A chronic disease, often very painful, which inflicts cruel deformities and mutilations, caused by bacteria closely related to those that cause tuberculosis. Biblical references to lepers probably concerned various repulsive skin diseases rather than leprosy as it is known today. About 12 million persons suffer from leprosy today. Most of them live in tropical or subtropical countries, but leprosy still occurs in Hawaii, Puerto Rico, and the southern United States. The disease affects the skin and nerves of all patients, but is usually classified according to which tissue is predominantly involved. Patients with "nerve" leprosy develop discolored skin areas, devoid of feeling because nerves are deadened. Ultimately, fingers, toes, or other parts may shrivel and drop off. Patients with "skin" leprosy develop thick, knobby growths which grossly distort the features. Drugs known as sulfones seem to prolong the lives of some patients but others appear to get worse after chemotherapy is begun. Close skin contact with a patient who has leprosy seems a likely route of entry of organisms into the body. Leprosy is generally thought not to be very "catching." Husbands and wives of patients with leprosy may remain apparently uninfected after living many years together. Some investigators feel that leprosy is a highly contagious disease but only to a few people who are highly susceptible.

Leptospirosis (*infectious jaundice; spirochetal jaundice*). An infectious disease caused by certain spirochetes (*leptospira*). The germs are spread in the urine of infected animals—rats, mice, dogs, cows, pigs—and most people who acquire the infection have had contact with animals or with water or moist soil to which animals have access. The disease is not exceptionally rare in the United States. Several local outbreaks have been traced to swimming or wading in ponds or slow-moving streams in rural areas where waste disposal is not properly screened. The germs enter the body through mucous membranes or minute breaks in the skin. Typically, the infection produces sudden fever, chills, headache, and muscle pains. In some cases there may be few if any symptoms; in others, jaundice may develop. Usually leptospirosis is a brief self-limited illness, but *Weil's disease* (51) is a severe form in which jaundice, kidney failure, hemorrhage, anemia and heart damage may become threatening complications.

Lesion. Alteration of tissue or function due to injury or disease. A pimple, fracture, abscess, scratch, wart, or ingrown toenail may be called a lesion.

Leukemia. Malignant disease of the blood-forming organs, sometimes called "cancer of the blood." The characteristic abnormality is gross overproduction of white blood cells. There are several acute and chronic forms of leukemia, so diverse that the word does not refer to a single specific disease but to a variety of "leukemic states" (164).

Leukocytes. White blood cells (142).

Leukocytosis. Abnormal increase in numbers of white blood cells. The cell count normally increases slightly after eating and in pregnancy, but the word implies an abnormal increase, often associated with bodily defenses against infection and inflammation. For instance, a high count may help to confirm a diagnosis of appendicitis. Disorders of the blood-forming organs may also induce leukocytosis.

Leukoderma. See VITILIGO.

Leukopenia. Abnormal scantiness of white blood cells. The condition may result from allergies, drug reactions, irradiation, certain kinds of infections or anemias.

Leukoplakia. Whitish, leathery patches on mucous membranes of the mouth (544) or vulva (441). No specific cause is known, but continued irritation is considered to be a factor. Patients with oral leukoplakia are forbidden to smoke and the white patches may regress if this and other irritations are removed. Leukoplakia by no means progresses inevitably to cancer, but it is considered to be a precancerous lesion and requires competent medical care and followup.

Leukorrhea. Whitish discharge from the vagina. Increased flow of mucus about midway between menstrual periods often accompanies OVULATION. The discharge is sometimes called "the whites." It may result from yeast or protozoal infection. See TRICHOMONIASIS and MONILIASIS.

Leydig cells. Interstitial cells of the testes which produce testosterone, the male hormone (and small amounts of female hormone). The cells are separate structures from those that produce SPERMATOZOA (335). Thus, infertile males whose production of spermatozoa is impaired may produce adequate amounts of male hormone and be entirely potent.

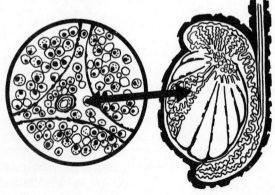

In circle, Leydig cells of the testis (right).

LH. Luteinizing hormone of the pituitary gland. It causes a GRAAFIAN FOLLICLE which has released a "ripened" egg to become a yellow body which produces *progesterone,* a hormone which helps to prepare the lining of the uterus for implantation of a fertilized egg (339).

Libido. Commonly means sexual drive; in Freudian psychology, the sum total of psychic energy.

Lichenification. Leathery thickening and hardening of the skin, usually the result of long-continued irritation from scratching and rubbing.

Lichen planus. An itching eruption of unknown cause; dull purplish-red spots appear on thin-skinned areas of the body (192).

Ligament. A band of tough, flexible fibrous tissue which connects bones or supports organs.

Ligate. To tie up; for example, a bleeding blood vessel. In surgery, a *ligature* is a thread of silk, catgut, wire, or other material used for tying vessels.

Lightening. The time around the middle of the last month of pregnancy when the baby's head settles more deeply into the pelvis preparatory to birth. This slightly decreases the mother's feeling of abdominal distention, "lightens" the load (374).

Limbus. A border; the edge of the cornea where it joins the white of the eye.

Lipids. A broad term for fats and fatlike substances. Lipids contain one or more fatty acids. Lipids include fats, cholesterol, phospholipids, and similar substances which do not mix readily with water.

Lipoid pneumonia. See ASPIRATION PNEUMONIA.

Lipoma. A compressible tumor composed of fat tissue, occurring chiefly on the trunk, back of the neck, forearms or armpits. Lipomas must be distinguished from other tumors by a physician. Lipomas usually stop growing after they reach a certain size and remain at that size indefinitely. True lipomas are painless, harmless, never become malignant, and are best left untreated unless they are so large and cosmetically objectionable as to justify surgical removal.

Lithiasis. Stones where they don't belong (gallstones, kidney stones); the condition of having stones.

Lithotomy. Cutting into the bladder to remove a stone (287). Structures are close to the surface, and because of this accessibility the operation has an ancient history. Mortality was high in the centuries before antiseptic surgery, but some patients did recover, notably Samuel Pepys, who spent a few shillings for a box "to hold the stone that I was cut of." Wandering surgeons who "cut for stone" in ancient times were not highly regarded by contemporary physicians, as is evidenced by a sentence from the Hippocratic Oath: "I will not use the knife, not even on sufferers from stone." This Hippocratic prohibition has long since fallen into desuetude.

Little's disease. Cerebral palsy of children affecting both sides of the body.

Liver. The largest organ of the body and the most versatile chemically (460, 476).

"Liver rot." A disease acquired by ingesting food or water contaminated with cysts of sheep liver flukes, a species of flatworm (67).

Lobotomy. Cutting into a lobe of an organ, especially a lobe of the brain. See PSYCHOSURGERY.

Lochia. The discharge from the vagina which continues for a week or two after childbirth. It is a normal aftermath of childbirth and ceases when the uterus returns to its pre-pregnancy state.

Locked knee. A painfully swollen knee joint which cannot be extended fully, due to torn CARTILAGE. Surgical removal of the injured cartilage is usually necessary (644).

Lockjaw. See TETANUS.

Locomotor ataxia. See ATAXIA.

Lordosis. Exaggeration of the normal forward curve of the spine at the small of the back. The general aspect is that of an abdomen thrust forward and shoulders thrust back. Lordosis usually reflects a feat of balancing abdominal weight to bring it into comfortable alignment with the body's center of gravity. The characteristic posture of late pregnancy, called "pride of pregnancy" because of the seemingly flaunted abdomen, is a temporary lordosis. Abnormalities of the hip joint sometimes cause lordosis.

Low blood sugar (HYPOGLYCEMIA). Less than normal amounts of GLUCOSE (sugar) in circulating blood. Blood sugar naturally drops if we go a long time between meals. Mild transient symptoms of hunger, weakness, faintness, are perfectly normal and no surprise at all to anyone who skips food long enough to deplete his reserves; a square meal restores the balance. *Chronic* hypoglycemia may be associated with various endocrine and other disorders. Insulin, which reduces abnormally high blood sugar levels, is only one agent in nature's complicated balancing scheme. A companion hormone, *glucagon*, also produced by the pancreas gland but by different cells than those which produce insulin, stimulates the liver to convert GLYCOGEN to blood sugar and raise low blood sugar levels.

LSD. Lysergic acid diethylamide. See Chapter 27.

Lues. Syphilis.

Lumbago. A general term for pain in the middle of the back, the lumbar region (618). Lumbago is not a specific disease but a symptom to be investigated.

Lumbar puncture. Withdrawal of CEREBROSPINAL FLUID through a hollow needle inserted between lumbar vertebrae of the small of the back (616). Withdrawal may be done for purposes of diagnosis, to relieve pressures, or the puncture may be made to introduce medication, as an anesthetic.

Lumen. The open space inside a tubular structure such as an intestine or blood vessel; the "hole of a tunnel" through which traffic passes.

Lumpy jaw. See ACTINOMYCOSIS.

Luxation. Dislocation.

Lymphangitis. Inflammation of lymph vessels due to spread of an infection, producing swelling and burning pain. Irregular, wavy red lines mark the path of inflamed vessels. There is danger of bacteria getting into circulating blood. Treatment is directed to overcoming the original infection.

Lymphedema. Swelling of a part of the body, especially the legs or arms, from a "back-up" of fluids because of obstruction or inadequacy of the lymphatic drainage system (143). The condition may cause huge enlargement of a part (ELEPHANTIASIS). Lymphedema of the arm sometimes occurs after breast removal surgery. Obstructive lymphedema is secondary to other conditions such as tumors or FILARIASIS. A less frequent, sometimes congenital form results from primary defects in the functioning of lymphatic channels in the skin and its deep layers. This type of lymphedema manifests itself as a grossly swollen leg in the teens or middle life. The unsightly swelling may be controlled to some degree by rest in bed, elevation of the limb to promote drainage, and wearing a firm rubber bandage over a white stocking when up and about.

However, this does not cure a chronic condition which tends to worsen with time, and surgery to remove the diseased tissue before extensive changes occur may be advisable.

Lymphogranuloma venereum. A disease produced by viruses transmitted by sexual contact (57).

Lymphosarcoma. A malignant tumor of lymphatic tissue (170). *Lymphogranulomatosis* is sometimes a synonym for HODGKIN'S DISEASE.

Lysozyme. A natural antibacterial substance contained in many bodily secretions, such as tears (558).

M

Maceration. Sodden; softening and deterioration of tissue soaking or in confined contact with fluids.

Macula lutea. A small, round, yellowish spot near the center of the retina, the area of color perception and most distinct vision (556).

Macule. A flat discolored spot on the surface of the skin.

Madura foot (*mycetoma*). A chronic fungus infection of the feet, occurring in tropical regions. The swollen foot becomes filled with connecting cyst-like areas from which fungus-containing pus drains. In the course of time the disease destroys muscle and bone and amputation may be necessary.

Magenstrasse. "Stomach street"; a groove along which food passes to the outlet of the stomach.

Maidenhead. The HYMEN.

Malabsorption syndrome. A descriptive term for several disorders resulting from defective absorption of foodstuffs in the small intestine (485). Certain diseases or surgical procedures may disturb previously normal assimilative processes, but the most common forms of the syndrome (variously called *celiac disease, sprue, idiopathic steatorrhea*) seem to involve hereditary defects in the absorptive surface of the small intestine, and deficient activity of intestinal enzymes. Large amounts of unabsorbed fat produce frequent, pale, loose stools (steatorrhea). *Celiac disease* in children is the same as *nontropical sprue* in adults. Symptoms in adults—diarrhea, weakness, loss of weight, anemia deceptively like pernicious anemia—are insidious and require careful diagnosis. Young children with celiac disease commonly have poor appetite, various signs of malnutrition, stunted growth, bulging abdomen, and frequent frothy stools containing excessive amounts of fat. Gluten, a wheat protein, has a toxic effect on the small bowel of many patients with malabsorption syndromes. Strict elimination of gluten from the diet often restores bowel function to normal and maintains it even though there is no structural improvement in the bowel. A gluten-free diet prohibits wheat, rye, oats, and their products such as bread, cookies, and crackers, as well as foods such as gravies and soups which have wheat flour added to them.

Malacia. Softening of part of an organ.

Malar. Pertaining to the cheek; the cheekbone, the *zygoma*.

Malaria. An infectious disease characterized by chills and intermittent or remitting fever, caused by parasites transmitted to man by the bites of mosquitoes (72).

Mal de mer. Seasickness; a form of MOTION SICKNESS.

Male climacteric. An indefinite "change of life" state in elderly men, analogous to the menopause in women but without a clearcut sign comparable to cessation of menstruation which marks the female climacteric. Some physical changes occur with age as the hormone output of the sex glands diminishes; it may be difficult to separate physical factors from psychological reactions to fears, worries, boring environment, retirement, decreased sexual function and opportunity, unrecognized illness, depression, apprehensive brooding on the passage of time. Vague symptoms self-attributed to the male climacteric call for a physical checkup by a physician, who may decide that hormone treatment is worth a trial, or who may find some condition that requires quite different treatment. Symptoms associated with diminished male hormone production (restorable to normal maintenance levels by replacement therapy) are decreased sexual potential, irritability, depression, lack of concentration, moderately diminished growth of beard and body hair.

Malaise. Listlessness, tiredness, irritability, depression, distress, general feeling of illness and of being "under par"; often is a forerunner of some feverish infection.

Malignant. Life-threatening; the usual medical meaning is "cancerous."

Malingering. The feigning of illness. The motive may be to avoid work, collect damages, escape military service, or gain sympathy. The deception can usually be exposed by tests and observations not recognized or understood by the malingerer.

Malleus. One of the three tiny bones (*ossicles*) of the middle ear which amplify vibrations of the eardrum and conduct them to the inner ear (584). "Malleus" means "hammer"; the "handle" of the hammer, attached to the eardrum, amplifies vibrations which are hammered onto the adjacent anvil-bone.

Malocclusion. Inharmonious meshing of the upper and lower teeth; poor "bite"; bad alignment of teeth and jaws (543).

Malpresentation. Any position of the fetus in the birth outlet other than the normal head-down position at childbirth; for example, breech, forehead, foot presentation.

Mammography. X-rays of the breast; several views are taken, to improve accuracy in detecting very small lesions (447, 785).

Mammoplasty. Plastic surgery of the breast; especially, an operation to correct sagging breasts. It is performed by excising tissue and fixing the glands in their normal position.

Mandible. The lower jawbone (545).

Manic-depressive psychosis. A severe form of mental illness (711). It is characterized by swings from intense elation and hyperactivity to blackest depression; between swings the patient may act quite normally. In the manic phase, the patient is enormously optimistic, overtalkative, physically busy, always on the go; his thoughts skip wildly from one subject to another; he is excited by grandiose projects. In the depressive phase, he may be hopelessly discouraged, have feelings of utter worthlessness, hear "voices" which nag him unmercifully, and have difficulty in performing the simplest mental and physical tasks.

Mantoux test. See TUBERCULIN TEST.

Manubrium. The uppermost handle-like part of the breastbone (617).

Marasmus. Wasting and emaciation of infants from no discoverable cause.

March foot. Painful swelling, even fracture of bones of the foot, not produced by acute injury but by excessive strain, as in marching.

Marfan's syndrome. A rare hereditary disorder, characterized by unusual flexibility of joints, disproportionately long legs, flabby tissues, funnel chest or pigeon breast, spider fingers, flat foot, displacement of the lens of the eye, and heart defects (98). The fundamental defect appears to be in connective tissue which breaks down or fails to produce normal amounts of strong fibers sufficiently strong to support body structures.

Marginal ulcer. A peptic ulcer occurring at the junction where the stomach and jejunum have been surgically united.

Marie-Strumpell disease (*ankylosing spondylitis*). A progressive disease of joints of the spine, related to but not identical with rheumatoid arthritis (666).

Marrow. Soft material which fills the cavities of bones. Formation of blood cells takes place in the *red marrow* of certain bones of adults and of all bones in early life. *Yellow marrow* is fatty material which does not perform any blood-making function.

Masseter. A "chewing" muscle that moves the lower jaw.

Mastectomy. Surgical removal of the breast, usually because of cancer (447, 756). In *simple* mastectomy, only the breast tissue is removed and underlying muscles are preserved. Usually, if cancer is present, *radical* mastectomy is performed, to remove not only the breast but lymph nodes near the collarbone and armpit, and sections of arm and chest muscles.

Mastitis. Inflammation of the breasts, from bacterial infection or other causes. The most common disease of the female breast is *chronic cystic mastitis;* the breasts contain nodules and small cysts of rubbery consistency, usually painful. Most patients with this condition can be treated satisfactorily by a physician in his office. A "lump" in the breast is not necessarily cancer, but it is imperative to have a physician determine its nature (445).

Mastodynia. Pain in the breast.

Mastoid. "Breast-shaped"; refers to mastoid air cells which surround the middle ear. Infection reaching these cells from the middle ear may require *mastoidectomy,* surgical removal of affected cells (597).

Materia medica. Substances used in medicine, and the science concerned with the origin, preparation, dosage and administration, and actions of such substances.

Maxilla. The upper jawbone.

Maxillary sinus. A pyramid-shaped cavity, largest of the nasal sinuses, located in the front of the upper jaw on either side of the nose (606). Also called the *antrum.* The floor of the cavity is close to the root of the eye-tooth.

Measles (*rubeola*). An infectious disease caused by viruses (418). Although most children recover from a natural attack of measles without suffering serious after-effects, the disease is treacherous and can be fatal. It can lead to ENCEPHALITIS and mental retardation. Immunizing vaccines of the live-virus type make it unnecessary for any child to be exposed to such risk. One injection of live-virus measles vaccine gives long-lasting, probably lifetime immunity. The U. S. Public Health Service recommends immunization against measles of all infants at one year of age, and immunization on entering school of all children not given measles immunization in infancy.

Meat grades. Except for products produced and sold within a state, all meat and meat products are inspected by experts of the U. S. Department of Agriculture. The inspection begins with the live animal and continues through the slaughtering operation. It applies to the meat through its many stages of processing and manufacture and to the many ingredients that are used and the processes employed. After the production of clean disease-free meat in the slaughtering department, production-control inspectors see that the clean meat stays wholesome and that it is handled under sanitary conditions. Recent legislation extends the protection of Federal inspection to meat and meat products produced within a state.

Meat *grading* by Federal inspectors is not compulsory. This is an evaluation of quality; some processors establish their own grading systems. Federal grades, however, give a uniform designation of quality of beef, veal, and lamb, useful to livestock dealers and consumers. About half of the beef, one-third of the lamb and mutton, and one-sixth of the veal produced by commercial slaughterers is Federally graded. There are six Federal grade marks stamped on the carcass: USDA Prime, USDA Choice, USDA Good, USDA Standard, USDA Commercial, and USDA Utility. A large part of the limited supply of Prime beef goes to hotels and restaurants and these cuts are not often available in retail stores. The top grade generally available from retailers is USDA Choice. USDA Good, the next grade, has less fat and less taste appeal. The lowest grades, Standard, Commercial, and Utility, may sometimes be found in retail markets but much goes into the preparation of meat product specialties. The lowest grades are perfectly wholesome but tougher and less flavorful, and they need additional care in cooking.

Meatus. An opening or passage, such as the external opening of the urethra.

Meckel's diverticulum. An outpouching from the small intestine, a blind tube two to five inches long (483). It is normally obliterated in the course of fetal development, but in some people it remains as a vestigial remnant. It may become inflamed and cause symptoms resembling appendicitis.

Meconium. Pasty, greenish material which fills the intestines of the fetus before birth and forms the first bowel movement of the newborn. *Meconium ileus,* obstruction of the intestines by sticky, viscid meconium, is the earliest manifestation of *cystic fibrosis* (407).

Mediastinum. The space in the middle of the chest between the lungs, breastbone, and spine, containing the heart, great blood vessels, esophagus, windpipe and associated structures.

Medicaid. Medical Assistance, sometimes referred to as Medicaid, is a program that pays medical care costs for people with low incomes. It differs from Medicare in that it is a State-administered program, aided by Federal funds. Each State decides for itself if it wants the program. Status of the program in a particular State can be learned by checking with the Department of Welfare of the State. More than half the States have initiated programs. Medicaid is designed to provide medical care for needy persons of all ages under a definition of need defined by each State. Eligibility of the individual or family is determined by State provisions. There are State by State differences in who is eligible and for what benefits.

Automatically eligible groups are (1) all persons who receive financial assistance from the federally aided public assistance programs for the aged, the blind, the disabled, and families with dependent children; (2) all persons who would be eligible for financial assistance except that they do not meet certain State conditions—durational residence requirements, for example; (3) all persons under age 21 who, except for a State age or school-attendance requirement, would be eligible for assistance through the program of aid to families with dependent children. A State may also include persons whose income is too high to permit eligibility for financial assistance to meet their daily living expenses but not high enough to meet their medical bills.

Anyone who wishes to apply can get full information about State regulations from the local public welfare agency.

Medical genetics. The science concerned with associations of heredity with defects and disease. See Chapter 25.

Medical specialists. A physician may limit his practice to any branch of medicine he is qualified for. A specialist does not necessarily have to be "Board Certified." Usually, however, after he completes a period of special training and experience in addition to his basic medical education, the physician who wishes to specialize takes written and oral examinations of the American Specialty Board concerned with his specialty. If successful, the candidate becomes a Diplomate of the Board—that is, he holds a diploma and is said to be Board Certified.

The need for a particular specialist cannot always or often be wisely self-determined by the patient, but is a matter for advice by his medical advisers. A reference book called Directory of Medical Specialists, primarily for physicians who wish to check a physician's qualifications, gives the biographies, affiliations, and backgrounds of Board Certified specialists. The book can be consulted at most public libraries.

Medicare. This broad system of health insurance, administered by the Social Security Administration, is for all citizens who have passed their 65th birthday. It is not necessary to have earned wages under Social Security. Persons over 65 who receive a Social Security pension automatically receive a Medicare card; other eligible persons must apply at an office of the Social Security Administration.

There are two parts to Medicare: *Hospital Insurance* (HI) and *Supplementary Medical Insurance* (SMI). HI is free. SMI coverage is voluntary; the subscriber must enroll for it and pay $5.80 a month.

HOSPITAL INSURANCE provides up to 90 days of hospitalization for one illness. The patient pays the first $40 of the hospital bill; after 60 days, he pays $10 a day. The limit is 90 days. But if another illness requiring hospitalization occurs 60 days or more after discharge from a hospital or nursing home, another 90-day period of benefits begins again.

What is covered: hospital room and board in a semi-private room; regular services of nurses, interns, resident physicians; operating room charge; drugs and appliances furnished by the hospital; diagnostic and therapeutic services.

Not covered: Private room, private duty nurses, cost of first three pints of blood for transfusions, extras such as room phone or TV.

Nursing home care. If a Medicare patient is transferred to a qualified nursing home after a hospital stay of at least three days, the cost of semi-private room, board, nursing and other care ordinarily furnished is paid for the first 20 days. For the next 80 days Medicare pays $5 a day. The limit for one illness is 100 days.

There are comparable benefits for hospital outpatients, covering diagnostic services, and for home care after a hospital stay.

SUPPLEMENTARY MEDICAL INSURANCE helps to pay medical bills. The subscriber pays premiums of $5.80 a month, matched by the government. It is important to apply for coverage several weeks before the 65th birthday.

What is covered: Reasonable charges of physicians and surgeons; services, tests, and supplies related to treatment; drugs not administered by the patient; home health services even if the patient is not hospitalized first. The patient pays the first $50 of medical expense in any calendar year; SMI pays 80 per cent of any additional doctor bills for covered services and the patient pays 20 per cent.

Not covered: Eyeglasses, hearing aids, drugs the patient can administer, dentures, routine physical checkups, routine dental care, immunizations, services of chiropractors, naturopaths, chiropodists or optometrists.

Regulations are *subject to change* and latest information should be obtained from a Social Security office well in advance of one's 65th birthday.

Medicare does not cover every penny of hospital and medical expense. Blue Cross and many commercial insurance companies offer policies to take care of costs that Medicare does not pay. These policies are paid for by the individual who must decide if they fit his needs and budget.

Medulla. The inside parts of certain organs, such as glands and bones, as distinguished from the cortex or surface layer of the organ. The word also means "marrow-like."

Medulla oblongata. The lowest part of the brain, where it merges with the spinal cord (241). It resembles a bulb at the end of the spinal cord. It contains vital nerve centers which control such functions as heart action, breathing, and swallowing.

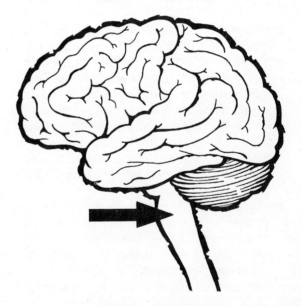

Medulla oblongata.

Megacolon. Gigantic colon. In a congenital form known as *Hirschsprung's disease,* the colon lacks nerve cells necessary for its emptying (486). The symptoms are a greatly enlarged abdomen and intractable constipation; days may go by without a bowel movement. An acquired type of megacolon usually has a psychologic basis; the child refuses to have a bowel movement and the rectum and colon become greatly distended from the mass of retained feces.

Megakaryocyte. A giant cell of the bone marrow. Fragments of this "mother cell" are blood PLATELETS, essential for normal coagulation of blood (159).

Meibomian glands. Sebaceous glands of the eyelid, subject to infection (*sty*) and obstruction (CHALAZION).

Melanin. A yellow to black pigment which is a factor in skin color. It is derived from an AMINO ACID, tyrosine, through the action of an enzyme; if the enzyme is missing the person is an albino. Its production is stimulated by a hormone of the pituitary gland (317). Suntan, freckles, and flat brown spots on the skin of elderly people are examples of melanin deposits.

Melanoma. A dark mole colored by melanin granules. The word often means *malignant melanoma*, a dangerous form of cancer, arising from pigment-producing cells. Many physicians recommend that blue or black moles be removed as a preventive measure. Moles that darken or increase in size or appear after age 30 can be dangerous and should be removed (194).

Melena. Black, tarry stools discolored by presence of blood altered in the intestinal tract, as in bleeding from the stomach or intestines. Melena of the newborn occasionally occurs from seepage of blood into the alimentary tract and is rarely a symptom of disease. Otherwise, passage of tarry stools calls for medical investigation.

Membrane. A thin layer of tissue which lines a part, separates cavities, or connects adjacent structures.

Menarche. The time of first occurrence of menstruation (429). The periods may be irregular while the menstrual cycle (339) is becoming established. In the U. S. the average age at onset of menses is about 13 years; variations of a year on either side of the average are not unusual. If menstruation is not established before or shortly after the sixteenth year, the cause should be investigated.

Meninges. Membranes which cover the brain and spinal cord (248).

Meningitis. Inflammation of the MENINGES (41, 418).

Menopause. Cessation of menses; the milestone which marks the end of a woman's reproductive years (346). The average age at menopause in the U. S. is 48 years, but it is not unusual for women to continue to menstruate up to or beyond 50 years of age. At menopause, menstruation may cease abruptly, or there may be a gradual increase in the number of days between menstrual periods over a year or two. The final menstrual cycles are usually *anovulatory*—that is, no egg cells are produced by the ovaries. Many cycles which occur long before the menopause are probably anovulatory, but this cannot be relied on as assurance against conception. The average menstrual life span is about 33 years, during which a mature egg cell is released from the ovaries every month. Over the years, fewer and fewer cells which develop into ova remain in the ovaries. Along with the dwindling numbers of such cells there is progressive decrease in production of ovarian hormones. "Hot flashes" and other symptoms of the menopause reflect this decline. Most women adjust to the menopause with little difficulty. Perhaps one out of four seeks medical attention for symptoms which are likely to be more annoying than incapacitating. However, symptoms occurring at this time may be wrongly blamed on "the change" and should be investigated to determine the cause, which may be quite unrelated to the menopause.

Menorrhagia. Excessive menstrual bleeding (340).

Merycism. Deliberate regurgitation, rechewing, and reswallowing of food; an innocent habit of some infants and a pernicious one engaged in by some mentally ill persons.

Mescaline. See HALLUCINOGENIC DRUGS.

Mesentery. The flat, fan-shaped sheet of tissue which carries nerves and blood vessels and supports the intestine, from the "handle" of the fan attached to the back wall of the abdomen (458, 728). The arrangement allows considerable freedom of intestinal movement within the abdomen.

Metabolism. The sum total of all the physical and chemical activities by which life processes are organized and maintained; the breakdown and buildup of complex substances by body cells, assimilation of nutrients, and transformations which make energy available to the living organism. *Basal metabolism* is the minimal amount of heat (energy) needed to sustain activities when the body is in a state of rest about 18 hours after eating.

Metaplasia. Alteration of one kind of tissue into another.

Metastasis. Spread of disease from one part of the body to an unconnected part, by transfer of cells or organisms via blood and lymph channels. Ability to metastasize is characteristic of invasive cancer.

Metatarsalgia. Foot pain in the instep area (647), usually due to weakness of muscles and ill-fitting shoes.

Metatarsals. The five long bones of the foot, overlying the longitudinal arch, between toe joints and heel (645).

Meteorism. "Gassiness"; inflation of stomach or intestines with gases. The term comes from a Greek word meaning "to lift off the ground," fairly descriptive of ballooning sensations.

Metritis. Inflammation of the uterus.

Metrorrhagia. Abnormal bleeding from the uterus at times other than the menstrual period.

Microtome. An instrument which cuts extremely thin slices of tissue which are placed on slides, stained, and studied by pathologists.

Micturition. The act of passing urine.

Middle ear. The air-filled bony box between the eardrum and the inner ear. It contains the chain of three tiny bones over which sound vibrations are conducted (583, 595).

Miliaria. Prickly heat, heat rash (190). Obstruction of sweat glands traps sweat under the skin, producing small pricking, burning, tingling, itching pimples. The condition disappears when the stimulus to sweating is removed, as by a cool environment.

Milk leg. A form of THROMBOPHLEBITIS which occasionally occurs a week or two after childbirth. The affected leg swells and the tensed skin has a white appearance, hence the name. Getting out of bed and moving around soon after delivery helps to prevent clot formation in veins. There is very little risk of EMBOLISM in this condition.

Milk line. "Extra" breasts or nipples are congenital anomalies that occur occasionally in men and women. Supernumerary nipples with little or no underlying breast tissue are more common than miniature out-of-place breasts. In some instances, superfluous breasts of women may attain considerable size and even produce milk. The most frequent site of accessory breasts is about three inches below the normal pair, but they may occur anywhere along an imaginary line running from the armpit to the groin on either side. This is called the "milk line," and marks the course of structures which permit the development of multiple breasts in mammals other than man. Development of accessory breasts along this line is determined

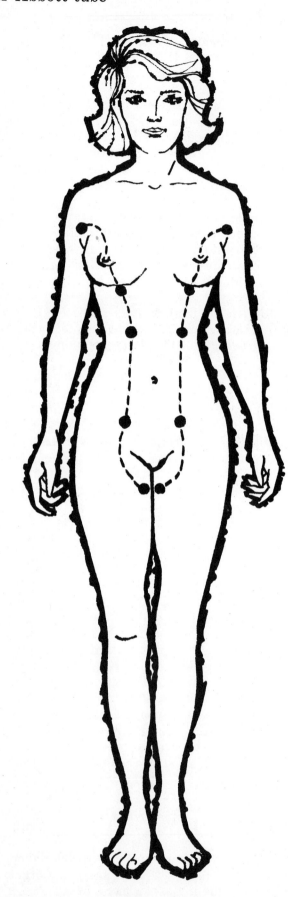

Milk line.

early in fetal life when traces of cells which will develop into distinct parts first appear.

Miller-Abbott tube. A double-channeled tube for insertion through the nose into the stomach to relieve distention of the small bowel. One channel has a small balloon at the end which is inflated in the stomach; peristaltic movements carry the tube farther down. Intestinal contents are withdrawn through the other channel.

Mineralocorticoids. Hormones of the cortex of the adrenal gland which regulate salt and water balances (330).

Minimal brain damage. The term is coming into use as a description of children who appear to lag in development, are hyperactive or listless, and exhibit inappropriate activity.

Miscarriage. Expulsion of the fetus before it is capable of independent life. See ABORTION (361).

Mitochondria. Infinitesimal sausage-shaped particles in body cells; "power plants" of the cell which contain the chemical machinery for generating energy. A typical mitochondrion has an outside membrane and numerous connecting internal folds. The outer membrane extracts energy from molecules derived from food and shunts it to inner membranes which make ATP (*adenosine triphosphate*), the form of energy that keeps life processes going.

Mitral valve. The valve on the left side of the heart which admits oxygenated blood to the main pumping chamber, the left ventricle (103). The valve has two peaked flaps shaped somewhat like a bishop's miter. The valve may be damaged by rheumatic fever so that it leaks, or is scarred and thickened and cannot open widely enough (106). An operation to slit the scarred valves open is called *mitral commisurotomy* (745).

Mittelschmerz. A sign of OVULATION; lower abdominal pain produced by escape of blood into the peritoneal cavity as a result of ovulation, about midway in the menstrual cycle. The nature of the pain is usually identified by absence of any signs of pelvic disease and onset of menses about 14 days later.

Molar pregnancy. See HYDATIDIFORM MOLE.

Molluscum contagiosum. A contagious viral infection of the skin, producing yellowish pulpy pimples containing cheesy material (193).

Mongolian spot. A bluish-dark spot or spots in the region of the lower back, seen in some newborn infants. The congenital spots usually disappear by the fourth or fifth year. Not related to MONGOLISM.

Mongolism. A congenital abnormality which gets its name from the somewhat Oriental appearance of the child (415). Mongoloid babies tend to have upward slanting eyes, broad face, flattened skull, short hands, feet and trunk, stubby nose. The average mongoloid seldom achieves a mental capacity beyond that of a 3 to 7-year-old

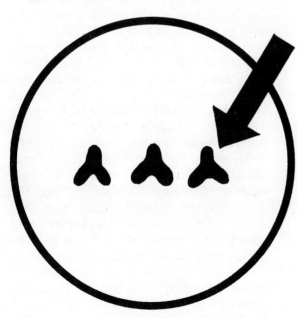

Three instead of the normal two chromosomes in a set (No. 21). This abnormality, called *Trisomy*, is characteristic of mongolism.

child, but is often lively and lovable. Life expectancy is not great. Placement in an institution is often recommended, especially if there are other children in the family. Mongolism results from a specific defect in CHROMOSOMES, called *trisomy*. One set of chromosomes (No. 21) is not a normal pair, but a triplet. The extra "mongolism chromosome" causes defects of physical and mental development. The mongoloid child has 47 instead of the normal complement of 46 chromosomes. The parents are in no way responsible for this accident, which occurs sporadically. See medical genetics, Chapter 25.

Moniliasis. Infection caused by yeastlike organisms, usually *Candida albicans*, which have a predilection for mucous membranes. Common sites of infection are the skin, nails, mouth, vagina, gastrointestinal tract. See vaginal yeast infections (434), in pregnancy (364), thrush (417).

Monocyte. A type of large white blood cell with a single central mass or nucleus (168). *Infectious mononucleosis* gets its name from an excess of such cells, arising from infection.

Monosodium glutamate. A substance used to enhance the flavors of foods. It is a concentrated source of sodium and would not be permitted in diets in which sodium intake must be kept low.

Monozygotic. Developed from a single fertilized egg, as identical twins (378).

Mons veneris. The rounded prominence of fatty tissue above the external female sex organs.

"Montezuma's revenge." A flip name for tourist diarrhea, the gastrointestinal upset of undetermined cause which frequently afflicts visitors to foreign countries until they become adapted.

Morning sickness. The simplest form of nausea of pregnancy (358, 515). Nausea and vomiting usually occur around breakfast time, then subside, only to recur the next morning. The symptom usually persists for two or three weeks and clears up without treatment. The cause is not known, but nothing serious can be afoot since it is estimated that 50 per cent of pregnant women experience a few episodes of morning sickness. A more serious form of vomiting of pregnancy (*hyperemesis gravidarum*) may go on for weeks, produce serious weight loss, and require medical treatment or a period of hospitalization.

Morphinism. Addiction to morphine.

Morton's toe. A form of METATARSALGIA; there is acute pain in the region where the fourth metatarsal bone, next to the little toe, joins the toe joint.

Motion sickness. Nausea and vomiting induced by forms of motion which rotate the head simultaneously in more than one plane (sea sickness, car sickness, train sickness, air sickness). The trouble originates in the labyrinth of the ear where organs of equilibrium are located (586). Confusing impulses reach the vomiting center in the brain. Motion sickness may sometimes be prevented or minimized to some extent by not overeating or overdrinking; by lying down; by taking a position where motion is least exaggerated, as amidships in a vessel; by not reading or looking out a car window or watching a rolling horizon from a boat. A number of drugs help to prevent or lessen motion sickness if taken according to a physician's directions.

Mottled enamel (*dental fluorosis*). Dappled yellow-brown discoloration of enamel of the teeth, produced by high concentrations of fluorides naturally present in drinking water in some parts of the country.

Mountain sickness. A temporary condition brought on by diminished amounts of oxygen in the air at high altitudes. Persons who live at high altitudes adapt to the thin air; their red corpuscles increase in number. Acute mountain sickness is most likely to affect persons who are suddenly transported to high altitudes and do strenuous work. Edward Whymper, the first man to climb the Matterhorn, described an attack of mountain sickness which overcame him and his companions on a trip to the Andes: "I was incapable of making the least exertion. We were feverish, had intense headaches, and were unable to satisfy our desire for air except by breathing with our open mouths. There was no inclination to eat. All found smoking too laborious and ceased the effort in a sort of despair." The symptoms usually abate in a few days to a week.

Mouth breathing. The habit of breathing through the mouth instead of the nose has a drying action on mouth tissues, which become inflamed, sometimes swollen and painful. Habitual mouth breathers may develop abnormal positions of the teeth because the upper teeth get no muscular support from the tongue and lower lip if the mouth is held open continually. Another risk of mouth breathing is an uncommon type of tooth decay, associated with large whitish spots around the gum line of the front teeth, a result of drying of foreign material that collects about the necks of the teeth. Mouth breathers usually have a high incidence of colds and upper respiratory infections because they do not have the normal protection of the filtering, warming, air-conditioning functions of the nose. Some children with short upper lips may keep their mouths partly open while breathing, although they actually breathe through the nose and are not true mouth breathers. Physical factors may encourage mouth breathing. Children with narrow nasal passages, easily "stuffed up" by a minor cold, tend to breathe through the mouth. Enlarged adenoid or tonsil tissue, which normally grows in excess up to about 10 years of age and then diminishes, may obstruct the airway and force the child to breathe through the mouth, which can easily become a habit. A physician or dentist can diagnose mouth breathing easily, determine if there is a physical cause, and help parents to help a child to overcome a harmful habit with unpleasant consequences.

Mucous colitis. Not an organic disease, but the overreaction of an easily irritated colon to various stimuli such as emotions or foods (486). Passage of large amounts of mucus with bowel movements is quite harmless.

Mucous membrane. Mucus-secreting tissue lining the inner walls of body cavities and passages which contain or may contain a certain amount of air and hence could dry out if not moistened. Mucous membranes are quite similar in general design but perform somewhat different functions in various parts of the body. Mucous membranes of the nose warm and moisten air before it reaches the lungs. Membranes of the windpipe are equipped with fine hairlike processes which sweep a thin film of mucus containing trapped particles of dust and dirt outward from the lungs. Membranes of the stomach have special glands concerned with digestion; the membrane of the uterus undergoes periodic changes of engorgement and recession linked with the menstrual cycle.

Mucus. Watery material secreted by mucous membranes, normally thin and unobtrusive, profuse in the presence of colds, and subject to thickening and stickiness if its water content becomes greatly reduced.

Multipara. A woman who has previously given birth to several children.

Multiple births. The statistical chance of a mother's giving birth to twins is about one in 90 and the odds against triplets, quadruplets, or quintuplets are very much greater (377). But averages are not very dependable; twins are more frequent in countries with high birth rates and more frequent among Negroes than white people. There is some tendency for fraternal (two-egg) twins to run in families. Women under age 20 have the lowest incidence of twins and women 35 to 39 the highest. Likelihood of having twins is greater if a woman has already borne children, and greater yet if any of those children were twins. Treatment with gonadotropin hormones to stimulate fertility seems to increase the likelihood of multiple births. Several women so treated have given birth to septuplets; all died within minutes of birth.

Mummification. Drying and shriveling of tissue to a mummy-like mass, a result of dry GANGRENE.

Mumps skin test. A test for susceptibility to mumps, carried out by applying mumps ANTIGEN to the skin of the forearm. It is helpful in determining whether persons in a family exposed to the disease are likely to catch it. A surprising percentage of adults who have no history of having had mumps are in reality immune to the disease.

Mumps vaccine. A new addition to the vaccine family. It is of the attenuated live virus type (see VACCINE) which gives durable and lasting immunity.

Muscae volitantes. "Spots before the eyes"; floating specks like flitting flies or stars (581).

Muscle. About half the body's weight is muscle, remarkable tissue which has one pre-eminent ability: to contract, shorten its length, pull its ends together. Muscle is not like iron, but more like jelly; it is about 80 per cent water and most of the rest is protein. We have three types of muscle, different in function and visibly different under a microscope. Muscles we are most aware of are the big ones that move our bones and make it possible to chew, walk, and execute all manner of graceful or clumsy movements. This type is called *striped*, *voluntary*, or *skeletal* muscle. It has dark and light crossbands giving a striped appearance. Voluntary muscles move when we will them to; their ends are connected to the parts they move. (The only notoriously voluntary muscle that is not attached at both ends is the tongue). Another type of muscle is called *smooth, visceral,* or *involuntary.* It has no cross-striping. It is present in the walls of the digestive tract, blood vessels, bladder, uterus, windpipe and other tissues, where it works without our conscious command. The pupil of the eye changes its size involuntarily; we are propelled into the world by the involuntary contractions of smooth uterine muscles. A third type of muscle is unique. It constitutes the heart muscle (*myocardium*). It is a firm network of fibers connected to one another to function as a unit, in continuous operation. Muscle contraction requires energy, produces heat, and is responsible for most of the body temperature. Even when "resting," muscles are in a constant state of mild contraction (*tonus*). *Muscle cramps* result from too-continuous nerve impulses which keep a muscle in a painful state of contraction. A "pulled muscle" results from tearing or stretching by some massive effort. Exercise increases the size of muscles by enlarging individual cells, not by adding more cells. (Muscle table, 639).

Mutation. A change in the hereditary material of an organism, producing a change in some characteristic of the organism; especially, alteration of the character of a GENE. Mutations may occur spontaneously or they may be induced by some external stimulus, such as irradiation.

Myasthenia gravis. A chronic debilitating disease characterized by rapid fatigue of certain muscles, with prolonged time of recovery of function. Muscles of the eyes and throat are most often affected, producing such symptoms as inability to raise the eyelids, difficulties of swallowing and talking, loss of chewing power, impairment of breathing. The muscles do not waste away. It is thought that the patient lacks some chemical concerned with nerve transmission. A drug called *neostigmine* acts at nerve and muscle fiber junctions to restore considerable muscle power quite rapidly. Many myasthenia gravis patients have an enlarged *thymus gland* (314) or tumors of the thymus. X-ray treatment or surgical removal of the gland has produced some remissions, but results of these treatments for individual patients are not predictable.

Mycetoma. See MADURA FOOT.

Mycoses. Infections caused by fungi (74).

Myelin. White, fatty material which covers most nerve AXONS, in the manner of insulation around an electric wire; it is essential to proper transmission of nerve impulses. Degeneration or disappearance of the myelin sheath is the characteristic lesion of *demyelinating diseases* (263).

Myelitis. Inflammation of the spinal cord or bone marrow. *Poliomyelitis* is inflammation of gray matter of the cord.

Myelogram. An x-ray film of the spinal canal made after injecting a contrast medium opaque to x-rays.

Myeloma, multiple. Malignant tumors of the bone marrow (174).

Myiasis. Infestation with larvae of flies which develop in the skin, eyes, or passages of the ear or nose.

Myocarditis. Inflammation of the heart muscle (105).

Myocardium. The heart muscle; a highly specialized, cross-layered, very powerful involuntary muscle (82). Shutting off of blood supply to a portion of the muscle, as in coronary thrombosis, results in local death of tissue (*infarction*), a common sequel of heart attack.

Myocyte. A muscle cell.

Myoglobin. A form of HEMOGLOBIN, slightly different from that of blood, which is present in muscles and serves as a short-time source of oxygen to tide muscle fibers from one contraction to another.

Myoma. A tumor composed of muscle elements; it is a rather common benign tumor of the uterus (435).

Myometrium. The muscle of the uterus.

Myopathy. Any disease of muscle.

Myopia. Nearsightedness (561).

Myositis. Inflammation of muscle.

Myringitis. Inflammation of the eardrum.

Myringoplasty. Surgical repair of a damaged eardrum.

Myringotomy. Incision of the eardrum to relieve pressure of pus and fluids behind it (595).

Myxedema. Thyroid deficiency, *hypothyroidism* in adults (324). Congenital thyroid deficiency in children is known as *cretinism*. The patient with untreated myxedema has dry, thick, puffy skin, thinning hair, low basal metabolism, is sensitive to cold, thick of speech and mentally sluggish.

Myxoma. A tumor derived from connective tissue.

Myxomatosis. A fatal virus disease of rabbits; no threat to human beings.

N

Narcissism. Self-love, undue admiration of one's own body; a psychologic term indicating self-admiration fixed at a level appropriate to infants but not to adults. The word comes from a character in Greek mythology who saw his image reflected in a pool and was forever after enamored of it.

Narcolepsy. Irrestible attacks of sleep, often with transient muscular weakness. Attacks occur during normal waking hours, not only under conditions conducive to drowsiness—after a heavy meal, during a dull lecture, riding on a train—but in inappropriate and even hazardous circumstances, as in driving a car. The affected person usually sleeps a few minutes, wakes refreshed, but may fall asleep again in a short time. The sleep does not differ from normal sleep except in its untimeliness; there are no signs of disease or physical abnormality. Treatment with amphetamine drugs is usually successful in warding off attacks of somnolence during the day.

Narcosis. A state of deep sleep, unconsciousness, and insensibility to pain. *Narcotics* are drugs that produce such effects. Such drugs are very important in medicine, but if misused can lead to true drug addiction.

Nares. The nostrils.

Narcosynthesis. A method of treating psychoneuroses by intravenous injection of a hypnotic drug which induces the patient to dredge up suppressed emotional material.

Nasopharynx. The top part of the throat behind the nasal cavity (607).

Nates. The buttocks.

Nausea of pregnancy. See MORNING SICKNESS.

Near point. The point closest to the eye where an object, such as fine print, is seen distinctly. The near point is too far away when a newspaper has to be held at arm's length to read it, at the time of life when the lens of the eye has lost some of its flexibility and glasses for efficient close vision become desirable.

Necropsy. Autopsy; a post-mortem examination.

Necrosis. Death of a localized portion of tissue surrounded by living tissue.

Negri bodies. Round or oval particles in certain cells of animals dead of *rabies* (56). Their presence is proof that the animal had rabies.

Neisserian infection. Usually means infection with gonorrhea germs, *Neisseria gonorrhoeae* (40).

Neonatal. Newborn; the first two or three days of life.

Neoplasm. Any abnormal new growth; a tumor which may be malignant or benign. "Neoplastic disease" is a common term for cancer.

Nephrectomy. Surgical removal of a kidney.

Nephritis. Inflammation of the kidney, not as a direct result of infection (292).

Nephrolith. Kidney stone.

Nephroma. Malignant tumor of the cortex of the kidney.

Nephron. The urine-forming unit of the kidney (283). It consists of a double-walled cup-shaped structure (*Bowman's capsule*) within which a tuft of tiny blood vessels (*glomerulus*) exudes blood constituents which pass as a dilute filtrate into the tubule of the capsule. Most of the water and some essential materials in the filtrate are reabsorbed and the remainder is concentrated as urine.

Nephropexy. Surgical anchoring of a "loose" or floating kidney.

Nephrosclerosis. Nephritis due to hardening of kidney blood vessels (293).

Nephrosis. Degeneration of the kidney without signs of inflammation; usually refers to nephrotic disease of children (293).

Nephrotoxic. Poisonous to the kidneys.

Nerve. Any of the cordlike bundles of fibers, composed of microscopic neurons, along which nerve impulses travel. See Chapter 7.

Nerve deafness. Impairment of hearing from partial or complete failure of auditory nerves to transmit impulses to hearing centers in the brain (589).

Nettlerash. Hives, urticaria (692).

Neuralgia. Severe pain in a nerve or along its course, without demonstrable change in the structure of the nerve (267). The pain is typically sharp, stabbing, excruciating, though short-lasting.

Neurasthenia. A somewhat out-of-fashion term for a state of great fatigability, listlessness, aches and pains, once attributed to depletion or exhaustion of nerve centers, but without any demonstrable abnormality of the nervous system. Nerves do not become screamingly twisted or come apart like frayed ropes, although such misbehavior is popularly attributed to them. Neurasthenic symptoms may have some organic cause and medical examination may disclose some treatable condition quite unrelated to nerves. If not, the label "neurasthenia" indicates a functional disorder with a psychic basis.

Neuritis. Inflammation of a nerve or its parts due to infection, toxins, compression, or other causes.

Neurodermatitis. A chronic skin condition of unknown cause, not related to infection or allergy. It occurs most frequently in nervous women and may have a neurotic basis. Itchy patches of thickened skin (see LICHENIFICATION) occur especially on the neck, the inner surface of the elbows, and the back of the knees. Treatment to relieve itching and discourage rubbing of the skin helps to alleviate the condition.

Neurofibromatosis. A condition of multiple, painless soft tumors in the skin along nerve pathways. The tumors, mainly composed of fibrous material, tend to increase in size and number. The growths are not cancerous, but very rarely may undergo malignant transformation. Frequently the tumors can be removed surgically, often permanently, although in some cases they have a tendency to recur. The disorder is thought to be hereditary.

Neurogenic. Of nervous origin.

Neuron. The complete nerve cell, including the cell body, *dendrites* which bring incoming impulses to the body, and the *axon* which carries impulses away from it (242).

Neuropsychiatry. The medical specialty concerned with both nervous and mental disorders and their overlappings.

Neurosis. See PSYCHONEUROSIS.

Neurosyphilis. A late stage of syphilis affecting the central nervous system (48).

Neutrophil. A type of white blood cell stainable by neutral dyes (142). *Neutropenia* is a condition of scarcity of such cells in the blood (162).

Nevus. A local area of pigmentation or elevation of the skin; a mole, a birthmark.

Nictitation. Winking.

Nidation. "Nesting"; implantation of a fertilized egg in the uterus.

Nidus. A nest; a point of origin or focus.

Nieman-Pick disease. A rare hereditary condition occurring almost exclusively in children of Jewish families (173). It is a disorder of LIPID metabolism (inability to handle fatlike substances) which progresses to anemia, emaciation, mental retardation, blindness and deafness. Affected children rarely survive their second year. There is no treatment. The disease is inherited as a recessive trait.

Night blindness (*nyctalopia*). Imperfect vision at night or in dim light; reduced dark adaptation. The symptom may result from deficiency of vitamin A, which is necessary for regeneration of nerve cells of the retina (rods) which do most of the work of seeing when light is poor (504, 556). Certain diseases of the retina can also cause night blindness.

Nitrogen balance. An expression of the body's PROTEIN balance, determined by measurements of its nitrogen constituents. If nitrogen intake exceeds excretion, the balance is positive. Excessive retention of nitrogen may indicate kidney disease or other conditions. Negative nitrogen balance may indicate inadequate dietary protein, excessive loss of protein due to toxic goiter, burns, draining wounds, etc., impaired absorption of protein, or defective metabolism of protein as in some liver diseases.

Nitrogen mustard. A drug used to destroy malignant cells in lymphomatous diseases.

Nitrous oxide. Laughing gas; an inhalant for producing brief anesthesia, as for tooth extraction.

Nocturia. Excessive urination at night.

Node. A small protuberance, swelling, rounded knob, knot of cells. A *nodule* is a small node.

Nodular goiter. Enlargement of the thyroid gland characterized by lumpy masses on the surface or in the substance of the gland (326).

Nonviable. Incapable of living.

Normotension. Normal blood pressure.

Nosocomial. Pertaining to a hospital.

Nuchal. Pertaining to or in the region of the nape of the neck.

Nuclear medicine. This young, developing, changing branch of medicine got a foothold when RADIOISOTOPES produced in nuclear reactors became available on a large scale. Radioisotopes of an element "decay" spontaneously—ultimately revert to a stable atom—and in the process give off energy in the form of radiation which is detectable by very sensitive devices. Thus, substances "tagged" or labeled with radioisotopes (for example, radioactive iodine, phosphorus, chromium) can be followed in their course through the body, giving information about chemical processes of life. Drugs can be tagged to gain new knowledge of how they work. There are now about 120 different tests and 60 clinical procedures that can be performed with radioactive materials. Recently developed *scintillation cameras* translate isotope emissions into dots on film, giving a pattern of radiation within a patient's body. Certain tissues are selective for certain elements; the thyroid gland, for instance, is avid for iodine. Radioisotopes which tend to concentrate in such tissues may be given with the object of destroying or reducing the functioning of cells. Diagnostically, radioisotopes help to measure the functional abilities of certain tissues, are useful in evaluating some blood disorders, and in locating and marking the boundaries of tumors.

Nucleus. The rounded central body of a cell, surrounded by cytoplasm. It contains the CHROMOSOMES and mechanisms of cell division and heredity.

Nummular eczema. Dry skin with coin-shaped plaques on the back of the hands and outer surfaces of the arms, legs, and thighs (188).

Nullipara. A woman who has never borne a child.

Nyctalopia. See NIGHT BLINDNESS.

Nymphomania. Insatiable sexual desire of a female (348).

Nystagmus. Involuntary, rhythmic oscillation of the eyeballs, horizontal, ver-

tical, or rotary. Most persons experience nystagmus if the body is whirled to produce dizziness and an attempt is made to fix the gaze on a stationary object. Simple forms of nystagmus can result from eye strain or refractive errors (561). Nystagmus may be a symptom of inner ear disturbance or disorder of the nervous system.

O

Obesity operations. Occasionally, a surgeon may deem it feasible to remove a huge apron of fat from an obese person. More drastic and controversial is the "intestinal bypass" operation for weight reduction. In principle, the operation permits an obese person to eat all he wants but still lose weight by preventing the assimilation of substantial amounts of food (and calories). This is accomplished by connecting a short part of the small intestine to the colon, leaving behind a non-functioning loop of the small intestine, thus bypassing a considerable area in which food assimilation normally occurs. A variation of the operation consists of cutting out a part of the small intestine, without leaving a bypassed loop. These procedures do lead to weight reduction by leaving the patient incapable of absorbing some of the food he eats, but there is risk of early and late complications. Liver degeneration, anemia, malnutrition, congestive heart failure and a variety of metabolic disturbances have been reported to have occurred sometime after a bypass operation. Until further study reveals why such complications occur and how they can be prevented, the bypass operation for obesity must be considered to be somewhat risky.

Obstetric forceps. Two curved flat blades (right and left) which are separately placed with great care around the head of the fetus in the birth passage; the handles are then interlocked (383). Used to assist extraction of the baby in difficult deliveries.

Occiput. The back part of the head.

Occlusion. Closure or shutting off, as of a blood vessel; also, the meeting position of upper and lower teeth when closed (533).

Occult. Hidden, not evident to the naked eye; as, occult blood in feces.

Ocular. Pertaining to the eye.

Ocular muscle imbalance. Disharmony of muscles which move the eyeball (552). Associated with such conditions as cross-eye, wall-eye, poor fusion of images, amblyopia (566).

Oculist. Same as OPHTHALMOLOGIST.

"Oil" pneumonia. See ASPIRATION PNEUMONIA.

Olecranon. A curved part of one of the forearm bones (*ulna*) at the elbow end. It is what we lean on when we rest an elbow on a table.

Olfactory bulb. A structure just above the thin bone which separates the top of the nasal cavity from the brain. It receives nerve fibers that pass upward through small holes in the bone from the "smell area" of the nose (604).

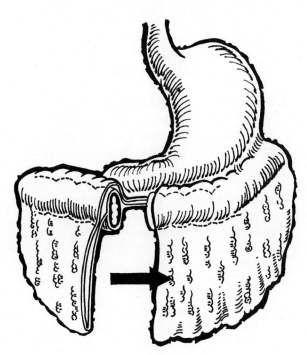

Omentum.

Oligomenorrhea. Scanty menstrual flow, or abnormally long time between menstrual periods.

Oligophrenia. Mental deficiency, feeble-mindedness.

Oligospermia. Abnormally few SPERMATOZOA in the semen.

Oliguria. Scanty secretion of urine; abnormal infrequency of urination.

Omentum. A layer of tissue, a fold of the peritoneum, that hangs from the stomach and transverse colon and covers the underlying organs like an apron. It forms a fat pad on the front of the abdomen, sometimes conspicuously thick.

Omphalic. Pertaining to the navel.

Omphalotomy. Cutting of the umbilical cord; for most people, their first surgical experience.

Onchocerciasis. A form of FILARIASIS occurring in tropical areas. Infection with threadlike worms produces tumors in the skin and sometimes blinding disease of the eyes.

Oncology. The science of tumors, new growths.

Onychia. Inflammation of the bed of a nail, often resulting in loss of the nail.

Onychophagy. Nail-biting.

Ophthalmia. Inflammation of the eye, especially with involvement of the conjunctiva (569).

Ophthalmologist. A doctor of medicine specializing in medical and surgical care of the eyes (559).

Ophthalmoscope. An instrument which gives a magnified view of structures of the eye (560).

Opiates. Narcotics derived from or related to opium; for example, morphine, heroin, codeine, paregoric, laudanum. In a broad sense the word applies to any sense-dulling, stupor-inducing drug.

Opisthotonos. A position of the body in which the head and lower legs are bent backward and the trunk arched forward, due to convulsive spasm of muscles of the back, such as is produced by strychnine poisoning.

Optic atrophy. Irreversible degeneration of optic nerve fibers.

Optic chiasm. An arrangement of nerve fibers in which the optic nerves of both eyes cross at a junction near the pituitary gland (557).

Optic disk. The area at the back of the eye where all the nerve fibers of the retina merge with the optic nerve (579). Because light is not perceived at the point where the optic nerve enters the eye, the area is a normal BLIND SPOT.

Optician. A skilled technician who fills the prescription of an ophthalmologist or optometrist for glasses or contact lenses; a manufacturer or designer of optical equipment.

Optic nerve. A bundle of a million or so nerve fibers which transmits impulses from the RETINA to the occipital lobe at the back of the head where they are transformed into vision.

Optometrist. An expert qualified to fit and prescribe glasses and contact lenses and give non-medical care of the eyes (559).

Oral contraceptives. STEROID compounds taken by mouth by women to prevent conception; "the pill" (347). The tablets contain combinations of estrogen-progestogen or they may be "sequential," furnishing estrogen alone on certain days of the cycle, followed by combined estrogen-progestogen. Regularity of dosage is very important.

Orbit. The bony socket that contains the eyeball (551).

Orchidectomy. Castration; surgical removal of the testicles. The operation leaves the patient sterile.

Orchitis. Inflammation of the testicles. It may be a complication of mumps.

Organ of Corti. The center of the sense of hearing in the inner ear. It contains feathery cells which oscillate in response to pulsating fluids, stimulating nerve endings which merge into the nerve of hearing that carries impulses to receiving centers in the brain.

Organic disease. Disease that has a physical cause, a lesion, disorder of an organ, as opposed to FUNCTIONAL DISEASE.

Orgasm. The climax of the sexual act, terminating in ejaculation of semen by the male and release of tension in the female (432).

Oriental sore (*cutaneous Leishmaniasis*). Single or multiple skin ulcers produced by infection with organisms transmitted by sandflies (73).

Orifice. The opening, entrance, or outlet of a body cavity or passage.

Ornithosis (*parrot fever, psittacosis*). A pneumonia-like disease produced by viruses from infected birds (57).

Orthodontics. "Tooth straightening"; the branch of dental science concerned with prevention and correction of irregularities of the teeth and jaws (543).

Orthopedics. The surgical and medical specialty concerned with correction of deformities, diseases, accidents and disorders of body parts that move us about—limbs, bones, joints, muscles, tendons, etc.

Orthopnea. The need to sit upright in order to breathe comfortably, manifested by persons with congestive heart failure (100).

Orthopsychiatry. A division of psychiatry concerned with "straightening out" disorders of behavior and personality, especially in children.

Orthoptics. Teaching, training, and exercise programs for improving the fusion of images from both eyes (as in cross-eyes), putting a "lazy eye" back to work, and generally making visual mechanisms more efficient (567, 581).

Orthostatic. Induced or intensified by standing upright; for example, *orthostatic hypotension,* a lowering of blood pressure brought on by changing from a lying-down to an upright position.

Osgood-Schlatter disease. Degeneration of a natural protuberance on the knee-end of the TIBIA, the long bone of the lower leg. A form of OSTEOCHONDRITIS, occurring most frequently in young persons.

Osmosis. The phenomenon of transfer of materials through a semipermeable membrane that separates two solutions, or between a solvent and a solution, tending to equalize their concentrations. *Osmotic pressure* is that exerted by the movement of a solvent through a semipermeable membrane into a more concentrated solution on the other side. This pressure is the driving force that causes diffusion of particles in solution to move from one place to another. Walls of living cells are semipermeable membranes and much of the activity of the cells depends upon osmosis.

Osseous. Composed of bone or resembling bone; bony.

Ossicle. One of the three tiny bones of the middle ear (*malleus, incus, stapes*) which conduct sound vibrations to the inner ear (584).

Ossification. The process of forming bone. CARTILAGE is made into bone by the process of ossification. Calcium and phosphorus are deposited in the cartilage, changing it into bone.

Osteitis. Inflammation of bone.

Osteitis deformans. A chronic process of bone overgrowth, destruction, and new bone formation, ultimately producing deformities; PAGET'S DISEASE (651). The skull and weight-bearing bones are most commonly affected.

Osteochondritis. Inflammation of both bone and CARTILAGE. *Osteochondritis dissecans* is a fairly common condition of late adolescence in which there is local death of a section of the joint surface of a bone (usually of the knee) and its overlying cartilage (643). *Osteochondritis deformans juvenilis* (Perthe's disease) is a degenerative condition of the upper end of the thigh bone in children three to eight years of age, which eventually heals but may leave some permanent deformity of the hip joint (640).

Osteogenesis imperfecta. A rare hereditary condition of defective formation of bony tissues, resulting in brittle bones which fracture easily.

Osteomalacia. Adult RICKETS; softening of bone, abnormal flexibility, brittleness, loss of calcium salts. Usually due to vitamin D deficiency or impaired absorption of nutrients; rare in the U. S. (650).

Osteomyelitis. Infection of bone and marrow due to growth of germs within the bone. Infection may reach the bone through the bloodstream or direct injury (38, 624).

Osteoporosis. Enlargement of canals or spaces in bone, giving a porous, thinned appearance. The weakened bone is fragile and may be broken by some minor injury or may fracture spontaneously. The condition is relatively common in women after the menopause and occurs to some degree in all aging persons (650). Recent evidence indicates that drinking water with adequate fluoride content helps to prevent the condition; see FLUORIDES.

Osteotome. A specialized surgical instrument used for cutting through bone.

Otalgia. Earache.

Otitis. Inflammation of the ear. *Otitis externa* is a bacterial or fungal infection of the ear canal (594). *Otitis media* is an acute or chronic infection of the middle ear (595).

Otoplasty. Plastic surgery for correction of malformed ears. See PROTRUDING EARS.

Otorhinolaryngologist. A medical specialist in diseases of the ear, nose, and throat. An *otologist* confines himself to the ear.

Otorrhea. Chronic, malodorous discharge from the ear (595).

Otosclerosis. Overgrowth in parts of the middle ear of spongy bone which "freezes" sound-conducting mechanisms to some degree, dampens vibrations, and impairs hearing (589). This type of hearing loss is often correctible by surgery which restores the vibration-transmitting system to good working order (591).

Otoscope. A funnel-ended instrument with a light source for inspecting the ear canal and eardrum (595).

Oval window. A membrane-covered opening to the inner-ear, to which the footplate of the STAPES is attached (584). Sounds conducted by the chain of bones in the middle ear are "hammered" against the oval window and transmitted to fluids behind it and thence to the inner ear.

Ovarian cyst. A sac containing fluid or mucoid material arising in the ovary (436, 735). A cyst with a stem may become twisted and produce sudden severe pain in the lower abdomen.

Ovariectomy. Surgical removal of one or both ovaries (735). Also called *oophorectomy.*

Oviducts. The tubes through which the egg cell is transported to the uterus, and in which fertilization usually occurs (367). Same as *Fallopian tubes.*

Ovulation. Release of a mature egg cell from the follicle in the ovary in which it develops (339). This is the time during the menstrual cycle when conception can occur. There are no infallible signs of ovulation that a woman can unfailingly recognize, but there are suggestive signs. Ovulation usually occurs about midway between menstrual periods in a normal menstrual cycle of approximately 28 days. Body temperature tends to rise sharply, though to small degree, at the time of ovulation. Abdominal pain and a pinkish discharge from the vagina may also occur at the time of ovulation; see INTERMENSTRUAL PAIN, "SHOW" and MITTELSCHMERZ.

Ovum. The female reproductive cell; an egg. The ovum is the largest human cell but it is barely discernible by the naked eye. It is about one-fourth the size of the period at the end of this sentence. It is a round cell with a clear shell-like capsule, with the consistency of stiff jelly, weighing about a 50-billionth of an ounce—the "original weight" of every human being (the weight of the much smaller fertilizing sperm scarcely counts). Like the sperm, the ovum contains only 23 CHROMOSOMES, which at conception "pair off" with those of the sperm to give the embryo a normal complement of 46 chromosomes. Although the ovum is about 85,000 times larger than the sperm, both contain the same number of GENES. The relatively huge size of the ovum is partly accounted for by its content of nutrient yolk globules. Only about 400 ova ripen to maturity and are released by ovulation during a woman's reproductive lifetime; of these, only a very few are fertilized.

Outpatient. A patient who comes to a hospital for treatment but does not reside there.

Oxyhemoglobin. HEMOGLOBIN carrying a full load of oxygen; the hemoglobin in bright red arterial blood.

Oxytocin. A hormone of the pituitary gland which stimulates the uterus to contract. It is frequently administered by slow drip into a vein in order to stimulate labor and insure effective contractions (383).

Oxyuriasis. Pinworm infection (71).

Ozena. A chronic disease of mucous membranes of the nose, giving off a very foul-smelling odor or discharge.

P

Pacemaker. A small knot of tissue in the right auricle of the heart which triggers the heartbeat (81). In certain heart disorders, battery-powered devices connected to the heart can take over the pacemaking function. See CARDIAC PACEMAKER.

Pachydermatous. Thick skinned.

Paget's disease. Two diseases bear this name. *Paget's disease of the breast* is manifested by thickened, eczema-like scaliness of the area around the nipple, with fissuring, oozing, and destruction of the nipple as the underlying disease (cancer of the central ducts of the breast) advances. The other Paget's disease, also known as *osteitis deformans*, is a chronic disease of bone metabolism. The skull, pelvis, spine, and long bones are especially affected. Calcium is lost from the bones, which become soft and bend easily. Irregular replacement of calcium causes thickening and deformity. Bone pain, impaired hearing, and muscle cramps are frequent symptoms. The disease progresses slowly and after many years may lead to chronic invalidism.

Painful menstruation, exercises. Primary dysmenorrhea (348) is characterized by pain, cramps, or mild to severe discomfort occurring at the onset of menstrual periods, in the absence of any organic disorder. Physical exercises may help to banish distress. Any exercise which involves systematic twisting, bending, and extending of the trunk is helpful. The following simple exercises can be performed in ordinary clothing without equipment: 1. Stand upright, arms raised sideward at shoulders, trunk turned to left. Keep the knees straight, twist and bend the trunk downward, touch left foot with right hand, try to touch outside of heel of right foot. Repeat with trunk turned to right— each side as a unit. 2. Stand upright, arms at sides, feet parallel. Swing both arms upward and forward, at the same time raising one leg vigorously backward. Repeat with other leg. Do the exercises three times a day, exercising each side several times at each session.

Painful shoulder syndrome. Limitation of motion and pain about the shoulder may arise from injury, calcium deposits, bursitis, osteoarthritis, degeneration of tissues, diseases of the chest, coronary heart disease. The predominant symptom is severe pain in the shoulder area and inability to raise the arm because of pain and weakness (654).

Painter's colic. LEAD POISONING.

Palliative. Relieving pain, suffering, or distressing symptoms of disease but without any curative action.

Palpation. A method of obtaining information about a patient's condition by manipulating or feeling a part of the body with the hand.

Palpebral. Pertaining to the eyelid.

Palpitation. Throbbing, "pounding," rapid or fluttery heartbeat, sufficiently out of the ordinary to make the patient aware of it. More often than not the condition is temporary and not of serious import, but there are many causes and if the symptom is repeated or alarming it should be investigated (108).

Palsy. Slight or moderate paralysis.

Pancreatitis. Inflammation of the pancreas gland. It occurs in acute and chronic forms (481).

Pandemic. A super-epidemic, one that occurs on a large scale over a very wide area of a country or of the world.

Panhypopituitarism. Severe loss of function of the anterior pituitary gland (320). See SIMMONDS' DISEASE; SHEEHAN'S DISEASE.

Panniculus. A layer of fat beneath the skin; the layer on the front of the abdomen sometimes expands the waistline quite noticeably.

Panophthalmitis. Pus-producing inflammation of all the tissues of the eye, threatening total and permanent blindness.

Papanicolaou smear (*"Pap test"*). A screening test for cancer of the cervix and the uterus, employing CYTOLOGIC DIAGNOSIS. Cell scrapings obtained painlessly from the surface of the cervix are spread on glass slides, stained, and examined under a microscope. Detection of cancer cells in the specimen, and confirmation of cancer of the cervix by other diagnostic measures, leads to prompt treatment of a form of cancer which in its early stages is almost invariably curable (440). (See illustration, opposite page).

Papilla. A small conical or nipple-shaped elevation, like a pimple. Papillae give the front of the tongue its velvety appearance, and orderly lines of papillae projecting into the upper skin layer give us our fingerprints.

Papilledema (*choked disk*). Non-inflammatory swelling of the optic nerve where it enters the eye, due to increased pressures within the skull or interference with flow of blood from veins of the eye. It occurs most frequently in patients with brain tumor, brain abscess, or meningitis; concussion or hemorrhage may also be responsible. Vision is good in early stages but gradually deteriorates. Treatment depends on detection of the underlying cause.

Papilloma. A tumor of surface-lining tissues—skin, mucous membranes, glandular ducts—composed of epithelial cells covering supporting papillae. It is usually benign.

Papule. A small solid elevation on the skin; a solid pimple containing no pus or fluid.

Paracentesis. Surgical puncture of a body cavity to withdraw fluid.

Paraffin packs. A way of heating body parts, especially painful arthritic hands, giving sustained deep penetration of heat. The hands are dipped into melted paraffin until a thick heat-retaining layer is built up (29).

Paralytic ileus. Intestinal obstruction resulting from decreased peristaltic activity of the bowel (483).

Paranoia. A form of mental illness characterized by suspiciousness, delusions, feelings of being persecuted, spied upon, endangered. The patient's delusions are so systematized and seemingly logical that they can be quite convincing to others, especially since the paranoid patient often seems quite sane and reasonable except on one or a few subjects. Mild paranoid trends are not uncommon in suspicious people who think others "have it in for them," put obstacles in their way, and are responsible for their failures, but the extreme paranoid, who may do violence to his supposed persecutors, has a severe mental illness (707).

Paraplegia. Paralysis of both legs, usually due to injury or disease of the spinal cord. The bladder, bowels and other organs may be paralyzed as well

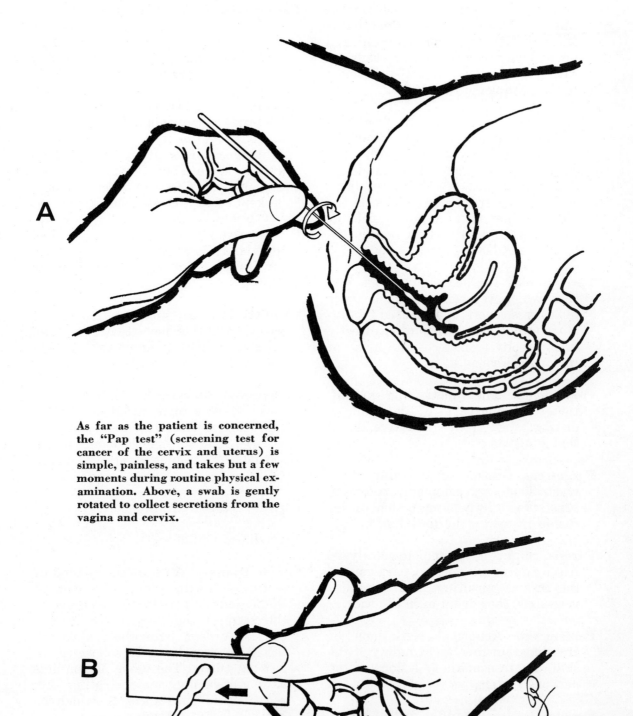

A

As far as the patient is concerned, the "Pap test" (screening test for cancer of the cervix and uterus) is simple, painless, and takes but a few moments during routine physical examination. Above, a swab is gently rotated to collect secretions from the vagina and cervix.

B

Secretions containing cast-off cells are transferred to a glass slide, stained, and examined under a microscope by cytologists trained to recognize normal and abnormal cells. If some cells appear to be malignant, other tests are done to rule out or confirm the presence of cancer.

as the legs, depending on the controlling part of the nervous system that is injured. Rehabilitation training and devices may restore a good measure of satisfying function and self-sufficiency to the paraplegic patient.

Parathyroid glands. Four bead-size glands embedded superficially on the back and side surfaces of both lobes of the thyroid gland. The glands secrete hormones which maintain a stable concentration of calcium in the blood. Either an excess or deficiency produces mild to serious bodily disturbances (328).

Paratyphoid. An acute infectious disease which resembles typhoid fever but is less severe. It is caused by *Salmonella* bacteria transmitted directly or indirectly from feces and urine of infected persons (420).

Parenchyma. The functioning, specialized, "working part" of an organ, as distinguished from connective tissue that supports it.

Parenteral. Outside of the alimentary tract. The word commonly refers to substances given by injection or infusion instead of by mouth.

Paresis. Slight or incomplete paralysis. Also, a term for general paralysis of the insane, resulting from syphilis, rare since the advent of antibiotics.

Paresthesia. Abnormal sensations of crawling, burning, and tingling of the skin, due to neuritis or lesions of the nervous system.

Parietal. Pertaining to the wall of a cavity; especially, the bones of the skull at the top and sides of the head behind the frontal bones (618).

Parkinson's disease (*parkinsonism*). A chronic progressive disease of which the chief symptoms are tremor, stiffness, and slowness of movement, resulting from disturbance of a small center at the base of the brain (251).

Paronychia. Pus-producing infection of tissues around the nails, caused by yeasts (200) or bacteria. Acute bacterial paronychia is usually treated by hot saline soaks and antibiotics administered by the physician. Surgical drainage may be necessary. Chronic bacterial paronychia may require prolonged treatment with hot soaks, drainage, and local application of an antibiotic ointment. During treatment the involved finger or fingers should be kept as dry as possible.

Parotid gland. One of the saliva-producing glands, located in the angle of the jaw in front of and below the ear (452).

Parotitis. Mumps; inflammation of the parotid gland. A new MUMPS VACCINE gives long-lasting immunity; a skin test detects susceptibility.

Paroxysmal tachycardia. Periodic attacks of extremely rapid beating of the heart, as many as 300 beats per minute. Attacks may last only a few seconds or as long as several hours (109).

Parrot fever. See PSITTACOSIS.

Parturition. Childbirth.

Passive transfer. An indirect method of testing for skin allergies. Serum of the patient is introduced into areas of the skin of another person, and a couple of days later these sites are tested for reactions to suspected allergens (683). The other person acts as a guinea pig, demonstrating skin reactions to substances to which he himself is not allergic.

Patch test. A method of identifying allergic sensitivities by applying suspected material to the skin, leaving it uncovered, or more often covering it with a bandage (683).

Patella. The kneecap (537).

Patent. Wide open.

Paternity tests. Blood groups (147) are determined by unvarying laws of HEREDITY. This is the basis of tests for excluding paternity. If a child's red blood cells contain substances called "factors" which are incompatible with the blood groups of its presumed parents, one of the couple cannot be the father or the other cannot be the mother. A person with AB blood cannot have a child of group O; a person of group O cannot have a child of group AB; a person of group M cannot have a child of group N. Presence or absence of a number of other factors follows the same hereditary rules. The blood factors of the mother, child, and putative father are determined by sensitive tests using antiserums and red blood cells known to contain A, B, O, M or N factors. If the factor tested for is present, the red cells clump together; if it is absent they do not. Tests cannot prove that a man *is* the father of a certain child. They can only prove that he cannot be, and they cannot always do that because by coincidence his blood may contain the same factors as the actual father. The chance that non-paternity can be proved is a little better than 50 per cent. Only three blood groups (ABO, MN, Rh-Hr) are used for medicolegal purposes, but several other factors are known and it is theoretically possible to distinguish 50,000 different blood group combinations. Indeed, it is believed that blood is as individual as fingerprints, a testament of personal uniqueness, and when its subtle chemical markers are more fully revealed it may become possible to determine that a child is the offspring of a particular couple.

Pathogenic. Having the capacity to produce disease. Many bacteria are harmless and even beneficial to man, but the vicious sorts that cause disease are pathogenic organisms.

Pathology. The science and study of the nature of disease: its processes, effects, causes, manifestations; changes from normal in structure and function. Pathology does not mean "disease," but its study. The word is often misused. Even the reports of some doctors, who mean to say that an examined patient is free from disease, state that "no pathology was found." *Pathologists* examine stained cells and tissues, do autopsies, and employ chemical and laboratory methods to assist in diagnosis of disease, identify normal and abnormal structures, and to add to scientific knowledge of disease processes in general.

Pectoral. Pertaining to the chest.

Pedicle graft. A flap of a patient's own skin attached to the body by a stalk or pedicle containing intact blood vessels that supply nourishment while the flap is "taking hold" in an area to which it is grafted (770).

Pediculosis. Infestation with body lice (201).

Pellagra. A DEFICIENCY DISEASE manifested by rough skin, sore mouth and tongue, sometimes mental disturbance (504).

Pelvimetry. Measurement of the dimensions of the bony pelvis, usually done to determine whether the outlet between the two bones that rim the birth passage is of sufficient size to permit the fetus to pass into the world (360).

Pelvis. A basin-shaped cavity, especially that formed by bones in the hip region. The bony pelvis supports the spinal column, rests on the legs, and contains structures of the lower end of the trunk (619). The *kidney pelvis* is a cavity which collects urine from the organ's filtration units and funnels the urine to the ureter and thence to the bladder (285). The female bony pelvis is slightly different and distinguishable from that of the male.

Pemphigus. An uncommon but serious disease manifested by crops of large blisters which rupture and leave raw surfaces (198).

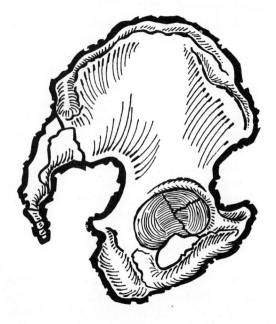

Side view of left half of the bony pelvis; the "tailbone" is at extreme lower left of drawing.

Penicillin reactions. The major single cause of systemic reactions to drugs is penicillin. Reactions occur in persons previously sensitized to the drug by therapeutic doses, or sometimes by indirect contact, as in milk products. The most serious and fortunately the most rare reaction is ANAPHYLAXIS; its most common pattern is acute breathing difficulty, swelling of the larynx threatening suffocation, profound shock. This reaction occurs within seconds or minutes after administration of penicillin to sensitized patients. Far more common and less serious, but distressing, are skin reactions such as rash, hives and itching. SCRATCH TESTS on persons with no previous history of penicillin sensitization may be performed before administering the drug, but if patients with past histories of penicillin sensitivity are to be tested, emergency treatment facilities should be immediately available.

Penis. The male sex organ.

Pepsin. A protein-digesting enzyme in gastric juices. It is active only in an acid environment, which the stomach provides (454).

Peptic ulcer. An ulcer associated with the digestive action of acid juices; it may be located in the stomach or duodenum, or at the site of surgical joining of the stomach and jejunum. The most frequent form is duodenal ulcer (475).

Percomorph. Refers to fish of the perch family. Percomorph oil, prepared from the livers of such fish, is a concentrated source of Vitamin D.

Percussion. A method of physical diagnosis. Short firm blows are tapped upon a body surface by a finger or small hammer to produce sounds or vibrations. Solid, fluid-filled, tense, empty, or congested organs have different resonances, just as an empty barrel sounds different when tapped than a barrel full of water. Percussion is most often applied in examinations of the chest and back.

Perennial allergic rhinitis. A condition similar to hay fever but running a more or less continuous course without seasonal variations (689).

Perforated eardrum. The eardrum may be punctured by direct injury (never stick hairpins or toothpicks into the ear canal!) or by infections of the middle ear which break through the drum. A punctured eardrum may heal itself, close the openings, but if not, a route of invasion of infectious material from the outside world is wide open. A person with a punctured eardrum should not dive or swim or get the head under water because of danger that infectious material may be forced into internal ear parts. Ear plugs do not give dependable protection. A perforated eardrum can be closed by an operation known as *tympanoplasty* (597).

Perianal. Situated around the anus.

Pericarditis. Inflammation of the PERICARDIUM from causes such as rheumatic fever or extension of infections from neighboring parts (104).

Pericardium. The sac of tough tissue that encloses the heart (82). It secretes lubricating fluids that permit free-sliding movements of the expanding, contracting heart.

Perimeter. An instrument for mapping the limits of the field of vision (560).

Perineum. The area between the anus and scrotum in the male, and the anus and the vulva in the female.

Periodontal disease. Inflammation of membranes that cover the roots of the teeth (532); laymen commonly call it PYORRHEA.

Periosteum. The tough, membranous covering of nearly all bone surfaces (622).

Peripheral. At or near an outer surface; for example, peripheral blood vessels, near skin surfaces.

Peristalsis. Wavelike movements of constriction and relaxation which propel materials along the digestive tube. Encircling muscle contracts to squeeze material forward while muscles in front of the material relax; the latter muscles constrict in their turn, and so on (452).

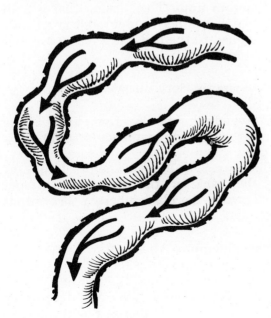

Peristalsis.

Peritoneum. The strong, smooth, colorless membrane which lines the abdominal wall and contains the abdominal organs.

Peritonitis. Inflammation of the PERITONEUM; the most frequent cause is a ruptured appendix, but infection can occur from other routes (486).

Perleche. Cracks at the side of the mouth, thickened, covered with whitish material. The condition is classically associated with deficiency of a vitamin, riboflavin, but this is rare in the U. S. Usually the patient has excessive folding of the skin at the corners of the mouth—perhaps congenital, or the result of missing teeth or poorly fitting dentures—and the moist opposing surfaces rub together, resulting in maceration, inflammation, possible infection. The patient licks the cracks, fostering further maceration; spicy or acid foods may be irritating. Perleche must be distinguished by a physician from other lesions that may resemble it. An ointment may be prescribed, together with appropriate measures to keep the area dry—correction of malocclusion, poorly fitting dentures, abstention from smoking, chewing gum, and chewing tobacco.

Perspiration. The refined person's sweat (180).

Perthe's disease. Degeneration of the upper end of the thighbone in young children (640).

Pertussis. Whooping cough (422).

Pessary. One of many devices of metal, rubber, or plastic, of different shapes and sizes, placed in the vagina or the uterus or parts of it to support sagging, tipped, slipping, or otherwise displaced pelvic structures.

Petechiae. Tiny pinpoint hemorrhages under the skin (159).

Petit mal. A relatively mild form of epileptic attack, consisting of sudden loss

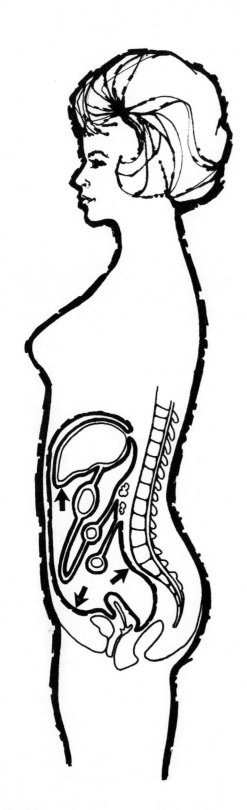

Peritoneum. As the small arrows indicate, the membrane is a continuous lining of the abdominal cavity and covers most of the organs contained in it.

of consciousness lasting only a few seconds (274).

Pets. See HOUSEHOLD PETS.

pH. Technically, a symbol expressing hydrogen ion concentration; practically, a scale of the acidity or alkalinity of substances. The neutral point is pH 7. Below 7, acidity increases. Above 7, alkalinity increases.

Phagocyte. A white blood cell which has the engaging property of engulfing, digesting, and generally eating up invading bacteria or other foreign particles (142).

Phalanx. One of the bones of the fingers or toes (617). The plural is *phalanges.*

Pharmacopoeia. An authoritative collection of formulas and methods of preparing and using drugs, which sets minimum standards of purity, safety, and potency. Some manufacturers exceed the standards. The U. S. Pharmacopoeia is recognized as the standard in this country. It is revised every few years, dropping some old drugs and adding new ones. A medicine with the initials "U.S.P." on the label conforms to Pharmacopoeia standards.

Phantom limb. The illusion that a limb which has been amputated is still attached to the body and feels pain and other sensations.

Pharyngitis. Sore throat.

Pharyngeal tonsils. Lymphoid tissue better known as *adenoids* (607).

Pharynx. The membrane-lined tube at the back of the nose, mouth, and larynx; the place where a sore throat hurts (607).

Phenylalanine. An essential AMINO ACID, present in protein foods.

Phenylketonuria (*PKU*). Hereditary inability to metabolize phenylalanine, an essential amino acid, because of a genetically determined lack of a necessary enzyme; an inherited "error of metabolism." Breakdown products of incompletely metabolized phenylalanine accumulate in the infant's body and impair brain function. The *Guthrie* test of an infant's blood gives evidence of the condition soon after birth (798). Institution of a diet of special foods, very low in phenylalanine, lessens the threat of damage to the developing nervous system.

Pheochromocytoma. A tumor, usually arising in the inner part of the adrenal gland, which secretes excessive amounts of hormones, producing such symptoms as tremor, cramps, palpitations, headache, nausea, and high blood pressure. Treatment is surgical removal (334).

Philadelphia chromosome. An abnormal CHROMOSOME which can be found in nearly 95 per cent of patients with chronic myelogenous leukemia (167). Its association with leukemia supports the hypothesis that specific GENE mutations may induce a high frequency of chromosome "breakage" and that chromosome rearrangements may be one of a number of mechanisms through which cancer-inducing factors are expressed.

Phimosis. Elongation and tightening of the foreskin of the PENIS, preventing retraction over the head of the organ.

Phlebitis. Inflammation of the walls of a vein, which may lead to formation of a clot, *thrombophlebitis* (137).

Phlebothrombosis. Formation of a clot in a vein (137).

Phlebotomy. "Bloodletting" by cutting into a vein; venesection. Irrational bloodletting for almost any state of ill health—the aspirin of its day—was practiced wholesale in the seventeenth and eighteenth centuries. The practice undoubtedly weakened and hastened the death of thousands of patients, including George Washington, and fell into highly deserved disrepute as a panacea. But there are some conditions for which bloodletting is recognized as a part of modern treatment; see HEMOCHROMATOSIS and POLYCYTHEMIA (153).

Phlegmasia alba dolens. See MILK LEG.

Phobia. An abnormal, excessive dread or fear. There are scores of specific phobias, each with its own medical name. Some of the more common are:

Phobia	Fear of
acrophobia	heights
agoraphobia	open places
aichmophobia	sharp objects
ailurophobia	cats
algophobia	pain
androphobia	men
bacteriophobia	germs
ballistophobia	missiles
belonephobia	needles, pins
claustrophobia	confined spaces
cynophobia	dogs
dipsophobia	drink
erythrophobia	blushing
genophobia	sex
gymnophobia	nakedness
hemophobia	blood
hypnophobia	falling asleep
lalophobia	talking
lyssophobia	becoming insane
melissophobia	bees
mysophobia	dirt, contamination
ochlophobia	crowds
osmophobia	odors
pedophobia	children
photophobia	light
pyrophobia	fire
siderodromophobia	railroads
sitophobia	eating
tocophobia	childbirth
triskaidekaphobia	number 13
xenophobia	strangers

Phocomelia. A type of congenital malformation in which the upper and lower limbs are absent or grossly underdeveloped but the hands and feet are present.

Photophobia. Intolerance of light or morbid fear of light.

Photoscanner. An instrument which measures the concentration of radioisotopes (measured doses of radiation) in a patient's body. It has a scintillator crystal which, when struck by radiation, energizes an amplified stream of high-speed electrons from a photomultiplier tube. This burst is employed in the simultaneous production of two records of the concentration of radioactivity. One record consists of dots produced on a moving sheet of paper; the more concentrated the radioactivity, the more concentrated the dots. The other record is produced on an x-ray film; here the increased concentration of radioactivity produces increased blackness of dots as well as an increase in the number of dots. The complete system enables doctors to differentiate areas of tissue with as little as 15 to 25 per cent more radiation than their surroundings. The instrument can scan a patient's body at a rate of 200 inches per minute and record diagnostic information in as little as ten minutes. See NUCLEAR MEDICINE.

Photosensitivity. A number of disorders are triggered or made worse by exposure to sunlight. Photosensitive reactions may result from certain drugs taken internally, from materials in cosmetics or substances applied to the skin, from contact with certain plants (parsnips, celery, carrots, dill, parsley), or from underlying disease which increases the sensitivity of the skin to sunlight. A clue to photosensitive reactions is the presence of lesions on exposed areas of the forehead, nose, rims of the ears and backs of the hands, while areas under the jaw not exposed to sunlight are not affected. Patients with *lupus erythematosus* (195, 666) are very sensitive to ultraviolet rays of sunlight.

Phototherapy. Treatment with light rays, including invisible ultraviolet and infrared wave lengths.

Phrenic nerve. The principal nerve of breathing which activates the great muscle of respiration, the *diaphragm* (214). The nerve also serves the PERICARDIUM and PLEURA.

Phthisis. An old term for pulmonary tuberculosis.

Physical allergy. Allergic reactions induced by purely physical factors such as heat, cold, or light (701).

Phytobezoar. A compact ball of vegetable matter in the stomach.

Pia mater. The innermost of the three membranes that cover the brain and spinal cord (265).

Pica. A craving to eat strange foods or unnatural substances—wood, clay, coal, dirt, chalk, starch, etc. Clay-eating is not uncommon in some parts of the country; it may lead to anemia and other ailments. Pica is particularly dangerous in children who swallow lead-containing flakes of paint or plaster, leading to LEAD POISONING.

Pigeon-breeder's lung. A recently recognized respiratory disease occurring in pigeon breeders or others in close contact with pigeons. Chills, fever, cough and shortness of breath develop a few hours after inhaling dusts in an environment of pigeons. The disease is not a bacterial or viral infection, but appears to be a hypersensitivity reaction to ANTIGENS in pigeon feathers and droppings, an allergic lung disease similar to FARMER'S LUNG.

Pigeon toe. Inward turning of the feet and toes when walking. Children in the early stages of walking are often pigeon-toed but usually outgrow the condition (647).

Piles. See HEMORRHOIDS.

"Pill rolling." Involuntary movement of thumb and fingers, as if a pill were being rolled, characteristic of Parkinson's disease (251).

Pilonidal cyst. A congenital hair-containing sac under the skin overlying the tailbone (*coccyx,* 619) at the top of the buttock crease. There may be only a dimpling of the skin or a hairy overlying tuft to mark the presence of the cyst until it becomes infected, swollen and painful, and perhaps develops a FISTULA through which fluids are excreted. Surgical removal of the cyst is usually necessary to accomplish a permanent cure.

Pimple. The ordinary term for what doctors call a *papule* or *pustule.*

Pineal gland. A cone-shaped structure about a quarter of an inch long which lies very nearly in the center of the brain. For centuries physiologists were unable to ascribe any function to it. Now there is evidence that the pineal is a sort of "biological clock" which sends out "ticks" to influence the activities of hormones. Experiments with animals indicate that in some way the pineal regulates the sex glands. Whether visible light, acting upon the pineal, is in some way translated into hormonal triggers of the human menstrual cycle is a speculation that challenges investigators.

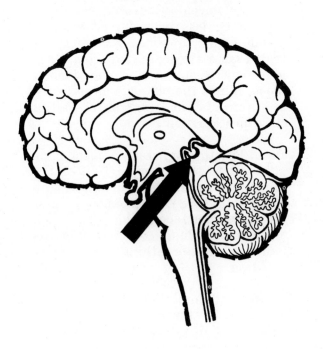

Pineal gland.

"Pink eye." Acute *conjunctivitis,* a highly contagious infection of the eye (568). Discharges contain the infectious organisms.

Pinna. The external ear; the obvious, protruding part of the hearing mechanism, mainly a sound collector.

Pinta. An infectious disease, most frequent in tropical America, characterized by white, blue, brown or red spots on the skin, produced by a *spirochete* very similar to the organism of syphilis (50).

Pinworm infection. Oxyuriasis (71).

Pityriasis rosea. A non-infectious, noncontagious skin disease of young adults, characterized by scaly spots which disappear in two or three months (192).

Placebo. An inert substance such as a sugar pill, without drug effect, given to please the patient. Oddly, seeming therapeutic benefits from placebos are not uncommon. This phenomenon, called the "placebo effect," has to be taken account of in treatment and evaluation of drug effects.

Placenta. The organ on the wall of the uterus through which the fetus receives nourishment and eliminates wastes (357). Structures of the implanted embryo grow into the uterine wall and the placenta develops until it occupies about half the area of the uterus at the fourth month of pregnancy. The fetus and placenta are connected by the UMBILICAL CORD. The placenta has a definite life span and is a senile organ by the time labor pains begin. It is expelled as the AFTERBIRTH shortly after the baby is born. The placenta gets its name from a Latin word for "a flat cake." It somewhat resembles a cake about an inch thick and six or seven inches in diameter. Complications of pregnancy may be caused by a mislocated placenta (*placenta previa,* 374) or by premature detachment.

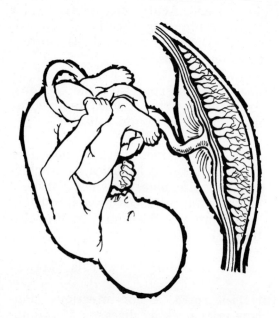

Placenta; umbilical cord connects with fetus.

Plague. An acute feverish disease caused by bacilli (*Pasteurella pestis*). It is primarily a disease of rats and other rodents, which tend to be inhabited by fleas, which can transmit the plague organisms to man (46). *Bubonic plague* is characterized by swellings (*buboes*) which may break down into bleeding ulcers. *Pneumonic plague* affects the lungs and has a high fatality rate. The black plague, or black death, which decimated Europe in the fourteenth century, was a form of bubonic plague with an exceptionally high incidence of hemorrhage.

Plantar. Pertaining to the soles of the feet. The most frequent affliction of this area is *plantar warts* which usually form at points of pressure on the ball of the foot (192).

Plaque. Tiny patches or unnatural formations on tissues such as on tooth surfaces and on inner arterial walls. *Atheroma*, plaques that are found in walls of arteries, contain some LIPIDS and some connective or scar tissue. They contribute to stiffening of blood vessel walls, closing of arteries, choking of circulation, and ruptured arteries, associated with heart attacks.

Plasma. The fluid part of the blood, minus the blood cells and clotting elements (140).

Plasma cell. A type of white blood cell closely related to *lymphocytes* (173). MULTIPLE MYELOMA and a form of leukemia are associated with plasma cell abnormalities.

Plasmodium. The genus of parasites that cause malaria, transmitted by the bites of mosquitoes (72).

Platelets (*thrombocytes*). Tiny, colorless formed elements of the blood, about one-fourth the size of a red blood cell, which help to initiate blood clotting (143). They are formed in the bone marrow. Platelets are quite fragile and short-lived outside of the circulation, and there are various methods of salvaging and transfusing them. *Platelet transfusions* may be necessary in some bleeding disorders such as *purpura* (159). Platelet transfusions may be of fresh whole blood, or of recently stored blood collected in specially treated glass containers or plastic bags. Since it is the platelets themselves rather than whole blood which the patient usually requires, a recently developed procedure promises to be less wasteful of hospital blood bank supplies. Platelets for transfusion are separated from blood given by a donor, and the donor's blood, minus the platelets, is returned to his circulation after a short wait in the collection room.

Pleura. The thin, glistening membrane attached to the outer surface of the lungs and the inner surface of the chest wall (208). The opposed fluid-lubricated surfaces glide over each other as the lung contracts and expands, so that breathing is a painless function.

Pleurisy. Inflammation of the pleura, heralded by knifelike pains aggravated by a deep breath or coughing. There are "wet" and "dry" forms of pleurisy (231).

Pleurodynia. Excruciatingly sharp pain in the muscles between the ribs. It is characteristic of DEVIL'S GRIP, an acute virus-caused epidemic disease, also called *epidemic pleudorynia* and *Bornholm disease*.

Plumbism. LEAD POISONING.

Pneumoconiosis. Chronic inflammation of the lungs due to long-continued inhalation of various kinds of mineral dusts (235).

Pneumoencephalogram. An x-ray film of the brain made after replacing the CEREBROSPINAL FLUID of the brain cavities with air or gas.

Pneumonectomy. Removal of an entire lung (740).

Pneumonia. Inflammation of the lungs caused by various organisms (35). In the past it was customary to classify pneumonias according to the part of the lung affected—*lobar pneumonia* if a lobe or lobes were involved (209), *bronchopneumonia* if infection was localized to air sacs connecting with bronchi. Now the trend is to classify pneumonia according to the organism that causes it. The terms *viral pneumonia* and *primary atypical pneumonia* came into vogue after World War II to describe pneumonias not caused by recognized bacteria. Viruses may be implicated, but it is now known that most cases of atypical pneumonia are caused by *mycoplasma*. These are strange organisms, like bacteria with their skins off. They lack the stiff outer covering that holds conventional bacteria in shape and are enveloped only in a flexible membrane. During the progress of research the organisms have been called *Eaton's agent* and *pleuropneumonia-like organisms* (PPLO), the latter because they resemble organisms which cause a respiratory disease of cattle called pleuropneumonia. They have recently been given a category of their own, the genus *mycoplasma*. Respiratory infection caused by these germs comes on gradually, producing fever, chills and cough. The patient does not appear to be very ill, and often does not consult a doctor, although he may stay home from work for a few days with a "bad cold." The organisms are sensitive to tetracycline, an antibiotic. Another form of pneumonia, of which the cause may not be immediately suspected, is parrot fever (*ornithosis, psittacosis*), an infection transmitted by parrots and other birds. Other unusual pneumonias may result from foreign material that gets into the lungs; see ASPIRATION PNEUMONIA.

Pneumothorax. Collapse of a lung due to air in the pleural cavity (233).

Podagra. Gout.

Podalic version. The maneuver of turning the fetus in the uterus to bring the feet through the birth canal for feet-first delivery.

Polyphagia. Voracious eating.

Poisonous plants. Any plant that is not a familiar food plant is poisonous if parts of it are eaten. That is the safest rule to follow, even though parts of some strange or common plants may be harmless. Children are particularly attracted by berries which look good to eat but may be highly poisonous. They should be taught never to chew or eat unknown berries, leaves, roots or barks. Many highly toxic plants are cultivated in gardens; others, some of them quite attractive, grow wild.

A partial list of toxic plants includes many cultivated for their beauty: foxglove leaves and seeds, poinsettia leaves, oleander leaves and branches, iris roots, larkspur and delphinium, lily of the valley, monkshood, yew, daphne, Christmas rose, bittersweet. Bulbs of hyacinth, narcissus and daffodil are toxic; as purchased, plant bulbs may be treated with toxic chemicals. Bloodroot, castor beans, Jimson weed, rhubarb leaves (the stalks are edible), Wisteria seeds, any part of laurels, rhododendrons and azaleas can produce serious poisoning. Play safe by never putting any part of a growing plant into the mouth. Immediate treatment of plant poisoning is emptying of the stomach by inducing vomiting, unless the victim is unconscious or convulsing, and calling a doctor who will know the specific antidote if the plant can be identified.

Pollen counts. Measurements of the number of pollen particles in the air at a given time, made by counting the number of particles adhering to a glass slide covered with sticky material and exposed to the atmosphere.

Pollinosis. A state of allergic reaction to inhaled plant pollens; for example, hay fever, bronchial asthma (675).

Polyarteritis. A rare disease characterized by inflammation and nodular swellings of artery walls, sometimes leading to local death of tissues. Also called *periarteritis nodosa* and *polyarteritis nodosa*. The cause is not known. Frequently there is an allergic background.

Polycystic kidney. A kidney filled with multiple bubble-like cysts; a congenital condition (290).

Polycythemia. Too many red cells in the blood (153).

Polydactyly. More than the normal number of five fingers or toes.

Polydipsia. Enormous thirst, characteristic of *diabetes insipidus* (316).

Polyps. Smooth outgrowths or tumors of mucous membranes which line body cavities. Usually the polyp hangs from a stem or stalk. Polyps occur most commonly in mucous tissues of the nose (609), uterus (435), and colon (490). They rarely cause symptoms, but nasal polyps may be associated with allergies, and some polyps, as of the colon, may be precancerous and are best removed when discovered. Surgical removal is relatively simple.

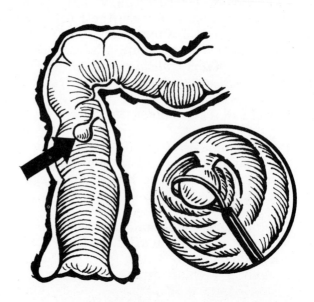

Rectal polyp indicated by arrow; in circle, relatively simple surgical removal by loop dissection.

Polyunsaturated fats. Much interest has been aroused by well-publicized knowledge that high levels of CHOLESTEROL in the blood may be reduced by increasing the proportion of polyunsaturated fats in the diet. The hope is that reduction of blood cholesterol may slow the process of *atherosclerosis* (86) which leads to heart attacks. It is not possible to speak with complete assurance about prevention of an extremely complex and incompletely understood process, but most authorities agree that it is unwise to flood the body with large amounts of saturated fats (89). "Saturated" is a technical word referring to bonds between carbon atoms of fatty acids which combine with glycerol to form fats and oils. These bonds in *saturated fats* contain all the hydrogen atoms they can hold. *Unsaturated* and *polyunsaturated* fatty acids have additional bonds between carbon atoms and can take on additional hydrogen atoms; thus they are more chemically active. Most of the animal fats and some of the vegetable oils (for example, coconut oil) are formed from fatty acids which are highly saturated. Fish oils, corn oil, safflower oil, cottonseed oil, and some other vegetable oils are highly unsaturated. The polyunsaturated fatty acid of principal nutritional importance is *linoleic acid*. Most of the fat stored in the adult human body is relatively unsaturated. The average human body contains about two pounds of linoleic acid in its fat storehouse.

Polyuria. Excessive output of urine.

Popliteal. Pertaining to the hind part of the knee joint.

Portuguese man-of-war. Creatures that people call "jellyfish" sometimes depopulate beaches in a hurry. The most formidable, not exactly a jellyfish, is the Portuguese man-of-war, a creature—actually composed of many separate organisms—which floats on the surface like an overturned toy boat and drapes scores of tentacles into the depths. The tentacles, as long as 50 feet, contain venom-injecting surfaces for killing prey. The "stingers" feel like a hot iron to the bather who comes in contact with them. There is immediate pain, burning, feeling of tightness in the chest, and nausea after a minute or so. The muscles cramp and it feels that every muscle of the body is contracted. The stung areas should be flushed with water while medical help is on the way. The skin may be rubbed with a cloth, or better yet, lathered and shaved with a safety razor to remove venomous particles. Antihistamine drugs seem to give the most rapid relief of pain, cramping and spasm. Persons with weak hearts may be dangerously affected by the man-of-war toxin and should have prompt medical care.

Postpartum. After childbirth.

Postprandial. After a meal. *Postcibal* has the same meaning.

Postural drainage. Use of gravity to assist in draining secretions from the lungs and chest. The patient lies face down over the edge of a bed or table, his head, shoulders and chest hanging down lower than the waist. In this position, gravity helps to drain secretions. Hawking, coughing, and thumping the back encourage drainage.

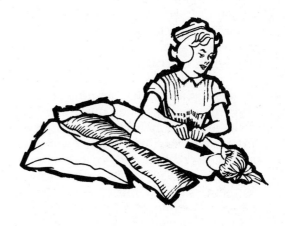

Postural drainage.

PPLO. Pleuropneumonia-like organisms. See PNEUMONIA.

Precordial. Pertaining to the area of the chest overlying the heart, approximately under the tip of the breastbone. Precordial pain may or may not come from the heart; there are many structures in this area.

Precursor. Forerunner; something that precedes. In biology, a compound that can be used by the body to form another compound. For example, the body converts vegetable *carotene* into Vitamin A.

Prematurity. Birth weight of 5½ lbs. is customarily and rather arbitrarily taken as the borderline between a premature and a mature baby.

Premenstrual tension. Cyclic occurrence of emotional symptoms associated with body changes about a week before onset of a menstrual period. Most women are aware of some change in disposition during the premenstrual week and learn to live with it, but some have sufficient distress to seek medical attention. Nervous symptoms such as irascibility, tension, fatigue, moodiness, weepiness, severe enough to upset domestic tranquillity, are not "all in the mind" but reflect subtle changes. Physical symptoms such as abdominal bloating, weight gain, puffing of the hands and swelling and tenderness of the breasts, indicate that the fundamental disturbance which provokes emotional irritability is cyclic EDEMA—transitory retention of fluids, which exert pressure on internal organs and have far-flung effects. The tension state ends quite abruptly at the onset of menstruation. A physician may prescribe diuretic medicines, sedatives, stimulants, or other measures according to individual need. Explanation that premenstrual tension is not abnormal is reassuring.

Prenatal. Before birth.

Prepuce. A fold of skin covering the glans (head) of the PENIS or CLITORIS; the foreskin; the part that is removed in circumcision.

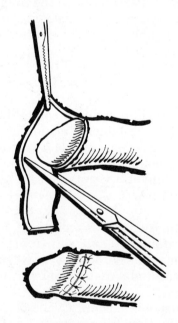

Circumcision.

Presbycusis. Normal diminution of acuteness of hearing that comes with increasing age (588). Mainly, sensitivity to the highest sound frequencies is reduced while sensitivity to lower frequencies—those most important in conversation and daily affairs—remains good.

Presbyopia. "Old sight"; not always so very old—it begins to come on in middle life when the crystalline lens of the eye loses some of its elasticity and power of ACCOMMODATION. Near objects have to be held farther away to see them distinctly. In a culture that puts a premium on reading, close vision, and paperwork, corrective glasses are a kindness and an aid to efficiency.

Priapism. Abnormal, painful, sustained erection of the PENIS, unrelated to sexual stimuli. It may result from obstruction of vessels that drain the organ, from injury to nerve centers, or from triggering stimuli such as bladder stones or PROSTATITIS.

Prickly heat. See MILIARIA.

Primary irritants. Caustic, acid, corrosive, or otherwise irritating substances which are harmful to anyone's skin on first exposure in sufficient concentration; no allergic reaction is involved (681).

Proctitis. Inflammation of membranes of the rectum (490).

Proctologist. A medical specialist in diseases of the anus and rectum.

Proctoscope. A tubular instrument with a light source which permits the inner lining of the bowel to be viewed directly (444).

Prodromal. Premonitory; early warning signs of an oncoming condition before overt symptoms appear.

Progeria. Premature aging; a child so afflicted looks like a very old little man.

Prognosis. A doctor's forecast of the course and duration of an illness based on the best information available to make a judgment.

Projectile vomiting. Ejection of stomach contents so forcefully as to hurl material a foot or two from the body (396).

Prolactin. A hormone of the pituitary gland which stimulates milk production (317, 320).

Prolapse. A falling downward of a part from its normal position; for example, *prolapsed uterus* (437).

Prophylaxis. Prevention of the spread or development of disease. A specific form of prophylaxis is the mechanical removal of tartar by a dentist.

Prostaglandins. A group of extremely potent hormone-like substances which occur in minute amounts in virtually all body tissues. The name, something of a misnomer, originated with discovery of the substances in semen, to which the prostate gland contributes. Different prostaglandins (at least 16 natural forms are known, and pharmaceutical chemists synthesize many analogs) have different and even opposite effects. Prostaglandins are so versatile that many investigators expect them to become major therapeutic agents if experimental and clinical trials prove their safety and effectiveness in a wide range of conditions. Prostaglandins stimulate or relax smooth muscle, appear to regulate cell behavior, and inhibit and potentiate hormones. Based on current clinical and experimental studies, specific prostaglandins may become very valuable drugs for: induction of labor at term; contraception; induced abortion; prevention and treatment of peptic ulcer (by shutting off gastric secretions); induction of delayed menstruation; control of high blood pressure; treatment of bronchial asthma, emphysema, even the common cold (by opening closed airways). Aspirin tends to halt production of prostaglandins, which sheds some light on the way aspirin works. Various prostaglandins can cause fever, inflammation, and headache, symptoms commonly relieved by aspirin.

Prostatectomy. Removal of all or part of the *prostate gland* by one of several surgical techniques (307, 747).

Prostatitis. Acute or chronic inflammation of the *prostate gland* (306).

Prosthesis. An artificial substitute for a missing part of the body; for example, artificial eye, limb, or denture.

Prosthodontics. The branch of dentistry that pertains to the replacement of missing teeth and oral structures by artificial devices.

Proteins. Large complex molecules built up of long chains of simpler AMINO ACIDS. Skin, hair, nails, most of us that is visible to the public, is largely protein. It is the characteristic stuff of life (the word means "of first importance"). Enzymes which trigger multitudes of living chemical processes of the body are proteins. About one half of the dry weight of the body is protein. Protein constituents of foods are broken down into their constituent amino acids by digestion, assimilated, and the separated parts are reassembled by body cells into specific and unique personal proteins (see GENES, HEREDITY). Incessant bodily synthesis of proteins is essential not only for growth and repair of tissues but for the continuance of the multitudes of chemical processes we live by. Protein elements of foods can be burned for energy if necessary, but carbohydrates and fats are superior energy providers and spare protein.

Prothrombin. A plasma PROTEIN, one of many elements necessary in the complicated step-by-step processes of blood coagulation. Tests of "prothrombin time" are used in patients having a tendency to hemorrhage and as a guide to treatment of patients receiving anticoagulant drugs (801).

Protoplasm. Living matter; the viscid, translucent material which is the essential stuff of living cells, never found in the inanimate world. The word was meaningful years ago when the best that scientists could do was to analyze the cell constituents—carbohydrates, proteins, fats, salts, water, etc.—of what they considered to be a homogeneous mixture. Today, many of the structures and activities of specific elements of protoplasm are known—mechanisms of heredity, protein synthesis, energy transformations, chemical directives of life—and the word is outliving its usefulness except as a very general term for living matter.

Protruding ears. Plastic surgery to correct protruding, flattened, or deformed ears is usually performed on children but is just as suitable for adults. The operation (*otoplasty*) is performed by means of incisions behind the ears. The procedure takes from an hour to an hour and a half. The patient may be discharged from the hospital as soon as 24 hours after surgery. A bandage is worn over the ears for about one week after surgery, and the ear is further protected during sleeping for another two weeks.

Protozoa. Single-celled organisms of the animal kingdom. Most protozoa do not cause disease, but those that do are responsible for malaria, amebic dysentery, and a number of other serious diseases (71).

Proud flesh. An excess of GRANULATION TISSUE.

Prurigo. A chronic skin ailment characterized by small, deep-seated, solid pimples that itch intensely.

Pruritus. Severe itching.

Psilocybin. See Chapter 27.

Psittacosis (*ornithosis, parrot fever*). A pneumonia-like disease transmitted by infected birds (57). The disease not only affects birds of the parrot family, but pigeons, chickens, ducks, turkeys and other birds.

Psoriasis. A chronic disease of the skin, of unknown cause, usually persisting for years with periods of remission and recurrence (190). It is characterized by elevated lesions in various

parts of the body—elbows, knees, scalp, nails, lower back—covered with dry silvery scales that drop off. General health is rarely affected, although *psoriatic arthritis,* a destructive form of arthritis in the fingers and toes, may develop in some patients.

Psychedelic. The word means "mind manifesting," from Greek words for "mind" and "clear."

Psychoanalysis. A system of mental therapy created by Sigmund Freud, originally as a research method to gain insight into mental processes. Essentially, the patient bares his soul to the psychoanalyst by speaking of whatever comes to mind, during a long series of half-hour to hour-long sessions which usually total several hundred hours for a complete analysis. Unconscious conflicts expressed through dreams, slips of the tongue, symbolism, etc., are interpreted by the psychoanalyst with the object of giving the patient insight into his conflicts and thus lessening their trauma. The therapeutic value of psychoanalysis is somewhat controversial (715).

Psychomotor seizure. A relatively mild form of epileptic attack which the patient never remembers (274). The person does not fall but may stagger, make restless movements and strange sounds, lose contact with his environment for a minute or two.

Psychoneurosis. Relatively mild, emotionally based disturbance of the personality, often severe enough to be handicapping, generally a defensive reaction to psychic threats and conflicts (710).

Psychosomatic disease. Disability, sometimes but not always without accompanying physical causes, in which disturbing emotions of the patient play an important part in inciting, worsening, or continuing the disability (710).

Psychosis. Serious mental illness, disabling, usually requiring treatment in a hospital for a period of time. Some psychoses have organic causes and others primarily psychological causes or possibly metabolic disturbances too subtle to be identifiable (711).

Psychosurgery. Operations on parts of the brain to improve a patient's mental state (716). *Prefrontal lobotomy*, an operation in which the frontal lobes of the brain are cut into, at one time had many advocates. Unmanageable, assaultive, manic patients subjected to this procedure usually became tractable and even amiable, but too often there was gross deterioration of personality to a vegetative level. Psychosurgery is a highly drastic procedure that is resorted to only when all other measures have failed.

Psychotherapy. Treatment of emotional and mental disorders by psychological methods as opposed to physical or medical methods (713).

Pterygium. A triangular growth of the conjunctiva in the corner of the eye nearest the nose, due to a degenerative process caused by long-continued irritation of the tissues, as from exposure to wind and dust.

Ptomaines. Putrid substances produced by decay of dead animal matter. Food poisoning is not caused by ptomaines, which are too repulsive for anyone to ingest. Food poisoning is commonly caused by salmonella or staphylococcus organisms.

Ptyalin. An enzyme in saliva which initiates the digestion of starch (466). It is what gives a sweetish taste to a piece of cracker held in the mouth for a while. *Ptyalism* is a condition of profuse drooling of saliva; salivation.

Puberty. The age at which the reproductive organs become functionally active. It occurs when a person is between 12 and 17 years old and is indicated in the girl by the beginning of menstruation and in the boy by seminal discharge and change of voice.

Pudenda. The external sex organs.

Puerperium. The time between childbirth and return of the uterus to its pre-pregnancy size and state, about six weeks (385).

Purpura. A disorder of blood coagulation; tiny blood vessels bleed into the skin and mucous membranes and cause purplish patches or pinpoint hemorrhages (159).

Purulent. Containing, exuding, or producing pus.

Pustule. A small elevation of the skin containing pus.

Pyelogram. An x-ray film of the pelvis of the kidney and the ureter, visualizing the entire urinary tract.

Pyelonephritis. Infection of the kidney and its urine-collecting pelvis (292).

Pyemia. Pus in the blood.

Pyloric stenosis. Congenital obstruction of the outlet of the stomach due to abnormal thickening of the pyloric muscle that encircles it. The condition is completely relieved by an operation which cuts some of the muscle fibers (416, 474).

Pylorospasm. Spasm of the circular muscle at the outlet of the stomach, manifested by PROJECTILE VOMITING of an infant shortly after birth (416). Usually the condition can be corrected by medication which relaxes the spastic muscle and permits normal passage of food to the intestines.

Pyogenic. Pus-producing.

Pyorrhea. Flow of pus; a common term for *periodontoclasia*, inflammation and gradual destruction of supporting tissues of the teeth. Pockets form and enlarge between the gum surface and tooth, bacteria and debris fill the pockets, pus forms, bone is resorbed, eventually the tooth becomes loose in its socket and is lost from lack of support. The condition can be arrested but lost tissue cannot be restored (532).

Pyrexia. Fever.

Pyridoxine. One of the B vitamins, commonly designated as Vitamin B₆.

Pyrosis. Heartburn.

Pyuria. Pus in the urine (292).

Q

Q fever. A self-limited RICKETTSIAL DISEASE resembling pneumonia, often mild and unrecognized (66).

Q.i.d. Four times a day.

Quadriceps. The large muscle which extends the thigh.

Quadriplegia. Paralysis of both arms and both legs.

Quartan. Occurring every fourth day, as, the fever of *quartan malaria*.

Quartipara. A woman who has borne four children. A *quadripara* is bearing or has borne her fourth child.

Queasiness. Nausea.

Quick. A tender, vital part, as the bed of a fingernail.

Quickening. The time around the middle of pregnancy when bumps, kicks and flutters within the uterus give unmistakable proof that lively life is present (371). Father may be invited to "meet" the baby via its abdominally communicated contortions.

Quincke's edema. ANGIONEUROTIC EDEMA (693).

Quinsy. An abscess in and around a tonsil, causing a very sore throat (38).

Quotidian. Recurring every day.

R

Rabbit fever (*tularemia*). An infection acquired from handling diseased rabbits or from the bites of ticks (46).

Rabbit test. A biologic test for determining pregnancy (358).

Rabies (*hydrophobia*). A lethal disease caused by viruses which have an affinity for brain and nervous tissue (58). The virus is transmitted to man by the bite of an infected (rabid) animal. Mere contact of saliva of an infected animal with abraded or scratched skin can transmit the disease. "Mad dogs" are not the only sources of rabies. A considerable reservoir exists in wildlife of the U.S. Bats, foxes, squirrels, raccoons, skunks and other rabid animals can transmit the disease directly by biting people or indirectly by infecting domestic animals which in turn can transmit the disease by their bites or saliva. This chain of transmission is broken if the family dog is properly immunized against rabies. The disease is invariably fatal but has an incubation period of a month to a year or more. The incubation period is shortest if bites are inflicted on the head, face, neck or arms, and are severe and numerous. Prompt "Pasteur treatment"—daily injection of rabies vaccine for two weeks—usually prevents rabies from taking hold. The treatments are painful and the type of vaccine cultivated in animal nerve tissue sometimes has bad side effects. A newer type of duck-embryo rabies vaccine greatly reduces the serious problem of nervous system reactions. Immediate preventive injections may not be necessary if the biting animal can be caught and kept under observation. If killed, the animal's body and particularly the head should be kept for laboratory studies which can determine whether or not the animal was rabid by the presence or absence of NEGRI BODIES in the brain tissue. If injections have been started, and the animal proves not to be rabid, they can be discontinued. The problem of what to do about the bite of a possibly rabid animal should be turned over immediately to the family physician and local health department.

Rachitic rosary. A beadlike row of nodules on the ribs of children with rickets, strung along the junctions of ribs and cartilage.

Radiation sickness. Illness resulting from intense or less intense but accumulative exposure to sources of radiation. Exposure to massive doses of radiation, as in the neighborhood of a nuclear explosion, is very rare, which is fortunate because an overwhelming dose of radiation is extremely serious if not fatal. Necessary therapeutic use of x-rays may sometimes be followed by mild radiation sickness—lassitude, nausea, vomiting—which usually disappears rather quickly and can be coped with effectively by the physician or radiologist. There is virtually no threat of radiation sickness from the use of diagnostic x-rays by an experienced physician or radiologist (791).

Radiculitis. Inflammation of a spinal nerve root.

Radiograph. An x-ray photo.

Radioisotopes. See NUCLEAR MEDICINE.

Radiologist. A physician who specializes in the making and interpretation of x-ray studies and applications of radiation (781).

Radiopaque. Not transparent to x-rays. Radiopaque substances (for example, BARIUM MEAL) are introduced into parts of the body to give clear delineation of structures which otherwise would not show up distinctly on an x-ray film or fluoroscopic screen.

Radiosensitivity. The capacity of tissues to react with different degrees of intensity to radiation. Radiosensitive tumors and cells are more susceptible to destruction by radiation than less sensitive ones.

Radiotherapy. Treatment of disease by x-rays, radium, radioisotopes, and other forms of ionizing radiation (788).

Radon. A colorless radioactive gas given off by the decay of radium. *Radon seeds* are tiny radon-containing tubes of gold or glass for implantation into tumors (788). The gas decays at a steady rate and after a week or so loses all of its radioactive power, so no harm is done if radon seeds remain in or are lost in tissues.

Rales. Abnormal sounds from the lungs or air passageways, heard over the chest. The sounds, described as coarse, medium, fine, wet, dry, etc., are not specific for specific diseases but help the trained ear to judge the condition of the patient.

Ratbite fever. Two varieties of infectious disease transmitted by the bites of rats (50). A type caused by bacteria (*Haverhill fever*) is sudden in onset, marked by a skin rash of arms and legs, headache, fever and joint pains. The other type, caused by spirochetes, is characterized by a relapsing type of fever, dusky skin rash, a hard ulcer and enlarged lymph nodes at the site of the bite. A bite by a rat or any other rodent should have prompt treatment by a physician.

Raynaud's disease. Intermittent blanching and reddening of the skin, especially of the fingers and toes, brought on by exposure to cold. Blood vessels first constrict, causing pallor and numbness, then expand and the affected area tingles and becomes very red or reddish-purple as large amounts of blood return. An attack may last for minutes or hours. The condition may be secondary to other diseases, but more often the peculiar blood vessel spasms occur without apparent cause; 90 per cent of patients are women. There is some evidence that affected persons may be unusually susceptible to collagen diseases such as SCLERODERMA in later life, but in itself Raynaud's disease is more of a nuisance than a serious condition. Patients are usually instructed to protect themselves well against cold, as by wearing lined gloves and overshoes, because a certain amount of exposure to cold is necessary to trigger attacks. Smoking, which tends to constrict superficial vessels, is forbidden. In its most extreme and rare form, Raynaud's disease may eventually lead to dry GANGRENE of fingers or toes. Surgical severing of nerve branches which serve blood vessels of affected areas may be resorted to in patients with severe symptoms.

Rectalgia. Pain in the rectum.

Rectocele. A bulging of the rectum through the rear wall of the vagina (438, 736).

Rectum. The terminal part of the bowel, about six inches long, ending in the narrow muscular anal canal and anus (459).

Red palms (palmar erythema). The palms often become deeply pink or reddish, like a sustained blush, during pregnancy. The reddening, caused by a high level of circulating hormones, fades after delivery and needs no treatment. A similar phenomenon occurs in some patients with cirrhosis of the liver.

Reed-Sternberg cell. A type of cell characteristic of HODGKIN'S DISEASE.

Referred pain. Pain that doesn't originate where it hurts. For instance, pain which originates in an acting-up gallbladder may be felt in the back under the shoulder blade.

Reflex. An action in response to a stimulus, occurring without conscious effort or thinking about it (244); for example, dilation or contraction of the pupil in response to different intensities of light. Some 300 different reflexes have been catalogued. They are useful in helping to diagnose or locate the sites

of disorders, infections, or injuries that may involve the nervous system.

Refraction. Bending of light waves from a straight line in passing through lenses or transparent structures of different densities. In ophthalmology, the measurement and correction by lenses of defects of the eye (*nearsightedness, far-sightedness, astigmatism*) which prevent light waves from being brought to sharp focus exactly on the retina (561).

Regional ileitis (*regional enteritis*). Inflammatory disease of the lower portion of the small bowel (484). The disease may be principally inflammatory, obstructive, or diffuse, with varied symptoms. Total recovery may be made after a single attack and there may be no symptoms for many years although abnormalities of the small bowel still exist. Medical treatment usually is effective but complications may require surgery.

Regurgitation. Effortless casting up of food from the stomach soon after eating; "spitting up" of food. Babies are adept at it (396). Not to be mistaken for vomiting. The word also means backflow of blood through a leaky heart valve (105).

Reiter's syndrome. A form of arthritis with inflammation of the mucous membrane of the eyes and of the urethra. It resembles rheumatoid arthritis but in many respects is less crippling and is self-limited.

Relapsing fever. Episodes of fever which subside spontaneously, then recur. Specifically, an acute infectious disease caused by organisms spread by lice and ticks (50).

Remedial reading. See DYSLEXIA.

Renal. Pertaining to the kidneys.

Renal insufficiency. Incapacity of the kidneys to filter toxins adequately from the blood (292).

Renin. A kidney protein capable of raising blood pressure by activating *angiotensin,* a powerful pressure-elevating agent (116).

Resect. To cut out a part of an organ or tissue; a term used by surgeons.

Residual urine. Significant amount of urine left in the bladder after urination. The symptom in the male may be associated with prostate trouble; in the female, with CYSTOCELE or pressure of tumors of the uterus.

Respiratory distress syndrome. See HYALINE MEMBRANE DISEASE.

Respirator. An "iron lung"; a mechanical breathing device for patients whose breathing muscles are paralyzed by disease or injury.

Resuscitation. Artificial respiration applied to a person threatened with death by asphyxia (823).

Reticulo-endothelial system. Pervasive mechanisms woven like a meshwork through the body, which defend against foreign invaders and carry oxygen and carbon dioxide to and from every cranny of the body (139).

Retina. The tissue-thin light-receiving structure at the back of the eye, composed of several specialized layers (555). Hundreds of thousands of nerve endings in the retina merge into the optic nerve which conveys impulses to the seeing part of the brain at the back of the head.

Retinal detachment. See DETACHED RETINA.

Retinitis pigmentosa. Hereditary degeneration and atrophy of the retina.

Retinoblastoma. A malignant tumor of the retina; a congenital form of cancer occurring in infants and young children. An early sign is a white pupil; this sign in an infant or young child has serious import and immediate medical diagnosis is imperative. Retinoblastoma is life-threatening, but improved methods of treatment, given as soon as the tumor is discovered, usually save life though sometimes at the cost of partial or total blindness. If only one eye is affected, it is usually removed. If both eyes are involved the more seriously affected one is usually removed and the other is treated in hope of destroying the tumor and preserving as much vision as possible. X-rays, radioactive applicators, photocoagulation and other measures may be used in an effort to save the eye. The disease is thought to be inherited as a dominant trait.

Retinopathy. Any abnormal condition of the retina.

Retractors. Instruments of varied design, to hold or pull back the edges of an incision or wound.

Retrobulbar. Behind the eyeball.

Retroflexion. Condition of being bent backward.

Retrolental fibroplasia. An ocular disease in which a mass of fibrous tissue forms in back of the lens of the eye, blocking vision; associated with premature birth and excessive oxygen in incubators (580).

Retroversion. A backward-tilted position of an organ, as a retroverted uterus (437).

"Rh disease." See ERYTHROBLASTOSIS.

Rheumatism. A general term for distressing, painful, disabling conditions affecting the joints and their surrounding structures (653).

Rheumatoid factor. An abnormal PROTEIN in the blood of about 70 per cent of patients with classic *rheumatoid arthritis* (660, 668). The rheumatoid factor acts like an ANTIBODY against one of the patient's own normal body proteins, with resulting inflammation and damage to tissue. This is much like an acquired allergy to a part of one's self. Mechanisms which produce the rheumatoid factor have not been proved to be a cause of rheumatoid arthritis, but better knowledge about the factor may throw light on the fundamental nature of the disease. Tests for the factor are commonly given in diagnosing a suspected case of rheumatoid arthritis.

Rhinal. Pertaining to the nose.

Rhinitis. Inflammation of mucous membranes of the nose. It may arise from something as common as the common cold or from infections or allergies (688).

Rhinophyma. Gross overgrowth of blood vessels, sebaceous glands, connective tissue, and skin of the nose, giving the enlarged organ a knobby, reddish, conspicuously bulbous appearance (611). The condition is sometimes associated with over-spirited indulgence in spirits. Correction is surgical.

Rhinoplasty. Plastic surgery of the nose, for cosmetic purposes or correction of deformities (611).

Rhinorrhea. Runny nose.

Rhinoviruses. A family of 30 or more viruses which are major causes of the common cold.

Rhodopsin. A purple pigment in rods of the retina. It is bleached on exposure to light and requires Vitamin A for regeneration.

Rhythm method (*calendar method*). A method of avoiding conception which relies on abstinence from sexual intercourse during the fertile phase of the menstrual cycle (343). OVULATION occurs around the mid-point of the menstrual cycle (339); the "fertile period" of about one week is assumed to span this midpoint, during which abstinence is practiced. If the menstrual cycle is regularly 28 days in length,

the fertile period can be counted as beginning 11 days after onset of menstruation and continuing through the 18th day (or for extra assurance, beginning on day 10 and continuing through day 20). Menstrual cycles are rarely of exactly the same duration month after month. Calendar records may give a reasonably good average over several months, but if swings are great the accuracy of calculations is lessened. Some subjective signs suggest but do not positively prove that an egg has been released and that conception is possible; see OVULATION. In general, for couples who adopt the rhythm method, the "safest" safe period when conception is unlikely is the few days just before and just after menstruation.

Rice diet. A diet furnishing about 10 ounces of boiled rice a day, with fruit juices and sugar, introduced in 1949 as an adjunct in treatment of patients with severe high blood pressure. Benefits of the diet have been attributed largely to its very low sodium (salt) content. Many physicians feel that low-sodium diets which offer a greater variety of foods (32), and restrict calories if weight loss is desirable, are just as effective and better tolerated than a monotonous rice diet. Since the introduction of anti-hypertensive and diuretic drugs, it is usually no longer necessary to restrict salt intake extremely (120).

Rickets. A vitamin DEFICIENCY DISEASE of infants, resulting from insufficient dietary vitamin D or insufficient exposure to sunshine which creates vitamin D from substances in the skin (503). Infantile rickets is manifested by distortion, softening, and bending of incompletely mineralized bones, and sometimes by nodules strung like beads over the ribs (*rachitic rosary*). Infantile rickets is rare in the U.S. because of vitamin D fortification of milk and prescription of vitamin supplements by a pediatrician if he deems it necessary. *Renal rickets* is not a deficiency disease but a congenital incapacity of the kidneys to reabsorb phosphate salts necessary for sturdy bone structure.

Rickettsiae. Disease-causing microbes smaller than bacteria but larger than viruses (64). They are transmitted to man via the biting activities of obnoxious fleas, ticks, and lice. Among the diseases they cause are *typhus, Rocky Mountain spotted fever, trench fever, Q fever, and rickettsialpox.*

Rickettsialpox. A mild non-fatal infection characterized by fever, chills, lymph node enlargement, headache, and chickenpox-like rash (66). It is caused by the bites of mites harbored by mice or small rodents.

Rifampin. The most recent addition to anti-tuberculosis drugs; a synthetic antibiotic which, in combination with at least one other well-known drug (isoniazid, streptomycin, ethambutol) is effective in eliminating tubercle bacilli from the sputum of most patients in about 20 weeks.

Ringworm. Not a worm at all, but infection by various fungi of "dead" tissues of the skin, hair, nails and scalp (199). The troubles they cause have a general medical name, DERMATOPHYTOSIS, and a general word, *tinea,* linked with a name for the affected area, as *tinea capitis, tinea barbae, tinea pedis* (the latter better known as "athlete's foot").

R.N. Registered nurse.

Rocky Mountain spotted fever. A feverish, eruptive infection transmitted by ticks, not limited to western parts of the country (65).

Rodent ulcer. A form of skin cancer (*basal cell epithelioma,* 194) which does not spread to other areas of the body but which, if long neglected, tends to penetrate deeply and erode soft tissues and bones. The ulcers usually occur on sun-exposed areas of the face, especially at margins of the eyes, lips, nose, and ear. The edges of the ulcer have a rolled appearance. The lesion usually begins as a single pinhead to pea-sized nodule, waxy or pearly, which slowly enlarges by development of other waxy nodules near it and coalescence with them. In early stages before undermining of skin and bones begins, surgical removal or x-ray is effective and leaves little scarring.

Rods. Cylindrical nerve structures in the retina, about 100,000,000 to each eye (556). The rods see only shades of gray but are extremely sensitive to faint light and are responsible for most of what we see in dim surroundings. Rods cover most of the cup-shaped RETINA and discern movements which we don't look at directly but perceive from the "corner of the eye." There are no rods in the small round spot near the center of the retina (*fovea*) where all color vision and fine discriminating seeing takes place. The fovea is composed of different, close-packed nerve structures called CONES.

Roentgen (*r*). A quantitative unit of x-radiation, used in calculating intensity of exposure.

Roentgenogram. An x-ray photo.

Rohrschach test. See INKBLOT TEST.

Rongeur. A type of forceps for cutting bone, shaped somewhat like pliers with sharp cupped edges.

Root canal. A small channel in the root of a tooth, continuous with the pulp chamber above it (522). A tooth dead or dying from injury to its pulp ("nerve") may sometimes be saved by root filling or root resection procedures (538).

Rosacea. See ACNE ROSACEA.

Rose fever. A form of hay fever due to sensitivity to rose pollens.

Roseola. Any rose-colored eruption of the skin. *Roseola infantum* is a viral infection of young children producing a fever which lasts three or four days, after which temperature drops to normal, a skin rash appears, and the child is well (420).

Roughage. Indigestible food residues in the intestinal tract, mostly composed of cellulose. A reasonable amount of bulky material is a mechanical aid to intestional functioning.

Roundworms. Several varieties of opprobrious worms that invade the human body if given a chance, gaining entrance via their eggs or larvae in contaminated soil or by hand-to-mouth transmission. The giant of the species is *Ascaris lumbricoides* (70); roundworms of lesser size, but just as repugnant, are HOOKWORMS, WHIPWORMS, PINWORMS. Good sanitation, shoe-wearing, handwashing, hygiene, and cooking are preventive measures.

"Royal jelly." A substance from the salivary glands of bees, fed by the worker bees to the queen bee. No important nutrient has been reported to be present in "royal jelly" that cannot be obtained readily from ordinary foods in our regular food supplies.

Rubefacient. Any agent that makes the skin red.

Rubella. See GERMAN MEASLES.

Rubeola. Measles. Preventable by measles vaccine.

Rubin test. A test of female fertility; also called *tubal insufflation*. It determines whether the OVIDUCTS through which egg cells are transported to the uterus are open or obstructed. A gas, usually carbon dioxide, is introduced through the cervix under pressure. An instrument records significant changes in pressure as the gas flows through. If the oviducts are open, bubbles of gas pass into the abdominal cavity and the patient experiences shoulder pain when she sits upright. The procedure takes but a few minutes (342).

Rugae. Wrinkles, folds, elevations, ridges of tissue, as of the linings of the stomach and vagina.

Runaround. Inflammation all around a nail; PARONYCHIA.

Rupture. See HERNIA.

Ruptured disk. Protrusion of the pulpy, cushioning pad between vertebrae through a rent in surrounding ligament (627).

S

Sabin vaccine. Oral poliovirus vaccine (OPV) for immunization against polio. It contains weakened live polio viruses which produce an inapparent infection that establishes long-lasting immunity, possibly for a lifetime. The American Academy of Pediatrics recommends the vaccine for routine immunization in infancy, as the most effective procedure for the prevention of polio.

Sac. A pouch or baglike covering of an organ or tissue; for example, the pericardial sac of the heart, the sac of a cyst or hernia or tumor.

Saccular. Sac-shaped.

Sacro-iliac trouble. Backache in the region of the sacro-iliac joints. The large sciatic nerve traverses this area (266) and ligaments and muscles are subject to injury. Many mechanisms can produce low back pain; correction depends upon determination of the cause (626).

Sacrum. A large, triangular, curved bone of the lower back, just above the tailbone, composed of five vertebrae that have fused together (618). The sacrum forms the back wall of the bony pelvis, is close to the surface, and can be just about covered by a hand placed on the back between the hips a little below the belt line. On either side of the sacrum is the big hipbone, the *ilium,* and their junction constitutes the site of the sometimes winceful *sacro-iliac joint.*

"Safe period." The days during the midpoint of menstrual cycle when conception is not likely to occur. See RHYTHM METHOD.

St. Anthony's fire. Erysipelas (38).

St. Louis encephalitis. A mosquito-transmitted infection producing feverish illness, headache, stiff neck, sleepiness, mental confusion (60).

St. Vitus' dance. See CHOREA.

Salicylism. A toxic condition produced by overdosage with drugs of the aspirin family (salicylates), causing ringing in the ears, rapid breathing, nausea, visual disturbances, dizziness.

Salivary glands. The three saliva-producing glands on each side of the face: the *parotid* gland in front of and below the ear (the one that is affected in mumps); the *sublingual* gland under the tongue; and the nearby *submaxillary* or *submandibular* gland (452).

Salivation. Excessive secretion of saliva. Ordinary MOTION SICKNESS, irritation of the nervous system, poisoning, local inflammations, certain infectious diseases, and disturbances of the stomach or liver can produce it.

Salk vaccine. A killed-virus vaccine for establishing immunity to polio. It is given in spaced injections; booster doses are recommended every two years. Oral polio vaccine (see SABIN VACCINE) is considered by the American Academy of Pediatrics to have clearcut superiority "from the point of view of ease of administration, immunogenic effectiveness, protective capacity, and potential for the eradication of poliomyelitis."

Salmonella. A family of bacteria which cause gastrointestinal infections (43). They are the most common causes of FOOD POISONING. There are some 400 varieties of Salmonella; one type produces typhoid fever. Most cases of Salmonella food poisoning are not definitely identified. The U. S. Public Health Service estimates that there are up to 2,000,000 cases a year and that the incidence is increasing. The most frequent symptom is gastroenteritis, ranging from a few cramps to fulminating diarrhea. A small percentage of recovered patients become carriers of the infection. The organisms are widely distributed in eggs, poultry, and other animal products. Thorough heating (above 165 degrees) destroys the organisms.

Salpingitis. Inflammation of one or both OVIDUCTS (Fallopian tubes). Symptoms are pain in the lower abdomen, tenderness, discharge from the cervix. The word also applies to inflammation of the Eustachian tube which connects the middle ear and the throat.

San Joaquin fever. *Coccidioidiomycosis* (74).

Sarcoidosis. A non-contagious disease of unknown cause, somewhat resembling tuberculosis. Small lumpy tumors arise in almost any tissue, but particularly in the lungs, skin, bones, eyes, lymphatic system, liver, muscle (236). The nodules may persist more or less unchanged for years or they may heal and recur. Symptoms vary with the organs affected. There is no specific treatment.

Sarcoma. A form of cancer arising mainly from connective tissue. *Osteogenic* sarcoma is a bone tumor, usually requiring amputation of the part. *Ewing's* sarcoma of children and young adults affects the shafts of long bones; the prognosis is poor. A somewhat similar tumor, *reticulum cell* sarcoma, is sensitive to x-rays and treatment by irradiation or amputation offers a good chance of survival.

Saturated fat. See POLYUNSATURATED FATS.

Satyriasis. Excessive and uncontrollable sexual desire in the male.

Scabies. "The itch"; infestation with female mites that burrow tiny tunnels in the top layer of the skin and lay eggs in them (201).

Scaphoid. A small boat-shaped bone of the wrist (635) or ankle.

Scapula. The shoulder blade (617).

Scheuermann's disease. Wedge-shaped deformation of parts of certain vertebrae; a relatively common cause of backache in adolescents (628).

Schick test. A skin test for immunity to diphtheria, performed by injecting a minute amount of diluted diphtheria toxin into the skin. If the injected area becomes red and swollen within a week, it indicates that the individual is not immune to diphtheria and should have protective shots (418).

Schistosomiasis (*bilharzia*). A parasitic disease of the tropics acquired by wading in fresh water where free-swimming forms of a blood fluke hook onto the skin and migrate to various organs via the bloodstream. Snails in which eggs of the parasite develop into free-swimming larvae are reservoirs of the disease (67).

Schlemm's canal. A small channel at the junction of the white of the eye and the cornea through which fluids drain from the chamber of the eye in front of the lens. Narrowing or blocking of the drainage channel builds up destructive pressures within the eye (*glaucoma*, 573). Damage wrought by glaucoma cannot be repaired. Glaucoma may be kept from progressing by eye drops, or surgery may be necessary to open channels.

Sciatica. Not a disease, but a symptom: pain in the back of the thigh and leg along the course of the sciatic nerve (266). Sciatica may be a form of neuritis (265) or severe forms may result from "disk trouble" (627).

Scirrhous. Hard.

Sclera. The strong, elastic outer coat of the eye, visible in front as the white of the eye (552).

Scleroderma. "Hidebound skin"; a connective tissue disease (660) of unknown cause. The first signs usually appear in skin of the hands and feet, in patchy areas which gradually involve more and more of the body. The skin slowly becomes hard, thickened, stiff, smooth and shiny. The face may become masklike because of loss of flexibility. Internal organs—lungs, heart, digestive tract, kidneys—are progressively affected. There is no specific treatment but measures to deal with manifestations in various organs are valuable.

Sclerosing agents. Substances injected to harden and obliterate vessels, as in varicose veins and hemorrhoids.

Sclerosis. Hardening of tissue, especially by overgrowth of fibrous tissue. The sclerosing process affects many kinds of tissues; for example, nerve tissue (*multiple sclerosis*) and linings of the arteries (*arteriosclerosis*). What iniates and perpetuates the process is not fully understood.

Scoliosis. Sidewise curvature of the spine (628).

Scorbutus. SCURVY.

Scotoma A dark spot, blind, or partially blind area in the field of vision, indicating some change in the optic nerve or retina requiring examination by an ophthalmologist. *Scintillating scotomas,* frequently colored, which have saw-toothed shimmering edges and spread out from a small spot to a large area and disappear in a few minutes, are often migraine-like phenomena.

Scratch test. A skin test for allergic sensitivity, especially to inhaled and contacted substances, done by scratching test materials lightly into the skin without drawing blood (682), If the patient is sensitive to the substance, a positive reaction appears within a very few minutes.

Scrofula. Tuberculosis of lymph glands of the neck. The affliction was once common but has almost vanished since the advent of modern methods of treating tuberculosis. A popular treatment used to be the "laying on" of a king's hands, and monarchs honored this regal obligation in ceremonies hopefully attended by the afflicted. One of the last patients to be treated in this manner in England was Dr. Samuel Johnson, the famous subject of Boswell's biography, who as a small child had a laying on of hands by Queen Anne—to no avail. He carried the scars left by the disease for the rest of his life.

Scrotum. The pouch covering the testicles (312).

Scrub typhus (*tsutsugamushi fever*). A feverish disease of eastern Asiatic regions, transmitted by mites (66).

Scuba diving. Diving with Self-Contained Underwater Breathing Apparatus. A physical examination once a year is essential to minimize the hazards of this popular sport. Persons with PERFORATED EARDRUM or acute or chronic infections of the respiratory tract should not dive. Increase and decrease in pressure associated with ascent and descent in diving can turn a simple cold into a serious ear, sinus, or lung infection. The teeth should be in good condition; a pressure-caused gas pocket in a tooth can be excruciating. Physical examination should give special attention to the ears, heart, and respiratory system and should include a chest x-ray. Scuba divers should be aware of the hazards of AIR EMBOLISM and CAISSON DISEASE.

Scurvy. A DEFICIENCY DISEASE due to lack of Vitamin C (503), easily preventable and curable by replacement of the vitamin. Advanced scurvy with its classic symptoms of spongy, bleeding gums, loose teeth, and hemorrhages under the skin is rare in this country, but mild scurvy due to monotonous diets, food aversions, or inadequate supplementation of infant foods is still encountered occasionally.

Seasickness. See MOTION SICKNESS.

Seatworms. Pinworms (71).

Sebaceous cyst. A wen; a skin tumor produced by obstruction of the outlet of an oil-secreting gland (206).

Sebaceous glands. "Oil wells" of the skin which secrete *sebum* or skin oil; usually associated with hair follicles (180).

Seborrhea. Overproduction or change in quality of skin oil secreted by sebaceous glands, producing "oily skin," crusts or scales; associated with acne, dandruff, seborrheic dermatitis (188).

Secundines. The placenta, umbilical cord, and membranes expelled from the uterus after a baby is born.

Sedimentation rate. The rate at which red blood cells settle out of a prepared specimen of blood under laboratory conditions; useful in diagnosis of certain diseases.

Self-limited. A disease that comes to an end all by itself in a limited time, such as an uncomplicated cold.

Semen. The viscid, whitish, mucoid secretion containing SPERMATOZOA which is ejaculated by the male during orgasm. It is a mixture of secretions of testicular organs and of the prostate gland which contributes most of it.

Semicircular canals. Three interconnecting, partially fluid-filled canals of the inner ear which lie in planes at right angles to each other (587). Our sense of balance is located here. Fluid in the canals responds to movements and sends information over nerve pathways to the brain.

Semilunar. Halfmoon-shaped, as the *semilunar valve* of the heart (80).

Seminal vesicles. Accessory glands of the male reproductive system, continuous with the prostate gland (305, 310). The two pouchlike vesicles lie behind the bladder and rectum. Each consists of a single tube much coiled upon itself. The vesicles are storage organs for spermatozoa and secrete a fluid which is added to secretions of the testes. Infection of the vesicles is rare.

Seminoma. A tumor of the testicle.

Sepsis. Fever, chills, and other reactions of the body to bacteria or their toxins in the bloodstream; the thing that antisepsis is against.

Septal defects. Abnormal openings between chambers of the heart which permit blood to "leak" from one side of the heart to the other (97, 745).

Septicemia. "Blood poisoning"; fever, prostration, reactions to living, growing bacteria in the blood. Septicemia is much less common, and much more controllable when it does occur, since doctors have had antibiotics to combat and prevent it.

Septum. A partition or wall between two compartments or cavities; for instance, the nasal septum which divides the left and right nostrils.

Sequestrum. A small piece of dead bone which has become detached from its normal position; for example, "joint mice" (643).

Serum. The amber-colored fluid of blood that remains after the blood has coagulated and the clot has shrunk. It contains disease-fighting ANTIBODIES of the host. This is the basis of serums and antitoxins for treatment of dis-

ease. Animals, commonly horses, are inoculated with gradually increasing doses of bacteria or toxins until they build up large amounts of corresponding antibodies. The animal's serum is withdrawn, purified, and injected to increase a person's resistance to a particular disease.

Serum sickness. A reaction to drugs (699). The most common symptom is HIVES. Some patients break out with a skin rash; some have fever, pain in the joints, enlarged lymph nodes. Serum sickness is closely related to ANAPHYLAXIS but much milder and symptoms do not appear until several days after contact with the offending drug, usually a serum product.

Sessile. Broad-based; said of a tumor that does not have a stem or stalk.

Sex determination. Although sex is almost always self-evident at birth, there are borderline cases where anomalies of development make the true sex difficult to determine (see HERMAPHRODITE). A guide to determination of genetic sex has been found to be the presence or absence in the subject's body cells of minute particles called *chromatin bodies*, which are visible under a microscope. Female cells contain chromatin bodies. Male cells do not, although the chromatin may be undetectable rather than absent. The sex chromatin method has been used to predict the sex of an infant before birth, by study of cells obtained from amniotic fluid which surrounds the fetus.

Sex-linked heredity. Certain traits such as COLOR BLINDNESS and HEMOPHILIA show a form of inheritance called *sex-linkage*. For example, mothers who do not themselves exhibit a trait may transmit it to their sons, who do exhibit it, but not to their daughters. However, the daughters may "carry" the trait, which is in turn manifested in their sons. There are many technical and complex differences in sex-linked transmission lines, but the general principle is fairly simple: sex-linked traits occur because the GENES for expressing them are located in the pair of sex CHROMOSOMES which all normal persons possess. A female has two X chromosomes, one from her mother and one from her father, in her pair (XX). A male has an X chromosome from his mother and a Y chromosome from his father (XY). The Y chromosome is smaller and contains fewer genes. Many genes in the X chromosome have no counterpart in the Y. If there is a defective gene in one X chromosome of a woman, she has another X which is likely to be normal and to suppress the defective gene trait (although she still carries it). But the same defective gene in a man's X chromosome is paired with a Y which has no complementary gene to neutralize the trait, which therefore is fully expressed.

Sheehan's disease. Much the same as SIMMOND'S DISEASE, but resulting from local deficiency of blood supply to the pituitary gland because of severe postpartum hemorrhage (320).

Shigellosis. See BACILLARY DYSENTERY.

Shingles (*herpes zoster*). A virus infection of nerve endings, manifested in the skin by crops of small blisters which follow nerve pathways (56). The chest, face, and upper abdomen are most often affected. Red patches appear and develop into fluid-filled blisters which become dry and scabby in four or five days and eventually heal. The skin should be kept clean and dry and a doctor can prescribe measures to relieve distress. Infection of a facial nerve may reach the eye and threaten to leave scars on the *cornea;* competent care by an eye physician is important. In older people, shingles is sometimes followed by painful, stubborn, long-lasting *neuralgia* that is difficult to treat. Viruses that cause shingles and chickenpox are thought to be identical. Some adults exposed to chickenpox have "come down" with a case of shingles.

Shoe dermatitis. Not all cases of dermatitis of the feet are "athlete's foot." Some cases which may be mistaken for common fungus infection of the feet are instances of shoe dermatitis —sensitization and reaction to rubber, leather, dyes, adhesives, and innumerable substances used in the manufacture of shoes. The affected skin may be dry and scaly, or it may be red and itchy and crops of little blisters may develop. Sweating and maceration of the skin promote sensitization by leaching irritant substances from the shoes and more or less bathing the feet in them. Shoe dermatitis may first be suspected when treatments for supposed "athlete's foot" do not give any benefit. Unlike fungus infection of the feet, shoe dermatitis does not affect the webs of the toes or cause crumbling of the nails. Shoe dermatitis may be suspected if both feet are affected in the same symmetrical pattern, which may correspond with the design of the shoes. If the irritation subsides when a particular pair of shoes is not worn, and flares up when they are worn again, some irritant in that pair of shoes may be suspected. Shoes are made of dozens of different materials and scores of different chemicals are used in processing these materials. Identification of a specific irritant depends upon a PATCH TEST done with samples taken from the patient's shoes. The only remedy is to cease wearing a particular pair of shoes that gives trouble.

Shoe fluoroscopes. Radiation devices in some shoe stores make the bones of the feet visible, ostensibly for better fitting of shoes. Unfortunately, some of the devices, or their excessive use by children for the fun of it, can deliver substantial amounts of quite unnecessary radiation. Many states and municipalities have outlawed the use of shoe-fitting fluoroscopes, and both the American Medical Association and the American College of Radiology have publicly condemned their use as hazardous (792).

"Show." A small amount of reddish or pink discharge from the vagina indicating the onset of labor (379).

Sickle cell anemia (*sicklemia*). An hereditary abnormality of hemoglobin. Crises marked by fever and attacks of pain occur (157).

Siderosis. A form of *pneumoconiosis* (235); chronic lung inflammation due to long inhalation of dusts containing minute particles of iron.

Sigmoid. S-shaped; especially, the *sigmoid flexure,* in the part of the colon above the rectum.

Silicosis. Lung inflammation caused by inhalation of high concentrations of very fine particles of silicon dioxide over a long period of time (235).

Simmond's disease. A severe form of *panhypopituitarism* (320); major damage of the anterior pituitary gland with loss of its function, due to atrophy, necrosis, or tumor. Simmond's disease in women is characterized by shrinkage of breasts and genital organs, loss of sexual hair, weakness, poor appetite, premature aging. Symptoms vary somewhat with the degree of secondary disturbance of the thyroid and adrenal glands.

Sims-Huhner test. A test of semen in the vaginal canal for viability of SPERMATOZOA, employed in diagnosis of infertility (342).

Singer's nodes. Nodules like calluses on the vocal cords of singers, orators, and others who use the voice to excess.

Singultus. HICCUPS.

Sinus. A hollow space, cavity, recess, pocket, dilated channel, suppurating tract. Of the scores of medically designated sinuses, the *paranasal sinuses*— "holes in the head," membrane-lined cavities in bones around the nose—are most familiar to laymen (606). *Sinusitis* (inflammation of the sinuses) is experienced to some degree by everyone who has a head cold, and more excruciatingly if drainage channels become blocked and congested and infection sets in.

Sippy diet. Originally, a diet for patients with acute peptic ulcer, providing a mixture of milk and cream every hour for three days, then gradually adding cereal and egg, and after ten days, other bland foods to replace the milk-cream mixture, until at the end of four weeks the patient is graduated to a low-residue diet. Modifications of the Sippy diet may alternate antacid powders with the milk-cream mixture at the beginning and after a few days add foods of a bland diet (32).

Situs inversus. Transposition of all the organs of the chest and abdomen from the "normal" side of the body to the opposite side. For example, the liver is on the left side instead of the right; organs are in mirror-image positions. Total transposition does not necessarily impair general health.

Sitz bath. Application of wet heat to relieve pain, congestion, spasm, etc., in the pelvic area, by sitting in a tub of warm water (110 degrees or a little more) which covers only the hips and buttocks.

Skene's glands. Two glands with ducts just inside the opening of the female urethra. *Skenitis* is an inflammation of the glands, which may involve the bladder and cause urgency of urination; the most common cause is gonorrheal infection.

Skin writing. See DERMOGRAPHIA.

Skipped beat. See EXTRASYSTOLE.

Sleep. New insights into patterns of sleep have come from studies with the ELECTROENCEPHALOGRAPH, but no researcher can yet say precisely what sleep "is." Brain waves of hundreds of experimental subjects show that we fall asleep in four stages, from Stage

1 (light sleep) to Stage 4 (deepest sleep), and awaken in reverse order. It takes about an hour and a half to go from light sleep to deep sleep and back again. There are about five such cycles in an average uninterrupted night's sleep of approximately eight hours. At the top or light sleep phase of each cycle, we are close to waking, and may even awaken and go back to sleep without remembering it. Perhaps this is the most critical time for insomniacs who fall asleep easily enough but wake in a little while and can't get to sleep again. The discovery that dreaming is accompanied by a peculiar but characteristic kind of rapid eye movements has given some new information about dreams. Hundreds of studies confirm that we generally have the first dream of the night after we ascend to light sleep from the first deep sleep. The average sleeper spends about two hours a night in dreams which occur in four or five cycles corresponding to light sleep. Experimenters believe that everybody dreams repeatedly every night but that dreams are almost immediately forgotten, remembered only unless we awaken while a dream is in progress, and then not usually remembered long.

Sleeping pills. See BARBITURATES.

Sleeping sickness. Untimely attacks of sleepiness do not necessarily imply organic disease (see NARCOLEPSY). "Sleeping sickness" usually refers to a symptom resulting from various injuries, infections, or inflammations of the brain, especially *encephalitis lethargica* (60). *African sleeping sickness* is a specific disease that is transmitted by the bite of an infected tsetse fly (73).

Sleepwalking (*somnambulism*). Parents are often concerned about sleepwalking in children; the condition is more rare in adults. Sleepwalkers may perform dangerous feats, but they may also injure themselves by falling out of windows or crashing against objects. Anxiety and tensions are often strong components of sleepwalking, and investigation of such factors is desirable if sleepwalking persists. The belief that it is dangerous to awaken a sleepwalker has no basis in fact. It is better to awaken him, to prevent injury to himself or others.

Slipped disk. See RUPTURED DISK.

Slit lamp. An instrument for examining structures of the front part of the eye. It produces a slender beam of light and has a microscope which magnifies structures.

Slough. A mass of dead tissue cast off from or contained in living tissue.

Smallpox vaccination. See VACCINIA.

Smears. Secretions or blood spread on a glass slide for examination under a microscope. Smears are often stained with various dyes to bring out fine details of structure.

Smegma. Thick, cheesy material that sometimes accumulates under the PREPUCE in men and around the CLITORIS in women (427).

Smell patch. A small area of tissue about a half inch square at the top of the nasal cavity, where receiving ends of nerves of the sense of smell are located (603).

Snellen chart. The familiar eye test chart consisting of block letters in diminishing sizes (561).

Snoring. If snoring is a "disease," it is one that does no injury to the snorer, only to those within earshot. A snorer almost never knows that he is snoring, even though he may occasionally be awakened by an especially vigorous snort. He knows of his affliction only through the testimony of others. The sounds of snoring—gasps, whistles, gurgles, buzzes, hisses—are produced by vibrations of air passing in and out over the soft palate and other soft structures. Symphonic variations are modified by the force of air flow, frequency of vibration, and the size, density, and elasticity of affected tissues. Sleeping on one's back is conducive to snoring, but some virtuosos can perform while sleeping on their sides. A few causes of snoring may be correctable; it is worth consulting a physician to find out. Most cases of snoring in children are associated with enlarged tonsils and adenoids. Snoring is often associated with mouthbreathing, and if blocked nasal passages or predisposing conditions are treatable there is hope of relief. Nasal polyps are readily removed, a deviated septum can be corrected, blockages associated with infections and allergies are treatable. However, many snorers have native skills that cannot be exorcised and often the best that can be done is to keep them from sleeping on their backs by sewing a rubber ball, or something else uncomfortable, into the back of their pajamas. The most practical remedy, useless to the snorer but of great value to his auditors, is ear plugs.

Soft contact lenses. Conventional contact lenses are made of optical glass or hard plastic. "Soft" lenses are made of water-absorbing plastic which stays soft and supple by absorbing moisture from the eye. Advantages claimed for soft lenses are: easier to fit (the lens molds to the shape of the cornea); greater comfort; less chance of falling out (soft lenses cover about twice as much eye surface as hard ones). Disadvantages are: greater routine care (daily sterilization rituals); inadequate correction of astigmatism; greater susceptibility to wear and damage; sometimes, alternate clearing and blurring of vision; higher cost, approximately $100 more than hard contacts. Progress in this field is quite rapid; improvement of materials and resolution of problems of sterilization are to be expected, as well as probable use of soft contacts as "bandages" for the eyes in certain conditions, and as carriers of medicines in conditions requiring frequent applications.

Solar urticaria. HIVES produced by exposure to sunlight.

Solitary kidney. A rare congenital condition; only one kidney is present.

Somatic. Pertaining to the body.

Somatotype. Body build, constitutional type. Somatotyping procedures most widely used today were developed by Dr. William H. Sheldon whose terms, *endomorph, mesomorph,* and *ectomorph* have entered the common language. Constitution-classifying is based on the three primitive cell layers of the embryo from which particular organs and systems develop. Skin and nervous system derive from the outside layer, the *ectoderm.* Bones, muscles and vascular system derive from the middle layer, the *mesoderm.* The lining of the gut derives from the inner layer, the *endoderm.* Everyone has all three components, but in varying proportions. The circus weight lifter, fat man, and living skeleton are extreme constitutional types. An extreme mesomorph has a predominance of muscle and bone and a hard, square build. An extreme endomorph has superb digestive tract, soft roundness of body, and great facility for getting fat. An extreme ectomorph with a preponderance of skin and nervous tissue has a slender "beanpole" build and great alertness to what is going on around him. Accurate somatotyping requires accurate measurements and photographing of the nude body.

Somniferous. Producing sleep.

Somniloquy (talking in sleep). It is quite common for children to talk in their sleep. Even some adults worry that they may babble secrets when sleeping. Words spoken in sleep are usually fragmentary, mumbled, even ludicrous, and probably indicate participation in dreams or remembered events of the previous day. Talking during sleep probably reflects decreased depth of sleep and is nothing to be alarmed about. See SLEEP.

Spasm. Sudden, severe, involuntary contraction of muscles, interfering with function and often causing pain. If tightening of muscle is steady and persistent, as in leg cramps, it is called *tonic* spasm. If contractions alternate with relaxations, causing jerky movements, the spasms are called *clonic*. Both voluntary and involuntary muscles can be affected, causing a variety of *spastic* conditions. Spasms of involuntary muscle may involve the bronchial tubes (ASTHMA), intestines, blood vessels (RAYNAUD'S DISEASE), and sphincters of the gallbladder and urethra, to mention a few conditions. Antispasmodic drugs such as belladonna may be prescribed to ease spastic conditions of involuntary muscle, such as spastic colon (486).

Speculum. An instrument for viewing the interior of a passage or body cavity; for instance, the vagina, rectum, nose, ear.

Spermatocele. A swelling of the SCROTUM caused by cystic dilation (fluid-filled sac) of the sperm-conducting tubules of the testicle (312). Surgical removal of the painless cyst is usually desirable if it is persistent.

Spermatocide. An agent that kills SPERMATOZOA.

Spermatozoa. Male germ cells; sperm (341). The sperm is the smallest human cell, and the only one capable of independent locomotion, by virtue of its tail which acts as a propeller. Sperms are produced in enormous numbers in the seminiferous tubules of the testicle. Primitive cells in the lining of the tubules develop into maturing sperms which fall off and are carried into a coiled tube, the *epididymis*, and thence into a straighter tube, the *vas deferens* (311, 335). The trip takes about two weeks, during which the sperms continue to mature. They do not move under their own power until they are suspended in SEMEN at the time of ejaculation. Sperm production is a continuous process from puberty to old age. The average man produces some 400,000 *billion* sperms in his lifetime, a number too vast to be comprehensible. The average ejaculate contains from 200 to 250 million sperms. An individual sperm has a head, neck, midpiece and a tail. The head carries the nucleus which contains 23 CHROMOSOMES, one of which is a sex chromosome—either an X (female-determining) or a Y (male-determining) chromosome. The sex chromosome of the human egg is always an X. Hence, it is the sperm that determines the sex of offspring. If the sperm contains a Y chromosome to pair with the X chromosome of the egg, the XY combination produces a boy. If the sperm contains an X chromosome to pair with the X of the egg, the combination produces a girl.

Sperm banks. Interest in storage facilities for frozen sperm has been stimulated by the growing popularity of vasectomy for male sterilization. Some men who undergo surgical sterilization may wish to take out "vasectomy insurance" by storing their sperm for later use in artificial insemination should they change their minds about fertility. Several sperm banks have been established around the country. The semen specimen is diluted with glycerol and placed in a dozen plastic vials which are put into a metal canister that is submerged in stainless steel barrels containing liquid nitrogen at −196° C. No guarantees can be given as to how long the frozen semen may remain viable, or what effect protracted storage may have on genetic adequacy, but normal pregnancies and offspring have resulted from artificial insemination after two years or more of frozen storage. There are few if any state laws regulating the operations of sperm banks. Current information about them can usually be obtained from urologists who perform vasectomies. The frozen sperm technique has been used for two decades to enhance the fertility of husbands with a poor sperm count, by adding several specimens together.

Sperm count. A laboratory procedure for calculating the numbers of SPERMATOZOA in a specimen of semen, useful in assessing male fertility. Although a count of 40,000,000 sperms per cubic centimeter of ejaculate is generally considered normal (counts two to three times greater are not unusual), conception can occur with a relatively low sperm population. Vigorous activity of sperms, and relative lack of abnormal forms, may be more significant to fertility than a relatively low sperm count. If sperms are vigorous and well-shaped, a sperm count of 20,000,000 per cubic centimeter is generally considered adequate for fertility. The volume of ejaculated semen ranges from two to six cubic centimeters.

Sphenoid. Wedge-shaped; especially, the *sphenoid sinuses* of the bone which lies behind the upper part of the nasal cavity (607).

Sphincter. A "purse string" muscle which surrounds and controls opening and closing of a natural orifice; for example, the anal sphincter.

Sphygmomanometer. The instrument that measures arterial blood pressure when a physician puts a rubber cuff around your arm and inflates it.

Spider (arterial). Dilation of small blood vessels in the skin, branching somewhat like the legs of a spider. "Spider bursts" may be associated with liver disease, pregnancy, varicose veins and other conditions but may also occur in normal persons.

Spider bite. The Black Widow spider (860) has been thought to be the only common American spider capable of inflicting an excruciating bite. A relative newcomer, the Brown Recluse spider, is now known to be even more venomous and to be expanding its habitat into many states. It is a shy brown spider that tries to stay away from people, but hides in shoes, blankets, rolled-up newspapers and similar haunts that people are always disturbing. When a brown spider bites, the victim may feel a mild sting or nothing at all. Pain soon occurs, followed by swelling, blistering, even hemorrhage and ulceration. A severe bite may require hospitalization. There is no specific treatment, but prompt injection of cortisone-like drugs, followed by two or three injections on alternate days, is recommended by some investigators. The brown spider's venom is more potent than cobra and other snake venoms, but fortunately the creature can inject only a small amount.

Spina bifida. A congenital malformation of the spine in which some of the vertebrae fail to fuse, so that a sac containing the covers of the spinal cord and even the spinal cord itself may protrude under the skin (272).

Spinal cord. The soft, fluted column of nerve tissue enclosed in the bony vertebral column (246, 617). *Spinal nerves* (all the nerves of the body except the 12 pairs of cranial nerves) enter or leave the spinal cord through openings in the vertebrae.

Spinal tap. Withdrawal of CEREBROSPINAL FLUID through a needle; used in diagnosis of diseases such as meningitis, tumors, polio. The procedure is also called lumbar puncture, since the needle is inserted into the lumbar (lower back) area. Medicines are not injected by this route except in emergency cases.

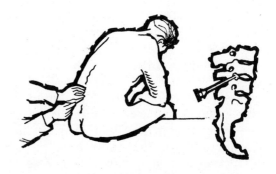

Spinal tap.

Spirochete. A microbe shaped like a corkscrew (47). Many kinds of spirochetes are quite harmless, but the more malicious ones cause syphilis, yaws, relapsing fever, tropical ulcer, ratbite fever, and a few other infections.

Splenomegaly. Enlargement of the spleen.

Split graft. A flap of skin from which the deeper layers have been cut away, leaving the outer layers for grafting (770).

Spondylitis. Inflammation of vertebrae (640).

Spondylolisthesis. Deformation of the lower spine, due to a slipping forward of a lumbar vertebra (627).

Spoon nail. A nail with a concave outer surface instead of the normal convexity, somewhat resembling a spoon.

Spore. An inactive form of a micro-organism that is resistant to destruction and capable of becoming active again. For example, TETANUS spores.

Sporotrichosis. Infection by a kind of fungus that is parasitic on plants. The disease produces nodules along the course of lymphatic vessels which enlarge, ulcerate, and discharge pus. Nurserymen, farmers, and persons in contact with plants and woods are most susceptible. The infection is stubborn and may persist for months but usually responds to treatment.

Spotting. A slight show of blood in the vaginal discharge at times other than menstruation. Slight spotting is not uncommon at the approximate time of OVULATION between menstrual periods. Spotting in pregnancy (364) or after the menopause (442) should be reported promptly to a doctor.

Sprain. Tearing or laceration of ligaments that hold bones together at a joint, a result of severe wrenching.

Sprains are sometimes difficult to distinguish from fractures; both may result from the same injury (850). Diagnosis should be left to physician.

Sprue. See MALABSORPTION SYNDROME.

Squint (*strabismus*). Failure of the two eyes to direct their gaze simultaneously at the same object because of muscle imbalance (566).

Staghorn calculus. A large stone which more or less fills the cavity of the kidney and has irregular projecting surfaces somewhat resembling antlers (289).

Stamp grafts. Small pieces of skin about the size of a postage stamp, used for grafting (771).

Stapes. A tiny, stirrup-shaped bone of the middle ear (584). "Freezing" of the footplate of the stapes by bone growing around it (*otosclerosis*) prevents free conduction of sound to the inner ear. Several types of operations aim to correct this form of hearing loss (592, 755). *Stapes mobilization* is a procedure to "unfreeze" the stirrup bone from its surroundings and restore free vibratory movements. In *stapedectomy*, the stirrup bone is removed and replaced by a plastic substitute.

Staphylococci. Spherical bacteria which tend to grow in clumps like a bunch of grapes (34). They are common inhabitants of the skin and nasal passages (13).

Stasis. Stagnation; slowing of normal flow of body fluids, blood, intestinal contents. *Stasis dermatitis* is an eczematous condition of the leg, common in elderly persons (204).

Status. A severe, refractory condition. *Status asthmaticus:* intractable asthma, extreme difficulty in breathing, cyanosis, exhaustion, lasting a few days to a week or longer (685). *Status epilepticus:* epileptic attacks coming in rapid succession, during which the patient does not regain consciousness.

Steapsin. An enzyme produced in the pancreas gland that aids in the digestion of fats and oils.

Steatorrhea. Stools containing large amounts of undigested fats.

Stein-Leventhal syndrome. A rare condition of sterility, absence of menstruation, and hairiness, in women having enlarged ovaries with many cysts. Treatment is surgical removal of a wedge-shaped section of tissue from each ovary.

Stenosis. Narrowing or constriction of a duct or aperture of the body.

Sterilization, human. Any procedure which leaves a man or woman incapable of having children; usually, a surgical procedure. See TUBAL LIGATION and VASECTOMY. Voluntary sterilization is legal in all 50 states and there are no restrictions on the purposes of the operation except in Connecticut and Utah, where it may be performed only for reasons of "medical necessity," not very sharply defined.

Sternum. The breastbone (617).

Sternutation. Sneezing.

Steroids. Natural hormones or synthetic drugs whose molecules share a common skeleton of four rings of carbon atoms (the steroid nucleus) but which have different actions according to the attachment of other atoms. Natural steroids include the male and female sex hormones and cortisone-like hormones of the cortex of the adrenal glands (330). Oral contraceptives ("the pill") are steroids. Many synthetic steroids developed by pharmaceutical research increase potency, enhance desired effects, minimize side effects or otherwise "improve" the actions of a molecule by shifting, attaching, or disattaching a few atoms.

Stethoscope. An instrument which conducts bodily sounds, especially those of the heart, but of other organs as well, to the ears of the examiner. It is the device that interns carry around their necks in television shows about the travails of doctors. A piece of paper rolled into a cylinder, one end of which is placed on the chest of the patient and the other at the ear of the listener, demonstrates the principle. The stethoscope was invented by Rene Laennec, a French physician, who was called upon to examine a young woman and found a way to listen to her chest sounds without offending her modesty.

Still's disease. A disease of children, like rheumatoid arthritis, affecting many different joints.

Stingray injuries. Stings inflicted by stingrays (it happens to about 750 people a year along our coasts) inject venom. Immediate treatment is to immerse the part in hot water, as hot as the patient can stand, and to keep it immersed for about an hour. Heat detoxifies the venom. This is an immediate first aid measure; afterward, the wound requires medical attention.

"Stomach flu." A term more current among griping patients than physicians. Usually the complaint is of queasiness, vomiting, and diarrhea, which run their course in a couple of days or even 24 hours and have nothing to do with influenza. Gastrointestinal viruses may cause such upsets but it is practically never possible to identify the viruses. Many cases of self-diagnosed "stomach flu" may actually be instances of unsuspected FOOD POISONING.

Stomatitis. Inflammation of soft tissues of the mouth. The inflammation may be limited to the mouth or it may be a symptom of some systemic disease. Viruses, bacteria, or fungi may infect mouth tissues, membranes may be sensitized to certain materials, some drugs may produce oral inflammation.

Stomatitis may be an aspect of blood disorders, vitamin deficiencies, mechanical injuries from jagged teeth or ill-fitting dentures, and skin diseases. Treatment is as varied as the causes.

Stool. The bowel evacuation; feces.

Strabismus. Cross-eyedness (566).

Stratum corneum. The topmost horny layer of the outer skin or epidermis, composed of dead cells that are shed and replaced from below (178).

Strawberry mark. A birthmark comprised of superficial blood vessels, present at birth or developing shortly thereafter, which has a tendency to disappear spontaneously in the course of time (194).

Strawberry tongue. A bright red tongue seen especially in scarlet fever; the blood-engorged papillae are enlarged and prominent.

Streptococci. Sphere-shaped bacteria which tend to grow like chains of little balls (34). They are responsible for scarlet fever, "strep throat," and many other infections.

Stria (pl. *striae*). A streak, line, stripe, narrow band. Whitish striations of the abdomen may appear as the skin is stretched during pregnancy and in the breasts after milk production ceases. Obesity or an excess of cortisone-like hormones (332) may produce "stretch marks" on the abdomen. Striations may appear temporarily in adolescent girls as hormone balances of sexual maturity are becoming established.

Stricture. Narrowing or tightening of the passageway of a duct or hollow organ; may result from inflammation, contraction, injury, scarring, or obtrusion of tissue.

Stroke. Apoplexy, cerebrovascular accident, paralytic stroke (123).

Stroma. The supporting tissue of an organ, as opposed to its active "producing" tissue.

Struma. Goiter.

Stupe. A cloth wrung out of hot water and applied to the skin; turpentine is sometimes sprinkled in the water as a counter-irritant.

Subacute. An almost acute condition; intermediate between chronic and acute illness.

Subclinical disease. A disease, usually mild, that has no definite symptoms or signs which can be recognized by the usual visual or clinical means.

Subcutaneous. Beneath the skin, as a hypodermic injection.

Subluxation. Partial or incomplete dislocation, sprain.

Substernal. Underneath the breastbone.

Sudorific. Sweat-inducing.

"Summer itch." A North American form of SCHISTOSOMIASIS, quite different from the serious tropical variety. It sometimes afflicts swimmers in northern fresh water lakes. Larvae which are parasites of snails in the lakes get into the skin, cause a prickling sensation, and itchy red spots and pimples develop (68). The condition clears up by itself but in the meantime, lotions to decrease itching are comforting.

Sunburn, Suntan. Too long exposure to intense sunlight will, as practically everyone has learned, cause sunburn, which is in every sense a burn. What most people want to acquire is a suntan, not a burn. The amount of sun that individuals can stand varies with thickness, pigmentation, and personal structure of the skin. For most of North America the sun usually is intense enough to affect the skin between 9:30 a.m. and 2:30 p.m. from

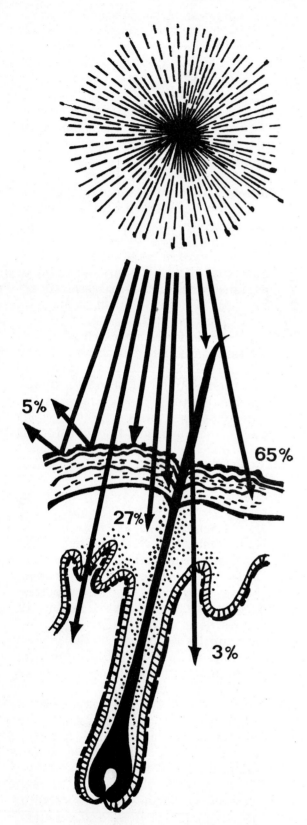

April through August. To develop a tan without a burn, the skin should be exposed gradually, starting with an exposure of no more than 20 minutes the first day, increasing exposure by about one-third each successive day. After a week the skin should have been conditioned sufficiently to permit a moderate amount of sunbathing through the summer. Suntan is produced by the darkening and moving toward the surface of melanin granules made by cells in deeper skin layers. Exposure to sun not only darkens the skin, but thickens it. The extra thickness gives much of the protection against sunlight. The extra thickness lasts only six weeks or so after exposure has ceased. Unlimited exposure to burning rays of the sun has undesirable long-term effects. Continued exposure ages the skin prematurely, thickens, wrinkles, and leatherizes it. This aging is irreversible, the delayed price of overexuberant tanning.

Superfluous hair. Hirsutism; especially, excessive hairiness of the lips, cheek, chin or legs of women. There may be an underlying endocrine disorder (340), a family tendency to hairiness, or hair may be unduly conspicuous in an area where it is normally present. Electrolysis performed by a skilled operator employs electric current to destroy the hair root permanently, but its application is tedious. Chemical depilatories remove hair satisfactorily but directions must be followed carefully to avoid skin irritation. A bleach may mask the condition if hair growth is fine.

Supernumerary. More than a normal number, as a sixth finger or toe.

Suppuration. Formation of pus.

Suprarenal glands. Adrenal glands (330).

Supraspinatus syndrome. A term for disorders of the shoulder region which make it painful or impossible to lift the arm completely (630).

Suntan-sunburn: 5% of ultraviolet rays reflected off skin surface, 65% absorbed by horny layers of skin, 27% absorbed by rest of epidermis, 3% reach dermis ("true skin").

Surfer's knots. Soft-tissue swellings on the instep and just below the knee, produced by continued kneeling on a surfboard. After a year or two of steady surfing the knots become hard and firm. Large knots over a joint may cause changes in small bones of the feet. The knots may be painful and sometimes require treatment. If surfing is discontinued the knots tend to disappear in a few months, but knots of several years' duration may disappear only partially after the sport is given up. Probably no greater permanent disability will be suffered than mild deformity or arthritis of the foot or possibly the knee.

Sympathectomy. Surgical removal of fibers of the sympathetic nervous system (248). The object is to modify for the better the activity of organs regulated by sympathetic nerve trunks, as in sympathectomy for reduction of high blood pressure (120).

Sympathetic ophthalmia. Inflammation of one eye due to injury of the other eye. Prompt treatment of an injured eye is important to prevent involvement of the other eye and possible blindness.

Symphysis. The junction of originally distinct bones which have grown together; for example, the lines of fusion of the sacrum and the coccyx, and of the pubic bones (619).

Suture. To sew up a wound, or the threadlike materials used for this purpose; catgut, linen, silk, wire, cotton, etc. *Absorbable* sutures such as catgut (actually, sheep's intestines) are often used to close wounds in deep tissues. Sutures used to sew surface tissues are usually non-absorbable and removable, to the considerable anguish of the patient.

Swimmer's ear. "Athlete's foot" of the ear canal; water incompletely drained from the ear sets up moist and soggy conditions favorable to fungus infection (594).

Swimming pool granuloma. A rare infection of the skin caused by acid-fast bacteria related to tuberculosis germs. The organisms apparently gain lodgment in cracks, fissures and rough surfaces of some swimming pools. The first sign of infection is the appearance of a group of small, red, tender pimples on the skin. Later the pimples merge to form a plaque or nodule which occasionally contains pus. The elbows are the most common site of infection. Lesions may also appear on the knees and feet. These are body areas most likely to be banged or scraped against rough pool surfaces. Pressure or rubbing against parts of a pool where germs are present apparently gives them entrance to the skin, although there may be no obvious sign of abrasion or injury. The infection is chronic and may persist for many weeks. Patients with swimming pool granuloma given TUBERCULIN TESTS commonly have a positive reaction. Adequate chlorination of the water and repair of broken tiles or concrete to produce smooth surfaces protect against outbreaks of the infection. It is not known where the germs come from or why they are peculiarly associated with swimming pools.

Sycosis. Inflammatory disease of the hair follicles, especially of the beard. Usually a STAPHYLOCOCCUS infection, characterized by pus-filled pimples perforated by hairs.

Sydenham's chorea. See CHOREA.

Synapse. A point of communication between processes of nerve cells which come close together but do not actually touch; a sort of "spark gap" for nerve impulses to jump (243).

Syncope. Fainting.

Syndactyly. Webbed or fused fingers or toes.

Syndrome. A set of symptoms which occur together and collectively characterize a disease.

Synovial fluid. The clear viscid fluid, resembling the white of an egg, which lubricates the movements of tendons and joints.

Systemic disease. One which affects the body as a whole, not limited to a particular part; for example, an infection spread through the bloodstream.

Systole. The period of blood-pumping contraction of the heart. Systolic pressure is the higher of the two figures (such as 120/80) by which doctors express blood pressure readings. See DIASTOLE.

Saphenous veins. Two large veins of the leg near the skin surface which sometimes become varicosed (133).

T

Tarry stools. Stools resembling tar in color and consistency; usually an indication of bleeding into the intestinal tract. Iron and other medications can produce similar stools.

Tachycardia. Rapid heart beat (108).

Talipes. Foot deformity; clubfoot (647).

Tarsus. The instep of the foot (645).

Tampon. A plug of absorbent material inserted into a body cavity, such as a pack for nosebleed or a vaginal tampon to absorb menstrual flow.

Taenia. TAPEWORM.

Tapeworm. A ribbonlike flatworm which may invade the intestines of consumers of undercooked beef, fish, or pork (68).

Tartar (*dental calculus*). Hard, mineralized deposits on surfaces of teeth, irritating to the gums and underlying bone (532). Toothbrushing helps to prevent the deposits when they are in a soft state, but they solidify quickly. Periodic removal by a dentist or dental hygienist is good insurance against disease of supporting tissues of the teeth, popularly called pyorrhea.

Tattooing. Insertion of permanent colors into the skin through punctures, as by a needle. "Tattoo parlors" whose operators decorate the skin with garish designs and sentiments have no relation to medicine, unless a customer who is emblazoned with the name of a girl friend he wants to forget asks a physician about the possibilities of erasure. Unclean tattoo needles can transmit viral HEPATITIS and other diseases, and for that reason many municipalities have banished the old-time tattoo artist. In competent medical hands, tattooing has recognized but limited value, primarily for minimizing skin discolorations. *Portwine stain*, a bluish-red birthmark (194), may be made less conspicuous by tattooing opaque skin-colored pigments into the affected area.

Tapping. Emptying fluids from a body cavity by surgical puncture; resorted to when accumulated fluids embarrass the functioning of the heart, lungs, abdomen, cranium, and other organs.

Tabes dorsalis. See ATAXIA.

Tay-Sachs disease. See AMAUROTIC FAMILIAL IDIOCY.

Tear gas. Increasing sale of tear gas pens, pencils, and gas shells causes some concern about possible burns or injuries of the eyes. The tear gas most commonly used (chloracetophenone) is ejected by a black powder propellant covered by wadding. If the gun is exploded so close to the eye that liquid or solid particles strike it directly, the eye may be seriously injured. Otherwise, there is little or no danger of permanent damage. Exposure to a fine spray or cloud of tear gas causes tears to flow copiously and the eyelids to close spasmodically. In fresh air these symptoms disappear and only a slight redness of the conjunctiva may remain for a short time.

Teflon. A coating applied to skillets to keep foods from sticking. The material is perfectly safe. Teflon does not decompose except at temperatures far greater than can be attained by any cooking procedure.

Temporal bone banks. This is a program by means of which persons with impaired hearing or other forms of ear disorders (head noises, Meniere's disease, etc.) can bequeath their inner ear structures for medical research. Temporal bones are those which contain the inner ear and its nerve structures inside the head. These cannot be examined directly during life and research into causes and prevention of deafness is severely handicapped. By relating a patient's history of ear disease to abnormalities observed in his bequeathed temporal bones, the Temporal Bone Banks Program aims to obtain information of scientific value in assessing the effectiveness of medical and surgical treatments and in the prevention and correction of ear disorders. Four regional Temporal Bone Banks Centers are located at the University of California, San Francisco; the University of Chicago; Johns Hopkins Hospital, Baltimore; and Baylor University, Houston. Information can be obtained from the Deafness Research Foundation, 366 Madison Ave., New York, N. Y. 10017.

Tenaculum. A long, slender type of forceps like tongs, with scissors handles, having teeth or hooks at the end to grasp a part, such as the cervix of the uterus. It is used especially in gynecologic surgery.

Tendon. A band of tough white fibrous tissue that connects a muscle to a bone. Muscle fibers merge into one end of a tendon, the other end of which is attached to a bone. Sometimes a tendon conveys muscle action over a considerable distance, as in the back of the leg, where a long tendon inserted into the rear of the ankle transmits the pull of calf muscles above it. This makes it unnecessary to have a huge mass of muscle around the ankle itself. Most tendons are covered by sheaths which secrete lubricating fluids for easy sliding. Tendons and their sheaths are subject to injury by tearing, stretching, twisting stresses ("pulled tendon" is a common athletic injury) and to inflammations, for which there are technical names such as *tenosynovitis* and *tenovaginitis*.

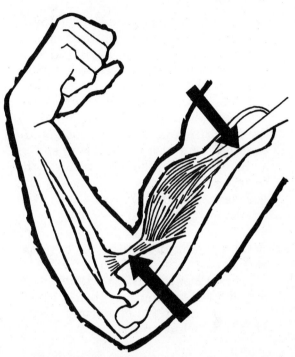

Tendons connecting biceps muscle to bones.

Tenesmus. Painful straining to empty the bowel or bladder, without success.

Tennis elbow. This painful condition of the outer side of the elbow joint can affect anyone who overvigorously uses a screwdriver as well as a tennis racquet. It is a form of BURSITIS produced by violent extension of the wrist with the palm downward or vigorous rotary movement of the forearm against resistance, putting severe stress on the elbow joint (633).

Tendinitis. Inflammation of tendons and their attachments.

Telangiectasis. Dilation of groups of small blood vessels, appearing as fine lines on the skin, sometimes associated with diseases of the skin, cirrhosis of the liver, and other disorders. The dilations may form hard, red, wartlike spots the size of a pinhead or pea. In *hereditary hemorrhagic telangiectasis*, a rare form, the dilated vessels become thin and fragile, rupture spontaneously, and bleed into the skin, intestines, or other parts of the body. It is inherited as a dominant trait; see Chapter 25.

Temperomandibular joint. The joint in front of the ear in which the hinge of the lower jaw fits into a socket in the base of the skull. Its close relationship to the teeth may bring about changes not common in other joints. Uneven bite, tooth-clenching habits, poorly fitting dentures or tooth restorations, may throw the joint out of joint, limit sidewise motion, limit the opening of the mouth, cause pain, soreness, clicking noises, and even headaches (545).

Teratology. The branch of science concerned with the study of malformations and monstrosities. A *teratoma* is a tumor containing hair, teeth, bones, or other material not normal to the part in which it grows.

Term (at term). The end of the normal period of gestation or pregnancy when birth occurs.

Testicle, testis. The primary male sex glands or gonads; paired organs, enclosed in the pouch of the SCROTUM, together with accessory structures (335).

Testosterone. The male hormone, a STEROID hormone produced by cells of the testicle independent from cells which produce SPERMATOZOA.

"Test tube babies." Popular term for offspring of ARTIFICIAL INSEMINATION.

Tetanus (*lockjaw*). A grave, often fatal infection caused by toxins of tetanus organisms which get into the body through perforating, penetrating, or deep wounds and thrive in the absence of oxygen (42, 848). The disease is easily prevented by harmless *tetanus toxoid* "shots." These are routinely given to infants and should be just as routine for adults who are as likely to suffer accidents as anybody (420).

Tetany. Painful muscle twitchings, spasms, especially of wrists and feet; sometimes convulsions. Insufficient calcium in the blood causes the muscular irritability and consequent symptoms. Insufficiency of circulating calcium may result from vitamin D deficiency or underactivity of the parathyroid glands (329). Treatment is with calcium salts, orally or by infusion if the condition is severe. Do not confuse with *tetanus*.

Tetralogy of Fallot. Congenital malformation of the heart, exhibiting four defects: aorta turned to the right, ventricular septal defect, constriction of the pulmonary artery or valve, hypertrophy of the right ventricle.

Thalassemia. Cooley's anemia (158).

Thelarche. Precocious growth of the female breast (319).

Thenar. Pertaining to the palm of the hand; especially, the padded thenar eminence that bulges at the base of the thumb.

Therapy. Treatment of disease. Anything that is therapeutic is designed to help or heal.

Thermography. Body surfaces emit slightly different amounts of heat because of local differences in underlying blood supply. This is the principle of thermography, which employs sensitive instruments to scan body areas and record slight heat differentials on sensitized paper. Thermography has been used to detect and localize very small breast tumors, to investigate blood vessel obstructions, and to localize the site of the placenta. It is a young technique, limited to a few medical centers.

Thoracentesis. Puncture of the chest wall with a hollow needle for withdrawal of fluids.

Thoracoplasty. Removal of several rib segments to collapse the chest wall and lung (221). A treatment for tuberculosis that has become less common since the development of effective anti-tuberculosis drugs.

Thorax. The chest.

Threadworms. Roundworms which in larval form can enter the body through the skin, usually of the feet, and migrate to the intestines, causing diarrhea and pain in the pit of the stomach (69).

Thrombin. An enzyme present in blood oozing from a wound, but not in circulating blood. It acts upon a blood protein to produce *fibrin,* which is the essential portion of a blood clot.

Thromboangiitis obliterans. See BUERGER'S DISEASE.

Thrombocytes. Blood PLATELETS which help to initiate blood clotting.

Thrombocytopenia. Deficiency of platelets necessary for blood coagulation, resulting in bleeding from tiny blood vessels into the skin and mucous membranes, known as PURPURA (159).

Thrombophlebitis. Presence of a blood clot (THROMBUS) in a vein, with inflammation; *venous thrombosis* (137). Veins of the leg are most commonly affected. If superficial, the affected vein may be felt as a very tender cord. Thrombosis of deep veins is serious because blood clots may break off and be carried in the bloodstream until they become "stuck" and plug vital vessels. A large particle (EMBOLUS) may reach the heart or lungs and cause death. The tendency of clots to form in slightly injured veins is greatly increased by physical inactivity such as prolonged bed rest. Getting the patient out of bed soon after surgery or childbirth, and encouraging bedridden patients to carry out frequent movements of the legs, are preventive measures. Treatment of active deep venous thrombosis includes such measures as elevation of the foot of the bed, warmth, and anticoagulant drugs which retard blood clotting.

Thrombosis. Formation of a clot in a blood vessel, and the partial or complete plugging of the vessel that ensues. The most familiar example is *coronary thrombosis* (88), but the process can occur in many vessels besides those which supply the heart.

Thrombus. A clot which forms in a blood vessel and remains at the site of attachment. If a fragment or the entire clot breaks off and is carried through the bloodstream, the free-moving particle is called an EMBOLUS.

Thrush. A fungus infection of the mouth, occurring in young infants. Whitish spots in the mouth become painful shallow sores (417).

Thymus gland. An organ in the chest (313) which for years puzzled anatomists who could find no function for it. Recent research has shown that immediately after birth, the thymus begins to activate the body's defenses against infections. The thymus is a self-starter which produces and sends out millions of tiny *lymphocytes* (145) to the spleen and lymph nodes, where they synthesize ANTIBODIES. Once these seedbeds are established with the aid of a hormone from the thymus, production of lymphocytes in lymphoid tissues continues throughout life. The thymus, having got things going, shrinks and retires. In infants the thymus is a large organ, relative to body size. It continues to grow for eight to ten years. By that time the body's immunity systems are running smoothly and the thymus which ignited them is no longer necessary. The gland begins to shrink and in adults is very small. At one time it was thought that an enlarged thymus was a cause of sudden unexplained deaths of infants, because the thymus of infants dead from infections was much smaller than the thymus of infants who died suddenly from unknown causes. It is now realized that the thymus of infants who die from infections is abnormally small because the gland shrinks rapidly in the presence of infections and stresses, and that a relatively large thymus is normal in infancy. There is some evidence that the thymus may play a part in the inception of AUTO-IMMUNE DISEASES.

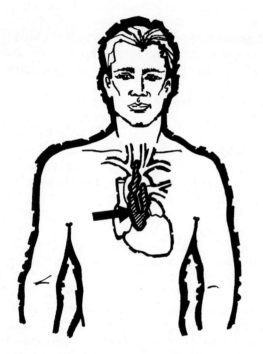

Thymus gland.

Thyroglobulin. An iodine-protein substance, the form in which thyroid hormone is stored in the gland (315).

Thyroid. The shield-shaped gland in the neck, covering the sides and front of the windpipe (315). It is a "governor" of metabolism, regulator of the rate at which body fires burn.

Thyroidectomy. Surgical removal of part of the thyroid gland (323, 751).

Thyroiditis. Acute or chronic inflammation of the thyroid gland (326).

Thyrotoxicosis. Hyperthyroidism; a toxic condition due to excessive activity of the thyroid gland, or to a tumor of the gland (322).

Thyroxine. The hormone released from the thyroid gland (321).

Tibia. The shinbone.

Tic douloureux (*trigeminal neuralgia*). Stabbing, excruciating pain in one side of the face along pathways of a cranial nerve, set off by touching a "trigger" area (267).

Tick paralysis. Muscular weakness, incoordination, or paralysis, beginning in the legs and ascending, caused by toxins which enter the blood through bites of woodticks or dog ticks. Symptoms give warning to search carefully for an imbedded tick which may be hidden in hairy parts of the body. Prompt removal of the tick (859) is usually followed by gradual disappearance of symptoms.

Tics. Habit spasms; quick, twitchy, repetitive movements of certain muscle groups, always in the same manner: pouting the lips, batting the eyelids, wrinkling the nose, making faces, shaking the head, shrugging a shoulder, tilting the neck, etc. The nervous habits develop most commonly in children and often disappear in the course of time if the child isn't constantly nagged about them. Usually the "ticky" youngster is pretty tense and tightened up inside to begin with; he may be a target of demands, expectations, and pressures that might make anyone twitchy if bottled up inside. A little loosening of the reins by those who hold them may help to relax a child who, after all, does not consciously decide to indulge in tics. Nervous habits should be distinguished from purposeless movements associated with some physical disorder. Genuine tics never appear during sleep.

T.i.d. Three times a day.

Timetable of fetal development. See pages 372-3.

Tinea. Ringworm; fungus infection of the skin (199).

Tine test. A form of TUBERCULIN TEST. A small disposable stainless steel disk with four prongs covered with dried *tuberculin* is pressed into the skin (219). The unit is used on only one patient, is never reused. The technique is advantageous in screening large population groups of school children and susceptible young adults for tuberculosis.

Tinnitus. Head noises; ringing, roaring, clicking or hissing sounds in the ears (597).

Tipped uterus. Forward, backward, or other displacement of the uterus from its theoretically ideal position (437).

Tissue culture. A method of growing cells in a suitable nutrient in flasks or test tubes outside of the body, and of propagating viruses in the cells. Polio viruses and some others are grown in tissue culture for manufacture of vaccines. Viruses can be identified by tissue-culture reactions under laboratory conditions. More than 100 "new" viruses have been isolated and identified by tissue culture techniques in the past decade and some have been associated with diseases.

Toad venom. Ordinary toads are harmless. But a giant tropical variety (*Bufus marinus*) which has invaded the Florida coast in the Miami Beach area exudes venom similar to a cobra's. Some small animals that have tangled with the toads have died from the venom's effects. The giant toad, weighing a pound or more, is yellowish brown with black markings. Its milk-colored venom is exuded from glands behind the eyes. The creatures breed in ponds and lakes but often come out on dry land at night to hunt insects. The giant toads should not be picked up or touched.

Tolerance. Ability to withstand abnormally large doses of a drug, induced by its continual use.

Tomograms. X-ray films of layers or planes of the body, like a layer cake. A tomogram shows a plane of the body about a half inch thick. The layer shows in fine detail but structures above and below it are fuzzy (784).

Tonometer. An instrument for measuring internal pressures of the eyeball, used in screening for *glaucoma* (577).

Tophi. Masses of urate deposits in the external ear, joints, and other structures composed largely of CARTILAGE; characteristic of *gout* (657).

Torticollis (*wry neck*). A condition in which muscles of one side of the neck are in a state of more or less continuous spasm, pulling the head into an unnatural position (270, 630).

Torulosis. A serious systemic fungus infection, occurring in eastern and southern parts of the U. S.; *cryptococcosis* (74). The infection most frequently attacks the central nervous system but may invade the bones, lungs, and skin.

Tourist's diarrhea. Mild to severe attacks of vomiting, nausea, diarrhea, afflicting unacclimatized visitors to foreign lands. Although popularly blamed on the water, spicy foods, oils, exotic cuisine, and the like, the specific causes remain a mystery. Common bacteria seem not to be responsible. Other forms of dysentery having specific causes should be ruled out. There is no certain preventive, but sensible eating helps. Eat two meals a day of familiar foods that you are accustomed to at home, if you can get them, and limit yourself to one meal a day of strange foreign foods until you become adapted. Go easy on sauces, gravies, salad oils containing mixtures of unknown ingredients. Cooked foods are safest to eat in unfamiliar places. If an attack comes on, take fluids to combat dehydration; plain warm tea is excellent. Applesauce, boiled rice, boiled chicken, and bland soups are good. Add other simple plain foods until recovery. Drugs do not attack the unknown cause of tourist's diarrhea but some help to control the symptoms.

Toxemia. A "poisoned" condition due to absorption into the blood of toxic substances produced by bacteria or body cells, but without the presence of bacteria in the blood. *Toxemia of pregnancy* is a disturbance of metabolism which in severe form (rare if the patient has good prenatal care) is attended by fever, headache, convulsions and rapid rise in blood pressure (375).

Toxic goiter. THYROTOXICOSIS, hyperthyroidism (322).

Toxin. A poisonous substance originating in cells of microbes, animals, or plants. Injection of a specific toxin into an animal stimulates the production of specific ANTIBODIES. This is the basis for pharmaceutical preparation of an antitoxin that neutralizes a particular toxin, for example: *botulinus, tetanus, diphtheria, snake venom.*

Toxoid. Resembling a toxin; a substance prepared by treating a toxin with agents which produce a *toxoid* that has the same immunity-stimulating ability as the toxin but is itself harmless and non-toxic. Tetanus and diphtheria toxoids are widely used in routine immunization.

Toxoplasmosis. A disease caused by infection with protozoan organisms (73). Inapparent infection of a pregnant woman may cause severe abnormalities in her baby.

Tracer elements. See RADIOISOTOPES.

Trachea. The windpipe.

Tracheobronchitis. Inflammation of the windpipe and bronchial tubes (406).

Tracheotomy. Cutting an artificial hole in the windpipe to bypass an obstruction and permit air to flow under it into the lungs (754).

Trachoma. A contagious disease of the eyes, caused by viruses which attack the lining membranes of the lids and eyes (570). Raspberry-like elevations on the inner eyelids rub against the CORNEA, leading to ulcers and blindness.

Tragus. The small lid of CARTILAGE over the external opening of the ear.

Tranquilizers. A popular, non-medical term for a variety of drugs which more or less selectively depress the central nervous system to produce calming, sedative effects but which do not dull consciousness or induce sleep, in proper doses. "Tranquilizer" is a broad term that includes many drugs of somewhat different individual actions, taken account of by a physician in prescribing a particular agent. The drugs are often categorized as *major* and *minor* tranquilizers.

The major tranquilizers, most of which belong to chemical families known as *phenothiazines* and *piperazines*, have their greatest use in treating severely disturbed psychotic patients. They tend to reduce agitation, excitement, panic, hostility and to quiet the wild, assaultive, destructive behavior associated with those emotional states, and there may be a reduction of psychotic symptoms such as hallucinations and delusions. This often makes the calmed patient more reachable by other forms of therapy. Many can be discharged from hospitals and returned to their communities relatively soon. Many patients must continue on the drugs for varying lengths of time, but this often can be supervised by the family physician, and recovery tends to be assisted by a comfortable environment of home and family.

The major tranquilizers are sometimes used in non-psychiatric patients for their secondary actions in pre-

Hypothetical mode of action of tranquilizing drugs. Drawing A shows *limbic system,* a border around the brain stem. The limbic cortex, hypothalamus, and associated structures are concerned with "non-thinking" activities of internal environment and of self-preservation, provocative of emotions—fear, rage, anxiety, agitation, sexual and defensive reactions. In a sense, emotions go round-and-round in the limbic system and are diffusely projected to other parts of the nervous system. Excessive, persistent reverberations of emotions are thought to be factors in neuroses, phychosomatic ailments, mental illnesses. Tranquilizing drugs are thought to dampen the stresses of disturbed emotions by disconnecting or interrupting reverberative circuits. Below, interacting structures of the limbic system. Colored lines suggest circuits, arrows suggest outward pathways of nerve impulses; actual pathways not known.

1. Limbic cortex.
2. Corpus callosum
3. Fornix system.
4. Thalamus.
5. Hypothalamus.
6. Amygdaloid nucleus.
7. Hippocampus.

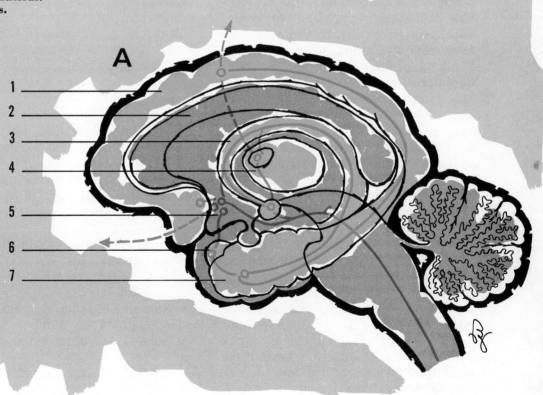

venting or arresting nausea and vomiting, and for intensifying the actions of anesthetics and pain-relievers so that smaller doses of the latter can be given.

The minor tranquilizers (sometimes called *atarctics* or "peace of mind" drugs) are mainly used to suppress mild to moderate manifestations of anxiety and tension in psychoneurotic patients as well as in normal persons who react tensely to stresses of their environment. Their action is quite similar to, and probably not superior to, that of the barbiturates in easing anxiety-tension states. However, the classic sedatives cause some drowsiness and loss of alertness; in correct doses, the minor tranquilizers produce mild sedation without dulling consciousness or impairing performance. Some of them have moderate muscle-relaxing action. The minor tranquilizers have considerably greater margin of safety than potent sedatives and massive overdosage is less likely to be serious or fatal, although huge overdoses, taken with suicidal intent, can lead to coma, shock, and even death. Patients who take excessive amounts of the drugs for long periods may become dependent upon them and suffer withdrawal reactions when they are discontinued.

Transillumination. Examination of a cavity or structure by means of light passing through it; for example, examination of nasal sinuses with the aid of a light in the patient's mouth.

Transplantation. Surgical techniques for transplanting an organ from one person to another are well advanced. The best known procedure is kidney transplantation (298), but the heart, lung, liver, and spleen have been transplanted in a very few human beings, demonstrating that surgical techniques of transplantation have been mastered. The major obstacle to permanent transplantation is the body's ultimate rejection of a donated organ as foreign tissue by the patient's immune mechanisms.

Trauma. Injury, wound.

Transvestism. Perverted desire to wear the clothes of the opposite sex; a person who does so is a *transvestite.*

Tremor. Involuntary quivering and trembling of muscle groups, other than from obvious causes such as shivering in the cold. Tremor is a symptom which may give information about a constitutional disease. A doctor may ask a patient to hold out the arms at shoulder level with palms down and fingers stretched; fine, rapid tremor of the fingers may suggest hyperthyroidism. There are fine, coarse, slow and rapid tremors; harmless but annoying hereditary tremors; tremors that appear when at rest; and "intention tremors" that appear when voluntary movement of a part is attempted. Tremors may or may not indicate a disorder of the nervous system; there are hysterical tremors that have no organic basis.

Trench fever. A louse-borne, typhus-like, non-fatal RICKETTSIAL INFECTION. Many cases occurred in World Wars I and II but the disease has since gone into hiding (66).

Trench mouth (*Vincent's infection*). Painful, swollen, malodorous inflammation of the mouth and gums (37, 535). The disease is not considered to be contagious. Susceptibility is increased by debilitating disease, malnutrition, poor mouth hygiene, and heavy smoking.

Trepanning. Cutting a button of bone out of the skull with a *trephine,* a circular instrument with sawlike edges.

Treponema. A tribe of spiral microbes responsible for a number of infectious diseases, including syphilis (47).

Triceps. The muscle that extends the forearm.

Trichinosis (*trichiniasis*). A parasitic disease due to ingestion of encysted larvae of worms present in raw or undercooked pork (69).

Trichobezoar. A ball of hair formed into a mass in the stomach.

Trichomoniasis. A quite common infestation of the vagina with minute pear-shaped creatures which have tiny propellers for getting about (434). Their presence produces vaginal irritation and a thin, white, watery, offensive discharge. Men may be affected too but often have no symptoms. Local methods of treatment by insufflation of powders, medicated douches, etc., give relief but the organisms are hard to eradicate. Infection may be re-transmitted by marital partners and for total eradication, both partners may be treated. A new oral drug, *metronidazole*, is highly effective in eradicating the infection.

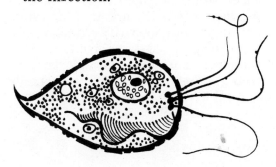

Trichomonad, the causative organism of trichomoniasis.

Trichophytosis. Ringworm of the scalp (199). The causative fungi fluoresce when exposed to a WOOD'S LIGHT. The condition, which is contagious, occurs in children before puberty.

Trichotillomania. A neurotic habit of pulling out one's own hair.

Tricuspid valve. A valve with three triangular-shaped leaflets through which blood moves from auricle to ventricle in the right side of the heart (80, 103).

Trigeminal neuralgia. See TIC DOULOUREUX.

Trigger finger. A condition in which efforts to unbend a finger are at first unsuccessful, but it is soon straightened with a snap or a jerk, like the release of a trigger. It is caused by a constriction which prevents free movement of a tendon in its sheath (636).

Trimester. Three months, or one-third of the nine months of pregnancy. The nine months of pregnancy are traditionally divided into the first, second, and third trimesters.

Trismus. Spasmodic tightening of muscles of the jaw, as in lockjaw.

Trocar. A perforating instrument for puncturing a cavity to release fluid; it fits inside a *cannula.*

Tropical ulcer. Chronic, tissue-destroying ulceration of the lower leg or foot, caused by a spirochete (50).

Trypanosomiasis. African sleeping sickness, produced by organisms transmitted to the blood by the bite of an infected insect (73).

TSH. Thyroid-stimulating hormone (305).

Truss. A device, usually a pad attached to a belt, designed to hold in place a HERNIA or internal organ which tends to protrude through the skin.

Trypsin. A protein-digesting enzyme produced by the pancreas gland.

Tryptophan. One of the essential AMINO ACIDS. It is frequently inadequate in food protein of plant origin.

Tsutsugamushi disease. See SCRUB TYPHUS.

Tubal ligation *(salpingectomy).* An operation for sterilization of women. The surgeon makes a small incision in the abdomen and cuts and ties the OVIDUCTS (343). This prevents the meeting of sperm and egg and makes conception impossible. The procedure is comparable to an appendix operation and is always performed in a hospital. It is frequently performed a few hours after delivery of a baby but can be done at any time for a non-pregnant woman. Tubal ligation does not interfere with menstruation or sexual capacity; the ovaries continue to produce hormones. The operation should not be undertaken unless permanent sterility is desired.

Tubal pregnancy. Implantation of a fertilized egg in the walls of the Fallopian tube instead of in the uterus; the most common form of ECTOPIC PREGNANCY (370).

Tubercle. A small nodule or prominence; especially, a mass of small spherical cells produced by tubercle bacilli that is characteristic of tuberculosis. The word also means a rough, rounded prominence on a bone.

Tuberculin test. A skin test for tuberculosis (219). There are several modifications of the test; the MANTOUX TEST is usually employed in routine case-finding. Tuberculin in various forms is a sterile fluid containing substances extracted from dead tuberculosis germs. Tissues of a person with tuberculous infection are hypersensitive to products of tubercle bacilli. Injection of a small amount of tuberculin under the skin gives a positive or negative reaction. A positive reaction, indicated by redness and swelling of the injected area within a few hours, indicates the presence of tuberculous infection but does not tell whether the infection is active or inactive. It merely indicates that tuberculous infection was acquired at some time, and appropriate measures can be taken.

Tubule. A little tube; any minute tubular structure, such as the kidney tubules or the semeniferous tubules of the testes.

Tularemia. Rabbit fever (46).

Tumefaction. Swelling.

Turbinates. Scroll-shaped bones of the outer sidewalls of the nasal cavity, covered by spongy tissue which moistens and "air conditions" inhaled air (601).

Turner's syndrome. A congenital condition in which the ovaries do not mature or produce egg cells (340). The affected girl develops along female lines but breast enlargement and menstruation do not occur at puberty, unless the condition is recognized early and treated with female hormones; however, the patient is permanently sterile. A woman with Turner's syndrome has only 45 instead of the normal 46 CHROMOSOMES. One sex chromosome is missing. A normal woman has two XX (female-determining) chromosones; in Turner's syndrome, one X chromosome is lacking. Its absence results in ovaries lacking egg-producing follicles, and there is retardation of body growth; ultimate stature is usually less than five feet. With judicious hormone therapy the affected woman can live a reasonably normal life but will be sterile and can never bear children.

Tussis. A cough.

Twins. See MULTIPLE BIRTHS.

Tympanites. Taut distention of the abdomen by intestinal gases or fluids; bloating.

Tympanoplasty. Plastic surgery of the middle ear, to close a punctured eardrum (597) or to clean out and reconstruct the cavity (755).

Tympanum. The middle ear and the eardrum, the *tympanic membrane* (583).

Typhoid fever. Acute feverish illness caused by germs of the Salmonella family, contained in the feces of infected patients and unknowing carriers; usually transmitted by contaminated water or food or poor personal hygiene (43). Modern sanitation, alert health departments, and medical progress have made typhoid fever a rare disease in the U.S. where it was once common, feared, disabling, and often deadly. An antibiotic, chloramphenicol, is very effective in treating typhoid fever. Vaccination against the disease (three inoculations a week or more apart, and an annual booster dose if one remains in an infected area) is recommended for travelers to regions where typhoid fever is endemic, but not for the general population in this country (420).

Typhus. A RICKETTSIAL DISEASE transmitted to man by infected lice and fleas, with rats and mice as intermediaries. There are several varieties of typhus (65). The disease has not existed in the U.S. for many years, but is endemic in parts of Asia, the near East, India, and other areas. Vaccination is recommended for travelers to such areas (52).

U

Ulcer. An open sore with an inflamed base; local disintegration of tissues of the skin or mucous membranes, leaving a raw, sometimes running surface. The cause may be infection, pressure (as in BEDSORES), erosive irritation (PEPTIC ULCER), varicosities, systemic disease, impaired circulation.

Ulcerative colitis. Inflammation of the colon and rectum, characterized by sores or ulcers inside the tube and bloody diarrhea. The disease may be mild and responsive to medical treatment or so severe as to require surgical removal of the affected part of the colon (490, 731).

Ulceromembranous stomatitis. TRENCH MOUTH.

Ulna. The bone on the side of the forearm opposite to the thumb; its companion bone is the RADIUS (617).

Ultrasound. Sound waves of high frequencies above the range of human

hearing. Ultrasonic devices of various and changing design have several medical uses. Instruments which register the "echoes" of ultrasound have been used to locate and define brain tumors, to locate the position of the placenta and fetus, and to identify the site and severity of arterial obstruction by registering the rate of blood flow in deep vessels. Therapeutically, ultrasonic equipment is used to clean tartar from teeth, to treat bursitis, and an ultrasound "probe" has had some success in destroying nerve endings in the inner ear, without damage to hearing and the sense of equilibrium, in patients with MENIERE'S DISEASE (269, 756) who have not responded to medical treatment.

Ultraviolet rays. Wavelengths of radiation too short to be seen as visible light. They lie between the wavelengths of visible light and x-rays. The spectrum of visible light runs from short violet rays to long red rays. The sequence of colors in a rainbow or sunlight scattered by a prism is incorporated in a memory-aiding word, VIBGYOR: violet, indigo, blue, green, yellow, orange, red. Beyond red lie the long, invisible and hot *infra-red rays*, emanated by special lamps sometimes used to deliver dry heat to parts of the body. Ultraviolet rays contained in sunshine or produced by ultraviolet lamps (sunlamps) act upon substances in the skin to make vitamin D. They also produce a skin tan (see SUNBURN). These are the only known benefits of ultraviolet rays in moderation. Excessive exposure to natural or artificial ultraviolet radiation can produce severe burns and age the skin prematurely. It is wise to ask for and follow a physician's advice about the use of sunlamps.

Umbilical cord. The long flexible tube which is attached to the PLACENTA at one end and to the abdomen of the fetus at the other (357). It is the lifeline of the fetus. Through vessels of the cord the fetus receives nutrients and disposes of wastes without effort. The cord allows considerable freedom of movement in the dark fluid cavern of the womb. The cord continues to function until it is tied and severed at birth. After that the newborn human being is on his own.

Umbilical hernia. A protrusion of the intestines through a weakness in the abdominal wall in the region of the navel, not uncommon in infants (411).

Umbilicated. Depressed like a navel.

Umbilicus. The navel, belly-button; a depressed round scar in the middle of the abdomen, permanent memorial to umbilical vessels that nourished the fetus via the placenta.

Uncinaria. HOOKWORMS (69).

Underweight. Body weight 10 per cent less than desirable weight (505) is usually considered to be underweight. However, healthy people vary in bone and muscle proportions and rates of energy expenditure. Underweight may be a symptom of some disease process and should be evaluated by a doctor; sudden unexplained loss of weight requires medical investigation. What is thought to be underweight may be only a mother's expectation that a child ought to eat more and be chubbier. Simple underweight should respond to an increase in food calories (511). In addition to calories, plenty of rest, relaxation, and easing of tensions may be necessary in energetic, restless, overcommitted, hard-driving underweight people who burn their candles at both ends.

Undescended testicles. See CRYPTORCHIDISM (311, 336).

Undulant fever. See BRUCELLOSIS.

Ungual. Pertaining to the nails.

Unguentum. An ointment.

Uniovular. Pertaining to or originating from a single egg, as identical twins.

Universal donor. A person with Type O blood does not have "factors" which would antagonize blood of Types A, B, or AB, and hence is presumably compatible with all blood types. However, there are many blood factors besides the ABO group (Rh, M, N, Lewis, Kell, Duffy, Lutheran, and others) which may make the blood of a Type O donor antagonistic to a recipient. A universal donor's blood may be given in an emergency, but cross-matching of blood is necessary for greatest safety in transfusions (148).

Unsaturated fats. See POLYUNSATURATED FATS.

Upper respiratory infection. Infection of nasal passages or throat above the lungs. An infection may extend from the original site of symptoms. See opposite page.

Urea. A nitrogen-containing substance in blood and urine, formed mainly from nitrogen groups removed in the liver from the AMINO ACIDS of protein foods. Some is formed from nitrogen released by the wear and tear of body tissues. Increasing the protein portion of the diet increases the output of urea in the urine. The *urea clearance test* of blood is a test of kidney function.

Uremia. Presence in the blood of toxic substances due to incapacity of the kidney to filter and excrete them in urine; *uremic poisoning* (292, 295). Symptoms may develop in a few hours or over a period of weeks: headache, dimness of vision, drowsiness, restlessness; later, diarrhea and vomiting, difficult breathing during the night, convulsions, coma, death. It is the way in which serious kidney disease usually terminates. It is this condition of dammed-up toxins that the ARTIFICIAL KIDNEY is designed to overcome (296).

Ureter. The narrow tube through which urine from the kidneys passes into the bladder (285). Urine is not drawn down the tube by gravity nor does it descend in a steady flow. The ureter

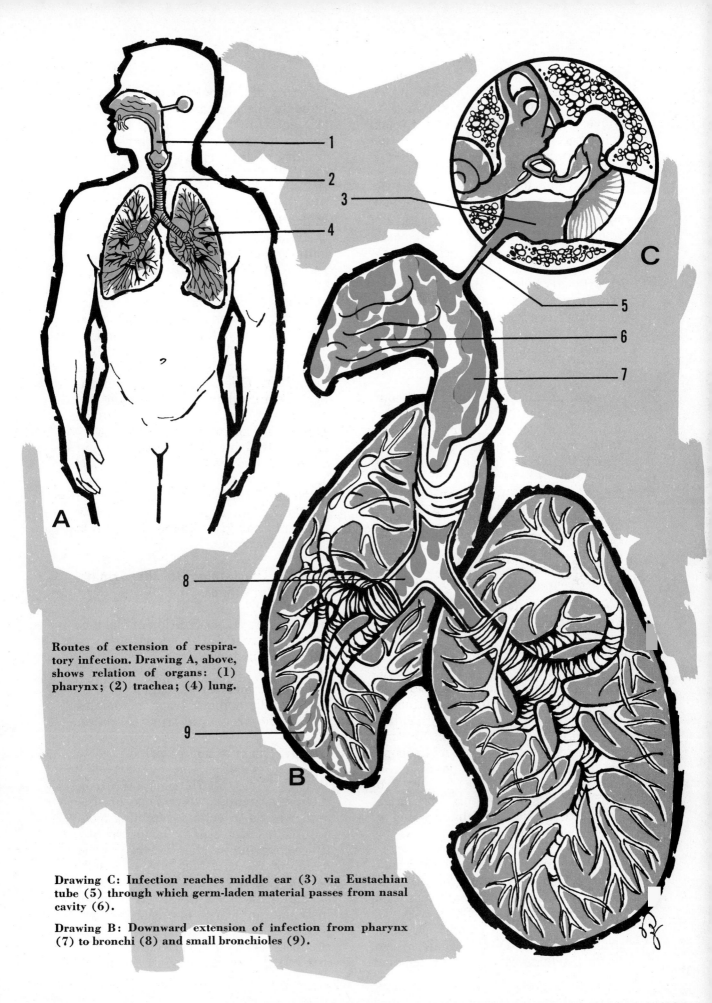

Routes of extension of respiratory infection. Drawing A, above, shows relation of organs: (1) pharynx; (2) trachea; (4) lung.

Drawing C: Infection reaches middle ear (3) via Eustachian tube (5) through which germ-laden material passes from nasal cavity (6).

Drawing B: Downward extension of infection from pharynx (7) to bronchi (8) and small bronchioles (9).

has walls of smooth muscle which contract in waves (PERISTALSIS) to move urine into the bladder in jets which occur from one to half a dozen times a minute.

Urethra. The canal from the neck of the bladder to the outside through which urine is passed. The female urethra is about an inch and a half long; the male urethra, eight to nine inches (281). Voiding of urine is regulated by circularly arranged sphincter muscles which in the adult are largely under voluntary control.

Urethritis. Inflammation of the URETHRA.

Uric acid. A nitrogen-containing compound present in normal blood and urine. It is derived from substances in the nuclei of cells called *purines*, in which liver, sweetbreads, kidney and other glandular meats are particularly rich. An excess of uric acid products is characteristic of GOUT (657), a disorder in which tiny, spiky urate crystals tend to be deposited in cartilage with "red hot" intimations of their presence.

Uricemia. Excessive amounts of URIC ACID in the blood.

Urinalysis. Inspection and chemical analysis of urine. The extent of analysis depends on what the doctor wants to find out. At the minimum, observations of color, clarity, specific gravity, acidity, sugar, and ALBUMIN content are usually made. More extensive microscopic or chemical analysis of possible constituents—pus, bile, blood cells, protein, crystals, casts—may be necessary to throw light on what is going on in the body (286).

Urine. The amber-colored, slightly acid fluid secreted by the kidneys. It is mostly water but normally contains about four per cent of dissolved materials such as salt, ammonia, urea, uric acid, hormones or their breakdown products. Excessive or deficient amounts of normal constituents may indicate disease, and abnormal constituents—fat, blood, pus, bacteria, spermatozoa, bile—almost always do. Acidity of the urine varies with the diet. Most fruits reduce the acidity of the diet; starvation or a high protein diet increases it. Acidity of the urine indicates that the kidneys are doing their job of maintaining the slight alkalinity of the blood (see ACID-BASE BALANCE). The average adult forms about three pints of urine a day. The volume of urine is reduced in hot weather, by strenuous muscular exercise or scanty fluid intake, and is greater on a high than a low protein diet. The most concentrated urine is passed after getting up in the morning. Doctors have good reason for specifying that a sample of urine should be taken at a certain time. Formation of urine is decreased during sleep; decided and persistent increase of volume of night urine, with many gettings-up, may be a sign of chronic kidney or other disease. The yellow pigment that gives urine its color is called *urochrome*.

Urogenital. Pertaining to the urinary and genital organs.

Urogram. X-ray visualization of the urinary tract made after injecting a radiopaque substance.

Urologist. A medical specialist in diseases of the urinary tract in females and of the urogenital tract in males.

Uroscopy. Examination of urine.

Urticaria (*hives, nettlerash*). Whitish, intensely itching elevations of the skin, wheals or welts, resembling mosquito bites but usually larger, sometimes covering patches as large as the palm (692). An attack may be a solitary event, never again experienced, subsiding in a few days, but in some instances urticaria is miserably repeated and persistent. Frequently the condition is an allergic reaction to certain foods (strawberries, shellfish, etc.), to drugs (700), to cold (701), to heat or sunlight (702).

Urushiol. The despicable oil in poison ivy and poison oak that causes distressing skin eruptions.

U.S.P. United States Pharmacopoeia.

Uterine displacements. "Tipped uterus"; backward, forward, or sideward shift of the uterus, or a "fallen womb" protruding into the vagina (437).

Uterine tubes. The Fallopian tubes; OVIDUCTS.

Uterosalpingography. X-rays of the uterus and tubes, following injection of iodized oil into the uterus, to determine whether the tubes are open (342).

Uterus. The womb; the pear-shaped, muscular, hollow, distensible nesting-place of the fetus in pregnancy (357). In the adult non-pregnant woman the uterus is about three inches long, two and a half inches wide near the top, tapering to a neck (*cervix*) about an inch wide, which occupies the upper part of the vagina. It has walls of smooth muscle like thick felt with a lining of mucous membrane (ENDOMETRIUM). Its triangular cavity, a mere slit, is continuous with a narrow canal through its neck which affords an entrance for SPERMATOZOA and an exit for menstrual discharges. The uterus lies between the bladder and the rectum, tilted forward, its upper part resting on the bladder. It is rather loosely supported by eight LIGAMENTS which allow freedom of motion and position in adjusting to pressures of surrounding organs and enlargement of pregnancy. The organ enlarges slightly during menstruation, enormously during pregnancy, and after childbirth returns almost to its previous size but its cavity is larger than before.

Uvea. Pigmentary layers of the eye: the IRIS, CILIARY BODY, and CHOROID coat, composed largely of interlaced blood vessels vital to the eye's nutrition (553).

Uveitis. Non-pus forming inflammation of the UVEA, the IRIS and associated eye structures (571). It is a serious condition that can cause blindness. It may be associated with systemic diseases (TOXOPLASMOSIS, HISTOPLASMOSIS, LEPTOSPIROSIS), but there are many types of uveal inflammation for which no specific cause can be found. One form is thought to be an AUTOIMMUNE DISEASE resulting from a patient's sensitization to tissues of the lens of his own eyes.

Uvula. The blob of tissue hanging like a big tear from the soft palate at the back of the mouth. You can see it with a mirror by opening your mouth wide and depressing the tongue (424). It rarely causes any trouble, except that it may be implicated in snoring, but generally that does not trouble the snorer, only his auditors.

V

Vaccine. The word derives from the Latin word for "cow," the source of cowpox virus used to vaccinate against smallpox. It has come to mean any bacterial or viral material for inoculation against a specific disease. Virus vaccines are of two types, *live virus* or *killed virus* vaccines. Live virus vaccines contain living viruses, so weakened that they cannot cause significant disease, but still can stimulate the body powerfully to make protective ANTIBODIES against a particular disease. For example, SABIN VACCINE contains live viruses, so weakened in the laboratory that they produce only unnoticeable infection but stimulate antibody production that persists for a long time, perhaps a lifetime. Killed virus vaccines contain viruses treated by physical or chemical means to kill or inactivate them so they cannot cause disease but nevertheless can stimulate immunity-producing mechanisms of the body. SALK VACCINE is of this type. In general, live virus vaccines are more potent and create longer lasting immunity than killed virus vaccines.

Vaccinia. Cowpox; a disease of cattle caused by viruses which, inoculated into man, create immunity to smallpox. Babies used to be vaccinated against smallpox before they were a year old but routine vaccination is no longer recommended (infants with eczema, impetigo, or skin rashes should not be vaccinated until the condition clears up, nor should they be in close contact with others who have just been vaccinated). About three days after smallpox vaccination a red pimple appears at the site of inoculation, enlarges, gets blistery, and is surrounded by a reddened area about the size of a quarter. The lesion begins to dry in a week to ten days. It forms a scab which falls off by the end of the third week or sooner, leaving a flat whitish vaccination mark which some persons prefer to have elsewhere than on the arm. Reaction to one's first smallpox vaccination is a "primary take." Reactions in persons who have been vaccinated previously are milder, but if there is no reaction at all it does not mean that one is naturally immune, but that the vaccine was weak or did not get through the skin.

Vacuole. A clear space in tissue.

Vacuum extractor. A cuplike device within which a partial vacuum is created when it is placed over the presenting part of a baby's head during childbirth. The adherent cup with its handle facilitates extraction of the baby and the device is sometimes used in delivery as a substitute for obstetric forceps.

Vagina. A sheath; the female organ of copulation, a muscular canal lined with mucous membrane which opens at the surface of the body and extends inward to the cervix of the uterus (428, 437).

Vaginal diaphragm. A contraceptive device consisting of a spring-rimmed rubber dome inserted into the vagina to cover the cervix.

Vaginal hysterectomy. Surgical removal of the uterus through the vagina (735).

Vaginismus. Painful, spastic constriction of female pelvic muscles, making sexual intercourse difficult or impossible (433).

Vaginitis. Inflammation of the vagina, characterized by discharge and discomfort; see MONILIASIS and TRICHOMONIASIS (434). A form occurring after menopause is called *atrophic* or *senile vaginitis*.

Vagotomy. Cutting of certain branches of the VAGUS nerve which communicates with many organs in the chest and abdomen. The object is to diminish the flow of nerve impulses, such as those which stimulate the stomach to produce acids (727).

Vagus. The "wandering" cranial nerve which arises in the brain and extends its fibers to the pacemaker of the heart, to the bronchi, esophagus, gallbladder, pancreas, small intestine and secretory glands of the stomach.

Valsalva maneuver. Originally a technique devised by an Italian anatomist for pushing air into the middle ear by exhaling forcibly while keeping the glottis closed, so that air cannot escape from the throat. A similar condition is produced by coughing or straining at the toilet. The maneuver is used by cardiologists as a diagnostic test of congestive heart failure. Buildup of pressure within the chest and abdomen prevents the return flow of blood from the head, hands, and feet. Heart output decreases and venous blood pressure increases. When the effort is ended, a surge of venous blood into the right side of the heart causes temporary overloading of the heart chambers. The mechanism explains why some persons feel light-headed or dizzy during bowel movements or while coughing.

Valve. A structure that prevents back-flow of fluids. There are valves in the heart (104), in many veins, at the stomach outlet, and at junctions along many tubular communication lines, to keep blood or fluid materials moving in the right direction.

van den Bergh test. A qualitative test of blood serum, useful in determining the origin of different types of JAUNDICE and measurements of liver function.

Varicella. Chickenpox (418).

Varices. VARICOSE VEINS.

Varicocele. Varicosed, dilated, twisted veins of the spermatic cord; a soft mass in the SCROTUM that feels like a bag of worms. The condition occurs most frequently in adolescence and tends to disappear with maturity. Usually it is a minor affliction, often undetected, causing no discomfort, or sometimes a slight draggy feeling relieved by wearing a suspensory. Varicocele does not significantly affect the health of the testes or lead to impotence or sterility. Only the most distressing cases warrant surgery.

Varicose veins. Swollen, dilated, knotted, tortuous veins (132). The sites most frequently affected are the legs and anus (HEMORRHOIDS). Varicose veins frequently develop during or are aggravated by pregnancy (363).

Variola. Smallpox.

Variola minor (*alastrim*). A mild form of smallpox. Symptoms are similar to those of virulent smallpox (420) but much less severe; fatalities are very rare. Standard smallpox vaccination protects also against this mild form of the disease.

Vas. A tube or vessel, usually but not always a blood or lymphatic vessel.

Vascular. Pertaining to or abundant in vessels, especially blood vessels. Well-vascularized tissues have abundant blood supply; *avascular* tissues such as the CORNEA have none at all.

Vas deferens. The duct through which SPERMATOZOA are transported from the testicle to the seminal vesicles and urethra (310).

Vasectomy. A relatively simple surgical procedure for sterilization of the male. The excretory duct of the testis (*vas deferens*, 310) is severed or a portion cut out of it to prevent SPERMATOZOA from entering into the SEMEN. The structures are close to the surface and the operation is usually done in the doctor's office under local anesthesia. There is no interference with sexual capacity since the hormone-producing tissues of the testicle are not affected. It is prudent to regard the sterilization as permanent, although in a few cases the severed ends of the ducts have been rejoined, with restoration of fertility.

Vasoconstrictor. A drug or natural body substance or mechanism that clamps down on small blood vessels, narrows their caliber and reduces the volume of blood flowing through them. This action, rather like that of myriads of tiny tourniquets, increases the amount of blood in the reservoirs of big expansible arteries and increases blood pressure until matters come into balance.

Vasodilator. An agent that dilates small blood vessels so that more blood flows through them; blood pressure is usually lowered. If it happens locally, one blushes. The opposite of VASOCONSTRICTOR.

Vasomotor. Pertaining to mechanisms that control dilation or constriction of walls of blood vessels, and thus the volume of blood flowing through them. Impulses from centers in the brain go to muscle fibers in walls of blood vessels over nerves of opposite action: constriction or dilation. Feedback mechanisms of the vasomotor system are exceedingly intricate. In hemorrhage, for instance, the fall in blood pressure caused by loss of blood triggers the vasomotor machinery to constrict blood vessels and speed the heart, which tends to restore blood pressure to normal.

VDRL test. A screening test for syphilis using blood serum (Venereal Disease Research Laboratory).

Vector. A carrier, spreader of disease; especially, an insect or animal host that carries disease germs and transmits them to human beings.

Veins. Thin-walled, strong, low-pressure vessels that collect dark "used" blood from tissues and carry it to the heart to be pumped through the lungs, where the blood dumps a load of carbon dioxide and takes on a load of oxygen. Blood from capillaries is collected into *venules* (very tiny veins) which enter into larger veins and finally into the *vena cava* which opens into the right auricle of the heart (79). When a vein is cut the blood wells out in a steady flow with no evident pressure. Veins can hold large reservoirs of blood (Vein chart, 135).

Venereal warts. CONDYLOMA ACUMINATA.

Venesection. Bloodletting; same as PHLEBOTOMY.

Venoclysis. Injection of fluids by vein. A vein of the wrist is preferred but is sometimes too small, inaccessible, or shrunken, and a vein of the leg, foot, or thigh may be used.

Ventral. The belly side; the aspect of a part directed toward the belly.

Ventricle. A small cavity or chamber; especially, the ventricles of the heart and brain. The lower part of the heart has a right ventricle which receives venous blood and pumps it to the lungs, and a left ventricle which receives oxygenated blood from the lungs and pumps it to the body (78).

The brain has several ventricles filled with CEREBROSPINAL FLUID (271). Increased volume and pressure of fluid in brain ventricles, due to impaired drainage, results in HYDROCEPHALUS (272).

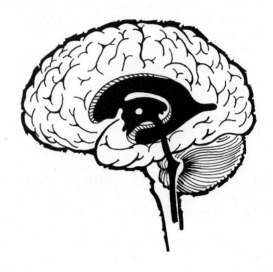

Ventricles of the brain.

Ventriculogram. An x-ray of the brain taken after introducing air or a contrast medium into certain ventricles.

Venules. The smallest veins, communicating with capillaries.

Vermiform. Worm-shaped.

Vermifuge. An agent that kills or expels intestinal worms.

Vernix caseosa. A greasy, cheesy substance that covers the skin of the fetus, removed at the first cleansing.

Verruca. A wart.

Version. Turning, manipulation of the fetus in the uterus to attain a better position for delivery, such as turning the feet in PODALIC VERSION.

Vertebra (pl., *vertebrae*). One of the 33 bones which constitute the backbone (617). Vertebrae are flat, roughly circular bones with knobs for muscle attachments and a hole in the middle for passage of the great nerve trunk, the spinal cord. Individual vertebrae, except the four which are fused to form the COCCYX, are separated by pads of elastic cartilage (*intervertebral disks*) which absorb shocks and give a certain amount of flexibility.

Vertex. The highest point of the skull, the topmost part of the head.

Vertigo. See DIZZINESS.

Vesicant. An agent that produces blisters, such as mustard gas.

Vesicle. A small sac containing fluid; a tiny bladder, like a skin blister.

Viable. Capable of living.

Vibrissae. Hairs in the nose. Also, a cat's whiskers.

Villi. Minute fingerlike projections from the surface of a mucous membrane. The small intestine contains millions of villi which increase the surface area in contact with foods and give the lining of the tract a velvety feel (456).

Vincent's infection. TRENCH MOUTH (37, 535).

Virilism. Development in a female of masculine characteristics (beard growth, deep voice, etc.), usually due to a masculinizing tumor of the ovary, overactivity of the cortex of the adrenal glands, or administration of androgenic hormones (340).

Viruses. Molecules that cause disease (53).

Visceroptosis. Sagging of abdominal organs from their normal position.

Viscid. Sticky, adhesive.

Viscus (pl., *viscera*). An internal organ, especially one of the great cavities of the body, such as the intestines, stomach, heart, lungs and kidneys, hence "visceral: to feel deeply."

Visual field. The area of physical space seen when the gaze is fixed straight ahead (558, 560).

Visual purple. A pigment produced by RODS of the RETINA, essential for good vision in dim light. The purplish pigment bleaches to yellow when exposed to light. A product of its breakdown is vitamin A, which is also needed for its regeneration. Severe deficiency of vitamin A causes night blindness because of inability of visual purple to regenerate adequately.

Visual radiations. Nerve fibers which fray out to the rear of the brain where what we see is actually seen (557).

Vitiligo (*leukoderma*). Piebald skin; irregular white patches of skin, sometimes streaks of white or gray hair, due to lack of pigment. Often there is a family tendency to develop the condition. The white patches are most conspicuous when surrounded by deeply tanned skin. No infallible way of inducing repigmentation of the spotty patches is known, but in some instances the taking of an oral drug, *methoxypsoralen*, followed by controlled exposure to sunlight, may produce some deposit of pigment. However, results are uncertain and the treatment may cause some irritation of affected areas and excessive pigmentation of surrounding skin. Vitiligo is not a systemic disease but a purely cosmetic defect which, if distressing, can usually be covered satisfactorily with a tinted preparation.

Vitreous humor. Transparent, colorless, soft gelatinous material which fills the eyeball behind the lens (551).

Volvulus. Twisting or knotting of the bowel, leading to intestinal obstruction and GANGRENE of the part (483).

Vomiting. Forcible ejection of stomach contents, triggered by a vomiting center in the brain; a protective mechanism for getting rid of toxic or irritating materials. Rats do not have a vomiting center and consequently may be poisoned by substances which vomiting mammals get rid of with ease. Ordinarily, vomiting is a transient event of no great significance in itself, provoked by gastric indiscretion, motion sickness, or some infectious illness accompanied by other symptoms. Simple vomiting from minor intestinal upsets can be managed rather simply (396). However, PROJECTILE VOMITING or COFFEE-GROUND VOMIT is a symptom requiring immediate investigation. Intractable, long-continued vomiting (or diarrhea) can seriously deplete body fluids and ELECTROLYTES, especially in infants who have small reserves. Common causes of "ordinary" infant vomiting are stomach dilation from *overfeeding* (too frequent feedings or too much at a time) or *underfeeding,* leading to hunger, crying, lots of air-swallowing and distention. Too hot feedings may induce vomiting. Formulas at room temperature are quite acceptable. Vomiting may be controlled by ice-cold feedings.

von Gierke's disease. GLYCOGEN STORAGE DISEASE with involvement of the liver and the kidneys.

von Recklinghausen's disease. See NEUROFIBROMATOSIS.

Vulva. The external female sex parts.

Vulvovaginitis. Inflammation of both the VULVA and VAGINA. A rare but severe gonorrheal form occasionally is transmitted to female infants and children by careless hygiene. See TRICHOMONIASIS and MONILIASIS.

W

Wall-eye. Outward turning of an eye; divergent squint, a condition of ocular muscle imbalance (566).

Warts. Harmless but unsightly small growths from the skin (191). Common warts of the hands, face, and feet, most frequent in children, are caused by viruses, are contagious, and the sufferer can re-inoculate himself over and over again. Common warts can be removed by a great variety of methods, including hocus-pocus, and they tend to disappear in time with no treatment at all. An isolated wart is probably best left alone, unless it is very disfiguring or painful, or is enlarging or changing its appearance, or is in a part of the body subject to constant irritation.

Warts at the edges of fingernails or underneath them are hard to treat; applications of cold—dry ice or liquid nitrogen—are commonly used. Warts in the scalp or beard area are especially troublesome because shaving and combing the hair tend to spread them. A man with warts in the beard area should use an electric shaver.

Wassermann test. The original blood test for syphilis. It is not specific for syphilis; "false positive" reactions may be produced by malaria, hepatitis, mononucleosis, and other unrelated diseases. Many newer tests (sometimes used in conjunction with Wassermann-type tests) have been developed: Kline, Kahn, Mazzini, Hinton, VDRL, Eagle, and others. One of the most specific tests for syphilis is the *treponema immobilization test* (TPI). Blood tests required by many states for issuance of a marriage license employ one or another of these testing procedures.

Waterhouse-Friderichsen syndrome. Overwhelming meningococcal infection in children, characterized by convulsions, collapse of the circulatory system, and bleeding into the adrenal glands.

Water on the brain. HYDROCEPHALUS (271).

Wax epilation. A method of removing superfluous hair, usually of the legs or lips. A waxy compound is warmed to make it fluid and a layer is applied in the direction in which the hair lies. After the layer has hardened, the sheet is pulled sharply against the direction of hair growth. Imbedded hairs are pulled out by the roots. The hair follicle is not permanently destroyed, as it is in ELECTROLYSIS. Fine hair tips reappear in two or three weeks, but wax epilation does not leave a stubble as shaving does. Repeated wax epilation tends to damage some follicles and in time to reduce the number of hairs. Slight irritation lasts for a few hours after wax epilation. The treatment is considered to be safe in competent hands, but the skin of some women will not tolerate it.

W.B.C. White blood cell count. If the count is high, infection is suspected.

Webbed fingers. Connection of adjacent fingers (or toes) by a thin fold of skin between them (647).

Weber test. A hearing test to determine which ear hears better by bone conduction. It is performed by touching a vibrating tuning fork to various parts of the head.

Weil's disease. An acute feverish illness caused by spirochetes (51), also called *infectious jaundice.* A severe form of LEPTOSPIROSIS.

Wen. A sebaceous cyst, a skin tumor ranging up to the size of a marble or larger, filled with cheesy material; movable, firm, rarely painful (206). Wens usually occur on the scalp, face, or back, and result from obstruction of an oil-secreting gland.

Wetzel grid. A chart for plotting, comparing, and projecting the height, weight, and other growth aspects of children.

Wheals. Hives; temporary skin swellings resembling mosquito bites, but often much larger (692). Wheals may result from allergies, drugs, irritants, or injection of substances in skin tests of sensitivities.

Whiplash injury. A popular term for injury sustained when the head is suddenly thrown forward and jerked backward, as in cracking a whip (630). The injury is something like a "sprained neck"; muscles and ligaments may be strained and torn but bones and nerves are rarely damaged.

Whipple's disease. A rare progressive disease of unknown cause characterized by multiple arthritis, fever, fatty stools, lymph gland enlargement, diarrhea, loss of weight and strength, and abnormalities of the small intestine. Antibiotic treatment continued for many months may reverse the course of the disease, which may possibly be of bacterial origin.

Whipworms. Slender worms which inhabit the CECUM of dogs, pigs, sheep and goats. Their eggs can be transmitted to man by contact with contaminated soil (69). The infection may be symptomless or it may produce diarrhea or acute appendicitis.

Whites. Vaginal discharge; see LEUKORRHEA.

Whitlow. See PARONYCHIA.

Whooping cough (*pertussis*). A serious but preventable disease of childhood, especially dangerous and sometimes fatal in young infants whom it readily attacks (422). Active immunization of all infants with an effective vaccine (often combined with *diphtheria* and *tetanus* toxoids) should be started between six and 12 weeks of age.

Widal test. An ANTIBODY test of blood for diagnosis of typhoid fever.

Wilms tumor. A malignant tumor of the kidney occurring in children (295). The tumor may first be noticed as an abdominal mass by mothers in caring for their babies. Early discovery and immediate treatment (surgery and radiation) give the best hope of permanent cure. Simultaneous administration of *dactinomycin,* an antibiotic which causes the tumor to regress, has recently been shown to improve the chances of cure.

Wilson's disease (*hepatolenticular degeneration*). A disease inherited as a recessive trait (see HEREDITY). Abnormal deposits of copper in many tissues, especially the brain, eyes, kidneys, and liver, cause damage producing various symptoms as the disease progresses: tremor, clumsiness, psychic disturbances, weakness, emaciation, blue half-moons of the nails, retraction of the upper lip exposing the upper teeth. Treatment is directed to decreasing the intake of copper-rich foods (chocolate, molasses, shellfish, kale, liver, peas, nuts, corn, whole-grain cereals, dried beans, mushrooms, lamb, pork, dark meat of chicken), and use of drugs to prevent absorption of copper and speed its excretion (512).

Witch's milk. A milk-like secretion, resembling COLOSTRUM, exuded from the breasts of newborn infants of either sex. If left alone, the secretion dwindles and disappears in a few days.

Withdrawal symptoms. Physical reactions to withdrawal of certain drugs (narcotics, barbiturates) from persons addicted to them, who have established physical dependence on the drug. The patient has nausea, diarrhea, a runny nose, watery eyes, chills, waves of gooseflesh. His arms and legs ache, muscles twitch, he perspires and even in hot weather may cover himself with a heavy blanket. Usually the worst is over within a week.

Womb. The UTERUS.

Wood's light. A device used in diagnosing ringworm of the scalp. Light passed through a special glass filter causes certain fungi to fluoresce.

Wool-sorter's disease. So named because of its occurrence in persons who handle raw animal hides and hairs; *anthrax* (47).

Wrist drop. Drooping of the hand at the wrist, inability to lift or extend it, due to paralysis or injury of muscles or tendons which extend the fingers and hands.

X

Xanthelasma. A form of XANTHOMA occurring as soft yellow-colored plaques on the eyelids (193).

Xanthoma. "Yellow tumor"; a yellowish nodule or slightly raised yellow-colored patch in the skin.

Xanthomatosis. A generalized condition attended by many deposits of yellowish fatty material in tissues, due to some disturbance of CHOLESTEROL and LIPID metabolism (173). An hereditary form characterized by masses of yellowish deposits around tendons, especially in the elbows, wrists, and ankles, may appear early in life. It is transmitted as a dominant trait (see HEREDITY). In this condition (*familial hypercholesterolemia*) blood levels of cholesterol are very high and patients have a tendency to develop premature hardening of the arteries. The inborn trait cannot be corrected but blood cholesterol levels may be lowered by stringent dietary restriction of saturated fats.

Xanthopsia. "Yellow vision," a condition in which objects look yellow. It sometimes accompanies JAUNDICE.

Xanthosis. Yellow discoloration of the skin, due to eating excessive amounts of carrots, squash, sweet potatoes and yellow vegetables which contain pigments (*carotenoids*) that are deposited in the skin. The condition clears up when yellow vegetable intake is restrained.

X chromosome. The female sex-determining chromosome: females have two of them, males only one. See CHROMOSOMES. The X chromosome is larger than the Y chromosome and contains some GENES for which there are no complements on the Y chromosome.

X disease. An epidemic form of encephalitis, first recognized in Australia, now called *Murray Valley encephalitis* (60).

Xeroderma. Dry skin; a mild form of "fish skin disease" (206). A rare form, *xeroderma pigmentosum*, begins in childhood. Pigmented spots, made worse by sunlight, appear in the skin, and there is scattered TELANGIECTASIS. The skin contracts and the lesions progress to warty growths which become malignant.

Xerophthalmia. Extreme dryness of membranes which line the eyelids and front of the eye. Lack of tears may cause infection and ulceration of the CORNEA. The condition is associated with NIGHT BLINDNESS and severe deficiency of vitamin A. Specific treatment consists of prescribed daily doses of the vitamin.

Xerostomia. Dryness of the mouth, due to deficient salivary secretion, drugs, dehydration, or secondary to fevers or other diseases.

Xiphoid. Shaped like a sword; applies to the structure at the lower tip of the breastbone.

X-rays (*roentgen rays*). Electromagnetic radiation of shorter wavelength than visible light. X-rays can penetrate "solid" substances, produce shadows of structures of different densities on film, and destroy living tissues (788). Some living cells, said to be RADIOSENSITIVE, are more easily destroyed by x-rays than others; this is the basis for therapeutic use of x-rays in cancer.

Y

Yaws. A tropical disease caused by *spirochetes* resembling syphilis organisms (40). It is non-venereal, possibly is transmitted by insect bites. It is characterized by fever, rheumatic pains, red skin eruptions, and destruction of skin and bones of the nose if not treated.

Yellow fever. An acute, infectious, feverish disease caused by viruses transmitted by the bites of mosquitoes (56). The disease does not exist in the U. S. but travelers to tropical America where yellow fever is endemic should be protected by a vaccine which is highly effective.

Yellow spot. The *macula lutea*, the small spot near the center of the RETINA which is the focus of all finely detailed seeing (556).

Y chromosome. The male sex-determining chromosome. See CHROMOSOME.

Yogurt. A milk product formed by the action of acid-producing bacteria. It has the same food value as the milk from which it is made. When made from partially skimmed milk, as it often is, yogurt is lower in fat, Vitamin A, and calories than when it is made from whole milk. Yogurt is good source of the other nutrients obtained from milk, however, especially calcium, riboflavin, and protein.

Z

Zonules. Tiny slinglike processes which suspend the crystalline lens of the eye (553). *Zonulysis* is a technique of dissolving the zonules with a specific enzyme to loosen the lens for extraction in selected cases of CATARACT surgery.

Zoonoses. Diseases of animals transmissible to man.

Zoster, zona. SHINGLES.

Zygoma. The cheekbone.

Zygote. The fertilized egg cell before it starts to divide.

INDEX

Index

Page numbers for the main treatment of a subject are in
bold face type when more than one reference is given.

A

Abortion, 361, 369-70, 880
  also see Miscarriage
Abrasions, 847
Abscess, 36, 37, 39, 72, 228,
  238, 625
Abuse, drug, 815
Accident prevention, children,
  398
Acetone, in diabetes, 353-54
Achalasia, 880
Achilles tendon, 126
Achondroplasia, 881
Acid and alkaline foods, 880
Acid-base balance, 881
Acid stomach, 882
Acne, 181-85, 333
  rosacea, 184
Acromegaly, 317-18
ACTH, 236, 317, 330, 332, 485,
  706
Actinomycosis, 74
Acupuncture, 883
Adams-Stokes syndrome, 883
Addison's disease, 331-32
Adenoids, 608
  removal, 424, 750
Adenoma, 318
Adenoviruses, 55
Adhesions, 126, 884
Adhesive tape removal, 884
Adipose tissue, 884
Adolescence, female, 429-32
Adrenal:
  glands, 116, 117, 314,
    330-334, 331
  hormones, 330, 332-33
Adrenalin, 330, 334, 688,
  705-06
Adrenocorticotrophic
  hormone, *see* ACTH
Aerophagia, 885
African sleeping sickness, 73
After-image, 885
Agammaglobulinemia, 885
Aged:
  diseases of, 35, 36
  and gallstones, 480
  heart disease in, 86

skin conditions of, 202
Agranulocytosis, 323
Air embolism, 885
Air-swallowing, 885
Air travel, 52, 885
Akinesia, 251
Albuminuria, 293
Alcohol, 130, 259, 471, 482, 818
Alcoholism, 818
Aldosterone, 116, 330, 332
Alkaline-ash diet, 886
Alkaptonuria, 886
Allergy and allergies, 185,
  187, 224, 403, 492, 518, 565,
  609, **671-706**
  allergens, 671, **675-681**
  detection and diagnosis,
    682-84
  drugs, 697-701
  gastrointestinal, 690-96
  insects, 696-97
  physical, 701-04
  treatment, 704-06
Alopecia, 196
Alveoli, 212
Amblyopia, 887
Amebiasis, 71-72, 478
Amebic dysentery, 71
Amenorrheas, 338
Amino acid, 156, 887
Aminopterin, 170, 191
Amniocentesis, 808
Amphetamines, 817
Amputations, 765
Amyotrophic lateral
  sclerosis, 264
Anabolic steroids, 887
Anaphylaxis, 888
Androgens, 333, 341
Anemia, 69, 103, 116, 139, 320,
  474, 484, 485, 504, 796
  Cooley's, 158
  hemolytic, 155-56
  iron-deficiency, 149
  sickle cell, 157
  states, 149-53
  pernicious, 150
Anesthesia, 381, 778, 780
Aneurysms, 124, 125-26,
  131-32

and stroke, 125
  arterial, 131
Angina pectoris, **91-93**, 118
Angiography, 123
Angioneurotic edema, 693
Animals:
  bites, 399-400, 860
  see also names of animals
Aniseikonia, 889
Anorexia nervosa, 890
Anoxia, 99
Anthrax, 47
Antibiotics, 38, 39, 41, 45, 46,
  56, 58, 100, 183, 185, 228,
  232, 255, 294, 385, 467, 485,
  625, 668, 797, 799
  see also names of antibiotics
Antibody, 671
Anticoagulants, 94, 124, 130,
  138, 890
Anticonvulsants, 890
Antidiuretic hormones, 317,
  321
Antidotes, for poisons, 855
Antihistamines, 55, 687-88,
  705-06, 890
Antihypertensive drugs, 120
Antimalarial drugs, 193
Anti-Rh serum, 891
Antithyroid drugs, 323
Antitoxins, 42-43, 891
Aorta, 96, 103, 132, 743
Apocrine glands, 180
Apoplexy, 123-28
  first aid for, 865
Appendicitis, 486, 489, 727
Appetite, loss of, 58, 69, 105,
  293, 316, 317, 329, 473
  depressants, 891
Arrhythmias, 81, **107**
Arteries, 82-83, 114, 118-19,
  129
  aneurysms, 131-32
  atherosclerotic disease of,
    128-131
  and cerebrovascular
    disease, 124-26
  and heart disease, 85-86
  table of, 110-111

Index

Arteriography, 125
Arterioles, 114, 118
Arteriosclerosis, 39, 86, 116, 125, 204, 254, 300, 355, 578-79, 580
Arthritis, 40, 634, 642, **653-70**, 796
  infection-caused, 667-68
  osteoarthritis, 655-57
  psoriatic, 666
  rheumatoid, 660-65
  spinal, 629-30
  suppurative, 625
  tests, 668-69
Arthroplasty, 765
Artificial heart, 892
Artificial insemination, 895
Artificial kidney, 296
Artificial respiration, 214, 823-27
Asbestosis, 236
Ascariasis, 70-1
Aspiration, pneumonia, 237, 895
Aspirin, 55, 56, 106, 256, 386, 387, 393, 630, 658, 662
Asthma:
  bronchial, 684-88
  cardiac, **100-101**, 187
Astigmatism, 562
Ataxia, 896
Atelectasis, 226, 239
Atheroma, 86
Atherosclerosis, 86-95, 128
Athetosis, 270, 896
Athlete's foot, 200
Athletic heart, 896
Atropine, 416, 473, 486
Aura, epileptic, 273
Australia antigen, 62
Autograft, 896
Auto-immune diseases, 896
Auto-intoxication, 897
Aversion therapy, 818
Axon, 242

B

Babies, see Infants
Bacillary dysentery, 45, 897
Bacilli, 34, 35, 45
Back pain, 26, 57, 58, 363, 626-28
  in pregnancy, 363
Backrests, 16
Backrub, 26
Bacteremia, 38, 44-5
Bacteria, 530, 568
  types of, 34
Bacterial diseases, 34-47
Bacterial endocarditis, 39, 795
Bag of waters, 379
Balance, 586
Baldness, 196-8
Ballistocardiograph, 84
Bandages and bandaging, 841

Banti's syndrome, 163
Barbiturates, 195, 817
Barium meal, 899
Barrel chest, 234
Bartholin glands, 899
Basal metabolism rate (BMR), 324, **799**
Bathing, 23, 25-6, 185
Bats, 58, 75
BCG, 899
Bearing down pains, 899
Bed: of home patient, 14, 17, 21
  making, 21-24
Bedpan, 27-28
Bed patient: see Home care of patient
Bedrest, 56, 130, 230, 374, 387, 479, 482
Bedsores, 26-27
Bed-wetting, 299, **400**
Bee stings, 400, **696**
Bejel, 50
Bell's palsy, 267
Bence-Jones protein, 174
Bends, see Caisson disease, 906
Beriberi, 504
Berlock dermatitis, 195
Berylliosis, 236
Bezoar, 900
Bifocals, 562
Bile, 461, 479
  duct, 349, 478, 483
Bilharzia, 67
Biliousness, 900
Bilirubin, 900
Biologic clocks, 900
Biopsy, 306, 441, 464-66, 470, 478, 545, 799, 801, 901
Birth control: see Contraception
Birth defects, 803
Birthmarks, 194, **402**
Bites, first aid for, 858
Blackheads, 182
Blackwater fever, 72
Black widow spider, 860
Bladder, 290, 303, 306, 310
  disorders, 68, 298-300, 307, 438, 749, 802
Blastomycosis, 74
Bleb, 233, 265, 488
Bleeding, 159-62, 303, 306, 318, 340, 348, 358, 364, 369, 374, 386, 387, 441, 470
  measures for stopping, 822, 830-34
  see also Hemorrhages
Blindness, 264, 272
Blisters, 179, 186, 198-99, 200, 847
Blood, 139-176
  cells, 140-46
    red, 140-43, 151, 154, 158

white, **142-43**, 164-70, 218, 323
circulation, 77-138
clotting, 124, **129-30**, 138, 154, 161-62, 363, 387
coagulation, 154, 160, 799
composition of, 140-43, 283
count, **143**, 323, 801
diseases, 149-174
groups, 139-40, 147, 360
loss, 149-50
plasma, **140**, 154, 161
platelets, **143**, 146, 150, 154, 160, 801
RH factor, 148, 376, 589, 801
tests, 47, **794**, 796, **799-802**, 902
transfusions, 148, 160, 331, 374, 472, 797-98
Blood donors, 148
Bloodletting, 154
Blood poisoning, 38
Blood pressure, 80-81, 87
  high, 114-122, 332, 333
  low, 122
Bloodstream, 38
Bloodsuckers, 71
Blood vessels, 92, 184
  atheroma formation in, 86
  and cerebral vascular disease, 123-28
Blue babies, 97
Body build, 903
Body lice, 201
Boeck's sarcoid, 236
Boils, 38, 46, 47, 201
Bone, 615-652
  age, 334, 391, 903
  banks, 903
  broken, first aid, 835-41
  diseases, 650-5
  infection in, 624
  structure and growth, **319**, 391, 622-25
  surgery, 762-65
  see also Marrow
Botulism, 42
Bowel, 72
  biopsy, 465-66
  diseases, 483-86
  movement, 387, 486, 723
Bowlegs, 642
Brain, 118, 248-49, 316
  diseases of, 60, 123-28, 272-73
  injuries, 262-63
  structure, 248-48
  surgery, 261, 262, 272, 278, 759-60
  tumor, 262
Brain waves, 277, 932
Breakbone fever, 58
Breast, 359, 429, 430, 514
  cancer, 444-50, 796, 799
  milk, 513
  prosthetic devices, 449

support, 904
surgery, 756-58, **798**
Breath, "bad," 547, 613-14
Breath-holding, 403, 904
Breathing, 206, 213-15, 234, 406
artificial respiration, 822, 823-27
Breech delivery, 384
Bright's disease, 116, **292-93**
Brill's disease, 65
Bromism, 904
Bronchial asthma, 684
Bronchiectasis, 226-229, 236
Bronchioles, 211, 212, 215, 224, 234-34, 795
Bronchitis, 224-26, 688
Bronchography, 226, 228-29
Bronchus, 210-12, 239
Bronze diabetes, 955
Brown spider, 905
Brucellosis, 45-46, 231, 478, 796
Bruises, first aid for, 847-50
Bruxism, 534
Bubonic plague, 46
Buerger's disease, 905
Bunion, 649
Burkitt's lymphoma, 905
Burns, first aid for, 852-3
Bursitis, 631, **654**
of shoulder, 631
Byssinosis, 906

C

Caffeine, 906
Caisson disease, 906
Calcitonin, 329, 642
Calcium, 329, 330, 546, 623, 799
Callus, 906
Calories, 351, **493,** 503, 518
table of, 507-09
Cancer, 240, 305, **811-14**
of bladder, 300
breast, 444
colon and rectum, 491, 766
esophagus, 470
eye, 578
female reproductive organs, 439
gallbladder, 481
larynx, 239, 613
liver, 478
lung, 236, **239-40**
mouth, 544
pancreas, 482
prostate gland, 308
skin, 194
stomach, 153, **473**
tests, 239, **795, 796, 799,** 800, 801, 802
urinary system, 749
Candidiasis, 75
Canker sore, 535, 907

Cannula, 907
Capillaries, 38
Carbohydrates, 89, 351, 493, 495
Carbon monoxide poisoning, 828
Carbuncles, 38, 47, 909
Carcinoma, 204, 336, 473
Cardiac asthma, 100
Cardiac catheterization, 84, 98
Cardiac pacemaker, 113
Cardiographs, 84
Cardiospasm, 469
Caries, dental, 505, 528-32
Carotene, 908
Castration, 314, 448
Cat: bite, 860
scratch disease, 64
Cataracts, 329, **576**
surgery, 771-72
Catarrhal jaundice: *see*
Hepatitis, infectious
Catatonia, 909
"Cat cry" syndrome, 909
Caterpillar dermatitis, 909
Catheter, 286-7
Catheterization, 84, 98
Causalgia, 910
Cells, 481
nerve, 241-43
Centipede bites, 910
Cerebral:
hemorrhage, 125
palsy, 270, 911
Cerebrospinal fluid, 911
Cerebrospinal meningitis, 41
Cerumen, impacted, 598
Cervical rib, 911
Cervix, 360, 428, 431
cancer of, 440-41, 799
cervicitis, 434-35
surgery, 737
Cesarean section, 385
Chagas' disease, 71
Chalazion, 912
Chancre, 41, 48
Chancroid, 41
Change of life: *see*
Climacteric, Menopause
Character disorders, 709-10
Charleyhorse, 912
Cheilitis, 190
Chemotherapy, 45, 167, 811
Chest, 59, 220, 240, 794, 799
Cheyne-Stokes respiration, 912
Chickenpox, 56, 185, 224, 226, 418
Chiggers, 65
Chilblain, 912
Child: care, 389-426
eyes, 565-67
foot problems, 647-48
nutrition, 514-15
teeth, 524-28

Childbirth, 379-88
preparation for, 366
Children's diseases: heart, 96-107
hemophilia, 161
infectious, 418-23
muscular dystrophy, 271-72
nephrosis, 293-94
purpura, 159
Chills, 33, 35, 36, 38, 45, 50, 51, 58, 72
Chloasma, 912
Choking, 828
Cholangitis, 480
Cholecystitis, 479, 795
Cholera, 45, 913
vaccination, 52
Cholesteatoma, 596, 913
Cholesterol, 87, 89-90, 193, 325, 794, 799, 913
and heart disease, 87
Chorea, 104, 105, 270
Choriocarcinoma, 336
Choroiditis, 573
Christmas disease, 162
Chromosomes, 311, 336, 804-07
Cilia, 216, 225, 231, 601
Cinefluorography, 287
Circadian rhythm, 900
Circulation, blood, 77-138
Circulatory system, 77-138
Cirrhosis of the liver, 231, 477-78, 795
Claudication, 129
Cleft palate and lip, 614
Climacteric, male, 337
Clubbed fingers, 915
Clubfoot, 647
Coagulation time, 915
Coarctation of aorta, 743
Cobalt bomb, 790, 915
Cocaine, 818
Cocci, 34, 41
Coccidioidomycosis, 74
Code, genetic, 804
Codeine, 386
Coitus: *see* Sexual Intercourse
—interruptus, 343
Cold: applications, 30
common, **55,** 255
exposure to, 864
hypersentitivity to, 701-02
Cold sores, 56, 690
Colic, 403-04, 691
Colitis, 45, 486, 490, 731, 795
Collagen, 915
Colloid baths, 185
Colloid goiter, 325
Colon, 459-60, 794
disorders, 486-92, 732
Color blindness, 581
heredity, 916
Colorado tick fever, 58
Colostomy, 732, 916
Colostrum, 917

Coma, 295
  diabetic, 354
Comedones: *see* Blackheads
Conception, 339, 340-41
Condom, 343
Congenital heart disease, 98
Congestive heart failure, 100
Conjunctivitis, **568-70**
  allergic, 689-90
Constipation, 122, 259, 325,
  329, 359, 362, **397-98**, **486-88**,
  489, 689
Consumption: *see*
  Tuberculosis
Contact: dermatitis, 185
  lenses, 563, 577
Contraception, 343, 376
Convulsions, 273-74, 295, 329,
  375, **404-06**
Cool enema, 393
Cooley's anemia, 158
Corneal ulcer, 572-73
  scars, 773
Coronary: arteries, 83, 92, 745
  artery disease, 85, **86-95**
  thrombosis, 87, 93-95, 795
Corneal transplant, 553, 918
Corns, 919
Corpus luteum, 919
Cortex, 315, 330
Corticosteroids, 156, 160, 168,
  170, 186, 188, 192, 199, 663
Cortisone, 106, 236, 478, 485,
  663, 706
Coryza: *see* Cold
Cosmetic, 188-90, 192, 194, 196
  allergy, 700-01
  dermatitis, 186, **188-190**
Coughing and coughs, 224,
  225, 226, **230-31**, 236, 237,
  406, 467, 684
Cowper's glands, 302
Coxsackie viruses, 59
"Crabs," 201
Cradle cap, 406
Cramps, 45, 72, 266, **269-70**,
  362, 431, 483, 484, 485
  leg, 269
  in pregnancy, 363
Cranial nerve, 920
Craniotomy, 759
Cretinism, 324
Crohn's disease, 484
Cross-eye, 566
Croup, 406
Cryosurgery, 920
Cryotherapy, 205
Cryptorchidism, **311-12**, 337
Curettage, 342, 360, 443, 736
Curvature of the spine, 628-29
Cushing's disease, 116, **332-33**
Cuts, first aid for, 847-850
Cyanosis, 922
Cystic fibrosis, 407, 922
Cystinuria, 287, 923
Cystitis, 299, 307

Cystocele, 438, 736
Cystoscope, 287-88, 800
Cysts, 340, 436, 437, 438, 478,
  756
  "chocolate," 437
  ovarian, 436, 735
  pilonidal, 619, 766
Cytomegalic inclusion, 56

D

Dandruff, 179, 182, 188
D & C, 736, 923
DDT, 65, 415
Deafness, 264 588-594, 590-98
Decibel, 590
Deficiency diseases,
  nutritional, 503
Deformity, 253-54
Dehydration, 45, 284, 924
Delirium, 72, 924
  tremens, 924
Demyelinating diseases, 263
Dengue fever, 58
Dental caries, 89, 505, **528-32**
Dental erosion, 535
Dentifrices, 546
Dentistry, 548
Dentures, 539
Deoxyribonucleic acid, 804-5
Depression, 717
Dercum's disease, 925
Dermabrasion, 183, 204-05
Dermatitis, 134, **185-88**, 204
  contact, 681
Dermatoglyphics, 925
Dermatology, 178
Dermatomyositis, 667
Dermis, 179
Dermographia, 926
Desensitization, 705
Desoxyribose nucleic acid,
  804-5
Detached retina, 773
Detergents, 186
Deviated septum, 610
Devil's grip, 59, 232
Devil's pinches, 926
Dhobie itch, 200
Diabetes, 87, 89, 103, 185, 204,
  240, **349-56**, 481, 517, 802
  and eyes, 578
  insipidus, 316, 317, **321**
  mellitus, 318, **349-56**, 796
Dialysis, 295
Diaper rash, 409
Diaphragm, **208**, 214, 234, 235,
  238
  vaginal, 343
Diarrhea, 44, 45, 50, 64, 69, 72,
  354, 362, **396-97**, 483, 484,
  488, 490, 491, 689, 691, 698
  tourist's, 1047
Diastole, 80
Diastolic pressure, 114, 116
Diathermy, 927

Diet
  and acne, 183
  adequate, 499
  alkaline ash, 886
  bland, 32, 472, 486
  bulk-forming, 31
  and constipation, 488
  diabetic, 350
  epilepsy, 278
  gluten-free, 949
  gout, 657-59
  heart disease, 88-89, 102
  and hypertension, 119-20
  ketogenic, 972
  light or convalescent, 31
  low salt (sodium), 32, 102,
    120, 375, **519-20**
  pregnancy, **361**, 375, 515
  reducing, 510
  special, for home patients,
    31
  therapeutic, 517-20
  and tooth decay, 529
Dietary allowances, 496
Digestion, 448, 453-54, **456-58**,
  485
Digestive system, 218, **451-492**
Digitalis, 102, 110
Dilation, 342, 360, 443, 736
  and curettage, 736
Diplopia, 928
Diphtheria, 796, 802
  vaccination, 394
Diseases
  bacterial, 34-47
  gastrointestinal, 463-492
  infectious, 33-72, 418-23
  intestinal, 43-44, **483-492**
  viral, **53-64**
  of women, 405-450
  see also names of diseases
Disk trouble, 627-8
Dislocations, 651
  first aid for, 851
Diuretic drugs, 102, 120-21,
  348, 478
Diverticulosis, 488
Diverticulum, 467, 476, 483,
  730
Dizziness, 269, 598A
DNA, *see* deoxyribonucleic
  acid
Dogs, 58, 69, 73
  bites 399, **860**
  hair, 679
Douches, 432
"Downers," 817
Down's syndrome: *see*
  Mongolism
Dropsy, 69, **101-02**
Drowning, 828
Drowsiness, 253, 259, 264
Drug: addicts, 72, 819
Drug eruptions, 190
Drug use and abuse, 815-19
Drugs: *see* names of drugs

Dry ice, 930
Dry socket, 542, 929
Dumping syndrome, 474
Duodenum, 141, 349, 453, 455-58, 482, 483, 794
  disorders, 475-76
  drainage, 466, 800
  ulcer, 475, 518
Dupuytren's contracture, 636
Dwarfism, 317, 318-19
Dysentery, 45, 71-72
Dyslexia, 931
Dysmenorrhea, 431
Dyspareunia, 433
Dystrophy, muscular, 271

E

Ear, 583-98
  disorders of, 588-594
  earache, 594
  foreign bodies in, infections, 594-98
  infections, 594-96
  structure and function, 583-88
  surgery, 753-56
EB virus, 63
Eccrine glands, 180
ECHO viruses, 59
Eclampsia, 375
Ectopic: kidney, 290
  pregnancy, 370
Eczema, 185-88, 195, 413
Edema, 101, 143, 199, 204, 262, 284, 477, 505, 932
EEG, see Electroencephalography
Ejaculation, 307
Elbow: disorders, 633-34
Electric shock, 828-29, 830
Electrocardiogram (EKG), 84, 91, 93, 104, 106, 109, 113, 800
Electrocardiograph, 93, 109
Electroencephalography, 250, 276
Electrolytes, 284, 933
Electromyography, 250
Embolus, 124
Emergency telephone numbers, 820
Emetic, 68
Emotion: disturbances of, 707-716
  and skin, 177-78, 183
Emphysema, 154, 224, 225, 234-35, 239
Empyema, 232
Encephalitis, 60, 116, 253, 262, 264
Endocarditis, bacterial, 39-40
Endocrine glands, 313-348, 794
Endocrinology, 314-15
Endometriosis, 436, 800

Endometrium, 342, 368, 441
Endothelium, 139, 145
Enemas, 30, 387, 393
Enteritis, 484, 492
Enterobiasis, 71
Enuresis, 299, 400
Enzymes, 45, 159, 244, 326, 451, 454, 458, 482, 512
Epidemic pleurodynia, 59
Epidemics, 36, 44, 45, 55, 58, 59, 72, 87, 104, 232, 253, 264
Epidermis, 178
Epididymis, 310, 311, 312
Epiglottis, 210
Epilepsy, 250, 273
Epinephrine, 330, 334, 688, 705-06
Epiphysis, 334
Episiotomy, 381, 387
Epispadias, 302
Epstein-Barr virus, 63
Equilibrium, 586
Equine encephalomyelitis, 60
Ergotism, 936
Erosion, dental, 535
Erysipelas, 38
Erythroblastosis, 376, 796
Erythrocytes, 140-42, 153-54, 158
Esophagus, 210, 452, 463, 467
  disorders, 467-70
  ulcer, 468
Estrogens, 334, 337, 340, 348, 436
Eunuchoidism, 314, 316, 336
Exercise, 88-89, 130, 351, 356, 364, 366, 387, 431, 581, 664-65
  in diabetes, 351
  isometric, 970
  in pragnancy, 364, 366
  therapeutic, 127-28, 260-61
Exhaustion, 359
Exostosis, 318
Exophthalmos, 323
Expectoration, 224, 226
  blood, 239
Exstrophy of bladder, 299
External cardiac massage, 937
Eye, 40, 45, 47, 56, 58, 253, 551-82
  bags under, 582
  bulging, 582
  care, 564-65
  detached retina, 578, 773
  disorders, 570-82
  examinations and tests, 251, 559-64, 794, 802
  exercises, 581
  floating spots, 581
  injuries, first aid, 861-63
  muscles, 551-56, 773
  refraction, 561
  structure, 551-59
  surgery, 771-75

  vision, 556-59
  wash, 565
Eyeglasses, 562, 577
Eyelids, 190, 193, 568

F

Face lift, 938
Face neuralgia, 267
Facet syndrome, 627
Fainting, 363, 571
  aid for, 866
Falciparum malaria, 72
Fallopian tubes, 338, 342, 367, 428, 442
False pregnancy, 939
Fanconi's syndrome, 174
Farmer's lung, 939
Farsightedness, 562
Fats, 89, 495
  polyunsaturated, 519
  see also Cholesterol
Favism, 158, 940
Feces, 32, 43, 466, 695
Feeble-mindedness, 272
Felty's syndrome, 163
Feminine hygiene, 432
Fenestration, 755
Fertile period, 339
Fertilization, 346, 368
Festination, 252
Fetus, 77, 272, 369
  timetable of development, 372-73
Fever, 18, 33, 51, 104, 105, 231, 264, 265, 393-94, 484, 485, 688, 940
  relapsing, 50
  types, 50
Fever blisters, 56
Fibrillation: atrial, 106
  ventricular, 112
Fibrinogen, 941
Fibroid tumors, 435
Fibrositis, 654
Filariasis, 71
Fimbria, 338, 368
Fingernails, 182
First aid, 821-863
  index to topics, 821
Fish,
  as allergens, 680
Fish hook removal, 849
Fissures, 239, 405, 490
Fistulas, 490, 766, 941
Flat feet, 646
Flatulence, 942
Floaters, 581
Flukes, 67
Fluorides, 360, 529, 530
Fluoroscopy, 783, 789, 791-92
Flutter, 109
Folic acid, 152-53, 169
Follicle, 181
Fontanel, 943

Index

Food
  allergies, 679-81
  fads and fallacies, 516-17
  groups, 499
  and hives, 694
  poisoning, 44, 944
  storage, refrigerator, 520
Food handling, 43-44
Foot, 126, 131
  clubfoot, 647
  and diabetes, 355
  disorders, 645-50
Foot-and-mouth disease, 58
Forceps delivery, 383
Formulas, infant, 395
Fractures, 651, 762, 796
Freckles, 196
Frigidity, 348
Froelich's syndrome, 315, 945
Frog test, 358
Frostbite, 864
Frozen section, 798, 945
Frozen shoulder, 632
Fungus infections, 74-75,
  190-200, 594
Funnel chest, 945
Funny bone, 945
Furuncles, 38

G

Galactosemia, 512, 946
Gallbladder, 333, 462-63, 794
  disorders, 479-81, 519, 800
  surgery, 732-34
Gallop rhythm, 946
Gallstones, 156, 479-80, 732
Gamma globulin, 52
Gamma rays, 788
Ganglia, 251, 252, 486
  ganglion of wrist, 634
Ganglionic blocking agents,
  946
Gangrene, 131, 355, 946
  in diabetes, 355
  gas, 42
Gas endarterectomy, 947
Gas poisoning, 828
Gastrectomy, 474
Gastric freezing, 356
Gastric juice, 454, 466
Gastritis, 471
  allergic, 690
Gastroenteritis, 44, 64
Gastrointestinal tract, 44, 154,
  429-92, 800
  allergies, 690-696
Gastroscopy, 463, 471, 800
Gaucher's disease, 172
Genes, 804
Genetic code, 804
Genitalia, 41, 48, 57, 200,
  300-312, 333, 337, 430
Geographic tongue, 948
Geotrichosis, 948

German measles, 99, 365, 418,
  589
Germs, staph, 13-14, 36
G.I. series, 786
Giantism, 318
Gingivitis, 532
Glands
  adrenal, 116-17, 314, 320,
    330-35
  Cowper's, 301, 302
  endocrine, 313-356
  lacrimal, 558-59
  pancreas, 141, 314, 349, **463**
  parathyroid, 314, 328-30
  parotid, 452
  pineal, 314, 1011
  pituitary, 309, 314-16,
    317-321
  prostate, 166, 301, 302, 304,
    305-10, 336, 745
  salivary, 451-52
  sebaceous, 180-82
  sweat, 179-81
  thymus, 314, 1045
  thyroid, 314-15, **321-28**
  urethral, 301
Glaucoma, 251, 571-75, 802
  surgery, 774-75
Glomerulonephritis, 116, **292**
Glomerulus, 283
Glottis, 238
Glucocorticoids, 330
Glucose, 350, 800
Glucose tolerance test, 949
Gluten, 485
  gluten-free diet, 949
Glycogen storage disease, 949
Goiter: colloid (simple), 325
  nodular, 326
  toxic, 322-24
Gold compounds, 662
Gonadotrophins, 317, 319, 336,
  337, 340
Gonads, 302, 320
Gonococci, 41
Gonorrhea, 40-41, 304, 306,
  667, 802
Goofballs, 817
Gout, 657, 802
Graafian follicles, 339
Grafts, skin, 770-71
Gram-positive, -negative, 950
Grand mal, 273
Granulation tissue, 950
Granulocytes, 142-43, 146, 162
Granuloma inguinal, 41
Graves' disease, 322-24, 327
Grippe: see Influenza
Growing pains, 951
Growth: infant and child, 389
  nutrition and, 513
Gums, 532
  Vincent's angina, 37
Gynecology, 427-50
Gynecomastia, 336, 952

H

**HAA antigen (hepatitis
  associated),** 62
Hair, 181-82
  dyes, 189
  gray, 202
  pubic, 201
  scalp, 197-98
  see also Baldness
Hair follicles, 38, 198
Halitosis, 547, 613
Hallucinations, 244
Hallucinogenic drugs, 817
Hammer toe, 649
Hand: disorders, 636-57
  eczema, 187
**Hand-Schuller-Christian
  disease,** 173
Hansen's disease: see Leprosy
Hashimoto's thyroiditis, 327
Haverill fever, 50
Hay fever, 187, 679, **688-90**
  map, 676
Headaches, 33, 36, 41, 43, 47,
  50, 58, 59, 69, 73, 76, 262,
  264, 265, **268-69,** 293, 295,
  318, 332, 347, 580, 698
Head noises, 597
Hearing, 584-86
  aids, 593, 952
  and heredity, 590
  impaired, 588-94
  loss, 753
Heart, 77-138
  arrhythmias, 81, **107-111**
  attack, 85, 87, **93-95,** 866
  block, 112
  congenital disorders, 96-103
  embryonic development, 95
  enlarged, 119
  functions, 78
  murmurs and sounds, 83,
    409-11
  rheumatic, 85, 103
  surgery, 98, 102, 106-7,
    741-46
  technical terms re, 82-83
  tests, 794-95
  transportation, 776
  valves, 35, 39, 78, 80, 104,
    105, 106
Heartbeat, 77, 80
  irregularities, 107-11
Heartburn, 362, 470-71, 957
  in pregnancy, 362
Heart disease, 154
  congenital, 95-103
  diagnosis, 83-84
  rheumatic, 103-107
  types, 85, 86
  see also Coronary artery
    disease, Coronary
    thrombosis
Heart failure, 86, **100**

Heart-lung machine, 107, 742, 954

Heart murmurs, 409, 953

Heat: hypersensitivity to, 702
  illnesses, first aid for, 864-65
  treatments, 28-29, 657, 665

Heberden's nodes, 657, 953-4

Height, 318, 390-91

Hemangiomas, 194, 402

Hematuria, 291

Hemiplegia, 123

Hemochromatosis, 955

Hemodialysis, 296, 298

Hemoglobin, 140-41, 149, 150, 151, 213, 800

Hemoglobinopathies, 156

Hemoglobinuria, 158

Hemolytic anemias, 155-56

Hemolytic streptococci, 36, 38, 104, 106

Hemophilia, 139, 161, 809

Hemorrhage, 57, 124, 125, 160, 262, 320, 472, 475, 580

Hemorrhagic fever, 64

Hemorrhoids, 149, 363, 477, 490
  surgery, 767-69

Hepatitis, infectious, 61
  serum, 61

Hepatoma, 478

Heredity, 87, 117, 146-47, 803-10
  and allergy, 674
  and blood, 146
  diabetes, 349-50
  and epilepsy, 275
  and heart disease, 87, 89
  sex-linked, 1030
  and tuberculosis, 223

Hermaphroditism, 310, 333

Hernias, 411-13, 438, 468-69
  surgery, 737-40

Heroin, 816

Herpangina, 59

Herpes: simplex, 56
  zoster, 56-7, 166, 265

Hiatus hernia, 468

Hiccup, 238, 957

High blood pressure: *see*
  Blood pressure

Hip, disorders of, 637, 764
  bent, 640
  congenital dislocation, 637

Hippocratic oath, 958

Hirschsprung's disease (*see*
  Megacolon)

Hirsutism, 340

Histamine, 334, **673-74,** 701

Histoplasmosis, 75

Hives, 195, **692-696,** 700, **701-704**

Hoarseness, 613

Hodgkin's disease, 170-71, 473, 796

Home care of patient, 11-32

bathing, 23, 25, 30
bed, 21
  making, 21-24
  comfort in bed, 14-17
  pulse and respiration, 27
  sickroom, 13, 19-21
  temperature, 17-19

Hookworm, 69

Hordeolum, 568

Hormones, 203, 309, 314, 342, 800
  adrenal cortex, 330, 332-33
    excesses, 332-33
  antidiuretic, 321
  cortisone: *see* Cortisone
  estrogens, 318, 320, 334, 337, 339, 346
  gonadotrophic, 317, 319, 336
  insufficiency, 331-32
  insulin: *see* Insulin
  lactogenic, 317, 320
  oxytocin, 317
  parathyroid, 329
  pituitary, 317, 383
  sex, 311, 314, 330, **333-34,** 335, 448
  tests, 796, 800
  therapy, 309-10
  thyroid, 315, 321-22
    deficiency, 324
  vasopressin, 317

Horseshoe kidneys, 291

House dust, 679

Household pets, 959

Housemaid's knee, 654

Housewife's eczema, 187

Hunger, 350, 404

Hunner's ulcer, 959

Huntington's chorea, 959

Hutchinson's teeth, 960

Hyaline membrane disease, 960

Hydatid disease, 69

Hydramnios, 960

Hydrocele, 312, 413, 960

Hydrocephalus, 272

Hydronephrosis, 297

Hydrophobia, 58-59
  first aid, 860-61

Hymen, 427

Hyperbaric therapy, 961

Hypercorticoidism, 332-33

Hyperopia, 562

Hyperparathyroidism, 329

Hyperplasia, 332

Hypersplenism, 160

Hypertension, 103, **114-122,** 305

Hypertensive heart disease, 85

Hyperthyroidism, 322-24, 326

Hyperventilation, 238

Hypnosis, 367, 961

Hypoglycemia, 350, 481

Hypoglycemic agents, 352

Hypoparathyroidism, 329-30

Hypospadias, 303

Hypotension, 122

Hypothalamus, 315

Hypothyroidism, 324-25

Hysterectomy, 443, **734**

I

Iatrogenic diseases, 962

Ichthyosis, 206

Idiopathic thrombocytopenic purpura (ITP), 160

Ileitis, 730

Immediate dentures, 540

Immunity, 963
  in cancer, 813

Immunization, 55, 56, 394-95, 418-23
  and allergy, 672
  for travel abroad, 52
  see also Vaccines

Imperforate hymen, 427

Impetigo, 206

Impotence, 964

Indigestion, 471
  allergies and, 692

Induction of labor, 384

Infant, 389-426
  development, 391-92
  feeding, **386, 395, 513-14**
  premature, 361
  sleep patterns, 964
  teeth, 523-24

Infantile dermatitis, 187

Infantile paralysis: *see*
  Poliomyelitis

Infantilism, 319, 338, 340

Infant sleep patterns, 964

Infarct, 93

Infection, 40, 130, 138, 143, 183, 185, 218, 231
  and allergy, 672-73
  and diabetes, 350, 356
  prostate gland, 306-07
  symptoms of, 33-34

Infections
  bacterial, 34-47
  during and after pregnancy, 363-64, 365, 387-88
  eye, 568
  kidney, 292
  mycoses, 74
  of nervous system, 264-69
  parasitic, **67-71, 191-92,** 694-95
  pelvic, 433
  protozoan, 71-74
  rheumatic, 105-6
  salmonella, 43-44
  skin, 198-202
  spirochetal, 47
  urethral, 304
  viral, 55-64

Infectious mononucleosis, 63, 965

Index

Infectious diseases: *see*
Diseases, infectious
Infectious hepatitis: *see*
Hepatitis, infectious
Infectious mononucleosis: *see*
Mononucleosis, infectious
Infertility, 320, 340-43, 796
Inflammation, 33, 183, 375
Influenza, 36, 55-56, 224, 226, 232, 253, 264, **418-19**
Ingrown hairs, 965
Injured, transporting, 846
Inkblot tests, 965
Insect bites, 400, **696-97,** 859
Insomnia, 346
Insulin, 314, 349, 481
types and use of, 351-52, 354
reactions, 354
Intercourse: *see*
Sexual intercourse
Interferon, 967
Intermenstrual pain, 339, 967
Intermittent claudication, 129
Intersex, 310
Intertrigo, 967
Intervertebral disks, 617, 627
Intestinal flora, 968
Intestines
diseases of, 43-44, 413-15
large, 458-60
obstruction, 483
operations, 726-30
parasites of, 67-71
small, 455-58
Intrauterine contraceptive devices, 345
Intrauterine transfusion, 968
Intrinsic factor, 150
Intussusception, 414, 483
Iodine, 321, 323, 324, 326, 505
tests, 800, 801
Ionizing radiation, 781
Iris, 555, 573
Iritis, 571
Iron, 148
deficiency, 149, 150, 340
lung, 214
test for, 800-01
Iron poisoning, 970
Irradiation therapy, 194, 300, 309, 312
Irritable colon, 486
Ischemia, 85
Isometric exercise, 970
Itch, 57, 68, 69, 71, 200, **201-02**
Itching, 185, 187-88, 200, 201, 203-04, 265, 295, 346, 350, 434
IUD, 344
Ivy, poison, 186

J

Jacksonian seizure, 274
Jaundice, 50, 56, 62, 476, 480, 483

tests, 795
hemolytic, 155-56
Jaw, 42, 74
fractures, 840
Jejunal ulcer, 971
Jet injection, 971
Jockey strap itch, 200
Joints, 126
diseases, 126, 653-70
tests, 794

K

Kahn test, 796, 801
Kala-azar, 73
Karyotype, 807
Keloids, 206
Keratin, 181, 187, 190, 195
Keto-acidosis, 353
Ketogenic diet, 972
Ketosis, 353, 972
Kidneys, 116, 117, 118, 218, 281-312, 582
artificial and transplanted, 295-96, 298, 776
diseases of, 116-117, 118, 287-290, 293-94
function, 281-84
infections: *see* Nephritis
stones, **287-90,** 329, **747-49,** 795
tests, 794, 795
tumors, 294-95
Kinesthesia, 972
Klebsiella pneumonia, 36
Klinefelter's syndrome, 310, **336**
Knee, disorders, 642
Koplik's spots, 973
Korsakoff's psychosis, 973
Kraurosis, 441
Kwashiorkor, 973
Kyphosis, 973

L

Labor, 379-81
stages in, 366, **379-80,** 384
Laboratory tests, 793
Lacrimal glands, 558
Lactation, 317, 320, **386,** 974
and nutrition, 516
persistent, 320
Laryngitis, 613, 688
Laryngotracheobronchitis, 406
Larynx, 210, **607**
Laser, 974
Laurence-Moon-Biedl syndrome, 976
Laxatives, 238, 488
Lead poisoning, 976
Leeches, 71
Left-handedness, 976

Leg, 186
cramps, 269
palsies, 266-67
Leishmaniasis, 73
Leprosy, 478, 977
Leptospirosis, 51
Letterer-Siwe's syndrome, 173
Leukemia, 139, **164-70,** 185, 204, 580
acute, 169
chronic, 165
monocytic, 168
myelogenous, 167
Leukocytes, 142-43, 801
Leukoplakia, 195, 544-45, 978
Leukorrhea, 434
Levodopa (L-dopa), 258
Lice, 50, 65, 66, 201, 415
Lichen: planus, 192
simplex chronicus, 188
Lightening, 374
Lightning, 829
Lipid endothelioses, 172
Lipoid pneumonia, 237
Lipoma, 978
Lipophagic granulomatosis, 173
Lips, 48, 56, 190
Lipstick dermatitis, 190
Lithium, 716
Lithotomy, 287, 979
Liver, 61, 254, 460-62, 478
biopsy, 464-65, 478
cirrhosis, 61, 231, **477-78,** 795
diseases of, 61, 476-79, 795
Lobectomy, 208
Lobes, of lungs, 209
Lockjaw, 42-43, 420
Lordosis, 979
Louse: *see* Lice
Low back pain, 626
Low blood pressure: *see* Blood pressure
Low blood sugar, 979
Low sodium diets: *see* Diets
LSD (lysergic acid diethylamine), 817
Lumbago, 980
Lumbar puncture, 980
"Lump in the throat," 469
Lumpy jaw, 74
Lung fluke disease, 67
Lungs, 207-40
abscess, 228
cancer, 236, 249, 795
collapse, 210, 220, 233
diseases, 216-24, 229, 231
physiology of, 208-216
surgery, 740
vital capacity, 214
Lunula, 182
Lupus erythematosus, 195
systemic (SLE), 666
test, 801

Lymph, 143, 145, 231
  nodes, 37, 47, 50, 57, 58, 142, 144, 145, 165, 170, 218, 236, 240
Lymphatic system, 143-45
  diseases, 170-74
Lymphedema, 143, 980
Lymphoblastoma, 172
Lymphocytes, 142, 145, 146, 165, 796
Lymphogranuloma venereum, 58
Lymphoma, 139, 170, 695
Lymphosarcoma, 170, 473

M

Madura foot, 980
Malabsorption syndrome, 485, 980
Malaria, 47, 56, 71, **180-81**
  tests for, 796
Male climacteric, 337, 981
Male reproductive system, 305
Malocclusion, 533
Malta fever, 45
Mammography, 447, 785
Manic-depressive psychosis, 711
Marfan's syndrome, 98, 982
Marie-Strumpell disease, 666
Marihuana, 816
Marriage, 432
Marrow, 140-42, 151, 154-55, 160, 162, 165, 166, 174, 622-23, 799
Massage, 26, 259, 306
Mastectomy, 447, 449, **757**
Mastitis, 445, 982
Mastoidectomy, 755
Mastoiditis, 597
Measles, 36, 60, 99, 224, 226, 395, 418, 589
Meat grades, 983
Meatus, 300, 302
Meckel's diverticulum, 483
Meconium, 407, 984
Medicaid, 984
Medical genetics, 803-10
Medicare, 984
Medicines, 12
  allergies to, 690, 700
Mediterranean anemia, **158**
Medulla, 214, 330, 334
Medulla oblongata, 214, 215, 249
Megacolon, 486
Megakaryocytes, 146, 160, 167
Melanin, 179
Melanoma, 194
Melena, 986
Meniere's syndrome, 269, 598A, 753
  surgery, 756
Meningitis, 40, 41-42, 44, 59,

250, 262, 264, 265, **418-19**
  tests, 796
Meningococcemia, 42, 56
Menopause, 188, 269, **346**, 658, 986
  post- complaints, 442-43
Menorrhagia, 340
Menstruation, 149, 316, 319, 320, 334, 337, 338, 340, 386, **429-32**, 582
  cycle, 338, 339, 341, 359
  disorders, 346
  onset, 429
Mental: illness, 223, **707-720**
  retardation, 711-12
Mescaline, 817
Mesenteric thrombosis, 731
Mesentery, 458, 728
Metabolism, 324, 512
  tests, 794-796
  see also Basal metabolism rate
Mice, 65, 74
  joints, 643
Migraine headache, 269
Miliaria, 190
Milk leg, 987
Milk line, 987
Mind, disorders of, 707
Miscarriage, 360, **361**, **369**
Mites, 46, 64, **201-02**
Mitochondria, 988
Mitral valve, 80, 102, 105, 106
  surgery, 744
Mittelschmerz, 988
Mold: *see* Fungi
Molecular diseases of blood, 156
Moles, 194, 360, 402
Molluscum contagiosum, 193
Mongolism, 98, 325, 415, 806-08
Moniliasis, 75, 364, 417, 434
Monocytes, 142, 146, 168
Mononucleosis, 63
Morning sickness, 358, 515
Morphine, 816
Mortality rate
  bronchitis, 224
  cholera, 45
  encephalitis, 60
  endocarditis, 40
  erysipelas, 38
  heart disease, 86, 87, 93
  hemorrhagic fever, 64
  meningitis, 42
  pneumonia, 35
  tuberculosis, 217, 223
  typhoid fever, 44
Mosquitoes, 56, 58, 60, 71, 72
  bites, 859
Motion sickness, 586
Motor nerves, 244
Mountain sickness, 990
Mouth, 37-38, 48, 56, 58,

451-52, 466, 607
  diseases, 544-46
Mouth breathing, 990
Mucous colitis, 486
Mucous membranes, 74, 160, 991
Multiple births, 377
Multiple myeloma, 174
Multiple sclerosis, 244, **264**
  test for, 796
Mumps, 60, 337, 418
Mumps skin test, 991
Murine typhus, 65
Murmurs, heart, 83, 409
Muscle, 991
Muscle table, 639
Muscles, 244, 391, **615-652**, 991
  rigidity, 252-53
Muscular dystrophy, 271
Myasthenia gravis, 314, 992
Mycosis infections, 74
Myelin, 242
Myeloblast, 146, 168
Myelofibrosis, 164
Myeloma, 174
Myocardial infarction, 89, 93, 94, 118
Myocarditis, 105
Myocardium, 82
Myomas, 435
Myopia, 561
Myringoplasty, 753
Myxedema, 324

N

Nails, 181, 182, 187, 191, 203
  see also Fingers, Toes
Narcissism, 993
Narcolepsy, 993
Narcotics, 816
Nausea, 33, 45, 47, 50, 58, 62, 259, 264, 265, 269, 293, 295, 329, 471, 477, 691, 698
  during pregnancy, 358-59
Nearsightedness, 561
Neck, 270
  broken, 840
Negri bodies, 56
Neoplasms, *see* Cancer
Nephritis, 38, 104, 204, **292-93**
  tests for, 795
Nephron, 283
Nephrosis, 293
Nerve
  cells, 241-43
  chart, 256
  cranial, 248
  impulse, 243
  motor, 244
  optic, 552-53, 558
  peripheral, 246, 248
  sensory, 244-45
  surgery, 759-62
Nerve deafness, 589

Nervous system, 241-80
autonomic, 247
disorders, 250-80
infections, 264-69
sympathetic, 120, 248
tests, 796
Nervous tension, and heart
disease, 90
Neuralgias, 57, **267**
Neurasthenia, 994
Neuritis, 265-67
in diabetes, 356
Neurodermatitis, 187, 994
Neurofibromatosis, 994
Neurons: *see* Nerve cells
Neuroses, 710
Neurosurgery, 759
Neurosyphilis, 48
Neutropenia, 162
Neutrophils, 218
Nevi, 194, 402
Nieman-Pick's disease, 173
Night blindness, 504, 556
Night sweats, 74
Nitrogen balance, 995
Nodular goiter, 326
Noise, 588, 590, 596-97
Noradrenalin, 330
Nose, 599-605
broken, 840
Nosebleed, 50, 105, **834**
Nuclear medicine, 995
Nummular eczema, 188
Nursing, home, 12, 28-31
Nutrition, 493-520
daily dietary allowances,
496
deficiencies 151-53
diseases, 503
Nymphomania, 348
Nystagmus, 561

O

Obesity, 117, 118, 120, 134,
505-06, 510-11
operation, 996
Obliterative arterial disease,
128
Obstructions, 297
Ocular muscle imbalance, 552,
566
Old people: *see* Aged
Operations, 40, 311, 381, 470,
721-780
adrenalectomy, 333-335
amputations, 765
bone, 625, 762-63
brain, 261, 262, 272, 278,
759-62
breast, 756-58
bronchiectasis, 228-29
cancer, 240, 300, 447, 749,
752
on children, 779

circulatory system, 124-25,
126, 131
colon, 732
ear, 591-93, 598A, **753-56**
eye, 771-775
female, 443, 734-35
gallbladder, 479, 480, 481,
732
goiter, 326, 327
heart, 98, 102, **106-7, 741-46**
hemorrhoids, 767-69
hernia, 737-740
hyperthyroidism, 323
intestines, 726-31
kidney and bladder stones,
289, 290, **747-49**
lung, 230, **740-41**
nerve, 247, 261, **759-62**
nose, 611
obesity, 996
orthopedic, 762-68
pancreas, 482
plastic surgery, 770-71
prostate, 307-08, 745
rectal, 766
spinal cord, 760-62
spleen, 156, 159, 160, 163,
166, **734**
stomach, 724-27
throat, 614
thyroid, 353, 751-52
tonsils and adenoids, 749-51
tuberculosis, 221
tumors, 751
ulcer, 473, 475, **724**
uterus, 436, 441, 443, **734-35**
varicose veins, 136
Opiates, 816
Oral contraceptives, 347
Organ transplantation, 775
Orgasm, 432
Oriental sore, 73
Ornithosis, 57
Orthodontics, 543
Orthopedic surgery, 762
Orthopnea, 100
Orthoptics, 567, 581
Osmosis, 998
Osteitis deformans, 651
Osteitis fibrosa cystica, 329
Osteoarthritis, 655
Osteochondritis, 643, 999
Osteomalacia, 650
Osteomyelitis, 38, **624**
Osteoporosis, 650
Otitis, externa, 594
media, 595
Otosclerosis, 589, 591
Ovaries, 314, 319, 320, 337-40,
367, 428
disorders, 338, 436, 441, 735
Overbreathing, 238
Overweight, 117, 118, 120, 134,
505-06, 510
diets, 510-11
Oviduct: *see* Fallopian tubes

Ovulation, 334, 339, 340-42,
431
Ovum, 1000
fertilization, 342, 368
Oxytocin, 317, 383

P

Pacemaker, 81
Paget's disease, 651, 1001
Painful menstruation, 431,
1001
Painful shoulder syndrome,
654
Palate, cleft, 614
Palpation, 297, 334
Palpitation, 108
Pancreas, 141, 314, 349, **463**
disorders, 481-83, 795
Pancreatitis, 481
Panhematopenia, 163
Panhypopituitarism, 320
"Pap smear" test, 360, 432,
440, 794
Papilla, 181
Paraffin baths, 29
Paralysis, 272
Paranoia, 707, 1002
Parasites: infections, 67-71,
201-02
intestinal, 694-95
Parathyroid glands, 314,
328-30
diseases, 329, 796
Paratyphoid fever, 420
vaccination, 52
Paresis, 49
Parkinson's disease, 250,
251-262
Paronychia, 200
Paroxysmal tachycardia, 109
Parrot fever, 57
Pasteur treatment, 58, 860
Pasteurella tularensis, 46
Pasteurization, home, 857
Patch test, 683
Patent ductus arteriosus, 85,
98, 99
Paternity test, 1005
Pathogens, 33
Pathologists, 798
Patient, home care of: *see*
Home care of patient
Pediculosis, 201, 415
Pedigrees, 809
Pellagra, 504
Pelvic examination, 360
Pelvis, 359, 360, 839-40
infections, 433
kidney, 282, 285
Pemphigus, 198
Penicillin, 35, 36, 37, 38, 40, 47,
49, 105, 568, 1006
Penis, 300, 301, 302, 303, 333,
336

Pentamidine, 73
Pep pills, 817
Peptic ulcer, 472, 475
Perforated eardrum, 597
Pericarditis, 104
Pericardium, 82
Perineum, 302
Periodontal disease, 532
Peripheral nerves, 246
Peristalsis, 452, 469, **486**
Peritoneoscopy, 464
Peritonitis, 43, 45, 486
Perleche, 1007
Pernicious anemia, **150**, 471, 580
Perspiration, 181, 200, 284
Perthes' disease, 640
Pertussis, 422
Pessaries, 439
Petit mal, 274
Peyer's patches, 142, 145
Peyote, 817
Phagocytes, 142, 143, 155
Pharynx, 607
Phenobarbital, 416
Phenol, 68, 791
Phenylketonuria, 798
Pheochromocytoma, 334
Phlebitis, 137, 204, 363
Phlebothrombosis, 137
Phlegmasia alba dolens, 138
Phobias, 1009
Phocomelia, 1009
Phosphorus, 154-55, 166, 167, 169, 329, 801
Photosensitivity, 195, 666
Phrenic nerve, 214
Phthisis: *see* Tuberculosis
Physical therapy, 271, 716
Physiotherapy, 126, 127-28, 259-60
Pica, 1010
Pigeon breeder's lung, 1010
Pigeons, 57, 60, 74
Pigeon toe, 647
Pigmentation, 206, 317, 331, 402
Piles, 363, 477
  surgery for, 766-69
"Pill," the, 344
Pilonidal cyst, 619, 766, 1011
Pimples, 193
Pineal gland, 314, 1011
Pink eye, 568, 690
Pinta, 50
Pinworm infection, 71
Pituitary gland, 309, 314, 315, 317-21, 796
Pityriasis Rosea, 192
Placenta, 337, 357, 374
  premature separation, 375
  previa, 374
Plague, 46

Plantar wart, 192
  vaccination, 52
Plasma cell diseases, 173
Plasminogen, 162
Plasmodia, 72
Plastic surgery, 334, 337, **770**
  of nose, 611
Platelets, 143, 146, 150, 154, 159, 801
Pleura, 208, 231
Pleural cavity, 208, 214, 230, 233
Pleurisy, 231, 239
Pneumococci, 35, 39
Pneumoconiosis, 235
Pneumonectomy, 208
Pneumonia, 33, 47, 55, 56, 795
  atypical, 36
  bacterial, **35-36**
  lobar, 56
Pneumothorax, 210, 220, 221, 233
Poisoning: antidotes, 853-58
  food, 44, 944
  iron, 970
  ivy, 186
  lead, 976
Poisonous plants, 1013
Poliomyelitis, 59, 250, 366, **420**
  tests for, 796
  vaccination, 52, 265, 395, 420
Pollen, 675-78
  hay fever map, 676
Polycystic kidneys, 290
Polycythemia, 153
Polymyositis, 667
Polyneuritis, 266
Polyps
  colon, 490
  nose, 609
  uterus, 435
Polyunsaturated fats, 89, 519
Portuguese man-of-war, 1015
Portwine stain, 194, 402
Postnasal drip, 609
Postpartum care, 387
Postural drainage, 1015
Posture, 625
Pregnancy, 99, 133-34, 194, 337, **357-88**, 535, 546, 675
  and allergy, 675
  care and examination, **360-65**
  course of, **369-378**
  diagnosis, 357-60, 796
  false, 939
  nutritional needs, 515-16
  tests, 357-8
  varicose veins in, 133
Premature birth, 371
Premature labor, 371
Presbyopia, 562
Prescriptions, 75-6
Prickly heat, 190
Primaquine, 72, 159

Proctoscope, 463-64, 490, 769, 801
Progesterones, 337, 340, 346, 358, 436
Projectile vomiting, 396
Prolactin, 317, 320
Prolapse of uterus, 438
Prostaglandins, 1017
Prostatitis, 306
Prostate gland, 301, 302, 304, **305-10**, 336
  cancer of, 308-10
  enlargement, 307-08
  examination, 306
  infections, 306-07
  surgery, 745
Prostheses, 125, 450, **756-66**
Prostration, 47, 55
  heat, 864
Proteins, 493, 495, 503, 699, 1017
  tests, 801
Prothrombin test, 154, 801
Protozoan infections, 71
Protruding ears, 1018
Pruritus, 185, **203-04**, 346
Pseudohermaphroditism, 333
Pseudomonas bacillus, 45
Psilocybin, 817
Psittacosis, 57
Psoriasis, **190-92**
Psychedelic drugs, 817
Psychoanalysis, 715, 1018
Psychological disorders, 707
Psychomotor seizure, 274
Psychoneurosis, 710
Psychosis, 711
Psychosomatic diseases, 710
Psychosurgery, 1019
Psychotherapy, 255, 713
Ptomaine poisoning, 44, 1019
Puberty, 319, 333, 337, 338, 391
Pubic hair, 201, 319, 333, 336, 337, 338, 429
Puerperium, 385
Pulmonary: stenosis, 743-44
  vein, 83
Pulse, **107-11**
  counting, 27
Purines, 167, 168, 169
Purpura, 159, 204, 691-92
  tests, 796
Pus, 33, 35, 38, 39, 41, 44, 45, 58, 72, 183, 224, 226, 229, 306, 409
Pyelonephritis, 116, 292, 305, 795
Pyloric stenosis 416, 474
Pylorospasm, 416
Pylorus, 453
Pyorrhea, 532
Pyrosis, 362, **470-71**

Q

Q fever, 66
Quackery, 669, 812
Quickening, 371
Quincke's edema, 693
Quinidine, 109
Quinine, 698
Quinsy sore throat, 38

R

Rabbit fever, 46
Rabbit test, 358
Rabies, 59, 1020
 first aid for, 860
Races, and tuberculosis, 222-23
Radiation sickness, 791
Radiation therapy, 788
Radioactive: iodine, 323, 325, 328, 790
 phosphorus, 154-55, 166, 167, 169, 801
Radiology, 781-792
 examinations, 784-788
Radium, 788
Ragweeds, 677
Rash, 41, 48, 58, 65, 66, 67, 105, 409, 418-23
Rat-bite fever, 50
Rats, 46, 50, 65, 74
Rauwolfia drugs, 120
Raynaud's disease, 1021
Recommended dietary allowances, 496
Rectocele, 439, 736
Rectum: disorders, 490, 492
 examination and tests, 766, 794, 795
 surgery, 766
Red blood cells, 140-42, 143, 151, 154, 159, 801
Red cell enzymes, 159
Red eye: see Iritis, Glaucoma
Reducing diets, 510
Reflex, 245, 250
Refraction, of eyes, 561
Regional ileitis, 484
Regurgitation, 102, 105, 106
Rehabilitation, 128
 see also various therapies
Reiter's syndrome, 1022
Relapsing fever, 50
Renal insufficiency, 295
Reproduction, 305-12
Reproductive system, 338
 tests, 794, 796
Reserpine, 323
Resorcin, 182
Respiration, 207
 artificial, 823
 counting, 27
 mechanism of, 212-13
Respiratory tract, 35, 218
 cancer of, 239-40

Resuscitation, 823
Reticulo-endothelial system, 139-40, 141, 143, 145, 146, 147
Retina, 555
 detached, 578
 surgery for, 773
Retinitis pigmentosa, 580
Retinoblastoma, 578, 1023
Retrolental fibroplasia, 580
Retroversion, of uterus, 437
Rh factor, 148, 360, 376, 589
 test, 801
Rheumatic diseases, 653-70
 tests, 668-69
Rheumatic fever, 37, 39, 103-107, 795
Rheumatic heart disease, 85, 103
Rheumatism, non-articular, 653
Rheumatoid arthritis (rheumatism), 660-665
Rheumatoid factor, 660, 668
Rhinitis, allergic, 688
Rhinophyma, 611
Rhinoplasty, 611
RhoGam, 376
Rhythm method, 339, 343, 1024
Rib, broken, 838
Ribonucleic acid, 805
Rice diet, 1024
Rickets, 503, 650
Rickettsia, 64
 diseases, 64-66
Rigidity, 251-53
Ringworm, 199
RNA, see Ribonucleic acid
Rocky Mountain Spotted Fever, 65, 420
Rodent ulcer, 194, 1025
Root canal, 522, 538
Rosacea, 184-85
Roseola infantum, 420
Roundworm infections, 70
Royal jelly, 1026
Rubella, see German measles
Rubin test, 342, 1026
Rupture, 411, 438, 468-69, 473, 475, 737-40
Ruptured disk, 627

S

Sabin vaccine, 59
Sacro-iliac trouble, 266, 626
St. Louis encephalitis, 60
St. Vitus' dance, 104
Salicylates, 195
Saliva, 451-52, 466, 547
Salk vaccine, 59
Salmonella infections, 43
Salt, 117, 118, 120, 284, 326, 409, 505

 see also Diets
San Joaquin fever, 74
Sandflies, 73
Saphenous veins, 133, 135
Sarcoidosis, 236
 tests, 796
Sarcoma, 168, 169, 172, 473, 1027
Scabies, 185, 201
Scalp, 183, 189-90, 191, 197-98, 201
Scarlet fever, 425
Scars, 183
Scheuermann's disease, 628
Schick test, 398, 1028
Schistosomiasis, 67
Schizophrenia, 711, 718
Schoenlein-Henoch purpura, 691
Sciatic nerve, 266
Sciatica, 266, 1028
Sclera, 552
Scleroderma, 1028
Sclerosis, 264, 579, 667
 multiple, 254, 264
Scoliosis, 628
Scotoma, 1028
Scratch test, 250, 682
Scrofula, 1029
Scrotum, 302, 312
Scrub typhus, 66
Scuba diving, 1029
Scurvy, 503
Seabright-Bantam syndrome, 330
Seafood, 183
Seasickness: see Motion sickness
Sebaceous: cyst, 206
 glands, 180
Seborrheic dermatitis, 188
Secretin, 314
Sella turcica, 317
Semen, 336, 341
Semicircular canals, 586-87
Seminal vesicle, 305, 310, 336
Septal defect, 745
Septate vagina, 427
Septicemia, 38-39, 625
Serum: hepatitis, 61
 sickness, 699
Sex determination, 1030
Sex: hormones, 311, 314, 448
 instruction, 431-32
Sex-linked heredity, 1030
Sexual: infantilism, 319-20
 intercourse, 40, 41, 57, 301, 302, 432-33
 precocity, 316, 317, 319
Sheehan's disease, 320
Sheep liver fluke disease, 67
Shingles, 56, 166, 265
Shock, 834, 852
Shoe dermatitis, 1031
Shoe fluoroscopes, 1031

Shoulder, 126
disorders, 630-34, 654-55
Sickle cell anemia, 157
Sickness at home: *see* Home
care of patient
Sickroom, 13, **19-21**
Siderosis, 235
Silicosis, 154, **235**
Simmonds' disease, 320
Sims-Huhner test, 342
Sinus, 81, 306, 606
Sinusitis, 190, 611
Sippy diet, 1032
Skeleton, 615
Skene's glands, 1032
Skin, **177-206**, 355
cancer of, 194-95
cosmetics and, **188-90**, 192,
194, 196, 700-01
diseases, 178, **182-202**
eruptions, 56, 58, 413
glands, 180-81
infections, 198-202, 409, 413
lesions, 38, 48, 50, 130, 191,
192, 193, 195, 200, 203
structure 178-181
sunburn and suntan, 195-
96, 1039
surgery and grafts, 770
tests, 58, 682-83, **801**
Skull fracture, 840
Sleep, 264, 363, 1032
infant, 964
Sleepiness: *see* Drowsiness
Sleeping pills, 817
Sleeping sickness, 60, 73
Sleepwalking, 1033
Smallpox, **420**
vaccination, 52
Smear test, 360, 432, **440-41**,
794
Smell, 603
Smoking, 37, 90, 117, 118, 120,
195, 235, 359, 365
Snake bites, 399, 858
Snellen chart, 561
"Sniffing," 818
Snoring, 1033
Sodium, 102, 120, 801
see also Diets
Soft contact lenses, 1034
Somatic therapy: *see*
Physical therapy
Somatotrophin, 317
Somatotype, 1034
Sore throat, 33, **36-37**, 59, 104,
105
Spasms, 270, 1035
Spastic colitis, 486
Sperm, 337, 801
Spermatocele, 312
Spermatozoa, 301, 305, 310-
11, 336, 341
Sperm banks, 1035
Sperm count, 1036
Sphygmomanometer, 114

Spider bite, 860, 1036
Spina bifida, 272
Spinal, cord, 35, 41, 151, 244,
246
anesthesia,
disorders of, 272-73
fluid, **250**, 796
nerves, 246
surgery, 760-62
test, 802
Spinal tap, 1036
Spine, 615
disorders, 625-31
Spirilla, 34
Spirochetal infections, 47
Spirochetes, 47
Spirometer, 214
Spitting, 224, 226
see also Sputum
Spleen, 155, 166
blood-producing role, 141-
42, 146, 155
diseases of, 155
hypersplenism, 160
surgery, 156, 158, 160, 163,
166, 734
Splinters, 849
Spondylitis, 666
Spondylolisthesis, 627
Spores, 42, 47
Sporotrichosis, 1037
Spotting, 364, 442
Sprains, 651, 850
Sprue, 485
tropical, 153
Sputum, 35, 36, 217, 224, 226,
229, 230, 240
tests, 802
Squamous cell, 195
Squint, 566
Staghorn calculi, 289
Stapes, operation 592, 755
Staph germs (staphylococci),
13, 34, 36, 38
infections, 36, 38, 667
Starches, 89
Stasis dermatitis, 188, 204
Steam: inhalation, 29, 55, **406**,
688
tent, 29, 231
Stein-Levinthal syndrome,
344
Stenosis, 102, 105, 106, 109,
416, 474, 743
Sterility, 40, 340-42
Sterilization, male and
female, 344
Steroid drugs, 106, 188, 192,
269, 294, 319, 333, 334, 689
Stimulants, 817
Stingray injuries, 1038
Stings, first aid for, 860
Stomach, **452-55**
disorders, 153, **470-75**
structure, 452

surgery, 724-27
tests, 795
Stomatitis, 37, **535**, 690, 1038
Stones, kidney, 287-90, 329,
747-49, 795
Stools, 43, 45, 61, 69, 323, 407,
414, 466, 474, 483, 486, 490,
695
tests, 802
Strabismus, 566
Strains, 851
Stratum corneum, 178
Strawberry mark, 194
"Strep throat," **36-37**, 103,
802
test for, 796
Streptococci, 34, 568
infections, **35-36**, 38, 39,
103, 105-06, 293
Streptomycin, 40, 41, 47, 50,
221-22
Stress, and hypertension, 119
and heart, 90
Stretchers, 846
Strictures, 303-4, 467-68
Stroke, apoplectic, 123-28,
796, 865
rehabilitation, 126-27
Strongyloides, 69
Stye, 568
Subdeltoid bursitis, 631, 655
Sugar, 89, 349, 512, 529
Sugar diabetes: *see* Diabetes
mellitus
Sulfonamide drugs, 39, 41, 42,
45, 485
Sulfonylurea drugs, 352
Sulfur, 182
Summer itch, 68
Sun: burn, 196, 1039
light, 218
and skin, 195-96
solar urticaria, 703
stroke, 864-65
Sunglasses, 563
Superfluous hair, 340, 1040
Supraspinatus syndrome, 630
Surfer's knots, 1041
Surgery: *see* Operations
Swallowed objects, 863
Sweat glands, 179-81
tests, 802
Sweating, 45, 50, 334, 347,
409, 571, 698
Swimmer's ear, 594
Swimming pool granuloma,
1041
Sympathectomy, 120, 121, 131
Sympathetic nerves, 120
Syncope, 866
Synovial fluid test, 802
Syphilis, 48-49, 132, 366, 794
tests, 47, 366, 796, 801, 802
Systemic lupus erythemato-
sus, 666

Systole, 80, 108
Systolic pressure, 114, 116

T

Tachycardia, 108
Talking in sleep, 1034
Tapeworm, 68
Tartar, emetic, 68
  teeth, 532
Taste, 603
  buds, 605
Tattooing, 1042
Tear ducts, 559
Tear gas, 1042
Teeth, 306, 360, **521-550**
  brushing, 529-30, 546-47
  decay, 89, 505, **528-32**
  development, 523-528
  diseases, 532-538
  extraction, 541-42
  false (dentures), 539-41
  fillings, 549-50
  gums, 532
  replacement, 538
  structure, 521-23
  tartar, 532
  toothache, 537-38
Teething, 417, 526
Telangiectasis, 1043
Temperature: body, **17-19,**
  359
  taking, **17-19,** 393
Temporal bone banks, 1043
Temporo mandibular joint,
  545
Tendon, 1043
Tennis elbow, 633
Tension: see Hypertension,
  Nervous tension
Testes, 59, 301, 302, 305, 310,
  311, 314, 317, 320, 334, **335-
  37**
  disorders of, 310-12, **336-37**
Testosterone, 335-36
Tests, laboratory, **793-802**
  definitions of major, 799-
  802
  disease diagnosis by organ
  systems, 795
  health evaluation by organ
  systems, 794
The following refer to pages
  in the text chapters:
  allergies, 682
  blood, **796,** 802
  body balance, 250
  bones and joints, 794
  cancer, 239, 795, 796, 799,
  800, 801, 802
  dye, 189, 479
  eye, 561, 575, 794, 802
  gastrointestinal diseases,
  463-66
  hearing, 590
  heart, 794

hormone, 796, 800
kidney, 794
liver, 62, 794
lungs, 794
metabolism, 470, 794, 796
  basal, 327
Metapirone, 332
neurologic, 250
pancreas, 795
patch, 683
phenylketonuria, 798
pneumonia, 795
pregnancy, 357, 796
reproductive system, 794,
  796
rheumatic diseases, 668
salt in body sweat, 409
scratch, 250, 682
skin, 58, 682, **801**
smear (Pap), 360, 432, **440-
  41,** 794
spinal cord, 796, 802
spleen, 796
stomach, 794
syphilis, 47, 158, 366, **796,**
  801, 802
thyroid, 324, **327-28,** 796,
  802
tuberculosis, 219-21, 795
ulcers, 795
urine, 286, 306, 334, 353-54,
  357, 360, 668-69, 795, 796-
  801, 802
uterus, 342, 796
virus, 796, 801, 802
Tetanus, 42-43, 420
  vaccination, 52, 395, 420,
  848
Tetany, 329
Thalamus, 241, 249
Thalassemia, 158
Therapies: see names of
  therapies, e.g. Drug,
  Physical, Physio-, Psycho-,
  Radiation
Thermography, 1044
Thermometers, 18-19, 20, 393
Threadworms, 69
Throat, 607-08
  streptococcal infections of,
  36-37, 802
Thrombocytes: see Blood
  platelets
Thrombophlebitis, 137
Thrombosis, 87, 93-95, 129,
  154, 731
  coronary, 93-95
  mesenteric, 731
  process, 129
Thrush, 74, 417
Thumbsucking, 547
Thymus gland, 313, 1045
Thyroid gland, 314, 315, **321-
  328**
  activity, 116, 322
  deficiency, 324

diseases, 322-328, 582, 796,
  802
hormones, 321-22
surgery, 751-52
tests of function, 324, 327,
  796
Thyroiditis, 326
Thyroxine, 321
Tic, 270, 1046
  douloureux, 267
Ticks, 46-47, 58
  bite, 860
Timetable, of fetal
  development, 372-73
  of tooth eruption, 524
Tine test, 219
Tinea, 199
Tinnitus, 597
Tipped uterus, 437
Tissue, connective, diseases,
  660
Tissue culture, 1047
Toad venom, 1047
Tobacco, 90, 103, 130
  see also Smoking
Toe, 131
  hammer, 649
  web, 647
Toenails, 200, 356
  ingrown, 650
Tomograms, 1047
Tongue-thrusting, 547
Tonsils, 37, 38, 59, 139, 306,
  607
  removal, 423, **749-50**
Tooth: see Teeth
Torticollis, 270, 630
Torulosis, 74
Tourist's diarrhea, 1047
Toxemia, 360, 375
Toxic goiter, 322
Toxins, 42, 43, 175, 293, 698
Toxoplasmosis, 73
Trachea, 210, 322, 740
Tracheotomy, 210, 753-54
Trachoma, 570
Tranquilizing drugs, 120, 121,
  195, 472, 486, 488, **1048**
Transfusion, blood, 148
Transplantation, organs, 775
Tremor, 250, 251-52, 254, 334,
  1050
Trench: fever, 66
  mouth, 37, **535**
Treponemes, 47-49
Trichinosis, 69
Trichomoniasis, 364, 434, 1051
Trichophytosis, 199
Trigeminal neuralgia, 267
Trigger finger, 636
Tropical: sprue, 153
  ulcer, 50
Trypanosomiasis, 73
Tsetse fly, 73
Tubal ligation, 344
Tubal pregnancy, 370

Tubercle bacillus, 217-19, 221, 231
Tuberculin, 219
Tuberculosis, 154, 168, 204, 216-24, 236, 237, 422-23, 478, 667
    eradication, 223-24
    pulmonary, 217-19
    tests, 219-21
Tuberculous pleurisy, 231
Tularemia, 46-47, 231
Tumors, 154, 198, 340
    adrenal, 332, 334
    bladder, 300
    bowel, 485
    brain, 262, 580, **759**
    colon, 490
    duodenum, 476
    esophagus, 470
    gallbladder, 481
    kidney, 294
    larynx, 613
    liver, 478
    mouth, 544
    ovaries, 436
    pancreas, 482
    prostate gland, 307
    reproductive organs, 428
    respiratory tract, 239
    stomach, 473
    surgery, 729, 751
    testes, 312, 336
    urethra, 303
    uterus, 435
Turner's syndrome, 340
Twins, 377
Tympanoplasty, 597, 755
Typhoid fever, 43-44
    tests for, 796, 802
    vaccination, 52, 420
Typhus fever, 65
    vaccination, 52

U

Ulcer, 41, 48, 50, 149, 204, 795
    duodenal, 475, 518
    esophagus, 468
    eye, 573
    mouth, 535, 545
    operations for, 724-27
    stomach, 472
Ulceration, 37, 185, 204, 490
Ulcerative colitis, 490, 731
Ulceromembranous stomatitis, 37
Ultrasound, 1053
Ultraviolet rays, 1053
Umbilical hernia, 411
Unconsciousness, 262, 264
    first aid for, 865
Underweight, 505, 511
Undescended testicles, 311, 336
Undulant fever, 45
Universal donor, 148, 1054

"Uppers," 817
Urea, 1054
Uremia, 292, **295**
Ureter, 282, 285, 297-99
Urethane, 167
Urethra, 285, 300-05
    female, 301, 304-05
    male, 300-04, 305
Urethritis, 299, 306
Urinalysis, 286, 360, 688, 795, 796, 801, 802
Urinary bladder: *see* Bladder
Urinary tract, 284, **298-312**
    diseases, 45, 68, **287-312**
Urination, 27-28, 40, 284, **299-300**, 302, 304, 306, 323, 329, 332, 348, 350, 359, 387, 434
Urine, 50, 72, 158, 218, 282, **283-84**, 288, 293, 295, 298-99, 302-03
    in diabetes, 353
Urticaria, 692, 700, **701-04**
Uterus, 42, 342, 386
    cancer of, 441, 796, 802
    disorders, 340, 342, 435-36
    prolapse, 438
    surgery, 443, **734-35**
Uveitis, 571
Uvula, 1057

V

Vaccinia, 1058
Vaccination, 55, 366, 395
    for travel abroad, 52
Vaccines, 44, 45, 46, 56, 58, 59, 265, **419-23**
Vacuum extractor, 1058
Vagina, 364, 427-28, 429
    cancer of, 442
    diaphram, 343
    disorders, 433-34, 438-39
Vaginal hysterectomy, 735
Vaginismus, 433
Vaginitis, 434
Vagotomy, 247, 727
Valsalva maneuver, 1058
Vaporizer, 29, 231
Varicella, 56
Varicose veins, 132, 204, 363, 469-70
    see also Hemorrhoids
Variola, *see* Smallpox
Vas deferens, 310
Vasectomy, 344
Vasodilators, 124
Vasomotor, 1059
Vasopressin, 317
VD Epidemic, 49
Veins, varicose, 132-34
    table of, 135
    stripping, 136
Venereal diseases, 40-41, 47, 49
    see also Gonorrhea, Syphilis

Venesection, 154
Venous stasis, 101-02
Ventilation, 20-21, 226, 238
Ventricle, heart, 78, 80-81, 95-97, 102, 109-11
    brain, 271
Vertebra, 617
Vertigo: *see* Dizziness
Verucca, *see* Warts
Vibrio, 34-35, 45
Vincent's infection, 37, 535
Viral hepatitis, 60
Virilism, 340
Virus, 36, 568
    and cancer, 812
    definition, 53-54
    diseases or infections, **55-64**
    influenza, 53, 56
    tests, 796, 801, 802
Vision: *see* Eye
Visual purple, 1061
Vitamins, 403, 496, 501, 580-81, 663-64
    A, 499, 500, 501, 504, 512, 515
    B, 153, 185, 500, 501, 504
    B12, 152, 153, 258, 454, 459, 472
    C, 153, 500, 501, 513
    D, 330, 498, 499, 500, 501, 503, 512, 513
    deficiency, 503-04
    food composition, 507-09
    K, 154
    table of, 498
Vitiligo, 206, 1061
Volvulus, 483
Vomiting, 45, 47, 50, 56, 59, 69, 72, 238, 264, 265, 269, 293, 295, 331, 334, 354, 414, 416, 468, 470, 471, 472, 474, 477, 479, 482, 483, 489, 571, 684, 689, 691
    during pregnancy, 358
    infants and children, 396
von Recklinghausen's disease, 329
Vulva, 441

W

Wall-eye, 566
Warts, 191
Wassermann test, 47, 158, 365, 796, 802
Water contamination, 43, 61, 67, 68, 72
Watercress, 65
Water diabetes: *see* Diabetes insipidus
Water on the brain: *see* Hydrocephalus
Wax epilation, 1062
Wax in ears, 598
Web-toes, 647

Weight, 88-89, 361, 375, 389-90, 515
  loss, 105, 350, 473, 477, 480, 484, 582
  overweight, 117, 118, 120, 134, **505-06**, 510-11
  underweight, 511-12
Weil's disease, 51
Wen, 206
Wheals, 311, 692
Whiplash injury, 630
Whipple's disease, 1063
Whipworm infection, 71
White blood cells, 142-43, 164-68, 218, 802
Whitfield's ointment, 200
Whooping cough, 36, 224, 395, 422-23
  test for, 796
Widal test, 802
Wilm's tumor, 295
Wilson's disease, 512, 1064
Windpipe: *see* Trachea
Witch's milk, 1064
Withdrawal symptoms, 1064
Women, diseases of, 427-50

Wood's light, 1064
Wool-sorter's disease, 47
Worms, 67-71, 695, 795
Wounds, first aid for, 847-50
Wrinkles, 204
Wrist, disorders, 634
Writer's cramp, 266
Wry-neck, 630

X

Xanthelasma, 193
Xanthomatoses, 173
Xeroderma, 206
Xerophthalmia, 1065
X-ray, 36, 125, 128, 231, 233, 236, 239, 250, 325, 334, 340, 781-92
X-ray diagnosis and examination, 783-88
The following are references from the text:
  cancer, 239-40
  chest, 220-21
  dental, 536
  digestive tract, 467, 470, 476, 477, 478, 481, 482, 483, 486, 488, 490, 492
  epilepsy, 276
  heart, 84
  joints, 655, 656, 658, 662, 666, **669**
  nephritis, 293
  ulcer, 472, 475, 476
  urinary tract, 287
X-ray therapy, 166, 167, 171, 174, 183, 300, 318, 470, 788-92

Y

Yaws, 49
Yeast, 200-01
Yellow fever, 56
  vaccination, 52
Yellow spot, 556
Yogurt, 1065

Z

Zonules, 553
Zoster (*see* Shingles)

FAMILY HEALTH RECORD

Enter the major events of family health in the following pages, as they occur. You will have a permanent, concise, accurate record of family medical matters that are easily forgotten with the passage of time. The record can be invaluable in jogging faulty memories, in filling out insurance, school, and industrial forms requiring medical histories, in assisting diagnosis and treatment by your physician, and in furnishing facts that could be significant to future generations.

CHILDREN'S BIRTH RECORD

Name	Date, hour	Blood Type	Circumstances (e.g., breech delivery, Cesarean, forceps, prematurity, complications)

IMMUNIZATIONS: Enter in Immunization Record, page 394.

SPECIAL MEDICAL INSTRUCTIONS AND ADVICE

List any individual problems, conditions calling for special awareness or alertness, such as: sensitization to penicillin, other drugs, bee stings; allergies; medications taken regularly; unusual reactions; disorders that may provoke crises (e.g., diabetes, epilepsy).

Name	Blood Type	Conditions

GENEALOGICAL RECORD: The Family Tree

Some diseases or defects occur more frequently in some families than in others (see Medical Genetics, Chapter 25). List any major or chronic disease that affects or did affect family members: diabetes; cancer; epilepsy; hypertension (high blood pressure); allergies; defects of eyes, ears, heart, other organs; mental retardation; psychiatric illness; congenital abnormalities; tuberculosis; blood diseases; obesity; pulmonary disease; seizures; cardiac disease; thyroid disease. Be as specific as you can. Remember that underlying conditions may manifest themselves in different ways; for example, atherosclerosis may manifest itself as a heart attack or stroke.

PATERNAL SIDE OF FAMILY

Name	Birth date	Diseases, operations, illnesses	If deceased, cause of death
HUSBAND			
Sisters			
Brothers			
Mother			
Father			
Grandmother			
Grandfather			

MATERNAL SIDE OF FAMILY

Name	Birth date	Diseases, operations, illnesses	If deceased, cause of death
WIFE			
Sisters			
Brothers			
Mother			
Father			
Grandmother			
Grandfather			

FAMILY ILLNESSES

Did you ever have German measles or mumps? Not everybody knows for sure—unless a parent or someone else made a permanent record at the time. Some diseases leave lifelong immunities; some may become chronic or have serious after-effects. Make a note of infectious diseases suffered by members of the family (see pages 418-422), as well as of diseases mentioned in the genealogical record on the opposite page, and of surgical operations and what was done, and of accidents resulting in broken bones or other injuries.

Name	Date	Diseases, operations, illnesses, injuries	Physician